a LANGE medical book

CURRENT
Diagnosis & Treatment: Occupational & Environmental Medicine

SIXTH EDITION

Editors

Joseph LaDou, MS, MD

Clinical Professor Emeritus
Division of Occupational & Environmental Medicine
University of California, San Francisco

Robert J. Harrison, MD, MPH

Clinical Professor of Medicine
Division of Occupational & Environmental Medicine
University of California, San Francisco

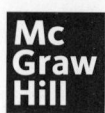

Mc
Graw
Hill

New York   Chicago   San Francisco   Athens   London   Madrid   Mexico City
Milan   New Delhi   Singapore   Sydney   Toronto

CURRENT Diagnosis & Treatment: Occupational & Environmental Medicine, Sixth Edition

Previous editions copyright © 2014 by McGraw-Hill Education; © 2007, 2004 by the McGraw-Hill Companies; © 1997 by Appleton & Lange.

· 1 2 3 4 5 6 7 8 9   LCR   26 25 24 23 22 21

ISBN 978-1-260-14343-0
MHID 1-260-14343-0
ISSN 1047-4498

Notice

Medicine is an ever-changing science. As new research and clinical experience broaden our knowledge, changes in treatment and drug therapy are required. The authors and the publisher of this work have checked with sources believed to be reliable in their efforts to provide information that is complete and generally in accord with the standards accepted at the time of publication. However, in view of the possibility of human error or changes in medical sciences, neither the authors nor the publisher nor any other party who has been involved in the preparation or publication of this work warrants that the information contained herein is in every respect accurate or complete, and they disclaim all responsibility for any errors or omissions or for the results obtained from use of the information contained in this work. Readers are encouraged to confirm the information contained herein with other sources. For example and in particular, readers are advised to check the product information sheet included in the package of each drug they plan to administer to be certain that the information contained in this work is accurate and that changes have not been made in the recommended dose or in the contraindications for administration. This recommendation is of particular importance in connection with new or infrequently used drugs.

This book was set in Minion Pro by KnowledgeWorks Global Ltd.
The editors were Kay Conerly and Kim J. Davis.
The production supervisor was Catherine Saggese.
Project management was provided by Parag Mittal, KnowledgeWorks Global Ltd.

This book was printed on acid-free paper.

Contents

---

*Deceased.

Section IV. Occupational and Environmental Exposures

Section V. Program Management

Authors

Carisa H. Adamson, PhD, MSPT, CPE
Associate Professor
Division of Occupational & Environmental Medicine
University of California, San Francisco (UCSF)
Director, UCSF/UC Berkeley Ergonomics Research & Graduate
    Training Program
San Francisco, California
Chapter 6

Sammy Almashat, MD, MPH
Occupational Medicine Physician
Dignity Health
Woodland, California
Chapters 24 & 25

Christina Armatas, MD, MPH
Public Health Medical Officer
Occupational Health Branch
California Department of Public Health
Richmond, California
Chapter 52

John R. Balmes, MD
Professor of Medicine
Division of Occupational & Environmental Medicine
Division of Pulmonary & Critical Care
Zuckerberg San Francisco General Hospital
University of California, San Francisco
San Francisco, California
Chapters 19 & 50

Rahmat Balogun, DO, MS, MPH
Assistant Clinical Professor of Medicine
Division of Occupational and Environmental Medicine
University of California, San Francisco
San Francisco, California
Chapter 31

Neal L. Benowitz, MD
Professor of Medicine Emeritus (Active)
Division of Cardiology
University of California, San Francisco
Zuckerberg San Francisco General Hospital
San Francisco, California
Chapter 20

Paul D. Blanc, MD, MSPH
Professor of Medicine
Division of Occupational & Environmental Medicine
University of California, San Francisco
San Francisco, California
Chapter 32

Sherry L. Burrer, DVM, MPH
Epidemiologist and Senior Veterinary Officer
Emergency Preparedness and Response Office
National Institute for Occupational Safety and Health
Centers for Disease Control and Prevention
Atlanta, Georgia
Chapter 45

John H. Cary, MD
Louisiana State University School of Medicine
New Orleans, Louisiana
Chapter 17

John R. Chamberlain, MD
Clinical Professor of Psychiatry
Department of Psychiatry and Behavioral Sciences
University of California, San Francisco
San Francisco, California
Chapter 36

David Claman, MD
Professor of Medicine
Director, UCSF Sleep Disorders Center
University of California, San Francisco
San Francisco, California
Chapter 37

Diana Coffa, MD
Associate Professor
Department of Family Community Medicine
University of California, San Francisco
San Francisco, California
Chapter 10

Margaret Cook-Shimanek, MD, MPH
Medical Director
Montana Department of Labor and Industry Employment
    Relations Division
Helena, Montana
Chapter 49

Caitlin R. Costello, MD
Health Sciences Associate Clinical Professor
Department of Psychiatry and Behavioral Sciences
University of California, San Francisco
San Francisco, California
Chapter 36

Carl F. Cranor, PhD, MSL
Distinguished Professor of Philosophy
Faculty Member, Environmental Toxicology
Distinguished Teaching Professor
University of California
Riverside, California
Chapter 4

Rupali Das, MD, MPH
Senior Vice President and California Medical Director
Zenith Insurance Company
Clinical Professor of Medicine
Division of Occupational & Environmental Medicine
University of California, San Francisco
San Francisco, California
Chapter 43

Lisa J. Delaney, CAPT, MS, CIH
Associate Director for Emergency Preparedness and Response
National Institute for Occupational Safety and Health
Atlanta, Georgia
Chapter 45

Alexis Descatha, MD, PhD
Associate Professor, Occupational Health
INSERM, Centre for Research in Epidemiology and
    Population Health
Garches, France
Chapter 8

Michael J. DiBartolomeis, PhD, DABT
Owner and Principal
Toxicology Research International
Haiku, Hawaii
Chapter 55

Robert Dobie, MD*
University of California
Department of Otolaryngology
Sacramento, California
Chapter 12

Timur S. Durrani, MD, MPH, MBA
Associate Clinical Professor of Medicine
University of California, San Francisco (UCSF)
Assistant Medical Director, San Francisco Division
California Poison Control System
Associate Director
UCSF Pediatric Environmental Health Specialty Unit
San Francisco, California
Chapters 14, 16, & 20

Judith Eisenberg, MD, MS
Medical Officer
National Institute for Occupational Safety and Health
Centers for Disease Control and Prevention
Cincinnati, Ohio
Chapter 45

Samuel M. Goldman, MD, MPH
Clinical Professor of Medicine & Neurology
Division of Occupational & Environmental Medicine
University of California, San Francisco
San Francisco, California
Chapter 23

Sandeep Guntur, MD, MPH
Associate Clinical Professor of Medicine
Division of Occupational & Environmental Medicine
University of California, San Francisco
San Francisco, California
Chapter 21

Robert J. Harrison, MD, MPH
Clinical Professor of Medicine
Division of Occupational & Environmental Medicine
University of California, San Francisco
San Francisco, California
Chapters 1, 2, 21, 24, 25, 30, 31, & 54

Camille Hawkins, MD, PA-C
Captain, U.S. Public Health Service
Health, Safety, and Work-Life, Operational Medicine
U.S. Coast Guard (Retired)
Portsmouth, Virginia
Chapter 44

German T. Hernandez, MD
Partner, El Paso Kidney Specialists
Clinical Associate Professor of Medicine
Division of Nephrology & Hypertension
Texas Tech University Health Sciences Center El Paso
El Paso, Texas
Chapter 22

Stephanie M. Holm, MD, MPH
Assistant Clinical Professor of Medicine
Co-Director of the Western States Pediatric Environmental
    Health Specialty Unit
Division of Occupational & Environmental Medicine
University of California, San Francisco
San Francisco, California
Chapters 48, 50, & Appendix A

John Howard, MD, JD
Director
National Institute for Occupational Safety and Health
Centers for Disease Control and Prevention
Washington, DC
Chapter 34

*Deceased.

Yang Hu, MD, PhD
Assistant Professor
Department of Ophthalmology
Stanford University School of Medicine
Palo Alto, California
Chapter 11

Leslie M. Israel, DO, MPH
Medical Director
Los Angeles Department of Water and Power
Los Angeles, California
Chapter 51

Sarah Janssen, MD, PhD, MPH
Assistant Clinical Professor
University of California, San Francisco
San Francisco, California
Chapters 27 & 28

Michael J. Kosnett, MD, MPH
Associate Clinical Professor
Division of Clinical Pharmacology & Toxicology
Department of Medicine
University of Colorado School of Medicine
Department of Environmental and Occupational Health
Colorado School of Public Health
Aurora, Colorado
Chapter 29

Robert Kosnik, MD, DIH
Professor of Medicine
Director, Occupational Health Program
University of California, San Francisco
San Francisco, California
Chapter 37

Ware G. Kuschner, MD
Professor of Medicine
Division of Pulmonary, Allergy, and Critical Care Medicine
Stanford University School of Medicine
Chief, Pulmonary Section
VA Palo Alto Health Care System
Palo Alto, California
Chapter 32

Joseph LaDou, MS, MD
Clinical Professor Emeritus
Division of Occupational & Environmental Medicine
University of California, San Francisco
San Francisco, California
Chapters 1, 3, & 47

Romain Lancigu, MD
Service de Chirurgie Orthopédique
CHU d'Angers
Angers, France
Chapter 8

A. Scott Laney, PhD, MPH
Workforce Screening and Surveillance Team
Surveillance Branch, Respiratory Health Division
National Institute for Occupational Safety and Health
Centers for Disease Control and Prevention
Morgantown, West Virginia
Chapter 41

Richard Lewis, MD, MPH
Site Occupational Medicine Director
AnovaWorks/Pacific Northwest National Laboratory
Richland, Washington
Chapter 29

Becky S. Li, MD
Department of Dermatology
Howard University Hospital
Washington, DC
Chapter 17

Jane Lipscomb, PhD, RN
Professor Emeriti
School of Nursing
University of Maryland
Baltimore, Maryland
Chapter 38

Matthew London, MS
Occupational Health Internship Program (OHIP)
Albany, New York
Chapter 38

Ulrike Luderer, MD, PhD, MPH
Professor of Environmental and Occupational Health,
   Developmental and Cell Biology, and Medicine
Department of Environmental and Occupational Health
University of California, Irvine
Irvine, California
Chapter 26

Anthony C. Luke, MD, MPH
Professor of Clinical Orthopedics
University of California, San Francisco
San Francisco, California
Chapters 7 & 9

C. Benjamin Ma, MD
Professor in Residence
Sports Medicine and Shoulder Surgery
Vice Chair, Adult Clinical Operations
Department of Orthopaedic Surgery
University of California, San Francisco
San Francisco, California
Chapters 7 & 9

Howard I. Maibach, MD
Professor of Dermatology
University of California, San Francisco Medical School
San Francisco, California
Chapter 17

Kathleen M. McPhaul, PhD, MPH, RN
Manager, Occupational Health Services
Smithsonian Institution
Washington, DC
Chapter 38

Wolf E. Mehling, MD
Professor of Clinical Family and Community Medicine
Department of Family and Community Medicine
Osher Center for Integrative Medicine
University of California, San Francisco
San Francisco, California
Chapter 10

Mark D. Miller, MD, MPH
Associate Clinical Professor of Medicine
Division of Occupational & Environmental Medicine
University of California, San Francisco
San Francisco, California
Chapter 48

Karen B. Mulloy, DO, MSCH
Associate Professor
Department of Family Medicine and Community Health
Department of Population and Quantitative Health Sciences
Mary Ann Swetland Center for Environmental Health
Case Western Reserve University School of Medicine
Cleveland, Ohio
Chapter 2

Lee S. Newman, MD, MA
Distinguished University Professor
Center Director
Center for Health, Work & Environment
Department of Environmental and Occupational Health and
    Department of Epidemiology
Colorado School of Public Health
Division of Pulmonary Sciences and Critical Care Medicine
School of Medicine
University of Colorado
Chapters 35 & 49

Michael O'Malley, MD, MPH
Associate Clinical Professor
Center for Health and Environment
Department of Public Health Science
University of California, Davis
Davis, California
Medical Consultant, Worker Health and Safety Branch
Department of Pesticide Regulation, California Environmental
    Protection Agency
Sacramento, California
Chapter 33

Kent R. Olson, MD
Clinical Professor of Medicine and Pharmacy (Retired)
University of California, San Francisco
San Francisco, California
Chapter 14

Karin A. Pacheco, MD, MSPH
Associate Professor
Division of Environmental & Occupational Health Sciences
National Jewish Health
Denver, Colorado
Colorado School of Public Health
Aurora, Colorado
Chapter 15

Joshua R. Potocko, MD, MPH
Commander, Medical Corps
U.S. Navy
Public Health Emergency Officer
Director, Public Health Services
Naval Health Clinic Quantico
Quantico, Virginia
Chapter 13

Glenn Pransky, MD, MOH
Associate Professor
University of Massachusetts Medical School
Departments of Family Medicine, Community Health and
    Quantitative Health Sciences
Worcester, Massachusetts
Chapter 5

Rajan Puri, MD, MPH
Clinical Assistant Professor of Medicine
Section of Occupational & Environmental Medicine
Associate Medical Director
SLAC National Linear Accelerator Laboratory
Director, Strategic Health Initiatives and Innovation
Director, Workplace Health Innovation Lab (WHIL)
Stanford University
Chapter 53

David M. Rempel, MD, MPH
Professor Emeritus
Department of Medicine
Division of Occupational & Environmental Medicine
University of California, San Francisco
San Francisco, California
Chapters 6 & 8

Jordan S. Rinker MD, MPH
Medical Consultant
Clinical Professor of Medicine
Division of Occupational & Environmental Medicine
University of California San Francisco
Corte Madera, California
Chapter 5

Rudolph A. Rodriguez, MD
Professor of Medicine
Division of Nephrology
University of Washington
Director of Hospital and Specialty Medicine
VA Puget Sound Medical Center
Seattle, Washington
Chapter 22

Jennifer B. Sass, PhD
Senior Scientist
Natural Resources Defense Council
Part-Time Faculty
George Washington University
Washington, DC
Chapter 55

Natalie V. Schwatka, PhD
Assistant Professor
Department of Environmental & Occupational Health
Center for Health, Work & Environment
Colorado School of Public Health
University of Colorado Anschutz Medical Campus
Aurora, Colorado
Chapter 35

James P. Seward, MD, MPP
Clinical Professor of Medicine
Division of Occupational & Environmental Medicine
University of California, San Francisco
San Francisco, California
Chapter 13

Michael Shahbaz, MD, MPH
Assistant Professor
Division of Occupational and Environmental Medicine
Mount Sinai Health System, Downtown Network
New York, New York
Chapter 27

Jill M. Shugart, MSPH, CP
CAPT, U.S. Public Health Service
Public Health Program Specialist
Center for State, Tribal, Local and Territorial Support
Centers for Disease Control and Prevention
Atlanta, Georgia
Chapter 45

Dennis J. Shusterman, MD, MPH
Professor of Clinical Medicine, Emeritus
Division of Occupational & Environmental Medicine
University of California, San Francisco
San Francisco, California
Chapter 18

Gina M. Solomon, MD, MPH
Clinical Professor of Medicine
Division of Occupational & Environmental Medicine
University of California, San Francisco
San Francisco, California
Chapter 46

Cecilia J. Sorensen, MD
Center for Health, Work & Environment
School of Public Health
Colorado Consortium on Climate Change and Human Health
Department of Environmental and Occupational Health
School of Medicine
University of Colorado
Aurora, Colorado
Chapter 49

Eileen Storey, MD, MPH
Senior Consultant (CTR)
Respiratory Health Division
National Institute for Occupational Safety and Health
Centers for Disease Control and Prevention
Morgantown, West Virginia
Chapter 41

Dana L. Thomas, MD, MPH
Rear Admiral, U.S. Public Health Service
Director of Health, Safety and Work-Life
United States Coast Guard
Washington, DC
Chapter 44

Nina Townsend, MPH, CSP, CIH
Associate Safety Engineer
Department of Industrial Relations
Division of Occupational Safety and Health
Oakland, California
Chapters 39 & 40

Laura S. Welch, MD
Professorial Lecturer
School of Public Health and Health Services
George Washington University
Washington, DC
Chapter 42

Lisa G. Winston, MD
Professor
Department of Medicine
Division of HIV, Infectious Diseases, and Global Medicine
University of California, San Francisco at Zuckerberg
    San Francisco General
San Francisco, California
Chapter 16

Richard Wittman, MD, MPH
Clinical Assistant Professor
Division of Primary Care and Population Health,
    Occupational Medicine
Stanford University
Stanford, California
Chapter 53

Preface

The sixth edition of *Current Diagnosis & Treatment: Occupational & Environmental Medicine* continues to serve as a concise yet comprehensive resource for health care professionals in all specialties who diagnose and treat occupational and environmental injuries and illnesses.

COVERAGE & APPROACH TO THE SUBJECT

The book provides a complete guide to common occupational and environmental injuries and illnesses, their diagnosis and treatment, and preventive measures in the workplace and community. Our aim is to help health care professionals understand the complexities of occupational and environmental health issues and provide useful clinical information on common illnesses and injuries. The book contains many new chapters, expanding the coverage of occupational and environmental medicine well beyond that of the earlier editions. To enhance the book's usefulness as a clinical resource, it is published in the Lange® Current series. The series consists of practical, concise, and timely books in core specialties and key subspecialties that focus on essential diagnostic and treatment information.

SPECIAL AREAS OF EMPHASIS

- Detailed coverage on the diagnosis and treatment of a broad spectrum of occupational and environmental injuries and illnesses.
- Chapters on how to conduct an occupational and environmental history, perform a physical examination, and prevent further injury.
- The important role that health care providers can play in preventing disability and in the provision of workers' compensation benefits, with ethical issues and principles.
- Practical information on the toxic properties and clinical manifestations of common industrial materials and environmental agents, with a new chapter on genetic toxicology.
- Techniques to prevent workplace-related injuries and illnesses through the application of ergonomic principles.
  - Emerging issues in occupational and environmental medicine, including climate change, the changing nature of work, total worker health and workplace violence
  - Basics of pediatric environmental health
  - Practical methods and principles in responder safety and health

ORGANIZATION & HIGHLIGHTS OF EACH SECTION

Section I (Chapters 1–5) defines the practice of occupational and environmental medicine and introduces the health care provider to the diagnosis of occupational injuries and illnesses. These chapters offer guidance for identifying workplace and community exposures to toxic materials—putting this information to immediate clinical use and applying it toward better health and safety practices in the workplace. This section presents a comprehensive discussion of disability management and prevention. An understanding of workers' compensation law and the physician's critical role in determining care and benefits can be gained from these chapters.

Section II (Chapters 6–13) concisely discusses common occupational injuries and their treatments. Noise-induced hearing loss and the impact of other physical hazards, such as heat, cold, and radiation, are examined. This section also discusses how ergonomic principles can be instituted in the workplace to minimize work loss associated with injury and illness. The chapter on management of chronic pain is a guide to the use of pain medication and to the prevention of misuse of therapeutics.

Section III (Chapters 14–28) is a comprehensive discussion of clinical toxicology arranged by organ system, with special emphasis on the environmental as well as workplace origins of toxic exposure. It thoroughly reviews commonly recognized environmental and occupational illnesses and highlights many clinical problems not often thought to be work related. A new chapter on genetic toxicology accompanies a review of occupational cancer.

Section IV (Chapters 29–33) presents the most common toxic materials encountered in the workplace and community with diagnostic and treatment recommendations. This section is designed to serve as an immediate reference source and clinical guide for the practicing health care professional. The discussion on pesticides emphasizes the environmental as well as occupational exposures that may lead to illness.

Section V (Chapters 34–45) presents chapters on occupational mental health and workplace violence, and substance use disorders present programs for controlling and treating these problems. It adds new chapters on sleep disorders and total worker health. These chapters present the roles and responsibilities of the industrial hygienist and the safety professional and serves as a guide for health care professionals to work with them.

Section VI (Chapters 46–55) provides a comprehensive discussion of environmental medicine and some of the complex societal issues that accompany industrialization and technologic advances throughout the world. Emphasis is placed on recognizing that some common "occupational" exposures are found also in homes and public locations and require the same high index of suspicion that is assumed when encountered in the workplace. A vital new chapter on climate change completes the discussion.

The Appendix A reviews biostatistics and epidemiology. These topics are important not only in research but also in clinical practice. Ultimately, all occupational and environmental physicians serve as clinical epidemiologists.

A quiz follows each chapter to allow readers to test their retention of key elements of the book. Answers to quiz questions are presented in Appendix B as true statements from the text.

ACKNOWLEDGMENTS

This book brings together many authors with unique experience in the clinical practice and the teaching of occupational and environmental medicine. We are grateful to these many authors and their institutions for their participation.

Joseph LaDou, MS, MD
Robert J. Harrison, MD, MPH
San Francisco, California
May 2021

The Practice of Occupational Medicine

Joseph LaDou, MS, MD
Robert J. Harrison, MD, MPH

Nearly 4 million work-related injuries and illnesses are reported each year in the United States. Due to limitations in the current injury reporting system and widespread under-reporting of workplace injuries, this number significantly understates the magnitude of the problem, with the true rate 20–60% higher.

Each year more than 5000 workers are killed on the job in the United States. Transportation incidents account for the largest number of these deaths. Significantly elevated rates are seen among agricultural, forestry, and construction industry workers, and among high-risk occupations such as roofers.

Violence is the second most common fatal event. One-sixth of fatal occupational injuries are violence-related, including homicides and suicides at work.

Each day, 150 workers die from hazardous working conditions. High fatality rates are reported from exposure to harmful substances or environments, fires, and explosions.

Overdoses from the nonmedical use of drugs or alcohol while on the job are increasing steadily. Drug-related deaths and suicides are important contributors to the long-term excess mortality of injured workers.

An estimated 50,000–60,000 workers die from preventable occupational diseases each year, a tragic number considering the use of safer substitutes and engineering controls that can reduce the risk.

Occupational injuries and deaths in the United States cost an estimated $250–$360 billion a year. Businesses pay between $180 billion and $360 billion annually in direct and indirect (overtime, training, and lost productivity) costs for workers' compensation benefits. The human costs associated with occupational injuries and illnesses are staggering. The medical and indirect costs of occupational injuries and illnesses are at least as large as the cost of cancer. Moreover, lost-time occupational injuries are associated with a substantially elevated mortality hazard.

The focus on prevention and enforcement of health and safety programs often hinges on the political climate and government policies toward worker safety and health.

Work-related injuries and illnesses can be prevented with organized labor advocating for strong government policies for worker safety and health, strengthening enforcement, issuing key safety and health standards, and improving anti-retaliation protections and other rights for workers. With moves toward populist politics, these gains are threatened. Across the globe, there are deregulatory agendas to repeal and delay worker safety and other rules and propose cuts in budgets for public health and enforcement, and the elimination of worker safety and health training and other programs.

FEDERAL AGENCIES

The Occupational Safety and Health Act of 1970 (OSHAct) ensures "every working man and woman in the United States safe and healthful working conditions." This act created the Occupational Safety and Health Administration (OSHA) and the National Institute for Occupational Safety and Health (NIOSH).

▶ Occupational Safety and Health Administration

The OSHAct created the OSHA to assure safe and healthful working conditions for working men and women by setting and enforcing standards and by providing outreach training, education, and assistance. OSHA is part of the U.S. Department of Labor. The administrator for OSHA is the Assistant Secretary of Labor for Occupational Safety and Health. The OSHA administrator reports to the Secretary of Labor, who is a member of the cabinet of the President of the United States. The OSHAct covers most private sector employers and their workers, in addition to some public sector employers and workers in the 50 states and certain territories and jurisdictions under federal authority.

The OSHA Strategic Partnership Program (OSPP) provides opportunities for OSHA to partner with employers, workers, professional or trade associations, labor organizations, and other interested stakeholders. OSHA Strategic Partnerships are unique agreements designed to encourage, assist, and recognize partner efforts to eliminate serious hazards and enhance workplace safety and health practices. They establish specific goals, strategies, and performance measures to improve worker safety and health and focus on improving safety and health in major corporations, government agencies, at large construction projects, and private sector industries where OSHA has jurisdiction.

Although it has been 50 years since the passage of the OSHAct, concerns continue about the adequacy of the nation's occupational injury and illness surveillance system. Greater resources are needed for OSHA to inspect and impose meaningful penalties for noncompliance with basic precautions, and for NIOSH to implement a nationwide system for tracking of occupational diseases.

▶ National Institute for Occupational Safety and Health

Workers are injured or killed every day as a result of preventable workplace accidents or exposures. The Health Hazard Evaluation Program helps employees, union officials, and employers learn whether health hazards are present at their workplace and recommends ways to reduce hazards and prevent work-related illness. NIOSH evaluations are done at no cost to the employees, union official, or employers. NIOSH research seeks to improve workplace safety and health through safe practices, policies, and procedures. NIOSH is involved in a range of occupational safety and health activities including surveillance, research, and technology transfer. The NIOSH Program Portfolio focuses on relevance, quality, and impact. This is achieved through strong involvement of partners and stakeholders throughout the entire research continuum (conceiving, planning, conducting, translating, disseminating, and evaluating research).

The OSHAct mandates that NIOSH provide an adequate supply of qualified personnel to carry out the purposes of the law. NIOSH Education and Research Centers (ERCs) have a key role in helping meet this mandate and contribute to the Institute's core mission of providing national and world leadership to prevent workplace injuries and illnesses. NIOSH supports academic degree programs and research training opportunities in the core areas of industrial hygiene, occupational health nursing, occupational medicine, and occupational safety. The NIOSH ERCs help translate scientific discoveries into practice through effective education, training, and outreach. The NIOSH Program Portfolio has been organized into Sector Programs that represent industrial sectors and seven health and safety Cross-Sector Programs organized around health outcomes based on the National Occupational Research Agenda (NORA).

In a landmark publication in 2020, **Envisioning the Future of Work to Safeguard the Safety, Health, and Well-being of the Workforce**, NIOSH stated that the complex "future of work offers numerous opportunities, while also presenting critical but not clearly understood difficulties, exposures, and hazards." NIOSH suggests an integrated approach to address worker safety, health, and well-being, one that offers an important role to occupational physicians and other health care providers in the work environments of the future. This is a challenging time for occupational and environmental medicine, one that requires a firm commitment to study, research, practice, and teaching of the many disciplines of the field.

OPPORTUNITIES IN OCCUPATIONAL MEDICINE

As a result of passage of the OSHAct and formation of OSHA and NIOSH, occupational medicine became the center of considerable attention by medical schools, hospitals, clinics, and physicians from many different specialties. The opportunities for public health practice, union-based clinical care, and independent consulting created new career opportunities for medical students. Medical schools received financial support for training from NIOSH, and OSHA gave occupational physicians a voice in the increasingly regulated industrial setting.

NIOSH estimates that the future national demand for occupational safety and health services will significantly outstrip the number of professionals with the necessary training, education, and experience to provide such services. The need for an adequate supply of trained professionals is particularly great as we anticipate that growing numbers of older professionals will retire over the next decade. As new technologies continue to enter the workplace, occupational safety and health professionals will require specialized skills and knowledge to meet the needs of workers in new work environments.

The Institute of Medicine (IOM) states that there is a critical shortage of specialty-trained occupational and environmental physicians in communities, in academic medical centers, and in public health and related agencies. Moreover, the IOM reports a severe shortage of frontline primary care physicians who are willing and able to care for patients with occupational and environmental illnesses. The IOM concludes that data from the Bureau of Labor Statistics (BLS) are significant underestimates of occupational diseases, which emphasizes the need for more and better diagnoses of occupational diseases by primary care practitioners.

Employers expect to hire almost 500 occupational physicians over the next 5 years and are looking for residency-trained specialists. Skills in evidence-based clinical evaluation and treatment, determining fitness for work, and worker and management communications are the most important technical skills needed by employers. The estimated number of occupational physicians that employers expect to hire over the next 5 years is substantially higher than the number estimated to be produced from current training programs. Opportunities in occupational medicine, and in the increasingly important specialty of environmental medicine, vary by region. There are many industrial areas with an established medical community serving their needs, yet in other areas there are growing industrial corridors very much in need of occupational physicians.

▶ Occupational Medical Practice

Occupational injuries and illnesses are among the five leading causes of morbidity and mortality in the United States and in most other countries. Injuries at work comprise a substantial part of the country's injury burden, accounting for nearly half of all injuries in some age groups. One-third of all injury cases result in loss of work. There are over 5000 traumatic occupational fatalities each year, ranking the workplace as the eighth leading cause of death. Since the early 1970s, more than 113,000 worker deaths have been attributed to pneumoconioses. This number represents only a small portion of the total deaths attributable to occupational lung disease. The number of deaths from asbestos-related mesothelioma has remained relatively constant in the same time period, as have deaths with hypersensitivity pneumonitis as an underlying or contributing cause. Asthma is now the most common occupational respiratory disease. Population-based estimates suggest that approximately 15% of new-onset asthma in adults is work-related.

Workers' compensation law places the occupational physician in a critically important role. The physician must determine that an injury or illness is caused by work, diagnose the condition, prescribe care, and assess the extent of impairment and the ability of the worker to resume work. In some instances, determinations that injuries or illnesses are the result of work may be contentious and require the physician to determine causation and provide an opinion in the legal setting.

Occupational physicians play an important role in prevention, recognition, and treatment of injuries and illnesses. In some regions, occupational physicians customarily are employed by corporations. More recently, it has become the practice of corporations to contract with occupational physicians to act as their consultants. These consultants increasingly become involved in issues of environmental as well as occupational health. Most workplace injuries and illnesses, however, are attended by private practitioners in clinic and hospital settings. This is a function of the framework of the workers' compensation systems within each state.

When a compensation case results in litigation, occupational health professionals become important experts in resolving disputes. The physician asked to evaluate the worker in most states is designated an independent medical examiner (IME). The evaluation by IME is often the highest level of evaluation the worker will encounter. Most requests for IME opinions come from insurers, but on occasion, plaintiffs' attorneys, judges, and others may initiate an IME evaluation. Many occupational physicians find a full-time practice in this highly specialized area of workers' compensation.

▶ Recognition of Occupational Injury & Illness

Workers' compensation insurance often fails to compensate most occupational injuries and illnesses, including fatalities. Only a small fraction of occupational diseases is covered by workers' compensation, and only a small fraction of individuals suffering from occupational illnesses ever receive workers' compensation benefits. Either by law or by practice, compensation in many states is particularly limited for occupational diseases. A recent study suggests that workers' compensation insurance absorbs only 21% of the true costs of occupational injuries and illnesses.

Many workers' compensation laws now prevent or discourage the recognition of occupational diseases. The efforts of many industries and their insurers to deny claims lead to the failure to compensate workers who have occupational diseases. Another important contributing cause is the limited information available to physicians. Of the tens of thousands of chemicals in common commercial use in the United States each year (3000 of them in quantities of > 1 million pounds per year), only 7% have been screened for toxicity, and fewer than half of those have been studied thoroughly. Although interest in occupational medicine is increasing across the country, the failure to diagnose occupational diseases and the lack of proper compensation of workers continue to be major social policy failures.

More than half a million chemicals are found in work settings, and many millions of workers are exposed to these substances. Yet only 10,000 workers' compensation claims for illnesses caused by chemical exposure are filed each year. Workplace exposure to carcinogens accounts for about 5–10% of all cancer cases, yet fewer than 1% of cancer patients ever receive any settlement from employers. For example, NIOSH estimates that 16–17% of lung cancer cases in men and 2% of cases in women are work-related. As many as 15,000 of the 100,000 commonly used industrial chemicals are carcinogenic to humans. Although occupational cancers are totally preventable, workers continue to be exposed to carcinogens, possibly because few cases are reported, are awarded benefits, or are successful in litigation. With the exception of cancers caused by exposure to asbestos, few occupational cancer cases ever receive workers' compensation benefits.

▶ Teaching Occupational Medicine

The majority of physicians who practice occupational medicine in the private practice setting do so with the knowledge gained by self-study, attendance at continuing education courses, and practice experience. A lack of training in occupational medicine may account for some of the failure to diagnose occupational diseases and eventually to compensate workers. Traditional public health approaches are infrequent in many such practices. Moreover, the long latency periods of many occupational diseases present a causation dilemma both for physicians and for insurers. Time constraints and knowledge may hamper the ability to recognize common work-related conditions, such as work-related asthma, and concerns regarding the effect of the diagnosis on the patient's job and income may discourage reporting.

Occupational and environmental medicine in recent years is receiving an increasing emphasis in medical schools. Faculty that had limited opportunity for research and teaching in occupational medicine at most medical schools now find a number of new positions through the avenue of environmental health. This dynamic advancement is largely the result of academic achievements in the United States where fundamental research in both fields appears to be expanding. The success of adding environmental medicine to occupational medicine is now beginning to be recognized throughout the world in both teaching and research venues.

▶ Residency and Other Training

NIOSH, in addition to its roles in supporting occupational health research and recommending occupational standards to OSHA, funds most training programs in occupational health and safety. NIOSH extramural funds support a network of 18 regional education and research centers located at universities in 17 states and approximately 30 individual training project grants in 20 states. The NIOSH extramural research and training programs include investigator-initiated research, mentored research scientist career development awards, training programs, and small business innovation research projects. Multidisciplinary education and research centers, state surveillance programs, and global occupational health initiatives complement the extramural research and training at NIOSH. In 2018–2019, 540 professionals graduated from NIOSH-funded training programs with specialized training in disciplines that include occupational medicine (53 graduates), occupational health nursing, industrial hygiene, occupational safety, and other closely related occupational safety and health fields of study.

Most training programs in occupational medicine are associated with universities that have schools of public health, but some programs are found within specific departments (eg, preventive medicine, community medicine, internal medicine, or family practice) within a medical school. There are 24 approved residency programs in the United States. The annual number of graduates from each residency program averages only slightly greater than two. This small number does not answer the requirement for academically trained occupational physicians, nor does it fill the vacancies in public health departments in many areas of the country.

▶ Board Certification

Board-certified physicians generally have more diverse practice activities and skills, with greater involvement in management, public health-oriented activities, and toxicology. The American Board of Preventive Medicine (ABPM) began board certification of specialists in occupational medicine in 1955. ABPM has certified a total of 4373 occupational physicians through 2018. Fewer than half of these board-certified occupational physicians are currently in practice. Although occupational medicine is the most popular of the ABPM certifications, it remains one of medicine's smallest specialties. Applicants for board certification peaked at 331 in 1996. Fewer than half that number now apply each year for board certification. Moreover, the number of occupational

physicians certified by ABPM is not replacing the losses to retirement or retreats from the field. In 2018, 75 of 82 physicians (a pass rate of 91%) passed the board certification examination. This small supply of new board-certified specialists is far below that which would be required merely to replace the loss by retirement of older board-certified physicians.

The ABPM approved a complementary pathway in 2010 to accommodate physicians who want to make a mid-career shift into the practice of preventive medicine and to achieve certification by the ABPM in one of three specialty areas—aerospace medicine, occupational medicine, or public health and general preventive medicine. A variety of distance learning opportunities are increasingly available for maintenance of certification for physicians with ABPM certification after 1998.

For details on certification, contact

American Board of Preventive Medicine
111 West Jackson Boulevard, Suite 1110
Chicago, IL 60604
(312) 939-2276
abpm@theabpm.org

REFERENCES

AFL-CIO. Death on the Job: The Toll of Neglect 2020. Report. Workplace Health and Safety. October 6, 2020. https://aflcio.org/reports/death-job-toll-neglect-2020.

Boden LI, O'Leary PK, Applebaum KM, Tripodis Y: The impact of non-fatal workplace injuries and illnesses on mortality. Am J Ind Med 2016;59(12):1061-1069 [PMID: 27427538].

Bureau of Labor Statistics Injuries, Illnesses and Fatalities: https://www.bls.gov/iif/.

Finkel AM: A healthy public cannot abide unhealthy and unsafe workplaces. Am J Public Health 2018;108(3):312-313 [PMID: 29412707].

Katie MA, Abay A, Paul K, Andrew B, Yorghos T, Leslie IB: Suicide and drug-related mortality following occupational injury. Am J Ind Med 2019;62(9):733-741 [PMID: 31298756].

National Academies of Medicine: A Smarter National Surveillance System for Occupational Safety and Health in the 21st Century, 2018.

NIOSH [2018]. NIOSH extramural research and training program: annual report of fiscal year 2017. Felknor SA, Williams DF, Grandillo P. Cincinnati, OH: U.S. Department of Health and Human Services, Centers for Disease Control and Prevention, National Institute for Occupational Safety and Health, DHHS (NIOSH) Publication No. 2019-122. https://doi.org/10.26616/NIOSHPUB2019122.

OSHA. About OSHA, 2020: https://www.osha.gov/about.html/.

Peckham TK, Baker MG, Camp JE, Kaufman JD, Seixas NS: Creating a future for occupational health. Ann Work Expo Health 2017;61(1):3-15 [PMID: 28395315].

Sara LT et al: Envisioning the future of work to safeguard the safety, health, and well-being of the workforce: A perspective from the CDC's National Institute for Occupational Safety and Health. Am J Ind Med Dec 2020;63(12):1063-1169 [PMID: 32926431].

■ SELF-ASSESSMENT QUESTIONS

Select the one correct answer for each question.

Question 1: Occupational injuries and illnesses
  a. are defined by workers' compensation law
  b. require an occupational physician to provide medical care
  c. are among the five leading causes of morbidity and mortality in the United States and in most other countries
  d. are declining in number as insurance settles claims

Question 2: Occupational physicians
  a. are primarily employed by public health agencies
  b. play an important role in prevention, recognition, and treatment of injuries and illnesses
  c. are prevented by law for acting as consultants to employers
  d. should endeavor not to become involved in issues of environmental and occupational health

Question 3: Independent medical examiners
  a. are required when a compensation case results in litigation
  b. are hired by workers to resolve disputes
  c. often provide the highest level of evaluation the worker will encounter
  d. are in most jurisdictions hired by plaintiff's attorneys

Question 4: Board-certified physicians
  a. generally have more diverse practice activities and skills, with greater involvement in management, public health-oriented activities, and toxicology
  b. make up the large majority of occupational physicians in private practice
  c. more than replace the losses to retirement or retreats from the field
  d. are unable to appear as expert witnesses in court cases

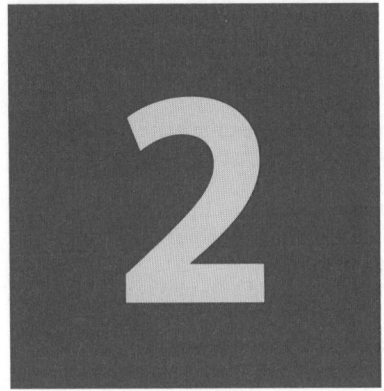

The Occupational & Environmental Medical History

Karen B. Mulloy, DO, MSCH

Robert J. Harrison, MD, MPH

The relationship between exposures at work and the development of injury or disease has been well documented throughout history. One of the earliest writings on lung conditions of miners was in the fourth century BC by Hippocrates. With the publishing of *De Morbis Artificium Diatriba* (Diseases of Workers) by Bernardino Ramazzini in 1700, the description of the health hazards of chemicals, dust, metals, and other agents encountered by workers in 52 occupations established occupational exposure as an important contributor to chronic disease. Ramazzini proposed that physicians should extend the list of questions that Hippocrates recommended they ask their patients by adding, "What is your occupation?"

The importance of the occupational and environmental medical history cannot be overemphasized. Occupational and environmental health and safety is an integral part of population health and is one of the social determinants of health. Working Americans spend greater than ½ of their waking hours at work, and the impact of the many exposures and stress factors encountered on the job can have significant effect on workers' health, both physical and mental. It can also profoundly influence the health of their families and communities and contribute to the social and economic costs to society as a whole. Moreover, with the advent of industrialization and the introduction of thousands of chemicals and other toxic substances into the environment, it is important for the medical practitioner to consider both occupational and environmental exposures when taking the medical history.

▶ Screening History

The relationship of injury or illness to work is often overlooked or even forgotten in the medical history. An accurate and complete occupational and environmental history is the most important tool in the evaluation and diagnosis of occupational and environmental injuries and illnesses. The patient who presents with wheezing may have asthma related to a long history of seasonal allergies, or the asthma may be related to exposure to isocyanates on the job. Without the occupational and environmental history, the correct diagnosis, treatment plan, and prevention may not be achieved.

Accurate diagnosis of occupational illnesses is important beyond the usual reasons for accuracy in medical diagnosis. There are public and population health, social, and economic implications of occupational disease and injury for the community of workers in the same workplace or in other workplaces with similar exposures. In many states, the diagnosis of an occupational illness triggers additional responsibility on the part of the clinician. These responsibilities are primarily those of timely notification: informing the worker regarding the potential legal and other implications of the diagnosis, informing the workers' compensation insurer of the diagnosis and the basis for the clinician's opinion, and reporting to the appropriate public health or labor-related governmental agencies. A differential diagnosis that appropriately includes occupational exposures as potential causes or exacerbating factors of the patient's presenting symptoms or suspected disease is a crucial first step in recognition (Figure 2–1).

With the passage of the 2009 Health Information Technology for Economic and Clinical Health (HITECH) Act, there has been an increase in the development and use of electronic health records (EHRs) within clinical practice. The EHR offers the ability for the clinician to have immediate access to a wide variety of significant information about their patients. Patients may already be asked to provide their job title or occupation for administrative and reimbursement purposes and integrating that information with clinical data will not only aid in the diagnosis of individual patients but will also improve health and safety conditions for groups of workers and expand public health surveillance of occupational illness and injury for prevention.

The chief complaint and history of present illness may suggest potential diagnostic possibilities that lead to specific etiologic hypotheses. For example, a history of headache while at work suggests potential solvent or carbon monoxide exposure, and cough and wheezing while at work or predictably delayed after leaving work may suggest irritant or triggering allergen exposure. A history of fevers and back pain in

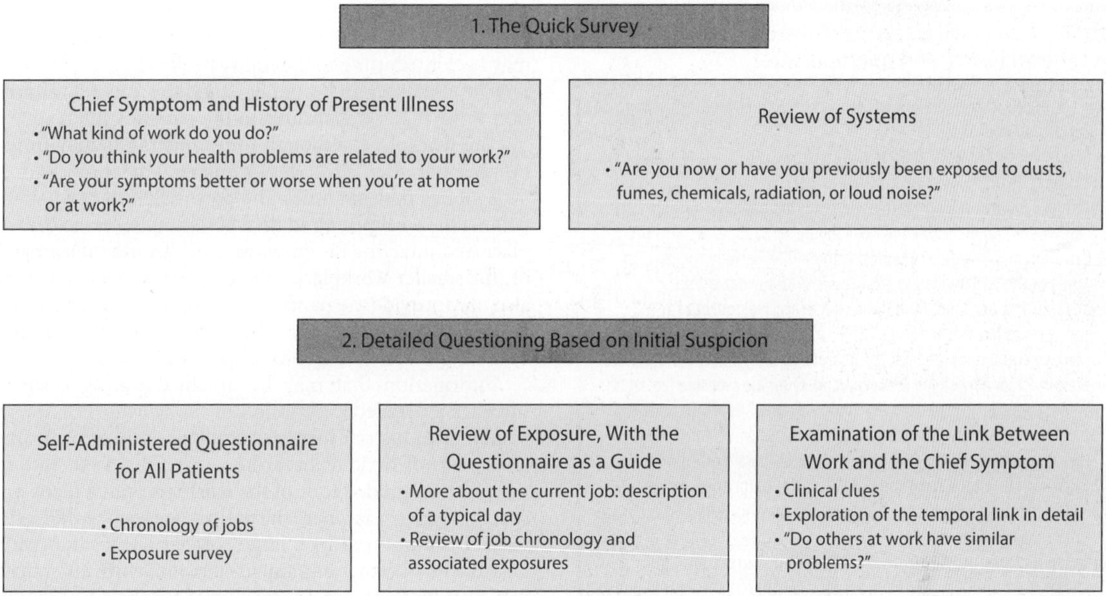

1. The Quick Survey

Chief Symptom and History of Present Illness
• "What kind of work do you do?"
• "Do you think your health problems are related to your work?"
• "Are your symptoms better or worse when you're at home or at work?"

Review of Systems

• "Are you now or have you previously been exposed to dusts, fumes, chemicals, radiation, or loud noise?"

2. Detailed Questioning Based on Initial Suspicion

Self-Administered Questionnaire for All Patients

• Chronology of jobs
• Exposure survey

Review of Exposure, With the Questionnaire as a Guide
• More about the current job: description of a typical day
• Review of job chronology and associated exposures

Examination of the Link Between Work and the Chief Symptom
• Clinical clues
• Exploration of the temporal link in detail
• "Do others at work have similar problems?"

▲ **Figure 2–1.** The initial clinical approach to the recognition of illness caused by occupational exposure.

a clinical laboratory worker or slaughterhouse worker suggests possible brucellosis. Additional sources of information may help to confirm or rule out hypothesized occupational or environmental etiology.

EXPANDED HISTORY

If answers to the occupational/environmental survey questions are positive, more detailed follow-up questioning is necessary (Table 2–1). It is also important to collect information about current and previous jobs in a systematic manner and inquire about possible environmental exposures at home and in the surrounding community and hobbies. The Agency for Toxic Substances and Disease Registry (ATSDR), a federal public health agency of the U.S. Department of Health and Human Services, provides health information to prevent harmful exposures and diseases related to toxic substances. In the ATSDR "Case Studies in Environmental Medicine," there is a case study of "Taking an Exposure History" that has an expanded "Exposure History Form" that may be used to capture an expanded and detailed occupational and environmental history.

▶ Prior Medical History

It is important to have access to the patient's entire medical history. Have the employee sign a release to obtain medical records from the treating or consulting clinicians. These records may provide important clues about prior diagnoses, history of exposures, predisposing factors for illness, and the course and progress of the illness.

▶ Exposure Assessment

When a patient's medical history suggests that occupational or environmental factors may be a primary or secondary cause or contributor to illness or injury, the clinician should identify all potentially toxic materials or hazards in the workplace, home, and/or environment. It is common in practice that the clinician does not have quantitative data about the patient's exposure, as contemporaneous measurements of air, water, or soil contaminants were not obtained during the period of relevant exposure. In this instance, the clinician must make a qualitative assessment of exposure based on the patient's occupational history, plausibility of the exposure pathway, information obtained from other sources (such as Safety Data Sheets, chemical supply data, and co-worker/manager work descriptions), and temporal relationship between exposure period and consistent symptom onset. This qualitative exposure assessment should be used to inform the clinician assessment of the likelihood that the work or environmental exposure was the cause of the patient's health condition.

Useful employee documents may include medical surveillance and/or job surveillance records from the employer. The employer or union may have reports from a safety inspection or an industrial hygienist that may provide insight into the exposures and risk for disease. The company health and safety manager should cooperate in answering questions about similar illnesses in coworkers. Working with the patient and obtaining permission to talk to the employer/union representative is an important step in the medical workup. Conducting a worksite evaluation will be invaluable

Table 2–1. Essential elements of the comprehensive occupational history and questionnaire.

Do the symptoms vary in relation to day of the week, or do they improve on vacations or weekends?

Current or most recent work and exposure history:

Job title; type of industry; name of employer

Duration of job; year/month started, year/month finished (if not currently employed); hours worked per day; hours worked per week; shift

Description of job (what is a typical workday), especially the parts of the job the patient believes may be potentially hazardous

Exposures to dust, fumes, radiation, chemicals, biologic hazards, or physical hazards

Protective equipment used (clothes, safety glasses, hearing protection, respirator, or gloves). Are these appropriate for the exposure (eg, latex gloves provide no protection from most solvents)? How often changed?

For exposures that are potentially relevant to the chief complaint, what was the duration and intensity of exposure? For example, was dust so thick that it impaired visibility? Was paint applied with brush, roller, or sprayer? Is there a temporal relationship between exposure and onset of symptoms?

Engineering controls (process enclosure, local exhaust ventilation, general ventilation, shielding, recent substitution of safer equipment or chemicals)

History of military service:

Were you in the military? If yes, where were you stationed? Which years did you serve? What was your job classification?

Membership in a union; safety climate; supervisory relations; recent organizational changes; work stress; layoffs; speedup

Epidemiologic evidence:

Other employees at the workplace who have similar health problems

Toxicologic evidence:

Do chemically analogous exposures cause similar disease symptoms, even though the chemical in question may have little known toxicity?

Participation in workplace medical monitoring (eg, blood, urine, respirator program, chest radiograph)

Occupational Safety and Health Administration (OSHA) inspection results, other industrial hygiene inspections; ergonomic workstation evaluations

Prior work history

Job chronology, working backward from the current or most recent job

Relevant information as above for each significant job previously held

Major types of exposures:

Based on your knowledge of the exposures associated with specific occupations, inquire into potential exposures to:

- Corrosive substances (acids, alkalis)
- Dusts
- Fibers (asbestos, fiberglass)
- Gases
- Heavy metals
- Pesticides, insecticides, herbicides
- Plastics (di-isocyanates, phthalates, acrylonitrile)
- Petrochemicals
- Physical agents (noise, heat, vibration, repetitive lifting or other motions)
- Radiation (electromagnetic, x-ray, ultraviolet)
- Solvents
- Workplace stress

into gaining insight into possible work exposures or work processes that the patient had not thought important but that may be contributing to the injury or illness.

The clinician can best understand the potential contribution of workplace exposures to the patient's illness by visiting the workplace, although time constraints may limit the number of patients for whom this may be performed. This necessitates first obtaining the permission of the patient to contact the workplace and then obtaining access to the workplace by contacting the employer's health and safety manager or, for smaller workplaces, the owner/manager. The patient also may provide the name of a union shop steward or health and safety committee member who may be of assistance in obtaining access to unionized worksites.

Information that may be obtained during a site visit includes a detailed description of the work processes, prior results of industrial hygiene sampling and medical surveillance, lists of toxic or hazardous materials used, and, most important, a guided tour of the work site with a focus on the specific work areas where the patient has been working. If the worker is employed by a large company with an organized health and safety program, discussion with an industrial hygienist on the company staff or, if unionized, at the international union may be useful for identifying other exposure information, control measures, and potential future monitoring to evaluate the effectiveness of control measures.

There may have also been an inspection performed by Occupational Safety and Health Administration (OSHA) or other safety and health regulatory agencies that can be accessed. An OSHA referral may be particularly useful in situations where the clinician suspects that potential violations of OSHA standards may be occurring. Additionally, the National Institute for Occupational Safety and Health (NIOSH) has a Health Hazard Evaluation (HHE) program that can perform public health investigations that may provide additional information. The HHE is a study of a workplace to determine if workers are exposed to hazardous materials or harmful conditions. Employees, union officials, or employers can request an HHE, and all employee information can be kept confidential.

Obtaining the assistance of a physical therapist, occupational therapist, or hand therapist experienced with workstation evaluation may be useful with ergonomic problems and repetitive-motion injuries in the workplace.

The most readily available source of information on chemical ingredients in compounds available commercially is the safety data sheet (SDS), previously called a material safety data sheet (MSDS). The SDS is a document that provides information on the properties of hazardous chemicals and how they affect health and safety in the workplace. The OSHA Hazard Communication Standard (HCS) requires chemical manufacturers, distributors, or importers to provide workers access to the SDS on all hazardous substances in a workplace.

There are other agencies and organizations that may help in the evaluation of a patient for both occupational and environmental exposures. The American Association of Poison

Control Centers offers free and confidential medical advice 24 hours a day, 7 days a week, and is a resource for advice on toxicological issues. The ATSDR has information on exposures and diseases related to toxic substances. There are also datasets readily available to research into specific exposures and chemicals.

▶ Sentinel Case Reporting

NIOSH defines the *sentinel health event (occupational)* (SHE[O])as "a disease, disability, or untimely death, which is occupationally related and whose occurrence may provide the impetus for epidemiologic or industrial hygiene studies; or serve as a warning signal that materials substitution, engineering control, personal protection, or medical care may be required." The SHE(O) sentinel cases can prove to be extremely useful in triggering regulatory or public health investigations that can lead to prompt control of new hazards, thereby preventing new cases of work-related disease from occurring. Each state has specific reporting requirements for suspected occupational injuries and diseases.

▶ Clinical Practice Guidelines

Since the 1970s, the summarizing of research to develop evidence-based clinical practice guidelines has been established across a range of medical specialties including occupational health. The incorporation of evidence-based medicine into clinical practice can reduce practice variation and improve quality. A clinical algorithm or flowchart often seen as a graphic format that sets forth a stepwise procedure for managing a clinical problem has been used in making decisions about diagnosis and treatment of clinical problems. A number of state workers' compensation bureaus have developed and/or adopted clinical practice treatment guidelines for work-related injury and illness. However, it is important for the clinician to remember that guidelines are only descriptions of normative data, observed best practices, expert consensus, or high-grade evidence, and that each clinical case must be evaluated and treated individually.

ENVIRONMENTAL HEALTH HISTORY

Pollution of air, soil, and water; contamination of food; releases from nearby industrial facilities or waste sites; and environmental hazards in the home environment are all common causes for concern among patients, community members, and public health officials. Physicians today are called on increasingly to address questions or problems related to environmental health. The environmental health history is becoming an important tool for evaluating patients, especially on initial clinical visits and for those with new-onset asthma or allergic rhinitis symptoms, dermatitis, symptoms suggesting potential lead or pesticide poisoning or exposure, as well as at least once during prenatal and well-baby visits. The CH^2OPD^2 mnemonic (**c**ommunity, **h**ome, **h**obbies, **o**ccupation, **p**ersonal habits, **d**iet, and **d**rugs) may be a useful starting point for a more focused environmental history. All physicians must understand the effects of common environmental exposures and the similarities and differences between environmental health and occupational health.

ESTABLISHING CAUSATION

There are two general rubrics for causation to be considered by the clinician: general and specific causation. General causation refers to the methodology by which scientists determine whether or not an agent is capable of causing a disease or disorder. The determination of general causation requires research in such fields of science as epidemiology, biostatistics, toxicology, pathology, molecular biology, carcinogenesis, cytogenetics, and other fields of medicine related to the particular disease of interest. In forming an opinion, the clinician should consider not just published epidemiologic reports but all relevant data, including human case reports, animal data, experimental studies, laboratory data, mechanistic data, and other types of data, as well including unpublished studies. Generally accepted methodology for determining general causation includes (1) identifying all relevant studies, (2) reading and critically evaluating all the relevant studies, (3) evaluating all the data based on recognized scientific factors (the Bradford Hill viewpoints) and other factors relevant to the chemical and the disease, (4) exercising best professional judgment in reaching a conclusion on the issue of whether a particular chemical or class of chemicals can cause a particular disease, and (5) explaining the factual basis and the reasoning supporting the conclusion.

In reaching an opinion regarding specific causation, the clinician considers whether exposure in the individual patient likely caused or contributed to the disease. In order to reach this determination, the clinician should abstract and evaluate medical records; evaluate the potential alternative causes for the claimed injury (differential etiology); analyze diagnostic errors, including highlighting failures of differential diagnosis; evaluate the extent of the exposure to the agent(s); and examine temporal relationships, including latency.

CASE PRESENTATIONS

▶ Case 1—Occupational or Environmental?

A 42-year-old woman comes to your clinic for her annual physical examination. She has no major medical illnesses, takes a multivitamin and calcium, and her only complaint is some mild fatigue in the last several months. Her laboratory tests were normal except for a mild anemia. Follow-up testing does not reveal a cause for the anemia. The patient states she wonders if the anemia is related to her work at an electronics assembly plant. You inquire about what she does at work and she tells you that her job is soldering conductive wires to printed circuit boards. You obtain permission from the patient to talk to the company safety professional.

The safety professional states that her exposures might include lead exposure and that he will request an industrial hygiene (IH) evaluation to see if the safety measures that have kept the patient free of lead exposure in the past are still working. In addition, the workers' compensation insurance company contacts you to discuss the case. You have received permission from the patient to talk with the safety personnel at the workers' compensation insurance company.

Following your discussion with the company safety professional, you have tested the patient for blood lead level and it comes back slightly elevated. It is your responsibility to notify the state Department of Health as a part of their lead poisoning prevention program. They inquire about your patient's employer, and if there are any children involved. The state has an occupational health surveillance program, and they will be contacting the company to see if the lead exposure is from the worksite and if other workers are involved.

You discover in the course of taking both occupational and environmental histories that the patient has a hobby of making stained glass windows. Your questions reveal that this is done in her basement without adequate ventilation. A private IH survey reveals lead deposits in the basement with wipe samples. The patient does not have any children in the house, but her husband is being tested for lead exposure.

The IH report from the workplace showed an area in her work station that needed further engineering controls, but that no other workers had elevated blood lead levels. The patient is instructed on proper IH measures in the home, and once the home environment is cleaned, she is allowed to return to her hobby with proper attention to safe practices when handling lead.

▶ Case 2—Sentinel Lung Disease

A 50-year-old man presents with a 3-month history of shortness of breath and nonproductive cough. He does not have medical insurance through his employer, and was examined in the local public hospital emergency room. Physical examination was normal. The chest x-ray shows bilateral fine moderate linear interstitial infiltrates. The computed tomography (CT) scan of the chest shows diffuse nodular opacities in upper and mid lung zones, with several foci of large parenchymal opacities, bilateral hilar, and mediastinal adenopathy with microfoci of calcifications. He is referred for occupational medicine consultation.

On additional history, you learn that he has worked for the past 6 years cutting, polishing, and grinding artificial (engineered) stone. He is a nonsmoker and has no history of tuberculosis exposure. His employer did not provide local exhaust ventilation or wet methods during his work tasks, and he did not routinely wear personal protective equipment (PPE). He recalls that there is always visible dust in the air and on work surfaces. He was trained by his employer about the hazards of dust on the job but was not specifically aware of the effects of silica dust on the lungs. There are four other employees in his shop who also do the same work; he thinks that one to two other workers sometimes have trouble breathing.

Additional workup includes a TB skin test (negative) and three sputa for acid fast bacilli (culture negative). Pulmonary function studies show reduced total lung capacity (72% predicted), with reduced diffusing capacity (61% predicted). Serologic testing (antinuclear antibody, anti-Scl-70, anti-centromere antibody, anti-RNA polymerase III antibody, anticitrullinated peptide antibodies, rheumatoid factors) is negative. You make the diagnosis of silicosis based on the occupational history and clinical presentation and advise that he should not return to work with silica dust exposure. However, no work is available at this employer, and your patient is off work while his claim for benefits is adjudicated.

As part of your public health and regulatory reporting responsibility, you notify local or state government authorities. They conduct a follow-up investigation of this workplace where silica sampling shows levels 10 times above the permissible levels. In addition, a government-wide inspection program of all artificial stone fabrication shops is implemented, with no-cost silica medical examinations for all workers with more than 1-year exposure to silica dust.

RESOURCES

Selected Agencies & Organizations

AFL-CIO Workplace Health and Safety: https://aflcio.org/issues/workplace-health-and-safety.

Agency for Toxic Substances and Disease Registry (ATSDR) Toxicological Profiles: http://www.atsdr.cdc.gov/toxprofiles/index.asp; Medical Management Guidelines (MMGs) for Acute Chemical Exposures: www.atsdr.cdc.gov/MMG/index.asp.

American Association of Poison Control Centers (AAPCC): http://www.aapcc.org/.

Association of Occupational and Environmental Clinics (AOEC): www.aoec.org.

ATSDR Case Studies in Environmental Medicine: https://www.atsdr.cdc.gov/csem/csem.html.

Canadian Center for Occupational Safety and Health: https://www.ccohs.ca/.

Center for Construction Research and Training: https://www.cpwr.com/.

EPA Integrated Risk Information System (IRIS): https://www.epa.gov/iris.

European Agency for Safety and Health at Work: https://osha.europa.eu/.

European Commission Registration, Evaluation, Authorisation and Restriction of Chemicals (REACH): https://ec.europa.eu/environment/chemicals/reach/reach_en.htm#.

International Labor Organization (ILO): https://www.ilo.org/global/topics/safety-and-health-at-work/.

Mine Safety and Health Administration (MSHA): www.msha.gov/.

National Council for Occupational Safety and Health: https://www.coshnetwork.org/

National Institute of Environmental Health Sciences (NIEHS): https://www.niehs.nih.gov/.

National Institute for Occupational Safety and Health (NIOSH): (www.cdc.gov/niosh/); Registry of Toxic Effects of Chemical Substances: www.cdc.gov/niosh/rtecs; State-Based Occupational Health Surveillance Clearinghouse: https://wwwn.cdc.gov/niosh-statedocs/.

Occupational Safety and Health Administration (OSHA): www.osha.gov/.

Pediatric Environmental Health Specialty Units: https://www.pehsu.net/health_professionals.html.

Safe Work Australia: https://www.safeworkaustralia.gov.au/.

World Health Organization (WHO): https://www.who.int/health-topics/occupational-health.

Other References

Baron S, Filios MS, Marovich S, Chase D, Ash JS: Recognition of the relationship between patients' work and health: a qualitative evaluation of the need for clinical decision support (CDS) for worker health in five primary care practices. J Occup Environ Med 2017;59(11):e245-e250 [PMID: 29116994].

Basu S, Poole J, Adisesh A: A model for teaching occupational medicine. Clin Teach 2016;13(5):363-368 [PMID: 27624198].

Boschman JS, Brand T, Frings-Dresen MH, van der Molen HF: Improving the assessment of occupational diseases by occupational physicians. Occup Med (Lond) 2017;67(1):13-19. [PMID: 27834225].

Eaton JL, Mohammad A, Mohr DC, Brustein DJ, Kirkhorn SR: Occupational medicine specialist referral triggers: mixed-methods analysis of teleconsult cases. Occup Med (Lond) 2017;67(9):718-721 [PMID: 29155960].

Garg A, Mulloy KB: Developing a problem-based learning approach to the integration of environmental and occupational health topics into medical school curriculum. J Occup Environ Med 2018;60(8):754-759 [PMID: 29557838].

Papali A, Hines SE: Evaluation of the patient with an exposure-related disease: the occupational and environmental history. Curr Opin Pulm Med 2015;21(2):155-162 [PMID: 25602803].

■ SELF-ASSESSMENT QUESTIONS

Select the one correct answer for each question.

Question 1: Occupational/environmental history
- a. should include information about current and previous jobs in a systematic manner
- b. need not include possible environmental exposures at home and in the surrounding community and hobbies
- c. must establish a pattern of symptoms or organ systems involved
- d. may ignore an exposure type, occupation, or industry

Question 2: Safety data sheets
- a. must be available to workers if represented by counsel
- b. provide information on the properties of hazardous chemicals and how they affect health and safety in the workplace
- c. are required by OSHA to be up-to-date, complete, and accurate
- d. discourage contact with a manufacturing company toxicologist

Question 3: Sentinel Health Event (Occupational) (SHE[O])
- a. is a disease, disability, or untimely death, which is legally established as caused by work
- b. must be substantiated by epidemiologic or industrial hygiene studies
- c. requires materials substitution, engineering control, personal protection, or medical care
- d. may trigger regulatory or public health investigations that can lead to prompt control of new hazards

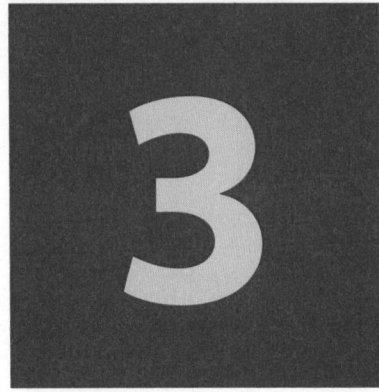

Workers' Compensation

Joseph LaDou, MS, MD

Virtually every industrialized country provides legislated entitlements to workers or their survivors to assist them in the event of an occupational injury or illness. Workers' compensation systems are designed to ensure that the injured worker receives immediate medical care, and that the injured worker also receives prompt but limited benefits to replace lost wages. Workers' compensation provides only part of the entitlement, with the rest—particularly for long-term disability—contributed indirectly through the country's social security system. Workers' compensation insurance assigns sure and predictable, "no-fault" liability to the employer.

Physicians and other health care providers who render care for work-related injuries and illnesses should understand the requirements of their jurisdiction's workers' compensation system. In addition to appropriate evaluation, diagnosis, and treatment, physicians are obligated to determine whether a worker's injury or disease claim was specifically caused by work activity—a process that often engenders an adversarial relationship between the physician, the patient, and the responsible party, that is, the employer. Physicians must provide services efficiently because they are accountable not only to their patient (the injured or ill worker) to alleviate suffering and to ensure the flow of benefits, but also to the insurer and the employer to minimize disability, lost work time, and costs associated with occupational injury or illness.

WORKERS' COMPENSATION LAW

The financial responsibility of the employer for the injury or death of an employee in the workplace was first established in Germany in 1884. Great Britain followed, in 1897, with legislation requiring employers to compensate employees or their survivors for an injury or death regardless of who was at fault. By the beginning of the twentieth century, all European countries had workers' compensation laws.

The German law provided a model of workers' compensation that was ultimately emulated by most European countries. The German system called for highly centralized administration of workers' compensation claims and disbursements. It provided for accident prevention, medical treatment, and rehabilitation. Its coverage was broad and compulsory by all employers. The law mandated that the insurance be proffered to employers by nonprofit mutual employers' insurance funds. The German system was closely linked to the rest of the nation's social insurance system.

The British law embodied a substantively different approach. Participation by employers was elective, administration was left to the judicial system, and insurance was offered to employers through private firms. The British system was not linked to the nation's social insurance system, and it did not provide for accident prevention, medical treatment, or rehabilitation. The British system was troubled from the outset by disputes over which jobs and what industries were to be covered, resulting in the very litigation that the law had been intended to replace.

There is a high degree of similarity between the basic criteria of the current workers' compensation systems in all European countries. Some European social security systems provide universal coverage for disability, regardless of whether it was caused or aggravated by work. Under this system, there is no specific insurance against employment injuries and occupational diseases. This form of social insurance provides wage replacement covering the loss of earnings due to old age, unemployment, temporary sickness, and/or permanent disability. For example, all workers in the Netherlands, Sweden, and Germany are covered against the risk of wage loss due to temporary sickness through government agencies. Coverage typically lasts up to 1 year, while transition is made to longer-term disability insurance programs if needed. In the Netherlands, partially disabled unemployed workers are given the same benefits as totally disabled workers.

US WORKERS' COMPENSATION

The workers' compensation movement did not begin in the United States until 1908, when a forerunner of the Federal Employees' Compensation Act (FECA) was passed. In the

United States, two separate and distinctly different workers' compensation systems, federal and state, function independently of one another.

▶ Federal Workers' Compensation

The FECA provides federal government employees who are injured in the performance of duty with workers' compensation benefits. These include wage-loss benefits for total or partial disability, monetary benefits for permanent loss of use of a body part, medical benefits, and vocational rehabilitation. FECA also provides survivor benefits to eligible dependents of workers who died as a result of a workplace injury or occupational disease.

The FECA is administered by the Office of Workers' Compensation Programs (OWCP) within the U.S. Department of Labor (DOL). FECA covers over 2.7 million federal employees in more than 70 different agencies, such as the U.S. Postal Service (USPS), the Department of Homeland Security, and the Department of Veterans Affairs. In addition, FECA covers a number of other worker groups adopted by Congress in various acts of expansion of the federal authority, namely military personnel, Longshore-Harbor workers, and specific high-risk workers (coal miners with black lung disease, energy employees exposed to certain materials such as beryllium, workers exposed to radiation, and veterans of military service). Military personnel constitute by far the largest federal program in workers' compensation. The federal system followed the German comprehensive model. FECA provides benefits without delay, and moves disabled workers to other government entitlement programs, including retirement, with relative ease. As a federally administered system, the FECA program operates without competition. The Secretary of Labor has exclusive jurisdiction over the entire program, including the various appeal and review processes. Most federal agencies include workers' compensation costs in their annual appropriations to Congress.

▶ State Workers' Compensation

Each of the 50 states, the District of Columbia, and the US territories has its own workers' compensation program. State workers' compensation programs vary in terms of who is allowed to provide insurance, which injuries or illnesses are compensable, and the level of benefits provided. When workers' compensation laws were gradually adopted by each state, they largely followed the less comprehensive British model. In 46 states, all or most workers' compensation insurance is currently provided by private insurance companies. Workers' compensation programs, with some important exceptions, are state-regulated, with laws determined by each state legislature and implemented by a state agency. The programs provide the payment of lost wages, medical treatment, and rehabilitation services to workers who have sustained an occupational injury or disease. Private insurers and self-insured employers administer the system on a day-to-day basis, accepting or denying claims, and paying benefits

to injured workers and medical providers. Some states give employers initial control of choice of physician, but limit the time of control. Some states give choice of physician to the worker. In either case, the choice of physician is ultimately split between worker and employer, even when one party is given de jure control.

▶ Characteristics of State Workers' Compensation Systems

A. No-Fault Principle and Exclusive Remedy

Employers' responsibility under the workers' compensation system for providing medical treatment and compensation benefits for employees injured at work or made ill from exposure to the workplace environment is based on a premise of liability without fault. Regardless of whether the worker, the employer, or neither is at fault, the employer is still responsible for providing medical treatment and compensation benefits to the injured employee.

A basic tenet of workers' compensation laws and the programs administered to implement them is that workers should receive quick and sure, though limited, payments for occupational injuries, and to assign to the employer sure and predictable liability for such payments. In return, benefits injured workers receive are their "exclusive remedy." The exclusive remedy principle is the quid pro quo under which the employer enjoys immunity from being sued, in exchange for accepting absolute liability for all occupational injuries and illnesses. The injured worker cannot sue his/her employer, however severe or permanent the work-related injury or illness, and regardless of the extent or circumstances of the extent of either the worker's or employer's culpability or negligence that led to the injury or illness.

B. Causation Test

To receive compensation under all state workers' compensation laws, a worker's injury or illness must "arise out of and in the course of employment" (AOE/COE). FECA uses the phrase "sustained while in the performance of duty." The success of the claimant largely depends on the validity, accuracy, and objectivity of the treating physician's evaluation and diagnosis. A work injury or illness that is determined to activate (accelerate) or aggravate a preexisting medical condition also is compensable in many states—though this definition varies by state and is subject to change with each elected legislature. Recurrence of an earlier compensable injury is also compensable. In some states, an injured worker may have a limited time period in which to "re-open" a closed claim, whereas in other states the worker is granted "lifetime reopening rights." Depending on the jurisdiction, judicial action may be necessary to resolve questions of liability for self-inflicted injuries and suicidal acts. Similar determinations may be necessary for injuries occurring under the influence of alcohol or drugs, during entirely personal activity (not AOE/COE), and for violence at work.

Table 3–1. Workers' compensation benefit costs.

	WC Claims	Benefits Paid
Medical-only cases	77%	8%
Indemnity (cash benefit) cases	23%	92%

C. Benefits

In the United States each year, more than 900,000 workers miss 1–4 days of work; more than 1 million experience temporary total disability (TTD); more than half a million have an injury that causes a permanent disability (partial in most cases); and more than 4000 experience a fatal injury on the job.

The vast majority of occupational injuries are minor sprains, strains, and abrasions. These minor injuries are self-limited in nature and readily treated in workers who are almost universally disposed to return to work. Many such cases involve a temporary assignment of modified or restricted duty, during which time the worker does not receive disability benefits. Well over 90% of occupational injuries are temporary disability cases.

Of the 8.5 million occupational injuries reported in a single year in the United States, the vast majority (> 6 million) do not involve time away from work. In these cases, the only benefits are payments made for medical care to physicians or other medical providers. Medical-only claims are not a major expense to the employer or insurer. Although they account for approximately 77% of workers' compensation claims, they constitute only 8% of all benefits paid (Table 3–1).

The remaining 23% of cases, which include the more serious injuries and some occupational diseases, account for 92% of worker benefits, medical care costs, and disability benefits.

1. Indemnity payments—Workers' compensation insurance for an accepted claim pays employees benefits (sometimes referred to a "cash benefits") for lost work time after a 3- to 7-day waiting period. Payment of benefits to workers or their families are of six types: (1) temporary partial disability (TPD), (2) temporary total disability (TTD), (3) permanent partial disability (PPD), (4) permanent total disability (PTD), (5) survivors' benefits, and (6) vocational rehabilitation benefits.

A. TEMPORARY PARTIAL DISABILITY—TPD occurs when a worker is injured to the degree that the worker cannot perform his or her usual work, but is still capable of working at some job during convalescence, usually with temporary restrictions or limitations ("modified duty," assigned by the treating physician). Under this category, the injured worker is compensated for the difference between wages earned before the injury and wages earned during the period of TPD, usually at two-thirds of the difference, assuming the modified duty work is significantly different than the regular job assignment.

Many insurers and employers view modified duty as a critical element of the treatment plan and rehabilitation of these injured workers. Modified duty may save the worker from wage differentials by preventing the TPD payment. When an employer does not have a job that can meet the restrictions imposed by the treating physician, or refuses to allow an injured worker to return to work until he/she is cleared by the physician for "full duty," the worker is entitled to receive TTD.

B. TEMPORARY TOTAL DISABILITY—The majority of injured workers receiving compensation are expected to recover with treatment and/or time, but are unable to work for some period of time. By law, these injured workers are entitled to receive TTD benefits. One million workers experience a TTD.

TTD benefits are paid during the recovery period on the basis of the worker's average earnings. Minimum and maximum limits apply, and benefits of as much as two-thirds of gross salary or 80% of take-home wages are paid until the individual is able to return to work or reaches maximum recovery. There is a waiting period for this type of compensation, but it is paid retroactively if the worker cannot work for a certain number of days or if hospitalization is necessary. The waiting period serves as an incentive to return to work after less serious injuries. Thus, it is like a deductible provision in other forms of health insurance in which the worker shares some of the cost, despite the "no-fault" principle.

Temporary disability benefits—TPD and TTD—account for 63% of claims involving cash benefits, yet they represent only 16% of the benefits incurred, with the preponderance of such benefits allocated to permanent disability (Table 3–2).

C. PERMANENT PARTIAL DISABILITY—PPD occurs when an injured worker is disabled to the point that he/she has lost some ability to compete in the open labor market. Injuries resulting in permanent impairments to body parts are typically compensated through the use of a "schedule," a list of injuries and well-recognized occupational diseases specified in workers' compensation statutes which are translated into a percentage of loss of total body function. For example, 100% loss of use of an arm entitles the worker to 500 weeks of benefits, and 50% loss of use of an arm to 250 weeks.

Nonscheduled PPD benefits are paid for injuries not on the schedule list. Injuries to the spine that are permanently disabling are typically not scheduled, nor are injuries to

Table 3–2. Indemnity (cash benefit) payments.

	WC Claims	Benefits Paid
Temporary partial disability plus temporary total disability	63%	16%
Permanent partial disability	36%	67%
Permanent total disability	1%	17%

certain internal organs, head injuries, and many occupational diseases. For unscheduled conditions, the approaches used can be categorized into four methods. Some states use an "impairment approach," which looks only at the medical consequences of the injury. The benefit is based entirely on the degree of impairment. In states that use the "loss of earning capacity approach," disability evaluation considers medical consequences as well as factors such as age, education, and job experience that affect the worker's earning capacity. Under the "wage-loss approach," benefits are paid only if the worker also has actual wage loss due to work injury, after it has been determined that maximum medical improvement has been achieved.

PPD cases account for more than half of all claims, with temporary disability typically lasting more than 7 days. PPDs account for 36% of claims that involve cash payments, but constitute 67% of benefit payments (Table 3–2).

D. **PERMANENT TOTAL DISABILITY**—PTD covers workers who are so disabled from an occupational injury or disease that they will not be able to work again in an open labor market, and for whom further treatment offers no hope of recovery. Most states compensate such individuals with two-thirds of their average wages, subject to minimum and maximum limits. Because benefits are not taxed, this can amount to approximately 85–90% of take-home wages. States also may provide additional funds for dependents. Although some states limit the duration of payments, others provide compensation for the remainder of the injured worker's life.

PTDs, together with fatalities, account for only 1% of all cases that receive cash benefits, yet they account for 17% of total cash benefit payments (Table 3–2). The medical costs per case are the highest by far for the 8200 who are permanently totally disabled by a workplace injury each year, averaging more than $680,000 per case.

E. **SURVIVORS' BENEFITS**—Dependent survivors of employees killed "on the job" are paid death benefits under workers' compensation. The method and size of payments vary widely among the various states, but all systems provide for a death benefit and some reimbursement for burial expenses.

Occupational diseases are responsible for more deaths than occupational injuries. However, many diseases that are probably associated with occupational exposures are either not recognized as such by the worker, his/her family, or the treating physician, or are disputed by the insurer or employer. Medical costs for deaths due to occupational diseases are sevenfold greater than the costs of injuries, estimated to be well over $20 billion.

F. **VOCATIONAL REHABILITATION BENEFITS**—Vocational and psychological counseling or retraining and job placement assistance are typical benefits. Some level of rehabilitation is provided in all states even if unspecified by statute. The goal is to return the injured worker to suitable, gainful employment.

2. Benefits from other sources—A number of benefits are available to workers from other sources.

A. **SOCIAL SECURITY DISABILITY INSURANCE (SSDI)**—In the United States, the social security system is the main funding source for workplace disabilities outside of the workers' compensation insurance system.

For permanently and totally disabled workers, SSDI supplements workers' compensation with monthly benefits for disability. Such benefits are available only after a 5-month waiting period and are calculated as if the disabled individual had reached social security retirement age. To be considered disabled, the injured person must be unable to work in substantial gainful employment. Furthermore, the disability must be expected to last more than 1 year or to result in premature death. SSDI combined with workers' compensation cannot exceed 80% of the worker's average earnings or the total family benefit under social security before the injury. If the combined compensation does exceed this amount, social security benefits are reduced accordingly, although some states will reduce workers' compensation benefits by all or part of the social security payments.

The SSA deems disabilities to be "total and complete" if applicants demonstrate that their impairments prevent them from earning at least $1180 a month. Presumptions of disability are based on age, education, work history, and other mitigating factors. Applicants are permitted to count the sum of multiple "non-severe" impairments as one "severe" disability. Nearly 9 million workers and 2 million dependents receive SSA disability payments each year.

B. **SECOND-INJURY FUNDS**—Second-injury (also called "subsequent injury") funds compensate workers for injuries that are exacerbated by a subsequent injury to the same body part or organ system. Some states' second-injury funds compensate workers for flare-ups that do not necessarily lead to total disability. These funds are established and maintained by most states, paid through employers' workers' compensation insurance premiums, in the hope that the outcome will encourage employers to hire the handicapped or previously injured workers. The employer's compensation carrier makes payments for the second injury, and the fund reimburses the carrier for any additional costs.

D. Apportionment

Apportionment is a legal device to deal with cumulative injury or illness such as low back pain or psychiatric conditions. It is intended to distribute financial responsibility to the insured employer versus previous employers, or to the worker him/herself. It is intended to ensure that employers are only responsible for the portion of injuries or illnesses that actually were caused in their workplace. Apportionment applies only to permanent disability.

Diagnostic assessment of causation must sometimes address the medical–legal question of apportionment. The compensability of a claim of occupational illness or injury is challenging in cases that involve multiple organ systems, or which present as a common symptom (eg, shortness of breath) that overlaps with many other common ailments or a preexisting condition, or which may be of a recurring nature (eg, asthma), or which could be caused or aggravated by both work-related and non-work-related factors that cannot be readily distinguished. Apportionment is an additional burden in the award of compensation, requiring the highest level of medical diagnostic skill and experience.

Apportionment is applicable in states where all or some injuries require something more than the traditional "contributing cause" standard. The most obvious examples are the "predominant cause" standard in Oregon for all claims, and the use of "predominant cause" in virtually all states that compensate mental-mental (purely psychological injury) claims. In this case, apportionment is really an "all or nothing" standard, excluding workers from any benefits if they fail the threshold.

E. Compromise and Release

Compromise and release (C&R) settlements are now accepted by workers' compensation for permanent disability in nearly all states. These agreements typically involve a partial or full release of the employer and insurer from further liability for the injury. These settlements allow the payment of benefits in a lump sum, rather than a series of payments over longer periods of eligibility. The settlement represents a compromise on the part of the claimant and the insurer or employer, releasing the employer from future medical obligations. The C&R may shift responsibility for future costs to other systems. The worker may require further treatment for an occupational injury under a health insurance policy long after the injury. In cases likely to overlap with Medicare, C&Rs are required to have a formal Workers' Compensation Medicare Set-Aside (WCMSA) which is a trust to pay future costs before Medicare becomes an option. In both these examples, the physician plays a key role in determining the value of future medical compromise, and the value of WCMSA for Medicare.

ROLE OF THE PHYSICIAN

Workers' compensation laws place the treating physician in a critically important role. The physician serves as the gatekeeper to benefits in the workers' compensation system, a health care system that is separate from mainstream medicine. Physicians must determine that an injury or illness is caused by work, diagnose it, prescribe care, and assess the extent of impairment and the ability of the worker to resume work.

Most physicians who participate in the workers' compensation system do not require specialized training in the diagnosis or treatment of occupational injuries, diseases, and related areas of disability. Primary care for work injuries is predominantly provided by emergency rooms, clinics, and medical practices devoted to worker injuries and other forms of urgent care. Orthopedic surgeons play a prominent role in workers' compensation because of the large number of musculoskeletal injuries. Residency-trained occupational medicine specialists ("occupational physicians") actually play a

relatively small role in workers' compensation injury care, as their training and specialization is focused more on occupational disease and cumulative trauma disorders where skills in history taking, exposure assessment, differential diagnosis, and causation assessment are required.

The WC system has changed dramatically in recent decades. In its early history, virtually all injuries were traumatic injuries. They clearly happened at work, usually in manufacturing industries, construction, and transportation/utilities. There were no other social insurance programs available to workers, such as contemporary health insurance or Social Security. In the current working environment, the large majority of occupational conditions, particularly for disabling conditions, are nontraumatic injuries and illnesses where work is not necessarily the single cause, or even the most important cause among many.

Determinations that injuries or illnesses are caused by work are increasingly contentious. The physician who takes a careful occupational health history, documenting the details of the events leading up to and including the event of the injury or illness, often will be the most important influence on the finder of fact (workers' compensation judge or referee) as to work-relatedness. The physician who provides treatment and follows the worker medically usually will be the most important influence on the finder of fact as to the nature and extent of the injury or illness.

All parties—the worker, the employer, and the insurer—benefit from an emphasis by the treating physician on early return to work. The proper determination of work restrictions acceptable to the employer and the worker draws on the physician's experience, his or her familiarity with the workplace and job description, and his or her rapport with both the worker and the employer. Moreover, through continuing care of the worker, the physician determines when the worker has reached maximal medical improvement (MMI) or maximal functional recovery (MFR).

Insurers also may ask the physician to determine work restrictions (eg, no overhead lifting for someone with shoulder problems, or no working around moving machinery or at unprotected heights for someone with a balance problem) in order to match the impairment to specific jobs. In some instances, the exact physical restrictions are best determined by a functional-capacity evaluation.

▶ Physician Selection

Workers in many states are permitted by state workers' compensation regulations to choose their own physicians. The choice may be any licensed physician or may be made from a list maintained by the employer or the state workers' compensation agency. The selection criteria for physician competence, qualifications, and experience vary with the jurisdiction.

The worker may be required to submit to periodic examinations by a physician of the employer's choice, or to an independent medical examination (IME), depending on the jurisdiction. If either the employer or the worker is dissatisfied with the progress under the chosen physician's treatment, either party can request, and often is allowed, to change physicians. Typically, an employee is permitted one such change for subjective reasons alone. In contrast, the employer can be required to prove to the state agency that a change is needed. Reasons for discharging a physician include incompetence, lack of reasonable progress toward recovery, inadequate or insufficient reporting by the physician, and inconvenience of the physician's practice location. If the employer selects the physician, and if the injured employee is not satisfied with the treatment and progress, he/she may be permitted consultation with another physician at the employer's (insurer's) expense.

Although the employer must cover the cost of medical treatment for the injured employee, if the employee refuses reasonable treatment or surgery without justifiable cause, the employer is relieved of responsibility for any benefits related to injuries caused by the delay in or refusal of any treatment. When the suggested treatment or surgery entails a significant risk, the worker's refusal usually is considered justified.

▶ Disability Determinations

Disability is defined as limitation in ability to work. Insurers in many states ask the physician to determine the degree of "impairment" (measured by anatomic or functional loss), which the insurers will give to disability raters, workers' compensation judges, commissioners, or hearing officers. These nonmedical people make the decision as to "disability" and to the degree of disability and its level of compensation. Disability, unlike impairment, depends on the job and one's ability to compete in the open job market. Impairment does not necessarily imply disability. It is important to discuss impairment and disability separately. An individual with carpal tunnel syndrome may be disabled when considered for a job with repetitive hand movements but not for a job that does not require extensive use of the hands.

In some states, an independent "rating physician" designated by the state workers' compensation governing agency examines the claimant to provide this determination. In other states, the treating physician examines and documents the injured worker's "objective" impairments, and a government administrator or tribunal makes the actual determination of the percentage of PPD. Fees for disability evaluations are often fixed by statute. Formal training for physicians who provide impairment and disability evaluations is offered by the American Board of Independent Medical Examiners (ABIME) and the American Academy of Disability Evaluating Physicians (AADEP).

The American Medical Association's (AMA) Guides to the Evaluation of Permanent Impairment is increasingly accepted as a standard for impairment and disability assessment in the United States by both state and federal programs. The AMA Guides emphasizes the fundamental skills physicians need to evaluate and communicate patient impairments. The sixth edition applies both terminology from and an analytical framework based on the International Classification of Functioning, Disability and Health (ICF), to generate five impairment classes which permit the rating of the patient from "no impairment" to "most severe."

Many workers' compensation cases are settled with "continuing medical treatment" provided either within limits or as a lifelong benefit. The opinion as to the value of continued medical treatment and for what purpose it is to be rendered should be stated, along with recommendations for current treatment should it be different from treatment already provided the employee by other physicians.

▶ Compensable Occupational Diseases

Occupational diseases affect 15–20% of all workers. Conservative estimates are that 5–10% of cancers, myocardial infarctions, strokes, and transient ischemia are caused by workplace factors. The vast majority of individuals with known or suspected occupational disease do not file claims for workers' compensation benefits. The suggestion to do so would be rarely encountered in most medical settings. Workers who develop occupational diseases following long latency periods seldom receive benefits.

Many states have rewritten their workers' compensation laws, making it even more difficult for injured workers to receive compensation for occupational diseases. The challenge with occupational disease, as with cumulative trauma such as low back pain, or psychiatric conditions, is that assigning cause can be more complex. Employers and their insurers, often with defense attorneys, take the position that there are multiple causes for most diseases. When multiple causes exist, it is not economically efficient to assign all responsibility to the employer. A cumulative injury where work is responsible for 10% of the cause requires the employer to pay 100% of the costs if it is recognized by workers' compensation. This explains, in part, why so much legislation is enacted each year to deal with workers' compensation programs in the various states. Because these conditions are subject to frequent dispute, they generate litigation and related friction costs, and often hurt the worker by fracturing the employment relationship. Nonetheless, the treating physician has an obligation to estimate work causation when caring for injured or ill workers.

▶ Employment Discrimination

There are over 24 million Americans underemployed or out of work. This includes a growing number of people often referred to as "no longer looking for work." In 1950, 14% of men were out of the labor force. Today, that figure stands at 31%. This group includes millions of workers who have been stigmatized by former injuries, illnesses, and claims for workers' compensation benefits. Many of them have been denied benefits by the state workers' compensation system, and few of them can meet the criteria for "total disability" imposed by the federal government. They receive no vocational rehabilitation or job training.

A past claim for workers' compensation is often used as an unspoken reason for denying job applicants. An employer may access digital information on workers' compensation claims history, use the data to company advantage, and leave no paper trail. The job applicant never knows a thing about it. Such abuse of the workers' compensation system should be reported and brought to the attention of relevant agencies.

▶ Independent Medical Examination

When a compensation claim determination is contested by the insurer, employer, or employee, physicians become important witnesses in resolving disputes. When a nontreating physician is requested to evaluate the worker, in most states this evaluation is designated as an IME. Requests for IME opinions from insurers, workers, plaintiffs' attorneys, judges, and others may initiate an IME evaluation, and typically require the insurer to cover the costs. The opinion of the IME likely will be the final opinion for the worker and determine the success or failure of his or her claim. The IME does not establish a legal doctor-patient relationship because the examination of the worker is not based on the worker's consent. The IME report should be complete and definitive and include diagnosis, cause of injury or illness, prognosis, MMI status, permanent impairment, work capacity, and opinion on further clinical management. The IME physician must be prepared to testify at a deposition and, on rare occasion, appear before a workers' compensation judge or referee. The IME physician seldom sees the worker again and ethically should not assume any responsibility for medical care. Physicians should strive to be unbiased, despite the presence of some perverse incentives.

EMPLOYERS' RESPONSIBILITIES

Workers' compensation insurance coverage is compulsory for most private employment. Workers' compensation laws cover approximately 87% of all wage and salary workers. Employees most likely to be exempt from coverage include self-employed people, domestic workers, agricultural workers, and casual laborers. Coverage also may be limited for workers in small companies with only a few employees, nonprofit institutions, and state and local governments.

A. Demonstration of Ability to Pay Benefits

Unless exempted by the law, employers must demonstrate their ability to pay workers' compensation benefits. There are three ways of accomplishing this: (1) insurance with a state fund, (2) insurance through a private carrier, or (3) self-insurance.

1. State insurance funds—The states have adopted two methods of meeting the problem of workers' compensation coverage. Some states require that employers insure through a state fund that operates as the exclusive provider of insurance. Other states operate their funds in competition with private carriers. A few states do not permit an employer to be self-insured. State funds are the third largest payer in workers' compensation. Nearly half of states pay some amount of workers' compensation benefits through a state fund. State funds serve as insurer of last resort for employers declined coverage by private carriers.

2. Private insurance carriers—Private workers' compensation insurance contracts have two purposes: (1) to satisfy the employer's obligation to pay compensation and (2) to ensure that the injured employee receives all the benefits provided by law. A contracted insurer is responsible for compensating the injured worker, and generally the employer is not involved in any claims administration, except to the extent of modified duty and return to work issues. The carrier's liability is not relieved by either the insolvency or death of the employer or any disagreement the carrier may have with the employer. Most state funds are similarly restricted.

3. Self-insurance—Larger employers, or groups of smaller employers in a common industry, may decide to serve as their own insurers. This approach includes the responsibility for adjusting claims and paying benefits. These tasks are contracted out to companies that provide such services (ie, third-party administrators). To qualify as a self-insurer, a company or group of companies must demonstrate that it has the financial ability to pay all claims that reasonably may be expected. The state agency usually has specific requirements that a bond or other security be posted. Because this form of insurance is both time-consuming and requires financial reserves, smaller companies seldom self-insure.

Companies choose to self-fund to reduce costs and to maximize cash flows. Because costs of benefits, claim reserves, litigation, and attendant administrative costs have spiraled in recent years, many companies have concluded that they could do as well as independent carriers while saving the cost of commissions and premium taxes, and take advantage of greater cash flow and increased investment income rates.

B. Penalties for Not Having Insurance

Workers' compensation insurance is mandatory in every state but Texas. There are heavy penalties for uninsured employers. They can be subject to fines, loss of common-law defenses, increases in the amount of benefits awarded, and payment of attorneys' fees. The biggest financial deterrent is that the employee may bring a civil suit against the employer. A number of states will force closure of an uninsured business. All states have an uninsured employer's fund(s) to which injured employees can apply for benefits. Applying to such a fund does not preclude the individual from also bringing legal action against the employer for penalties and legal fees. The uninsured employer is also required to reimburse the fund for benefits paid to injured workers.

▶ Claim Filing Requirements

The injured or ill employee is required to report the injury or illness as soon as he or she becomes aware that it has occurred. For overt accidents, this requirement is straightforward, whereas for cumulative injuries or diseases, a correct diagnosis may be delayed, the problem may be misdiagnosed, or may not be readily attributable to a work-related cause.

A statute of limitations limits the employer's liability when an injury or illness is not reported within a specified period, typically 1 week. The claim itself requires a written "notice of injury" in nearly all states. Employees who verbally inform their employer of a possible injury but do not put it in writing are thus vulnerable to loss of compensation benefits. In some states, the requirement is met if the employer is informed by someone other than the injured worker. Once a notice of injury has been filed, the employer then must provide all medical care reasonably required to alleviate the problem. If a claim is later denied by an insurer, there may develop a financial liability for the injured worker and/or physician for the care rendered in all but emergency situations.

MEDICAL COST CONTAINMENT

Total workers' compensation benefits to injured workers exceed $60 billion each year. However, that sum represents only 1.1% of the country's total health care costs. The public and its legislators view workers' compensation as a social insurance system paid for by employers, thus not a direct burden on taxpayers. For this reason, the ever-expanding bureaucracies of workers' compensation at federal and state levels evade reform efforts that affect the rest of the country's health care system.

In reality, all funds for health services ultimately come from private households, regardless of whether they flow through government, business, or charities. Employers' premiums, government disbursements, and charities' largesse are all extracted from households as payroll deductions, taxes, and donations. The costs and efficiency of workers' compensation are a necessary consideration of all participants.

Medical care now accounts for more than half of total workers' compensation costs. Physicians in private practice and in major health services corporations participate in a fee-for-service payment system widely accepted by employers and insurance carriers. Among larger occupational health services providers, there are incentives for cost containment as a part of the "business model" to gain contracts. In some states, the establishment of selected panels under the aegis of the insurance company has restricted access to specialists such as psychiatrists, neurologists, cardiologists, pulmonary specialists, oncologists, and dermatologists.

In most states, there are no statutory limitations on the length of time for or the cost of treatment. Most state laws allow for treatment even when recovery is not possible; that is, palliative care that does not cure but only relieves. States and private insurers are implementing a number of cost-containment strategies. These include (1) utilization review of inpatient and outpatient care, (2) hospital bill auditing of inpatient services, (3) medical bill auditing of practitioner and other services, (4) preferred provider networks for inpatient care where fees are discounted, and (5) care where the emphasis is on use of treatment guidelines, independent medical review (IMR), and optimization of outcome measures.

REFERENCES

American Medical Association. *Guides to the Evaluation of Permanent Impairment* 6th ed, amended, 2012.
World Health Organization (WHO): International Classification of Functioning, Disability, and Health, 2018: http://www.who.int/classifications/icf/en/.

■ SELF-ASSESSMENT QUESTIONS

Select the one correct answer for each question.

Question 1: Workers' compensation law
  a. is intended primarily to assign liability
  b. existed in the United States before European countries followed suit
  c. was first enacted by the states, then the Federal government
  d. requires the employer to provide compensation benefits to the injured employee

Question 2: Workers' compensation systems
  a. avoid lengthy and costly legal action
  b. provide an injured employee with medical treatment only when the incident is the fault of the employer
  c. compensate work injuries that activate or aggravate a preexisting condition
  d. do not compensate earlier compensable injury

Question 3: Occupational injuries
  a. are mostly temporary disability cases
  b. occur in fewer than 1 million workers each year in the United States
  c. are defined as injuries that involve time away from work
  d. are being erased through modern technology

Question 4: Temporary total disability
  a. encompasses the majority of occupational injuries
  b. benefits are paid during the recovery period on the basis of the worker's average earnings
  c. entails a waiting period, but it is paid retroactively if the worker cannot work for a certain number of days or if hospitalization is necessary
  d. is the costliest category of workers' compensation benefits

Question 5: Permanent total disability
  a. occurs in more than 10% of all compensable workers' compensation claims
  b. covers those workers who are so disabled that they will not be able to work again in an open labor market
  c. in most states is compensated with half of the workers' average wages
  d. does not provide additional funds for dependents

Question 6: Impairment
  a. is seldom determined by the physician
  b. is measured by anatomic or functional loss
  c. is another term for disability
  d. depends on the job and one's ability to compete in the open job market

Question 7: Occupational disease
  a. is present in half of all Americans
  b. claims result in benefits for most all workers with delayed illnesses

  c. claims for workers' compensation benefits are increasingly common
  d. does not include repetitive trauma disorders and mental disabilities

Question 8: Apportionment
  a. is a legal device for determining probable cause
  b. is intended to ensure that employers are responsible for all injuries or illnesses
  c. applies only to permanent disability
  d. no longer determines financial responsibility

Question 9: Compromise and release settlements
  a. are accepted by workers' compensation in only a few states
  b. allow the payment of benefits in a lump sum, rather than a series of payments over longer periods of eligibility
  c. represent a compromise only on the part of the insurer or employer
  d. do not overlap with Medicare

Ethics in Occupational Medicine

Carl F. Cranor, PhD

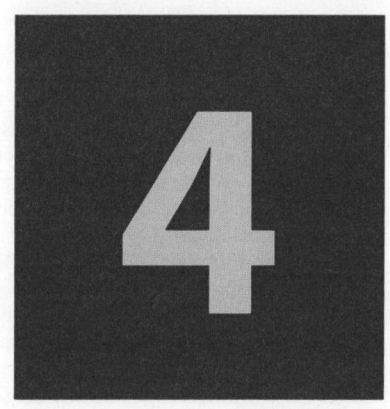

Among the central institutions of civilized society are those that seek to protect and ensure the health of people in the workplace. For most individuals, the workplace accounts for the majority of serious injuries and harmful exposures. If workers are properly protected, they receive a major contribution toward a healthier and likely longer life. In contrast, if workers are not protected, the workplace becomes a significant source of harm, loss of both physical and mental health, and may result in a shorter and less satisfying life.

The Justice Case for Preventing and Treating Occupational Diseases

Preventing occupational diseases is of primary concern because of their prevalence and the harm they inflict. Moreover, toxic exposures to workers can be brought into the home where they affect spouses and children. If the harm inflicted on adults or children is sufficiently great, it can arbitrarily interfere with lifelong well-being.

Health protection and health care institutions, along with educational institutions, are strategically important for securing and fostering *fair* opportunities. Everyone in the community, regardless of talents, abilities, and motivations, should have a fair opportunity to develop their endowments to the best of their ability in order to achieve life goals. This is the fair equality of opportunity aspect of justice.

Three precepts of justice generically guide the prevention and treatment of disease. Justice requires

1. Preventing diseases in the first place

2. Providing adequate and timely treatment for those who contract diseases or other workplace harms

3. Maintaining people as close as possible to a lifetime of good health

A just health protection and health care system would have institutions to prevent and treat diseases at all life stages.

Major Laws Protecting Worker Health

The federal institutions providing for workplace health protections in the United States are the *Occupational Safety and Health Administration* (OSHA) and the *National Institute for Occupational Safety and Health* (NIOSH).

The Occupational Safety and Health Act of 1970 (OSHAct) has several provisions for workplace protections. The main and legal authority for employee protections are OSHA-issued health standards addressing toxic materials or harmful physical agents. In order to protect employee from these toxicants the OSHAct requires the Secretary of Labor to issue health standards

> which most adequately [assure], to the extent feasible, on the basis of the best available evidence, that no employee will suffer material impairment of health or functional capacity even if such employee has regular exposure to the hazard dealt with by such standard[s] for the period of his working life.

When researchers have identified a toxicant, OSHA issues a proposed regulation following the substantive requirements and subject to administrative procedures specified in the law. The health standards must be based on the "latest available scientific data in the field, the feasibility of the standards, and experience gained under this and other health and safety laws" to attain "the highest degree of health and safety protection for the employee."

The proposed regulation is next posted in the Federal Register to elicit public comment. Once comments have been received OSHA holds an open hearing at which additional written or oral comments, subject to cross-examination, may be presented. Taking into account all the written and oral comments on the proposed health rule, OSHA then issues a final rule. This rule, provided it is not challenged in court, then has the force of law authorized by Congress in the OSHAct. If the final rule is challenged, it goes to a federal circuit court of appeals for adjudication. At that point the rule may be upheld in its entirety, partially upheld and partially overturned, or in the extreme overturned in its entirety. If it is overturned in part or as a whole, OSHA must go back to the administrative drawing board to revise or in the extreme drop the proposed law.

This substantive requirement of the OSHAct would be clearly endorsed by the prevention-of-disease component of justice. If a person is employed in a particular workplace, the law authorizes OSHA and pertinent companies to prevent "material impairment of health or functional capacity" even if a worker has regular exposure during a working lifetime, assumed to be 45 years. If the law were fully and justly implemented with follow-up enforcement to protect employees' health, in principle an individual could be employed in one workplace for a lifetime without suffering material impairment of health as a result of employment. If a person were to change jobs within a profession or change places of employment as long as the law was fully implemented and enforced across all industries, this too in principle would prevent initiation of occupational diseases.

While the OSHAct arguably measures up to an appropriate standard of justice to prevent occupational diseases, two qualifications should be noted. First, the health standard goal—that no employee suffers material impairment of health or functional capacity—must be "feasible." This vague requirement may attenuate fully adequate health protections but recognizes the extent to which health protections must be technologically and (to some extent) economically feasible, although this has not been fully clarified legally. This practical consideration potentially poses a barrier for health protections in industries whose health-threatening contaminants may be especially difficult to control or whose economic viability is borderline. The tension between good protective health standards and their "feasibility" may pose difficult choices for OSHA—to enforce standards for all companies even though some may be at risk economically, or have to declare bankruptcy (one appellate court has considered this possibility), or to fail to provide sufficient protections for some employees put at health risk by economically marginal workplaces. The permissible exposure limit in the OSHA lead standard is significantly in excess of safe levels, based on current toxicologic data. OSHA "protections" are heavily influenced by corporate economic interests.

A second qualification is that this 1970s law fails to protect *the children of employees* who can be harmed as a result of parental workplace exposures to toxicants. Such exposures may or may not result in harm to adults. However, recent research under the general title of the *developmental origins of health and disease* has revealed that a parent's exposures to toxicants if passed on to children in sufficient concentrations could cause them harm. Generically, this "is the theory that what happens to children during their development from embryonic and fetal life through infancy, early childhood, and the teenage years into adulthood can substantially influence their health and disease status, sometimes immediately but also even later in life."

A pregnant woman's toxic body burden, if sufficiently high, may contaminate a fetus developing *in utero* or a nursing newborn. Pregnant women's exposures to toxicants (or even exposures prior to pregnancy) would be the most obvious route by which adult exposures to toxic products could cause diseases in children, but even men's exposures to some toxicants can adversely affect developing fetuses. The problem of adult workplace exposures causing childhood diseases or pregnancy miscarriages will likely need to be addressed by either a new law specific to this purpose or by reducing exposures to toxicants in the workplace.

Sometimes workers can bring home toxicants that contaminate spouses or children, as has occurred with asbestos, a concern expressed in the OSHAct. Adult exposures to lead, mercury, methylmercury, other neurotoxicants, pesticides such as DDT, various xenoestrogens, for example, diethylstilbestrol (DES), radiation, tobacco smoke, solvents, dyes, and paints can trigger children's maladies or cause miscarriages. Animal data suggest that a much wider range of adult exposures can put offspring at risk of diseases. Exposed fathers may well cause miscarriages of fetuses or other prenatal or neonatal problems.

Standards for exposures to toxic materials and harmful physical agents must be established, properly implemented, and enforced. Merely having laws aimed at toxic substances or harmful physical agents identified by NIOSH, and having OSHA issue health standards to protect employees is not sufficient. Both NIOSH and OSHA must have sufficient funding and staffing to ensure that their respective tasks are carried out as envisioned by the law. Administrators of these public institutions have ethical responsibilities to ensure that the laws are properly implemented.

A second major component of the OSHAct that provides some protection for employees' health is its *general duty clause*. Even if OSHA has not issued a health standard, employers are responsible for complying with the general legal duty clause. Accordingly, companies must furnish employees with "employment and a place[s] of employment which are free from recognized hazards that are causing or are likely to cause death or serious physical harm."

This provision seems to be frequently used but difficult to implement. OSHA may apply it only when it has issued no formal health standard. The hazard must be recognized by an employer's industry, evidence of an employer's actual knowledge, or evidence that would be apparent to any reasonable person. The hazard must be causing or likely to cause death, and correcting it must be "feasible." According to those familiar with the procedures these conditions are difficult to use, but the general duty clause is nonetheless frequently utilized. Despite this, the general duty clause could be seen as a backup to the main substantive clause for health protections in extreme cases in which there is potential for death or serious physical harm.

Derivative Duties of Justice for Occupational Physicians

Beyond legal requirements and institutions for protecting worker health, individuals within NIOSH, OSHA, companies, and workers' compensation programs have roles in making these institutions function well to protect employees. A number of clearly identified ethical duties articulated in national or international codes of ethics for occupational physicians or health professionals more generally point to individual behavior to act or refrain from acting in order to protect employees from and to treat occupational diseases.

The considerations of justice, along with the Hippocratic Oath ("First do no harm") make prevention of occupational diseases preeminently important and support the design of institutions to implement many of the same protections. Moreover, these ethical duties are particularly important because occupational physicians are unusually subject to pressures that could frustrate just health goals.

While some ethical duties are prominent and obvious (eg, the duty to prevent harm to employees and promote their health), others are subsidiary to that and largely serve to facilitate and support the duty of prevention. Additionally, while there could be some temptation to underrate the importance of ethical duties, considerations of justice, which provide a foundation for many of the ethical duties, call attention to substantial adverse consequences to exposed workers if ethical duties are not adhered to. If diseases originating in the workplace are not prevented, the affected individuals will be harmed to one extent or another, either temporarily or permanently, depending on the disease.

Codes of Conduct

Organizations that represent occupational physicians and related specialists have developed Codes of Conduct for their members. The International Commission on Occupational Health (ICOH) has an extensive document, the International Code of Ethics for Occupational Health Professionals. The American College of Occupational and Environmental Medicine (ACOEM) Code of Ethics provides a similar guiding document for its members. The professional societies of industrial hygiene have similar codes. There are both ethical duties of occupational physicians and of scientific researchers that study occupational settings to determine whether or not workers are at risk.

The preeminent duty of an occupational physician, according to the International Code of Ethics for Occupational Health Professionals, is "to safeguard and promote the health of workers, to promote a safe and healthy working environment, to protect the working capacity of workers, and their access to employment." The American College of Occupational and Environmental Medicine concurs: the first duty is to "promote a safe and healthy workplace environment."

Protection of the health of employees might be either *generic* for a workplace or *specific* to particular individuals found to be at risk. An occupational physician might have to carry out either kind of prevention. The administrators of OSHA and NIOSH have legal and ethical duties to see to it that generic health protections are provided. NIOSH should carry out its responsibilities to identify occupational diseases that merit regulatory action by OSHA, and OSHA

should conduct as expeditiously as possible any appropriate additional research into hazardous exposures and issue health protections that are warranted. In addition, officials of private companies and their occupational physicians would also have a responsibility to provide generic workplace protections. Occupational physicians additionally have ethical duties to provide specific health protections for any individual identified as being at risk of occupational disease.

The major duty to safeguard and promote the health of workers is also supported by a number of subsidiary considerations or separate duties that assist in its implementation. For example, a physician can better serve generic prevention goals by being "proactive in terms of improving health and safety at work on the basis of their professional competence and ethical judgment." To carry out this task they need to "be familiar with the work and the working environment . . ." in order to be properly informed about any risks employees might face and how best to address them.

Moreover, proactive efforts to improve health and safety are well served by health surveillance to detect early onset of diseases or other injuries. Surveillance provides for ongoing health checks of employees who may be exposed to potentially hazardous substances. It can assist in detecting adverse health effects at an early stage, which serves both the generic health interests of employees and employers as well as more specifically any employee who shows early signs of occupational disease. It also helps employers to better evaluate any risks, institute any controls that might be needed, and may help identify lapses in health protections.

Properly conducted surveillance must be "consistent with available scientific evidence and relevant good practice." This includes being reliable and having "sufficient predictive value in relation to the requirements of the work assignment." Surveillance not based on good scientific evidence and practice is much less likely to reveal health risks that might be present.

In order for surveillance to have specific payoffs for employees it should be followed up with appropriate interpretations and adapted to the workplace for early detection of risks. Because it typically involves examinations of employees for early signs of disease, it should also be carried out with "non-coerced informed consent of the workers" with the import of any findings properly explained to them.

When surveillance and circumstances reveal an urgent health issue, physicians should rapidly implement "simple preventive measures [to reduce potential risks] which are technically sound" and properly followed up to determine "whether the measures are effective and whether more complete solutions" should be sought to provide needed protections from harm.

If individual workers are found to be at risk, a physician should, "communicate effectively and in a timely manner to an individual all significant observations about the health and health risk of that person and provide advice about interventions available to restore, sustain, and improve health or prevent illness."

As part of identifying health risks to employees a physician should communicate to an at-risk individual "significant observations about the health and health risk of that person," providing advice about potential interventions. This ethical provision reinforces the idea that an employee at risk should not remain ignorant of risky conditions or at the mercy of an employer who is sluggish to act on his or her behalf. With proper information an at-risk employee is empowered to make better life decisions. Importantly the physician should also report the same findings in individuals and populations to decision makers who are "in a position to take appropriate [individual or workplace wide protective] actions."

The International Code of Ethics for Occupational Health Professionals recognizes the importance of treating injured or diseased persons and maintaining them so that they can return to work. "Occupational health professionals should assist workers in obtaining and maintaining employment notwithstanding their health deficiencies or their handicap. It should be duly recognized that there are particular occupational health needs of workers as determined by factors such as gender, age, ethnicity, physiological condition, social aspects, communication barriers or other factors." This duty implicitly appears to recognize the importance of maintaining people as close as possible to normal biological functioning (perhaps even with some decrement in their workplace functioning), which in turn facilitates both their gainful employment and ideally their on-going opportunities that could last well beyond working years.

Conflicts of Interest

Codes of ethics call attention to resisting conflicts of interest in carrying out the ethical mandates for occupational medicine. The ACOEM strongly urges physicians to recognize, acknowledge, and appropriately address "any secondary interests that might in reality distort the integrity of judgments or be perceived to do so. Ethical practice must ensure that harm does not accrue as a result of such conflicts." The ICOH echoes this in strong language:

> Occupational health professionals must under no circumstances allow their judgment and statements to be influenced by any conflict of interest, in particular when advising the employer, the workers or their representatives in the undertaking on occupational hazards and situations which present evidence of danger to health or safety. Such conflicts may distort the integrity of the occupational health professionals who must ensure that the harm does not accrue with respect to workers' health and public health as a result of conflicts.

Ethical admonitions concerning conflicts of interest are especially critical given the myriad contexts in which occupational physicians must carry out their tasks as company doctors employed by corporations, consultants to corporations, or as private practitioners treating ill or injured workers. This group of physicians, including physicians in the employ of workers' compensation insurance companies or who act as "agreed medical examiners" for insurers and lawyers, face pressures to "manage patient care to promote the financial well-being of third parties." There may be substantial financial pressures to overlook or ignore diseases caused by the workplace to save companies money, to reduce workers' compensation payouts, or to protect one's income stream as a consultant.

Occupational physicians may also have a role in designing workplace health and safety programs, or in conducting research to determine whether or not a workplace likely is causing diseases or other harms. This can pose substantial conflicts when a company employs the professional or contacts with the physician or scientist as a consultant. Moreover, the consultant to a company may have a major conflict of interest under contract language, often including non-disclosure agreements to protect the company from litigation. The physician or scientist may also be influenced to show compliance to the company agenda in hopes of future consulting contracts awarded by a satisfied corporate client.

Occupational physicians face substantial financial pressures to "manage patient care to promote the financial well-being of third parties," not worker-patients, thus putting workers at risk of unidentified diseases, nondiagnosed diseases, or uncompensated diseases. These diseases, depending on their severity and longevity, may well cause lasting harm, truncated opportunities, and financial hardship.

Failures to properly promote a safe and healthy workplace would clearly constitute generic failure to prevent harm and be in violation of these codes. If diseases and dysfunctions occurred as a result, it would be unjust. Of course, failure to take prompt preventive action when a physician is aware of risks to employees or refusal or unwillingness to take remedial actions that would remove an undue risk would pose a comparatively direct threat to workers' health.

Failure to act in accordance with some indirect or *subsidiary duties* that support the central ethical obligation to promote a safe and healthy workplace from toxic exposures would not necessarily cause harm to employees, but this shortcoming likely would enhance or increase the risk of harm. For example, failure to use validated methods of risk assessment and health promotion and appropriate preventive measures with proper follow-up puts employees at risk and would be unjust if diseases or dysfunctions consequently occur.

Failure to maintain professional competence and expertise, while not necessarily causing harm, may put employees at risk of harm as a consequence. If harm occurs, that would be unjust. Similarly, physicians would need to communicate well with employees concerning that the hazards to which they are exposed, while recognizing language and cross-cultural barriers, in order to foster harm-prevention and keep employees informed about risks they face. Doing so would assist individual decision-making and perhaps empower workers to make choices to preclude or reduce risks. Again, a failure of this ethical duty may increase health risks to those not properly informed of them. Of course, conveying to employers the results of examinations of an employee's fitness for work or a particular task serves both generic prevention as well as more specific disease prevention for the individual involved.

Compliance

Ethical duties conveyed in codes of conduct are not always honored by occupational physicians and workplace researchers. In many cases, the funding source for scientific research influences the outcome. All too often there is a clear demarcation between studies done by a company that sponsors them and research done by nonprofit groups. Occupational physicians may face pressures to distort their diagnoses or data collection and interpretation to favor a sponsor instead of providing an accurate, impartial study of a workplace and its workers.

Compounding the problem are the ethical issues raised by scientific journals that favor industry research over more objective studies. Occupational physicians need to examine the ethical conflicts inherent in participation in biased editorial and peer-review schemes, improper presentation of findings, and distorted facts presented as science approved by editors and editorial boards that favor industry as a result of their conflicts of interest.

Studies may be designed and funded to not find adverse effects from exposures, or, in the extreme, specify what scientific results would be before the studies are even conducted. Examples such as these have become sufficiently common that investigative journalists have labeled as "scientists for hire" researchers and private companies that conduct studies often contrary to university, nonprofit, and consensus scientific conclusions, and typically are in business to confound more independent and impartial research. There is sufficient profit in such enterprises that a number of companies and individuals have strong incentives to carry them out.

In other instances, scientists or their employers have modified studies to show that there are no, fewer, or lower risks from their products. The consequence is that this can confuse and corrupt scientific fields, scientists, and physicians. In these instances, the "ethics" of commerce takes precedence over the workplace health protections, public health agencies, and other scientists.

The *International Network for Epidemiology in Policy* (INEP) provides a global forum at the interface of research and policy. It strives to protect public health by promoting ethical conduct in research. The 2020 INEP Position Statement **Conflict-of-Interest and Disclosure in Epidemiology** identifies where failure to disclose conflicting interests occurs, and where unethical tactics in epidemiologic research and publication are used to distort science.

The choices that lead to misleading science are in likely violation of scientific codes of ethics. Clearly such practices are unjust, should be condemned as wrong, and stand in substantial need of reform.

Conflicts of interest do not disappear because a professional organization publishes a Code of Conduct. At best, ethical codes are reminders to physicians and scientists that they need to continually examine their behavior and its impact on society.

REFERENCES

ACOEM: Medical Review Officer Code of Conduct, 2005: https://www.mrocc.org/code.pdf.

ACOEM: The Seven Ethical Principles of Occupational and Environmental Medicine, 2010. https://www.acoem.org/uploadedFiles/About_ACOEM/Code%20of%20Ethics%20-%20Condensed%20Version.pdf.

ACOEM: Confidentiality of Medical Information in the Workplace, position paper, 2018. www.acoem.org/guidelines.aspx?id=3558.

American College of Occupational and Environmental Medicine Code of Ethics, 2009: https://www.acoem.org/codeofconduct.aspx.

American Industrial Hygiene Association: Member Ethical Principles, 2018. https://www.acgih.org/membership/other/member-ethical-principles.

ICOH: International Code of Ethics for Occupational Health Professionals. 3rd ed. 2014: www.icohweb.org/site/multimedia/code_of_ethics-en.pdf.

International Network for Epidemiology in Policy (INEP) Position Statement Series: Conflict-of-Interest and Disclosure in Epidemiology, 2020. https://epidemiologyinpolicy.org/coi-d-position-statement

International Occupational Hygiene Association: Code of Ethics, 2012. https://ioha.net/files/2015/11/IOHA-Code-of-Ethics-2012.pdf.

■ SELF-ASSESSMENT QUESTIONS

Select the one correct answer for each question.

Question 1: The main and legal authority for employee protections are
   a. State workers' compensation systems
   b. OSHA-issued health standards addressing toxic materials or harmful physical agents
   c. NIOSH-issued directives to industry and labor
   d. OSHA directives to the individual states to issue health standards

Question 2: Protection of the health of employees
   a. might be either *generic* for a workplace or *specific* to particular individuals found to be at risk
   b. requires an occupational physician to carry out industry-supported research
   c. is the sole responsibility of the administrators of OSHA and NIOSH
   d. are legal and ethical duties of company safety and security officers

Disability Management & Prevention

Jordan Rinker, MD, MPH

Glenn Pransky, MD, MOH

Disability is commonly defined as a decrease in or inability to perform some or all functions related to personal, social, or workplace demands due to a physical or mental impairment. This view is distinct from impairment, defined as a reduction in normal function. Impairment should not necessarily imply that work disability is present, unless there is a functional limitation that precludes the worker from performing some or all of the tasks required in their job, after considering available work accommodations.

The American Medical Association's (AMA) *Guides to the Evaluation of Permanent Impairment* states that its impairment ratings are not intended to be used to rate disability because disability reflects a combination of medical and nonmedical factors. Critics point out that the numeric quantification of impairment, the aspect of the guides that encourages its expanding use, is not based on substantial evidence for validity and reliability. State workers' compensation programs may use the impairment ratings as a proxy for the extent of disability; although there is some relationship between impairment ratings and ability to work, the relationship is variable.

Work disability has not been consistently defined nor measured, and thus population data on incidence, prevalence, and causes are inconsistent. In developed countries, around one in six workers has or develops a significant health-related limitation in ability to work each year, and one-third have a period of work absence as a result—mostly short-term absences due to temporary conditions. A small but important group develops long-term work disability and accounts for the majority of total days lost from work due to health conditions.

Nearly one in four US adults is at least partially disabled from work due to mental and behavioral disorders, musculoskeletal problems, or neurologic conditions. About one-half of the disabled are severely limited and unable to work. Musculoskeletal disorders are the most frequent type of disability, but in some working age groups mental health disorders are now more frequent. The relationships between work, disability, and mental health are interrelated with each one having a potential impact on the other.

Work disability is a complex issue that can involve multiple participants and concerns beyond a particular health-related condition and its treatment. Personal, workplace, medical, and societal issues can affect the extent of a disability and how return to work (RTW) may succeed or fail. Social and environmental factors usually have a greater impact on disability and its prevention than health-related dimensions. The organizational work environment with supervisors, coworkers, unions, and management roles along with insurers, family, and society are recognized as major potentially modifiable influences on disability and RTW; the immediate workplace response to a worker with a potentially disabling condition is especially important. Health care providers must understand and address within and their medical systems (facilities, staff, insurers, administrators, medical records) these influences and be able to collaborate with and at times influence nonmedical personnel, to achieve optimal prevention and management of work disability.

The clinician's role in identifying and managing work disability should include early problem recognition, effective case management, and communication as needed with all involved parties with the goal of a safe return to full or partial functioning at work as quickly as possible. The holistic approach may need to consider multiple aspects of disability including medical, psychological, and social dimensions to assist those persons who are at high risk for long-term disability to stay at, return to, and remain in work.

RETURN TO WORK

All clinicians who evaluate and treat potentially disabling injuries and medical conditions must consider the importance of work. After a significant injury or illness, returning to work may require a stepwise process, with a continuum in the management of the individual and workplace to maximize functional capacity and productivity. The following evidence-based concepts should be integrated into their management of and advocacy for these persons.

1. Work can be therapeutic, promote recovery, and is an important part of rehabilitation.

2. Long periods out of work can cause or contribute to poor physical and mental health including excess mortality.

3. Advice to stay off work is a major clinical intervention with potentially serious long-term iatrogenic consequences.

4. Common health problems, such as musculoskeletal, cardiorespiratory, and mental health conditions, can often be accommodated at work, with appropriate modifications and support when needed.

5. Planning and supporting staying at or returning to work is an important part of the clinical management of disability.

Clinicians must also be aware of the larger workplace issues that can affect the RTW process. The emphasis should be on staying at work and shifting the focus to establish a collaborative environment between employee and employer that maintains productive employment. The Canadian Institute for Work and Health identified seven principles associated with successful RTW. These workplace-based interventions can include

1. Workplace commitment to health and safety by top management and labor across the organization.

2. Workplace offer of suitable early and safe modified work.

3. Coordination of RTW that ensures support for the returning worker without inconveniencing coworkers and supervisors.

4. Supervisors educated in safety and ergonomics and included in early communication and RTW planning.

5. Early and considerate contact with the injured or ill worker by the supervisor/employer.

6. Appointment of an RTW coordinator to facilitate planning, communication, and coordination among the involved parties.

7. Communication between employers and health care providers about workplace demands and RTW issues as needed, and with the approval of the injured or ill worker.

A successful stay at work and RTW process involves an understanding of all of these factors related to the recovery process in the person and the workplace. Interventions involving multiple strategies with work accommodation, health-focused, and service coordination and attention to worker cognition are most effective for reducing lost time. It is also important to recognize influences that facilitate staying at work once a person has returned. These may include perceptions that the work is appropriate with supportive workplace relationships, and a sense of job satisfaction. It is important to create a work environment in which the injured or disabled worker will feel successful and protected.

▶ Workplace/Employer Roles

Early and positive contact by the employer has shown to be a strong predictor of earlier RTW. It is also most beneficial for the employer to have a people-oriented culture with training in supporting the employee, attempting to avoid adversarial reactions, and encouraging the worker to not only seek proper medical care, but also make workplace modifications available for some form of RTW (ie, part-time, graded increase in activity, or other modified work program—see below). Training supervisors at the workplace to respond positively to reports of potentially disabling conditions has been shown to significantly decrease the number of disabling episodes, and the length of disability in those who have to leave work due to injury or illness. The employer should communicate with the clinician(s) and provide employment/workplace-related information that can help guide their understanding of work-related tasks. Ultimately, the decision to have an injured or disabled worker RTW in a temporary or permanently modified position is the responsibility of the employer. With the proper communication and support from the employer, the physical and psychological demands of work and any work restrictions can be addressed and possibly modified for a successful RTW process.

▶ Modified Work Programs

Modified work programs encompass a diverse set of work-related changes, including changed work hours, (eg, flexible or reduced hours) reduced tasks performed, or more permanent workplace alterations such as modifying workstations or equipment. Similar to physical conditioning programs, they may incorporate a gradual exposure to work-related tasks to increase workload over time. Numerous studies have shown benefit with modified work programs in specific workplaces. In most instances, modified work is informally arranged by workers and supervisors, and the most successful arrangements are those where work modifications are adjusted as needed to ensure that the worker has appropriate tasks that are within their current capabilities.

In addition, the employer may provide ergonomic worksite modifications and training, as well as consulting with an RTW coordinator. Ergonomic changes to the work environment may be preferable to the injured worker than worker-focused rehabilitation strategies. The ultimate goal of modified work programs is for the person to RTW as soon as possible in a safe environment that promotes recovery and prevents repeat injury or disability. Therefore, a balance must be met with returning to work and activity limitations, as the person should perform the duties within his or her functional abilities, with the appropriate workplace adaptations and social support.

▶ Factors Affecting Return to Work

Studies have shown that there are over 100 different factors that may affect RTW and have been studied to determine predictors of RTW. These factors fall into different domains or categories including individual worker characteristics (sociodemographic, psychological, attitudes and beliefs, health behaviors, clinical measures), injury descriptors and severity (pain and function), rehabilitation interventions and health care referrals, physical and psychosocial job characteristics, employer/employment factors, employer- or insurer-based disability prevention and disability management interventions, and administrative and legal factors, as well as social policy, legislative, and economic factors.

The management of an injured or disabled person may involve assessing for individual psychosocial and workplace factors that are obstacles to recovery and return to function. One approach to identifying these prognostic factors is using the concept of "flags," which stemmed from the medical use of "red-flags" for the presence of signs and symptoms of a possible serious medical condition. In essence, the presence of a "flag" is best seen as a potential obstacle to recovery and working that might need to be addressed before a person can successfully RTW. The term "Yellow Flags" was initially coined to assist clinicians in recognizing individual psychosocial factors (such as perceptions about symptoms, recovery, and the workplace) that have shown to be correlated with poor clinical outcomes and increased likelihood of persistent disability. In time, "blue flags" and "black flags" were developed to further identify and separate personal and injury-related factors from workplace and other prognostic factors. The blue and black flag system represents a refinement from the yellow flag screening approach to draw clinical attention to both individual psychosocial and workplace factors contributing to disability.

Individual perceptions about work are categorized as blue flags. Black flags are related to the context in which the person functions, such as organizational, social, financial, and family issues as well as the physical demands and tasks of the job. Blue flags mark worker perceptions of a job that may be stressful, unsupportive, highly physically demanding, or unfulfilling. While black flags include objective measures of job characteristics that may be amenable to interventions such as ergonomics, their broad context of work, social, and insurance organizational structures are not as easily influenced by a clinician as are blue flags. The presence of these flags, often in combination, may explain why one worker with acute back pain will recover with no work absence while another will experience significant periods of work disability.

Individual-level factors that may predict prolonged work disability (blue flags):

- Perception of heavy physical demands
- Perceived inability to modify work
- Stressful work demands
- Lack of workplace social support
- Job dissatisfaction and perceived injustice
- Poor expectation of recovery and RTW
- Fear of reinjury

Some workplace conditions that may predict prolonged disability (black flags) are

- Minimal availability of adjusted duties and graduated RTW pathways
- Lack of satisfactory disability management system (absence of reporting system, reporting discouraged, employer not interested)
- Job involving manual work or significant biomechanical demands that cannot be temporarily altered
- Job involving shift work or working unsociable hours
- Family or others unsupportive of RTW

There is inconsistent evidence of predicting RTW due to sex, education, use of nonnarcotic pain medication, and mental health issues other than secondary depression in the shorter term setting. Psychosocial risk factors are greater predictors overall of delayed RTW and persistent disability than biomedical or ergonomic factors. The factors affecting RTW in the chronic phase may be different than those identified in the short term. As work disability becomes prolonged, secondary depression, loss of supportive workplace relationships, and physical deconditioning can become additional RTW barriers.

Two methods to identify risk factors for delayed RTW in the context of low back pain include (1) using the clinical interview scenario or (2) using questionnaires, such as the Orebro Musculoskeletal Pain Questionnaire (OMPQ). The OMPQ is a self-report screening instrument that detects individual-level factors that predict work disability such as fear of reinjury, poor expectation of recovery or RTW, stress, job dissatisfaction, and heavy physical demands. Other individual-level factors and workplace conditions that may predict work disability from the preceding list may be identified through clinical interview or by conducting a workplace visit.

The Back Disability Risk Questionnaire (BDRQ) is another self-report questionnaire with a focus on workplace factors. It is designed to be administered within the first 14 days after the onset of work-related back pain. The BDRQ has been shown to have moderate validity to predict 1-month RTW. Six of the 16-item BDRQ questions (injury type, work absence preceding medical evaluation, job tenure, prior back surgery, worries about reinjury, expectation for early RTW, and stress) have been shown to predict presence of persistent pain, functional limitation, or impaired work status. An additional validated tool for screening persons for targeting interventions, based on identified risks for persistent disability due to low back pain, is the Keele Start Back Screening Tool.

Research suggests that the use of these patient questionnaires can also help identify persons in greatest need of early intervention to alleviate acute emotional distress. For back pain, there is strong evidence for the role of psychological distress/depressive mood in the transition from acute to chronic low back pain. Emotional distress has been shown to be a salient factor in delayed functional recovery even when measured in the first few days after pain onset.

Table 5–1. Workplace factors (Blue Flags) important for RTW, and suggestions for interview questions and possible actions.

Workplace Factor	Sample Interview Question	Possible Actions
Heavy physical demands	Are you concerned that the physical demands of your job might delay your return to work?	• Assemble list of problem job tasks • Conduct work site walk-through • Identify temporary sources of help
Inability to modify work	Do you expect your work could be modified temporarily so you could return to work sooner?	• Modified or alternate duty program? • Brainstorm with injured worker • Assess job flexibility
Stressful work demands	Are there stressful elements to your job that might be difficult when you first return to work?	• Modify speed or time pressures • Recognize stressful job elements • Assess usual coping strategies
Lack of workplace social support	What kind of response do you expect from coworkers and supervisors when you return?	• Establish more contact with coworkers • Encourage employer communication • Involve trusted coworkers
Job dissatisfaction	Is this a job you'd recommend to a friend?	• Assess whether career goals have changed • Clarify worker options and responsibilities • Motivational interviewing
Poor expectation of recovery and return to work	Are you concerned that returning to work may be difficult given your current circumstances?	• Clarify nature of concerns • Realistic messages conveyed by all medical providers? • Employer encouragement and reassurance
Fear of reinjury	Are you worried about any repeat episodes of back pain once you return to work?	• Develop action plan if symptoms recur • Plan for a more gradual return to work • Counter belief that activity is dangerous

Health care providers can be instrumental in helping a person at risk of chronic disability or work loss. A stratified approach to management of RTW interventions should be considered by screening earlier on to determine which persons are at greater risk of delayed RTW and prolonged disability with the tools previously mentioned. Once potential individual and workplace obstacles have been identified, health care providers can help develop an individualized plan of action to target each obstacle or flag and implement the plan. These high-risk persons may need additional evaluations for planning workplace and other appropriate interventions. Table 5–1 lists workplace factors (blue flags) that have been identified to be important for RTW, and some suggestions for possible questions and actions that may be coordinated among the employee, employer, and health care provider.

CLINICAL MANAGEMENT

Work disability should be addressed as a separate and important issue from a worker's medical condition. A discussion about the nonmedical factors that may prevent RTW, possible solutions, and how the clinician may help within the context of RTW is an important goal of their medical care.

Poor disability management by the health care team may result in a significant risk of long periods away from work and protracted disability. Health care factors adversely affecting RTW include fragmented and poorly coordinated care, delayed or inappropriate diagnostic workups, excessive and unnecessary treatment, prolonged and inappropriate activity restrictions, and long wait time for consultations. It has been recommended that improved communication between primary care providers and occupational medicine physicians or rehabilitation specialists may improve RTW decisions. Some health care providers lack the knowledge, awareness, and familiarity with disability and RTW issues, and are unable to determine proper activity limitations, restrictions, and outcome expectations. Primary care providers should consider referral to a source of RTW expertise (occupational medicine physician, physical therapist, occupational therapist, RTW coordinator) if a significant barrier to RTW develops between the employer and employee or other potential risk factors for prolonged disability arises.

The goal of disability management is to assist the person to maintain or return to their maximum functional work status as soon as possible after an injury, illness, or chronic medical condition. Depending on the resources available, many people may be involved in disability management, to various degrees. In the majority of the developing world, disability management is usually self-directed with few available resources. There is good evidence from developed countries that early intervention with appropriate treatment, reassurance about activity, and staying at or returning to work with workplace accommodation is sufficient management for most people. It is important to encourage the injured or disabled person to continue as a productive member of the community by focusing on returning to their daily activities and work, as there are significant psychosocial and economic benefits. In addition, a large aspect of disability management lies in preventing further injury and disability.

In the injured worker setting, the fundamental goal of the clinical evaluation of work capacity is to determine whether a worker can stay at or return to some form of work, and if so, what specific tasks or duties they can perform. The longer they remain away from work, the less likely the chance of ever returning to work, and the more likely they will remain on permanent disability or unemployed. If a worker has been off work for 12 weeks, there is only a 50% chance of ever returning to work. By 12 months, the likelihood of returning to work is only about 2%. A coordinated approach including all involved parties, and especially the health care provider(s), worker, and employer, has shown optimal results in staying at or returning to work.

Distinguishing impairment from disability is an important aspect when evaluating a person who has been injured or out of work due to a medical condition. A person may experience an impairment that does not result in disability, such as a below the knee amputation, where they have learned to walk and run with a prosthesis or a paraplegic who is fully independent in a wheelchair who works as an accountant. On the other hand, one can experience significant disability or activity limitations in the absence of significant physical impairment, such as a vascular surgeon or concert pianist who requires great hand dexterity with an injury to the median nerve of the hand.

The history can provide important information in limitations in function as well as extrapolating information for work functional capacity from their ability to perform common daily activities such as driving, sitting, walking, standing, bending over, lifting groceries or children, and climbing stairs. During the physical examination, the clinician can test range of motion, strength, sensation, and ask the person to demonstrate difficult activities. Level of effort and pain can be assessed while observing the person. A prediction of work function can then be made based on the clinical encounter along with a general understanding of the workplace.

The American College of Occupational and Environmental Medicine (ACOEM) has updated its consensus document that outlines the issues and roles that a health care provider should consider when dealing with stay at work or RTW concerns. The following components should be considered:

- Early in the course of treatment, discuss the expected healing and recovery times, as well as the positive role an early, graduated increase in activity has on physical and psychological healing.

- Ask about the impact of the medical condition on their ability to perform responsibilities at home and at work, and the availability of family and community support systems.

- Promote feelings of self-efficacy and earlier recovery by instructing that their behavior can determine the extent of their future recovery.

- When an injured or disabled person is able to stay at work or to return safely to some form of productive work, explain that resuming normal activities while symptoms continue to resolve is an important part of the rehabilitation process.

- Look for potential obstacles (flags) to the recovery of function and RTW as soon as practical. The care and RTW plans may need to be reevaluated and adjusted.

- Identified obstacles may need to be referred to appropriate parties involved in their health care and employment situation who can assist in addressing particular issues, such as benefits or claims payers, case managers, occupational health and safety professionals, human resources professionals, or workplace supervisors.

- Support direct communication between worker and employer early in treatment or rehabilitation in order to reduce social isolation and maintain the bond with the world of work.

- At each visit, provide guidance to the worker (and employer with authorization or as permitted by law) about what job functions are safe to do and realistic to expect. These "activity prescriptions" will naturally change over time. Encourage the worker to self-manage a gradual increase in work activity as tolerated.

- If the worker is able to do something productive but no work is available because of statutory prohibitions or employer policies, business practices, unwillingness or inability to make accommodations, or mitigate workplace risks, offer to contact the employer on the worker's behalf.

In high-risk persons and those who feel unable to work, a clinician or physical therapist evaluation may be able to direct or suggest additional resources within the workplace and refer those who need it the most to outside therapies (ie, physical, behavioral, social services focused on work issues). By targeting appropriate and timely resources to these persons, the clinicians, therapists, and workplace may prevent prolonged sick leaves, long-term disability, and promote health care cost savings within the community and workplace. Delaying assessment of RTW risk factors until several months of work absence have occurred provides much less opportunity to consider simple interventions that can prevent prolonged disability.

▶ Activity Prescriptions for Work

Providing workers, disabled persons, and employers with advice about work and activity is critical to their recovery, RTW, and prevention of prolonged disability. Clinicians can find resources for RTW assistance at Helping Workers

Get Back to Work and Work Safe BC's What Health Care Providers Need to Know, websites that include an activity prescription form and typical physical limitations for common injuries.

Whenever the clinical evaluation does not provide adequate information to determine specific physical activity or work limitations, the clinician may need to supplement the clinical information with other evaluations. In addition to workplace evaluations, one of the tools used to assist in translating impairment to job-relevant functional limitations are functional capacity evaluations.

▶ Functional Capacity Evaluations

Functional capacity evaluations (FCEs) have been purported to assess physical functional abilities for job placement, rehabilitation, work capacity, and disability evaluations. FCEs are performed in numerous ways and by a variety of practitioners. The two most widely used methods of determining functional capacity are performance-based tests, often using specific equipment and physical measurement instruments or job simulation, and self-assessments using questionnaires.

The typical performance-based FCE is a battery of standardized assessment measures addressing range of motion, strength, endurance, lifting, pushing, pulling, climbing, and other tasks designed to systematically measure a person's physical functional capacity. Because these FCEs often use general standardized measures, there are significant limitations in predicting work ability, RTW, and disability. The predictive value of FCEs remains low partly due to the fact that it is difficult to accurately assess specific on the job physical requirements, and the predictive value of these standardized tests for job performance is low. An accurate job assessment is necessary to develop a job-specific FCE that simulates the actual physical demands of the job.

Another method of determining functional capacity is through self-report or using a standardized questionnaire. Studies have demonstrated that performance-based measures assess different aspects of functional capacity than self-reported measures. Individual self-reports appear to provide a broader assessment of functional capacity related to not only physical attributes but also psychosocial aspects such as self-efficacy and may provide a wider scope of information than the performance-based measures. Four questionnaires used for FCEs have had high levels of both reliability and validity. These are the Pain Disability Index, Oswestry Disability Index, Roland-Morris Disability Questionnaire, and the Upper Extremity Functional Scale. The questionnaires mostly focus on issues of activities of daily living, and therefore their value in assessing ability to perform work-related duties is uncertain at best. The combination of performance and nonperformance tests might have a greater predictive value for work participation, but this has not been demonstrated yet.

There remains debate as to the predictive value of FCEs in most RTW settings. In persons with musculoskeletal disorders, the overall predictive quality of FCEs for work participation is modest to poor. Some specific functional measures such as lifting tests have been shown to be predictive of greater work participation. However, their value for sustained RTW has not been demonstrated. Demographics (gender) and work status (amount of time off work) have been shown to be stronger predictors of RTW than the FCE. Job simulations are consistently more valid and reliable as a means of evaluating work capacity.

The lack of evidence showing strong predictability of most FCEs (especially those lacking valid job simulations) for RTW reflects the complexity of predicting disability and its multifactorial nature. There are likely many factors that affect performance on FCEs, including both physical and psychosocial elements. Similarly, successful RTW depends not only on physical capacity, but psychological, social, and other factors. The performance on FCEs should not solely be used to assess an individual's functional capacity.

▶ Physical Conditioning Programs

Physical conditioning programs including work conditioning, work hardening, and functional restoration programs should be focused on RTW or improvement in current work status for those on modified duties. All typically involve some form of physical activity such as structured exercise to either simulate or duplicate a work or functional task in a safe, supervised environment. They can involve a gradual and graded-activity process set to the person's level of tolerance, which helps build strength, endurance, and confidence. These programs can occur either in a clinic or workplace-based environment. There is some evidence that physical conditioning in the workplace compared to the clinic-based environment has improved RTW outcomes in persons with musculoskeletal disorders. The workplace-based rehabilitation may be more effective by improving psychosocial well-being, especially by maintaining connection with the workplace and not being separated from the work routine. However, the effectiveness of these programs in disability management remains limited with only small effects seen in the long term and for limited types of conditions, namely subacute and chronic musculoskeletal disorders.

▶ Vocational Rehabilitation

Since the 1970s vocational rehabilitation (VR) programs have been assisting people with injuries, and with various states of disability to RTW as contributing members of society. VR has many definitions and connotations, depending on the locale, resources, work laws, and regulations in effect. The broadest scope includes "whatever helps someone with a health problem to stay at, return to, and remain in work." The proposed definition for VR from the International Classification of Functioning, Disability and Health is a "multi-professional evidenced-based approach that is provided in different settings, services, and activities to working age individuals with health-related impairments, limitations, or restrictions with work functioning and whose primary aim is to optimize work participation." This definition encompasses the expansion of all services participating in the rehabilitation of the person. This approach includes both work-focused health care and employer-based accommodations, which is broader than the typical US program of vocational counseling and rehabilitation planning by a rehabilitation counselor for unemployed or permanently disabled workers. This wider emphasis also shifts the model from returning-to-work to staying-at-work.

There are a wide variety of VR services, depending on individual needs and resources available. The majority of persons with health issues does not need comprehensive VR interventions and can be properly managed by the primary health care provider with minimal additional resources. When more complicated scenarios arise, a comprehensive stepwise approach may be necessary. VR services can assist persons with many needs, including obtaining appropriate treatments earlier on, determining activity limitations, and recommending workplace modifications after the first few weeks of disability. For those persons on disability for several months or years, VR can involve providing job support services, educating employers, communicating between health care providers and employers, as well as finding and entering training programs, job placement, finding new employment opportunities, determining alternate job options based on individualized skills and attributes, and even planning withdrawal from work. The programs can be at the individual or group level and can include counseling, planning, and proactive methods of maintaining and obtaining proper employment. VR can address work instability and incongruity, where there may be a mismatch between the skill of the individual and the duties required by the job description. If the person is still employed, VR may include a case manager or RTW coordinator who can assist with an evaluation of the work and work environment. Depending on the evaluations, the person may either return to the same work, return to the same work with modified duties or environment, or need to change jobs and find a new one that is more congruous with the capacity of the person.

VR has been shown to be effective in helping persons address the difficulties of work disability. On average approximately 60% of disabled persons who use VR programs become employed, though there is significant variability in employment based on the type of disability. There is strong evidence for effective VR interventions (when defined broadly) that improve work outcomes in musculoskeletal conditions.

Several strategies have been tested to manage work disability in those with chronic, serious mental disorders. The most effective approach is based on an individual placement and support model. Features include early resolution of medical issues, and a subsequent multidisciplinary team approach that deemphasizes medical aspects; career exploration in the job market based on client interests and motivation rather than sheltered workshops; and ongoing peer support with secondary vocational assistance, rather than a traditional train-and-place approach. Other innovations attempt to circumvent the link between health benefits and permanent disability certification, by providing full health insurance to persons with serious medical problems who wish to work. This allows persons with serious medical problems to take more flexible jobs (often part-time) that do not provide health insurance.

Persons and workplaces with complex cases or barriers to RTW may require closer supervision to help manage the interrelated risk factors and interventions, and may benefit greatly from a case manager or RTW coordinator. The case manager can assist in integrating the care plans and coordinating interparty communication, progress, and follow-up. Involvement of RTW coordinators has been shown to lead to significantly improved outcomes in cases with prolonged work disability. In addition, disabled persons may need to be monitored for compliance with the treatment plan. Interdisciplinary collaboration and involvement of worker and workplace is usually necessary to achieve a smooth transition back to work.

PREVENTION

Studies suggest that much of health-related work disability is preventable. The question of how best to prevent disability is an important one because a healthy workforce is an essential part of a vital nation. The ACOEM urges the adoption of a preventive-based paradigm centered at the workplace. They recommend primary prevention strategies that help people stay healthy and productive (like healthy workplace programs), secondary prevention strategies that catch problems before they manifest as work disability (like screening, health coaching, improved supervisor response and proactive work disability prevention programs), and tertiary prevention strategies (like disability and disease management and RTW programs) that limit the disability impact of an injury or illness and minimize obstacles to work for disabled persons.

Evidence shows that good physical health, good mental health, positive health behaviors, and absence of chronic disease and its complications are all associated with low occupational and general injury rates and decreased health-related work disability. Efforts that help workers and those seeking work attain and maintain good physical and mental health and that prevent chronic disease or its complications can be viewed as interventions to prevent disability. Awareness of factors that put a worker or disabled person at risk for sustaining an injury and factors that, once an illness or injury has occurred, put them at risk for prolonged disability is an important first step for any action that aims to prevent disability.

Factors that put a person at risk for sustaining an injury or developing work disability include

- Obesity
- Smoking
- Drug and alcohol abuse
- Taking certain prescription medications
- Fatigue and burnout

- Sleep disorder or sleep deprivation
- Poorly controlled diabetes
- Fair or poor eyesight
- Fair or poor hearing
- Low levels of physical activity
- Conflicts at work (with coworkers or supervisors)
- Depressive symptoms

These risk factors can be identified through discussions during a clinical encounter that include both personal and workplace issues, and through screening tools like health risk appraisals or assessments, or early disability risk prediction questionnaires.

Health care providers who seek to prevent disability must include a focus on work aspects in their clinical encounter. Studies on shiftwork, for example, show that changes aimed at sleep deprivation as a safety issue have also demonstrated improvements in health conditions such as obesity, diabetes, and cardiovascular disease. In order to address work-related health risks, they must be elucidated in a work history or work analysis. Governments, insurers, and employers can use these population data to design their health plans to respond to the risks that exist among their workers and the community.

Studies of morbidity in populations with differing risk factors often use self-report functional status instruments like the Health Assessment Questionnaire (HAQ) Disability Index to measure disability. Longitudinal studies that used the HAQ Disability Index as a metric conclude that self-reported disability was postponed by 14–16 years in vigorous exercisers compared with controls and postponed 10 years in low-risk compared with higher-risk cohorts (risk based on current smoking, overweight/obesity, and inactivity). A "low-risk" person who does not use tobacco, is not overweight or obese, and is physically active may postpone disability, as defined by self-reported functional status, and is less likely to develop a chronic disease or sustain a work-related injury.

Secondary prevention strategies such as health coaching and proactive work disability prevention programs can be employed once risk factors for disability have been identified. Evidence shows that health coaching, particularly health coaching that engages participants with motivational interviewing, is an effective strategy to help people with behavior change. One-on-one coaching that focuses on health factors, work-related factors, and social/psychological factors is particularly valuable for those identified at higher risk for early work loss. Research indicates that workers who receive such care show better work ability, less burnout, and better quality of life.

Health coaches can be trained to deliver cognitive-behavioral–based programs. Cognitive-behavioral interventions have been shown to enhance the prevention of long-term disability; one randomized controlled trial looking at persons with acute back pain showed that the risk for developing long-term sickness-related disability leave was

more than fivefold higher in the minimal intervention group compared to the cognitive-behavioral intervention group. The cognitive-behavioral intervention in this study included weekly group meetings with: (1) practice with problem solving, (2) skills training to give participants the opportunity to improve their coping skills, and (3) the development of a personal coping program.

While research shows that mental disorders like depression and anxiety are associated with impaired work functioning and long-term sick leave, and controlled trials demonstrate the effectiveness of cognitive-behavioral therapy (CBT) in improving mental health, CBT as typically delivered in outpatient settings lacks a focus on work. The integration of work-directed interventions with CBT components is a more effective strategy to prevent prolonged work absence for people who are on sick leave with mental health problems like depression or anxiety. A comparative outcome study that examined a work-focused CBT intervention and a regular CBT intervention among employees on sick leave due to common mental disorders (including depression and anxiety) concludes that employees who received work-focused CBT resumed work earlier than those who received regular CBT.

Work-focused CBT uses work and the workplace as a framework for customary CBT exercises and a context to reach treatment goals like activation, social contact, and increased self-esteem. Work-focused CBT can, for example, engage the participant in work-focused behavioral experiments to challenge dysfunctional thoughts. In addition to addressing behavioral and psychological risk factors, work-focused cognitive-behavioral interventions can help injured or disabled workers shift the way they perceive their work environment so perception-based risks (blue flags) can be addressed as well.

Occupational safety and health interventions are designed to minimize workers' exposures to job-related risks while workplace health promotion interventions aim to promote healthy behaviors. The evidence is lacking for worksite health promotion programs alone for preventing long-term work disability. Approaches that integrate occupational safety and health with organizational policies and programs around well-being (work organization and environment, benefits, community) in the workplace are being studied. Total Worker Health is the NIOSH strategy to integrate occupational safety and health protection with health promotion to prevent worker injury and illness and to advance health and well-being. According to this strategy, a worker is best kept safe and healthy in an atmosphere where management is fully engaged in the well-being of its staff, where the environment is hazard-free and supportive, and where workplace policies, interventions, and the work environment all encourage healthier choices.

Research priorities for disability prevention include studying (1) the effectiveness of comprehensive workplace health promotion and health protection initiatives, and ways to maximize participation (and minimize selection bias), (2) early interventions targeting specific disability risk factors,

(3) enhanced disease self-management programs that include a work disability prevention component, (4) the impact of positive supervisor responses with both formal and informal workplace accommodations, and (5) proactive interventions designed to optimize the emotional well-being of the entire workforce. As more studies document the prevalence of presenteeism, research is needed to determine who is at risk for a transition to work absence, and how this can be prevented through focused interventions.

REFERENCES

Awang H, Tan LY, Mansor N, Tongkumchum P, Eso M: Factors related to successful return to work following multidisciplinary rehabilitation. J Rehabil Med 2017;49(6):520 [PMID: 28617522].

Brendbekken R, Vaktskjold A, Harris A, Tangen T: Predictors of return-to-work in patients with chronic musculoskeletal pain: a randomized clinical trial. J Rehabil Med 2018;50(2):193-199 [PMID: 29206274].

CDC: Workplace Health Program. https://www.cdc.gov/workplacehealthpromotion/about/index.html.

Ervasti J, Joensuu M, Pentti J, et al: Prognostic factors for return to work after depression-related work disability: a systematic review and meta-analysis. J Psychiatr Res 2017;95:28-36 [PMID: 28772111].

NIOSH: Total worker health. www.cdc.gov/niosh/twh/.

Steenstra IA, Munhall C, Irvin E, et al: Systematic review of prognostic factors for return to work in workers with subacute and chronic low back pain. J Occup Rehabil 2017;27(3):369-381 [PMID: 27647141].

Washington Labor and Industry: Help Your Employee Return to Work. https://lni.wa.gov/claims/for-employers/help-your-employee-return-to-work.

Washington Labor and Industry: Helping Workers Get Back to Work. http://www.lni.wa.gov/ClaimsIns/Providers/Treating-Patients/RTW/default.asp.

Wickizer TM, Franklin GM, Fulton-Kehoe D: Innovations in occupational health care delivery can prevent entry into permanent disability: 8-year follow-up of the Washington State Centers for Occupational Health and Education. Med Care 2018;56(12):1018-1023 [PMID: 30234763].

Work Safe BC: What Health Care Providers Need to Know. https://www.worksafebc.com/en/claims/recovery-work/what-health-care-providers-need-to-know.

■ SELF-ASSESSMENT QUESTIONS

Select the one correct answer for each question.

Question 1: Disability
   a. is internationally defined as a decrease in or inability to perform some or all functions related to personal, social, or workplace demands due to a physical or mental impairment
   b. is synonymous with impairment
   c. presumes that impairment is present
   d. in just a less percent of all workers with health-related work limitations accounts for the majority of total days lost from work due to health conditions

Question 2: Functional capacity evaluations (FCEs)
   a. precisely determine physical functional abilities for job placement, rehabilitation, work capacity, and disability evaluations
   b. are performed solely by occupational physicians
   c. include performance-based tests, often using specific equipment and physical measurement instruments or job simulation, and self-assessments using questionnaires
   d. must include a battery of standardized assessment measures addressing range of motion, strength, endurance, lifting, pushing, pulling, climbing, and other tasks designed to systematically measure a person's physical functional capacity

Question 3: Vocational rehabilitation (VR)
   a. is required for the majority of persons with occupational injuries
   b. typically involves providing job support services, educating employers, communicating between health care providers and employers, as well as finding and entering training programs
   c. programs are at the individual but not the group level and include counseling, planning, and proactive methods of maintaining and obtaining proper employment
   d. can address work instability and incongruity, where there may be a mismatch between the skill of the individual and the duties required by the job description

Question 4: Cognitive-behavioral therapy (CBT)
   a. is required by workers' compensation to improve mental health in workers
   b. as typically delivered in outpatient settings has a focus on work
   c. intervention among employees on sick leave due to common mental disorders (including depression and anxiety) has no measurable value
   d. that is work-focused returns employees to work earlier than those who received regular CBT

Question 5: Individual factors that are associated with prolonged work disability (blue flags)

    a. do not explain why one worker with acute back pain will recover with no work absence, while another will experience significant periods of work disability

    b. include strong evidence of predicting RTW due to age, sex, education, use of nonnarcotic pain medication, and primary mental health issues

    c. may be identified in the context of low back pain by using the clinical interview scenario or questionnaires such as the OMPQ

    d. include minimal availability of adjusted job duties and lack of a satisfactory disability management system at work

Ergonomics & the Prevention of Occupational Injuries

Carisa Harris Adamson, PhD, MSPT, CPE

David M. Rempel, MD, MPH

Ergonomics—also called *human factors engineering*—is the study of the physical and cognitive demands of work to ensure a safe and productive workplace. The function of specialists in ergonomics is to design or improve the workplace, workstations, tools, equipment, and procedures of workers so as to limit fatigue, discomfort, and injuries while also efficiently achieving personal and organizational goals. The goal is to keep the demands of the job within the physical and cognitive capabilities of the people performing those job functions.

Approach to Job Design

Ergonomists, industrial engineers, occupational health and safety professionals, and most importantly, the people doing and supervising the job can work together to improve the design of jobs and workstations that have unsafe characteristics or have caused injury. Controlling errors, eliminating wasted movements, minimizing tool and/or material damage, and improving quality of work are also important goals. The principles of job design discussed in this chapter are relevant to all industry sectors, and examples are drawn from office, health care, and manufacturing. This chapter presents ergonomic approaches that can be applied in the workplace for the prevention and management of musculoskeletal disorders (MSDs) and facilitate stay-at-work and return-to-work approaches that prevent disability.

Approach to Prevention of Occupational Injuries

Health professionals should seek frequent opportunities to tour work areas and familiarize themselves with job procedures, equipment, and working conditions. The concepts presented here should be kept in mind during these workplace visits, and problem areas and activities should be noted for later study and possible job redesign. Such tours should focus on work areas and tasks with high injury rates, high turnover, excessive absenteeism, high error rate, or other signs of a mismatch between worker capabilities and demands of their jobs.

One way to redesign unsafe and unhealthy jobs is to restructure a job at a new level of skill or mechanization. This may involve job simplification (reduction of complexity of the job) or job enlargement (broader use of skills or a greater variety of tasks); the aid of an ergonomist or an industrial engineer will likely be necessary. These professionals prioritize employee health and safety while optimizing productivity because the two are closely interrelated. For example, eliminating unnecessary steps through the application of lean management techniques can also reduce repetitive motions and risk of associated MSDs.

Structure of an Ergonomics Program

Most ergonomic programs contain the elements, in one form or another, set out in Figure 6–1. Active and passive surveillance techniques can be used to identify and prioritize high-risk jobs for further analysis and intervention. Passive surveillance, also called health surveillance, is the review of existing data (eg, workers' compensation data, Occupational Safety and Health Administration [OSHA] logs, and clinic logs) that identifies high-risk jobs based on prior recordable incidents. These are often referred to as lagging indicators. Active surveillance, also called job-risk factor surveillance, utilizes walkthroughs and risk-assessment checklists to identify jobs that should be analyzed in more detail. These are often referred to as leading indicators. There are numerous risk-assessment checklists available (Figure 6–2; see list at the end of chapter); specific checklists should be chosen based on ease of use and specificity to the work being performed. Discussing problematic job tasks with employees and supervisors is another way to identify demanding jobs and tasks. After identifying problematic jobs, the next step is to perform a more detailed analysis of its high-risk tasks to quantify exposures and estimate risk of MSDs. Then specific engineering or administrative strategies to reduce exposures and related risk are identified, discussed with

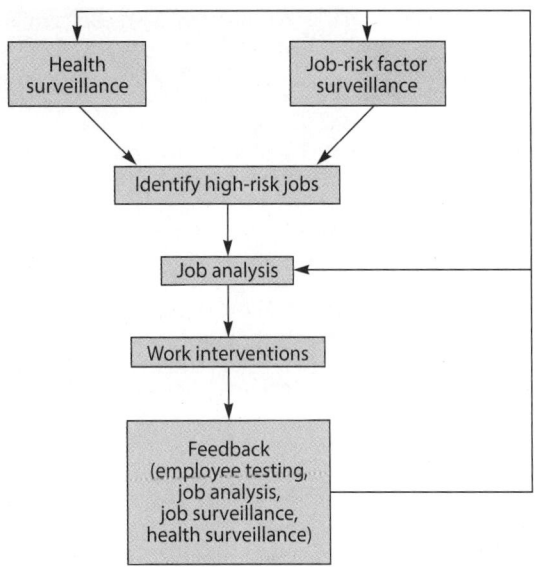

▲ **Figure 6–1.** Components of an ergonomics program. (Source: http://personal.health.usf.edu/tbernard/ HollowHills/WISHA_Checklist_20.pdf.)

stakeholders (workers, supervisors, engineering, facilities and maintenance, and management), and implemented on a pilot basis. The pilot intervention, which should last for 2 weeks to 2 months, is intended to ensure that the intervention is effective and does not cause new health problems or interfere with quality or productivity of work. Often a mock-up or prototype of the proposed workstation layout can be instrumental in uncovering potential problems as tasks are simulated (Figure 6–3).

In addition to the components in Figure 6–1, training in the components of an effectively managed program and basic ergonomic methodologies should be provided to relevant stakeholders including employees, supervisors, engineers, and health and safety staff. Easy to follow work organization and design guidelines (Figure 6–4) can be useful training tools and empower stakeholders to be proactive in making changes that reduce physical exposures and risk of MSDs. The training should include case studies based on recent tasks of concern from the company or from the same industry. Training that simply presents abstract principles of good ergonomics is less effective than job-specific, problem-solving discussions. Problem-solving discussions that include the workers and supervisors are effective ways to develop their understanding of physical exposures-related risk and common strategies used to mitigate such risk; this approach allows them to be actively involved in the identification and resolution of high-risk tasks in the future. Effective trainings also highlight the importance of early identification of workers' musculoskeletal symptoms and a process to immediately address the symptoms and the work that may have contributed to them. Supervisors and managers should be trained on how to effectively respond to symptom/injury reports to facilitate quick resolutions and recoveries.

The health professional should also work with a committee within the organization to plan health and safety reviews and follow-up activities and to act as a resource for management. These committees should include ergonomists, industrial or process engineers, health and safety personnel, maintenance and facilities personnel, the affected employees, supervisors, and risk management personnel. A successful management system makes assignments of job risk analysis, risk prioritization, and interventions to individuals on the committee with expected completion dates.

Various regional and national governmental and nongovernmental organizations have drafted ergonomics

2

Low Back Posture		Overall: None	Caution	Hazard
Working with the back bent forward more than 30° (without support or the ability to vary posture)		More than 2 hours total per day		Caution ☐
		More than 4 hours total per day		Hazard ☐
Working with the back bent forward more than 45° (without support or the ability to vary posture)		More than 1 hour total per day		Caution ☐
		More than 2 hours total per day		Hazard ☐

▲ **Figure 6–2.** Sample job risk factor surveillance checklist.

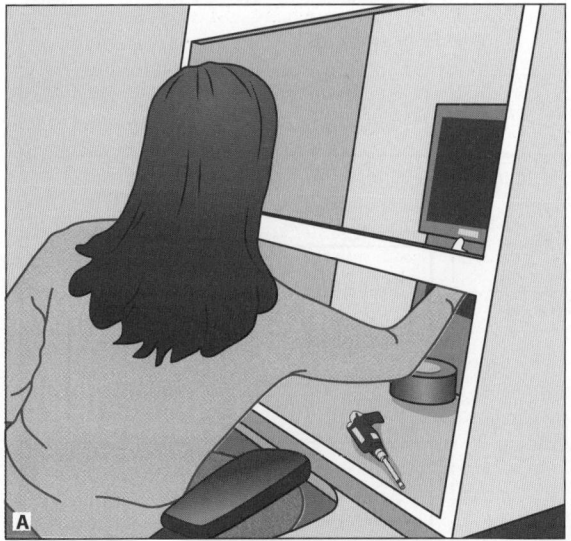

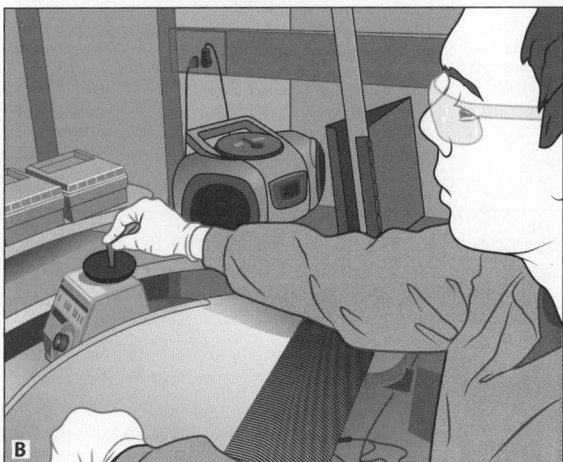

▲ **Figure 6–3.** A. Ergonomist, supervisor, and technician test mock-up of a new lab workstation design to identify barriers to task completion and awkward reaches. B. Final design, with recessed area and tilted receptacles, reduces awkward wrist postures and wasted motion and rounded front edge supports and protects forearms.

standards and guidelines for employers; Table 6–1 lists them. Many other countries and regions (eg, Japan, Australia, and Canada) have also developed standards and guidelines related to ergonomics.

Cost-Effectiveness of Preventive Activities

Management support is critical for success; managers should be informed of the expected cost, productivity, and quality impacts of an ergonomics program. Managers should be

warned that the initial trainings may lead to increased injury reports, but all evidence indicates that the long-term impact of ergonomics programs is a reduction of the overall cost and severity of work-related injuries such as MSDs.

The indirect costs of MSDs, such as replacement-employee wages (indemnity), training costs for replacement workers, productivity reduction, and quality reduction are typically three to four times as much as the direct costs of medical and rehabilitation expenses. Improvements in workstation or tool design and procedures often have a payback period of less than 1 year when the costs of the intervention are compared with the total costs of MSDs. Although job redesign usually focuses on reducing risk factors for common MSDs (eg, wrist tendinitis or low back pain), secondary benefits may include a reduction in acute injuries (eg, fractures, lacerations, bruises, and strains) and an improvement in product quality. For example, an analysis of injuries in a petrochemical plant revealed that many of the contusions, burns, and strains/sprains occurred while operating valves that were in close proximity to structural steel and steam lines. Subsequent measurements indicated that operating these valves required awkward postures and high forces. Most of these valves exceeded generally accepted civilian and military guidelines recommending an upper limit of 50 lb (23 kg) of tangential force applied to the hand wheel. Injuries often occurred when a worker's hands slipped off the hand wheel or valve wrench while attempting to operate the valve and came in contact with nearby hazards. Therefore, improving the ergonomics of the task not only reduced the high forces and awkward postures thereby reducing the risk of a MSD, but it also reduced the risk of contusions and burns associated with operating the valve.

PHYSICAL EXPOSURES ASSOCIATED WITH RISK OF MUSCULOSKELETAL DISORDERS

The National Institute for Occupational Safety and Health (NIOSH) and the National Academy of Sciences have reviewed the physical exposures (stressors) that are associated with increased risk of upper extremity and neck disorders and low back pain. These include

- The application of sustained or high forces
- Sustained (particularly awkward) postures
- Rapid, repeated motions
- Contact stress
- Environmental exposures such as vibration, cold temperatures, or excessive light and noise

Quantitative exposure-response information for each of these exposures and risk of specific MSDs is limited. However, some data do exist to help identify injury thresholds. Table 6–1 includes some risk-assessment models (eg, NIOSH Lift Equation, Strain Index, or ACGIH TLV for Hand Activity) that can be used to interpret levels of exposure and risk of MSDs; they are particularly useful before and after an

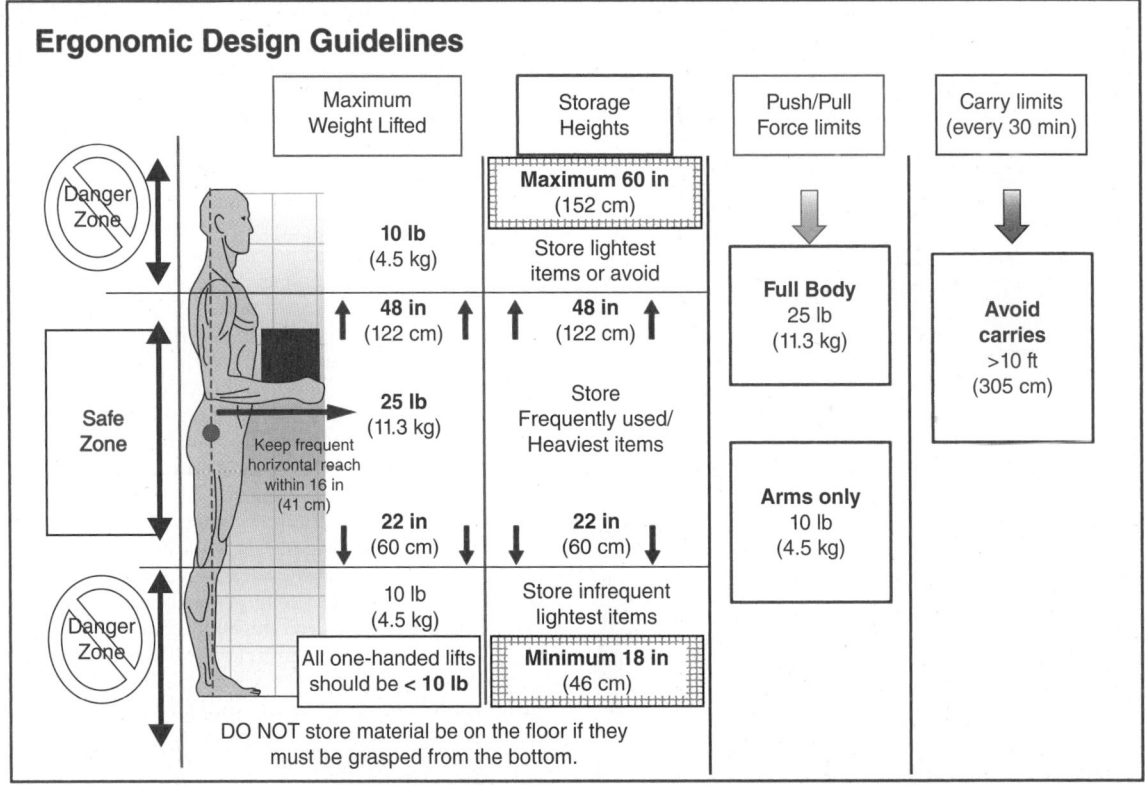

Ergonomic Design Guidelines

▲ **Figure 6–4.** Design guidelines that can be used in trainings of employees, supervisors, engineers, and health and safety staff to help them be proactive in making workplace changes that reduce risk of musculoskeletal disorders. (Provided by Meg Honan, UC Ergonomics Research & Graduate Training Program Senior Consultant.)

intervention to assess the effect of the intervention on risk of MSD.

WORKSTATION DESIGN PRINCIPLES

Reduce Sustained or High Forces

The forces required to perform a task should be kept as low as possible with efforts focused on balancing the demand of the task with the capacity of workers. Lifts associated with high compression, torsion, or shear forces on the spine have a greater potential to cause low back pain. High peak hand forces (≥ 2 on a 0–10 CR-10 BORG Scale) and those that exceed 1 kg of pinch or 5 kg of grip that last for more than 11% of the task cycle have been associated with increased risk of distal upper extremity MSDs. Such hand forces can be due to using inadequate or inappropriate tools or poor design of work tasks. Reducing sustained or high forces exerted by the upper extremity and back should be a primary focus in the design of acceptable work. Thus, more detail is outlined in the following discussion in the design of hand tools and manual material handling tasks.

Reduce Sustained Postures

Tasks, tools, and workstations should be designed to prevent sustained postures, particularly if they are awkward (far from neutral joint position). There is nothing wrong with occasionally moving joints through their full range of motion at work. However, postures that are sustained over several hours or repeated throughout the workday can pose a problem, particularly if they deviate from neutral position. Neutral joint position is typically where the load on noncontractile tissues is the lowest and contractile tissues (muscles) are at an optimal length to produce muscle force. Working with the hands above shoulder height for long periods, particularly when exerting high hand forces, can lead to shoulder, upper back, and neck disorders. Such sustained awkward shoulder postures may occur during construction work, automobile assembly and repair, or warehouse work. Sustained trunk flexion is seen often in agricultural or construction work. Work should be designed to prevent sustained

- Neck or trunk flexion, extension, or rotation
- Squatting

Table 6–1. State, national, and international ergonomics guidelines or standards.

Standard/Guideline	Organization	Issues
Hand Activity Level TLV 2012	ACGIH	Hand intensive work
Lifting TLV 2012	ACGIH	Repetitive lifting tasks
Hand-Arm Vibration TLV 2012	ACGIH	Vibrating hand tools
Whole Body Vibration TLV 2012	ACGIH	Heavy equipment
ANSI/HFES 100-2007	ANSI & HFES	Computer workstations
ANSI/HFES 200	ANSI & HFES	Software user interface
B11	ANSI	Design of machine tools
NIOSH Lifting Equation	NIOSH	Lifting limits
CCR Title 8, Section 5110	California OSHA	All industries
AB 1136	California OSHA	Patient handling
Guidelines	Federal OSHA	Meatpacking; nursing homes; grocery stores; poultry; shipyards; beverage distribution
MIL-STD-1472G, 2012	US DOD	Human engineering design criteria
Directive 90/269/EEC	European Union	Manual handling
Directive 90/270/EEC	European Union	Display screen
Directive 2002/244/EC	European Union	Vibration
Directive 2006/42/EC	European Union	Safety of machinery
ISO 9241, 9355, 14738	ISO	VDT, machine design
ISO 28927	ISO	Hand-transmitted vibration (tools)
ISO 2631, 5007, 25398	ISO	Whole-body vibration (vehicles)
ISO 11228	ISO	Manual handling
ISO 12296	ISO	Patient handling
Ergonomic Checkpoints- Practical and easy-to-implement solutions for improving safety, health and working condition	International Labour Organization	All Industries
Principles and Guidelines for Human Factors/Ergonomics Design and Management of Work Systems.	International Labour Organization	All Industries

Abbreviations: ACGIH, American Conference of Government Industrial Hygiene; ANSI, American National Standards Institute; DOD, Department of Defense; HAL, hand-activity limit; HFES, Human Factors and Ergonomics Society; ISO, International Standards Organization; MIL-STD, military standard; TLV, threshold limit value.

- Shoulder elevation, abduction, flexion, or external rotation
- Elbow flexion
- Wrist extension, flexion, or ulnar or radial deviation
- Finger extension or abduction

Awkward postures occur as a result of the interaction between the worker's size and shape (anthropometry) and the hand locations of the task or the visual target. Nearby machinery or material may get in the way of legs or arms, increasing reach distances. In general, the point of operation (the primary hand location for work) should be between waist and shoulder height and between the shoulders (Figure 6–4). The point of operation should be in the lower area of this envelope if the materials or tools handled are large or heavy, or if the hands have to be held in one area for a long period.

Sustained postures such as standing or sitting continuously have been associated with increased low back pain. Based on a scientific review of literature, standing for more than 1 hour continuously in combination with 4 hours cumulatively per day has been identified as unsafe with associations to leg swelling, discomfort of the low back and legs, increased risk of cardio/cerebrovascular strain, muscle fatigue, and preterm delivery. Allowing for the alternation of posture through sit-stand workstations and intermittent walking is an excellent way to mitigate the negative health outcomes associated with sustained (prolonged) sitting or standing.

Reduce Rapid or Forceful Repeated Motions

Repeated motions can be problematic if they are rapid, include awkward postures, and/or include high forces. Repeated forceful motions of the upper extremity have been associated with increased risk of distal upper extremity MSDs in multiple prospective cohort studies. The use of appropriate hand tools, reducing wasted motions or mechanizing tasks that include rapid or repeated forceful exertions are important strategies to consider when repetitive work is required.

Reduce Contact Stress

Hard surfaces and edges may make convenient sites to rest the arms, but they can put pressure on tendons, nerves, bones, or bursa and lead to sore spots or soft-tissue disorders. If support surfaces are necessary (eg, supporting arms during prolonged microscope use), the support should be rounded and padded to minimize the risk of contact stress and located so that it does not apply pressure on sensitive body regions (eg, wrist or elbow). With good arm support, a worker has more options for posture and movement that would otherwise be uncomfortable or injurious (Figure 6–5).

Design of Work Based on Anthropometric Data

One reason for increased musculoskeletal loads on the job is the mismatch in size between the worker and the workplace, equipment, or tools. This mismatch may result in prolonged forward bending to reach for tools or materials, having to hold a heavy tool at some distance from the body, or having to sit in a position that is too low or too high for the hands.

Figures 6–6 and 6–7 show the critical body dimensions of adult men and women in the United States, respectively. Workplaces and machines should be designed so that larger workers (up to the 95th percentile) and smaller workers (down to the 5th percentile) can easily complete their tasks. That is, a well-designed work space accommodates the larger worker's body size but also keeps supplies and control levers within comfortable reach for the smaller worker.

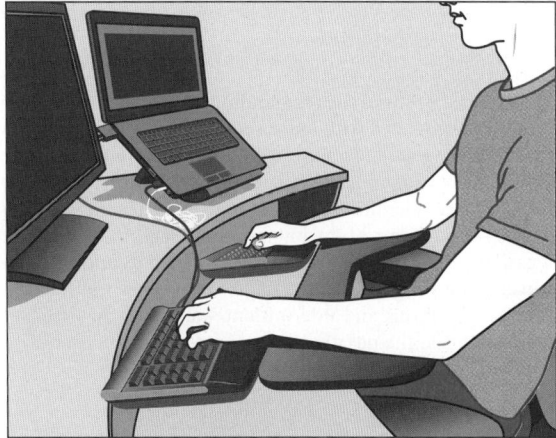

▲ **Figure 6–5.** Forearm support for sustained work at the computer.

The most important physical design rule for a sedentary job at a desk or workbench is that the operator be able to reach all frequently used items (eg, parts, supplies, keyboards, tools, and controls) without leaning, bending, or twisting at the waist. Frequent reaching should be restricted to moderate movements of the arm, if possible. Figure 6–8 illustrates the forearm-only (preferable) and full-arm (acceptable for occasional) reach limits for a North American population of men and women. Task designs that require movements outside the full-arm reach limits tend to increase the risks of shoulder, neck, and low back problems.

A. Example

Women of average dimensions (50th percentile) can reach horizontally about 74 cm (29 in), and short women (5th percentile) can reach horizontally about 68 cm (27 in), as measured from the backrest of the chair when they are seated in an upright position. If a shelf of supplies or a panel of controls is 91 cm (36 in) in front of them (also measured from the backrest of the chair), they will have difficulty obtaining supplies or manipulating controls even when bending and twisting at the waist. Productivity will be reduced. The work area should be redesigned to reduce the reach distances to frequently used items or controls to within a comfortable range.

The reach-envelope rules are particularly important if heavy items (> 10 kg) or high forces are applied. The heavier the tool or work piece, the closer it should be to elbow height and to the body. For repeated or continuous use, a heavy work piece or tool should be supported on a jig or work surface.

Work that involves high precision and visually demanding tasks should consider the location of the visual target (eg, part, tool). The visual targets should be prioritized and located based on frequency of viewing. Frequently viewed targets should be directly in front of the operator and between eye level and 45 degrees below eye level.

Logically Locate Controls & Displays

Machine operation is most productive and least stressful when the machine does the work and the operator does the thinking. Controls (eg, levers, switches, joysticks, and pedals) enable the operator to give a machine "orders" or feed it information. They also can provide feedback to the operator. Primary controls—those of greatest importance or used most often—should be located within the forearm-only reach limits (eg, near reach zone) and between the shoulders; infrequently used controls can be located within the full-arm (satisfactory) reach limits of the workstation, as shown in Figure 6–8.

The location of controls, displays, and other visual targets should be integrated with each other on a logical basis. Logical linkages and proximity suggest intuitive responses to the information displayed to the operator. In this manner, the control-display relationships can reduce the information

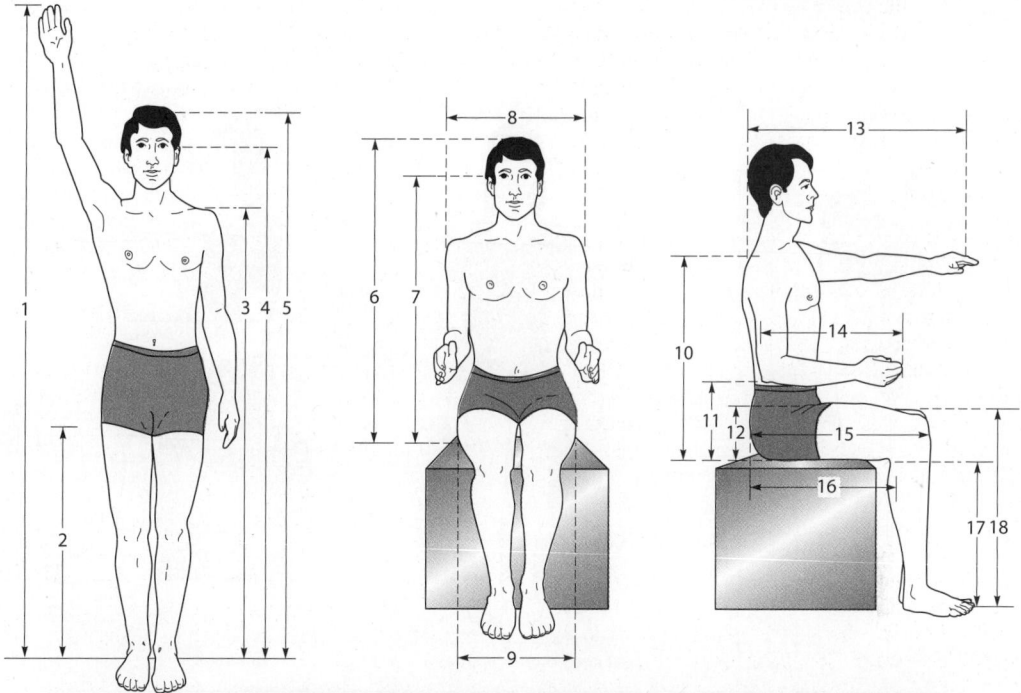

Male Body Dimensions (cm)

Dimension Number	Dimension Name	5th Percentile	50th Percentile	95th Percentile	Standard Deviation
1	Vertical reach	195.6	209.6	223.5	8.46
2	Crotch height	75.4	83.1	90.7	4.67
3	Shoulder height	133.6	143.6	154.1	6.22
4	Eye height	152.4	163.3	175.0	15.29
5	Stature	163.8	174.4	185.6	6.61
6	Height, sitting	84.5	90.8	96.7	3.66
7	Eye height, sitting	72.8	78.8	84.6	3.57
8	Shoulder breadth	41.5	45.2	49.8	2.54
9	Hip breadth, sitting	30.7	33.9	38.4	2.38
10	Shoulder height, sitting	57.1	62.4	67.6	3.18
11	Elbow height, sitting	18.8	23.7	28.0	2.78
12	Thigh clearance	13.0	14.9	17.5	1.36
13	Thumb tip reach	74.9	82.4	90.9	4.85
14	Elbow-fingertip length	44.3	47.9	51.9	2.31
15	Buttock-knee length	54.9	59.4	64.3	2.85
16	Buttock-popliteal length	45.8	49.8	54.0	2.50
17	Popliteal height	40.6	44.5	48.8	2.50
18	Knee height, sitting	49.7	54.0	58.7	2.73

▲ **Figure 6–6.** Body dimensions for men. Corresponding weights are as follows: 5th percentile, 57.4 kg (126.3 lb); 50th percentile, 71 kg (156.2 lb); and 95th percentile, 91.6 kg (201.5 lb). Appropriate dimensions (allowances) must be added for clothing and shoes.

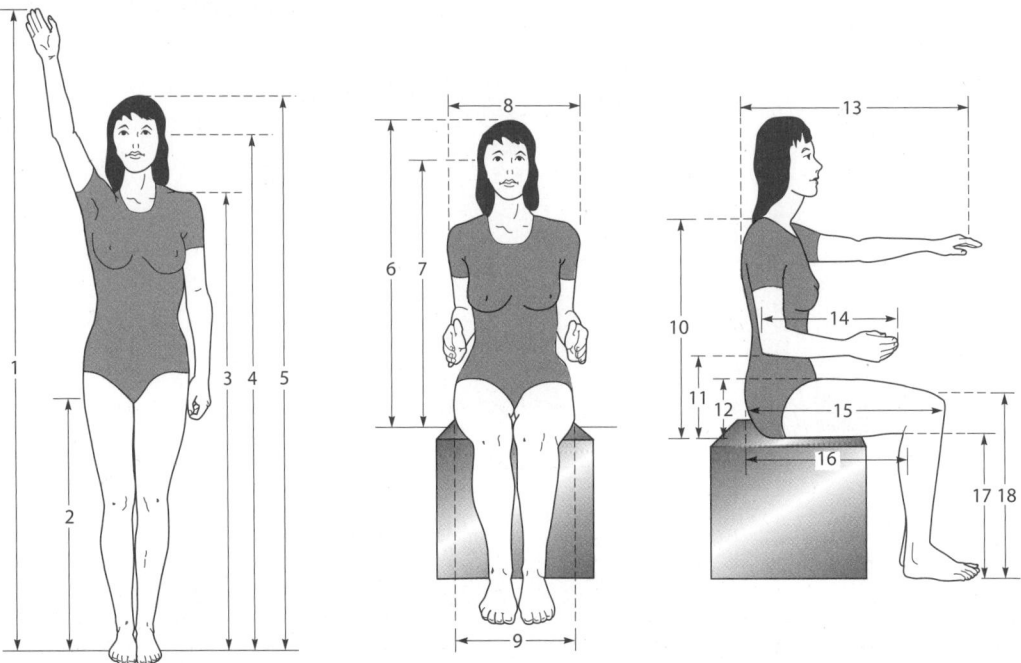

Female Body Dimensions (cm)					
Dimension Number	Dimension Name	5th Percentile	50th Percentile	95th Percentile	Standard Deviation
1	Vertical reach	185.2	199.1	213.4	8.64
2	Crotch height	68.1	74.4	81.3	4.06
3	Shoulder height	123.9	133.3	143.7	6.00
4	Eye height	142.2	149.9	158.8	6.35
5	Stature	152.6	162.8	174.1	6.52
6	Height, sitting	79.0	85.2	90.8	3.59
7	Eye height, sitting	67.7	73.8	79.1	3.46
8	Shoulder breadth	38.4	42.0	45.7	2.24
9	Hip breadth, sitting	33.0	38.2	43.9	3.27
10	Shoulder height, sitting	53.7	57.9	62.5	2.66
11	Elbow height, sitting	16.1	20.8	25.0	2.74
12	Thigh clearance	13.2	15.4	17.5	1.31
13	Thumb tip reach	67.7	74.2	80.5	3.88
14	Elbow-fingertip length	40.0	43.4	47.5	2.28
15	Buttock-knee length	53.1	57.7	63.2	3.06
16	Buttock-popliteal length	43.5	47.5	52.6	2.76
17	Popliteal height	38.0	41.6	45.7	2.35
18	Knee height, sitting	46.9	50.9	55.5	2.60

▲ **Figure 6–7.** Body dimensions for women. Corresponding weights are as follows: 5th percentile, 46.6 kg (103.5 lb); 50th percentile, 59.6 kg (131.1 lb); and 95th percentile, 74.5 kg (163.9 lb). Appropriate dimensions must be added for clothing and shoes.

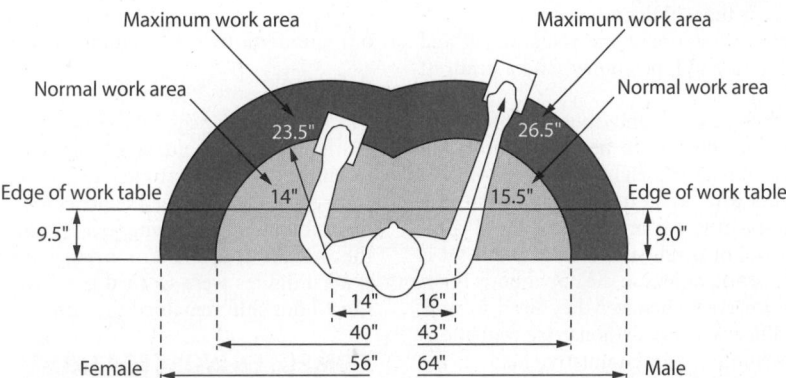

▲ **Figure 6–8.** Forearm-only (preferable) and full-arm (satisfactory) reach limits for men and women in working areas shown in the horizontal and vertical planes.

processing, for example, cognitive, load on the operator and thus reduce stress and the rate of errors.

A. Example

If a steam turbine is to be monitored and operated, the primary displays should be in front of and just below the eye level of the operator, and the turbine controls generally will be in front of and near the operator's hands. However, the control for rotational speed should be in proximity to and linked logically with its speed indicator display (eg, the control and display should both be contained in a common area on the panel or linked by means of a color-coded line). Movement of the speed control upward or to the right also should move the speed indicator display upward or to the right. This will increase the stimulus-response compatibility of the two devices and improve the control capability of the operator.

Proper Design of Chairs

Common complaints that stem from improper seating include fatigue or ache in the back or lower parts of the body. The primary purpose of a chair is to provide comfortable but stable support for the weight of the body without localized pressure points. The chair must support the employee in the posture best suited for the task (eg, slightly reclined for computer work or slightly forward-leaning for writing). Shifting body position over the course of the day is a natural way to distribute loads on the spine and maintain circulation in the buttocks and thighs; chair and workstation design should accommodate these postural variations.

If the seat pan is too deep (> 41 cm [16 in]), the front edge can press against the back of the knees, particularly in short women. A shallow seat or a smoothly curved "waterfall design" front edge can eliminate this contact stress for shorter people. The seat pan should not be so concave that it restricts occasional changes of position. Many chairs have size adjustment features for better fit (eg, sliding seat pans

offering a range of depths, or a choice of different size seat pans). The seat should be soft enough to be comfortable but not so soft that changing posture or standing up is difficult.

Chair design should also provide sufficient lumbar support to maintain a comfortable degree of lumbar lordosis and assist in supporting the weight of the trunk. A chair should be easily adjustable while the operator is seated to offer a full range of seat heights, lumbar support height, and backrest slope. Without good support, general fatigue is more likely, and back pain may result.

The base of chairs should have five legs to reduce the likelihood of tipping over if the occupant leans backward. If the environment allows, the texture of material on the back and seat should be porous and slightly rough or nubby to allow air circulation between the material and the body. If the chair has armrests, they should fit the employee or be adjustable in height and distance apart to provide appropriate arm support while the occupant performs work tasks. Care should be taken in selecting furniture so that armrests do not strike parts of the work surface during normal chair movements, resulting in increased reach distances. For example, desks in which the user is facing into a corner or a curved surface increase the chances that the armrests will bump against the desk and increase reach distances to the telephone and paperwork.

If it is necessary to adjust the chair height so that some employees' feet do not touch the ground, then a large, sturdy footrest must be provided to prevent the legs from dangling. Without stable foot support, a chair seat that is too high restricts circulation in the lower legs and makes it difficult to lean forward.

Types of Chairs

Chairs Versus Stools Versus Perch Support

Most adults can be accommodated by a chair that is adjustable from a seat height of 38–48.3 cm (15–19 in). Reclining the back support to more than 20 degrees from vertical can lead to increased neck loading unless the visual target and controls of input devices are well positioned and a headrest is provided.

Brief periods of sitting, for a highly mobile worker (eg, laboratory or production work), are best done on a tall stool or perch support with a seat height range of 53–72 cm (22–30 in). For workers who are at a workstation but also have to walk about frequently, it is more efficient and comfortable to use a tall stool or perch support whose height is nearly the length of the workers' legs so the upper body is not repeatedly raised and lowered whenever they need to walk or stand. Studies of office workers demonstrate reductions in lower extremity swelling and in cumulative load on the spine when employees alternate between sitting and standing so that each position is adopted for a total of at least 2 hours during the workday.

Proper Selection of Chairs

There are many well-designed chairs, but they must fit the task as well as the user. Some jobs involve paperwork or high precision visually demanding work, requiring "forward sitting." Others allow upright or reclining postures (eg, writing computer code). The employer or ergonomics committee should obtain samples of two or three chairs appropriate for the task (with appropriate seat, backrest, and armrest adjustments and forearm support if needed) and meet the requirements of the workers (appropriate seat pan depth, backrest shape, casters versus glides, etc.) and have the workers try them out for at least a week. A briefer period for chair testing is usually insufficient because initial impressions often differ from long-term satisfaction. The opinion of those performing the work, the workstation design, and the visual and physical demands of the tasks performed should all be considered when a supply of new chairs is ordered.

Avoid Static Body Positions: Task Variation

Workers who operate computers and some types of equipment may hold their bodies in a fixed position for long periods in order to maintain a consistent physical relationship with the equipment. For example, keyboard use requires a fixed spatial relationship between the seat, torso, hands, and the keyboard in order to strike the proper key without looking. In addition, computer users often maintain a rigid neck position for long periods to view the computer monitor. Laboratory technicians working at microscopes, hoods, or in biosafety cabinets are often in static postures for hours, performing visually demanding high-precision tasks.

In jobs of this sort, measures should be taken to prevent pain and fatigue in the shoulders, neck, and back due to static load. Padded forearm support can reduce shoulder and neck loads. Breaking up static tasks with alternative work every 20–60 minutes can reduce discomfort. These can be brief tasks (eg, retrieving printouts or supplies, obtaining new hard copy or samples, or filing) that involve a few minutes of walking and standing. It may be necessary to use a timer or reminder software to remind the worker to take the break.

A. Example

The usual break schedule of data-entry operators was two 15-minute breaks plus a 30-minute lunch break. This was modified to add a 5-minute break every hour. The employees were encouraged to use the break to take a short walk. With more frequent breaks, employees reported less discomfort in the shoulders, upper arm, neck, and back. Even though 20 fewer minutes were worked per day, the productivity over the 8-hour shift remained the same.

COMPUTER WORKSTATIONS

Computer operators often complain of pain and fatigue in the neck, upper back, shoulders, forearms, or wrists, especially when they use the computer for more than 4 hours per day. They also can experience visual fatigue or eyestrain from long-term viewing of the computer monitor. Appropriate setup and use of the computer workstation can help to reduce these aches and pains.

Adjust Chair First

The first step in adjusting a computer workstation is to adjust the seat, especially if the work surface is height-adjustable. The seat height should be adjusted low enough so that the operator's feet are firmly supported on the floor but not so low that the operator's weight is not evenly distributed over the seat pan. A large and stable footrest can be used when it is not possible to adjust the chair and workstation low enough to accommodate the short worker. Arm supports, which may be on the chair or the work surface, should comfortably support the forearms and prevent contact stress at the wrist or elbow (eg, ulnar nerve). Some computer users prefer to switch from sitting to standing during the day to promote posture changes; this requires workstations that adjust easily and rapidly in height (Figure 6–9) or rotation to a variety of tasks. Employees with neck, shoulder, or back problems may benefit from the ability to alternate between sitting and standing.

Proper Placement of Monitor & Documents

Primary visual targets (screens and hard copy) should be located in front of the operator, between 0 to 30 degrees below eye level, and approximately 48–72 cm (20–30 in) away. If hard copy is used, a document holder should be placed either to one side of the screen or between the monitor and the keyboard. This will allow the operator to view the monitor with a minimum of neck flexion, extension, or rotation. Bifocal lens users are an exception to this recommendation; they usually need the primary display lower, approximately 30–45 degrees below eye level. Bifocal lens users may benefit from prescription monofocal or occupational bifocal lenses for computer use; these lenses permit

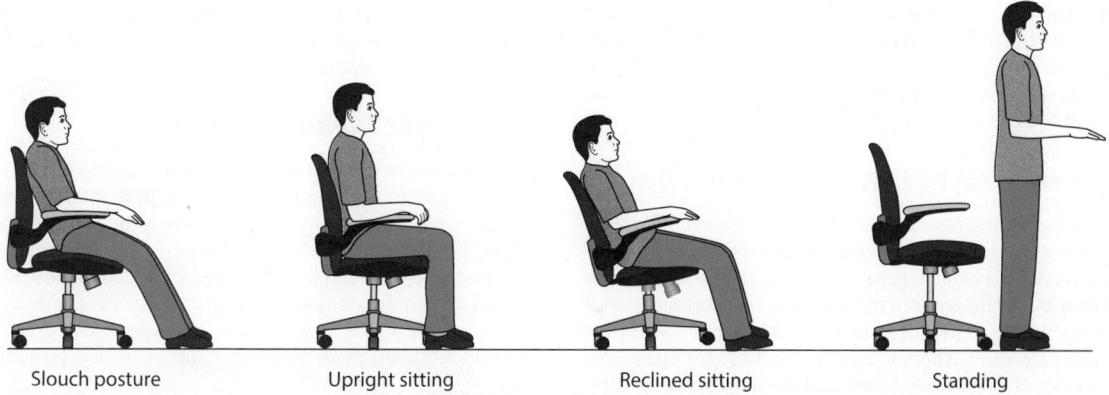

| Slouch posture | Upright sitting | Reclined sitting | Standing |

▲ **Figure 6–9.** The sitting posture during work can vary from forward sitting (visually demanding task) to upright sitting, reclined sitting (writing computer code), or standing.

a greater range of head postures. Optometrists should be informed of the type of work performed and the typical distance and location of the visual targets for consideration in the lens prescription. Computer users who lean forward to see the screen may need the font size increased, their vision checked, or the monitor moved closer.

A. Example

Workers in a call center reported experiencing increasing shoulder pain toward the end of the day and the end of the workweek. Forearm supports, attached to the front of the keyboard/mouse work surface, were provided and adjusted to the worker's body size. The workers who used the forearm support reported a steady decline in shoulder pain over the next few weeks.

Eliminate Glare

The computer monitor should be positioned so that glare is minimized. For example:

1. Change the location of the monitor so that the bright light source is to the side of (eg, window) or above (eg, ceiling light) the computer user, not directly behind or in front. Move the monitor so that it is more than 2 m (80 in) from windows.

2. Reduce the general illumination in the room to about 500 lux. This can be achieved by reducing the amount of overhead lighting (eg, removing every other bulb or fluorescent tube), installing indirect lighting to direct light upward toward the ceiling, installing parabolic louvers for the fluorescent lights to direct the illumination straight downward, or controlling window illumination with shades, louvered blinds, and/or tinted window film.

3. Provide more illumination where needed with desk lamps ("task lighting") directed at the appropriate visual

target. The goal is to have lighting as uniform as possible with a maximum ratio of 1:3 between the brightness of the computer screen and its immediate surroundings.

4. If steps 1 through 3 fail, use glare-reducing filters on computer screens. These filters are available in several designs, although the most effective are coated filters (eg, polarized filters).

Position of Input Devices

The height of keyboard and pointing device should be adjusted so that the shoulders are not elevated and the wrists are relatively straight during use. The slope of the keyboard can be adjusted so that the wrists are not held in extension during mousing or keying. A thin keyboard will reduce wrist extension. If elevated forearm supports are used, a thin keyboard or mouse may need to be slightly raised by placing one or more mouse pads under them to achieve a straight wrist.

Workers who use the computer for long hours and do not touch type should take typing lessons. This will reduce the neck flexion associated with looking at the keyboard during typing. Alternatively, they may benefit from moving the keyboard and mouse closer to the screen and supporting the forearms on the work surface to reduce load on the shoulders.

The use of a wrist rest has been associated with increased hand pain. If a wrist rest is used, it should be used occasionally during keyboard use, not constantly. It is better to provide support to the forearms with the chair armrests, the desk surface, or a forearm support.

Most software used today requires a pointing device (mouse, touchpad, trackball) to be used more than a keyboard. The mouse may require some type of forearm support to reduce wrist extension and shoulder loading. Mini-keyboards that do not have numeric keypads can reduce shoulder external rotation and reach to the mouse. Keyboard shortcuts can be used for frequently used commands (eg, copy and paste; repeated character sequences). In addition, alternative input devices can allow shortcuts to be assigned to extra keys.

Alternative Keyboards & Pointing Devices

Alternative keyboards or pointing devices can reduce awkward wrist and forearm postures; however, there are limited empirical data to guide recommendations. Keyboard designs that split the keyboard in half, with some separation and tilt between the two halves, can reduce wrist ulnar deviation and forearm pronation. There is some evidence that a fixed-split keyboard can reduce hand pain and disorders among computer users in comparison with a conventional keyboard, but the beneficial effect may take weeks to be noticed. As with chairs, it is suggested that employees evaluate a different keyboard or mouse for at least a week while performing their usual tasks before making a decision about whether or not to use the device. A systematic evaluation by an ergonomics committee can be used to identify an appropriate set of input devices for use at the employer.

Patients with pain in their mousing hand can switch to mousing with the other hand; however, pain may develop on both sides. Another solution is to provide several different types of pointing devices and have the employee alternate between them on a weekly basis. If the work involves frequent combinations of mouse click and simultaneous movement ("click and drag"), the use of a mouse with each hand, one to hold a button down and the other to move the cursor, can significantly reduce upper extremity strain. Additionally, hot key buttons can be used to reduce the amount of click and drags on the mouse and/or the number of keystrokes to perform common tasks.

HAND INTENSIVE TASKS & TOOL DESIGN

Reduce High Hand Force Exertions

The repeated or sustained application of high-pinch (> 1 kg) or high-grip (> 5 kg) force to hold parts or to grip power tools is associated with tendon disorders of the forearm, muscle fatigue, and carpal tunnel syndrome. A classic example of a high-risk task is the sustained grip maintained by meat packers on a wet and slippery knife. Sustained or repeated pinch grip puts tendons at even greater risk than a power grip. A pinch grip occurs when most of the force is applied between the fingers and the thumb (Figure 6–10). In a power grip, the force is applied evenly through the palm (Figure 6–11). Tasks and tools should be redesigned to reduce the force required to perform the tasks and to reduce the time duration that force is applied during the task cycle. Tools can also be redesigned to convert use from a pinch grip to a power grip.

Assembling parts with screws is usually performed with inline drivers. The high force required to hold and stabilize a powered driver when the screw tightens can be reduced by using a driver adjusted to the proper torque, the use of antitorque clutches or bars, and the selection of screws or other fasteners appropriate for the task.

Avoid Static Holding Positions

A production task might involve holding a work piece or tool continuously in one hand and working on it with the other. Reduction of fatigue may be accomplished by using a rapid-release holding clamp or vise. When sustained holding is still necessary, the tool can be suspended from cables with a balancing system or articulated with antitorque bars to decrease grip force. Heavy parts can be held with a jig or clamp so that the nondominant hand is not applying a constant grip force.

A. Example

In a quality-control task, each part being checked was picked up and held by the worker's left hand while testing clamps were attached and adjustments made. The job was redesigned so that each part was placed on a small, waist-high rolling jig, then the worker made attachments and adjustments with both hands.

Reduce Rapid, Repetitive Motions

Tasks that require very rapid hand and shoulder movements or movements that are repeated every few seconds throughout the day have been associated with hand and arm disorders. Exposures to these tasks can be controlled by limiting the number of hours per day that an employee performs these movements or by rotating employees between different tasks so that the same muscles are not repeatedly loaded all day.

Consideration also should be given to redesigning the task so that the distance moved is minimized, thereby reducing the speed necessary to complete the task. Experienced workers often know how to perform these tasks with smooth motions that reduce wasted energy and sudden impacts. Therefore, the experienced workers should be involved in teaching new hires the best work techniques.

Avoid Contact Pressures

The palm of the hand should not be used as a hammer. Even frequent light tapping with the hypothenar, "heel" region of the hand can cause injury to the ulnar nerve or artery (eg, hypothenar hammer syndrome). In sheet metal work, for example, the palm of the hand may be used to force parts together. A rubber mallet should be used instead.

Proper Design of Tool Handles

To avoid contact stress in the hands, tool handles should be designed so that the force-bearing area is as large as practicable and there are no sharp corners or edges. This means that handles should be either round or oval. Handles should have a high coefficient of friction in order to reduce hand-gripping

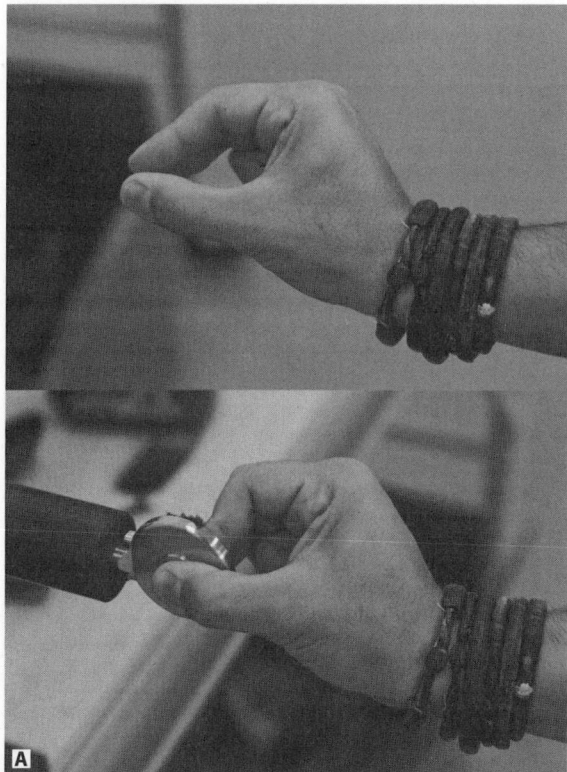
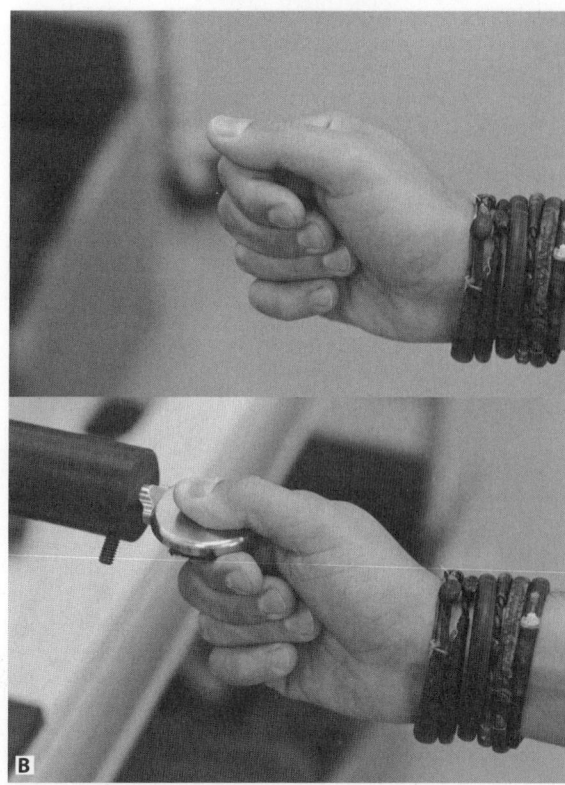

▲ **Figure 6–10.** Hand posture: pulp to pulp pinch and lateral/key pinch grips.

forces needed for tool control. Pinch points should be eliminated or guarded.

Rigid, form-fitting handles with grooves for each finger usually do not improve the grip function unless they are sized to the individual's hand. Formfitting, scalloped handles, which are often designed for the hand of a worker in the 50th percentile, will spread the fingers of a small (5th percentile) hand too far apart for efficient gripping and will cause uncomfortable ridges under the fingers of a large (95th percentile) hand.

Many power tools (eg, drills, sanders, and chain saws) are operated and controlled with two hands, and there is generally a primary handle with a trigger to provide for gripping by the dominant hand. If there is a secondary, stabilizing, or antitorque handle, it should be usable on either side of the tool to permit use by either left-handed or right-handed people and permit the user to change the trigger hand from time to time to reduce fatigue.

Excessive use of a single finger for operating triggers on hand tools causes local fatigue and may result in a stenosing tenosynovitis, or "trigger finger." Triggers can be designed to be operated by two or more fingers at once or by a switch triggered by the foot. Locking buttons also can reduce sustained

loading. Exposure to tool vibration will be addressed later in this chapter.

A. Example—Pipette Usability Study

A company had experienced pipette users complete a standardized pipetting task with five manual and five electronic pipettes. Each pipette was rated on key attributes of comfort and usability. Features associated with greater hand and arm comfort were lower tip ejection force, lower blowout force, and better pipette balance in the hand. The usability study was used to guide the purchasing of future pipettes.

EVALUATING HAND INTENSIVE TASKS

The Revised Strain Index

The Revised Strain Index (RSI) is another exposure assessment tool for the distal upper extremity. It is based on a model that incorporates tensile and compressive stress as well as recovery; thus, it includes intensity of exertion (I), frequency of exertion (E), duration per exertion (D), hand/wrist posture (P), and the overall duration (H) that a task is performed throughout the day/workshift. Equations allow each

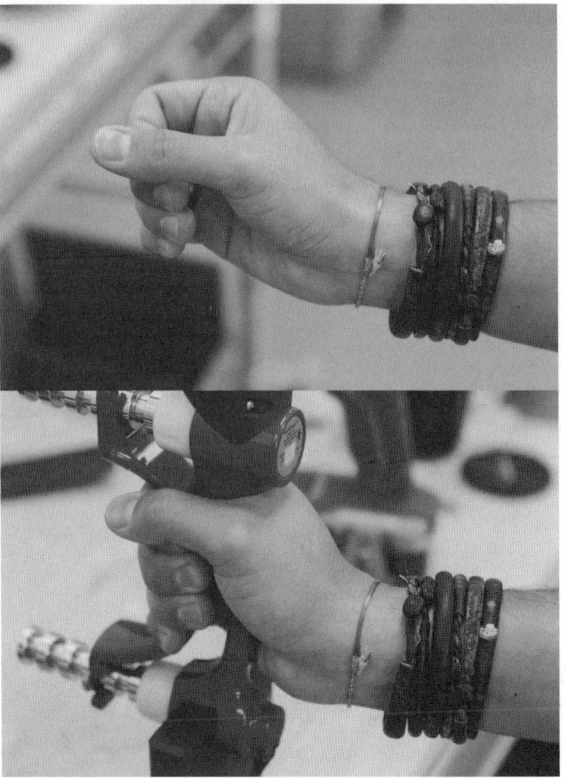

▲ **Figure 6–11.** Hand posture: power grip.

multiplier to be quantified on a continuous scale offering improved discrimination between exposures, particularly of intensity of exertion, which drives the overall risk score. The RSI score of 10 or less is considered safe, whereas scores above 10 are considered hazardous. The RSI is best used to determine risk of distal upper extremity MSDs in a cohort of individuals versus one worker and can be used as a tool for task analysis, intervention, and design. One benefit of the RSI is that there are methods to apply it when exposures vary within a task (Composite Strain Index) and methods to integrate physical exposure across multiple tasks (Cumulative Strain Index). The RSI equation is:

$$RSI = IM \times EM \times DM \times PM \times HM$$

The multipliers above are calculated using the following equations:

- The Intensity of Exertion Multiplier (IM) is a measure of force. The intensity of exertion can be measured subjectively using the BORG CR-10 scale by an analyst using the Moore-Garg Analyst Scale, or objectively using force matching or surface electromyography to estimate the percent of Maximum Voluntary Contraction (MVC). Intensity (I) is a 0–1.0 scale, where % MVC is expressed numerically from 0 to 1.0 or the Borg CR-10 rating is divided by 10.

$$IM = 30 \times I^3 - 15.60 \times I^2 + 13.00 \times I + 0.40 \qquad [0.0 < I \le 0.4]$$

$$IM = 36 \times I^3 - 33.30 \times I^2 + 24.77 \times I + 1.86 \qquad [0.4 < I \le 1.0]$$

- The Exertions per Minute Multiplier (EM) is a measure of frequency of exertions per minute. E is a frequency count of exertions per minute.

$$EM = 0.10 + 0.25 \times E \qquad [E \le 90/m]$$

$$EM = 0.00334 \times E^{1.96} \qquad [E > 90/m]$$

- The Duration per Exertion Multiplier (DM) is a measure of the average duration of exertion in seconds. D is a measure of duration in seconds.

$$DM = 0.45 + 0.31 \times D \qquad [D \le 60s]$$

$$DM = 19.17 \times \log_e(D) - 59.44 \qquad [D > 60s]$$

- The Hand/Wrist Posture Multiplier (PM) is a measure of wrist posture in degrees. It includes only postural deviations in the sagittal plane (flexion and extension) and decreases the penalty when in wrist extension up to and including 30°. P is a measure of wrist extension or flexion in degrees.

$$PM = 1.2 \times e^{(0.009 \times P)} - 0.2 \qquad [P = \text{Degrees of wrist flexion}]$$

$$PM = 1.0 \qquad [P \le 30° \text{ of wrist extension}]$$

$$PM = 1.0 + 0.00028 \times (P - 30)^2 \qquad [P > 30° \text{ of wrist extension}]$$

- The Duration of Hours per Day Multiplier (HM) includes a measure for the overall duration a task is engaged in over the course of a workshift and can accommodate workshifts greater than 8 hours. H is a measure of hours.

$$HM = 0.20 \qquad [H \le 0.05 \text{ h}]$$

$$HM = 0.042 \times H + 0.090 \times \log_e(H) + 0.477 \qquad [H > 0.05 \text{ h}]$$

The ACGIH TLV for Hand Activity

- The American Conference of Governmental Industrial Hygienists (ACGIH®) Threshold Limit Value (TLV®) for Hand Activity (ACGIH TLV HA 2018) evaluates job risk factors associated with musculoskeletal disorders of the hand and wrist. The tool assesses hand activity and level of effort for a typical posture while performing a short-cycle monotask job that lasts more than 4 hours a day. A monotask job is defined as a job requiring the same set of motions and/or repeated exertions. There are three steps:

1. *Determine hand activity level (HAL):* The rater first identifies the frequency of hand exertions or HAL on a scale from 0 to 10. On this scale, 0 represents virtually no activity (hands idle most of the time; no regular exertions), and 10 represents the highest imaginable hand activity (rapid, steady motion/difficulty keeping up or continuous exertion). HAL includes both effort

from repetition and duration and can also be calculated from the following equation:

$$HAL = 6.56 \ln D \, (F^{1.31} / (1 + 3.18 \times F^{1.31}))$$

where D is the duty cycle (0–100) and F is the frequency of exertions per second (Hz).

2. *Determine normalized peak force (NPF):* The rater characterizes the level of effort associated with typical high force within the work cycle. The NPF is the relative level of effort on a scale of 0–10 that a person of average strength would exert in the same posture required by the task. Methods for assessing hand force include worker and observer ratings using a subjective scale from 0 to 10 of perceived exertion (0: nothing at all; 10: extremely strong), biomechanical analyses, force gauges, or surface electromyography, in terms of percent of MVC (% MVC).

3. *Determine ergonomic risk of the task by combining both the HAL and NPF values on a TLV chart:* After determining the HAL and the NPF, draw a vertical line from the hand activity value and a horizontal line from the NPF value on the TLV chart. The intersection of these two lines, with respect to the TLV and action limit (AL) lines, determines the ergonomic risk of the task. Alternatively, the following equation can be used:

   ACGIH TLV for HA: NPF = 5.6 − 0.56 × HAL

   ACGIH Action Limit for HA: NPF = 3.6 − 0.56 × HAL

4. If the intersection point falls below the AL, the monotask job is likely safe. If the intersection point falls above the AL and below the TLV line, then the job likely has a greater risk of injury. If the intersection point falls above the TLV line, then the job should be modified. See the ACGIH website for further details: www.acgih.org.

5. It should be noted that recent epidemiologic studies have found that applying the ACGIH TLV for HA across multiple tasks using a time-weighted-average approach is associated with increased risk of distal upper extremity tendinopathies and entrapment disorders such as carpal tunnel syndrome. Because summarizing job-level exposure using a time-weighted-average approach may underestimate exposure and using peak exposure often overestimates risk, some prefer to use the most typical task (greatest duration) to represent job-level exposure. Currently, there is not a gold standard approach to summarizing the ACGIH TLV for HA across tasks to describe exposure at the job level.

ACGIH Upper Limb Localized Fatigue TLV

• The ACGIH Upper Limb Localized Fatigue TLV, first published in 2015, is another tool useful for the design of hand-intensive tasks. It applies to cyclical work that is

performed for 2 hours or more per day, and the intent is to prevent persistent upper extremity symptoms related to regional fatigue. The TLV is based on measurement of mean force applied over a cycle as a percent of MVC (% MVC) and the percent of time over a work cycle that force is applied (duty cycle, % DC). The TLV is represented by the inverse equations:

% MVC = (100%) × (−0.143 ln(DC/100%) + 0.066)

% DC = (100%) × e^((0.066 − (% MVC/100%))/0.143)

BIOMECHANICS OF LIFTING, PUSHING, & PULLING

Principles of Lifting

Figure 6–12 illustrates the estimated forces on the base of the spine (L5–S1) that would result from two different methods of lifting a load of 150 N (approximately 15 kg [34 lb]; 1 lb force = 4.44 N). When the lifting is done with the legs relatively straight (lifting in a "stooped" position), there is an estimated anterior shear force at L5–S1 of approximately 500 N and a spinal compression force of 1800 N. When the lifting is done with the knees bent (lifting in a squatting position, or "lifting with the legs"), the L5–S1 shear force is only 340 N, but the spinal compression force rises to 2700 N. This assumes that the load is too bulky to fit between the knees, as is often the case in practice. A commonly repeated safety rule is to "lift with the legs" and keep the load close to the body, but a deep squat often makes it difficult, if not impossible, to do both. In the example illustrated in Figure 6–12, the horizontal distance H from the spine to the center of gravity of the load is longer in the squatting position than it is with a stooped lift. This causes the load to exert more torque on the spine, increasing the compressive force on the lower lumbar disks. Workers tend to avoid deep squats when lifting because squatting takes more time, requires more energy, is hard on the knees, and often results in reduced ability to balance on the feet. Optimal lifting styles (Figure 6–13) are those that

• Allow the load to be kept as close as possible to the spine

• Offer a broad base of support for good balance

• Allow the worker to see ahead and avoid obstacles

• Allow the worker to retain a comfortable position ("neutral posture") of the spine, avoiding extremes of bending or twisting

If possible, twisting should be avoided by turning the shoulders and hips together as a unit. Figure 6–14 offers several suggestions and guidelines for reducing the risk of injury with lifting tasks.

Principles of Pushing & Pulling

The estimated forces involved in pushing and pulling loads are illustrated in Figure 6–15. Pulling with a force of 350 N

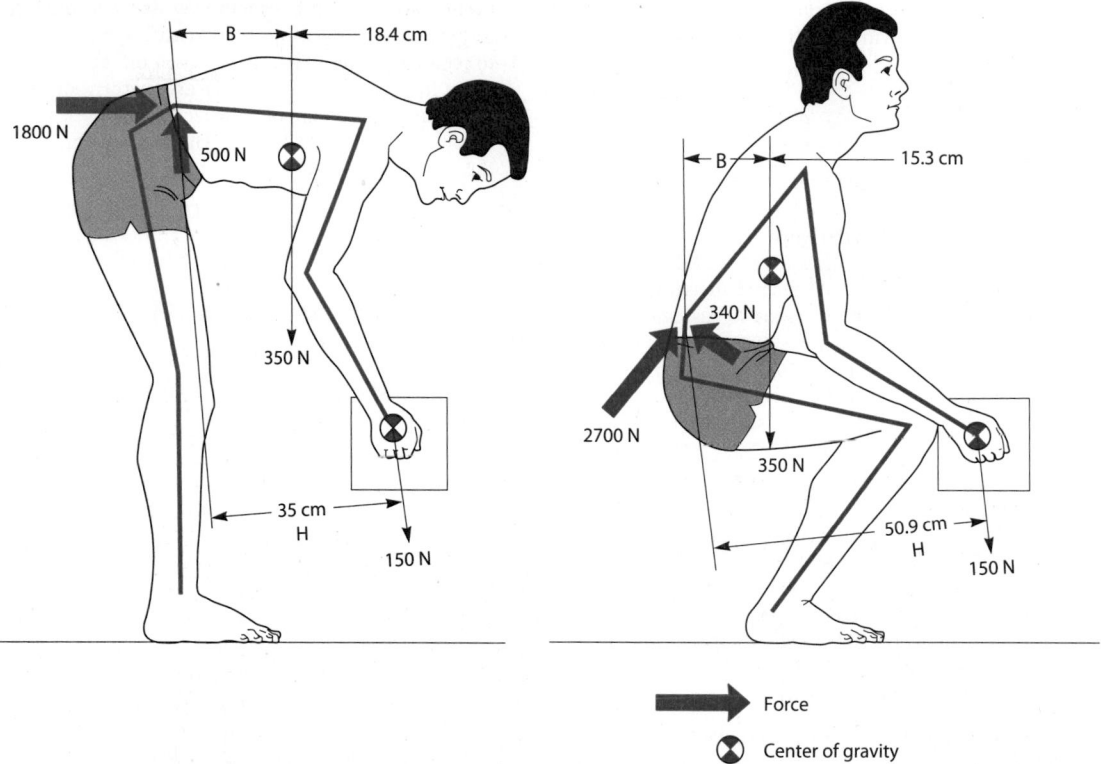

▲ Figure 6–12. Forces on the base of the spine (L5–S1 forces) that result from two different methods of lifting a load weighing 150 N. When the lifting is done with the legs relatively straight, there is an L5–S1 shear force of 500 N and a spinal compression force of 1800 N. When the lifting is done with the knees bent, the L5–S1 shear force is only 340 N, but the spinal compression force is 2700 N. B = horizontal distance from the L5–S1 joint to the body's center of gravity; H = horizontal distance from the L5–S1 joint to the load's center of gravity.

(80 lb) (the weight of the loaded cart times its coefficient of rolling friction) at a height of 66 cm (26.4 in) above the floor would result in a compressive force on the lumbar spine of about 8000 N, which is substantially above the U.S. NIOSH-recommended limit of 3400 N and even above the highest value (6400 N) that most workers can tolerate without injury.

The following are general guidelines to prevent injuries when pushing or pulling heavy loads: (1) Make certain that the area ahead of the load is level, offers adequate traction, and is clear of obstacles. If it is not level, some system of braking should be available. (2) Push the load, rather than pull it. This often will reduce spinal stress and, in most cases, will improve the visibility ahead. (3) Wear shoes that provide good foot traction. The coefficient of friction between the floor and the sole of the shoes should be at least 0.8 wherever heavy loads are moved. (4) When starting to push a load, brace the rear foot and shift the body weight forward. If the load does not start to move when a reasonable amount of force is applied, get help from a coworker or use a powered

vehicle. (5) Pushing or pulling is easier when the handles of the loaded cart are at about hip height (81–114 cm [about 32–47 in] for a mixed-gender population) than when they are at shoulder height or above. Handles lower than the hips are awkward and difficult to use. Two vertical handles, or two sets of handles at different heights, allow workers of different stature to grasp the load at optimal points (Figure 6–16).

EVALUATING MANUAL MATERIALS HANDLING TASKS

Despite our entry into the "information age," manual materials handling is still a major cause of low back pain and shoulder injuries. Efforts to address these with training programs directed at workers have largely failed. Although some of these injuries are associated with slips, trips, and falls while moving an object, most occur because the instantaneous or the cumulative load on the worker has exceeded his or her capabilities. Repeated lifting of heavy objects, especially with

• Test the load; get help if needed.
• Plan the lift and the path you will take.
• Keep the load as close to the body as possible.

• Pivot and move your feet with a broad base of support to avoid twisting.
• Try to keep your movements smooth and coordinated.
• Keep the back in a straight line from "head to tail."

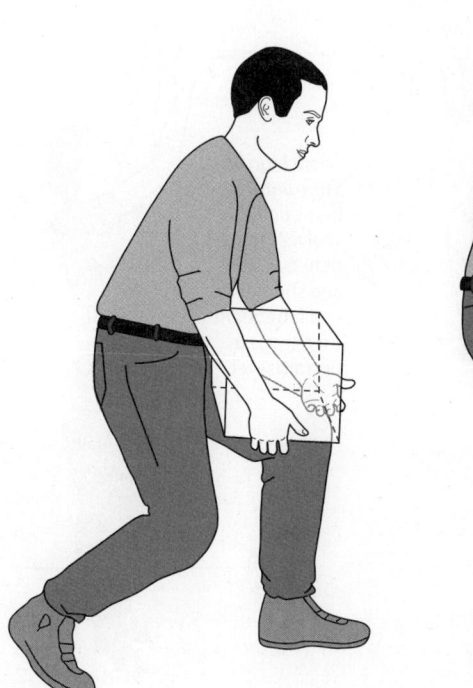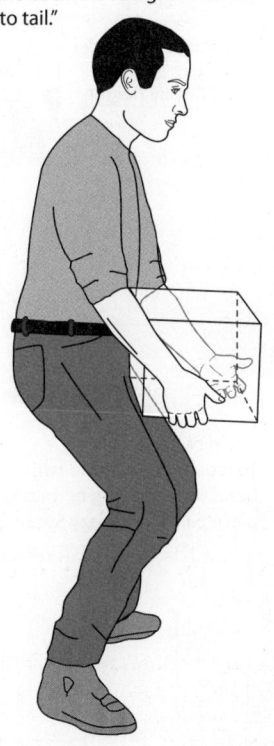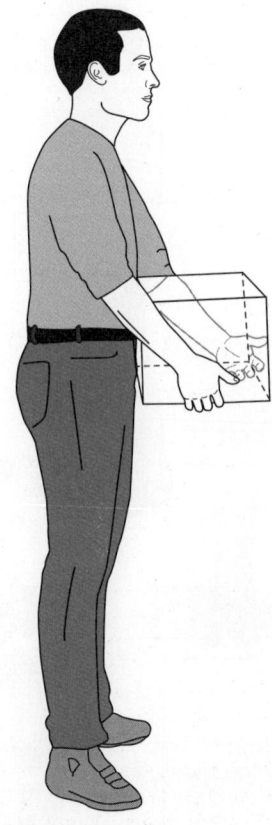

▲ **Figure 6–13.** With good lifting technique, the spine is kept stable even when it must be tilted forward.

spine twisting, is associated with low back pain. Psychosocial factors, such as work schedules, relations with coworkers, and work satisfaction, can influence low back pain reporting and disability.

The attempt to set safe limits for manual material handling can be approached in four ways:

1. *Epidemiologic:* Identifying the risk factors by analyzing the distribution of injuries in a population.

2. *Biomechanical:* Estimating the forces applied to the body by manual materials handling tasks and comparing those with tissue tolerances derived from cadaver studies.

3. *Physiologic:* Estimating the energy requirements of manual materials handling tasks compared with the aerobic capacity of workers.

4. *Psychophysical:* Simulating a manual materials handling task in a controlled environment and recording the subjects' acceptance of fatigue or discomfort. These should be done with subjects who are representative of

the population of interest in terms of age, physical condition, and gender. Maximum acceptable weights, forces, or distances for manual materials handling tasks can be estimated through this approach, although data on subsequent injuries usually are not collected because the study periods are so short (typically 1 day to 1 week).

NIOSH LIFTING EQUATION

Jobs in which lifting (as opposed to pushing, pulling, or carrying) is the predominant activity can be analyzed by using the U.S. NIOSH lifting equation (http://www.cdc.gov/niosh/docs/94-110/). It considers that a person's ability to lift may be limited by either biomechanical or metabolic factors; that is, the limiting factor may be the resulting forces on the body (biomechanical) or the energy expenditure (endurance) demanded by repeated lifting. The equation attempts to synthesize the results of biomechanical, physiologic, psychophysical, and epidemiologic studies.

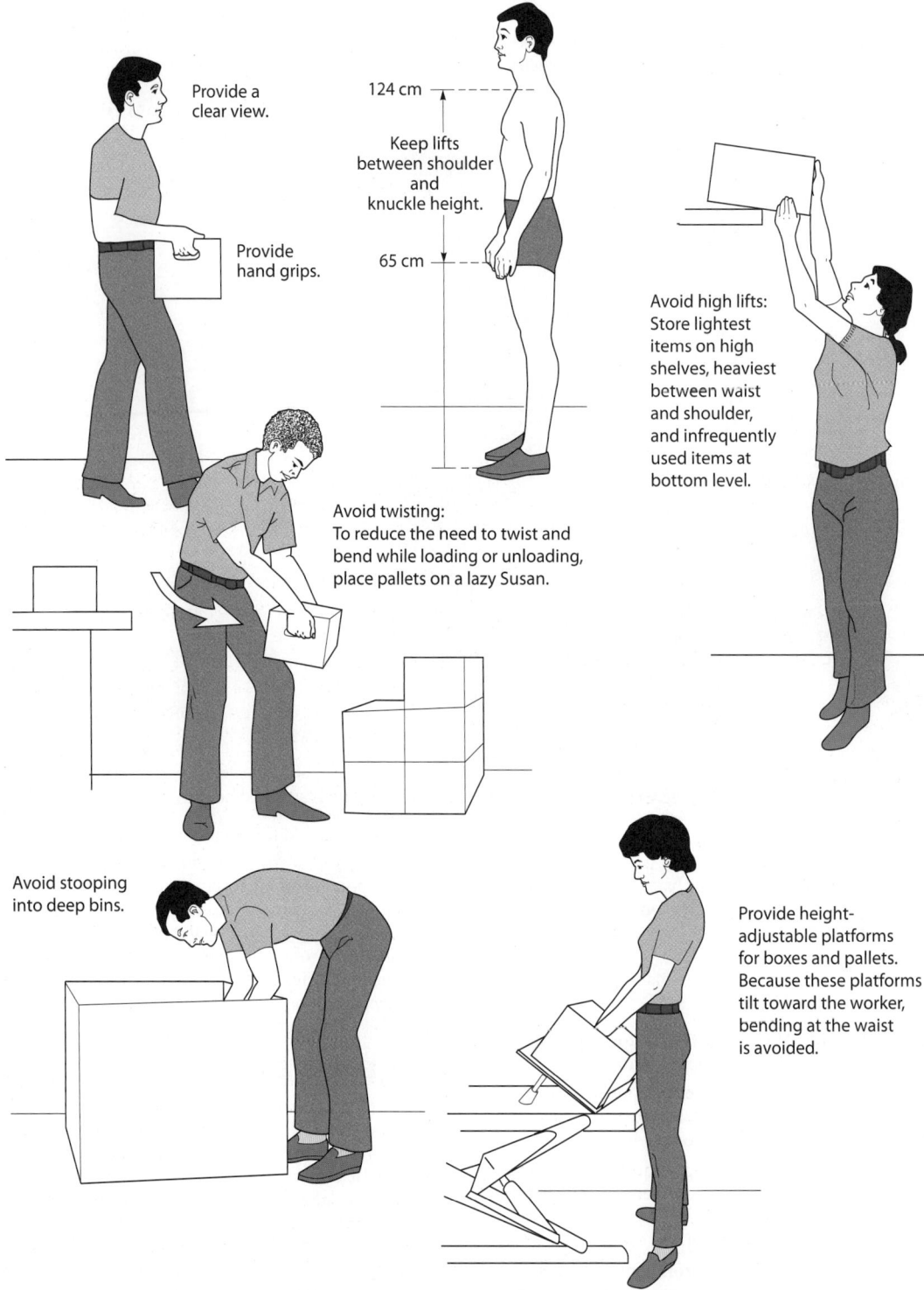

Provide a clear view.

Provide hand grips.

124 cm

Keep lifts between shoulder and knuckle height.

65 cm

Avoid high lifts: Store lightest items on high shelves, heaviest between waist and shoulder, and infrequently used items at bottom level.

Avoid twisting: To reduce the need to twist and bend while loading or unloading, place pallets on a lazy Susan.

Avoid stooping into deep bins.

Provide height-adjustable platforms for boxes and pallets. Because these platforms tilt toward the worker, bending at the waist is avoided.

▲ **Figure 6–14.** Suggestions for safe lifting.

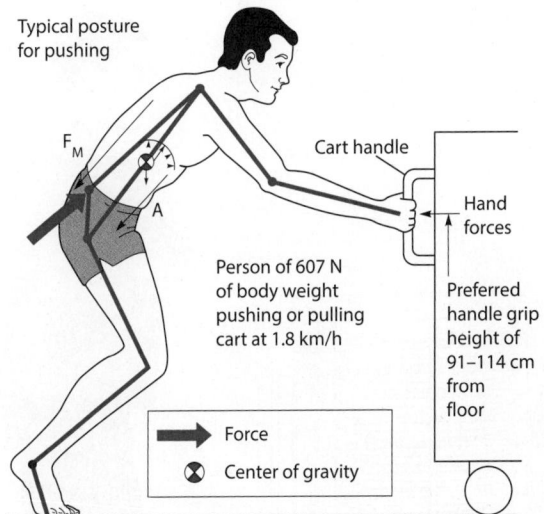

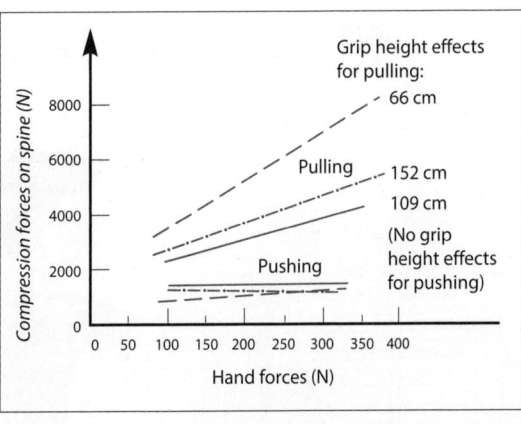

▲ **Figure 6–15.** Forces involved in pushing and pulling loads. Pulling a force of 350 N (the weight of the cart times its coefficient of rolling friction) at a height of 66 cm above the floor causes a compression force on the lower spine of about 8000 N, which is substantially above the highest value (6400 N) that most workers can tolerate without injury.

The NIOSH lifting equation (NLE) aims to provide recommended weight limits (RWLs) that are protective of at least 75% of working women and 99% of working men. Even lifts falling within the RWL may exceed the capabilities of some workers, especially older women. The NLE provides a ratio called the *lifting index,* which is calculated by dividing the actual weight lifted by the RWL. A lifting index of less than 1.0 is considered relatively safe for most workers.

The *load constant* (23 kg [51 lb]) is the highest RWL that would be possible, under ideal circumstances of good location (close to the worker), good coupling (good hand holds), and low repetition rate. The NLE considers that the following factors, or "modifiers," reduce a worker's ability to lift and therefore would reduce the RWL. Each of these modifiers is a number between 0 and 1 that, when multiplied by the load constant, reduces the acceptable lifting weight. Figure 6–17 provides an example of dimensions used in the formula.

- The horizontal modifier (HM) considers the leverage exerted by the load being lifted from the fulcrum, the L5–S1 disk, to the center of gravity of the load. It should be determined at both the origin and destination of the lift. Greater horizontal distances reduce the weights that are safe to lift.
- The vertical modifier (VM) takes into account the amount of trunk bending necessary to perform the lift. Lifts that originate or end below or above knuckle height from the floor (76 cm [30 in] for the average person) are more difficult, so the recommended weight is reduced accordingly.
- The distance modifier (DM) is the vertical travel distance from the origin to the destination of a lift. Higher travel distances tend to increase both the biomechanical and metabolic loads of the lift.

- An asymmetry modifier (AM) takes into account the twisting of the torso while moving the object. The greater the amount of twisting, the higher is the probability of an injury. This modifier should be calculated at both the beginning and the end of the lift.
- The frequency modifier (FM) is calculated based on the average frequency of the lift, in lifts per minute, and is used to incorporate fatigue into the equation.
- A coupling modifier (CM) characterizes the grip as good, fair, or poor. A poor coupling, for example lifting a bag of potatoes, would result in a modifier of 0.90, which would reduce the RWL by 10%.

ACGIH LIFTING GUIDELINES

The ACGIH has established a threshold limit value (TLV) for lifting. This TLV recommends upper limits for repetitive lifting, with the goal of allowing the majority of workers to perform the task without developing back and shoulder disorders. It is intended to apply to two-handed lifts in which lifting is without more than 30 degrees of rotation away from the sagittal plane. There are three tables used to calculate the TLV, chosen based on duration and lifting frequency per day. Each table is divided into four vertical zones of hand location ranging from floor level to 30 cm (12 in) above shoulder height. The three horizontal zones are defined in terms of distance of hand location in front of the midpoint between the observed worker's ankles.

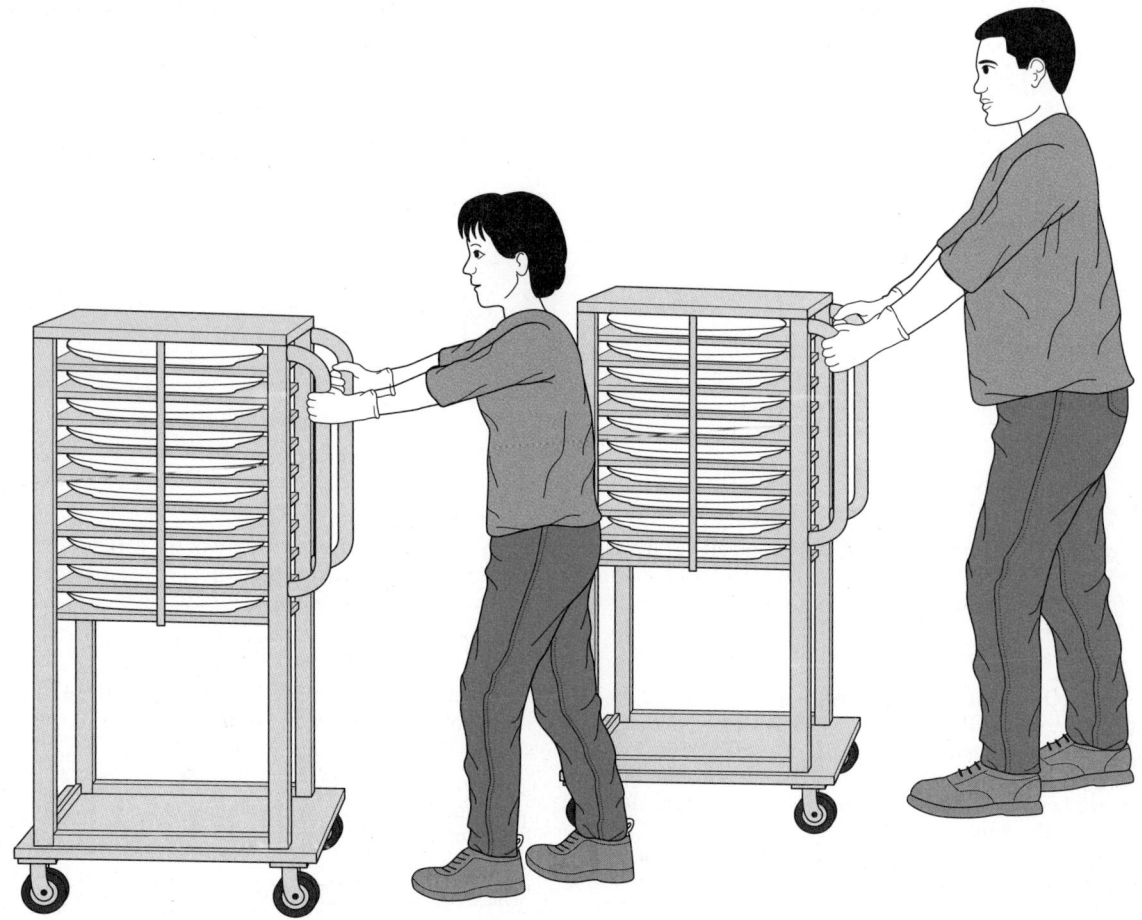

▲ **Figure 6–16.** An example of a design of handles on a cart that will both accommodate large and small employees.

Table 6–2 provides an example of the ACGIH TLV limits applied to moderate-frequency lifting. The NLE is based on a lower maximum permissible weight than the ACGIH lifting TLV (23 versus 34 kg) and allows for consideration of a smaller range of horizontal locations (ie, distance from the load). However, the NLE considers trunk flexion and trunk twisting beyond 30 degrees and lifting frequencies greater than 360 per hour, and includes consideration of grip quality (coupling) and vertical travel distance in its calculations. Neither approach is applicable to one-handed lifting, lifting in constrained postures, lifting in ambient high temperatures or humidity, poor traction underfoot, or lifting unstable objects with shifting loads, such as liquids. A comparison of the recommended weights for each approach by vertical location indicates that the ACGIH TLV tends to allow somewhat heavier lifts except near floor level.

PSYCHOPHYSICS & LIFTING

Substantial research has been done over many decades to develop recommended limits for a variety of lifting, pushing, and pulling tasks based on psychophysical testing. Psychophysical testing involves having uninjured workers replicate a task for a few hours a day or all day and report to the researchers what they feel they could comfortably perform over an 8-hour shift for a 5-day week (Table 6–3). These data can be used along with the other approaches or when a rough estimate of limits for lifting, pushing, and pulling tasks is needed. Unless otherwise noted, the applicability of psychophysical tables is limited to

- Task frequencies of no more than 4.3 lifts per minute
- Maximum acceptable forces for one-person manual handling
- Using carts, bins, or boxes with good handles

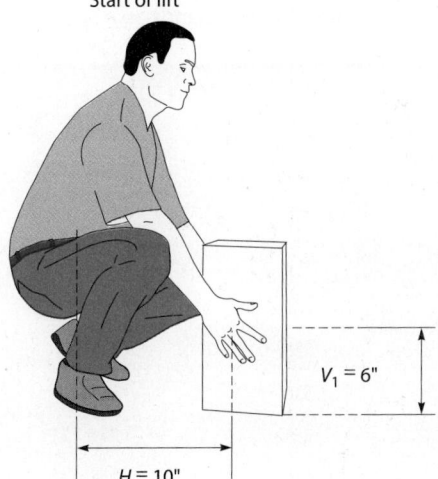

Start of lift

$V_1 = 6"$

$H = 10"$

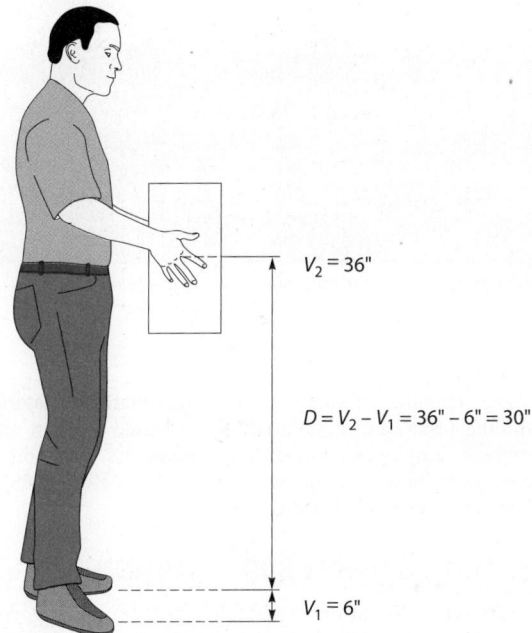

End of lift

$V_2 = 36"$

$D = V_2 - V_1 = 36" - 6" = 30"$

$V_1 = 6"$

▲ **Figure 6–17.** Example of a lifting task and measurements used in the NIOSH lifting equation. The origin of H is taken from the point halfway between the ankles. $D =$ distance modifier (in this case $D = 30$ in); $H =$ horizontal modifier; $V =$ vertical modifier.

Table 6–2. Moderate-frequency lifting > 2 h/d & < 30 lifts/h (kg/lb).

Horizontal Location/ Vertical Location	Close	Intermediate	Far
Shoulder & above	14/31	5/11	No known safe load
Knuckle to shoulder	27/59	14/31	7/15
Shin to knuckle	16/35	11/24	5/11
Floor to shin	9/20	No known safe load	No known safe load

Source: Based on American Conference of Governmental Industrial TLVs and BEIs, Cincinnati, OH, 2014.

- Distance of object handled from the front of the worker's body between 34 and 75 cm
- Vertical location of lift between 25 and 76 cm

As in the NLE and ACGIH lifting TLV, there is no consideration of specific body mechanics or lifting technique because these can be expected to vary from worker to worker. Teaching workers a "safe" way of lifting has not been demonstrated to prevent low back injuries.

The University of Michigan has published three-dimensional biomechanical models that are designed to make lifting, pushing, and pulling analyses easy to calculate on a personal computer (3D Static Strength Prediction Program, https://c4e.engin.umich.edu/tools-services/3dsspp-software/). The compression on the lower lumbar spine is estimated, as is the proportion of the industrial population capable of exerting a given force in a given direction. This model is static and does not consider the additional force required to accelerate the object or the fatigue generated by repeating the material

Table 6–3. Psychophysical limits for load lifting.

	Sagittal Plane Box Dimensions (cm)	Mean Lifting Limits[a] (N)	
		Men	Women
Floor-to-knuckle height when erect	30.5	296	194
	45.7	261	171
	61.0	236	152
Knuckle-to-shoulder height when erect	30.5	263	141
	45.7	233	129
	61.0	205	127
Shoulder-to-reach height when erect	30.5	221	120
	45.7	204	110
	61.0	195	112

[a]The values represent acceptable lifting limits (N) based on lifting per minute sustained for 8 hours.

Table 6–4. Static strengths demonstrated by workers when lifting, pushing, and pulling with both hands on a handle placed at different locations relative to the midpoint between the ankles on the floor.

Test Description	Handle Location[a] (cm)		Mean Strength[b] (N)	
	Vertical	Horizontal	Men	Women
Lift—legs in partial squat	38	0	903	427
Lift—torso stooped over	38	38	480	271
Lift—arms flexed	114	38	383	214
Lift—shoulder high and arms out	152	51	227	129
Lift—shoulder high and arms flexed	152	38	529	240
Lift—shoulder high and arms close	152	25	538	285
Lift—floor level, close (squat)	15	25	890	547
Lift—floor level, out (stoop)	15	38	320	200
Push down—waist level	118	38	432	325
Pull down—above shoulders	178	33	605	449
Pull in—shoulder level, arms out	157	33	311	244
Pull in—shoulder level, arms in	140	0	253	209
Push out—waist level, stand erect	101	35	311	226
Push out—chest level, stand erect	124	25	303	214
Push out—shoulder level, lean forward	140	64	418	276

[a]Handle locations are measured in midsagittal plane, vertical from the floor and horizontal from the midpoint between the ankles.
[b]1 lb = 4.45 N.

handling over time. It is based on static strength testing of a large sample of working men and women (Table 6–4).

Example: Patient Handling

A large hospital system had high rates of serious shoulder, back, and wrist injuries among nurses associated with patient lifting, transferring, and repositioning. They invested in a hospital-wide risk reduction process that included identification of high-risk patients, widespread installation of overhead lifts, lift maintenance and supply inventory, training of nurses, and use of patient handling algorithms based on patient mobility levels. The investment led to a dramatic decline in injury rates and improvement in employee morale and productivity.

Note: Spinal loads during patient transferring and repositioning consistently approach or exceed tissue tolerance limits, even with two caregivers moving a patient. In addition, the use of permanent overhead lifts is preferred over portable patient lifts because compliance with portable patient lifts is poor.

The maximal allowable limits for manual material handling tasks can be summarized and used to train and empower employees, supervisors, managers, and other stakeholders how to design work that reduces risk of MSDs by staying below the identified limits.

ESTIMATING WHOLE BODY EXERTION

For workers who must expend high levels of energy (eg, distribution center order selectors, fire fighting, and some types of agricultural work), the limiting factor regarding work capacity may be aerobic capacity relative to the demands of the job. The proportion of a worker's maximum aerobic capacity being used on the job can be estimated by measuring heart rate or oxygen uptake. Since heart rate and energy expenditure relate in a linear fashion except near the upper and lower levels of a person's capacity, heart rate monitoring of employees can be used to estimate the energy requirements of a job (Table 6–5). The heart rate at rest (HR_{rest}) is subtracted from the estimated maximum heart rate ($220 - age$) to yield heart rate reserve. The resting heart rate also is

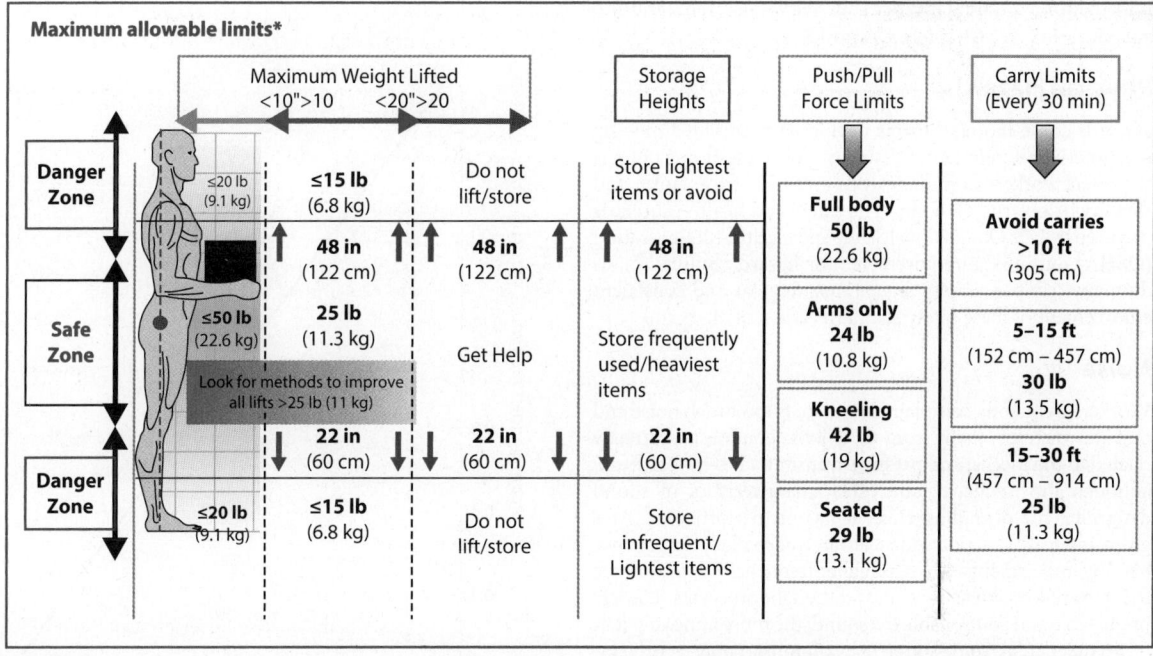

▲ **Figure 6–18.** A summary of maximal allowable limits that can be used to train and empower stakeholders to be pro-active in identifying exposures that may increase risk of MSDs by exceeding limits. (Provided by Meg Honan, UC Ergonomics Research & Graduate Training Program Senior Consultant.)

subtracted from the mean heart rate during working periods (HR_{work}) to form a ratio as in the following formula:

$$\%\text{HR range} = \% \text{ maximal aerobic capacity}$$
$$= [100\%(HR_{work} - HR_{rest})]/(HR_{max} - HR_{rest})$$

If there is ever a question about whether an observed employee is exceeding his or her maximum work capacity on a given job, attention also should be paid to modifying the task, improving the work environment (especially ambient temperature), or both.

A. Example

The manual harvesting of wine grapes involves rapidly and repetitively lifting heavy tubs. In the 1980s, the tubs used in to collect grapes were filled to an average of 57 lb (26 kg), had uncomfortable handles, and required high forces to slide from one vine to the next during the filling process. A team of ergonomists and engineers evaluated a plastic tub with a 46 lb (21 kg) average load, better handles, and a smooth bottom requiring lower forces to slide. The new tub was associated with lower physiologic and biomechanical risk, and workers reported less fatigue and pain when using the tub. The new tubs were widely adopted throughout Napa Valley "Wine Country" in California.

ENVIRONMENTAL FACTORS

The environment affects worker performance, health, and safety in a variety of ways. This discussion focuses primarily on physical aspects of the environment, although the social characteristics of the workplace (eg, isolation versus overcrowding, being undervalued versus being appreciated, and organizational flexibility versus rigidity) often play a significant role in stress-related problems. For additional

Table 6–5. Maximum heart rate and oxygen uptake for men and women in average physical condition.

Age (y)	Heart Rate (beats/min)		Oxygen Uptake (mL/kg/min)	
	Men	Women	Men	Women
20–29	190	190	34–42	31–37
30–39	182	182	31–33	25–33
40–49	179	179	27–35	24–30
50–59	171	171	25–33	21–27
60–69	164	164	23–30	18–23

information regarding injuries caused by noise, temperature, and vibration, see Chapters 12 and 13.

Physical Hazards

Hazards come in many forms, including unguarded moving machinery or equipment, missing or poorly designed railings to protect workers from dangerous areas, electrical faults, and slippery or obstructed floors. The safety and health standards prepared by U.S. Occupational Safety and Health Administration (OSHA) outline the requirements for hazard elimination, as do many company safety regulations. Regular and consistent enforcement of these safety standards is essential.

Noise

Workers frequently complain that there is too much noise and that this distracts them from their jobs. Loudness is directly related to the mechanical pressure transmitted to the eardrum, although the frequency and other characteristics of sound determine the degrading effect it has on performance. At a given intensity, lower frequencies are more likely to produce hearing impairments, whereas higher frequencies are more apt to interfere with concentration and thought processes. The less predictable and controllable the sound, the more annoying it is.

In quiet areas, some sound (eg, soft music) may be preferable as a means of masking nearby conversations that otherwise might be distracting. *White noise* (sound spread uniformly over the full hearing spectrum) is sometimes used successfully in lieu of music but occasionally is found to be objectionable.

Sound levels above 50 dB may become increasingly intrusive, objectionable, and fatiguing depending on their frequency and predictability. For example, the rate of complaints of low back pain among material handlers increases with higher ambient noise levels. Sound levels that exceed 85 dBA (as recorded on a sound level meter's A-weighted scale of frequency bands) and continue for as long as 8 hours may cause hearing loss. If noise levels routinely exceed 85 dBA, it is necessary to control the sound source or provide other means of hearing protection. Figure 6–19 shows the recommended maximum duration of human exposure to various noise levels. Workers should not be exposed to sounds above 115 dBA. Table 6–6 lists examples of the sound levels satisfying various communications needs.

Lighting

The amount of light required to perform a specific task without feeling visual fatigue is a function of the visual difficulty of the task at the desired work speed and quality and the visual acuity of the worker. Degree of visual difficulty typically is determined by (1) the contrast between the target and its background, (2) the spatial resolution, and (3) the size of the target. Visual acuity, even with corrected vision, varies with age. Table 6–7 shows the recommended ranges of illumination for various types of tasks.

As with computer work, it is critical to reduce objectionable glare in all workplaces. Glare may emanate directly from

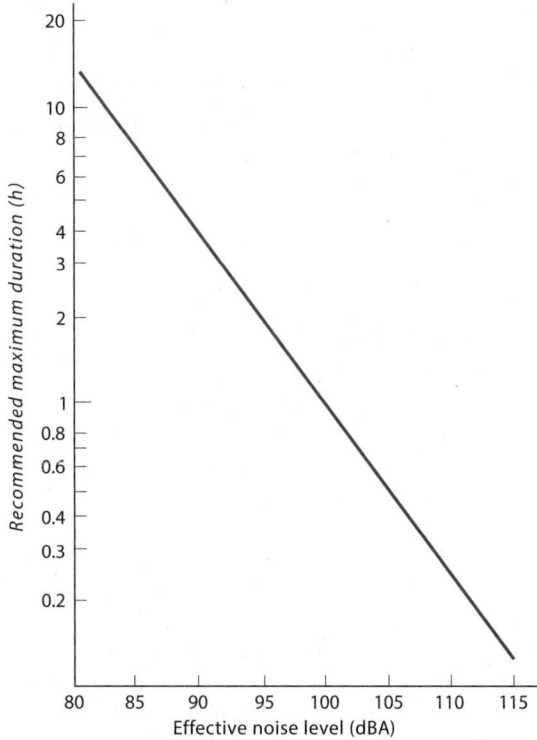

▲ **Figure 6–19.** Recommended maximum duration of human exposure to various noise levels. Workers should not be exposed to sounds above 115 dBA. (ACGIH: *Threshold Limit Values for Chemical Substances and Physical Agents in the Work Environment.* American Conference of Governmental Industrial Hygienists, 2014.)

a bright light source or may be reflected off the shiny surfaces of machines, worktables, windows, displays, or tools. It can be reduced or eliminated by limiting light from the source or covering shiny surfaces with dull or nonreflective coatings.

A. Example

In a garment plant, sewing machine operators complained of headaches and tired and itching eyes after lamps were installed on the far side of each machine. The purpose of the lamps was to improve visibility, but they had the opposite effect because their light reflected off the polished wood and metal sewing tables and the shinier material. Repositioning the lamps eliminated the glare and relieved the visual symptoms and headaches.

Temperature & Humidity

An elevated ambient temperature or humidity level increases the cardiovascular load of jobs requiring sustained heavy effort (repetitive materials handling), whereas a low

Table 6–6. Preferred noise criterion (PNC) curves and sound pressure levels recommended for several categories of activity.

	PNC Curve[a]	Approximate Sound Pressure Level (dBA)[b]
Listening to faint musical sounds or using distant microphone pickup	10–20	21–30
Excellent listening conditions	≤ 20	≤ 30
Close microphone pickup only	≤ 25	≤ 34
Good listening conditions	≤ 35	≤ 42
Sleeping, resting, relaxing	25–40	34–47
Conversing or listening to radio or TV	30–40	38–47
Moderately good listening conditions	35–45	42–52
Fair listening conditions	40–50	47–56
Moderately fair listening conditions	45–55	52–61
Just acceptable speech and telephone communication	50–60	56–66
Speech not required but no risk of hearing damage	60–75	66–80

[a]PNC curves are used in many installations for establishing noise spectra.
[b]Voice sound frequencies are used to determine the approximate sound pressure levels. These levels are to be used only for estimates because level does not give an indication of the spectrum.

Table 6–7. Recommended ranges of illumination for various types of tasks.

Type of Activity or Area	Range of Illumination[a]	
	Lux	Footcandles
Public areas with dark surroundings	20–50	2–5
Simple orientation for short temporary visits	> 50–100	> 5–9
Working spaces where visual tasks are only occasionally performed	> 100–200	> 9–19
Performance of visual tasks of high contrast or large size: reading printed material, typed originals, handwriting in ink, good xerography; rough bench and machine work; ordinary inspection; rough assembly	> 200–500	> 19–46
Performance of visual tasks of medium contrast or small size: reading pencil handwriting, poorly printed or reproduced material; medium bench and machine work; difficult inspection, medium assembly	> 500–1000	> 46–93
Performance of visual tasks of low contrast or very small size: reading handwriting in hard pencil on poor-quality paper, very poorly reproduced material; very difficult inspection	> 1000–2000	> 93–186
Performance of visual tasks of low contrast and very small size over a prolonged period: fine assembly, highly difficult inspection, fine bench and machine work	> 2000–5000	> 186–464
Performance of very prolonged and exacting visual tasks: the most difficult inspection, extra fine bench and machine work, extra fine assembly	> 5000–10,000	> 464–929
Performance of very special visual tasks of extremely low contrast and small size: some surgical procedures	> 10,000–20,000	> 929–1858

[a]The choice of a value within a range depends on task variables, the reflectance of the environment, and the individual's visual capabilities.

temperature can reduce finger flexibility and accuracy sub-stantially. The thermal comfort zone (Figure 6–20) is characterized by the ideal temperature and humidity conditions for work. The comfort zone is affected by a number of factors in addition to temperature and humidity. Among these are air velocity (producing a windchill effect), workload, radiant heat sources, and amount and type of clothing. In general, the body's core temperature should not vary by more than 1°C (1.8°F) in either direction, and the preceding factors should be adjusted to accommodate this range.

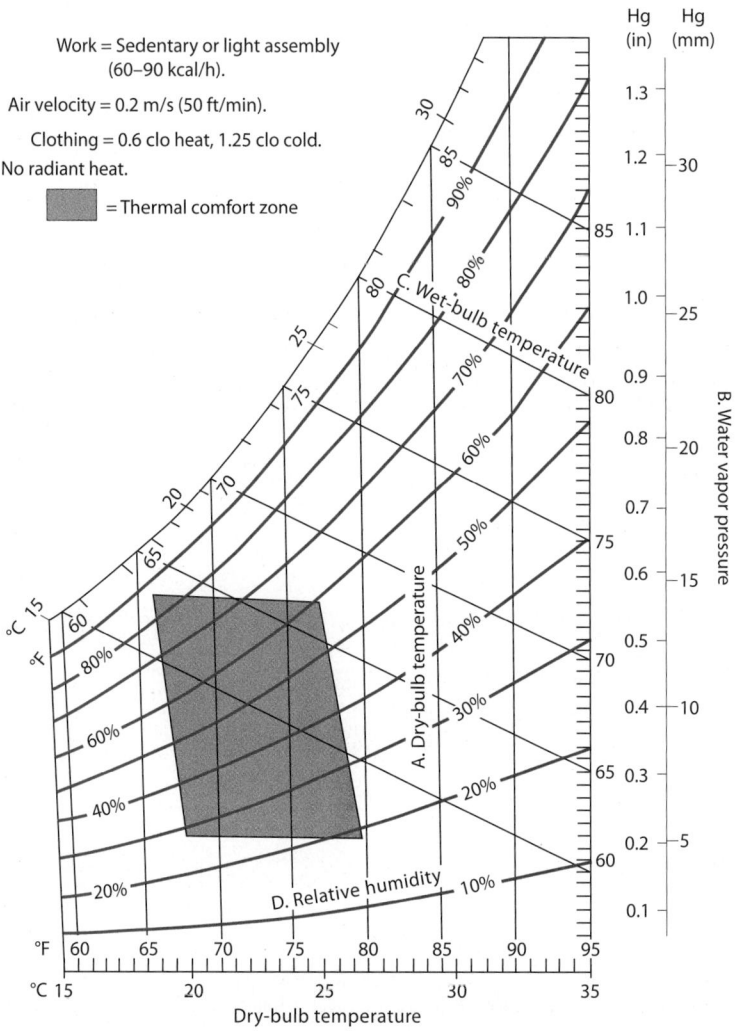

▲ **Figure 6–20.** Thermal comfort zone. The dry-bulb temperature and humidity combinations that are comfortable for most people doing sedentary or light work are shown as the shaded area on the psychometric chart. The dry-bulb temperature range is 19–26°C (66–79°F), and the relative humidity range (shown as parallel curves) is 20–85%, with 35–65% being the most common values in the comfort zone. On this chart, ambient dry-bulb temperature *(A)* is plotted on the horizontal axis and indicated as parallel vertical lines; water vapor pressure *(B)* is on the vertical axis. Wet-bulb temperatures *(C)* are shown as parallel lines with a negative slope; they intersect the dry-bulb temperature lines and relative humidity curves *(D)* on the chart. In the definition of the thermal comfort zone, assumptions were made about the workload, air velocity, radiant heat, and clothing insulation levels. These assumptions are given in the top left corner of the chart. (ACGIH: *Threshold Limit Values for Chemical Substances and Physical Agents in the Work Environment.* American Conference of Governmental Industrial Hygienists, 2014.)

Vibration

Vibration can be a hazard to the hands or spine. With the increasing interaction between workers and high-power tools, vibration at critical frequencies and accelerations has become an important source of injury and is associated with loss of equilibrium, nausea, hand-arm vibration syndrome (HAVS), and carpal tunnel syndrome. In addition, truck drivers and heavy equipment operators have an elevated risk of lumbar spinal disorders, hemorrhoids, hernias, and digestive and urinary tract problems, which may be a result of a combination of vibration, extended sitting, and truck loading and unloading.

Vibration of the hand and arm for extended periods, as occurs in the operation of hand power tools, such as chain saws, riveting hammers, sanders, pneumatic rock drills, power chisels, and grinders, may be a source of recurrent hand pain, numbness, and finger blanching or HAVS. HAVS involves damage to the small blood vessels and nerves of the fingers and is exacerbated by exposure to vibration and cold. Workers also may have a decrease in touch sensitivity, fine finger dexterity, and grip strength. Continued exposure with severe disease can lead to gangrene of the fingertips. Even after removal of vibration exposure, reversal of the disease will occur in only 50% of workers. Diagnosis, prevention, and treatment of HAVS are discussed in Chapter 13. The ACGIH and ISO have developed guidelines for vibration exposure from hand tools.

The types of whole-body vibration that are of most concern to occupational health and safety analysts are those associated with operation of vehicles (eg, buses, forklifts, and heavy construction equipment) and with operation of machinery (eg, large punch presses, conveyors, and furnaces). The effect of vibration depends on its acceleration, duration, frequency, and direction (vertical or lateral) (Figure 6–21). Lower-intensity exposure (measured by surface-mounted accelerometers) can be tolerated for longer periods without pain or injury than the high intensities; low-intensity vibrations of less than 1 Hz in fact may have a soothing effect.

Whole-body vertical vibration is a continuing problem for vehicle operators. The critical range of the torso's natural resonant frequency is 3–5 Hz, but discomfort can occur in the range of 2–11 Hz. Well-designed seats for bus and truck drivers will diminish the vibration in this critical frequency range by as much as 50%. However, older, stiffer seats can have an amplification effect of as much as 20%. In some buses or trucks, the lateral acceleration intensity may be twice the vertical intensity. Visual performance generally is impaired in the range of 10–25 Hz. Truck and bus seats usually do not transmit vertical vibrations in this frequency range, but other equipment (eg, overhead cranes, lumber mill saws, and conveying machinery) may.

A. Example

Construction workers building structural upgrades to a bridge were required to drill 10,000 holes into concrete by hand using 30-lb (14-kg) pneumatic rock drills. The vibration levels and forces were such that they were fatigued after only 40 holes per day. A jig was built that supported the drill,

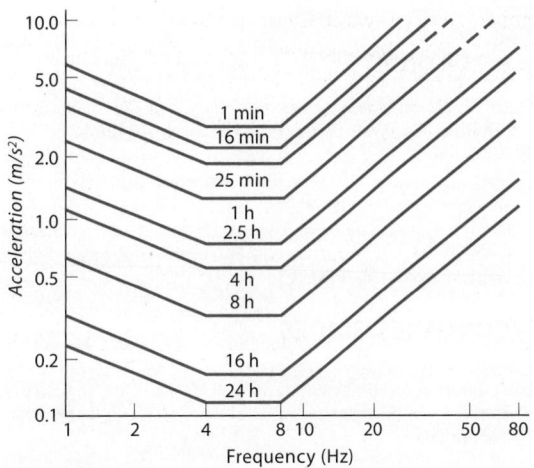

▲ **Figure 6–21.** Maximum acceptable whole-body vertical vibration exposure times to various frequencies and accelerations. The shorter the vibration exposure, the higher the acceleration levels that can be tolerated. The least-acceptable range of frequencies at all accelerations and durations of exposure is from 4 to 8 Hz. (ACGIH: *Threshold Limit Values for Chemical Substances and Physical Agents in the Work Environment.* American Conference of Governmental Industrial Hygienists, 2006.)

isolated the drill vibration, and reduced force applied by the worker. The work productivity doubled and workers were able to perform the task all day without fatigue.

REFERENCES

WEBSITES

American Conference of Governmental Industrial Hygienists (ACGIH): www.acgih.org.
Human Factors and Ergonomics Society (HFES): www.hfes.org.
International Ergonomics Association https://iea.cc/
MSD Prevention Guideline for Ontario: https://www.msdprevention.com/.
National Institute for Occupational Safety and Health (NIOSH): www.cdc.gov/niosh.
Safe Work Australia: https://www.safeworkaustralia.gov.au.
The Liberty Mutual Manual Materials Handling Guidelines for lifting, lowering, pushing, pulling: https://libertymmhtables.libertymutual.com/

SURVEILLANCE CHECKLISTS

Health & Safety Executive HSE Risk Assessment Worksheets http://www.hse.gov.uk/msd/pdfs/worksheets.pdf
Kodak Ergonomics Checklist: http://www.mhi.org/downloads/industrygroups/ease/checklists/ergonomic-checklist-for-material-handling.pdf.

MSD Preliminary Risk Assessment Checklist: https://www.msd-prevention.com/resource-library/view/msd-preliminary-risk-assessment-checklist.htm.

Quick Ergonomic Checklist: https://www.msdprevention.com/resource-library/quick-exposure-checklist-qec-.htm.

Washington State Caution & Hazard Zone Checklist https://www.lni.wa.gov/safety-health/preventing-injuries-illnesses/sprains-strains/evaluation-tools.

Washington State Safe Patient Handling Gap Analysis Checklist: http://www.wsha.org/wp-content/uploads/Worker-Safety_Gap_Analysis_Checklist.pdf.

ERGONOMICS GUIDES

Back Injury Prevention Guide in the Health Care Industry for Health Care Providers: www.dir.ca.gov/dosh/dosh_publications/backinj.pdf.

Ergonomics in Action: A Guide to Best Practices for the Food-Processing Industry. www.dir.ca.gov/dosh/dosh_publications/Erg_Food_ Processing.pdf.

Ergonomics: Guidelines for Nursing Homes. www.osha.gov/ergonomics/guidelines/nursinghome/index.html.

Ergonomics: Guidelines for Poultry Processing. www.osha.gov/ergonomics/guidelines/poultryprocessing/index.html.

Ergonomics: Guidelines for Retail Grocery Stores. www.osha.gov/ergonomics/guidelines/retailgrocery/index.html.

Keys to Success and Safety for the Construction Foreman: www.dir.ca.gov/dosh/dosh_publications/foremanweb.pdf

NIOSH Resources on Ergonomics: http://www.cdc.gov/niosh/topics/ergonomics/.

US Federal OSHA Ergonomics: www.osha.gov/SLTC/ergonomics/index.html.

■ SELF-ASSESSMENT QUESTIONS

Select the one correct answer for each question.

Question 1: The primary determinant of head posture when sitting is
a. the height of the work surface
b. the height of the chair
c. the location of the visual target
d. the back-support angle

Question 2: The ACGIH TLV for hand activity level
a. estimates the risk of nonoccupational injury
b. can be applied to a task of 1-hour duration
c. estimates the risk for wrist disorders
d. considers temperature in the risk model

Question 3: The most important physical design rule for a sedentary job at a desk or workbench is to
a. provide extensive movements of the arm
b. allow frequent reaching
c. encourage bending and twisting at the waist
d. careful layout to allow the operator to easily reach all frequently used items

Question 4: Tool handles should be designed so that
a. the force-bearing area is as small as possible
b. there are no sharp corners or edges
c. they are neither round nor oval
d. they fit the 95th percentile male hand

Question 5: Bifocal wearers who use a computer should
a. have their screen lower than other computer users
b. move the screen so it is further away than other computer users
c. remove glasses while at work
d. have their screen higher than other computer users

Question 6: The U.S. NIOSH lifting equation
a. considers that a person's ability to lift may be limited only by biomechanical factors
b. fails to consider physiologic, psychophysical, and epidemiologic studies
c. aims to provide recommended weight limits (RWLs) that are protective of at least 75% of working women and 99% of working men
d. provides a ratio called the *lifting index,* which is calculated by dividing the RLW by the actual weight lifted

Question 7: The ACGIH TLV for lifting
a. has the goal of allowing the majority of workers to perform the task without developing back and shoulder disorders
b. recommends no upper limits for repetitive lifting
c. is a recommended weight limit, unlike the NIOSH lifting equation
d. allows significantly heavier lifts than the NIOSH lifting equation

Question 8: Hand-arm vibration syndrome (HAVS)
a. involves damage to the small blood vessels and nerves of the fingers
b. is not exacerbated by exposure to cold
c. does not result in a decrease in touch sensitivity, fine finger dexterity, and grip strength
d. resolves in 90% of workers by limiting exposure

Question 9: Under ideal conditions (low repetitions and best lifting biomechanics) what is the maximum recommended weight a worker should lift based on the 1991 NIOSH lifting equation?
  a. 31 lb
  b. 41 lb
  c. 51 lb
  d. 61 lb

Question 10: Risk factors for neck/shoulder pain among computer users include
  a. center of computer monitor above eye height
  b. keyboard below elbow height
  c. reaching for the mouse with forearm support
  d. resting forearms on desk when using the keyboard

Question 11: Carpal tunnel syndrome is associated with
  a. working with sustained wrist extension of 10 degrees
  b. exposure to vibrating hand tools
  c. repeated power grip with more than 1 kg of force
  d. workplace transfers

Question 12: In the application of anthropometry principles, a 75% female height means that
  a. this is the mean height for 75% of the female population
  b. 75% of the female population are taller than this height
  c. this is the mean height for 25% of the female population
  d. 75% of the female population are shorter than this height

Musculoskeletal Injuries*

Anthony C. Luke, MD, MPH

C. Benjamin Ma, MD

GENERAL APPROACH TO MUSCULOSKELETAL INJURIES

ESSENTIALS OF DIAGNOSIS

▶ History is most important in diagnosing musculoskeletal problems.

▶ The mechanism of injury can explain the pathology and symptoms.

▶ Determine whether the injury is traumatic or atraumatic, acute or chronic, high or low velocity (greater velocity suggests more structural damage), or whether any movement aggravates or relieves pain associated with the injury.

▶ General Considerations

Musculoskeletal problems account for about 10–20% of outpatient primary care clinical visits. Fifty-three percent of adults older than 65 years complain of bothersome pain each month usually with multiple sites of pain and decreased physical function. Orthopedic problems can be classified as traumatic (ie, injury-related) or atraumatic (ie, degenerative or overuse syndromes) as well as acute or chronic. The history and physical examination are sufficient in most cases to establish the working diagnosis; the mechanism of injury is usually the most helpful part of the history in determining the diagnosis. The onset of symptoms should be elicited. With acute traumatic injuries, patients typically seek medical

attention within 6 weeks of onset. The patient should describe the exact location of symptoms, which helps determine anatomic structures that may be damaged. If the patient is vague, the clinician can ask the patient to point with one finger only to the point of maximal tenderness.

CLINICAL FINDINGS

A. Symptoms and Signs

The chief musculoskeletal complaints are typically pain (most common), instability, or dysfunction around the joints. Since symptoms and signs are often nonspecific, recognizing the expected combination of symptoms and physical examination signs can help facilitate the clinical diagnosis. Patients may describe symptoms of "locking" or "catching," suggesting internal derangement in joints. Symptoms of "instability" or "giving way" suggest ligamentous injury; however, these symptoms may also be due to pain causing muscular inhibition. Constitutional symptoms of fever or weight loss, swelling with no injury, or systemic illness suggest medical conditions (such as infection, cancer, or rheumatologic disease).

Typical evaluations in the clinic follow the traditional components of the physical examination and should include **inspection, palpation**, and assessment of **range of motion** and **neurovascular status**.

Inspection includes observation of *s*welling, *e*rythema, *a*trophy, *d*eformity, and (surgical) *s*cars (mnemonic, "SEADS"). The patient should be asked to move joints of concern. If motion is asymmetric, the clinician should assess the passive range of motion for any physical limitation.

There are special tests to assess each joint. Typically, **provocative tests** recreate the mechanism of injury with the goal to reproduce the patient's pain. **Stress tests** apply load to ligaments of concern. Typically, 10–15 lb of force should be applied when performing stress tests. **Functional testing**, including simple tasks performed during activities of daily living, is useful to assess injury severity.

*Chapter adapted, with permission, from Luke A, Ma CB: Sports medicine and outpatient orthopedics. In: Papadakis MA, McPhee SJ, Rabow MW, eds. *Current Medical Diagnosis and Treatment.* 59th ed. New York: McGraw-Hill, 2020.

B. Imaging

Magnetic resonance imaging (MRI) has become the best imaging test for many orthopedic diagnoses, although other modalities such as ultrasonography and computed tomography (CT) are still used. Bony pathology can be assessed using standard radiographs, although there also may be characteristic soft tissue findings. CT scans are an effective method for visualizing any bony pathology, including morphology of fractures. Nuclear bone scans are now less commonly used but are still valuable for identifying stress injuries, infection, malignancy, or multisite pathology. Positron emission tomography (PET) scans are useful in identifying metastatic malignant lesions. MRI provides excellent visualization of ligaments, cartilage, and soft tissues. High-field 3.0 Tesla MRI allows higher image resolution and decreased examination times compared to the more common standard 1.5 Tesla machines. Gadolinium contrast can be injected as an MRI arthrogram to increase sensitivity of detecting certain internal derangements in joints such as labral injuries. Musculoskeletal ultrasound, where available, can be useful for identifying superficial tissue problems, including tendinopathies and synovial problems.

C. Special Tests

Arthrocentesis must be performed promptly to rule out an infection when acute knee pain with effusion and inflammation are present and the patient is unable to actively flex the joint. The joint fluid should be sent for cell count, crystal analysis, and culture. Arthrocentesis and joint fluid analysis demonstrating crystals can lead to the diagnosis of gout (negatively birefringent, needle-shaped crystals) or pseudogout (positively birefringent, rectangular-shaped crystals). In large, uncomfortable knee joint effusions, removal of excessive joint fluid may improve joint range of motion (flexion) and patient comfort. To avoid infecting the joint, arthrocentesis should not be performed when there is an active cellulitis or abscess overlying the joint. It appears the risk of bleeding after arthrocentesis or joint injection is extremely low even if the patient is taking anticoagulants. Caution should be practiced if the INR is greater than 3.0; however, even a supratherapeutic INR did not suggest an increased risk of hemarthrosis in one study. Markers of inflammation such as complete blood cell count, erythrocyte sedimentation rate, and C-reactive protein, and rheumatologic tests are useful in evaluating for infectious, oncologic, or rheumatologic processes. Electrodiagnostic studies such as electromyography and nerve conduction studies are useful when there are neurologic concerns; they can also help with prognostication in chronic conditions.

TREATMENT

Conservative treatment includes physical therapy, assistive devices, and pain management. Most surgeries are performed arthroscopically to be less invasive than open procedures. While most outpatient musculoskeletal problems are best treated conservatively, the first consideration is whether there is an immediate surgical need. Surgical treatment is chosen when the outcome promises better health, restoration of function, and improved quality of life. During surgery, the musculoskeletal problem is usually repaired, removed, realigned, reconstructed, or replaced (eg, joint replacement).

If surgery is not immediately indicated, conservative treatment in the outpatient setting usually includes *m*odification of activities, *i*ce, *c*ompression, and *e*levation (remembered by the mnemonic, "MICE"). Controlling pain is an early concern for most patients. Commonly prescribed medications are analgesics (nonsteroidal anti-inflammatory drugs [NSAIDs], acetaminophen, or opioids). Other medications that may also be prescribed, albeit less commonly, are muscle relaxants or co-analgesics for neuropathic pain (which include the calcium channel alpha-2-delta ligands [eg, gabapentin] or tricyclic antidepressants). Topical medications, such as capsaicin cream or patch, lidocaine patches, and NSAID patches or gels, can help provide superficial local pain relief.

Immobilization by casting, slings, and braces is helpful to protect an injured limb. Crutches are useful to reduce weight bearing. Rehabilitation and physical therapy are frequently needed. Other modalities commonly used by patients include chiropractic manipulation, massage therapy, acupuncture, heat, and osteopathy.

Local injections can deliver treatments directly to the affected areas as well as create mechanical stimulation for healing. Common medications to inject include corticosteroid injections and hyaluronic acid (for osteoarthritis). Current popular interventions include platelet-rich plasma (PRP) injections and stem cell technology, which may show promise but lack conclusive evidence of benefit.

PRP injections have increased in use, especially by musculoskeletal specialists. PRP is hypothesized to augment tissue repair and regeneration after musculoskeletal injury. PRP is prepared after centrifuging several milliliters of autologous whole blood separating the plasma layer that is concentrated with platelets and several biologically active molecules and proteins from the red and white blood cells. Several growth factors have been identified to be concentrated in PRP including vascular endothelial growth factor (VEGF), insulin-like growth factor-1 (IGF-1), fibroblast growth factor (FGF), platelet-derived growth factor (PDGF), and transforming growth factor-β1 (TGF-β1). This injectant can be administered under ultrasound guidance toward injured tendons through an area of chronic tendinopathy or a partial tear. An additional procedure that can be performed alone or combined with the injections is percutaneous needle tenotomy. This involves passing the treatment needle several times through the tendon, referred to as fenestration. This treatment is hypothesized to disrupt chronic degeneration and encourage anabolic processes involving fibroblastic proliferation, leading to organized collagen synthesis and proper tendon healing. There are limited clinical data on the benefits of percutaneous needle tenotomy.

WHEN TO REFER

Indications for *emergency* referral (immediate)

- Neurovascular injury
- Fractures (open, unstable)
- Unreduced joint dislocation
- Septic arthritis

Indications for *urgent* referral (within 7 days)

- Fractures (closed, stable)
- After reduction of a joint dislocation
- "Locked" joint (inability to fully extend a joint due to mechanical derangement, usually a loose body or torn cartilage)
- Tumor

Indications for *early* orthopedic assessment (2–4 weeks)

- Motor weakness (neurologic)
- Constitutional symptoms (eg, weight loss, fever not due to septic arthritis)
- Multiple joint involvement

Indications for *routine* orthopedic assessment (for further management)

- Failure of conservative treatment (persistent symptoms for more than 3 months)
- Persistent numbness and tingling in an extremity

■ SELF-ASSESSMENT QUESTIONS

Select the one correct answer to each question.

Question 1: Functional testing
- a. recreates activities of daily living
- b. is seldom useful to assess injury severity
- c. is synonymous with stress testing
- d. replaces the need for stress testing

Question 2: CT scans
- a. are the most effective method for visualizing any bony pathology
- b. are of limited use in visualizing fractures
- c. are superior to MRI in visualizing ligaments, cartilage, and soft tissues
- d. have replaced musculoskeletal ultrasound for identifying superficial tissue problems

Question 3: Arthrocentesis
- a. must be performed promptly to rule out an infection with any acute knee pain
- b. is indicated with knee pain when effusion and inflammation are present
- c. should be performed even if there is an active cellulitis or abscess overlying the joint
- d. presents a serious risk of bleeding

Question 4: Cumulative trauma
- a. is unrelated to repetitive trauma
- b. affects bone, but not the tendon, muscle, capsule, or the nerve
- c. is seldom painful
- d. may involve the extremity

Shoulder, Elbow, & Hand Injuries

Alexis Descatha, MD, PhD

Romain Lancigu, MD

David M. Rempel, MD, MPH

INJURIES OF THE SHOULDER

Conditions of the neck or upper thoracic spine may cause referred pain to the shoulder. The comprehensive evaluation of shoulder pain includes careful examination of the cervical and thoracic spine.

1. Impingement Syndrome, Rotator Cuff Tendinosis or Tears, Supraspinatus Tendinitis, Subacromial Bursitis

The term *impingement syndrome* has replaced more diffuse diagnostic terms such as *bursitis* and *tendonitis* in the definition of shoulder pain following either repeated overuse or sudden overload. This pathology accounts for most shoulder pain that occurs spontaneously or with occupational loads.

In the normal shoulder, the coracoacromial ligament crosses the supraspinatus tendon of the rotator cuff. In some individuals, when a hand is brought from the side to an overhead position in forward flexion or abduction, there may be contact pressure or impingement of the acromion and coracoacromial ligament on the rotator cuff or the intervening bursa. The pathology starts with a subacromial bursitis and may progress to an irritation of the supraspinatus tendon or tendonitis. Further progression leads to the beginning of ulceration (partial-thickness tear) of the tendon, which can lead to a full-thickness discontinuity or rupture of the rotator cuff. The long head of the biceps projecting across the joint beneath the cuff to its origin on the supraglenoid tubercle may be damaged. Paralleling these soft-tissue changes, the anteroinferior aspect of the acromion develops osteophytic lipping with further encroachment on the subacromial space.

The onset of anterior shoulder pain may be gradual or acute. Occasionally, the onset coincides with the start of new repetitive work activities, especially overhead work. Patients may be unaware of the inciting activity. The pain may be expressed generally over some aspect of the anterior shoulder. In some cases, pain is limited to the lateral arm about the deltoid insertion on the humerus. Occasionally, pain is referred to the elbow and rarely, to the hand.

All levels of pain occur, including severe pain at rest caused by a tense subacromial bursa. Night pain is a common complaint that brings the patient to medical treatment.

Posttraumatic impingement syndrome may occur after a minor injury to the arm or shoulder. The self-imposed immobilization of the shoulder predisposes the patient to the impingement syndrome because of imbalanced rotator cuff muscle function secondary to painful inhibition of normal motion.

▶ Clinical Findings

On physical examination, patients begin to experience anterior shoulder pain when the arm is abducted to 30–40 degrees or flexed forward to 90 degrees or more. With the elbow flexed at 90 degrees, active external rotation usually does not cause discomfort. However, active internal rotation (when the patient attempts to place his or her thumb on the opposite inferior angle of the scapula) is painful. With significant disruption of the rotator cuff, a patient may have weakness on external rotation or no active flexion past 90 degrees. However, patients can have full-thickness tears of the rotator cuff without lost motion. Point tenderness anterior to the acromion over the subacromial bursa is common. Two common tests for impingement are the *supraspinatus isolation test* (empty can test) and the *Hawkins-Kennedy test* (Figure 8–1).

▶ Differential Diagnosis

Angina caused by myocardial ischemia may be confused with primary shoulder disease. Cervical radiculopathy can also present as pain radiating into the shoulder. Acute shoulder sepsis may mimic acute bursitis because of the

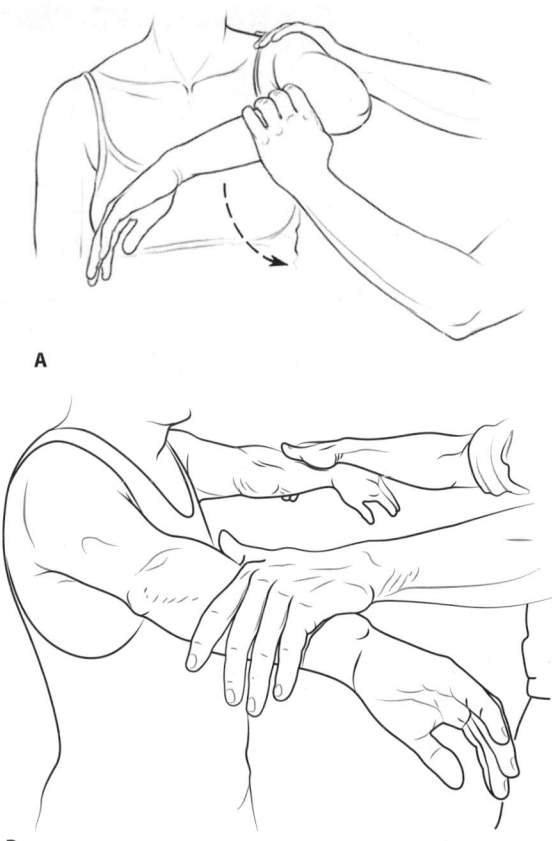

▲ **Figure 8–1.** A. For the *Hawkins-Kennedy test*, the arm is passively flexed forward to 90 degrees and the elbow is flexed to 90 degrees. When the examiner internally rotates the shoulder, pain indicates impingement of the supraspinatus tendon. B. For the *supraspinatus isolation test*, downward resistance is applied to the arm after the shoulder is abducted to 90 degrees and forward flexed 30 degrees and the straight arm is rotated so that the thumb is pointing to the ground. Weakness, when compared to the opposite side, indicates disruption of the supraspinatus tendon.

comparable severity of pain. Disorders related to macrocalcification of the shoulder are usually very painful, with potentially other sites of calcification and pain, and plain x-rays confirm diagnosis (and localize treatment). Sepsis usually is associated with systemic signs, such as an elevated erythrocyte sedimentation rate and white blood cell count, but is, in fact, quite rare. Osteoarthritis of the glenohumeral joint is not common and may be indistinguishable from some aspect of the impingement syndrome until plain radiographs are obtained. Pain from symptomatic degenerative arthritis

of the acromioclavicular (AC) joint may be diagnosed or resolved by steroid injection into the joint.

▶ Imaging & Diagnostic Studies

Plain x-rays include an anteroposterior (AP) view of the shoulder taken in internal and external rotation and an axillary and an outlet view. These may show some sclerotic change at the greater tuberosity or evidence of AC joint degenerative arthritis. With massive disruptions of the cuff, the humeral head may be elevated in relationship to the glenoid cavity.

An magnetic resonance imaging (MRI) can determine the state of the cuff, as well as the presence of bicipital tendon pathology, labral tears, muscle atrophy indicating nerve injury, subluxation, dislocation, and other soft-tissue changes. However, it is not necessary to make a specific diagnosis of cuff tear if the patient's symptoms improve. Computed tomography (CT) scan with arthrogram may be requested prior to surgery. There is an age-related increasing incidence of asymptomatic partial- or full-thickness cuff tears such that, after 70 years of age, most people will have cuff tears.

▶ Prevention

Avoidance of prolonged or repeated overhead work, high shoulder loads including hand-force exertion and hand-arm transmitted vibration may lessen the incidence of impingement type pain. In addition, rotator cuff strengthening exercises can sometimes improve the symptoms associated with pathology in this area.

▶ Treatment

The goals of treatment are to resolve the patient's pain and restore normal function and muscle balance around the shoulder. This usually can be accomplished with nonoperative treatment, beginning with rest, and, when pain is controlled, progressive resistance exercises. Patients with less severe symptoms can be started on anti-inflammatory medications, pendulum exercises, and shoulder rotator cuff exercises. Pendulum exercises are performed with the individual flexing at the waist, relaxing all shoulder girdle musculature, and dangling the involved arm in a pendulum-like fashion. This reduces the pressure on the impinged area and may increase the circulation to the tendon. Selective contraction of the internal and external rotator cuff muscles depresses the humeral head and reduces the pressure in the subacromial space. Patients are taught to do this using resistance exercises such as with an elastic band (Thera-Band), with the arm at the side, elbow flexed 90 degrees, applying force in internal and external rotation.

The fastest way to resolve impingement symptoms is to inject the subacromial space with corticosteroid and local anesthetic (eg, triamcinolone 40 mg and 1% lidocaine 4 cc). This mixture is injected with a no. 25 needle directed at the point of the shoulder toward the greater tuberosity 2.5 cm inferior to the anterolateral quarter of the acromion. The diagnosis is made when the patient's symptoms are relieved immediately. The patient then is started on progressive resistance exercises.

Patients who respond only temporarily to the injection or who develop recurrence after two or three injections and who have participated in proper exercises may be candidates for surgery or arthroscopic surgery to decompress the subacromial space. This includes removal of bone from the undersurface of the acromion and AC joint, bursectomy, and cuff debridement and repair as necessary.

2. Bicipital Tendinosis

The biceps brachii muscle has two heads, a short head that originates from the coracoid process and a long head that originates from the supraglenoid tubercle. The long head then passes along the intertubercular groove of the humerus. The tendon can become inflamed within this groove resulting in pain and stiffness.

▶ Clinical Findings

Patients will have anterior shoulder pain that is often worse with overhead activity. On physical examination, the patient will have point tenderness in the area of the intertubercular groove anteriorly over the humerus.

▶ Differential Diagnosis

Bicipital tendinosis or tendinitis must be differentiated from other causes of anterior shoulder pain such as impingement or rotator cuff pathology.

▶ Imaging & Diagnostic Studies

The diagnosis of bicipital tendinosis can be made clinically. Plain x-rays are often normal but ultrasound or MRI may show thickening of the tendon or fluid around the tendon. MRI may be useful to identify other pathology around the shoulder.

▶ Prevention

Strengthening the muscles of the rotator cuff and the scapular stabilizers may help prevent bicipital tendinosis, as can avoidance of repetitive or sustained overhead activity.

▶ Treatment

Initial treatment involves rest and nonsteroidal anti-inflammatory drugs (NSAIDs) followed by rehabilitation consisting of scapular stabilization techniques and rotator cuff strengthening. Ultrasound-guided steroid injection around the tendon can also be effective. Finally, surgery consisting of debridement, biceps tenodesis, or tenotomy can be considered in refractory cases.

3. Labral Tears

The glenohumeral joint is surrounded by a fibrocartilaginous rim that helps to deepen and stabilize the joint. This labrum can be torn with either an acute injury or from repetitive overhead activity such as in a throwing athlete. Tears that occur over the superior part of the labrum are known as *SLAP* lesions, or superior labral anterior to posterior lesions, and are often seen in throwing athletes such as pitchers. Bankart lesions involve tearing of the labrum and a portion of the inferior glenohumeral ligament from the anterior and inferior portion of the joint. This type of lesion is seen with traumatic dislocation of the shoulder.

▶ Clinical Findings

Complaints associated with SLAP lesions can be vague. Patients may have a deficit of internal rotation compared to the other side. The **O'Brien test** may be used to aid in diagnosis. With the shoulder 90 degrees flexed, adducted adduction, and full internal rotation the patient is asked to further flex and adduct the shoulder against resistance by the examiner. This maneuver causes pain in the presence of a SLAP tear. The pain is improved when the test is repeated with the arm in full external rotation. Patients with Bankart lesions will often have a history of a shoulder dislocation and injury and may show signs of anterior apprehension on examination.

▶ Differential Diagnosis

Other causes of shoulder pain including impingement, tendonitis, and rotator cuff pathology should be considered. MRI is useful in differentiating these conditions.

▶ Imaging & Diagnostic Studies

Plain x-rays are usually not useful in making this diagnosis and even a simple MRI cannot detect all labral tears. An MRI with arthrogram is more sensitive in assessing the labrum.

▶ Prevention

Careful adherence to proper mechanics with throwing can help prevent SLAP type lesions.

▶ Treatment

Therapy consisting of strengthening the dynamic stabilizers of the shoulder as well as proprioceptive feedback may be helpful in chronic instability. However, large labral lesions that are symptomatic often require arthroscopic repair with bicipital tenotomy or tenodesis.

4. Shoulder Osteoarthrosis

Osteoarthritis at the shoulder joint may occur at the glenohumeral and/or AC joints.

▶ Clinical Findings

Patients will present with decreased range of motion of the shoulder and pain with shoulder motion. They may also have tenderness and swelling over the AC joint.

Differential Diagnosis

Osteoarthritis of the shoulder has a similar presentation to adhesive capsulitis but the two are distinguishable by x-ray.

Imaging & Diagnostic Studies

Plain x-rays, including an AP view of the shoulder taken in internal and external rotation as well as an axillary and an outlet, will show narrowing of the glenohumeral or AC joint with subchondral cysts and osteophyte formation. For advanced disorders, CT scan is useful when surgery is considered.

Prevention

Massive rotator cuff tears may be associated with progression to arthritis, and patients with this condition should be advised that treatment of the tear may help prevent the development of arthritis.

Treatment

Conservative treatment includes rest, NSAIDs, and therapy. Steroid injection can also be performed into the glenohumeral or AC joint. Injection into the glenohumeral joint is often done under fluoroscopic guidance. Surgery for AC joint arthritis may consist of arthroscopic or open distal clavicle resection. The glenohumeral joint can be treated with arthroplasty.

5. Frozen-Shoulder (Adhesive Capsulitis)

In patients with frozen-shoulder syndrome, there is marked restriction of glenohumeral joint motion, presumably in response to diffuse capsular inflammation. The etiology is unknown but the condition may be associated with diabetes or other endocrine or autoimmune conditions.

Clinical Findings

These patients may be comfortable at rest, and symptoms are produced when they attempt to move the glenohumeral joint beyond that allowed by the inflammation and adhesions. All ranges of motion are limited. Loss of axial humeral rotation (internal and external rotation) with the elbow at the side is diagnostic. Adhesive capsulitis frequently is confused with loss of motion from rotator cuff pathology. In the latter situation, there is no loss of axial rotation.

Differential Diagnosis

Plain radiographs and MRI can be used to differentiate this condition from osteoarthritis of the glenohumeral joint.

Imaging & Diagnostic Studies

Standard radiographs are normal in this condition but may be ordered to rule out underlying arthritis.

Prevention

There is no known method of prevention. Though not a work-related disease, work restriction may be required temporarily for pain control.

Treatment

Resolution of pain from a frozen shoulder requires a short period of sling immobilization for pain relief. However, after this, patients should undergo a dedicated program of rehabilitation and therapy. Shoulder motion will recover gradually with therapy over 6–18 months. Recovery of motion can be facilitated initially by distension of the glenohumeral joint with 30 cc fluid, saline with lidocaine, and triamcinolone diacetate 0.5 cc, and in some cases under arthroscopic arthrolysis. This is followed by gentle manipulation of the arm into external rotation. Many treatments have been tried but without consistent results.

6. Shoulder Dislocations

The anatomy of the shoulder contributes to the ease with which shoulder dislocations can occur. Stability of the large humeral head in the shallow 5 cm × 2.5 cm glenoid depends on the shoulder capsule and specific ligament attachments to the margins of the glenoid. Excessive force applied in any direction may cause a dislocation. With forces applied to the arm held in a position of abduction and external rotation, the humeral head is driven forward, tearing the anterior and middle glenohumeral ligaments and capsule from the margin of the glenoid. The humeral head is driven out anteriorly and rests in a position anterior and inferior to the glenoid. Rarely, the humeral head can dislocate posteriorly with automobile accidents, grand mal seizures, or electroshock therapy. In young people with lax ligaments and psychiatric disabilities, it may be dislocated intentionally.

Clinical Findings

Acute anterior shoulder dislocation results from a specific injury and is associated with severe anterior shoulder pain. The patients may be aware of a configurational change in the shoulder. Patients guard against shoulder motion by holding the elbow flexed with the ipsilateral forearm in the opposite hand. Any attempt at motion is associated with severe pain. Posterior dislocations are less obvious.

Differential Diagnosis

Other injuries to the shoulder area such as fractures or acute rotator cuff or labral tears should be considered.

Imaging & Diagnostic Studies

AP and axillary radiographs are obtained in all suspected dislocations. Anterior dislocations will show the humeral head displaced inferiorly to the glenoid, confirming the diagnosis. In posterior dislocations, the humeral head is at the same level as the glenoid on the AP radiograph. The diagnosis can be confirmed with an axillary view, which shows the head posterior to the glenoid. Posterior dislocations may be missed in initial screening radiographs in the absence of an axillary view. Confirmation is obtained by arthrogram with CT scan or MRI.

Prevention

General fall prevention and good seizure control may help prevent dislocations. Strengthening of the dynamic stabilizers of the shoulder may be helpful in chronic dislocators.

Treatment

Anterior and posterior dislocations are reduced by closed techniques immediately. Anterior dislocations can be reduced by various methods, including the Hippocratic maneuver. This technique involves gradual axial distraction to the arm in a position of forward flexion. Countertraction is applied to the axilla with the patient under intravenous analgesia (such as 40–100 mg meperidine HCl [Demerol]). Gentle rotation of the arm into internal rotation frequently assists reduction. Confirmatory radiographs are obtained after reduction.

Following reduction, patients are immobilized with the elbow at the side and the arm in a position of 10 degrees of external rotation for 3 weeks. This position, as compared with a sling and the arm in internal rotation, is a new concept based on better anatomic contact between the torn labrum and the glenoid. However, some patients do not tolerate this position; then a traditional jacket is used. Patients are allowed to return to their usual activities at 6–8 weeks. Long-term rates of success with this position of immobilization are unknown. If patients have recurrent dislocations then repair of the torn capsular attachment from the labrum of the glenoid anteriorly can be done either arthroscopically or with open surgery. Some surgeons use a bone transfer. Acute posterior dislocations usually require temporary immobilization in a position of slight abduction, shoulder extension, and external rotation to keep the humeral head reduced.

7. Multidirectional Instability

Individuals with ligamentous laxity may have shoulder joints that sublux easily in the anterior, posterior, or inferior direction. In the absence of injury, patients are asymptomatic. Following a minor injury in which the shoulder joint is subluxed forcibly, patients may continue to have shoulder pain with daily activities and symptoms of instability with different positions of the shoulder and arm.

Clinical Findings

Physical examination may demonstrate evidence of ligamentous laxity in the wrists, elbows, and knees. Shoulder examination will reveal laxity and excessive translation of the humeral head in the anterior and posterior directions. Patients may demonstrate the instability voluntarily.

Differential Diagnosis

SLAP lesions and other labral tears can have a similar presentation.

Imaging & Diagnostic Studies

MRI may be helpful to rule out labral pathology.

Prevention

There is no known method of prevention, but shoulder strengthening as stated below may improve the symptoms.

Treatment

Treatment is directed at educating the patient to adjust to the problem, altering his or her lifestyle, strengthening the shoulder, and delaying symptomatic activities. In some patients, surgical repair is directed at correcting the dominant directional instabilities.

8. Clavicular Fractures

Clavicle fractures usually occur from a direct blow to the shoulder and rarely from falling on an outstretched hand. Middle-third fractures are most common. Distal-third fractures are infrequent.

Clinical Findings

The proximal fragment of the clavicle is elevated by the action of the sternocleidomastoid; the weight of the shoulder displaces the distal fragment downward. Local swelling occurs from bleeding from the fracture site. The patient supports the involved extremity with the opposite hand. Rarely, a proximal fragment can perforate the skin, producing an open fracture.

Differential Diagnosis

Dislocations at the AC joint can have a similar presentation.

Imaging & Diagnostic Studies

Plain radiographs of the clavicle are sufficient for diagnosis.

Prevention

Prevention includes avoidance of falls and workplace safety.

Treatment

Immobilization of the fracture is provided by the application of a figure-of-eight bandage or a sling and swath. It is doubtful that a figure-of-eight sling or even a plaster bolero will influence the fracture position. Some mild cosmetic deformity usually is present. Surgery consisting of open reduction with internal fixation may be indicated for distal-third fracture, highly displaced fractures, fractures with tenting of the skin, or for early return to work or sporting activity. Open fractures are considered surgical emergencies.

9. Proximal Humeral Fractures

Isolated fractures of the proximal humerus can occur after a direct fall onto the arm or elbow.

Clinical Findings

Clinical symptoms include pain experienced over the proximal shoulder region or radiating the length of the arm. Local swelling is noted on examination from bleeding at the fracture site. Dissection of the hematoma may be noted onto the anterior chest after a few days.

Differential Diagnosis

Dislocation of the glenohumeral joint can have a similar presentation.

Imaging & Diagnostic Studies

Evaluation is with plain radiographs of the scapula and shoulder. These include AP radiographs of the scapula and proximal humerus and a lateral scapular view. An axillary view is necessary to rule out a dislocation of the head fragment, and CT scan is routinely performed to assess the number of bone fragments.

Prevention

Fall prevention and the treatment of osteoporosis may help decrease the incidence of these fractures.

Treatment

The four-part classification of proximal humeral fractures of Neer is helpful in deciding treatment. Nondisplaced or minimally displaced fractures of the surgical or anatomic neck or of the greater or lesser tuberosities can be treated by temporary immobilization. Displaced fractures of one or both tuberosities are indicative of a rotator cuff tear. Displaced fractures may require surgical treatment by open reduction and internal fixation. Four-part fractures can result in lost blood supply to the humeral head and may require prosthetic replacement. Dislocation of the fractured humeral head requires reduction, usually by operative methods.

Instruction in early shoulder motion is required both for unfixed and for operated fractures. The goal of physical therapy is to restore normal range of motion and strength around the shoulder. Patients should be progressed from active range-of-motion to resistive exercises beginning with isometrics and progressing to isotonic exercises.

10. Acromioclavicular Joint Separation

AC joint injuries may result from falls or from direct trauma to the arm or shoulder. They are common in contact sports such as ice hockey and football. Stability across the AC joint is provided primarily by the conoid and trapezoid ligaments. These ligaments, which are connected to the undersurface of the clavicle, suspend the scapula in the upright position by their attachment at the base of the coracoid process. The less robust AC ligaments and the attachments of the deltoid musculature between the clavicle and the arm provide additional stability. In minor injuries, the ligaments of the AC joint are stretched, and with increased force, the coracoacromial ligaments are injured as well. In severe injuries, the deltoid can be partially avulsed from its origin at the clavicle or acromion.

Clinical Findings

Signs and symptoms include pain and tenderness over the AC joint and deformity.

Differential Diagnosis

Clavicle fractures have a similar clinical appearance and can be differentiated by plain radiographs.

Imaging & Diagnostic Studies

Radiographs of the injured shoulder will rule out a fracture of the clavicle or proximal humerus. Displacement of the AC joint usually can be demonstrated on an AP view of the joint. Shoulder radiographs can be taken with the patient holding a weight or with traction.

Prevention

Fall avoidance and workplace safety can prevent these injuries.

Treatment

Treatment for most injuries consists of relieving symptoms by using a sling to immobilize the shoulder and support the weight of the arm. Patients may resume activity as comfort returns. Once the shoulder is stable in terms of decreased pain (4–6 weeks), physical therapy may be helpful for increasing strength. The usual residual of AC injuries is a mild cosmetic deformity caused by prominence of the distal end of the clavicle. If there is severe disruption of the AC joint with detachment of the deltoid or tenting of the skin, surgery may be indicated.

11. Brachial Plexus Neuropathy—Thoracic Outlet Syndrome

Thoracic outlet syndrome (TOS) is a set of symptoms and signs caused by compression of the neurovascular structures passing out of the chest and neck and beneath the clavicle to the axilla. Compression of the vessels and nerves of the brachial plexus and/or subclavian vessels occurs in the interscalene triangle, behind or below the clavicle or subcoracoid space, or more distally at the pectoralis minor. Cervical ribs or congenital fibrous bands and rarely a nonunion or malunion of the clavicle can lead to thoracic outlet compression.

Women are affected more frequently than men, usually between the ages of 20 and 50.

Clinical Findings

The neurogenic disorder is more common than the vascular. Patients report pain and/or paresthesia radiating from the neck or shoulder and down to the forearm and fingers. Symptoms can be aggravated by overhead activities. The hand may feel swollen or heavy. The lower trunk of the brachial plexus is involved more commonly, producing signs of numbness, tingling, and weakness in the ulnar-innervated intrinsic muscles and symptoms on ulnar side of the forearm and hand. Patients also may have venous compression or arterial insufficiency from the outlet.

Differential Diagnosis

The diagnosis can be confused with cervical disk disease at the C7–T1 level (which is rare), which may produce a C8 radiculopathy. Entrapment of the ulnar nerve in the cubital tunnel or Guyon canal usually can be distinguished by the physical examination or appropriate electromyography (EMG). Provocative maneuvers (Figure 8–2) such as overhead exercise or standing in the *military brace position* will obliterate the ipsilateral radial pulse and produce symptoms. More important, one should look for the reproduction of symptoms with specific controlled *neural tension maneuvers*, for example, controlling the stretch on the brachial plexus through scapular depression, shoulder abduction (to 90 degrees) and external rotation, wrist/finger extension, followed by either elbow extension with forearm supination (median nerve) or elbow flexion with pronation (ulnar nerve). Other maneuvers, held for 60 seconds, may also reproduce symptoms, for example, Adson maneuver, Wright test, Roos Test or shoulder hyperabduction to 180 degrees. With these maneuvers, also observe the palm for pallor indicating an accompanying vascular compromise.

Imaging & Diagnostic Studies

Plain radiographs of the cervical spine should be studied for congenital differences such as cervical ribs and long transverse processes or even hypoplastic first ribs. Apical lordotic chest views are indicated to rule out Pancoast-type tumors. Sophisticated MRI and angiographic or high-resolution CT scans may be helpful. EMG may be useful, especially if muscle weakness is present.

Prevention

This condition may be secondary to an anatomic abnormality, but the symptoms can be triggered by overhead work, working on a computer with a forward head posture, and professional playing of string instruments. Identification and correction of postural triggers are an important part of management.

Treatment

The initial treatment is conservative and depends on appropriate postural strength training to reduce the mechanism of thoracic outlet compression. The reduction of obesity and general physical fitness are encouraged.

Patients should be taught that certain postures are a primary cause of impingement and begin postural training and general upper extremity and shoulder exercise. Overhead activities or carrying heavy loads should be minimized. Computer users may benefit from lowering the keyboard and mouse to elbow height and moving the monitor closer and to an appropriate height (eg, top of monitor at eye level). They may also benefit from a standing workstation. Progress is measured in weeks or months.

Vascular TOS may require surgery to release the anterior scalene muscles and resect of the first rib or fibrous band. When symptoms caused by a clavicular malunion do not respond to conservative treatment, clavicular osteotomy is indicated.

INJURIES OF THE ELBOW

Elbow pain and disability is common in the workplace; mean rates are 1% per year among workers. The clinical evaluation should differentiate between acute traumatic injuries and chronic injuries due to repetitive strain. The context,

Disorders	Key Element of Diagnosis
Lateral epicondylitis	Mechanical pain located at **lateral** epicondyle +/− weakness
Radial tunnel entrapment at elbow	Pain just distal to **lateral** epicondyle with paresthesias on the dorsal hand surface
Medial epicondylitis	Mechanical pain located at **medial** epicondyle +/− weakness
Ulnar nerve entrapment at elbow	Neuropathic symptoms in ulnar distribution of hand or forearm with **medial** elbow tenderness
Anterior interosseous syndrome	**Diffuse** weakness (OK sign)
Pronator syndrome	Carpal tunnel syndrome–like symptoms in the hand increased by resisted pronation
Olecranon bursitis	**Posterior** swelling at the elbow
Osteoarthritis	**Diffuse** progressive pain and stiffness
Ulnar collateral ligament injury	**Medial** pain in throwing sports
Elbow fracture	**Major trauma with point tenderness**
Elbow dislocation	Major trauma (high energy) and **posterior** displacement

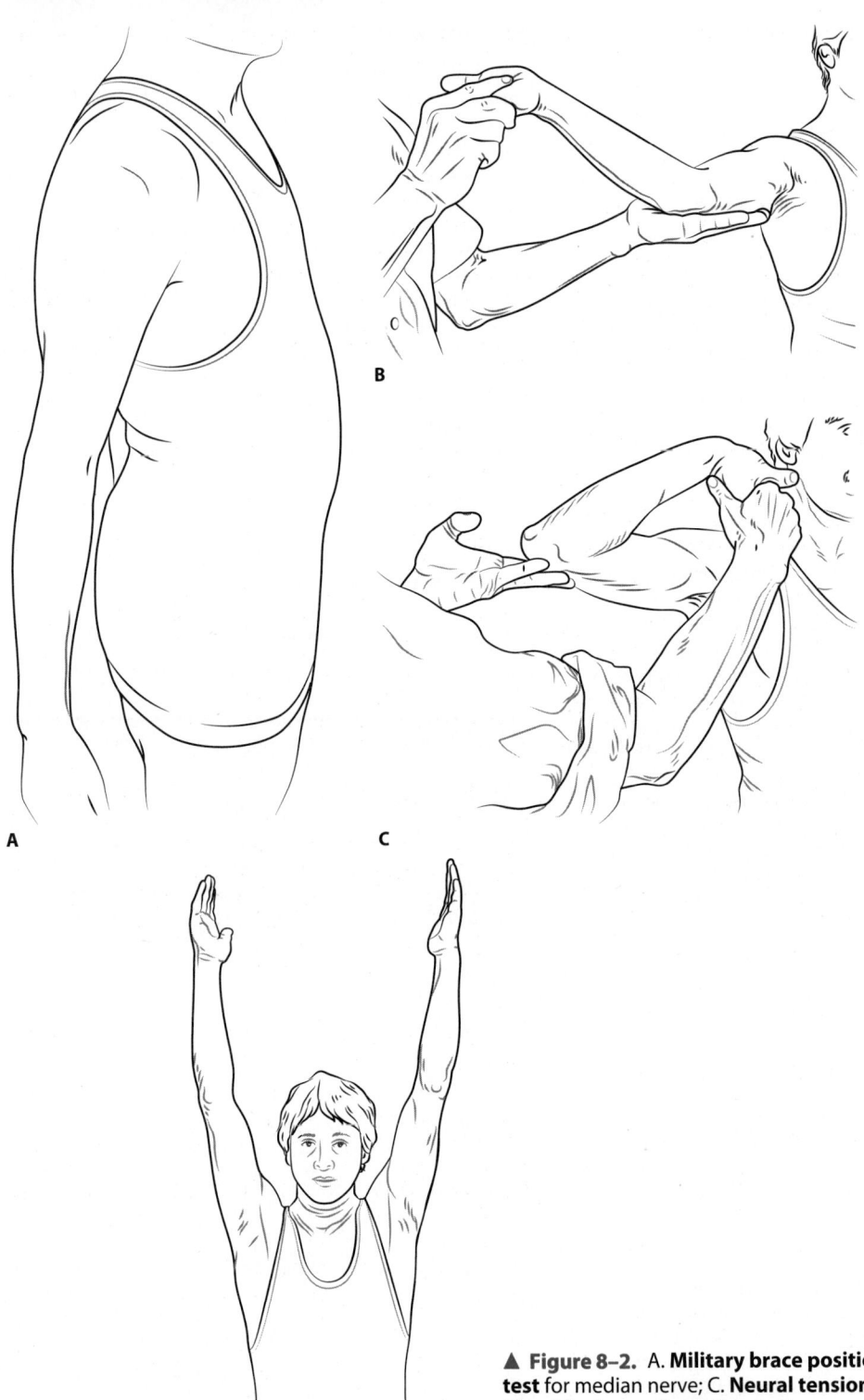

▲ **Figure 8–2.** A. **Military brace position**; B. **Neural tension test** for median nerve; C. **Neural tension test** for ulnar nerve; D: **Shoulder hyperabduction test**.

location, and type of symptoms combined with the physical examination are adequate for the diagnosis of most elbow disorders. Imaging and nerve conduction studies should be considered for possible fractures or peripheral neuropathies that are not responsive to conservative management. Treatment and prevention should be guided by workplace risk factors such as repeated high-force pinching or gripping, contact stress at the elbow, and awkward elbow postures.

1. Lateral Epicondylitis (Tennis Elbow)

Lateral humeral epicondylitis is also called "tennis elbow" because it is a common problem among tennis players. It can occur among workers who perform repeated forceful pinching or power grasps, work with the wrist in sustained extension, or repeatedly move the wrist forcefully in extension. The pathologic process involves tendon tears and necrosis at the attachment of the extensor carpi radialis brevis (ECRB) to the lateral humeral epicondyle and the extensor carpi radialis longus origin along the supracondylar line. The injury may be more proximal at the ECRB tendon muscle junction. The term *epicondylitis* is a misnomer because the pathology is related more to fibrosis and degenerative changes to the tendon than an acute inflammatory process.

▶ Clinical Findings

Patients may have ill-defined elbow symptoms or pain radiating into the dorsal aspect of the forearm. Symptoms may occur at night and at rest, but usually they are mechanical and related to activity, especially pinching, grasping (eg, steering wheel), wrist dorsiflexion or supination (eg, turning a door knob).

On examination, there is local tenderness over the lateral epicondyle or distal along the common extensor origin. Sometimes there is a pain at the distal third of the humerus at the origin of the ECRB. Because pain occurs with grasping, patients may complain of weakness. Symptoms can be reproduced by asking the patient to straighten the elbow then extend the wrist against resistance (Cozen test) (Figure 8–3);

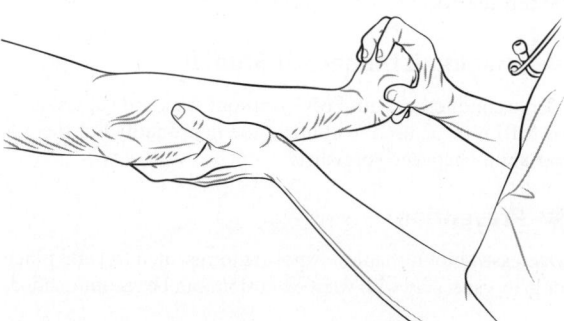

▲ **Figure 8–3. Cozen test**: Physician testing dorsiflexion of a patient's wrist against resistance. Resulting lateral humeral epicondylar pain suggests tennis elbow.

or extend the middle finger against resistance with the wrist straight; or grasp the back of a chair with the elbows straight and attempt to lift it (Chair test).

▶ Differential Diagnosis

The symptoms of radial head osteoarthritis, which is rare, can resemble those of tennis elbow. A plain-film radiograph will usually distinguish the two disorders.

A fractured radial head or neck, caused by falling on an outstretched hand, may cause similar symptoms. The history of trauma and anterior and lateral plain-film radiographic views will establish the diagnosis of a fracture.

Radial tunnel syndrome, caused by entrapment of the posterior branch of the radial nerve, may be considered in refractory cases although symptoms are usually more distal. Pain may be aggravated with resisted supination with the elbow slightly flexed.

Referred pain from C6 radiculopathy or a shoulder tendinopathy may be ruled out by an examination of the upper arm, shoulder, and neck.

▶ Imaging & Diagnostic Studies

Diagnosis is based on the clinical examination. With major trauma or refractory symptoms, imaging studies can be considered to rule out fracture or arthritis, ultrasonography with Doppler or MRI may be useful to rule out intra-articular pathology, confirm inflammation, and guide the steroid injection (if needed, see **Treatment**).

▶ Prevention

General strengthening of elbow and forearm musculature and proper instruction in the use of hand tools and/or modification of the hand tool may prevent lateral humeral epicondylitis in workers at risk. The intervention should be to eliminate high-force pinching or gripping and repeated forceful wrist extension.

▶ Treatment

Treatment of lateral epicondylitis is a matter of debate considering the slow natural history of healing after the aggravating activity is eliminated.

Removing or modifying the offending activities is fundamental for chronic disorders or temporarily for acute episodes. Patients should be instructed to avoid forceful pinching or gripping especially with wrist extension. Forearm muscle strengthening is helpful after the acute pain has resolved. Strengthening should be initiated with low loads with slow progression. For example, start with wrist curls using 250 g weights (or equivalent rubber tubing) and increasing the load each week or two. Although there is no evidence of long-term effectiveness of counterforce braces, there may be a temporary benefit and as a reminder to reduce grip force.

NSAIDs and ice can be considered for painful episodes especially with night pain, but there is no evidence that they are useful when taken continuously.

Steroid injections can reduce the pain for short durations (eg, weeks), but there is little evidence of long-term value. The steroid can be injected in multiple small doses into the most tender areas of the epicondyle or common extensor origin. Occasionally, a second injection is necessary. Complications include fat necrosis, local skin atrophy, and loss of pigmentation (usually temporary) in darker-skinned patients.

Injections with platelet-rich plasma (PRP) demonstrated no benefit in randomized controlled trials.

Physical therapy including stretching of the extensor origin and isometric and concentric exercises are often suggested. There is little evidence of value of eccentric muscle training or extracorporeal shock therapy.

Surgical debridement of the common extensor origin or ECRB, with or without repair, is rarely necessary, but remains a possibility for recalcitrant and confirmed lateral epicondylitis.

2. Medial Epicondylitis (Golfer's Elbow)

Medial epicondylitis can occur in golfers and baseball pitchers as well as in manual workers who do repeated forceful pinching or gripping or wrist flexion or pronation, especially when the elbow is flexed. Patients have pain on the medial aspect of the elbow radiating to the forearm. Many similarities exist between lateral and medial epicondylitis, including risk and prognosis factors, diagnosis strategy, prevention, and treatment.

▶ Clinical Findings

Physical examination findings include local tenderness over the medial epicondyle or common proximal flexor origin. The symptoms can be reproduced by resisted wrist flexion.

▶ Differential Diagnosis

As with lateral epicondylitis, osteoarthritis, other intra-articular pathologies, and referred pain of cervical radiculopathy are on the differential list.

Ulnar nerve entrapment at the elbow is sometimes associated with medial epicondylitis. The tissue swelling associated with medial epicondylitis can compress the ulnar nerve.

Referred pain from C8–T1 radiculopathy or a shoulder tendinopathy may be ruled out by an examination of the upper arm, shoulder, and neck.

▶ Imaging & Diagnostic Studies

Diagnosis is based on the clinical examination. With major trauma or refractory symptoms, imaging studies can be considered to rule out fracture or arthritis. Fluid accumulation can be observed with ultrasonography and MRI (increased T2 signal) may be useful to rule out intra-articular pathology. A nerve conduction study can rule out ulnar neuropathy.

▶ Prevention

General strengthening of elbow and forearm musculature and proper instruction in the use of hand tools and/or modification of the hand tool may prevent medial epicondylitis in workers at risk. The intervention should be to reduce high-force pinching or gripping or repeated forceful wrist or finger flexion.

▶ Treatment

Treatment involves rest of the involved tissues and modified activity. Steroid injection is generally not recommended due to the risk of ulnar nerve damage. Extracorporeal shock therapy has provided conflicting results. The need for surgical relief is rare.

3. Radial Nerve Entrapment at the Elbow (Radial Tunnel Syndrome)

Radial nerve entrapment at the elbow, also called radial tunnel syndrome, can be considered in cases of resistant lateral epicondylitis. The posterior (motor) branch of the radial nerve is compressed at the arcade of Fröhse, in the inferior portion of supinator muscle, or when crossing the extensors carpi muscles. Risk factors are similar to lateral epicondylitis, but it is not considered a common disorder.

▶ Clinical Findings

Patients typically present with pain that is 4–8 cm distal to the lateral epicondyle. The pain is aggravated by resisted supination and/or extension of the middle finger. However, none of these tests is specific for radial nerve entrapment. In severe disorders, radial deviation and weakness may be detected with extension of the first digit at the metacarpal joint.

▶ Differential Diagnosis

Lateral epicondylitis and referred C6 radiculopathy should be considered.

▶ Imaging & Diagnostic Studies

Nerve conduction with EMG (without standard values) and/or MRI may be used to confirm the neuropathy but there is variability between specialists.

▶ Prevention

Decreased biomechanical exposure to repeated forceful pinch or grip, especially with wrist extension, can be recommended.

▶ Treatment

Treatment consists of pain relief by ice or anti-inflammatory medications, relative rest with wrist splinting, and physical therapy. Activity modification includes avoiding frequent provocative maneuvers that may increase the symptoms, such as prolonged elbow extension with forearm pronation and wrist flexion.

Steroid injection with anesthetic can be considered if performed by an experienced hand or plastic surgeon. If conservative treatment fails to improve patients' symptoms after 6 months, surgical treatment may be considered.

4. Ulnar Neuropathy at the Elbow (Cubital Tunnel Syndrome)

Ulnar nerve entrapment at the elbow, also called *cubital tunnel syndrome*, is considered the second most common nerve entrapment disorder after carpal tunnel syndrome (CTS). The ulnar nerve may be trapped, irritated, or subluxed in its anatomic course through the ulnar tunnel (ie, cubital tunnel), at its entrance into the forearm through the cubital tunnel retinaculum (arcuatum or Osborne ligament) or at the arch of origin of the flexor carpi ulnaris. Compression of the nerve in the tunnel may be related to old elbow injuries with enlarging osteophytes, cubitus valgus deformity at the elbow, or subluxation of the nerve out of the groove. Work-related medial epicondylitis, contact stress (eg, truck driving), or sustained elbow flexion (eg, phone use) may cause localized edema, nerve compression, ischemia, fibrosis, and neuropathy.

▶ Clinical Findings

Patients present with neuropathic symptoms (eg, numbness, tingling, aching, burning, shooting, or stabbing pain) in the ulnar innervated fingers (eg, small and ring fingers) and less frequently in the medial aspect of the forearm and elbow. They may also experience allodynia (eg, normal touch is perceived as painful) or weakness. Symptoms are frequently aggravated by elbow flexion or resting the elbow on a work surface.

On physical examination, there may be a Tinel sign or tenderness over the ulnar nerve in the cubital tunnel or the tenderness may be localized proximally near the distal triceps or distally at the cubital tunnel retinaculum. Full elbow flexion for 60 seconds with the wrists straight (elbow flexion test) may trigger the symptoms (Figure 8–4). Sensory examination in the ulnar distribution on the fingers may be abnormal (eg, 2-point discrimination, Semmes-Weinstein monofilament testing, pin prick). Weakness and atrophy of the interossei/thumb adductor muscles indicates a more severe condition.

▶ Differential Diagnosis

The differential diagnosis includes compression of the ulnar nerve in Guyon canal at the wrist (uncommon), cervicothoracic C8–T1 radiculopathy, or brachial plexus neuropathy (eg, TOS). The physical examination or nerve conduction studies should be able to identify the location of the entrapment.

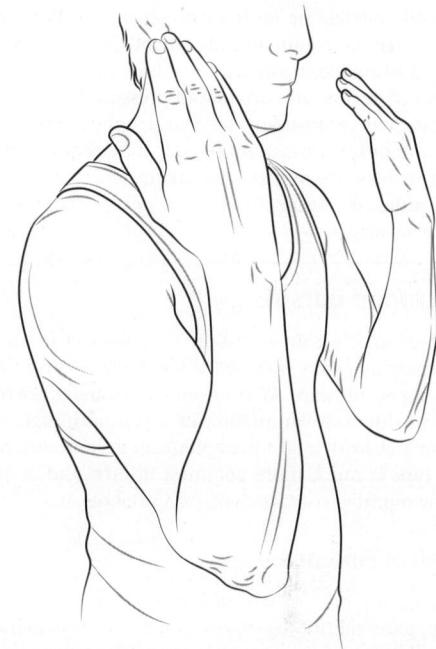

▲ **Figure 8–4.** Elbow flexion test for 60 seconds. With ulnar neuropathy at elbow tingling or numbness may occur in fourth and fifth digits. It can be useful to follow progress of treatment by recording the time to onset of symptoms.

Medial epicondylitis may be the inciting factor and should always be considered with possible ulnar neuropathy at the elbow.

▶ Imaging & Diagnostic Studies

Diagnosis of cubital tunnel syndrome is made from a combination of clinical data and nerve conduction studies of the ulnar nerve across the elbow. Recently, ultrasound and MRI have shown some value in identifying morphological changes of the nerve within the cubital tunnel.

▶ Prevention

Occupational risk biomechanical factors for medial epicondylitis should be minimized. Work practices should be modified to eliminate sustained elbow flexion, for example, use of head set instead of handheld phone. In addition, sustained contact stress, such as resting the arm on a chair arm-rest that presses on the ulnar groove, should be avoided.

▶ Treatment

Treatment is conservative initially. In addition to pain relief, the most commonly described methods of conservative treatment are activity modification, such as avoiding elbow flexion of 90 degrees or more or pressure over the medical epicondyle region. Night-time elbow splints should be used that are comfortable, maintain the elbow in approximately 45 degrees of flexion, and do not put pressure on the nerve.

Patients with interosseous muscle atrophy or who do not respond to conservative management may require surgical decompression of the nerve in the canal, medial epicondylectomy, or anterior transposition of the nerve subcutaneously or submuscularly.

5. Olecranon Bursitis

Olecranon bursitis is an irritation and swelling in the normally occurring bursa between the olecranon prominence and the overlying skin. Acute forms are usually not work-related but due to inflammation or sepsis, although a sudden trauma at work might precipitate an inflammation. The chronic type is much more common in men and is usually caused by repeated contact stress on the elbow.

▶ Clinical Findings

Patients usually present with a history of gradual swelling and pain, although these symptoms may occur acutely after a direct blow to the olecranon process. Signs of increased warmth suggest a septic process or another cause of inflammation. Localized fluctuant swelling will be present with or without sepsis/inflammation. Pressure exacerbates the pain.

▶ Differential Diagnosis

Sepsis and inflammatory diseases, like rheumatoid disease, crystalline deposits, or CREST (calcinosis, Raynaud phenomenon, esophageal dysmotility, sclerodactyly, and telangiectasia) syndrome are the main differential diagnoses.

▶ Imaging & Diagnostic Studies

Aspiration of the bursa and specific blood tests are useful depending on the differential suspected. Aspiration is best performed by introducing the needle at least 2.5 cm away from the bursa and then tunneling beneath the skin before actual penetration. This technique may prevent secondary infection of a sterile bursa. MRI in complex cases may be indicated (hypointensity on T1-weighted images).

▶ Prevention

Prevention is based on protection of repetitive trauma on the posterior face of the elbow. Use of a protective pad in specific jobs highly exposed to elbow trauma is usually effective.

▶ Treatment

In addition to the use of a protective pad to prevent reinjury, simple immobilization is adequate in most cases. For acute and painful cases, an elastic bandage and steroid injection (after infection is ruled out with an aspiration of the bursal fluid) may be used. For recurrent bursitis, arthroscopic bursal resection may be required.

6. Anterior Interossei & Pronator Syndrome

The median nerve can be compressed in the proximal forearm just distal to the antecubital fossa between the two muscular heads of the pronator teres. The anterior interosseus branch of the median nerve may be also compressed. This branch innervates the radial half of the flexor digitorum profundus, the flexor pollicis longus, and the pronator quadratus. These entrapments are rare and only case studies have been reported. The biomechanical risk factors may be forceful pronation, thumb adduction, or wrist flexion.

▶ Clinical Findings

In both cases, patients present with hand weakness, but those with pronator syndrome may present with paresthesia similar to CTS but with pain in the proximal volar forearm. These symptoms may be aggravated by repetitive pronation movements and are not reproduced by provocative median nerve testing at the wrist. Pronation against a resistance (hold patient's distal forearm) may reproduce symptoms.

With anterior interosseus syndrome, patients have difficulty pinching between the thumb and index finger. The thumb and index finger form a flat and triangular shape instead of normal round "OK" sign.

▶ Differential Diagnosis

CTS, brachial plexus neuropathy, and C6 radiculopathy are the primary differential diagnoses.

▶ Imaging & Diagnostic Studies

Nerve conduction studies with EMG can establish both diagnoses and rule out other neuropathies. In cases of significant motor loss, MRI may be useful to assess a particular anatomical variation that should to be treated.

▶ Treatment

The tension in the involved muscles must be reduced to decrease the impingement. Conservative management includes avoidance of aggravating activities, such as forceful pronation, thumb adduction, and wrist flexion curls. If conservative treatment is unsuccessful or if motor loss is significant, surgical decompression may be needed.

7. Elbow Osteoarthritis

Elbow osteoarthritis (OA) is a relatively rare condition that occurs almost exclusively in males, and has a strong association with repetitive strenuous use of the arm in activities ranging from weight lifting to operating heavy vibrating machinery. Elbow OA is marked by osteophyte formation whereas OA secondary to a trauma, with intra-articular fracture, includes osteophyte formation and joint space narrowing, bone sclerosis, and subchondral cysts. Sometimes, the OA associated with repetitive use is called primary OA of elbow to differentiate it from OA secondary to a prior trauma.

▶ Clinical Findings

Progressive diffuse pain is not specific. During the early course of the disease, when the joint space is still maintained, osteophytes in the olecranon fossa and the proximal portion of the olecranon cause pain in maximal extension. Similarly, if osteophyte formation occurs in the trochlea or in the coronoid process, impingement pain may be noted in extreme flexion. Patients may complain of pain throughout the arc of motion, but this is typically a late finding when the disease is more advanced.

▶ Differential Diagnosis

The differential includes secondary OA or rheumatoid arthritis.

▶ Imaging & Diagnostic Studies

Imaging is necessary to confirm the diagnosis. Plain radiograph or computed tomography (CT) of the elbow are usually adequate and show evidence of OA with osteophytes.

▶ Treatment

Conservative management includes decreased biomechanical exposure, pain relief, intra-articular steroid injections, physical therapy, and splinting. If conservative treatment fails or the OA is advanced, surgery should be considered. In young working patients, synovectomy, arthroscopic debridement, and interpositional arthroplasty can be tried. In others, cases, total elbow arthroplasty may be necessary.

8. Major Elbow Trauma: Elbow Fractures, Elbow Dislocation

Major trauma at the elbow can damage ligaments, bones, and joint. These disorders are not specific for workers and might occur in any circumstance of trauma.

▶ Clinical Findings

Continuous pain or pain with motion after a sudden trauma is the most frequent presentation. Patients may have a large amount of swelling or obvious deformity. Patients with an elbow dislocation are unable to bend the elbow and usually have a posterior displacement of the olecranon, often with an associated fracture.

▶ Differential Diagnosis

Pathological fractures should be considered in the case of minor trauma and deterioration of the patient's general health status.

▶ Imaging & Diagnostic Studies

Plain radiographs are usually sufficient for diagnosis but a CT scan is routinely performed before surgery.

▶ Prevention

Prevention is based on safe practices in the workplace and vehicles.

▶ Treatment

Conservative treatment is considered if fracture is not displaced but surgery is necessary in most cases. Conservative therapy includes PRICE (protection, rest, ice, compression, and elevation) before and during medical evaluation. Acute dislocations should be reduced in the emergency room under adequate sedation and splinted until evaluation by a surgeon. Rehabilitation should be performed as soon as possible with early range of motion exercise.

INJURIES OF THE WRIST & HAND

Injuries or pain in the hand and wrist are common in the workplace, particularly in occupations that involve a forceful and repetitive pinching or gripping. Careful assessment of symptoms and a focused physical examination are necessary to make the proper diagnosis since the symptoms can often be vague and difficult to reproduce.

1. Nonspecific Forearm, Wrist, or Hand Pain

Workers sometimes present to the occupational medicine clinic with nonlocalizing ache or pain in the distal upper extremities or symptoms that change in quality and location with time. Approximately half of these have a normal physical examination. These patients may have an early preclinical condition that has yet to declare itself with no localizing symptoms or physical findings. These patients can be rewarding or frustrating to manage depending on the approach to treatment.

One approach is to treat these as somatizations and try to identify and address underlying psychological or psychosocial factors that may be triggering symptoms. This approach should be considered if the symptom location and quality change with time and there is no apparent aggravation by specific tasks or biomechanical activities. Psychosocial factors at work can be explored by enquiring about relationships with coworkers and supervisors; concerns of job loss; the patient's pattern of wellbeing and energy level through the workweek; etc. Talking through constructive approaches to difficult work or home life may be very useful. A poor sleep pattern may also suggest psychosocial factors. The poor sleep pattern and symptoms respond well to daily exercises as simple as nondirected walks. Or they may respond to low-dose pm antidepressants or other mood-altering medications. These patients may benefit from a referral to a therapist.

Another approach is to try to identify the specific tasks and biomechanical activities at work or home that aggravate the symptoms. This approach is most useful if the symptom location does not change over time and the patient can identify specific aggravating activities. The physician should consider the ergonomic risk factors that might affect tissues in the location of the symptoms. For example, pain in the elbow region may be due to the repeated forceful pinching or gripping; sustained wrist extension; or contact stress at the elbow. For pain at the wrist, consider sustained wrist extension or ulnar deviation; sustained forearm pronation; repeated wrist motion; or prolonged contact stress on the volar surface of the wrist. Interventions should be proposed that directly address the aggravating activities. For example, some computer users are symptomatic using a conventional keyboard or mouse because their symptoms are aggravated by forearm pronation. They may respond well to a split keyboard and an asymmetrical mouse. The patient should be warned that their symptoms may take several weeks to resolve after the intervention is implemented. A number of workplace intervention studies have demonstrated a benefit of symptom reduction following the introduction of new tools or changes in work practices that address ergonomic risk factors.

In general, physicians should avoid using the terms repetitive strain injury or cumulative trauma disorder as a diagnosis but should instead identify the specific disorder or disorders, when possible. If there are no localizing physical examination findings, it is appropriate to use "hand pain" or "elbow pain." Effective treatments and prognoses are different between the specific disorders and the use of generic terms can cloud effective management.

2. Ganglion Cyst

Ganglion cysts are the most common soft tissue tumor of the hand. These mucin-filled cystic lesions can be asymptomatic or produce pain with direct pressure or during certain wrist motions. Patients seek care when they increase in size or become painful.

▶ Clinical Findings

Ganglion cysts can be associated with a joint capsule or tendon sheath. They are most commonly found over the dorsum of the wrist but can also occur on the volar side. They are well circumscribed and feel fluid filled. If they are large enough, then they can be transilluminated with a small penlight. When they occur in the hand, they are typically found on the volar surface and may present as a small, round, "BB-like" firm mass near the base of the digits.

▶ Differential Diagnosis

Other types of soft tissue masses should be considered, particularly if the mass feels more solid than cystic.

▶ Imaging & Diagnostic Studies

The diagnosis can be made clinically. Radiographs can be useful if the mass feels bony or calcified in nature. The diagnosis can also be confirmed with an MRI, CT scan, or ultrasound if the physical examination is inconclusive.

▶ Prevention

A few workplace studies link ganglion cysts to work involving repeated wrist motions, but the evidence is limited.

▶ Treatment

Asymptomatic lesions can be observed and will occasionally resolve on their own, particularly if they are small and have been present for less than a year. Avoiding weight-bearing with wrist extension can help decrease pain associated with dorsal wrist ganglia. Aspiration can be performed in the clinic although recurrence rates after aspiration have been reported to be 50–70%. Use of a large-bore needle (eg, 18 gauge) to puncture the cyst walls may decrease recurrence. Injection with steroid has been shown to have an increased incidence of skin depigmentation and subcutaneous fat atrophy. Surgical excision can be performed for symptomatic ganglia that do not respond to conservative treatment.

3. De Quervain Tenosynovitis (First Dorsal Wrist Extensor Compartment Tenosynovitis)

De Quervain tenosynovitis involves the first dorsal compartment of the wrist. The involved tendons include the abductor pollicis longus and the extensor pollicis brevis. The onset is usually associated with overuse of the thumb particularly with radial deviation, as in repetitive hammering, lifting, or pipetting. The tenosynovial lining will show low-grade inflammation.

▶ Clinical Findings

Patients performing new, hand intensive job activities or those who engage in repetitive lifting may complain of pain in an ill-defined area along the radial side of the base of the thumb, occasionally extending as far distally as the interphalangeal joint. This condition is also seen in new or nursing mothers. There is usually very localized tenderness over the radial side of the distal radius and swelling may be present. When the patient grasps the fully flexed thumb into the palm and then ulnar deviates the hand at the wrist, exquisite pain develops and reproduces the patient's complaint (Finkelstein test) (Figure 8–5).

▶ Differential Diagnosis

Chronic nonunion of the scaphoid bone occasionally produces similar symptoms. Pain associated with OA of the first carpometacarpal (CMC) joint, which occurs in approximately 25% of white women older than 55 years of age, may mimic De Quervain tenosynovitis, which occurs in younger patients.

▶ Imaging & Diagnostic Studies

This is primarily a clinical diagnosis and there are no specific radiographic findings. However, radiographs of the wrist

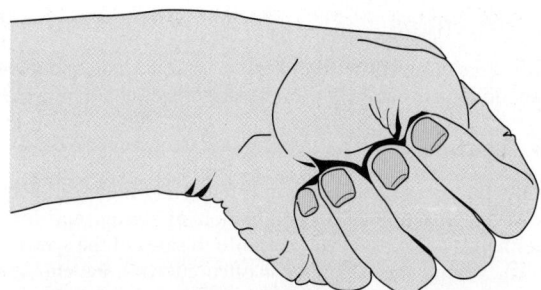

▲ **Figure 8–5. Finkelstein test.** With the thumb clasped in the palm as shown, the wrist is deviated toward the ulna, producing pain over the first dorsal extensor compartment.

and CT scan can rule out CMC OA and nonunion of the scaphoid bone.

▶ **Prevention**

Patients are instructed to lift with the palm facing upwards (full supination) rather than with the palm down, and avoid forceful repeated pinching with the thumb. Tools can be modified to reduce repeated forceful thumb flexion especially with the wrist in a nonneutral posture.

▶ **Treatment**

The first line of treatment can be activity modification including lifting with the palm in supination, avoiding repetitive pinching and thumb abduction, and use of a thumb spica splint to immobilize the thumb. NSAIDs can be helpful for pain management.

Steroid injection is often successful at curing this condition. Injection is generally performed with a combination of local anesthetic and steroid given into the tendon sheath over the area of the radial styloid with a single injection using a 25-gauge needle. Every attempt should be made to place the injection within the sheath and avoid subcutaneous injection of steroid that can cause skin depigmentation and fat atrophy. Only 1–2 cc of total fluid will fit into the tendon sheath.

In patients who do not respond to local injection, surgical decompression of the common extensor sheath by incision may be necessary. Patients who have certain anatomic variations, such as a separate subsheath for the extensor pollicis brevis tendon or multiple slips of the abductor pollicis longus, may be less likely to respond to injection. Unfortunately, there is no reliable way of distinguishing these patients clinically or radiologically.

4. Other Extensor Tendinopathies of the Wrist

Tendonitis can occur at five other specific sites on the extensor side of the wrist (Figure 8–6). The common sites are intersection syndrome (ECR, third compartment), extensor

digitorum communis (EDC, fourth compartment), and extensor carpi ulnaris (ECU, sixth compartment). Intersection syndrome (ECR travels beneath muscles of APL and EPB) and fourth extensor compartment tenosynovitis (EDC) can occur with repeated or sustained wrist extension or other overuse. ECU tendonitis occurs after a twisting injury and presents as vague or deep pain over the ulnar side of the wrist. EDC synovitis with swelling and fluid is unusual outside the setting of inflammatory or crystalline arthropathy, and patients with these findings should be evaluated for these conditions.

▶ **Clinical Findings**

It is useful to localize the tendonitis to the specific compartment. There may be very localized tenderness or pain with resisted loading of the tendon/muscle. Patients with tendonitis over the ECU tendon have ulnar-sided wrist pain that can often extend from the insertion point over the base of the fifth metacarpal bone, over the distal ulna, and into the distal forearm. The pain is often worse with resisted wrist extension and ulnar deviation. Similarly, tendonitis of the ECR tendons creates pain at the second and third metacarpal that also can extend into the forearm. Pain with this condition tends to be worse with resisted wrist extension and radial deviation. Intersection syndrome occurs at the distal forearm where the muscle bellies of the tendons of the first dorsal compartment cross over the radial wrist extensors, causing compression in this area.

▶ **Differential Diagnosis**

ECU tendonitis must be distinguished from a tear of the triangular fibrocartilage complex (TFCC). ECR tendonitis can be confused with De Quervain or scaphoid fractures or nonunions as well as radiocarpal arthritis.

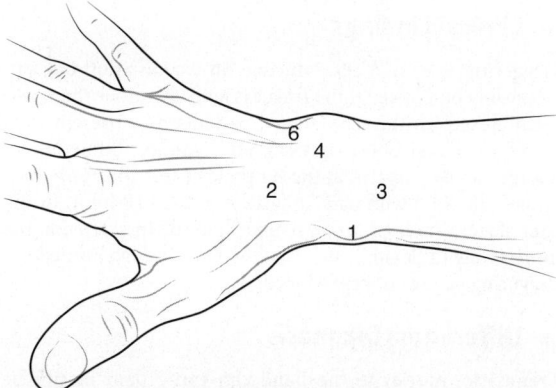

▲ **Figure 8–6.** Extensor tendon entrapment sites: First is De Quervain tenosynovitis (ABL and EPB), second is ECR insertion on carpal bones, third is intersection syndrome (ECR travels below ABL and EPB muscles), fourth is EDC, and sixth is ECU.

▶ Imaging & Diagnostic Studies

Tendonitis is primarily a clinical diagnosis. However, MRI studies will sometimes show fluid or inflammatory changes around the affected tendon.

▶ Prevention

Reduction of duration of forceful gripping and repeated wrist motion may prevent these conditions for hand intensive work. For computer users, ergonomic modifications can reduce wrist extension with keyboard and mouse use.

▶ Treatment

The primary treatments include activity modifications, wrist splints, NSAIDs, and, if indicated, ergonomic evaluation of work tasks and tools. Corticosteroid injections can be done but should be limited in number to prevent the risk of tendon rupture. Surgery is only indicated in very rare instances of refractory pain.

5. Trigger Digit (Stenosing Tenosynovitis)

Stenosing tenosynovitis of the flexor tendon to a finger or of the flexor pollicis longus to the thumb may produce pain when the digit or thumb is forcibly flexed or extended. Motion of the proximal interphalangeal (PIP) joint of the finger or the interphalangeal (IP) joint of the thumb produces the symptoms, which is a painful snap. This causes the joint to collapse suddenly much like a trigger.

The cause of the tenosynovitis may be repetitive finger flexion. It is also associated with systemic diseases such as diabetes, thyroid dysfunction, and rheumatoid arthritis. The patient's work history may reveal a cause of the disorder; however, most cases are idiopathic.

▶ Clinical Findings

Triggering is usually reproducible on examination but can often only be noticed if the finger is actively rather than passively flexed. In the early stages, patients may present with pain over the A1 pulley only and no triggering. Sometimes a nodule can be palpated at the A1 pulley (near the MCP joint on palmar side) with passive flexion of the PIP joint. In the later stages, the digit may become "locked" in extension (or more rarely in flexion) such that the motion is so limited the triggering cannot be reproduced.

▶ Differential Diagnosis

Traumatic injuries to the hand can cause pain in similar areas.

▶ Imaging & Diagnostic Studies

Imaging studies are not needed to make this diagnosis and are usually normal.

▶ Prevention

Avoidance of repetitive digit flexion against a load and good diabetic control can help prevent triggering.

▶ Treatment

At the early stages, splinting in extension at night can help. However, injection of a combination of steroid and local anesthetic (1–2 cc total volume) into the area of the synovial sheath around the A1 pulley is often curative. Patients not responding to injection or developing recurrent symptoms may require surgical release of the tendon sheath.

6. Carpal Tunnel Syndrome

CTS is an entrapment or pressure neuropathy of the median nerve as it passes through the carpal tunnel volar to the nine flexor tendons. The canal boundaries are the rigid transverse carpal ligament on the volar side and the carpal bones on the dorsal side.

CTS affects workers of any age but is more common in women. Pregnancy, increasing age, and obesity increase the risk. Symptoms may appear after an injury, such as a direct blow to the dorsiflexed wrist or with a Colles fracture. Rheumatoid arthritis, which causes inflammation in the sheath surrounding the flexor tendons, is one example of a space-occupying lesion that produces the encroachment. Rare hypothyroid patients with myxomatous tissue in this area are at risk for bilateral symptoms. While the cause of the syndrome is unknown in many cases, repeated or sustained forceful pinching or gripping has been associated with CTS.

▶ Clinical Findings

In the absence of an acute injury, patients can develop paresthesias in the median nerve distribution (volar surface of the thumb, index, and long fingers as well as the radial half of the ring finger). With progression of the syndrome, patients may be awakened at night with pain, tingling, burning, or numbness in this area of the hand. Characteristically, patients tend to stand up and massage the area or shake the hand. Symptoms may also occur with driving or sustained gripping (eg, cleaning, cooking, bicycle riding). Further progression may lead to hand weakness. Untreated CTS with progressively worsening symptoms may result in permanent damage to the median nerve with persistent sensory deficit and thenar muscle atrophy and weakness.

When patients are seen early, there is no evidence of thenar atrophy and sensation (2-point discrimination at 4 mm) remains intact. Patients who hold their wrists maximally flexed for 60 seconds (*Phalen sign*) may develop symptoms. Direct pressure over the carpal tunnel area can also recreate symptoms (carpal compression test) (Figure 8–7A). Tapping with a reflex hammer at the volar wrist may recreate shooting pains into the tips of the digits (Tinel sign). There may be diminished abductor pollicis brevis strength (Figure 8–7B). The diagnosis is confirmed by median nerve

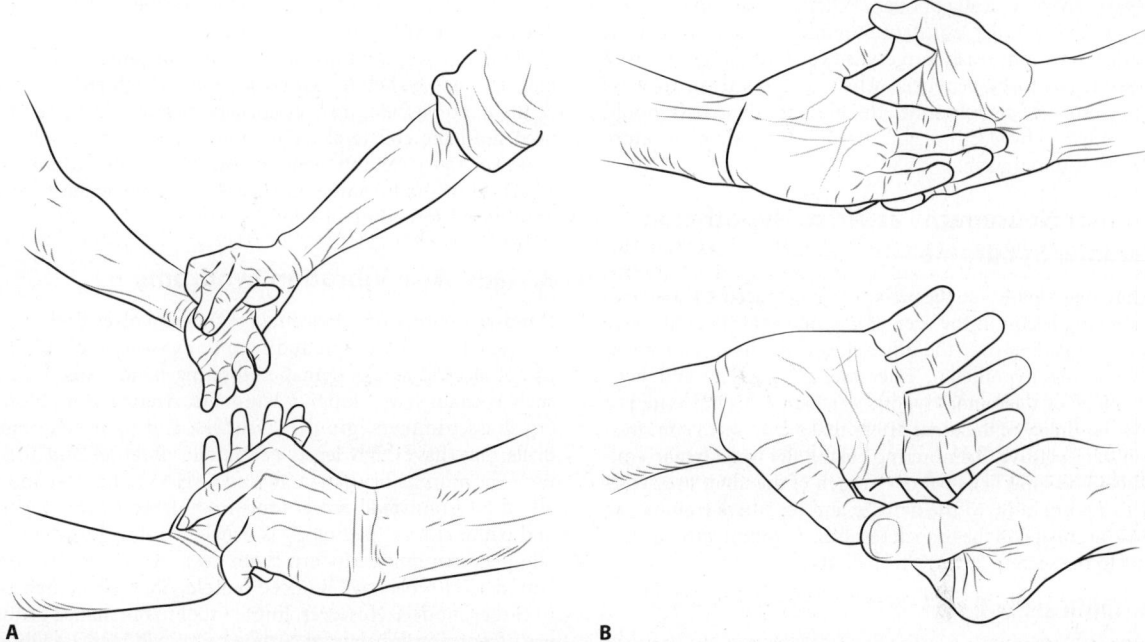

▲ Figure 8–7. A. Carpal compression test—wrists are flexed to 45 degrees and examiner's fingers press over carpal tunnel for 30 seconds; B. Strength testing of APB (median nerve innervated)—patients are instructed to raise up the tip of thumbs against examiner's thumbs.

electrodiagnostic studies (nerve conduction studies and EMG).

▶ Differential Diagnosis

Pain in the median nerve distribution with entrapment at the carpal tunnel should be distinguished from median nerve compression occurring proximally. Occasionally, cervical radiculopathy (C5, C6, C7) or pronator teres syndrome may resemble this condition, but neurologic examination should distinguish between these.

▶ Imaging & Diagnostic Studies

Plain imaging studies are not needed to make this diagnosis. Nerve electrodiagnostic studies are helpful in both confirming the diagnosis and estimating the severity of nerve dysfunction. The nerve conduction study should be temperature adjusted. In some cases, ultrasound and MRI are used to evaluate morphological change of the median nerve in the carpal tunnel prior to surgery.

▶ Prevention

Avoidance of repeated or sustained forceful pinching or gripping or repetitive wrist and finger movements, prolonged wrist flexion or extension, or direct pressure on the carpal tunnel can help prevent symptoms. There are many examples of tools or jigs that allow work to be performed with less forceful pinch or grip. Some examples are the use of anti-torque bars on inline screwdrivers; tool clutch adjustment to minimally effective torque; tools with lower force switches; and tool balancers that support the weight of the tool. Tools that reduce sustained posture extremes such as split keyboards or those that reduce extreme pronation such as asymmetrical computer mice may also be useful.

▶ Treatment

Underlying conditions, such as rheumatoid arthritis or hypothyroidism, that may cause carpal tunnel should be treated. In the absence of signs of neuropathy, patients are instructed in reducing provocative or repetitive activities. Wrist splints holding the wrist in neutral are effective in alleviating symptoms. Splinting consistently at night for a period of 4–6 weeks can be curative in the early stages. CTS associated with pregnancy usually responds to splinting and the symptoms resolve after delivery. For patients not responding to rest and splinting, injections of cortisone into the carpal tunnel (with care to avoid injection into the median nerve) can be beneficial. Patients who fail to respond to these measures or whose symptoms recur may require carpal tunnel release surgery, endoscopically or open. When patients present with signs of nerve injury, constant numbness, loss of sensibility, or thenar atrophy, early surgery is preferred. Surgery is well documented to be beneficial when performed on patients with confirmed carpal tunnel, therefore the diagnosis should be confirmed by electrodiagnostic studies or imaging before surgery is undertaken.

7. Ulnar Neuropathy at Wrist, Hypothenar Hammer Syndrome

Ulnar neuropathy at the wrist can be caused by a space-occupying lesion in the area of Guyon canal. Patients have loss of sensation over the ulnar side of the hand and weakness of the hypothenar, interosseous muscles, and even "clawing" of the hand. Hypothenar hammer syndrome is a vascular injury of the ulnar artery that occurs with compression or repetitive "hammering" using the hypothenar eminence. The superficial palmar branch of the ulnar artery lies in close proximity to the hamate and repetitive trauma can cause occlusion of the branch resulting in diminished arterial flow to the second through fifth digits.

▶ Clinical Findings

Callousing over the hypothenar eminence may be present. With ulnar neuropathy at the wrist, the patient may have diminished sensation of the small finger and ulnar border of the ring finger. At later stages, atrophy of the hypothenar muscles and the interosseous muscles can develop as well as clawing of the hand. Patients with hypothenar hammer syndrome present with signs of ischemia such as cold sensitivity, decreased capillary refill, discoloration, or tip necrosis. The Allen test may be useful to evaluate ulnar artery blood flow.

▶ Differential Diagnosis

Systemic causes of neuropathy, cubital tunnel syndrome, T1 radiculopathy, and Raynaud's syndrome should all be considered on the differential diagnosis.

▶ Imaging & Diagnostic Studies

MRI or CT scan may be helpful to identify an occult lesion in Guyon canal or elsewhere adjacent to the ulnar nerve. Neurodiagnostic studies can also be used to determine the area of compression and degree of dysfunction. Arteriography is very useful in confirming the diagnosis of hypothenar hammer syndrome.

▶ Prevention

Repetitive hammering with the hypothenar eminence of the hand should be avoided. Sheet metal workers should use a rubber mallet.

▶ Treatment

Ulnar neuropathy at the wrist due to an occult mass should be surgically treated. Release of Guyon tunnel can also be done in the absence of a mass. The treatment of hypothenar hammer syndrome is more controversial. Avoidance of smoking, keeping the digits warm, and calcium channel blockers may be helpful. Often there is enough redundancy in the hand vasculature that conservative treatment can be used until the collateral circulation becomes more robust. However, surgical interventions such as embolization or resection of the thrombosed segment with or without vein grafting are sometimes needed.

8. Hand-Arm Vibration Syndrome

Hand-arm vibration syndrome (HAVS) involves both neurologic and vascular signs and symptoms associated with the use of electric and pneumatic vibrating hand tools. Tools, such as chain saws, chipping hammers, riveting guns, blowers, grass trimmers, grinders, sanders, and rotary hammer drills may have high levels of handle vibration and their use over months or years may lead to HAVS. Because most vibration from small power tools is absorbed by the fingers and palm, clinical pathology is usually confined to the distal upper extremity. Modern chain saws and many vibrating commercial tools have reduced handle vibration compared to earlier models. However, limited tool maintenance or the use of worn or imbalanced cutting heads will increase vibration exposure. The clinical expression of HAVS occurs most commonly with outside work performed in colder climates. However, the underlying pathology is caused by the tool vibration not cold temperature.

▶ Clinical Findings

The classic presentation, which is the basis for hand tool vibration standards, is cold-provoked blanching of the fingers, thus the term vibration white fingers (VWF) or occupational Raynaud phenomenon. At lower exposures, neurologic symptoms predominate. These symptoms usually begin as problems of hand coordination and fine manipulation. Hand and arm pain and hand paresthesias are common in frequent hand tool users, and may be related to nerve compression or chronic soft tissue injury. Accordingly, differentiation of exposures and precise diagnosis of the medical condition are essential. At earlier stages, vascular signs and symptoms can be stabilized and reversed if vibration exposure is minimized or stopped. Because neurologic symptoms may involve either mechanoreceptors or trunk nerves, the prognosis is more variable. The most severe cases that involve skin trophic changes and gangrene are rarely seen. Their presence requires more extensive investigation for a major comorbidity, such as a collagen vascular disease or obstructive arterial disease. The examination should include skin perfusion evaluation digit sensory testing where available, such as with monofilaments or 2-point discrimination, and provocative maneuvers for distal nerve compression, as in the CTS. Each hand should be evaluated separately for the three stages of the clinical classification of vascular and neurological HAVS. For the vascular component, Raynaud type blanching is confirmed by a validated photograph with blanched skin clearly demarcated from unaffected skin; blanching score is calculated from the photographs as 3 for proximal, 2 for middle and 1 for distal phalanx of each affected finger. For the neurological component, neurosensory symptoms are considered pathological if lasting > 20 min; sensory perception is assessed on the pulp of two or more digits supplied by the median and ulnar nerves and standardized methods of testing must be followed for all (see revised International consensus criteria for diagnosing and staging hand-arm vibration syndrome).

▶ **Differential Diagnosis**

Raynaud disease and entrapment neuropathies, such as CTS and TOS should be considered, as well as microvascular disorders (eg, scleroderma). CTS and digital nerve pathologies may accompany HAVS due to biodynamic workplace factors. In addition, because HAVS is a vasospastic disorder, routine noninvasive vascular imaging will usually be normal. TOS can be a confounding diagnosis because of its independent effects on large arteries and the brachial plexus. However, vascular expressions of TOS are unusual and can be visualized by Doppler, angiography, MRA, or multidetector CT.

▶ **Imaging & Diagnostic Studies**

Sensory function can be evaluated with the vibration and thermal perception threshold tests (VPT and TPT), but these types of quantitative sensory tests (QSTs) have limited availability. Nerve conduction studies may be useful for evaluating digital nerve function and to rule out or rule in CTS. The value of using finger systolic blood pressure or laser Doppler to evaluate vasospasm, under conditions of cold provocation, has a long-established acceptance, but application is highly specialized. Routine noninvasive vascular tests are not useful, unless an obstructive pathology is under consideration. Capillaroscopy may be useful to rule out scleroderma or other microvascular disorders.

▶ **Prevention**

Use of power tools with lower levels of handle displacement (mm) or acceleration (m/s^2) can reduce the incidence and even prevent HAVS. The handle vibration level of vibrating hand tools should be available from the manufacture and compared to national (ANSI; ACGIH, EU) and international (ISO) standards. Exposure can also be reduced by reducing the minutes of tool use per day to below thresholds set by national and international standards. Monitoring of exposure duration and symptoms is especially important for tools with high levels of handle vibration. Vibration exposure levels can also be reduced with jigs or tool balancers that support the tool and isolate the vibration from the worker or reduce the grip force required to use the tool. The use of antivibration gloves or tape wrapped around tool handles can effectively reduce vibration exposure levels at higher frequencies. However, their utility under different working

conditions, patterns of tool use, and grip force characteristics remains undetermined. Smoking cessation is highly beneficial because it reduces arterial vasospasm.

▶ **Treatment**

Treatment involves minimizing exposure to vibrating hand tools. If CTS is also present it should be treated.

9. Wrist Sprain

Wrist sprains are common and usually involve a fall onto an outstretched hand with stretching of the dorsal wrist capsule or high-force loads such as occurs when a high-torque drill binds and twists the hand and forearm. The patient presents with pain and swelling over the dorsal wrist.

▶ **Clinical Findings**

Patients will have dorsal wrist pain over the radiocarpal joint and may have swelling and ecchymosis in this area as well.

▶ **Differential Diagnosis**

Fractures of the radius or carpus must be ruled out. Any patient with tenderness in the anatomic snuffbox should be assumed to have an occult scaphoid fracture and treated accordingly. Patients may also have a tear of the scapholunate (SL) ligament.

▶ **Imaging & Diagnostic Studies**

Imaging studies including a PA, lateral, and oblique of the wrist can be used to rule out fracture. Patients with snuffbox tenderness should be further evaluated with a scaphoid view. Clenched-fist views of the wrist can be helpful to evaluate for widening of the SL joint, which suggests injury to the SL ligament. An MRI can be obtained to look for a ligament injury or occult fracture.

▶ **Prevention**

Safe work practices to prevent falls and use of wrist guards during high-risk sporting activities can help prevent these common injuries. High-torque hand tools such as drills should have the clutch or torque limiter engaged. High-torque drills should be used with two hands instead of one.

▶ **Treatment**

Rest, wrist splinting, and NSAIDs are the mainstay of treatment for wrist sprains.

10. Ulnar Collateral Ligament Injury of the Thumb (Skier's or Gamekeeper's Thumb)

Forcible radial deviation of the thumb can cause partial or complete disruption of the ulnar collateral ligament with or without fracture. This condition can be seen in skiers when the thumb is injured forcibly against the ski pole. Scottish gamekeepers were thought to develop chronic attenuation of the same ligament by breaking the necks of ducks and other game by gripping the neck with both hands and rotating the forearms. Splinting can be used for stable injuries or nondisplaced avulsion fractures. Open surgical repair should not be delayed when there is instability.

▶ Clinical Findings

Rupture of the ulnar collateral ligament will cause pain and tenderness over the ulnar border of the thumb metacarpophalangeal (MP or MCP) joint (the three joints of the thumb are CMC, MCP, and IP). The ligament sometimes retracts proximal to the insertion of the adductor pollicis insertion and a lump (known as a Stener lesion) can be felt in this area. The thumb MCP joint should be evaluated for stability by gentle radial deviation in full extension and 30 degrees of flexion. Increased laxity or a "soft" endpoint in both positions when compared to the normal side suggests a complete tear.

▶ Differential Diagnosis

Fractures in the area as well as simple sprains of the MCP joint and radial collateral ligament injuries are on the differential.

▶ Imaging & Diagnostic Studies

Radiographs of the thumb can be used to diagnose avulsion injuries. MRI can be helpful for differentiating full from partial tears if the examination is equivocal.

▶ Prevention

Avoidance of repetitive forced radial deviation can prevent chronic attenuation of the ligament.

▶ Treatment

Partial tears or nondisplaced avulsion injuries can be treated with thumb spica casting for 6 weeks. Compliant patients can be treated with a hand-based thumb spica splint to include the MCP joint, but they must be cautioned to wear this full-time except for skin care and avoid any thumb radial deviation when the splint is off. Full-thickness tears with instability or those with a Stener lesion are treated with surgical repair or reconstruction.

11. TFCC Tears

The TFCC consists of ulnocarpal ligaments, the subsheath of the extensor carpi ulnaris tendon, the radioulnar ligaments, and a central fibrocartilagenous disk similar to the meniscus in the knee. The TFCC provides stability at the distal radioulnar joint (DRUJ). It can be torn from a fall onto an outstretched hand or other causes of high-force wrist loading.

▶ Clinical Findings

Patients with an acute tear will have pain over the ulnar portion of the wrist. It can be vague and is often described as "deep" in this area. They will be tender just distal to the ulnar head. Passive ulnar deviation of the wrist may worsen their pain. The DRUJ may be unstable and should be tested by stabilization of the radius with one hand and moving the distal ulna dorsally and volarly with the other and checking for laxity. The joint should be checked with the forearm in full pronation, neutral, and full supination and compared to the other side. Rotation of the wrist may produce a painful catch or clunk.

▶ Differential Diagnosis

A TFCC tear can be difficult to differentiate from ECU tendonitis. Patients with ECU tendonitis will be tender at the ECU insertion at the base of the fifth metacarpal and may have radiating pain up the forearm, whereas the pain is more localized with a TFCC tear. Mechanical symptoms such as a painful catch or clunk in certain positions are more suggestive of a TFCC tear.

▶ Imaging & Diagnostic Studies

Radiographs of the wrist may show an ulnar styloid avulsion; however, most of these injuries are not thought to be associated with TFCC tears. 3T MRI images or MR/arthrogram can be useful in the diagnosis of TFCC tears.

▶ Prevention

Fall prevention is important in preventing TFCC tears, as is the use of wrist splints in high-risk sporting activities. Patients with an "ulnar positive" wrist where the ulna is longer than the radius may be more prone to a central chronic TFCC tears.

▶ Treatment

Chronic central tears can often be treated conservatively with rest, ice, and splinting. Acute tears without DRUJ instability can also be treated conservatively but may require casting for 4–8 weeks until the symptoms improve. Tears associated with mechanical symptoms or DRUJ instability are often treated with arthroscopic surgery, as are other types of tears that fail conservative treatment.

12. Kienböck Disease

Kienböck disease is avascular necrosis (AVN) of the lunate. The condition is often idiopathic but can be associated with other conditions causing AVN such as chronic steroid use. It may be bilateral. A similar condition, called Preiser disease, can occur in the scaphoid. AVN of both carpal bones has been associated with very high levels of exposure to vibrating or percussing hand tools but the evidence is not strong.

Clinical Findings

Patients will have wrist pain centered over the lunate but it may be vague in nature. They may also have swelling and synovitis of the wrist. Stiffness with wrist flexion and extension may be present.

Differential Diagnosis

Wrist sprains, scaphoid nonunions, and OA of the wrist all have similar presentation. Kienböck tends to present in young men.

Imaging & Diagnostic Studies

PA, lateral, and oblique views of the wrist are needed to make the diagnosis and stage the disease. Typical findings include sclerosis of the lunate, lunate collapse or loss of lunate height, lunate fragmentation, and eventually degenerative changes in the radiocarpal and midcarpal joints. Stage 1 Kienböck is diagnosed on MRI only where T1 images will show decreased vascularity of the lunate. The disease occasionally occurs bilaterally and radiographs of the opposite side should also be performed.

Prevention

This condition is generally considered idiopathic but there may be an association with high levels of exposure to vibrating or percussing hand tools.

Treatment

Treatment depends on stage of the disease. Patients at the earlier stages of the disease and those with open physes can be treated with casting or splinting and can show revascularization of the lunate over 1–2 years. Patients with significant lunate collapse are often treated surgically. Those who are radial positive (radius longer than the ulna) can be treated with radial shortening or other "joint leveling procedures." Revascularization procedures can also be done. Once degenerative changes have begun in the wrist, salvage procedures including proximal row carpectomy or partial or total wrist arthrodesis may be needed.

13. Dupuytren Contracture

Dupuytren contracture is thickening of the palmar fascia, which is the layer of tissue between the skin and the underlying tendon sheath. It typically begins as a small nodule or nodules on the palmar surface near the MCP joint that can grow over time to form cords. The cords eventually lead to flexion contracture of the digit at the PIP and MCP joints. This condition is more common at the small and ring fingers. It is often seen in individuals of Northern European descent, is more common in males, and has a hereditary predisposition.

Clinical Findings

At the early stages, subcutaneous, nonmobile nodules can be felt at the palm. At later stages, palpable subcutaneous cords can be felt and may extend into the digits and cause puckering of the overlying skin. Patients may have relatively fixed contractures of the MP and PIP joints and an inability to lay the hand flat on a table.

Differential Diagnosis

Other causes of contracture, such as joint sprains, missed fractures, and tendon injuries, should be considered. Other masses of the hand such as ganglion cysts or nerve sheath tumors can have a similar appearance to Dupuytren nodules.

Imaging & Diagnostic Studies

No imaging is needed to make the diagnosis. Radiographs of the involved digits may be helpful in assessing underlying arthritis. MRI can be useful in differentiating Dupuytren nodules from other types of masses.

Prevention

The disease is thought to be primarily genetic in nature although there are some studies that suggest an association with alcohol abuse, smoking, and very high levels of physical exposure (vibration and force) during the working life.

Treatment

Patients who are asymptomatic can be observed. However, when the contractures reach around 30 degrees, patients may have some functional deficits. Splinting and therapy have not been shown to be particularly effective. Collagenase injections are effective in breaking the cords. Surgical options include needle fasciotomy or open partial fasciectomy, with the open procedure remaining the gold standard.

14. OA of the Fingers or Wrist

OA of the first (thumb) CMC joint occurs in about 25% of women older than 55 years of age. OA of the DIP and PIP joints is also extremely common with advancing age, affecting nearly 100% of women older than the age of 80. OA of the fingers and wrist has been linked to stereotypical use of the hand with tasks performed in the same way over 10–20 years.

Clinical Findings

Although the condition is frequently asymptomatic, some patients are aware of pain at the base of the thumb when grasping, such as when unscrewing large glass jars, and there may be a clinical deformity of "squaring" or a "shoulder sign" with subluxation of the base of the thumb at the CMC joint. In addition, there may be crepitus with pressure over the CMC joint. Patients may also have a positive *grind test* with reproduction of pain with axially loading of the thumb metacarpal onto the trapezium. The fingers may show bone spurs or synovitis at the DIP or PIP joints and patients often have limited flexion or extension at these joints.

Differential Diagnosis

The differential diagnosis of thumb CMC arthritis includes De Quervain tenosynovitis (discussed earlier) in which the tenderness and swelling are more proximal.

Imaging & Diagnostic Studies

Plain-film radiographs will demonstrate osteoarthritic changes in the joint.

Prevention

Smoking has been shown to increase cartilage degeneration. For jobs that involve repeating the same hand activities many times an hour, job rotation to other tasks involving other types of hand motions may reduce the risk.

Treatment

Most patients will respond to instructions to avoid repetitive painful activities such as extreme positions of thumb abduction. Wearing an orthosis to immobilize the thumb can minimize symptoms. For the digits, avoidance of repetitive gripping can help.

Anti-inflammatory drugs are helpful for patients who experience pain at night. Steroid injection can be done into the thumb CMC joint. The DIP and PIP joints are often so small that they can be difficult to inject with a steroid. Patients refractory to conservative treatment may benefit from surgery. At the thumb CMC joint, surgery usually consists of resection arthroplasty (removal of the trapezium) with or without ligament reconstruction and/or tendon interposition. Arthritis at the DIP and PIP joints is usually treated with arthrodesis, although arthroplasty at the PIP joint can be performed for limited indications.

15. Scaphoid Fractures

Scaphoid fractures typically occur from a fall on the outstretched hand. In elderly patients with osteoporosis, the same mechanism of injury may produce a Colles (distal radius) fracture. Any patient with an acute fall and snuffbox tenderness should be treated as if they have a scaphoid fracture since early diagnosis and immobilization play a key role in healing of these fractures. Scaphoid fractures that go on to nonunion almost invariably result in degenerative changes at the wrist.

Clinical Findings

Patients will have tenderness over the anatomic snuffbox or volarly over the distal pole of the scaphoid. They may also have swelling, ecchymosis, and limited range of motion.

Differential Diagnosis

Fractures of the radial styloid, De Quervain's tenosynovitis, and CMC arthritis can cause pain in the same area.

Imaging & Diagnostic Studies

PA, lateral, oblique views of the wrist as well as a scaphoid view should be obtained if a scaphoid fracture is suspected. Often the fracture is only visible on one of these three views. Nondisplaced scaphoid fractures are often not apparent on initial plain radiographs and may require repeat radiographs 1–2 weeks later or advanced imaging such as an MRI or CT scan.

Treatment

Any patient in whom a fracture is clinically suspected should be immediately immobilized with a thumb spica splint or cast until radiographs can be repeated in 1–2 weeks or advanced imaging obtained. A scaphoid fracture that is nondisplaced can be treated in a short arm thumb spica cast. Immobilization is continued until fracture union is seen radiographically, usually at least 12 weeks. The restrictions imposed by cast immobilization can be partially avoided by percutaneous screw fixation of the scaphoid. For displaced fractures, open reduction and internal fixation usually are indicated. Symptoms from a scaphoid nonunion may occur long after the original injury. Surgical treatment with bone grafting is necessary to repair a scaphoid nonunion.

16. Mallet Finger

Mallet fingers are injuries to the extensor tendon of the finger near the DIP joint. They typically occur after a high-velocity load to the end of the digit, such as when a ball hits the end of the finger leading to a stretch or rupture of the extensor tendon.

Clinical Findings

Pain at the DIP joint with inability to actively extend the DIP joint is the usual presentation (Figure 8–8). Fractures may or may not be present.

Imaging & Diagnostic Studies

A lateral view of the phalanges can identify fractures and will determine if the joint is subluxated.

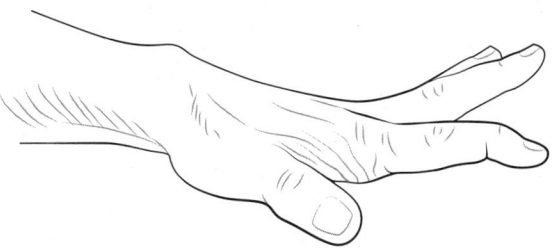

▲ **Figure 8–8.** Mallet finger. Patient is asked to extend the fingers and is unable to extend the injured DIP joint.

Treatment

Most injuries do well with conservative treatment even if they are several months old. The DIP joint is splinted in extension full-time with a Mallet splint for 6–8 weeks. The splint allows time for the tendon to recover; if the finger is flexed during this time the splint period may have to be restarted. In the case of a fracture with joint subluxation, surgical pinning may be indicated.

17. Phalangeal & Metacarpal Fractures

Fractures of the phalanges and metacarpals can occur after falls, a direct blow (such as punching a wall), or a twisting injury.

Clinical Findings

Pain, swelling, ecchymosis, decreased range of motion, and deformity are common with these fractures. Patients should be carefully assessed for malrotation. In a normal hand, gentle flexion of the digits into the palm should result in no digital overlap and all the tips of the fingers should point to the area of the scaphoid. Fractures of the metacarpals or phalanges can result in loss of this normal "cascade" of the tips of the fingers, or malrotation, with overlap or scissoring onto the neighboring digits or deviation of the border digits away from the palm.

Differential Diagnosis

Sprains, soft tissue contusions, and dislocations can have similar presentations and are readily distinguishable on radiographs.

Imaging & Diagnostic Studies

PA, oblique, and lateral views of the hand should be taken to diagnose metacarpal fractures. Fractures of the phalanges are better visualized on dedicated views of the involved finger.

Treatment

Treatment can vary depending on the displacement and type of fracture. Simple avulsion fractures can be treated with splinting or buddy-taping for pain. Nondisplaced metacarpal fractures or metacarpal fractures without malrotation or extensor lag can be treated with splinting or casting for 4–6 weeks. Phalangeal fractures treated conservatively are usually not immobilized for longer than 3–4 weeks because of the risk of permanent stiffness. Splinting or casting should be in the intrinsic plus position with the IPs extended and the MPs flexed 60–90 degrees, and should include the joint above and below the injury as well as the bordering digit(s). Fractures with malrotation, significant displacement, an unstable fracture pattern, significant shortening, joint involvement, or multiple fractures in the same hand are often treated surgically with closed reduction and pinning or open reduction and internal fixation.

18. Radius or Ulnar Fractures

Fractures of the ulnar or radius usually result from a fall or trauma. In young patients, the trauma is usually fairly high energy. In osteoporotic patients it is often a fall from standing.

Clinical Findings

Patients present with pain, swelling, ecchymosis, and deformity of the forearm or wrist. The skin should be carefully checked for any breaks that may indicate an open fracture. A careful neurovascular examination should also be performed.

Differential Diagnosis

Sprains and soft tissue injuries can have a similar presentation.

Imaging & Diagnostic Studies

PA and lateral views of the forearm or PA, lateral, and oblique views of the wrist should be obtained depending on the site of injury.

Prevention

Osteoporotic patients should be carefully treated and monitored to prevent these types of injuries. Forearm guards may be used in high-risk sporting activities such as martial arts.

Treatment

Almost all fractures of the radial shaft are treated surgically in adults. Isolated ulnar fractures can be treated with casting or splinting depending on location, displacement, and age of the patient. Distal radius fractures are treated with either casting or surgery again depending on the age of the patient, activity level, displacement of the fracture, and intra-articular involvement.

REFERENCES

Coombes BK: Effect of corticosteroid injection, physiotherapy, or both on clinical outcomes in patients with unilateral lateral epicondylalgia. JAMA 2013;309:461 [PMID: 23385272].

Freedman M: Electrodiagnostic evaluation of compressive nerve injuries of the upper extremity. Orthop Clin North Am 2012;43:409 [PMID: 23026456].

Gaskill TR: Management of multidirectional instability of the shoulder. J Am Acad Orthop Surg 2011;19:758 [PMID: 22134208].

Gruson KI: Workers' compensation and outcomes of upper extremity surgery. J Am Acad Orthop Surg 2013;21:67 [PMID: 23378370].

Harrison AK: Subacromial impingement syndrome. J Am Acad Orthop Surg 2011;19:701 [PMID: 22052646].

Jones NF: Common fractures and dislocations of the hand. Plast Reconstr Surg 2012;130:722 [PMID: 23096627].

McAuliffe JA: Tendon disorders of the hand and wrist. J Hand Surg Am 2010;35:846 [PMID: 20438999].

Palmer BA: Cubital tunnel syndrome. J Hand Surg Am 2010;35:153 [PMID: 20117320].

Poole CJM et al: International consensus criteria for diagnosing and staging hand-arm vibration syndrome. Int Arch Occup Environ Health 2019;92:117-127 [PMID: 30264331].

Popinchalk SP: Physical examination of upper extremity compressive neuropathies. Orthop Clin North Am 2012;43:417 [PMID: 23026457].

Robinson CM: Frozen shoulder. J Bone Joint Surg Br 2012;94:1 [PMID: 22219239].

Shiri R: Lateral and medial epicondylitis: role of occupational factors. Best Pract Res Clin Rheumatol 2011;25:43 [PMID: 21663849].

Sluiter BJ, Rest KM, Frings-Dresen MH: Criteria document for evaluating the work-relatedness of upper-extremity musculoskeletal disorders. Scand J Work Environ Health 2001;27 Suppl 1:1-102 [PMID: 11401243].

van der Molen HF et al: Work-related risk factors for specific shoulder disorders: a systematic review and meta-analysis. Occup Environ Med 2017;74:745-755 [PMID: 28756414].

Virtanen KJ: Operative and nonoperative treatment of clavicle fractures in adults. Acta Orthop 2012;83:65 [PMID: 22248169].

■ SELF-ASSESSMENT QUESTIONS

Select the one correct answer for each question.

Question 1: SLAP (superior labral anterior to posterior) lesions
a. are tears that occur over the superior part of the labrum of the glenohumeral joint
b. may be called Bankart lesions if they have a positive O'Brien test
c. result from repetitive lifting motions
d. present with a deficit of internal rotation compared to the other side

Question 2: Shoulder dislocations
a. are caused by excessive force applied in any direction
b. are reduced by closed techniques with no particular urgency
c. are reduced solely by the Hippocratic maneuver
d. prevent full work for only a few days

Question 3: Acromioclavicular joint injuries
a. result from falls or from direct trauma to the arm or shoulder
b. stretch the ligaments of the acromioclavicular joint but spare the coracoacromial ligaments
c. cause pain and tenderness over the acromioclavicular joint but no deformity
d. have a distinctly different clinical appearance from clavicle fractures

Question 4: Thoracic outlet syndrome
a. is common but the diagnosis is missed frequently
b. is a set of symptoms and signs caused by compression of the neurovascular structures passing out of the chest and neck and beneath the clavicle to the axilla
c. affects men more frequently than women
d. usually occurs between the ages of 40 and 60

Question 5: Lateral humeral epicondylitis
a. is an acute inflammatory process
b. is an inflammation at the attachment of the extensor carpi radialis brevis to the lateral humeral epicondyle
c. can occur among workers who perform repeated forceful pinching or power grasps
d. occurs in those who work with the wrist in sustained flexion, or repeatedly move the wrist forcefully in flexion

Question 6: Radial nerve entrapment at the elbow
a. occurs when the sensory branch of the radial nerve is compressed
b. is characterized by pain that is 4–8 cm proximal to the lateral epicondyle
c. results in pain that is aggravated by flexion of the middle finger
d. can be considered in cases of resistant lateral epicondylitis

Question 7: Ulnar nerve entrapment at the elbow
a. is less common than lateral humeral epicondylitis
b. is more common than carpal tunnel syndrome
c. may be related to old elbow injuries with enlarging osteophytes, cubitus valgus, or subluxation of the nerve out of the groove
d. is seldom work-related

Question 8: De Quervain tenosynovitis
a. causes pain in an ill-defined area along the ulnar side of the base of the thumb
b. results in localized tenderness over the ulnar side of the distal radius
c. is ruled out with a positive Finkelstein test
d. is usually associated with overuse of the thumb and wrist particularly with radial deviation, as in repetitive hammering, lifting, or pipetting

Question 9: Stenosing tenosynovitis of the flexor tendon to a finger or the flexor pollicis longus to the thumb
  a. is usually caused by repetitive finger extension
  b. is unrelated to systemic diseases such as diabetes, thyroid dysfunction, and rheumatoid arthritis
  c. heralds the onset of osteoarthritis
  d. may produce pain when the digit or thumb is forcibly flexed or extended

Question 10: Carpal tunnel syndrome
  a. is an entrapment or pressure neuropathy of the ulnar nerve as it passes through the carpal tunnel
  b. affects workers of any age but is more common in men
  c. is not affected by pregnancy, increasing age, or obesity
  d. is associated with repeated or sustained forceful gripping or repetitive wrist and finger movements involved in work

Question 11: Carpal tunnel syndrome
  a. shows early evidence of thenar atrophy and loss of sensation
  b. may lead to hand weakness if thyroid disease is present
  c. is ruled out by a negative Phalen sign but a positive Tinel sign
  d. is confirmed by median nerve electrodiagnostic studies

Question 12: Ulnar neuropathy at the wrist
  a. causes weakness of the hypothenar, interosseous muscles, but no "clawing" of the hand
  b. causes diminished sensation of the small finger only
  c. can be caused by a space-occupying lesion in the area of Guyon canal
  d. due to an occult mass rarely needs to be surgically treated to relieve the symptoms

Question 13: Hand-arm vibration syndrome (HAVS)
  a. is associated with the use of electric and pneumatic vibrating hand tools
  b. clinical pathology is seldom confined to the distal upper extremity
  c. occurs most commonly with outside work performed in warm climates
  d. pain may be related to nerve compression or chronic soft tissue inflammation

Back & Lower Extremity Injuries*

Anthony C. Luke, MD, MPH

C. Benjamin Ma, MD

SPINE PROBLEMS

1. Low Back Pain

ESSENTIALS OF DIAGNOSIS

▶ Nerve root impingement is suspected when pain is leg-dominant rather than back-dominant.

▶ Alarming symptoms include unexplained weight loss, failure to improve with treatment, severe pain for more than 6 weeks, and night or rest pain.

▶ Cauda equina syndrome is an emergency; often presents with bowel or bladder symptoms (or both).

▶ General Considerations

Low back pain remains the number one cause of disability globally and is the second most common cause for primary care visits. The annual prevalence of low back pain is 15–45%. Annual health care spending for low back and neck pain is estimated to be $87.6 billion. Low back pain is the condition associated with the highest years lived with disability. Approximately 80% of episodes of low back pain resolve within 2 weeks and 90% resolve within 6 weeks. The exact cause of the low back pain is often difficult to diagnose; its cause is often multifactorial. There are usually degenerative changes in the lumbar spine involving the disks, facet joints, and vertebral endplates (Modic changes).

Alarming symptoms for back pain caused by cancer include unexplained weight loss, failure to improve with

*Chapter adapted, with permission, from Luke A, Ma CB. Sports medicine and outpatient orthopedics. In: Papadakis MA, McPhee SJ, Rabow MW, eds. *Current Medical Diagnosis and Treatment.* 59th ed. New York: McGraw-Hill; 2020.

treatment, pain for more than 6 weeks, and pain at night or rest. History of cancer and age older than 50 years are other risk factors for malignancy. Alarming symptoms for infection include fever, rest pain, recent infection (urinary tract infection, cellulitis, pneumonia), or history of immunocompromise or injection drug use. The **cauda equina syndrome** is suggested by urinary retention or incontinence, saddle anesthesia, decreased anal sphincter tone or fecal incontinence, bilateral lower extremity weakness, and progressive neurologic deficits. Risk factors for back pain due to vertebral fracture include use of corticosteroids, age older than 70 years, history of osteoporosis, severe trauma, and presence of a contusion or abrasion. Back pain may also be the presenting symptom in other serious medical problems, including abdominal aortic aneurysm, peptic ulcer disease, kidney stones, or pancreatitis.

▶ Clinical Findings

A. Symptoms and Signs

The physical examination can be conducted with the patient in the standing, sitting, supine, and finally prone positions to avoid frequent repositioning of the patient. In the standing position, the patient's posture can be observed. Commonly encountered spinal asymmetries include scoliosis, thoracic kyphosis, and lumbar hyperlordosis. The active range of motion of the lumbar spine can be assessed while standing. The common directions include flexion, extension, rotation, and lateral bending. The one-leg standing extension test assesses for pain as the patient stands on one leg while extending the spine. A positive test can be caused by pars interarticularis fractures (spondylolysis or spondylolisthesis) or facet joint arthritis, although sensitivity and specificity of the test is limited.

With the patient sitting, motor strength, reflexes, and sensation can be tested (Table 9–1). The major muscles in the lower extremities are assessed for weakness by eliciting a resisted isometric contraction for about 5 seconds.

Table 9–1. Neurologic testing of lumbosacral nerve disorders.

Nerve Root	Motor	Reflex	Sensory Area
L1	Hip flexion	None	Groin
L2	Hip flexion	None	Thigh
L3	Extension of knee	Knee jerk	Knee
L4	Dorsiflexion of ankle	Knee jerk	Medial calf
L5	Dorsiflexion of first toe	Babinski reflex	First dorsal web space between first and second toes
S1	Plantar flexion of foot, knee flexors or hamstrings	Ankle jerk	Lateral foot
S2	Knee flexors or hamstrings	Knee flexor	Back of the thigh
S2–S4	External anal sphincter	Anal reflex, rectal tone	Perianal area

Comparing the strength bilaterally to detect subtle muscle weakness is important. Similarly, sensory testing to light touch can be checked in specific dermatomes for corresponding nerve root function. Knee (femoral nerve L2–L4), ankle (deep peroneal nerve L4–L5), and Babinski (sciatic nerve L5–S1) reflexes can be checked with the patient sitting.

In the supine position, the hip should be evaluated for range of motion, particularly internal rotation. The straight leg raise test puts traction and compression forces on the lower lumbar nerve roots (Table 9–2).

Finally, in the prone position, the clinician can carefully palpate each vertebral level of the spine and sacroiliac joints for tenderness. A rectal examination is required if the cauda equina syndrome is suspected. Superficial skin tenderness to a light touch over the lumbar spine, overreaction to maneuvers in the regular back examination, low back pain on axial loading of spine in standing, and inconsistency in the straight leg raise test or on the neurologic examination suggest nonorthopedic causes for the pain or malingering (Waddell signs).

B. Imaging

In the absence of alarming "red flag" symptoms suggesting infection, malignancy, or cauda equina syndrome, most patients do not need diagnostic imaging, including radiographs, in the first 6 weeks. The Agency for Healthcare Research and Quality guidelines for obtaining lumbar radiographs are summarized in Table 9–3. Most clinicians obtain radiographs for new back pain in patients older than 50 years. If done, radiographs of the lumbar spine should

Table 9–2. Spine: back examination.

Maneuver	Description
Inspection	Check the patient's posture in the standing position. Assess for hyperlordosis, kyphosis, and scoliosis.
Palpation	Include important landmarks: spinous process, facet joints, paravertebral muscles, sacroiliac joints, and sacrum.
Range of motion testing	Check range of motion actively (patient performs) and passively (clinician performs) especially with flexion and extension of the spine. Rotation and lateral bending are also helpful to assess symmetric motion or any restrictions.
Neurologic examination	Check motor strength, reflexes, and dermatomal sensation in the lower extremities.
Straight leg raise test	The patient lies supine and the clinician elevates the patient's leg. A positive test for sciatica pain is classically described as "electric shock"-like pain radiating down the posterior aspect of the leg from the low back. This can occur in the setting of a disk herniation or degenerative conditions causing neural foraminal stenosis. Cross-over pain, where sciatica symptoms occur down the opposite leg during a straight leg raise, usually indicates a large disk herniation.
Indirect straight leg raise test	The patient sits on the side of the exam table with the knees bent. The clinician extends the knee fully. A positive test for sciatica pain is classically described as "electric shock"-like pain radiating down the posterior aspect of the leg from the low back. Cross-over pain, where sciatica symptoms occur down the opposite leg during a straight leg raise, usually indicates a large disk herniation.

Table 9–3. AHRQ criteria for lumbar radiographs in patients with acute low back pain.

Possible fracture
Major trauma
Minor trauma in patients > 50 years
Long-term corticosteroid use
Osteoporosis
> 70 years

Possible tumor or infection
> 50 years
< 20 years
History of cancer
Constitutional symptoms
Recent bacterial infection
Injection drug use
Immunosuppression
Supine pain
Nocturnal pain

AHRQ, Agency for Healthcare Research and Quality.

include AP and lateral views. Oblique views can be useful if the neuroforamina or bone lesions need to be visualized. Magnetic resonance imaging (MRI) is the method of choice in the evaluation of symptoms not responding to conservative treatment or in the presence of red flags of serious conditions.

C. Special Tests

Electromyography (EMG) or nerve conduction studies may be useful in assessing patients with possible nerve root symptoms lasting longer than 6 weeks; back pain may or may not also be present. These tests are usually not necessary if the diagnosis of radiculopathy is clear.

▶ Treatment

A. Conservative

Nonpharmacologic treatments are key in the management of low back pain. Education alone improves patient satisfaction with recovery and recurrence. Patients require information and reassurance, especially when diagnostic procedures are not necessary. Discussion must include reviewing safe and effective methods of symptom control as well as how to decrease the risk of recurrence with proper lifting techniques, abdominal wall/core strengthening, weight loss, and smoking cessation. Tai chi, mindfulness-based stress reduction, and yoga have shown benefit for chronic low back pain patients. Exercise, psychological therapies, and multidisciplinary rehabilitation have been shown to be modestly effective for acute low back pain (strength of evidence, low).

Physical therapy exercise programs can be tailored to the patient's symptoms and pathology. A randomized controlled trial demonstrated that individualized physical therapy was clinically more beneficial than advice alone with sustained improvements at 6 months and 12 months. Strengthening and stabilization exercises effectively reduce pain and functional limitation compared with usual care. Heat and cold treatments have not shown any long-term benefits but may be used for symptomatic treatment. The efficacy of transcutaneous electrical nerve stimulation (TENS), back braces, and physical agents is unproven. Spinal manipulation, massage, and acupuncture have limited, low-strength evidence for chronic low back pain. Improvements in posture including chair ergonomics or standing desks, core stability strengthening, physical conditioning, and modifications of activities to decrease physical strain are keys for ongoing management. Radiofrequency denervation of facet joints, sacroiliac joints, or intervertebral disks did not result in clinically important improvement in chronic low back even when combined with a standardized exercise program in randomized controlled trials.

Nonsteroidal anti-inflammatory drugs (NSAIDs) are effective in the early treatment of low back pain. Acetaminophen and oral corticosteroids are relatively ineffective for chronic low back. There is limited evidence that muscle relaxants provide short-term relief; since these medications have addictive potential, they should be used with care.

Muscle relaxants are best used if there is true muscle spasm that is painful rather than simply a protective response. Opioids alleviate pain in the short term, but have the usual side effects and concerns of long-term opioid use. Treatment of more chronic neuropathic pain with alpha-2-delta ligands (eg, gabapentin), serotonin-norepinephrine reuptake inhibitors (eg, duloxetine), or tricyclic antidepressants (eg, nortriptyline) may be helpful. Epidural injections may reduce pain in the short term and reduce the need for surgery in some patients within a 1-year period but not longer. Therefore, spinal injections are not recommended for initial care of patients with low back pain without radiculopathy.

B. Surgical

Indications for back surgery include cauda equina syndrome, ongoing morbidity with no response to more than 6 months of conservative treatment, cancer, infection, or severe spinal deformity. Prognosis is improved when there is an anatomic lesion that can be corrected and symptoms are neurologic. Spinal surgery has limitations. Patient selection is very important and the specific surgery recommended should have very clear indications. Patients should understand that surgery can improve their pain but is unlikely to cure it. Surgery is not generally indicated for radiographic abnormalities alone when the patient is relatively asymptomatic. Depending on the surgery performed, possible complications include persistent pain; surgical site pain, especially if bone grafting is needed; infection; neurologic damage; nonunion; cutaneous nerve damage; implant failure; deep venous thrombosis; and death.

▶ When to Refer

- Patients with the cauda equina syndrome
- Patients with cancer, infection, fracture, or severe spinal deformity
- Patients who have not responded to conservative treatment

2. Spinal Stenosis

ESSENTIALS OF DIAGNOSIS

- ▶ Pain is usually worse with back extension and relieved by sitting.
- ▶ Occurs in older patients.
- ▶ May present with neurogenic claudication symptoms with walking.

▶ General Considerations

Osteoarthritis (OA) in the lumbar spine can cause narrowing of the spinal canal. A large disk herniation can also cause stenosis and compression of neural structures or the spinal artery resulting in "claudication" symptoms with ambulation. The condition usually affects patients aged 50 years or older.

Clinical Findings

Patients report pain that worsens with extension. They describe reproducible single or bilateral leg symptoms that are worse after walking several minutes and that are relieved by sitting ("neurogenic claudication"). On examination, patients often exhibit limited extension of the lumbar spine, which may reproduce the symptoms radiating down the legs. A thorough neurovascular examination is recommended.

Treatment

Exercises, usually flexion-based as demonstrated by a physical therapist, can help relieve symptoms. Physical therapy showed similar results as surgical decompression in a randomized trial, though there was a 57% crossover rate from physical therapy to surgery. Facet joint corticosteroid injections can also reduce pain symptoms. While epidural corticosteroid injections have been shown to provide immediate improvements in pain and function for patients with radiculopathy, the benefits are small and only short term. Consequently, there is limited evidence to recommend epidural corticosteroids for spinal stenosis, and they are not without potential risk. In 2012, there was a fungal meningitis outbreak during spinal injections related to contamination of injectable methylprednisolone prepared in a single compounding pharmacy.

Surgical treatments for spinal stenosis include spinal decompression (widening the spinal canal or laminectomy), nerve root decompression (freeing a single nerve), and spinal fusion (joining the vertebra to eliminate motion and diminish pain from the arthritic joints). However, a Cochrane review showed surgery was not clearly better than nonsurgical treatment and had complication rates of 10–24% compared to 0% for nonoperative treatments. Thus, the role of surgery for spinal stenosis is limited. In one multicenter randomized trial, subgroups initially improved significantly more with surgery than with nonoperative treatment. Variables associated with greater treatment effects included lower baseline disability scores (Oswestry Disability Index), not smoking, neuroforaminal stenosis, predominant leg pain rather than back pain, not lifting at work, and the presence of a neurologic deficit. However, long-term follow-up of the patients with symptomatic spinal stenosis who received surgery in the multicenter randomized trial showed less benefit of surgery between 4 and 8 years, suggesting that the advantage of surgery for spinal stenosis diminishes over time. A Cochrane review of 24 randomized controlled trials of treatments for lumbar spinal stenosis showed that various surgeries including decompression plus fusion and interspinous process spacers were not superior to conventional spinal decompression surgery alone. Some evidence suggests that instrumentation (adding surgical hardware to a spinal fusion) leads to a higher fusion rate, but there is no evidence that it makes any difference to clinical outcomes.

When to Refer

- If a patient exhibits radicular or claudication symptoms for longer than 12 weeks.
- MRI or computed tomography (CT) confirmation of significant, symptomatic spinal stenosis.
- However, surgery has not been shown to have clear benefit over nonsurgical treatment for lumbar spinal stenosis.

3. Lumbar Disk Herniation

ESSENTIALS OF DIAGNOSIS

▶ Pain with back flexion or prolonged sitting.
▶ Radicular pain into the leg due to compression of neural structures.
▶ Lower extremity numbness and weakness.

General Considerations

Lumbar disk herniation is usually due to bending or heavy loading (eg, lifting) with the back in flexion, causing herniation or extrusion of disk contents (nucleus pulposus) into the spinal cord area. However, there may not be an inciting incident. Disk herniations usually occur from degenerative disk disease (desiccation of the annulus fibrosis) in patients between 30 and 50 years old. The L5–S1 disk is affected in 90% of cases. Compression of neural structures, such as the sciatic nerve, causes radicular pain. Severe compression of the spinal cord can cause the cauda equina syndrome, a surgical emergency.

Clinical Findings

A. Symptoms and Signs

Discogenic pain typically is localized in the low back at the level of the affected disk and is worse with activity. "Sciatica" causes electric shock-like pain radiating down the posterior aspect of the leg often to below the knee. Symptoms usually worsen with back flexion such as bending or sitting for long periods (eg, driving). A significant disk herniation can cause numbness and weakness, including weakness with plantar flexion of the foot (L5/S1) or dorsiflexion of the toes (L4/L5). The cauda equina syndrome should be ruled out if the patient complains of perianal numbness or bowel or bladder incontinence.

B. Imaging

Plain radiographs are helpful to assess spinal alignment (scoliosis, lordosis), disk space narrowing, and OA changes. MRI is the best method to assess the level and morphology of the herniation and is recommended if surgery is planned.

Treatment

For an acute exacerbation of pain symptoms, bed rest is appropriate for up to 48 hours. Otherwise, first-line treatments include modified activities; NSAIDs and other analgesics; and physical therapy, including core stabilization and McKenzie back exercises. The **McKenzie method** identifies the mechanical direction of motion in the back that causes more or less pain, using careful history and physical examination to guide the treatment approach. An exercise protocol is carefully designed to centralize or alleviate the pain. Following nonsurgical treatment for a lumbar disk for over 1 year, the incidence of low back pain recurrence is at least 40% and is predicted by longer time to initial resolution of pain. In a randomized trial, oral prednisone caused a modest improvement in function at 3 weeks, but there was no significant improvement in pain in patients with acute radiculopathy who were monitored for 1 year. The initial dose for oral prednisone is approximately 1 mg/kg once daily with tapering doses over 10–15 days. Analgesics for neuropathic pain, such as the calcium channel alpha-2-delta ligands (ie, gabapentin, pregabalin) or tricyclic antidepressants, may be helpful. Epidural and transforaminal corticosteroid injections can be beneficial. A systematic review demonstrated strong evidence that fluoroscopic-guided epidural injections gave short-term benefit (< 6 months) in acute radicular pain for individuals. However, epidural injections have not shown any change in long-term surgery rates for disk herniations.

The severity of pain and disability as well as failure of conservative therapy were the most important reasons for surgery. A large trial has shown that patients who underwent surgery for a lumbar disk herniation achieved greater improvement than conservatively treated patients in all primary and secondary outcomes except return to work status after 4-year follow-up. Patients with sequestered fragments, symptom duration greater than 6 months, higher levels of low back pain, or who were neither working nor disabled at baseline showed greater surgical treatment effects. Microdiskectomy is the standard method of treatment with a low rate of complications and satisfactory results over 90% in the largest series. A minimally invasive technique is percutaneous endoscopic diskectomy, which involves using an endoscope to remove fragments of disk herniation (interlaminar or transforaminal approaches) under local anesthesia, although results are less successful than with microdiskectomy. Disk replacement surgery has shown benefits in short-term pain relief, disability, and quality of life compared with spine fusion surgery.

When to Refer

- Cauda equina syndrome
- Progressive worsening of neurologic symptoms
- Loss of motor function (sensory losses can be followed in the outpatient clinic)

4. Neck Pain

ESSENTIALS OF DIAGNOSIS

▶ Chronic neck pain is mostly caused by degenerative joint disease; whiplash often follows a traumatic neck injury, responds to conservative treatment.

▶ Cervical radiculopathy symptoms can be referred to the shoulder, arm, or upper back.

▶ Poor posture is often a factor for persistent neck pain.

General Considerations

Most neck pain, especially in older patients, is due to mechanical degeneration involving the cervical disks, facet joints, and ligamentous structures and may occur in the setting of degenerative changes at other sites. Pain can also come from the supporting neck musculature, which often acts to protect the underlying neck structures. Posture is a very important factor, especially in younger patients. Many work-related neck symptoms are due to poor posture and repetitive motions over time. Acute injuries can also occur secondary to trauma. Whiplash occurs from rapid flexion and extension of the neck and affects 15–40% of people in motor vehicle accidents; chronic pain develops in 5–7%. Neck fractures are serious traumatic injuries acutely and can lead to OA in the long term. Ultimately, many degenerative conditions of the neck result in cervical canal stenosis or neural foraminal stenosis, sometimes affecting underlying neural structures.

Cervical radiculopathy can cause neurologic symptoms in the upper extremities usually involving the C5–C7 disks. Patients with neck pain may report associated headaches and shoulder pain. Both peripheral nerve entrapment and cervical radiculopathy, known as a "double crush" injury, may develop. Thoracic outlet syndrome, in which there is mechanical compression of the brachial plexus and neurovascular structures with overhead positioning of the arm, should be considered in the differential diagnosis of neck pain. Other causes of neck pain include rheumatoid arthritis, fibromyalgia, osteomyelitis, neoplasms, polymyalgia rheumatica, compression fractures, pain referred from visceral structures (eg, angina), and functional disorders. Amyotrophic lateral sclerosis, multiple sclerosis, syringomyelia, spinal cord tumors, and Parsonage-Turner syndrome can mimic myelopathy from cervical arthritis.

Clinical Findings

A. Symptoms and Signs

Neck pain may be limited to the posterior region or, depending on the level of the symptomatic joint, may radiate segmentally to the occiput, anterior chest, shoulder girdle, arm, forearm, and hand. It may be intensified by active or passive neck motions. The general distribution of pain and paresthesias corresponds roughly to the involved dermatome in the upper extremity.

The patient's posture should be assessed, checking for shoulder rolled forward or head forward posture as well as scoliosis in the thoracolumbar spine. Patients with discogenic neck pain often complain of pain with flexion, which causes cervical disks to herniate posteriorly. Extension of the neck usually affects the neural foraminal and facet joints of the neck. Rotation and lateral flexion of the cervical spine should be measured both to the left and the right. Limitation of cervical movements is the most common objective finding.

A detailed neurovascular examination of the upper extremities should be performed, including sensory input to light touch and temperature; motor strength testing, especially the hand intrinsic muscles (thumb extension strength [C6], opponens strength (thumb to pinky) [C7], and finger abductors and adductors strength [C8–T1]); and upper extremity reflexes (biceps, triceps, brachioradialis). True cervical radiculopathy symptoms should match an expected dermatomal or myotomal distribution. The Spurling test involves asking the patient to rotate and extend the neck to one side (Table 9–4). The clinician can apply a gentle axial load to the neck. Reproduction of the cervical radiculopathy symptoms is a positive sign of nerve root compression. Palpation of the neck is best performed with the patient in the supine position where the clinician can palpate each level of the cervical spine with the muscles of the neck relaxed.

Table 9–4. Spine: neck examination.

Maneuver	Description
Inspection	Check the patient's posture in the standing position. Assess for cervical hyperlordosis, head forward posture, kyphosis, scoliosis, torticollis.
Palpation	Include important landmarks: spinous process, facet joints, paracervical muscles (sternocleidomastoid, scalene muscles).
Range of motion testing	Check range of motion in the cervical spine, especially with flexion and extension. Rotation and lateral bending are also helpful to assess symmetric motion or any restrictions. Pain and radicular symptoms can be exacerbated by range of motion testing.
Neurologic examination	Check motor strength, reflexes, and dermatomal sensation in the upper (and lower if necessary) extremities.
Spurling test	Involves asking the patient to rotate and extend the neck to one side. The clinician can apply a gentle axial load to the neck. Reproduction of the cervical radiculopathy symptoms is a positive sign of nerve root compression.

B. Imaging

Radiographs of the cervical spine include the AP and lateral view of the cervical spine. The odontoid view is usually added to rule out traumatic fractures and congenital abnormalities. Oblique views of the cervical spine can provide further information about arthritis changes and assess the neural foramina for narrowing. Plain radiographs can be completely normal in patients who have suffered an acute cervical strain. Comparative reduction in height of the involved disk space and osteophytes are frequent findings when there are degenerative changes in the cervical spine. Loss of cervical lordosis is commonly seen but is nonspecific.

MRI is the best method to assess the cervical spine since the soft tissue structures (such as the disks, spinal cord, and nerve roots) can be evaluated. If the patient has signs of cervical radiculopathy with motor weakness, these more sensitive imaging modalities should be obtained urgently. CT scanning is the most useful method if bony abnormalities, such as fractures, are suspected.

EMG is useful in order to differentiate peripheral nerve entrapment syndromes from cervical radiculopathy. However, sensitivity of electrodiagnostic testing for cervical radiculopathy ranges from only 50% to 71%, so a negative test does not rule out nerve root problems.

▶ Treatment

In the absence of trauma or evidence of infection, malignancy, neurologic findings, or systemic inflammation, the patient can be treated conservatively. More frequent observation of individuals in whom very severe symptoms are present early on after an injury is recommended because high pain-related disability is a predictor of poor outcome at 1 year even if individuals decline care. Ergonomics should be assessed at work and home. A course of neck stretching, strengthening, and postural exercises in physical therapy have demonstrated benefit in relieving symptoms. A soft cervical collar can be useful for short-term use (up to 1–2 weeks) in acute neck injuries. Chiropractic manual manipulation and mobilization can provide short-term benefit for mechanical neck pain. Although the rate of complications is low (5–10/million manipulations), care should be taken whenever there are neurologic symptoms present. Specific patients may respond to use of home cervical traction. NSAIDs are commonly used and opioids may be needed in cases of severe neck pain. Muscle relaxants (eg, cyclobenzaprine 5–10 mg orally three times daily) can be used for short-term if there is muscle spasm or as a sedative to aid in sleeping. Acute radicular symptoms can be treated with neuropathic medications (eg, gabapentin 300–1200 mg orally three times daily), and a short course of oral prednisone (5–10 days) can be considered (starting at 1 mg/kg). Cervical foraminal or facet joint injections can also reduce symptoms. Surgeries are successful in reducing neurologic symptoms in 80–90% of cases, but are still considered as treatments of last resort. Common surgeries for cervical degenerative disk disease include anterior cervical diskectomy with fusion and cervical disk arthroplasty. A meta-analysis of 18 randomized controlled trials showed that cervical disk arthroplasty was superior to anterior diskectomy and fusion for the treatment of symptomatic cervical disk disease, with better success and less reoperation rates.

When to Refer

- Patients with severe symptoms with motor weakness
- Surgical decompression surgery if the symptoms are severe and there is identifiable, correctable pathology

HIP

1. Hip Fractures

ESSENTIALS OF DIAGNOSIS

▶ Internal rotation of the hip is the best provocative diagnostic maneuver.

▶ Hip fractures should be surgically repaired as soon as possible (within 24 hours).

▶ Delayed treatment of hip fractures in older adults leads to increased complications and mortality.

General Considerations

Approximately 4% of the 7.9 million fractures that occur each year in the United States are hip fractures. There is a high mortality rate among older adult patients following hip fracture, with death occurring in 8–9% within 30 days and in approximately 25–30% within 1 year. Osteoporosis, female sex, height greater than 5-ft 8-in, and age older than 50 years are risk factors for hip fracture. Hip fractures usually occur after a fall. High-velocity trauma is needed in younger patients. Stress fractures can occur in athletes or individuals with poor bone mineral density following repetitive loading activities.

Clinical Findings

A. Symptoms and Signs

Patients typically report pain in the groin, though pain radiating to the lateral hip, buttock, or knee can also commonly occur. If a displaced fracture is present, the patient will not be able to bear weight and the leg may be externally rotated. Gentle logrolling of the leg with the patient supine helps rule out a fracture. Examination of the hip demonstrates pain with deep palpation in the area of the femoral triangle (similar to palpating the femoral artery). Provided the patient can tolerate it, the clinician can, with the patient supine, flex the hip to 90 degrees with the knee flexed to 90 degrees. The leg can then be internally and externally rotated to assess the range of motion on both sides. Pain with internal rotation of the hip is the most sensitive test to identify intra-articular hip pathology. Hip flexion, extension, abduction, and adduction strength can be tested.

Patients with hip stress fractures have less pain on physical examination than described previously but typically have pain with weight-bearing. The Trendelenburg test can be performed to examine for weakness or instability of the hip abductors, primarily the gluteus medius muscle; the patient balances first on one leg, raising the nonstanding knee toward the chest. The clinician can stand behind the patient and observe for dropping of the pelvis and buttock on the nonstance side (Table 9–5). Another functional test is asking the patient to hop or jump during the examination. If the patient has a compatible clinical history of pain and is unable or unwilling to hop, then a stress fracture should be ruled out. The back should be carefully examined in patients with hip complaints, including examining for signs of sciatica.

Following displaced hip fractures, a thorough medical evaluation and treatment should be pursued to maximize the patients' ability to undergo operative intervention. Patients who are unable to get up by themselves may have been immobile for hours or even days following their falls. Thus, clinicians must exclude rhabdomyolysis, hypothermia, deep venous thrombosis, pulmonary embolism, and other conditions that can occur with prolonged immobilization. Delay of operative intervention leads to an increased risk of perioperative morbidity and mortality.

Table 9–5. Hip examination.

Maneuver	Description
Inspection	Examine for the alignment of the lower extremity, consider lumbar spine exam
Palpation	Include important landmarks: ASIS and AIIS (proximal quadriceps muscle insertions), greater trochanter (gluteal tendon insertions and bursa), anterior femoral triangle (hip joint and hip flexion insertion), ischial tuberosity (hamstring tendon insertion), sacroiliac joints
Range of motion testing	Check range of motion passively (clinician performs) especially internal and external rotation of the hip
Hip strength testing	Test resisted hip flexion, extension, abduction, and adduction strength manually
Trendelenburg test	The patient balances first on one leg, raising the nonstanding knee toward the chest. The clinician can stand behind the patient and observe for dropping of the pelvis and buttock on the nonstance side

AIIS, anterior inferior iliac spine; ASIS, anterior superior iliac spine.

B. Imaging

Useful radiographic views of the hip include AP views of the pelvis and bilateral hips and frog-leg-lateral views of the painful hip. A CT scan or MRI may be necessary to identify the hip fracture pattern or to evaluate nondisplaced fractures. Hip fractures are generally described by location, including femoral neck, intertrochanteric, or subtrochanteric.

▶ **Treatment**

Almost all patients with a hip fracture will require surgery and may need to be admitted to the hospital for pain control while they await surgery. Surgery is recommended within the first 24 hours because studies have shown that delaying surgery 48 hours results in at least twice the rate of major and minor medical complications, including pneumonia, pressure injuries (formerly pressure ulcers), and deep venous thrombosis. High-volume centers have multidisciplinary teams (including orthopedic surgeons, internists, social workers, and specialized physical therapists) to comanage these patients, which improves perioperative medical care and expedites preoperative evaluation leading to reduced costs.

Stress fractures in active patients require a period of protected weight-bearing and a gradual return to activities, although it may take 4–6 months before a return to normal activities. Femoral neck fractures are commonly treated with hemiarthroplasty or total hip replacement. This allows the patient to begin weight-bearing immediately postoperatively. Peritrochanteric hip fractures are treated with open reduction internal fixation, where plate and screw construct or intramedullary devices are used. The choice of implant will depend on the fracture pattern. Since fracture fixation requires the fracture to proceed to union, the patient may need to have protected weight-bearing during the early postoperative period. Dislocation, periprosthetic fracture, and avascular necrosis of the hip are common complications after surgery. Patients should be mobilized as soon as possible postoperatively to avoid pulmonary complications and pressure injuries. Supervised physical therapy and rehabilitation are important for the patient to regain as much function as possible. Unfortunately, most patients following hip fractures will lose some degree of independence. Patients with hip fracture surgery when compared with elective total hip replacement have been shown to have higher risk of in-hospital mortality.

▶ **Prevention**

Bone density screening can identify patients at risk for osteopenia or osteoporosis, and treatment can be planned accordingly. There is strong evidence that bisphosphonates, denosumab, and teriparatide reduce fractures compared with placebo, with relative risk reductions of 0.60–0.80 for nonvertebral fractures. Nutrition and bone health (bone densitometry, serum calcium, and 25-OH vitamin D levels) should be reviewed with the patient. However, there is no evidence that increasing calcium intake prevents hip fractures. For patients with decreased mobility, systemic anticoagulation should be considered to avoid deep venous thrombosis. Fall prevention exercise programs are available for older adult patients at risk for falls and hip fractures. Hip protectors are uncomfortable and have less use in preventing fractures.

▶ **When to Refer**

- All patients in whom hip fracture is suspected
- All patients with hip fracture or in whom the diagnosis is uncertain after radiographs

2. Osteoarthritis

ESSENTIALS OF DIAGNOSIS

▸ Pain deep in the groin on the affected side.
▸ Swelling.
▸ Degeneration of joint cartilage.
▸ Loss of active and passive range of motion in severe OA.

▶ **General Considerations**

In the United States, the prevalence of OA will grow as the number of persons older than age 65 years doubles to more than 70 million by 2030. Cartilage loss and OA symptoms are preceded by damage to the collagen-proteoglycan matrix. The etiology of OA is often multifactorial, including previous trauma, prior high-impact activities, genetic factors, obesity, and rheumatologic or metabolic conditions. Femoroacetabular impingement, which affects younger active patients, is considered an early development of hip OA.

▶ **Clinical Findings**

A. Symptoms and Signs

OA usually causes pain in the affected joint with loading of the joint or at the extremes of motion. Mechanical symptoms—such as swelling, grinding, catching, and locking—suggest internal derangement, which is indicated by damaged cartilage or bone fragments that affect the smooth range of motion expected at an articular joint. Pain can also produce the sensation of "buckling" or "giving way" due to muscle inhibition. As the joint degeneration becomes more advanced, the patient loses active range of motion and may lose passive range of motion as well.

Patients complain of pain deep in the groin on the affected side and have problems with weight-bearing activities such as walking, climbing stairs, and getting up from a chair. They may limp and develop a lurch during their gait, leaning toward the unaffected side as they walk to reduce pressure on the arthritic hip.

B. Imaging

An anterior-posterior weight-bearing radiograph of the pelvis with a lateral view of the symptomatic hip are preferred views for evaluation of hip OA. Joint space narrowing and sclerosis suggest early OA, while osteophytes near the femoral head or acetabulum and subchondral bone cysts are more advanced changes. However, not all patients with radiographic hip OA have hip or groin pain; the converse is also true. Radiographs have low sensitivity for hip pain (sensitivity 36.7%, specificity 90.5%, positive predictive value 6.0%, and negative predictive value 98.9%). Findings of femoroacetabular impingement are commonly reported on radiograph reports with arthritic changes and anatomic variations involving the acetabulum and femoral head-neck junction. After age 35, MRI of the hips already show labral changes in almost 70% of asymptomatic patients.

▶ Treatment

A. Conservative

Changes in the articular cartilage are irreversible. Therefore, a cure for the diseased joint is not possible, although symptoms or structural issues can be managed to try to maintain activity level. Conservative treatment for patients with OA includes activity modification, proper footwear, therapeutic exercises, weight loss, and use of assistive devices (such as a cane). A 2014 randomized study found that physical therapy did not lead to greater improvement in pain or function compared with sham treatment in patients with hip OA. In a large cohort, running significantly reduced OA and hip replacement risk possibly since running is associated with lower BMI. Analgesics may be effective in some cases. Corticosteroid injections can be considered for short-term relief of pain; however, hip injections are best performed under fluoroscopic, ultrasound, or CT guidance to ensure accurate injection in the joint.

B. Surgical

Joint replacement surgeries are effective and cost-effective for patients with significant symptoms and functional limitations, providing improvements in pain, function, and quality of life. Various surgical techniques and computer-assisted navigation during operation continue to be investigated. A review of nine randomized controlled trials concluded that a direct anterior approach for hip replacement was associated with a shorter incision, lower blood loss, lower pain scores, and earlier functional recovery. However, there was no significant difference in complication rates between groups for the direct anterior or posterior approaches.

Hip resurfacing surgery is a newer joint replacement technique. Rather than using a traditional artificial joint implant of the whole neck and femur, only the femoral head is removed and replaced. Evidence to date suggests that hip resurfacing is comparable to total hip replacement and is a viable alternative for younger patients. The cumulative survival rate of this implant at 10 years is estimated to be 94%. Concerns following resurfacing surgery include the risk of femoral neck fracture and collapse of the head. In a systematic review of national databases, the average time to revision was 3.0 years for metal-on-metal hip resurfacing versus 7.8 years for total hip arthroplasty. Dislocations were more frequent with total hip arthroplasty than metal-on-metal hip resurfacing: 4.4 versus 0.9 per 1000 person-years, respectively.

Guidelines recommend prophylaxis for venous thromboembolic disease for a minimum of 14 days after arthroplasty of the hip or knee using warfarin, low-molecular-weight heparin, fondaparinux, aspirin, rivaroxaban, dabigatran, apixaban, or portable mechanical compression.

▶ When to Refer

Patients with sufficient disability, limited benefit from conservative therapy, and evidence of severe OA can be referred for joint replacement surgery.

KNEE

1. Knee Pain

ESSENTIALS OF DIAGNOSIS

▶ Effusion can occur with intra-articular pathology (eg, OA, meniscus, and cruciate ligament tears).

▶ Acute knee swelling (due to hemarthrosis) within 2 hours may indicate ligament injuries or patellar dislocation or fracture.

▶ General Considerations

The knee is the largest joint in the body and is susceptible to injury from trauma, inflammation, infection, and degenerative changes. The knee is a hinge joint. The joint line exists between the femoral condyles and tibial plateaus. Separating and cushioning these bony surfaces is the lateral and medial meniscal cartilage, which functions as a shock absorber during weight-bearing, protecting the articular cartilage. The patella is a large sesamoid bone anterior to the joint. It is embedded in the quadriceps tendon, and it articulates with the trochlear groove of the femur. Poor patellar tracking in the trochlear groove is a common source of knee pain especially when the cause is atraumatic in nature. The knee is stabilized by the collateral ligaments against varus (lateral collateral ligament [LCL]) and valgus (medial collateral ligament [MCL]) stresses. The tibia is limited in its anterior movement by the anterior cruciate ligament (ACL) and in its posterior movement by the posterior cruciate ligament (PCL). The bursae of the knee are located between the skin and bony prominences. They are sac-like structures with a synovial lining. They act to decrease friction of tendons and muscles as they move over adjacent bony structures.

Excessive external pressure or friction can lead to swelling and pain of the bursae. The prepatellar bursae (located between the skin and patella) and the pes anserine bursa (which is medial and inferior to the patella, just below the tibial plateau) are most commonly affected. Joint fluid, when excessive due to synovitis or trauma, can track posteriorly through a potential space, resulting in a popliteal cyst (also called a Baker cyst). Other structures that are susceptible to overuse injury and may cause knee pain following repetitive activity include the patellofemoral joint and the iliotibial band. OA of the knees is common after 50 years of age and can develop due to previous trauma, aging, activities, alignment issues, and genetic predisposition.

▶ Clinical Findings

A. Symptoms and Signs

Evaluation of knee pain should begin with general questions regarding duration and rapidity of symptom onset and the mechanism of injury or aggravating symptoms. Overuse or degenerative problems can occur with stress or compression from sports, hobbies, or occupation. A history of trauma, previous orthopedic problems with, or surgery to, the affected knee should also be specifically queried. Symptoms of infection (fever, recent bacterial infections, risk factors for sexually transmitted infections [such as gonorrhea] or other bacterial infections [such as staphylococcal infection]) should always be elicited.

Common symptom complaints include the following:

1. Presence of grinding, clicking, or popping with bending may be indicative of OA or the patellofemoral syndrome.

2. "Locking" or "catching" when walking suggests an internal derangement, such as meniscal injury or a loose body in the knee.

3. Intra-articular swelling of the knee or an effusion indicates an internal derangement or a synovial pathology. Large swelling may cause a popliteal (Baker) cyst. Acute swelling within minutes to hours suggests a hemarthrosis, most likely due to an ACL injury, fracture, or patellar dislocation, especially if trauma is involved.

4. Lateral "snapping" with flexion and extension of the knee may indicate inflammation of the iliotibial band.

5. Pain that is worsened with bending and walking downstairs suggests issues with the patellofemoral joint, usually degenerative such as chondromalacia of the patella or OA.

6. Pain that occurs when rising after prolonged sitting suggests a problem with tracking of the patella.

A careful history coupled with a physical examination that includes observation, palpation, and range of motion testing, as well as specific tests for particular anatomic structures is frequently sufficient to establish a diagnosis. When there is a knee joint effusion caused by increased fluid in the intra-articular space, physical examination will demonstrate swelling in the hollow or dimple around the patella and distention of the suprapatellar space.

Table 9–6 shows the differential diagnosis of knee pain, and Table 9–7 outlines possible diagnoses based on the location of pain.

B. Laboratory Findings

Laboratory testing of aspirated joint fluid, when indicated, can lead to a definitive diagnosis in most patients.

Table 9–6. Differential diagnosis of knee pain.

Mechanical dysfunction or disruption
Internal derangement of the knee: injury to the menisci or ligaments
Degenerative changes caused by osteoarthritis
Dynamic dysfunction or misalignment of the patella
Fracture as a result of trauma
Intra-articular inflammation or increased pressure
Internal derangement of the knee: injury to the menisci or ligaments
Inflammation or infection of the knee joint
Ruptured popliteal (Baker) cyst
Peri-articular inflammation
Internal derangement of the knee: injury to the menisci or ligaments
Prepatellar or anserine bursitis
Ligamentous sprain

Table 9–7. Location of common causes of knee pain.

Medial knee pain
Medial compartment osteoarthritis
Medial collateral ligament strain
Medial meniscal injury
Anserine bursitis (pain over the proximal medial tibial plateau)
Anterior knee pain
Patellofemoral syndrome (often bilateral)
Osteoarthritis
Prepatellar bursitis (associated with swelling anterior to the patella)
"Jumper's knee" (pain at the inferior pole of the patella)
Septic arthritis
Gout or other inflammatory disorder
Lateral knee pain
Lateral meniscal injury
Iliotibial band syndrome (pain superficially along the distal iliotibial band near lateral femoral condyle or lateral tibial insertion)
Lateral collateral ligament sprain (rare)
Posterior knee pain
Popliteal (Baker) cyst
Osteoarthritis
Meniscal tears
Hamstring or calf tendinopathy

C. Imaging

Knee pain is evaluated with plain (weight-bearing) radiographs and MRI most commonly, but CT and ultrasound are sometimes useful.

An acute hemarthrosis represents bloody swelling that usually occurs within the first 1–2 hours following trauma. In situations where the trauma may be activity-related and not a result of a fall or collision, the differential diagnosis most commonly includes ACL tear (responsible for more than 70% in adults), fracture (patella, tibial plateau, femoral supracondylar, growth plate [physeal]), and patellar dislocation. Meniscal tears are unlikely to cause large hemarthrosis.

2. Anterior Cruciate Ligament Injury

ESSENTIALS OF DIAGNOSIS

▸ An injury involving an audible pop when the knee buckles.

▸ Acute swelling immediately (or within 2 hours).

▸ Instability occurs with lateral movement activities and going downstairs.

▶ General Considerations

The ACL connects the posterior aspect of the lateral femoral condyle to the anterior aspect of the tibia. Its main function is to control anterior translation of the tibia on the femur. It also provides rotational stability of the tibia on the femur. ACL tears are common with sporting injuries. They can result from both contact (valgus blow to the knee) and noncontact (jumping, pivoting, and deceleration) activities. The patient usually falls down following the injury, has acute swelling and difficulty with weight-bearing, and complains of instability. ACL injuries are common in skiing, soccer, football, and basketball among young adolescents and middle-aged patients. Prepubertal and older patients usually sustain fractures instead of ligamentous injuries.

▶ Clinical Findings

A. Symptoms and Signs

Acute ACL injuries usually lead to acute swelling of the knee, causing difficulty with motion. After the swelling has resolved, the patient can walk with a "stiff-knee" gait or quadriceps avoidance gait because of the instability. Patients describe symptoms of instability while performing side-to-side maneuvers or descending stairs. Stability tests assess the amount of laxity of the knee while performing these maneuvers. The Lachman test (84–87% sensitivity and 93% specificity) is performed with the patient lying supine and the knee flexed to 20–30 degrees (Table 9–8). The clinician grasps the distal femur from the lateral side

and the proximal tibia with the other hand on the medial side. With the knee in neutral position, stabilize the femur, and pull the tibia anteriorly using a similar force to lifting a 10- to 15-lb weight. Excessive anterior translation of the tibia compared with the other side indicates injury to the ACL. The anterior drawer test (48% sensitivity and 87% specificity) is performed with the patient lying supine and the knee flexed to 90 degrees (Table 9–8). The clinician stabilizes the patient's foot by sitting on it and grasps the proximal tibia with both hands around the calf and pulls anteriorly. A positive test finds ACL laxity compared with the unaffected side. The pivot shift test is used to determine the amount of rotational laxity of the knee. The patient is examined while lying supine with the knee in full extension. It is then slowly flexed while applying internal rotation and a valgus stress. The clinician feels for a subluxation at 20–40 degrees of knee flexion. The patient must remain very relaxed to have a positive test.

B. Imaging

Plain radiographs are usually negative in ACL tears but are useful to rule out fractures. A small avulsion injury can sometimes be seen over the lateral compartment of the knee ("Segond" fracture) and is pathognomonic of an ACL injury. An ACL injury that avulsed the tibial spine can be seen in radiographs. MRI is the best tool to diagnose ACL tears and associated articular and meniscal cartilage issues. It has greater than 95% sensitivity and specificity for ACL tears.

▶ Treatment

Most young and active patients will require surgical reconstruction of the ACL. Some data suggest that reconstruction within 5 months of the tear has better outcomes. However, a small randomized trial suggested that acute ACL injuries can be treated nonoperatively and delayed ACL reconstruction had similar outcomes to acute ACL reconstructions but patients for whom the reconstruction is delayed have more cartilage or meniscus problems at the time of surgery. Common surgical techniques use the patient's own tissue, usually the patellar or hamstring tendons (autograft) or a cadaver graft (allograft) to arthroscopically reconstruct the torn ACL. Different patient groups experienced improved results with specific surgical graft choices. However, allografts do have a higher failure rate when compared with autografts. Recovery from surgery usually requires 6 months.

Nonoperative treatments are usually reserved for older patients or those with a very sedentary lifestyle. Physical therapy can focus on hamstring strengthening and core stability. An ACL brace can help stability. Longitudinal studies have demonstrated that nonoperative management of an ACL tear can lead to a higher incidence of meniscus tears. Cost-analysis studies have shown that early ACL reconstruction can be more beneficial than nonoperative treatment and delayed subsequent surgeries.

Table 9–8. Knee examination.

Maneuver	Description
Inspection	Examine for the alignment of the lower extremities (varus, valgus, knee recurvatum), ankle eversion and foot pronation, gait, SEADS.
Palpation	Include important landmarks: patellofemoral joint, medial and lateral joint lines (especially posterior aspects), pes anserine bursa, distal iliotibial band, and Gerdy tubercle (iliotibial band insertion).
Range of motion testing	Check range of motion actively (patient performs) and passively (clinician performs), especially with flexion and extension of the knee normally 0–10 degrees of extension and 120–150 degrees of flexion.
Knee strength testing	Test resisted knee extension and knee flexion strength manually.
Ligament stress tests	
Lachman test Fix femur	Performed with the patient lying supine, and the knee flexed to 20–30 degrees. The examiner grasps the distal femur from the lateral side, and the proximal tibia with the other hand on the medial side. With the knee in neutral position, stabilize the femur, and pull the tibia anteriorly using a similar force to lifting a 10–15 lb weight. Excessive anterior translation of the tibia compared with the other side indicates injury to the anterior cruciate ligament.
Anterior drawer	Performed with the patient lying supine and the knee flexed to 90 degrees. The clinician stabilizes the patient's foot by sitting on it and grasps the proximal tibia with both hands around the calf and pulls anteriorly. A positive test finds anterior cruciate ligament laxity compared with the unaffected side.

(continued)

Table 9–8. Knee examination. (Continued)

Maneuver	Description
Pivot shift 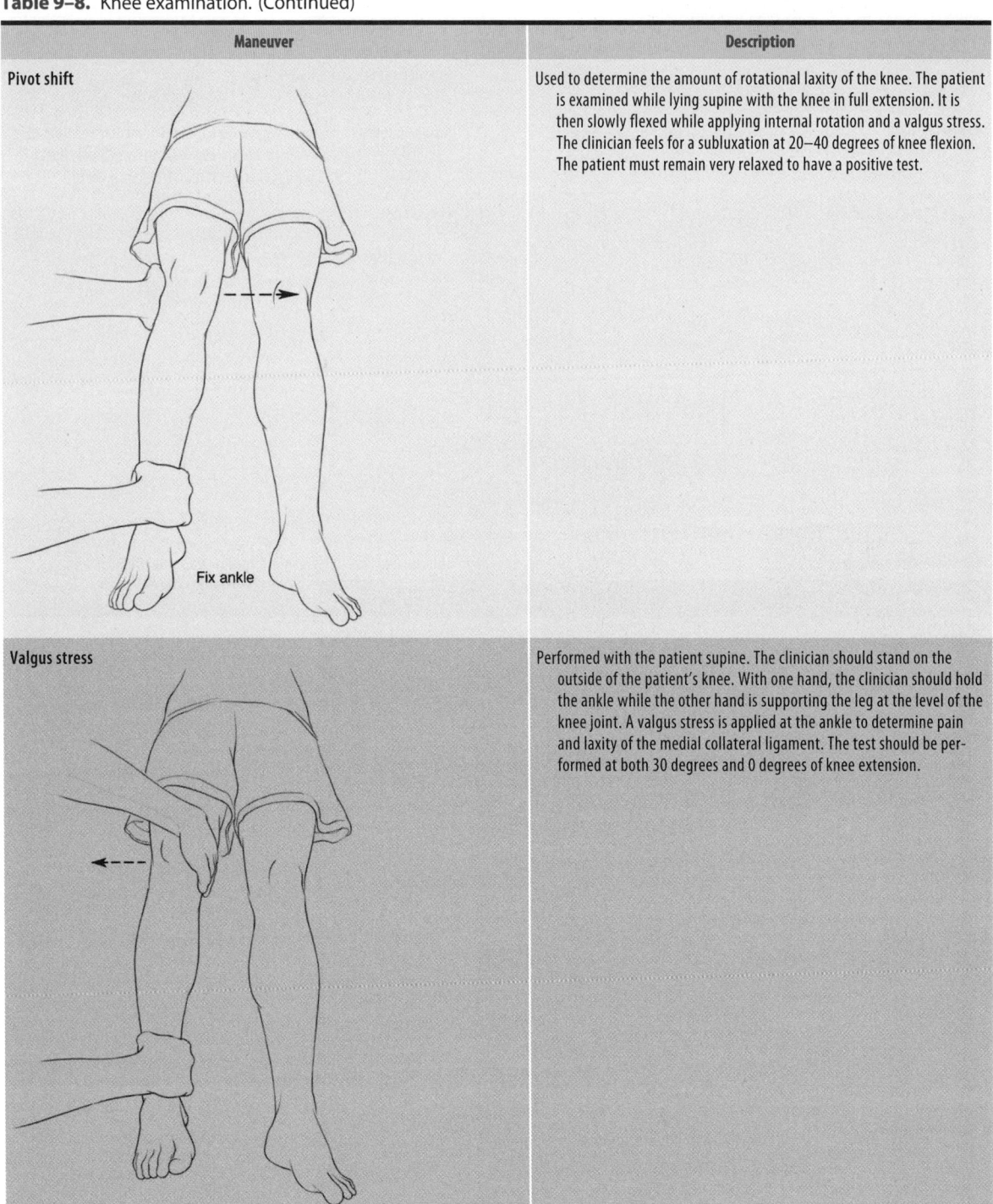 Fix ankle	Used to determine the amount of rotational laxity of the knee. The patient is examined while lying supine with the knee in full extension. It is then slowly flexed while applying internal rotation and a valgus stress. The clinician feels for a subluxation at 20–40 degrees of knee flexion. The patient must remain very relaxed to have a positive test.
Valgus stress	Performed with the patient supine. The clinician should stand on the outside of the patient's knee. With one hand, the clinician should hold the ankle while the other hand is supporting the leg at the level of the knee joint. A valgus stress is applied at the ankle to determine pain and laxity of the medial collateral ligament. The test should be performed at both 30 degrees and 0 degrees of knee extension.

(continued)

Table 9–8. Knee examination. (Continued)

Maneuver	Description
Varus stress 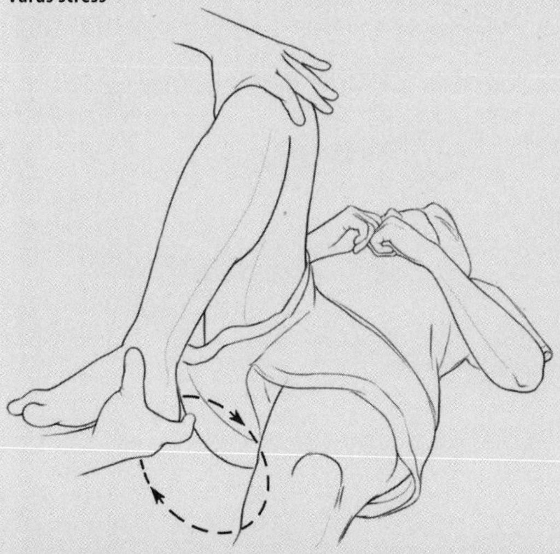	The patient is again placed supine. For the right knee, the clinician should be standing on the right side of the patient. The left hand of the examiner should be holding the ankle while the right hand is supporting the lateral thigh. A varus stress is applied at the ankle to determine pain and laxity of the lateral collateral ligament. The test should be performed at both 30 degrees and 0 degrees of knee flexion.
The sag sign	The patient is placed supine and both hips and knees are flexed up to 90 degrees. Because of gravity, the posterior cruciate ligament-injured knee will have an obvious set-off at the anterior tibia that is "sagging" posteriorly.
Posterior drawer	The patient is placed supine with the knee flexed at 90 degrees (see Anterior drawer figure above). In a normal knee, the anterior tibia should be positioned about 10 mm anterior to the femoral condyle. The clinician can grasp the proximal tibia with both hands and push the tibia posteriorly. The movement, indicating laxity and possible tear of the posterior cruciate ligament, is compared with the uninjured knee.
Meniscal signs	
McMurray test	Performed with the patient lying in supine. The clinician flexes the knee until the patient reports pain. For this test to be valid, it must be flexed pain-free beyond 90 degrees. The clinician externally rotates the patient's foot and then extends the knee while palpating the medial knee for "click" in the medial compartment of the knee or pain reproducing pain from a meniscus injury. To test the lateral meniscus, the same maneuver is repeated while rotating the foot internally (53% sensitivity and 59–97% specificity).

(continued)

Table 9–8. Knee examination. (Continued)

Maneuver	Description
Modified McMurray 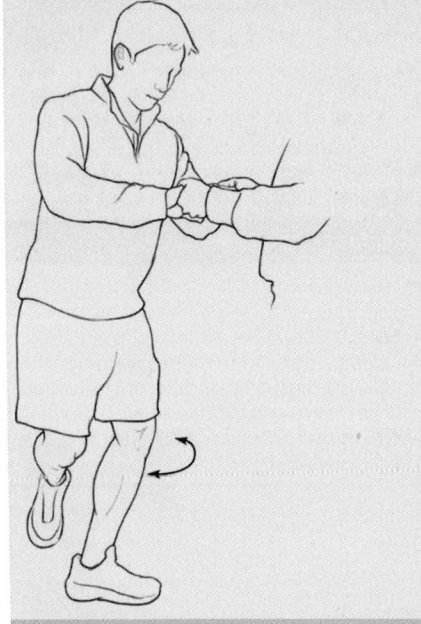	Performed with the hip flexed to 90 degrees. The knee is then flexed maximally with internally or externally rotation of the lower leg. The knee can then be rotated with the lower leg in internal or external rotation to capture the torn meniscus underneath the condyles. A positive test is pain over the joint line while the knee is being flexed and internally or externally rotated.
Thessaly test	Performed with the patient standing on one leg with knee slightly flexed. The patient is asked to twist the knee while standing on one leg. Pain can be elicited during twisting motion.
Patellofemoral Joint Test	
Apprehension sign	Suggests instability of the patellofemoral joint and is positive when the patient becomes apprehensive when the patella is deviated laterally.

SEADS, swelling, erythema, atrophy, deformity, and (surgical) scars.

When to Refer

- Almost all ACL tears should be referred to an orthopedic surgeon for evaluation.
- Individuals with instability in the setting of a chronic ACL tear (> 6 months) should be considered for surgical reconstruction.
- Patients with an ACL tear and associated meniscus or articular injuries may benefit from surgery to address the other injuries.

3. Collateral Ligament Injury

ESSENTIALS OF DIAGNOSIS

- ► Caused by a valgus or varus blow or stress to the knee.
- ► Pain and instability in the affected area.
- ► Limited range of motion.

General Considerations

The MCL is the most commonly injured ligament in the knee. It is usually injured with a valgus stress to the partially flexed knee. It can also occur with a blow to the lateral leg. The MCL is commonly injured with acute ACL injuries. The LCL is less commonly injured, but this can occur with a medial blow to the knee. Since both collateral ligaments are extra-articular, injuries to these ligaments may not lead to any intra-articular effusion. Affected patients may have difficulty walking initially, but this can improve when the swelling decreases.

Clinical Findings

A. Symptoms and Signs

The main clinical findings for patients with collateral ligament injuries are pain along the course of the ligaments. The patient may have limited range of motion due to pain, especially during the first 2 weeks following the injury. The best tests to assess the collateral ligaments are the varus and valgus stress tests. The sensitivity of the tests is as high as 86–96%.

The **valgus stress test** is performed with the patient supine (Table 9–8). The clinician should stand on the outside of the patient's knee. With one hand, the clinician should hold the ankle while the other hand is supporting the leg at the level of the knee joint. A valgus stress is applied at the ankle to determine pain and laxity of the MCL. The test should be performed at both 30 degrees and at 0 degrees of knee extension.

For the **varus stress test**, the patient is again placed supine. For the right knee, the clinician should be standing on the right side of the patient. The clinician's left hand should be holding the ankle while the right hand is supporting the lateral thigh. A varus stress is applied at the ankle to determine pain and laxity of the LCL. The test should be performed at both 30 degrees and at 0 degrees of knee flexion.

The test results can be graded from 1 to 3. Grade 1 is when the patient has pain with varus/valgus stress test but no instability. With grade 2 injuries, the patient has pain, and the knee shows instability at 30 degrees of knee flexion. In grade 3 injuries, the patient has marked instability but not much pain. The knee is often unstable at both 30 degrees and 0 degrees of knee flexion.

B. Imaging

Radiographs are usually nondiagnostic except for avulsion injuries. However, radiographs should be used to rule out fractures that can occur with collateral ligament injuries. Isolated MCL injuries usually do not require evaluation by MRI, but MRI should be used to evaluate possible associated cruciate ligament injuries. LCL or posterolateral corner injuries should have MRI evaluation to exclude associated injuries and to determine their significance.

Treatment

The majority of MCL injuries can be treated with protected weight-bearing and physical therapy. For grade 1 and 2 injuries, the patient can usually bear weight as tolerated with full range of motion. A hinged knee brace can be given to patients with grade 2 MCL tears to provide stability. Early physical therapy is recommended to protect range of motion and muscle strength. Grade 3 MCL injuries require long leg braces to provide stability. Patients can weight-bear, but only with the knee locked in extension with a brace. The motion can then be increased with the brace unlocked. Grade 3 injuries can take up to 6–8 weeks to heal. MCL injuries rarely need surgery. LCL injuries are less common but are usually associated with other ligament injuries (such as ACL and PCL). LCL injuries do not recover well with nonoperative treatment and usually require urgent surgical repair or reconstruction.

When to Refer

- Symptomatic instability with chronic MCL tears or acute MCL tears with other ligamentous injuries.
- LCL or posterolateral corner injuries require urgent surgical repair or reconstruction (within 1 week).

4. Posterior Cruciate Ligament Injury

ESSENTIALS OF DIAGNOSIS

- ► Usually follows an anterior trauma to the tibia, such as a dashboard injury during a motor vehicle accident.
- ► The knee may freely dislocate and reduce.
- ► One-third of multi-ligament injuries involving the PCL have neurovascular injuries.

General Considerations

The PCL is the strongest ligament in the knee. PCL injuries usually represent significant trauma and are highly associated with multi-ligament injuries and knee dislocations. More than 70–90% of PCL injuries have associated injuries to the posterolateral corner, MCL, and ACL. Neurovascular injuries occur in up to one-third of all knee dislocations or PCL injuries. There should be high suspicion for neurovascular injuries and a thorough neurovascular examination of the limb should be performed.

Clinical Findings

A. Symptoms and Signs

Most patients with acute injuries have difficulty with ambulation. Patients with chronic PCL injuries can ambulate without gross instability but may complain of subjective "looseness" and often report pain and dysfunction, especially with bending. Clinical examinations of PCL injuries include the "sag sign"; the patient is placed supine and both hips and knees are flexed to 90 degrees. Because of gravity, the posterior cruciate ligament-injured knee will have an obvious set-off at the anterior tibia that is "sagging" posteriorly. The PCL ligament can also be examined using the **posterior drawer test;** the patient is placed supine with the knee flexed to 90 degrees. In a normal knee, the anterior tibia should be positioned about 10 mm anterior to the femoral condyle. The clinician can grasp the proximal tibia with both hands and push the tibia posteriorly. The movement, indicating laxity and possible tear of the PCL, is compared with the uninjured knee (90% sensitivity and 99% specificity). A PCL injury is sometimes mistaken for an ACL injury during the anterior drawer test since the tibia is subluxed posteriorly in a sagged position and can be abnormally translated forward, yielding a false-positive test for an ACL injury. Pain, swelling, pallor, and numbness in the affected extremity may suggest a knee dislocation with possible injury to the popliteal artery.

B. Imaging

Radiographs are often nondiagnostic but are required to diagnose any fractures. MRI is used to diagnose PCL and other associated injuries.

Treatment

Isolated PCL injuries can be treated nonoperatively. Acute injuries are usually immobilized using a knee brace with the knee extension; the patient uses crutches for ambulation. Physical therapy can help achieve increased range of motion and improved ambulation. Many PCL injuries are associated with other injuries and may require operative reconstruction.

When to Refer

- If the lateral knee is also unstable with varus stress testing, the patient should be assessed for a posterolateral corner injury, which may require an urgent surgical reconstruction.
- Isolated PCL tears may require surgery if the tear is complete (grade 3) and the patient is symptomatic.

5. Meniscus Injuries

ESSENTIALS OF DIAGNOSIS

- ▶ Patient may or may not report an injury.
- ▶ Joint line pain and pain with deep squatting are the most sensitive signs.
- ▶ Difficulty with knee extension suggests an internal derangement that should be evaluated urgently with MRI.

General Considerations

The menisci act as shock absorbers within the knee. Injuries to a meniscus can lead to pain, clicking, and locking sensation. Most meniscus injuries occur with acute injuries (usually in younger patients) or repeated microtrauma, such as squatting or twisting (usually in older patients).

Clinical Findings

A. Symptoms and Signs

The patient may have an antalgic (painful) gait and difficulty with squatting. He or she may complain of catching or locking of the meniscal fragment. Physical findings can include effusion or joint line tenderness. Patients can usually point out the area of maximal tenderness along the joint line. Swelling usually occurs during the first 24 hours after the injury or later. Meniscus tears rarely lead to the immediate swelling that is commonly seen with fractures and ligament tears. Meniscus tears are commonly seen in arthritic knees. However, it is often unclear whether the pain is coming from the meniscus tear or the arthritis.

Provocative tests, including the **McMurray test,** the **modified McMurray test,** and the **Thessaly test**, can be performed to confirm the diagnosis. Most symptomatic meniscus tears cause pain with deep squatting and when waddling (performing a "duck walk").

B. Imaging

Radiographs are usually normal but may show joint space narrowing, early OA changes, or loose bodies. MRI of the knee is the best diagnostic tool for meniscal injuries (93% sensitivity and 95% specificity). High signal through the meniscus (bright on T2 images) represents a meniscal tear.

Treatment

Conservative treatment can be used for degenerative tears in older patients. The treatment is similar for patients with mild knee OA, including analgesics and physical therapy for strengthening and core stability. A randomized controlled trial showed that physical therapy compared to arthroscopic partial meniscectomy had similar outcomes at 6 months. However, 30% of the patients who were assigned to physical therapy alone underwent surgery within 6 months.

Randomized studies have shown that arthroscopic surgery has no benefit over sham operations in patients who have degenerative meniscal tears, especially with imaging showing signs of OA. Another randomized controlled trial found that patients with degenerative meniscus tears but no signs of arthritis on imaging treated conservatively with supervised exercise therapy had similar outcomes to those treated with arthroscopy at 2-year follow up. There is crossover between the groups; patients can be treated with supervised exercise therapy first, and if they do not respond to nonoperative treatment, they can undergo meniscus surgeries. Acute tears in young and active patients with clinical signs of internal derangement (catching and swelling) and without signs of arthritis on imaging or patients with acute mechanical locking with a displaced meniscus can be best treated arthroscopically with meniscus repair or debridement. There is also growing evidence that untreated meniscus root tears can lead to accelerated osteoarthritic changes. Surgical treatment before cartilage breakdown is recommended for acute meniscus root injuries.

▶ When to Refer

- If the patient has symptoms of internal derangement suspected as meniscus injury. The patient should receive an MRI to confirm the injury.
- If the patient cannot extend the knee due to a mechanical block, the patient should be evaluated as soon as possible. Certain shaped tears on MRI, such as bucket handle tears, are amenable to meniscal repair surgery.
- If the patient has not responded to physical therapy and nonoperative treatment and continues to have symptoms related to the torn meniscus.
- If the patient has MRI confirmation of acute meniscus root injuries.

6. Patellofemoral Pain

ESSENTIALS OF DIAGNOSIS

- ▶ Pain experienced with bending activities (kneeling, squatting, climbing stairs).
- ▶ Lateral deviation or tilting of the patella in relation to the femoral groove.

▶ General Considerations

Patellofemoral pain, also known as anterior knee pain, chondromalacia, or "runner's knee," describes any pain involving the patellofemoral joint. The pain affects any or all of the anterior knee structures, including the medial and lateral aspects of the patella as well as the quadriceps and patellar tendon insertions. The patella engages the femoral trochlear groove with approximately 30 degrees of knee flexion. Forces on the patellofemoral joint increase up to three times body weight as the knee flexes to 90 degrees (eg, climbing stairs), and five times body weight when going into full-knee flexion (eg, squatting). Abnormal patellar tracking during flexion can lead to abnormal articular cartilage wear and pain. When the patient has ligamentous hyperlaxity, the patella can sublux out of the groove, usually laterally. Patellofemoral pain is also associated with muscle strength and flexibility imbalances as well as altered hip and ankle biomechanics.

▶ Clinical Findings

A. Symptoms and Signs

Patients usually complain of pain in the anterior knee with bending movements and less commonly in full extension. Pain from this condition is localized under the kneecap but can sometimes be referred to the posterior knee or over the medial or lateral inferior patella. Symptoms may begin after a trauma or after repetitive physical activity, such as running and jumping. When maltracking, palpable and sometimes audible crepitus can occur.

Intra-articular swelling usually does not occur unless there are articular cartilage defects or if OA changes develop. On physical examination, it is important to palpate the articular surfaces of the patella. For example, the clinician can use one hand to move the patella laterally, and use the fingertips of the other hand to palpate the lateral undersurface of patella. Patellar mobility can be assessed by medially and laterally deviating the patella (deviation by one-quarter of the diameter of the kneecap is consider normal; greater than one-half the diameter suggests excessive mobility). The **apprehension sign** suggests instability of the patellofemoral joint and is positive when the patient becomes apprehensive when the patella is deviated laterally. The **patellar grind test** is performed by grasping the knee superior to the patella and pushing it downward with the patient supine and the knee extended, pushing the patella inferiorly. The patient is asked to contract the quadriceps muscle to oppose this downward translation, with reproduction of pain or grinding being the positive sign for chondromalacia of the patella. There are two common presentations: (1) patients whose ligaments and patella are too loose (hypermobility); and (2) patients who have soft tissues that are too tight, leading to excessive pressure on the joint.

Evaluation of the quadriceps strength and hip stabilizers can be accomplished by having the patient perform a one-leg squat without support. Patients who are weak may display poor balance, with dropping of the pelvis (similar to a positive hip Trendelenburg sign) or excessive internal rotation of the knee medially. Normally, with a one-leg squat, the knee should align over the second metatarsal ray of the foot.

B. Imaging

Diagnostic imaging has limited use in younger patients and is more helpful in older patients to assess for OA or to evaluate patients who do not respond to conservative treatment. Radiographs may show lateral deviation or tilting of the patella in relation to the femoral groove. MRI may show thinning of the articular cartilage but is not clinically necessary, except prior to surgery or to exclude other pathology.

▶ Treatment

A. Conservative

For symptomatic relief, use of local modalities such as ice and anti-inflammatory medications can be beneficial. If the patient has signs of patellar hypermobility, physical therapy exercises are useful to strengthen the quadriceps (especially the vastus medialis obliquus muscle) to help stabilize the patella and improve tracking. There is consistent evidence that exercise therapy for patellofemoral pain syndrome may result in clinically important reduction in pain and improvement in functional ability. Lower quality research supports that hip and knee exercises are better than knee exercises alone. Strengthening the quadriceps and the posterolateral hip muscles such as the hip abductors that control rotation at the knee should be recommended. Support for the patellofemoral joint can be provided by use of a patellar stabilizer brace or special taping techniques (McConnell taping). Correcting lower extremity alignment (with appropriate footwear or over-the-counter orthotics) can help improve symptoms, especially if the patient has pronation or high-arched feet. If the patient demonstrates tight peripatellar soft tissues, special focus should be put on stretching the hamstrings, iliotibial band, quadriceps, calves, and hip flexors.

B. Surgical

Surgery is rarely needed and is considered a last resort for patellofemoral pain. Procedures performed include lateral release or patellar realignment surgery.

▶ When to Refer

Patients with persistent symptoms despite a course of conservative therapy.

7. Osteoarthritis

ESSENTIALS OF DIAGNOSIS

▶ Degeneration of joint cartilage.

▶ Pain with bending or twisting activities.

▶ Swelling.

▶ Loss of active and passive range of motion in severe OA.

▶ General Considerations

In the United States, the prevalence of OA will grow as the number of persons older than age 65 years doubles to more than 70 million by 2030. The incidence of knee OA in the United States is 240 per 100,000 person-years.

Cartilage loss and OA symptoms are preceded by damage to the collagen-proteoglycan matrix. The etiology of OA is often multifactorial including previous trauma, prior high-impact activities, genetic factors, obesity, and rheumatologic or metabolic conditions.

▶ Clinical Findings

A. Symptoms and Signs

OA usually causes pain in the affected joint with loading of the joint or at the extremes of motion. Mechanical symptoms—such as swelling, grinding, catching, and locking—suggest internal derangement, which is indicated by damaged cartilage or bone fragments that affect the smooth range of motion expected at an articular joint. Pain can also produce the sensation of "buckling" or "giving way" due to muscle inhibition. As the joint degeneration becomes more advanced, the patient loses active range of motion and may lose passive range of motion as well.

As the condition worsens, patients with knee OA have an increasingly limited ability to walk. Symptoms include pain with bending or twisting activities, and going up and downstairs. Swelling, limping, and pain while sleeping are common complaints with OA, especially as it progresses.

B. Imaging

The most commonly recommended radiographs include bilateral weight-bearing 45-degree bent knee posteroanterior, lateral, and patellofemoral joint views (Merchant view). Radiographic findings include diminished width of the articular cartilage causing joint space narrowing, subchondral sclerosis, presence of osteophytes, and cystic changes in the subchondral bone. MRI of the knee is most likely unnecessary unless other pathology is suspected, including ischemic osteonecrosis of the knee.

▶ Treatment

A. Conservative

Changes in the articular cartilage are irreversible. Therefore, a cure for the diseased joint is not possible, although symptoms or structural issues can be addressed to try to maintain activity level. Conservative treatment for all patients with OA includes activity modification, therapeutic exercises, and weight loss. Lifestyle modifications also include proper footwear and avoidance of high-impact activities. Optimal exercise programs for knee OA should focus on improving aerobic capacity, quadriceps muscle strength, or lower extremity performance. Ideally, the program should be supervised and carried out three times a week.

Use of a cane in the hand opposite to the affected side is mechanically advantageous. Knee sleeves or braces provide some improvement in subjective pain symptoms most likely due to improvements in neuromuscular function. If patients have unicompartmental OA in the medial or lateral compartment, joint unloader braces are available to offload the degenerative compartment. Cushioning footwear and appropriate orthotics or shoe adjustments are useful for reducing impact to the lower extremities.

There are several oral and intra-articular pharmacologic options. Treatments that have been studied include oral acetaminophen, diclofenac, ibuprofen, naproxen, celecoxib, and intra-articular corticosteroids and hyaluronic acid. All treatments except acetaminophen showed clinically significant improvement in pain. If a traditional NSAID is indicated, the choice should be based on cost, side-effect profile, and adherence. The cyclooxygenase (COX)-2 inhibitor celecoxib is no more effective than traditional NSAIDs; it may offer short-term, but probably not long-term, advantage in preventing gastrointestinal complications. Due to its cost and potential cardiovascular risk, celecoxib should be reserved for carefully selected patients. Topical NSAIDs or capsaicin can be effective in the treatment of OA, since they avoid many of the traditional NSAID complications. Opioids can be used appropriately in patients with severe OA. Glucosamine and chondroitin sulfate are supplements that have been widely used and marketed for OA. Despite some initial promise, the best-controlled studies indicate these supplements are ineffective as analgesics in OA. However, they have minimal side effects and may be appropriate if the patient experiences subjective benefit.

Knee joint corticosteroid injections are options to help reduce pain and inflammation and can provide short-term pain relief, usually lasting about 6–12 weeks. Viscosupplementation by injections of hyaluronic acid-based products is controversial. Because reviews suggest that viscosupplementation has a questionably clinically relevant effect size, and has an increased risk of adverse events, the American Academy of Orthopedic Surgeons has recommended that viscosupplementation should not be used in the treatment of knee OA. However, the American College of Rheumatology's 2012 OA guidelines recommend the use of intra-articular hyaluronic acid injection for the treatment of OA of the knee in adults. Platelet-rich plasma injections contain high concentration of platelet-derived growth factors, which regulate some biologic processes in tissue repair. A meta-analysis of 10 studies demonstrated that platelet-rich plasma injections reduced pain in patients with knee OA more efficiently than placebo and hyaluronic acid injections. However, 9 of the 10 studies had a high risk of bias, and the underlying mechanism of biologic healing is unknown. An FDA safety and efficacy study showed that leukocyte-poor PRP autologous conditioned plasma improved overall Western Ontario and McMaster Universities Arthritis Index scores by 78% from the baseline score after 12 months, compared to 7% for the placebo group, though the sample size was small (30 patients).

B. Surgical

Two randomized trials demonstrated that arthroscopy does not improve outcomes at 1 year over placebo or routine conservative treatment of OA. Joint replacement surgeries are effective and cost-effective for patients with significant symptoms or functional limitations, providing improvements in pain, function, and quality of life. The number of total knee arthroplasty procedures jumped 162% from 1991 to 2010, along with an increase in complications and hospital readmissions. Minimally invasive surgeries and computer-assisted navigation during operation are being investigated as methods to improve techniques (eg, accurate placement of the hardware implant) and to reduce complication rates; however, major improvements have yet to be demonstrated.

Knee realignment surgery, such as high tibial osteotomy or partial knee replacement surgery, is indicated in patients younger than age 60 with unicompartmental OA, who would benefit from delaying total knee replacement. Knee joint replacement surgery has been very successful in improving outcomes for patient with end-stage OA. Long-term series describe more than 95% survival rate of the implant at 15 years.

▶ When to Refer

Patients with sufficient disability, limited benefit from conservative therapy, and evidence of severe OA can be referred for joint replacement surgery.

ANKLE INJURIES

1. Inversion Ankle Sprains

ESSENTIALS OF DIAGNOSIS

▶ Localized pain and swelling.

▶ The majority of ankle injuries involve inversion injuries affecting the lateral ligaments.

▶ Consider chronic ankle instability or associated injuries if pain persists for longer than 3 months following an ankle sprain.

▶ General Considerations

Ankle sprains are the most common sports injuries seen in outpatient clinics. Patients usually report "turning the ankle" during a fall or after landing on an irregular surface such as a hole or an opponent's foot. The most common mechanism of injury is an inversion and plantar flexion sprain, which injures the anterior talofibular (ATF) ligament rather than the calcaneofibular (CF) ligament. Other injuries that can occur with inversion ankle injuries are listed in Table 9–9. Women appear to sustain an inversion injury more frequently than men. Chronic ankle instability is

Table 9–9. Injuries associated with ankle sprains.

Ligaments
Subtalar joint sprain
Sinus tarsi syndrome
Syndesmotic sprain
Deltoid sprain
Lisfranc injury
Tendons
Posterior tibial tendon strain
Peroneal tendon subluxation
Bones
Osteochondral talus injury
Lateral talar process fracture
Posterior impingement (os trigonum)
Fracture at the base of the fifth metatarsal
Jones fracture
Salter fracture (fibula)
Ankle fractures

defined as persistent complaints of pain, swelling, and giving way in combination with recurrent sprains for at least 12 months after the initial ankle sprain. Chronic ankle instability can occur in up to 43% of ankle sprains even with physical therapy, which makes appropriate attention to acute ankle sprains important.

▶ Clinical Findings

A. Symptoms and Signs

The usual symptoms following a sprain include localized pain and swelling over the lateral aspect of the ankle, difficulty weight-bearing, and limping. The patient's ankle may feel unstable. On examination, there may be swelling or bruising over the lateral aspect of the ankle. The anterior, inferior aspect below the lateral malleolus is most often the point of maximal tenderness consistent with ATF and CF ligament injuries. The swelling may limit motion of the ankle.

Special stress tests for the ankle include the **anterior drawer test** (Table 9–10). The clinician keeps the foot and ankle in the neutral position with the patient sitting, then uses one hand to fix the tibia and the other to hold the patient's heel and draw the ankle forward. Normally, there may be approximately 3 mm of translation until an endpoint is felt. A positive test includes increased translation of one foot compared to the other with loss of the endpoint of the ATF ligament.

Another stress test is the **subtalar tilt test,** which is performed with the foot in the neutral position with the patient sitting. The clinician uses one hand to fix the tibia and the other to hold and invert the calcaneus. Normal inversion at the subtalar joint is approximately 30 degrees. A positive test consists of increased subtalar joint inversion greater than 10 degrees on the affected side with loss of endpoint for the CF ligament. In order to grade the severity of ankle sprains,

no laxity on stress tests is considered a grade 1 injury, laxity of the ATF ligament on anterior drawer testing but a negative tilt test is a grade 2 injury, and both positive drawer and tilt tests signify a grade 3 injury. Difficulty jumping and landing within 2 weeks from the acute ankle sprain, abnormal postural or hip muscle control, or ligamentous laxity noted 8 weeks after injury are poor prognostic signs.

B. Imaging

Routine ankle radiographic views include the AP, lateral, and oblique (mortise) views. Less common views requested

Table 9–10. Ankle examination.

Maneuver	Description
Inspection	Examine for the alignment of the ankle. (SEADS)
Palpation	Include important landmarks: Ottawa Ankle Rules (medial and lateral malleolus, base of fifth metatarsal and navicular area), anterior tibiofibular ligament, posterior talus; tendons (Achilles, peroneals, posterior tibialis, flexor hallucis longus).
Range of motion testing	Check range of motion actively (patient performs) and passively (clinician performs), especially with flexion and extension of the spine. Rotation and lateral bending are also helpful to assess symmetric motion or any restrictions.
Ankle strength testing	Test resisted ankle dorsiflexion, plantarflexion, inversion and eversion strength manually.
Ankle anterior drawer	The clinician keeps the foot and ankle in the neutral position with the patient sitting, then uses one hand to fix the tibia and the other to hold the patient's heel and draw the ankle forward. Normally, there may be approximately 3 mm of translation until an endpoint is felt. A positive test includes increased translation of one foot compared to the other with loss of the endpoint of the anterior talofibular ligament.
Subtalar tilt test	Performed with the foot in the neutral position with the patient sitting. The clinician uses one hand to fix the tibia and the other to hold and invert the calcaneus. Normal inversion at the subtalar joint is approximately 30 degrees. A positive test consists of increased subtalar joint inversion greater than 10 degrees on the affected side with loss of endpoint for the calcaneofibular ligament.
External rotation stress test	Performed when the clinician fixes the tibia with one hand and grasps the foot in the other with the ankle in the neutral position and then dorsiflexes and externally rotates the ankle, reproducing the patient's pain.

SEADS, swelling, erythema, atrophy, deformity, and (surgical) scars.

include the calcaneal view and subtalar view. The **Ottawa Ankle Rules** remain the best clinical prediction rules to guide the need for radiographs and have an 86–99% sensitivity and a 97–99% negative predictive value. If the patient is unable to bear weight immediately in the office setting or emergency department for four steps, then the clinician should check for (1) bony tenderness at the posterior edge of the medial or lateral malleolus and (2) bony tenderness over the navicular (medial midfoot) or at the base of the fifth metatarsal. If either malleolus demonstrates pain or deformity, then ankle radiographs should be obtained. If the foot has bony tenderness, obtain foot radiographs. An MRI is helpful when considering the associated injuries.

▶ **Treatment**

Immediate treatment of an ankle sprain follows the MICE mnemonic: *m*odified activities, *i*ce, *c*ompression, and *e*levation. Subsequent treatment involves protected weight-bearing with crutches and use of an ankle stabilizer brace, especially for grades 2 and 3 injuries. Early motion is essential, and patients should be encouraged to do home exercises or physical therapy. Proprioception and balance exercises (eg, "wobble board") are useful to restore function to the ankle and prevent future ankle sprains. Regular use of an ankle support with activities can reduce the risk of lateral ankle sprains. Chronic instability can develop after acute ankle sprain in 10–20% of people and may require surgical stabilization with ligament reconstruction surgery.

▶ **When to Refer**

- Ankle fractures
- Recurrent ankle sprains or signs of chronic ligamentous ankle instability
- No response after more than 3 months of conservative treatment
- Suspicion of associated injuries

2. Eversion ("High") Ankle Sprains

ESSENTIALS OF DIAGNOSIS

▶ Severe and prolonged pain.
▶ Limited range of motion.
▶ Mild swelling.
▶ Difficulty with weight-bearing.

▶ **General Considerations**

A syndesmotic injury or "high ankle" sprain involves the anterior *tibio*fibular ligament in the anterolateral aspect of the ankle, superior to the ATF ligament. The injury mechanism often involves the foot being turned out or externally

rotated and everted (eg, when being tackled). This injury is commonly missed or misdiagnosed as an ATF ligament sprain on initial visit.

▶ **Clinical Findings**
A. Symptoms and Signs

Symptoms of a high ankle sprain include severe and prolonged pain over the anterior ankle at the anterior tibiofibular ligament, worse with weight-bearing. This is often more painful than the typical ankle sprain. The point of maximal tenderness involves the anterior tibiofibular ligament, which is higher than the ATF ligament. It is also important to palpate the proximal fibula to rule out any proximal syndesmotic ligament injury and associated fracture known as a "maisonneuve fracture." There is often some mild swelling in this area, and the patient may or may not have an ankle effusion. The patient usually has limited range of motion in all directions. To perform the **external rotation stress test,** the clinician fixes the tibia with one hand and grasps the foot in the other with the ankle in the neutral position. The ankle is then dorsiflexed and externally rotated, reproducing the patient's pain. (**Note:** The patient's foot should have an intact neurovascular examination before undertaking this test.)

B. Imaging

Radiographs of the ankle should include the AP, mortise, and lateral views. The mortise view may demonstrate loss of the normal overlap between the tibia and fibula, which should be at least 1–2 mm. Asymmetry in the joint space around the tibiotalar joint suggests disruption of the syndesmotic ligaments. If there is proximal tenderness in the lower leg especially around the fibula, an AP and lateral view of the tibia and fibula should be obtained to rule out a proximal fibula fracture. Radiographs during an external rotation stress test may visualize instability at the distal tibiofibular joint. MRI is the best method to visualize injury to the tibiofibular ligament and to assess status of the other ligaments and the articular cartilage.

▶ **Treatment**

Whereas most ankle sprains are treated with early motion and weight-bearing, treatment for a high ankle sprain should be conservative with a cast or walking boot for 4–6 weeks. Thereafter, protected weight-bearing with crutches is recommended until the patient can walk pain-free. Physical therapy can start early to regain range of motion and maintain strength with limited weight-bearing initially.

▶ **When to Refer**

If there is widening of the joint space and asymmetry at the tibiotalar joint, the patient should be referred urgently to a foot and ankle surgeon. Severe or prolonged persistent cases that do not heal may require internal fixation to avoid chronic instability at the tibiofibular joint. Screw fixation remains the gold standard, although newer techniques with bioabsorbable constructs are emerging.

REFERENCES

Abolhasani M et al: Effects of kinesiotaping on knee osteoarthritis: a literature review. J Exerc Rehabil 2019;15(4):498-503 [PMID: 31523668].

Arnold E et al: The effect of timing of physical therapy for acute low back pain on health services utilization: a systematic review. Arch Phys Med Rehabil 2019;100(7):1324-1338 [PMID: 30684490].

Badri A et al: Clinical and radiologic evaluation of the posterior cruciate ligament-injured knee. Curr Rev Musculoskelet Med 2018;11(3):515-520 [PMID: 29987531].

Bagley C et al: Current concepts and recent advances in understanding and managing lumbar spine stenosis. F1000Res 2019;8:137 [PMID: 30774933].

Barrey CY et al: French Society for Spine Surgery. Chronic low back pain: relevance of a new classification based on the injury pattern. Orthop Traumatol Surg Res 2019;105(2):339-346 [PMID: 30792166].

Benner RW et al: Knee osteoarthritis: alternative range of motion treatment. Orthop Clin North Am 2019;50(4):425-432 [PMID: 31466659].

Black DM et al: Atypical femur fractures: review of epidemiology, relationship to bisphosphonates, prevention, and clinical management. Endocr Rev 2019;40(2):333-368 [PMID: 30169557].

Bolgla LA et al: National Athletic Trainers' Association Position Statement: management of individuals with patellofemoral pain. J Athl Train 2018;53(9):820-836 [PMID: 30372640].

Brosseau L et al: The Ottawa panel clinical practice guidelines for the management of knee osteoarthritis. Part two: strengthening exercise programs. Clin Rehabil 2017;31(5):596-611 [PMID: 28183213].

Brosseau L et al: The Ottawa panel clinical practice guidelines for the management of knee osteoarthritis. Part three: aerobic exercise programs. Clin Rehabil 2017;31(5):612-624 [PMID: 28183194].

Bruyère O et al: An updated algorithm recommendation for the management of knee osteoarthritis from the European Society for Clinical and Economic Aspects of Osteoporosis, Osteoarthritis and Musculoskeletal Diseases (ESCEO). Semin Arthritis Rheum 2019;49(3):337-350 [PMID: 31126594].

Bunt CW et al: Knee pain in adults and adolescents: the initial evaluation. Am Fam Physician 2018;98(9):576-585 [PMID: 30325638].

Butler AJ et al: Endoscopic lumbar surgery: the state of the art in 2019. Neurospine 2019;16(1):15-23 [PMID: 30943703].

Bydon M et al: Degenerative lumbar spondylolisthesis: definition, natural history, conservative management, and surgical treatment. Neurosurg Clin N Am 2019;30(3):299-304 [PMID: 31078230].

Chan AK et al: Summary of guidelines for the treatment of lumbar spondylolisthesis. Neurosurg Clin N Am 2019;30(3):353-364 [PMID: 31078236].

Chen ET et al: Ankle sprains: evaluation, rehabilitation, and prevention. Curr Sports Med Rep 2019;18(6):217-223 [PMID: 31385837].

Cohen SP et al: Advances in the diagnosis and management of neck pain. BMJ 2017;358:j3221 [PMID: 28807894].

Cook CJ et al: Systematic review of diagnostic accuracy of patient history, clinical findings, and physical tests in the diagnosis of lumbar spinal stenosis. Eur Spine J 2020;29(1):93-112 [PMID: 31312914].

Crossley KM et al: Rethinking patellofemoral pain: prevention, management and long-term consequences. Best Pract Res Clin Rheumatol 2019;33(1):48-65 [PMID: 31431275].

Dadabo J et al: Noninterventional therapies for the management of knee osteoarthritis. J Knee Surg 2019;32(1):46-54 [PMID: 30477045].

Delahunt E et al: Risk factors for lateral ankle sprains and chronic ankle instability. J Athl Train 2019;54(6):611-616 [PMID: 31161942].

Devitt BM et al: Isolated posterior cruciate reconstruction results in improved functional outcome but low rates of return to pre-injury level of sport: a systematic review and meta-analysis. Orthop J Sports Med 2018;6(10):2325967118804478 [PMID: 30386804].

Doherty C et al: Treatment and prevention of acute and recurrent ankle sprain: an overview of systematic reviews with meta-analysis. Br J Sports Med 2017;51(2):113-125 [PMID: 28053200].

Donohue MA et al: Meniscus injuries in the military athlete. J Knee Surg 2019;32(2):123-126 [PMID: 30630210].

Dreizin D et al: Imaging acetabular fractures. Radiol Clin North Am 2019;57(4):823-841 [PMID: 31076035].

Driban JB et al: Accelerated knee osteoarthritis is characterized by destabilizing meniscal tears and pre-radiographic structural disease burden. Arthr Rheumatol 2019;71(7):1089-1100 [PMID: 30592385].

Drobnič M et al: Treatment options for the symptomatic post-meniscectomy knee. Knee Surg Sports Traumatol Arthrosc 2019;27(6):1817-1824 [PMID: 30859265].

Elkin JL et al: Combined anterior cruciate ligament and medial collateral ligament knee injuries: anatomy, diagnosis, management recommendations, and return to sport. Curr Rev Musculoskelet Med 2019;12(2):239-244 [PMID: 30929138].

Filbay SR et al: Evidence-based recommendations for the management of anterior cruciate ligament (ACL) rupture. Best Pract Res Clin Rheumatol 2019;33(1):33-47 [PMID: 31431274].

Fort NM et al: Management of acute injuries of the tibiofibular syndesmosis. Eur J Orthop Surg Traumatol 2017;27(4):449-459 [PMID: 28391516].

Gadjradj PS et al: Management of symptomatic lumbar disk herniation: an international perspective. Spine (Phila Pa 1976) 2017;42(23):1826-1834 [PMID: 28632645].

Galliker G et al: Low back pain in the emergency department: prevalence of serious spinal pathologies and diagnostic accuracy of red flags—a systematic review. Am J Med 2020;133(1):60-72 [PMID: 31278933].

Georgiev T et al: Modifiable risk factors in knee osteoarthritis: treatment implications. Rheumatol Int 2019;39(7):1145-1157 [PMID: 30911813].

Grawe B et al: Lateral collateral ligament injury about the knee: anatomy, evaluation, and management. J Am Acad Orthop Surg 2018;26(6):e120-e127 [PMID: 29443704].

Guyen O: Hemiarthroplasty or total hip arthroplasty in recent femoral neck fractures? Orthop Traumatol Surg Res 2019;105(1S):S95-S101 [PMID: 30449680].

Honvo G et al: Update on the role of pharmaceutical-grade chondroitin sulfate in the symptomatic management of knee osteoarthritis. Aging Clin Exp Res 2019;31(8):1163-1167 [PMID: 31243744].

Horvath A et al: Outcome after anterior cruciate ligament revision. Curr Rev Musculoskelet Med 2019;12(3):397-405 [PMID: 31286413].

Hunter DJ et al: Osteoarthritis. Lancet 2019;393(10182):1745-1759 [PMID: 31034380].

Jin J et al: JAMA patient page. Patellofemoral pain. JAMA 2018;319(4):418 [PMID: 29362797].

Johnson SM et al: Imaging of acute low back pain. Radiol Clin North Am 2019;57(2):397-413 [PMID: 30709477].

Juch JNS et al: Effect of radiofrequency denervation on pain intensity among patients with chronic low back pain: the Mint randomized clinical trials. JAMA 2017 Jul 4;318(1):68-81. Erratum in: JAMA. 2017;318(12):1188 [PMID: 28672319].

Kaminski TW et al: Prevention of lateral ankle sprains. J Athl Train 2019;54(6):650-661 [PMID: 31116041].

Kaplan Y et al: When is it safe to return to sport after ACL reconstruction? Reviewing the criteria. Sports Health 2019;11(4):301-305 [PMID: 31136725].

Karia M et al: Current concepts in the techniques, indications and outcomes of meniscal repairs. Eur J Orthop Surg Traumatol 2019;29(3):509-520 [PMID: 30374643].

Karsy M et al: Surgical versus nonsurgical treatment of lumbar spondylolisthesis. Neurosurg Clin N Am 2019;30(3):333-340 [PMID: 31078234].

Kellett JJ et al: Diagnostic imaging of ankle syndesmosis injuries: a general review. J Med Imaging Radiat Oncol 2018;62(2):159-168 [PMID: 29399975].

Kurzweil PR et al: Meniscus repair and replacement. Sports Med Arthrosc Rev 2018;26(4):160-164 [PMID: 30395058].

Lee B et al: Injection alternatives for the management of knee osteoarthritis pain. Surg Technol Int 2019;34:513-519 [PMID: 30888679].

Lee JS et al: Comparison of percutaneous endoscopic lumbar diskectomy and open lumbar microdiskectomy for recurrent lumbar disk herniation. J Neurol Surg A Cent Eur Neurosurg 2018;79(6):447-452 [PMID: 29241269].

Lemmers GPG et al: Imaging versus no imaging for low back pain: a systematic review, measuring costs, healthcare utilization and absence from work. Eur Spine J 2019;28(5):937-950 [PMID: 30796513].

Mandegaran R et al: Beyond the bones and joints: a review of ligamentous injuries of the foot and ankle on (99m)Tc-MDP-SPECT/CT. Br J Radiol 2019;92(1104):20190506 [PMID: 31365277].

Martel JW et al: Evaluation and management of neck and back pain. Semin Neurol 2019;39(1):41-52 [PMID: 30743291].

McAlindon TE et al: Effect of intra-articular triamcinolone vs saline on knee cartilage volume and pain in patients with knee osteoarthritis: a randomized clinical trial. JAMA 2017;317(19):1967-1975 [PMID: 28510679].

Medina McKeon JM et al: The ankle-joint complex: a kinesiologic approach to lateral ankle sprains. J Athl Train 2019;54(6):589-602 [PMID: 31184957].

Metcalfe D et al: Does this patient have hip osteoarthritis? The rational clinical examination systematic review. JAMA 2019;322(23):2323-2333 [PMID: 31846019].

Migliorini F et al: Total hip arthroplasty: minimally invasive surgery or not? Meta-analysis of clinical trials. Int Orthop 2019;43(7):1573-1582 [PMID: 30171273].

Mora JC et al: Knee osteoarthritis: pathophysiology and current treatment modalities. J Pain Res 2018;11:2189-2196 [PMID: 30323653].

Neal BS et al: Risk factors for patellofemoral pain: a systematic review and meta-analysis. Br J Sports Med 2019;53(5):270-281 [PMID: 30242107].

Nickless JT et al: High ankle sprains: easy to miss, so follow these tips. J Fam Pract 2019;68(3):E5-E13 [PMID: 31039220].

Pache S et al: Meniscal root tears: current concepts review. Arch Bone Jt Surg 2018;6(4):250-259 [PMID: 30175171].

Paik J et al: Triamcinolone acetonide extended-release: a review in osteoarthritis pain of the knee. Drugs 2019 Mar;79(4):455-462. Erratum in: Drugs 2019;79(5):587 [PMID: 30847805].

Peng B et al: Cervical discs as a source of neck pain. An analysis of the evidence. Pain Med 2019;20(3):446-455 [PMID: 30520967].

Porrino J et al: An update and comprehensive review of the posterolateral corner of the knee. Radiol Clin North Am 2018;56(6):935-951 [PMID: 30322491].

Price AJ et al: Knee replacement. Lancet 2018;392(10158):1672-1682 [PMID: 30496082].

Purohit N et al: Surgical management of patellofemoral instability. I. Imaging considerations. Skeletal Radiol 2019;48(6):859-869 [PMID: 30542758].

Ramlall Y et al: Examining pain before and after primary total knee replacement (TKR): a retrospective chart review. Int J Orthop Trauma Nurs 2019;34:43-47 [PMID: 31272918].

Raterman HG et al: Current treatments and new developments in the management of glucocorticoid-induced osteoporosis. Drugs 2019;79(10):1065-1087 [PMID: 31201710].

Richardson C et al: Intra-articular hyaluronan therapy for symptomatic knee osteoarthritis. Rheum Dis Clin North Am 2019;45(3):439-451 [PMID: 31277754].

Richmond JC: Anterior cruciate ligament reconstruction. Sports Med Arthrosc Rev 2018;26(4):165-167 [PMID: 30395059].

Rigoard P et al: Optimizing the management and outcomes of failed back surgery syndrome: a consensus statement on definition and outlines for patient assessment. Pain Res Manag 2019;2019:3126464 [PMID: 30911339].

Saltychev M et al: Effectiveness of conservative treatment for patellofemoral pain syndrome: a systematic review and meta-analysis. J Rehabil Med 2018;50(5):393-401 [PMID: 29392329].

Shon OJ et al: Current concepts of posterolateral corner injuries of the knee. Knee Surg Relat Res 2017;29(4):256-268 [PMID: 29172386].

Skou ST et al: Physical therapy for patients with knee and hip osteoarthritis: supervised, active treatment is current best practice. Clin Exp Rheumatol 2019;37(Suppl 120):112-117 [PMID: 31621559].

Sobolev B et al: Canadian Collaborative Study of Hip Fractures. Mortality effects of timing alternatives for hip fracture surgery. CMAJ 2018;190(31):E923-E932 [PMID: 30087128].

Sterling M: Best evidence rehabilitation for chronic pain part 4: neck pain. J Clin Med 2019;8(8):E1219 [PMID: 31443149].

Stirton JB et al: Total hip arthroplasty for the management of hip fracture: a review of the literature. J Orthop 2019;16(2):141-144 [PMID: 30886461].

Strauss MJ et al: The use of allograft tissue in posterior cruciate, collateral and multi-ligament knee reconstruction. Knee Surg Sports Traumatol Arthrosc 2019;27(6):1791-1809 [PMID: 30824979].

Strudwick K et al: Review article: best practice management of neck pain in the emergency department (part 6 of the musculoskeletal injuries rapid review series). Emerg Med Australas 2018;30(6):754-772 [PMID: 30168261].

Tassignon B et al: Criteria-based return to sport decision-making following lateral ankle sprain injury: a systematic review and narrative synthesis. Sports Med 2019;49(4):601-619 [PMID: 30747379].

Teirlinck CH et al: Prognostic factors for progression of osteoarthritis of the hip: a systematic review. Arthritis Res Ther 2019;21(1):192 [PMID: 31443685].

Tucker HR et al: Harms and benefits of opioids for management of non-surgical acute and chronic low back pain: a systematic review. Br J Sports Med 2020;54(11):664 [PMID: 30902816].

Urits I et al: Low back pain, a comprehensive review: pathophysiology, diagnosis, and treatment. Curr Pain Headache Rep 2019;23(3):23 [PMID: 30854609].

Urits I et al: Minimally invasive interventional management of osteoarthritic chronic knee pain. J Knee Surg 2019;32(1):72-79 [PMID: 30500975].

Vincent P: Intra-articular hyaluronic acid in the symptomatic treatment of knee osteoarthritis: a meta-analysis of single-injection products. Curr Ther Res Clin Exp 2019;90:39-51 [PMID: 31289603].

Vuurberg G et al: Diagnosis, treatment and prevention of ankle sprains: update of an evidence-based clinical guideline. Br J Sports Med 2018;52(15):956 [PMID: 29514819].

Wang Z et al: A systematic review and meta-analysis of direct anterior approach versus posterior approach in total hip arthroplasty. J Orthop Surg Res 2018;13(1):229 [PMID: 30189881].

Webster KE et al: What is the evidence for and validity of return-to-sport testing after anterior cruciate ligament reconstruction surgery? A systematic review and meta-analysis. Sports Med 2019;49(6):917-929 [PMID: 30905035].

Yedavally-Yellayi S et al: Update on osteoporosis. Prim Care 2019;46(1):175-190 [PMID: 30704657].

Yuen CP et al: Distal tibiofibular syndesmosis: anatomy, biomechanics, injury and management. Open Orthop J 2017;11:670-677 [PMID: 29081864].

■ SELF-ASSESSMENT QUESTIONS

Select the one correct answer for each question.

Question 1: Low back pain
  a. seldom resolves within 2 weeks
  b. nearly always resolves within 6 weeks
  c. is not a presenting symptom in other serious medical problems
  d. is unrelated to degenerative changes in the lumbar spine

Question 2: Spinal stenosis
  a. is a narrowing of the spinal canal unrelated to osteoarthritis
  b. is typically the result of a disk herniation
  c. causes pain that worsens with flexion
  d. may present with neurogenic claudication symptoms with walking

Question 3: Lumbar disk herniation
  a. is the most common occupational injury
  b. must have a plausible history of an inciting incident
  c. does not occur from degenerative disk disease
  d. nearly always affects the L5–S1 disk

Question 4: Hip fractures
  a. should be surgically repaired as soon as possible (within 24 hours)
  b. can be entirely prevented with exercise programs
  c. can be entirely prevented with hip protectors
  d. should not be subjected to internal rotation of the hip

Question 5: Osteoarthritis
  a. should never be treated with corticosteroids
  b. can be reversed with anti-inflammatory drugs
  c. involves a degeneration of the joint cartilage
  d. is not affected by repetitive trauma

Question 6: Anterior cruciate ligament injury
  a. impacts rotational stability of the tibia on the patella
  b. is usually a painless buckling of the knee
  c. causes instability going up more than downstairs
  d. leads to acute swelling immediately (or within 4 hours)

Question 7: Collateral ligament injury
  a. is caused by a valgus or varus blow or stress to the knee
  b. is usually caused by a valgus stress to the partially extended knee
  c. seldom presents with pain along the course of the ligaments
  d. is assessed by the varus and valgus stress tests despite their lack of sensitivity

Question 8: Inversion ankle sprains
  a. may result in chronic instability
  b. never require surgical stabilization with ligament reconstruction
  c. require MRI to rule out associated injuries
  d. are treated in the same manner as eversion (high) ankle sprains

10

The Management of Chronic Pain

Diana Coffa, MD
Wolf Mehling, MD

Chronic pain is variously defined as (1) pain lasting more than 3 months, (2) pain lasting more than 6 months, and (3) pain lasting beyond the period of expected healing or persisting in the absence of injury. Chronic pain is distinguished from acute pain in a number of ways. Most concretely, it lasts longer. In many cases, though, what is genuinely unique about chronic pain is that it seems to persist even when a physical insult is not occurring, or it is out of proportion to the physical damage that has occurred.

In the first part of this chapter, we will explore some of what is known about the nature of chronic pain and try to understand how it is perpetuated and, ideally, how it can be interrupted. In the second part of this chapter, we will discuss specific therapies that are effective in the management of chronic pain.

Pain is an extraordinarily complex phenomenon. At first glance, it appears to be a simple sensation, a message passed to the brain by a peripheral nerve that has received a signal of tissue injury. Upon further examination, though, it becomes clear that what most people describe as pain is much more than a simple sensation. When people say the word "pain," they are generally referring to the *suffering* that is associated with a particular physical sensation. In the case of chronic pain, when the sensation often is not an accurate signal that a physical injury is occurring ("hurt does not equal harm"), the distress or the aversion to the sensation might accurately be described as the actual problem with pain. The pain sensations, as real as they are, are created in the brain. They do not simply represent nociception of a peripheral injury. They are better explained as a signal that the body feels it needs to protect itself. The pain sensations themselves can be translated in the brain in any number of ways and can lead to a wide array of emotions. These emotions typically lead to associations and thoughts. If the evaluation of a sensation is aversive and appraised as a threat, the emotions that arise in response to it will typically be unpleasant emotions including fear, anxiety, anger, despair, frustration, or hatred. The related thoughts, which can often become catastrophic stories about the future, then perpetuate the suffering of

the individual independent of the original sensation. These thoughts and emotions then lead to coping behaviors, which, in sufferers of chronic pain, often include decreased physical activity, social isolation, and avoidant behaviors, all of which themselves deepen the suffering.

This complex web of phenomena: sensation, translation, emotion, thoughts, and behavior patterns, provides the treatment team with a multitude of potential therapeutic targets. Treatment might target the origin of the physical sensation itself, the transmission of the signal, the interpretation of the sensation in the central nervous system, the emotional reaction to that interpretation, the thought patterns that result, or the habitual behaviors. Each of these areas is an independent source of suffering, and improvements in any of them will address at least some part of the patient's distress.

There are many kinds of chronic pain. In some disorders, the primary source of suffering appears to originate in a clear pain-generating pathophysiology. Inflamed joints, such as in rheumatoid arthritis, or invasive cancer are examples of this category of chronic pain. In other disorders, such as somatoform disorder or conversion disorder, the primary source of suffering appears to be almost entirely emotional or cognitive. In between these extremes lie the majority of chronic pain conditions. They are frequently initiated by some injury, neurologic disorder, or pain-processing dysfunction, but they seem to evolve so that psychological processes begin to play a greater role in the patients' suffering and in the perpetuation of pain. The distinction between psychologic and neurologic phenomena blurs, especially as we learn more about the specific neurologic correlates of the chronic pain experience.

NEUROLOGY OF PAIN

Recent research into the neurology of pain has dramatically changed our understanding of pain. Pain, whether acute of chronic, has commonly been interpreted as an aspect of the somatosensory system: Either a nociceptive stimulus hitting pain-specific receptors (nociceptive pain) or a damage to the nerve (neuropathic pain) creates a bottom-up nerve impulse that is transmitted through distinct anterolateral spinothalamic pain pathways and perceived in its discriminative (location and intensity) aspects in somatosensory cortex areas (SI) and in its affective aspects in limbic brain regions (anterior cingulate cortex, ACC). The last decades of pain research have widened that view and furthered our understanding of pain and its regulation. Some of the key findings pertinent to its management are briefly reviewed here.

First, the insular cortex is not only the terminal region for the ipsilateral ascending visceral pain pathway, but it now has been described as the key organ of interoception, that is, the perception of the inner milieu of the body. Interoceptive afferents including pain signals are transmitted through a lateral spinothalamic tract to the posterior insular cortex and are filtered to reach our awareness of the entire internal milieu of the body, pleasant or unpleasant, in the anterior insula (Figure 10–1). Pain perception relies on thick transmission cables to the somatosensory cortex for discrimination and sensorimotor integration and on thin-cabled homeostatic pathways to ACC and insula. Evolution provided only humanoids with this high-definition, topographically organized anterior insular cortex for re-representation of our internal milieu, which includes the felt aspects of emotions and pain. Therefore, with the discovery of the interoceptive homeostatic pathway, it is no longer a surprise that pain shares most qualities with emotions: it has a felt, sensory quality and an affective aspect, demands our mind's

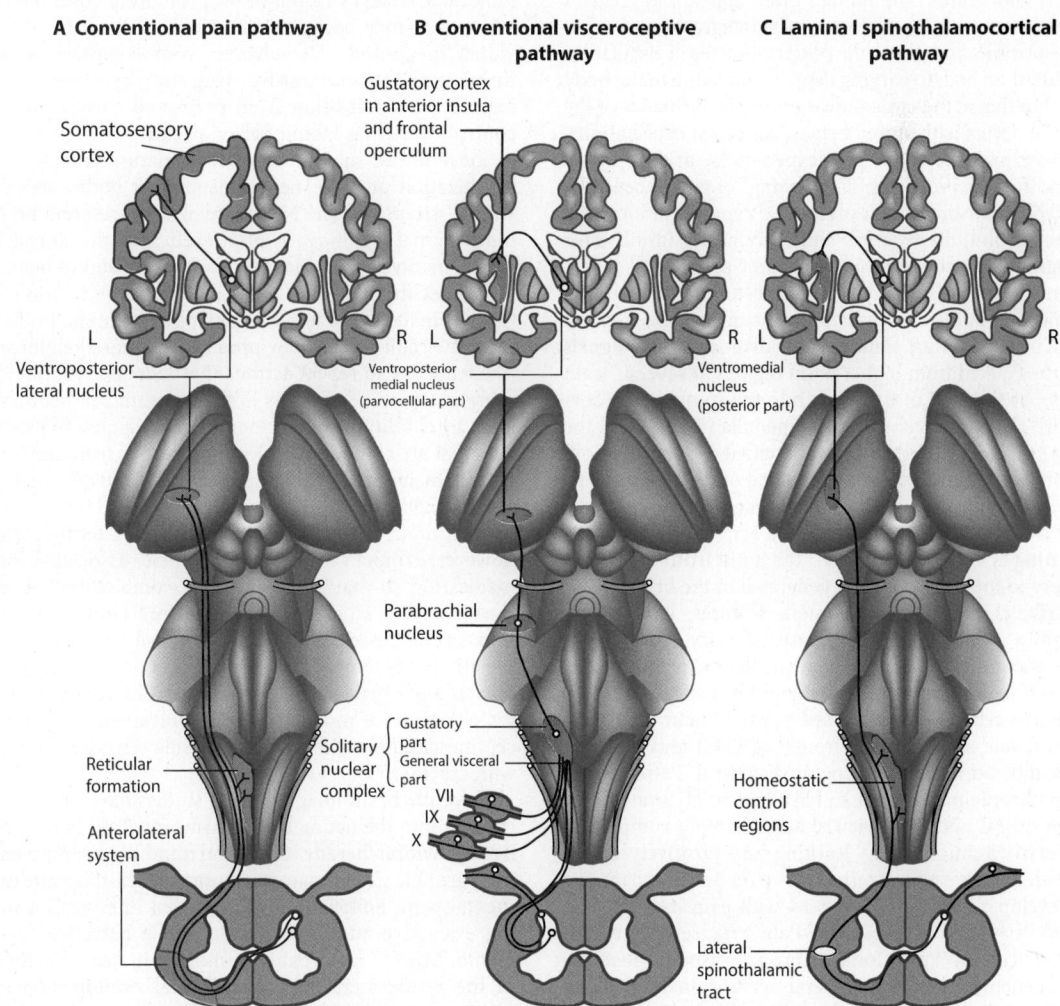

▲ **Figure 10–1.** Pathways of pain perception. (Reproduced with permission from Craig AD: How do you feel? Interoception: the sense of the physiological condition of the body. Nat Rev Neurosci 2002;3(8):655–666. Review. [PMID: 12154366].)

attention, and includes a strong behavioral drive toward homeostasis. The evolutionary gain of a more refined and graded emotion perception, however, comes with a price, namely the increased ability to be aware of and suffering from unpleasant emotions including pain. Pain regulation is conceptually and neurologically intriguingly similar to emotion regulation.

Second, the discovery in the 1930s that electrodes placed in specific cortical areas can elicit pain sensations projected into, for example, a peripheral limb, without any pain stimulus ascending from that limb itself, necessarily lead to the logical conclusion that "pain is all in your brain." This discovery implies that we may have preformed representations in our brain only waiting to be selected or modified by afferent nociceptive stimuli. This is similar to the current conceptualization of interoception which includes pain as one of its key modalities. The human brain appears to create a simulation copy, an "as-if" loop of the integrated and organized sensations brought to the posterior insula, a simulation that is based on and, to varying degrees, analogue to the body proper, but that at the same time is under the influence of the prefrontal cortex with stored beliefs, concepts, expectations, and predictions based on past experiences, and appraisal and conditioning processes. The "feeling" of pain is centrally generated in our brain with preformed representations that have been evolutionary useful. This usefulness is intuitive for acute pain but much less clear for chronic pain.

Third, key elements of the long postulated descending pathways for top-down regulation of pain have been elucidated. The bottom-up transmission of nociceptive signals can be modulated from higher brain regions at several "train stations," at the level of the entry into the spinal cord (dorsal horn), the rostral ventromedial medulla (RVM), and the nucleus cuneiformis. In the latter, specified cells have opioid receptors and perform top-down graded on or off functions on the ascending neurons, thereby decreasing or increasing the stream of bottom-up neuronal activity, filtering and modulating at each "train station" the input from the body's periphery to the pain sensation generated in the brain.

Fourth, chronic pain has unique features. It is associated with a reduction in brain matter density over time in nucleus accumbens (NAc), insula, and sensorimotor cortex (SC). Both developing chronic pain and its perceived intensity are associated with decreased negative neural connectivity of insula and SC to prefrontal (dlPFC) and thalamic regions, indicating impaired cognitive control. Patients who develop chronic pain appear to have increased connectivity between mPFC and NAc, viewed as underlying rumination and aversive reinforcement learning and positively correlated with affective pain intensity. As pain persists, pain circuits develop a hypersensitive state, with pain itself being a pain predictive conditioning cue. Pain hypersensitivity and its chronicity is an expression of neuronal plasticity, an *active* process generated in the peripheral nerve, spinal cord, and corticolimbic brain areas, rather than the passive consequence of the bottom-up transfer of peripheral nociceptive input to a cortical pain center.

Fifth, placebo research has elucidated the interaction of complex mental activities, such as expectancy, beliefs, and values with neuronal systems and pain. Placebo analgesia from conscious expectations or unconscious conditioning functions through the top-down modulation circuit, effectively modulating pain through opiate receptors at all "train stations," from pain-modulating cortical structures (ACC) through the brainstem, all the way down to the dorsal horn. The striking parallel between brain regions involved in the placebo response with pain and with aversive emotions (eg, depression) suggests that the placebo response is part of a neurobehavioral homeostatic self-regulation system that applies to both emotions and pain.

Sixth, opioid pain medications, in addition to their pain relief, particularly effective for acute pain, are both rewarding and behaviorally reinforcing. Repeated use can lead to molecular changes in the brain promoting continued drug taking that may become increasingly difficult for the individual to control. The change from voluntary drug use to habitual and compulsive drug use corresponds neurologically to a transition from prefrontal cortical to striatal control over drug taking behavior and from ventral (NAc) to more dorsal subregions of the striatum and depend on sensitization and the neuroplasticity in both cortical and striatal structures. The NAc is involved in responding to the motivational significance of stimuli, and the dorsal striatum is involved in the learning and execution of behavioral sequences that permit an efficient response to those cues. Opiates increase the levels of synaptic dopamine in the NAc reward circuit and thereby produce behavioral reinforcement (the tendency to repeat actions that increase synaptic dopamine). Dopamine neurons in the striatum can habituate, or learn by conditioning and then fire in response to predictive cues that are carried by projection neurons from the cerebral cortex (including insula), hippocampus, and amygdala, thus associating reward with external context and interoceptively felt emotional and physiologic states. Long-term opiate use, however, dampens the reward experience associated with the medication so that an unfortunate combination of several factors weaken an individual's behavioral control into addiction: (a) decreased reward circuit sensitivity, (b) enhanced sensitivity of memory circuits to conditioned expectations to opiates and opiate-related predictive cues, (c) stress reactivity, (d) negative mood, and (e) involvement of the interoception circuitry with increased insula sensitivity associated with craving.

Seventh, brain imaging fMRI studies have provided new insights into the neural mechanisms involved in how cognitive behavioral therapy (CBT) and mindfulness interventions (MI) are able to alter pain perception, at least in acute experimental pain. Following CBT, a verbal intervention involving evaluative attention to pain and a narrative cognitive mental process, pain patients showed increased activations in the ventrolateral prefrontal/lateral orbitofrontal cortex with experimental pain stimuli. These regions are associated with executive cognitive control. This suggests that CBT changes the brain's processing of pain by increasing access to executive brain regions for reappraisal of pain. In MI, quite differently, an increased *sensory* attention to the discriminatory aspects of pain coupled with decreased evaluative *thinking* about pain results in decreased affective pain (less bothersome) and is neurologically associated with increased insular cortex activity for interoceptive awareness and decreased lateral prefrontal cortex activity, interpreted as decreased cognitive control and less cognitive-evaluative reactivity. CBT directs attention away from pain and increases cognitive appraisal activity (reframing); MI refines attention toward the pain region and facilitates detachment from cognitive appraisal activity. However, both approaches—in real life—include numerous methods, and CBT for pain has integrated aspects of mindfulness into its modules, whereas MIs have integrated elements of CBT as mindfulness-based cognitive therapy (MBCT).

The above neurologic findings may help us in the understanding of the psychosomatics of pain and its regulation and management.

PSYCHOLOGY OF PAIN

On psychological personality profile tests, patients with chronic pain have been described as expressing exaggerated concern over body feelings, developing bodily symptoms in response to stress, and either often failing to recognize their own emotional state (eg, depression) or being demanding and complaining. Clinical studies have shown that these psychological attributes can improve with reduction in pain and are seen as a consequence of chronic pain rather than antecedent and predictive to it. However, the prognosis of both acute and chronic pain is more strongly dependent on psychological and occupational than on physical or medical factors. Although studies vary widely in inclusion criteria (duration of pain, primary care, workers compensation claims) and outcome parameters (return to work, pain or disability reduction, perceived recovery), several factors stand out and are now widely accepted as risk factors for (a) the transition from acute to chronic pain and (b) the persistence of chronic pain. These factors are modifiable by the nonpharmacologic interventions presented as follows:

1. Depression: Depression is more common in chronic pain patients than in healthy controls, and pain is more common in depressed patients than in nondepressed individuals. Whereas some researchers believe that depression is frequently overlooked in pain patients, others emphasize that depression is a consequence rather than an antecedent of chronic pain. Distress (complaining of physical symptoms associated with depression and anxiety), depressive mood, and somatization are all implicated in the transition to chronic low back pain. Although numerous studies show a strong cross-sectional association between pain and depression, longitudinal studies have yielded contradictory results regarding depression as a risk factor for onset of new

pain or for the progression to or persistence of chronic pain. Some researchers postulate that this is because people with chronic pain can be divided into two categories. In one group pain symptoms, nonpain somatic symptoms, and symptoms of depression and anxiety tend to cluster, with heightened stress reactivity and a tendency to overwhelm self-regulatory homeostatic systems. The second category, sometimes labeled "happy endurers," form a separate cluster by ignoring symptoms of discomfort and pain and making a nondepressed, "happy face" in response to stress or pain. These persons are equally at risk of pain chronification and longer pain duration but do not exhibit depressive symptoms.

When depression is comorbid with chronic pain, both are frequently seen as a dyad that requires a combined therapy, although systematic reviews have found no evidence that antidepressants are more effective for chronic low back pain than placebo.

2. Pain catastrophizing: Catastrophizing, a maladaptive coping style, is a construct with three components: magnification or amplification of pain, ruminating thoughts about pain, and perceived helplessness in the face of pain. It appears to be the strongest and most consistent psychosocial factor associated with persistence of pain and poor function in persons with chronic pain, even after controlling for depression. Catastrophizing is modifiable and, if treated by psychosocial interventions, pain improves with a decrease in catastrophizing.

3. Fear avoidance: Fear avoidance is another maladaptive coping behavior, the avoidance of work, movement, or other activities due to fear that they will damage the body or worsen pain. Pain patients high in fear avoidance have worse long-term outcomes. Fear avoidance is associated with catastrophic misinterpretations of pain, hypervigilance, increased escape and avoidance behaviors, and increased pain intensity and functional disability. Although it has not been shown that fear-avoidance leads to decreased physical fitness or deconditioning as a mediator for developing chronic pain, sufficient evidence has accumulated that pain-related fear may increase the risk for developing new-onset back pain, for its chronification, and for its persistence. The value of changing beliefs about pain early in its course has been shown in studies involving patient education in physician's offices and over the public radio.

4. Job satisfaction: Although supervisor support may be a factor in duration of sick leave, there is strong evidence that job satisfaction is *not* a prognostic factor for duration of sick leave. Studies assessing the effects of job demands, job control, job strain, skill discretion, decision authority, job security, co-worker support, supervisory support, psychological demands, physical demands, and work flexibility on duration of work absenteeism can be summarized as inconclusive. There is strong evidence, however, that heavy work is a predictor for longer duration of sick leave. Although assignment to light duties as

commonly used for a rapid return to work appears *not* to shorten sick leave in workers with acute low back pain, staying active and modified work are supported.

5. Distraction: Distraction is a coping style that generally is favored by patients. It's opposite, a hypervigilant attention style toward pain, is related to anxiety and is maladaptive. In research studies, distraction appears to have no consistent proven benefits for chronic pain, though evidence does exist that music, either by providing distraction or by increasing positive effect and inducing relaxation, may diminish pain. An attention focus toward pain can be either beneficial or maladaptive, a distinction that is likely mediated by the attention style. An anxiety-driven and hypervigilant attention style is likely maladaptive, while accepting and mindful attention may be beneficial. Research on this question is underway.

6. Ignoring/Endurance: Ignoring pain is generally considered an adaptive coping style, particularly with the use of cognitive distraction. This represents a focused approach to diverting attention from pain and is consistent with the aims of traditional CBT for pain. Yet, suppressing the perception of pain to avoid interruptions in daily activities, a more disorganized and nonfocused search for distraction that often fails and causes feelings of emotional distress, is a form of distressed endurance behavior and task persistence that has been shown to lead to chronic pain, possibly via physical overload. There are, however, studies indicating that the opposite of ignoring and suppression, an in vivo exposure approach such as with acceptance and mindfulness training, or CBT with added interoceptive exposure therapy, can be effective in pain patients.

7. Adverse life events are a risk factor for the onset of chronic multisite musculoskeletal pain. Individuals with multiple stressful experiences in childhood are at increased risk of developing chronic back problems. Adverse childhood experiences (ACE) such as abuse and neglect are common, can have cumulative effects on health, and increase the risk for chronic pain disorders and maladaptive coping strategies that can intensify patients' experience of pain and prolong treatment. Screening for ACE ideally is done when referrals for specific treatment options are available.

8. Recovery expectation: Recovery expectation is one of the strongest predictors of work outcome for patients with pain. Recovery expectations measured within weeks of new-onset of pain can identify people at risk of poor outcome. Expectation is a complex construct composed of numerous variables such as concerns about pain exacerbations, recurrent pain, financial security, support at work, and self-confidence. Practitioners may need to further inquire why patients have beliefs of delayed recovery and address specific concerns.

Using a combination of physical and psychological variables, feasible prediction tools have been developed in the United Kingdom and Sweden (Örebro Musculoskeletal Pain Questionnaire and STarT Back screening tool) for return to work as primary outcome after a first office visit for low back pain. The nine-item STarT Back tool has recently been validated in a primary care sample with mostly chronic pain in the United States. However, work-related low back pain was excluded, and no studies have been published testing the above tools in the United States in an occupational medicine setting. They are public and can be downloaded from the internet (https://startback.hfac.keele.ac.uk/).

CHRONIC PAIN MANAGEMENT

Chronic pain is a long-term condition that can always be managed and sometimes cured. The primary goal of therapy is generally management and coping rather than complete obliteration of the pain. Patients who have realistic expectations about pain treatment tend to have better outcomes than those that do not. Pain management programs are most effective when they emphasize self-management on the part of the patient and enhance the patient's sense of self-efficacy and confidence in their ability to cope with pain.

It is important to monitor the effectiveness of a given pain management program in order to make changes as appropriate. Unlike acute pain, which can often adequately be measured using numerical rating scales or visual analog scales, chronic pain requires more complex measurement tools. In addition to aiming to decrease the experience of pain, chronic pain treatment must also be focused on the improvement of function. Functional improvement can be measured in terms of physical function, emotional function, social function, or work function. Particularly when high risk or addictive substances are being used to control pain, it is critical that the prescriber have an objective measure to show that the strategy is in fact improving the patient's function rather than diminishing it.

Examples of tools for measuring pain and its impact on function include the pain, enjoyment, and general activity (PEG) scale (Figure 10–2) or the brief pain inventory (Figure 10–3). In general, both pain and function should be assessed at the initiation of treatment and at regular intervals as treatment progresses.

Because the suffering that arises from chronic pain can have its source in the physical sensations, emotions, thoughts and beliefs, or coping behaviors and their consequences, each of these domains needs to be addressed by a comprehensive pain management strategy. It is no surprise that multidisciplinary and multimodal approaches to chronic pain appear to be most effective. Treatment teams that include occupational therapists, physical therapists, psychotherapists, pharmacists, complementary medicine practitioners, and a physician, nurse practitioner, or physician's assistant are likely to be most effective.

What follows is a brief review of treatment modalities that can be effective in chronic pain. No one modality can be expected to suffice for a given patient, and an optimal treatment strategy will combine therapies from multiple

1. What number best describes your <u>pain on average</u> in the past week:

0	1	2	3	4	5	6	7	8	9	10

No pain   Pain as bad as you can imagine

2. What number best describes how, during the past week, pain has interfered with your <u>enjoyment of life?</u>

0	1	2	3	4	5	6	7	8	9	10

Does not interfere   Completely interferes

3. What number best describes how, during the past week, pain has interfered with your <u>general activity?</u>

0	1	2	3	4	5	6	7	8	9	10

Does not interfere   Completely interferes

▲ **Figure 10–2.** The pain, enjoyment, and general activity (PEG) scale.

categories. For chronic low back pain, current recommendations by the American College of Physicians (2017) emphasize nonpharmacologic modalities as first-line approach. These include exercise, multidisciplinary rehabilitation, acupuncture, yoga, tai chi, mindfulness-based stress reduction (MBSR), and CBT.

▶ Pharmacologic Therapies

In general, medications can be expected to reduce pain scores by 20–50%, depending on the type of pain and the type of medication. They are rarely sufficient alone for the management of chronic pain.

See Table 10–1 for a description of common classes of medication used to treat chronic pain.

In past years, it had become increasingly common to treat chronic pain with opioid medications. This was despite the absence of evidence for effectiveness with opioids beyond a 6-month period and consistent evidence that they do not improve function. Simultaneously, there has been a marked increase in the number of overdose deaths from prescription opioids and the incidence of prescription opioid addiction. For most patients, the risk of developing addiction to prescribed opioids remains low but real. In addition, if some people with preexisting addictions present to care stating that they are in pain and, in an attempt to treat pain, the prescriber inadvertently may contribute to the disease of addiction. In recent studies, up to 60% of patients prescribed opioids do not take them as prescribed. Some opioids that are prescribed for pain are given or sold to people to whom they are not prescribed, contributing significantly to the national epidemic of opioid overdose. For this reason, specific guidelines for safe opioid prescribing have been developed. These guidelines are designed to decrease the risk of overdose of opioid misuse and to assist the clinician in identifying signs a patient may be coming to harm from the medications. These CDC recommendations include

Determining When to Initiate or Continue Opioids for Chronic Pain

1. Nonpharmacologic therapy and nonopioid pharmacologic therapy are preferred for chronic pain. Clinicians should consider opioid therapy only if expected benefits for both pain and function are anticipated to outweigh risks to the patient. If opioids are used, they should be combined with nonpharmacologic therapy and nonopioid pharmacologic therapy, as appropriate.

2. Before starting opioid therapy for chronic pain, clinicians should establish treatment goals with all patients, including realistic goals for pain and function, and should consider how therapy will be discontinued if benefits do not outweigh risks. Clinicians should continue opioid therapy only if there is clinically meaningful improvement in pain and function that outweighs risks to patient safety.

3. Before starting and periodically during opioid therapy, clinicians should discuss with patients known risks and realistic benefits of opioid therapy and patient and clinician responsibilities for managing therapy.

Opioid Selection, Dosage, Duration, Follow-Up, and Discontinuation

1. When starting opioid therapy for chronic pain, clinicians should prescribe immediate-release opioids instead of extended-release/long-acting (ER/LA) opioids.

2. When opioids are started, clinicians should prescribe the lowest effective dosage. Clinicians should use caution when prescribing opioids at any dosage, should carefully reassess evidence of individual benefits and risks when increasing dosage to =50 morphine milligram equivalents (MME)/day, and should avoid increasing dosage to =90 MME/day or carefully justify a decision to titrate dosage to =90 MME/day.

STUDY ID #: _ _ _ _ _ _ _ _ _ _   DO NOT WRITE ABOVE THIS LINE   HOSPITAL #: _ _ _ _ _ _ _ _ _ _

Brief Pain Inventory (Short Form)

Date: _ _ _ _ / _ _ _ _ / _ _ _ _   Time: _ _ _ _ _ _ _

Name: _ _ _ _ _ _ _ _ _ _ _ _ _ _ _ _ _ _ _   _ _ _ _ _ _ _ _ _ _ _ _ _ _ _ _ _ _   _ _ _ _ _ _ _ _ _ _ _ _ _ _ _

            Last   First   Middle Initial

1. Throughout our lives, most of us have had pain from time to time (such as minor headaches, sprains, and toothaches). Have you had pain other than these every-day kinds of pain today?

     1. Yes   2. No

2. On the diagram, shade in the areas where you feel pain. Put an X on the area that hurts the most.

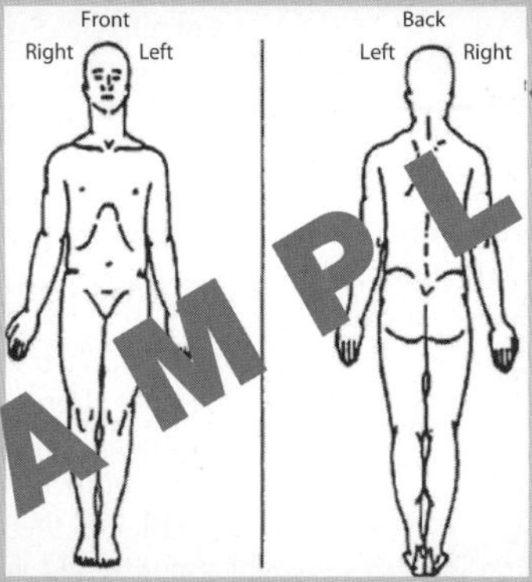

3. Please rate your pain by circling the one number that best describes your pain at its worst in the last 24 hours.

0	1	2	3	4	5	6	7	8	9	10
No Pain										Pain as bad as you can imagine

4. Please rate your pain by circling the one number that best describes your pain at its least in the last 24 hours.

0	1	2	3	4	5	6	7	8	9	10
No Pain										Pain as bad as you can imagine

5. Please rate your pain by circling the one number that best describes your pain on the average.

0	1	2	3	4	5	6	7	8	9	10
No Pain										Pain as bad as you can imagine

6. Please rate your pain by circling the one number that tells how much pain you have right now.

0	1	2	3	4	5	6	7	8	9	10
No Pain										Pain as bad as you can imagine

Page 1 of 2

THE UNIVERSITY OF TEXAS
MD Anderson
~~Cancer~~ Center

▲ **Figure 10–3.** Brief pain inventory. (Reproduced with permission from the University of Texas MD Anderson Cancer Center, Department of Symptom Research, Houston, TX. Copyright ©1991 Charles S. Cleeland, PhD, Pain Research Group. All rights reserved.)

STUDY ID #: _____   DO NOT WRITE ABOVE THIS LINE   HOSPITAL #: _____

Date: ___ / ___ _/ ____   Time: _____
Name: _____   _____   _____
                    Last   First   Middle Initial

7.   What treatments or medications are you receiving for your pain?

_____
_____

**8.   In the last 24 hours, how much relief have pain treatments or medications
       provided? Please circle the one percentage that most shows how much relief
       you have received.**

0%	10%	20%	30%	40%	50%	60%	70%	80%	90%	100%
No Relief										Complete Relief

**9.   Circle the one number that describes how, during the past 24 hours, pain has
       interfered with your:**

A.   General Activity

0	1	2	3	4	5	6	7	8	9	10
Does not Interfere										Completely Interferes

B.   Mood

0	1	2	3	4	5	6	7	8	9	10
Does not Interfere										Completely Interferes

C.   Walking Ability

0	1	2	3	4	5	6	7	8	9	10
Does not Interfere										Completely Interferes

D.   Normal Work (includes both work outside the home and housework)

0	1	2	3	4	5	6	7	8	9	10
Does not Interfere										Completely Interferes

E.   Relations with other people

0	1	2	3	4	5	6	7	8	9	10
Does not Interfere										Completely Interferes

F.   Sleep

0	1	2	3	4	5	6	7	8	9	10
Does not Interfere										Completely Interferes

G.   Enjoyment of life

0	1	2	3	4	5	6	7	8	9	10
Does not Interfere										Completely Interferes

Page 2 of 2

THE UNIVERSITY OF TEXAS
MD Anderson
Cancer Center®

▲ **Figure 10–3.** (*Continued*)

Table 10-1. Pharmacologic pain therapies.

Drug Class	Examples	Mechanism	Type of Pain	Safety
Acetaminophen	Acetaminophen	Unclear, multiple central CNS effects	All types	Can cause hepatic injury if taken in high doses.
Nonsteroidal anti-inflammatory drugs (NSAIDs)	Oral: Nonselective: Ibuprofen Naproxen Ketorolac Diclofenac Selective: Celecoxib Topical: Diclofenac	Inhibit production of COX-1 and 2 — Inhibit production of COX-2	All types. Particularly useful in inflammatory conditions.	Can cause gastritis, peptic ulcer, and renal damage. Increases risk of cardiac event, worsens congestive heart failure. — Topical forms are safer than oral forms.
Anti-epileptic medications	Gabapentin Pregabalin Carbamazepine Topiramate	Unclear, though likely through inhibition of pain pathways either via GABA receptors or decreased nerve conduction.	Neuropathic pain. Also used as adjuvant treatment in other types of pain.	Can cause sedation, dizziness, weight gain. Each drug has a different side effect profile.
Tricyclic antidepressants (TCAs)	Amitriptyline Nortriptyline	Decreased norepinephrine and serotonin reuptake activates descending pain pathways that inhibit pain signals.	Neuropathic pain. Also used as adjuvant treatment in other types of pain. In higher doses, useful to treat concurrent depression.	Anticholinergic side effects include drowsiness, dry mouth, and constipation. Should be avoided in suicidal patients, as lethal in overdose.
Serotonin-norepinephrine reuptake inhibitors (SNRIs)	Venlafaxine Duloxetine	Decreased norepinephrine and serotonin reuptake activates descending pain pathways that inhibit pain signals.	Neuropathic pain and depression.	Fewer side effects than TCAs, though may cause withdrawal symptoms.
Muscle relaxants	Cyclobenzaprine Baclofen Carisoprodol Methocarbamol	Variable. Most act in the CNS and inhibit muscle contraction.	Not clearly effective in chronic pain. Cyclobenzaprine is effective in fibromyalgia, possibly because of improved sleep.	Sedation. Carisoprodol in particular is a popular drug of abuse and is metabolized to the Schedule IV drug, meprobamate.
Anesthetics	Lidocaine Benzocaine	Inhibit nerve signal transduction.	Neuropathic pain. Used transdermally either as cream or patch.	Minimal. In very high doses, may cause cardiac arrhythmias, but this is extremely rare with topical formulations.
Capsaicin cream	Capsaicin cream	Inhibits signal transport through nociceptive nerve fibers.	Primarily neuropathic, though can be used for any pain.	Burning pain can occur for the first few applications. With time, this diminishes.
Opioids	Hydrocodone Codeine Morphine Oxycodone Hydromorphone	Bind endorphin receptors.	Not generally indicated in chronic pain. When used as a drug of last resort, generally most effective in non-neuropathic pain. Contraindicated for headache, full body pain, fibromyalgia, or somatoform disorders.	Constipation and hypogonadism are very common. Physical dependence is virtually inevitable and psychological dependence, or addiction, can develop. Sedation and death by overdose are increasingly common. Opioid-induced hyperalgesia may lead to worsening pain in the presence of opioids.

3. Long-term opioid use often begins with treatment of acute pain. When opioids are used for acute pain, clinicians should prescribe the lowest effective dose of immediate-release opioids and should prescribe no greater quantity than needed for the expected duration of pain severe enough to require opioids. Three days or less will often be sufficient; more than 7 days will rarely be needed.

4. Clinicians should evaluate benefits and harms with patients within 1–4 weeks of starting opioid therapy for chronic pain or of dose escalation. Clinicians should evaluate benefits and harms of continued therapy with patients every 3 months or more frequently. If benefits do not outweigh harms of continued opioid therapy, clinicians should optimize other therapies and work with patients to taper opioids to lower dosages or to taper and discontinue opioids.

Assessing Risk and Addressing Harms of Opioid Use

1. Before starting and periodically during continuation of opioid therapy, clinicians should evaluate risk factors for opioid-related harms. Clinicians should incorporate strategies in the management plan to mitigate risk, including considering offering naloxone when factors that increase risk for opioid overdose, such as history of overdose, history of substance use disorder, higher opioid dosages (=50 MME/day), or concurrent benzodiazepine use, are present.

2. Clinicians should review the patient's history of controlled substance prescriptions using state prescription drug monitoring program (PDMP) data to determine whether the patient is receiving opioid dosages or dangerous combinations that put him or her at high risk for overdose. Clinicians should review PDMP data when starting opioid therapy for chronic pain and periodically during opioid therapy for chronic pain, ranging from every prescription to every 3 months.

3. When prescribing opioids for chronic pain, clinicians should use urine drug testing before starting opioid therapy and consider urine drug testing at least annually to assess for prescribed medications as well as other controlled prescription drugs and illicit drugs.

4. Clinicians should avoid prescribing opioid pain medication and benzodiazepines concurrently whenever possible.

5. Clinicians should offer or arrange evidence-based treatment (usually medication-assisted treatment with buprenorphine or methadone in combination with behavioral therapies) for patients with opioid use disorder.

Standard of practice for chronic pain is moving away from monotherapy with opioids and toward a multimodal approach. The following sections describe nonpharmacologic pain treatment options that are recommended for patients with chronic pain.

▶ Psychologically Based Therapies

Regardless of whether a particular patient's pain has its source in psychosocial suffering, it will inevitably result in this type of suffering. For that reason, almost all patients with chronic pain benefit from psychosocial interventions. There is evidence that these therapies reduce pain intensity, improve function and quality of life, and reduce depression. What follows is an inexhaustive list of evidence-based psychosocial interventions for chronic pain. Which approach is the appropriate for a given patient may vary.

A. Self-Management Support

Chronic pain is in many ways analogous to other chronic illnesses. It can be expected to wax and wane in severity, and the degree to which a patient tolerates the illness is related to the degree to which the patient takes responsibility for managing it. Self-management support programs can take many different forms. Some programs take the form of classes that teach patients exercises, distraction techniques or mindfulness, muscle relaxation practices, and communication skills, while other programs involve coaches assigned to help patients manage pain at home, and others involve peer-led support groups. Each of these models has been found to reduce pain and some of them improve function and decrease disability. The fundamental components of a self-management program include

- Medication management training
- Emotional management, including education about the role of anger and depression and strategies for managing difficult emotions
- Social support management, including communication training and strategies for maximizing social support
- Sleep management, including sleep hygiene training and discussion of the impact of sleep on pain
- Pain coping practices, including distraction, muscle relaxation, visualization, meditation, and breathing exercises

B. Cognitive Behavioral Therapy

There is significant overlap between CBT and self-management support programs. Often, the two occur simultaneously. CBT is based on the understanding that habitual thoughts and beliefs, or cognition, alter patients' behaviors in ways that can either be productive or destructive. The goal of CBT is to help patients identify destructive thought patterns and learn to generate more constructive thought patterns. The focus of pain-based CBT will generally be on restructuring the patient's relationship with pain from one of helpless victim to one of active agent, learning to use self-management skills such as pacing, relaxation, and problem solving, and fostering self-confidence and hope. More recently CBT for chronic pain has included a mindfulness module. On a neurologic level, CBT supports neural connectivity associated with improved cognitive executive control.

CBT can be provided in both group and individual settings. Group therapy has the advantage of providing social support to patients who are often socially isolated, and also increases access to programs by allowing clinicians to see multiple patients simultaneously. Individual therapy has the advantage of being more tailored to the patient's specific needs and may be more appropriate for patients with significant co-occurring psychopathology.

C. Acceptance and Commitment Therapy

Acceptance and Commitment Therapy (ACT) is different from CBT in that it teaches acceptance and "just noticing" of one's present situation, including pain and suffering. ACT teaches patients to disentangle the perception of pain from its accompanying thoughts and emotions but does not teach patients to attempt to control and change these thoughts and feelings. Distraction from pain is viewed as experiential avoidance and as maladaptive, whereas mindful discrimination of pain is considered adaptive. Improved psychological flexibility is then combined with goal setting and commitment to take action. ACT has shown efficacy in the treatment of chronic pain, addiction, and anxiety disorders by reducing psychological risk factors for chronic pain: catastrophizing, fear-avoidance, and expectations of poor outcome. Many clinical psychologists combine CBT and elements of ACT.

D. Mindfulness Meditation

Mindfulness meditation has been adapted to and studied in the treatment of chronic pain since the 1980s. It has become a popular approach to chronic pain management not only because of its impact on pain, but because it also seems to address many patients' more global, even existential forms of suffering. Mindfulness is characterized by a nonjudgmental compassionate awareness of the present moment. Patients who are trained in mindfulness learn to minimize the narrative and emotional overlay of pain and to just experience the physical sensations of pain as more neutral, discriminate, and less personally loaded physical sensations. The goal is to learn to create space between the sensing pain and the emotional and mental reactivity that tends to follow, with the understanding that this mental and emotional reactivity is usually the source of much of a person's suffering. "Pain is part of life, suffering is optional." In medical settings, mindfulness meditation is usually taught in the MBSR format pioneered by Jon Kabat-Zinn. The MBSR format has been studied extensively and found to reduce pain intensity, increase physical activity, improve quality of life, and improve mood in patients with chronic pain. On the neurologic level, MBSR-related neuroplasticity changes are associated with increased interoceptive awareness (insula activation), improved attention regulation, and decreased rumination and cognitive-evaluative control. Based on MBSR and originally developed

for preventing relapse in depression, MBCT has recently been adapted for chronic pain.

E. Hypnotherapy and Guided Imagery

Hypnotherapy begins with the induction of a deep state of relaxation. Patients who are skilled in relaxation can induce this state themselves, or they can be guided into the state by a hypnotherapist. Once the relaxed state has been induced, the hypnotherapist speaks with the patient, providing useful suggestions to the patient's own imagery, cognitive frameworks, or narratives to help the patient develop more productive behaviors or cognitions about their pain. For example, a patient with shoulder pain might be guided to feel the hand relax and become easeful, or to see the bones and muscles of the shoulder realign in a healthful, comfortable alignment. Patients are generally taught to induce these states for themselves so that they can become part of the patient's self-management toolkit.

F. Biofeedback

Biofeedback refers to a variety of systems designed to give patients direct, visual feedback about internal psychophysical processes. A device can be used to provide feedback about muscle tension in target muscles (eg, suboccipital muscles and scalenes in tension headache), heart rate, respiratory rate, temperature, or skin conductance and how these immediately respond to stressful thoughts. The goal is to develop an awareness of these more subtle interoceptive physiologic phenomena so that they come under direct voluntary control by the patient. Biofeedback can therefore help patients learn to relax both physically and psychologically and has been shown to be effective in the management of pain conditions, particularly chronic headaches.

▶ Movement-Based Therapies

A. Physical and Occupational Therapy

It is beyond the scope of this chapter to describe physical and occupational therapies for each chronic pain condition. Broadly speaking, the goal of physical and occupational therapy for these patients is to teach them self-management skills and assist them in learning to function within the constraints of their limited abilities. The therapist working with chronic pain patients will find that overcoming fear-avoidance and catastrophizing cognitive patterns are of paramount importance. Gentle, playful, but persistent coaching and education are critical. In studies of physical therapy for patients with pain, physical therapy is generally as effective as or more effective than pharmacologic treatments for reducing pain scores, and is clearly superior at improving function.

B. Aerobic Exercise

Even absent a formal physical therapy program, engagement in regular physical activity is beneficial for patients with chronic pain. Exercise reduces chronic inflammation, improves mood, and improves strength and mobility. Patients who exercise regularly note decreased pain scores and increased sense of self-efficacy.

C. Tai Chi and Yoga

Both approaches have become very popular and are here jointly discussed, as both are essentially complex exercise interventions with a strong focus on postural correction and kinesthetic body awareness. The development of muscular strength, positive effect, reduced catastrophizing, and improved self-efficacy occur as products of these practices. Particularly yoga has been clinically studied in patients with chronic low back pain and is included in the guideline recommendations by the American Pain Society and American College of Physicians for its treatment. Yoga exercises may need to be individualized to the particular needs of patients, as some back-pain patients may be constitutionally hypermobile and experience worsened pain with extreme postures or may have either flexion or extension-sensitive back pain. Tai chi has been found to be effective for fibromyalgia pain, presumably because it is gentle enough to be tolerated by patients with significant pain sensitivity.

D. Pacing

Along with strategies for enhancing mobility and strength, patients with chronic pain can benefit from learning to pace themselves appropriately. Because of the waxing and waning nature of chronic pain, most patients will find that they have days or moments in which they feel minimal pain and other times in which they have increased pain. It is common for patients to become less physically active during periods of pain, sometimes failing to get out of bed or spending entire days sitting down. Conversely, on days with less pain, patients will often overextend themselves, rushing to complete all of the tasks and errands that they failed to accomplish on previous days. Both behavior patterns can lead to increased pain, one through increased stiffness, weakness, and depression, the other through soreness, increased inflammation, and even injury.

Pacing techniques prevent these periods of over- or under-activity by teaching patients to measure out task in advance and plan the amount of time they intend to spend on an activity. For example, the patient may plan in advance to spend 5 minutes on dishes, rest for 5 minutes, and restart the dishes again after rest. If a patient knows that 3 minutes of loading the laundry machine causes pain, one limits laundry to 2 minutes at a time with 3-minute breaks. Pacing can feel slow at first, but allows patients to remain active. Another pacing technique involves measuring one's pain score before starting an activity and periodically checking the pain score throughout. If the pain score rises more than 2 points, the patient is instructed to pause and rest.

▶ Interventional Therapies

Depending on the specific source of a patient's pain, a wide variety of mechanical or surgical interventions may be available. Joint injections with steroids are effective for arthritis, and can be performed in most medium to large joints in the body. Trigger point injections, which target points of muscular tension and aim to release them with local anesthetics, can be helpful for patients with chronic myofascial pain. Anesthesiologists and physiatrists are able to inactivate offending nerves with nerve blocks. If the patient's pain can be tracked to a single nerve or nerve plexus, nerve ablation can sometimes be performed. For intractable pain, intrathecal medication pumps or neural stimulators implanted in the spinal cord may provide relief. Finally, for some conditions, such as advanced osteoarthritis, surgical removal and replacement of the painful joint is appropriate and highly effective.

▶ Complementary Therapies

A. Acupuncture

A Cochrane meta-analysis (2005) found that acupuncture, the insertion and manual or electrical stimulation of thin needles (Gauge 30 and higher) inserted into specific, anatomically defined acu-points chosen according to diagnostic principals from traditional Chinese medicine (TCM), adds to other conventional therapies, relieves pain, and improves function better than conventional therapies alone. However, effects are small and vary. TCM is an entire system of applications including acupuncture, moxibustion, massage, exercises, herbs and verbal counseling. How it may work on a molecular, tissue, peripheral, and central neural level is the subject of numerous recent publications. Effects are strongest when in concordance with patient expectations. When self-management strategies for pain do not help, three to six sessions of acupuncture in addition to conventional treatments (PT, nonnarcotic pain medication) can provide a reasonable trial and clarify whether the patient will benefit. Licensed nonphysician acupuncturists have a much more extensive training than physicians who have taken shorter acupuncture courses.

B. Chiropractic Therapy and Osteopathic Manipulative Therapy

Manual therapy-trained physical therapists, chiropractors, and osteopaths are three professions which can apply a variety of mobilizing and manipulating techniques to patients with musculoskeletal pain summed up under the label of "manual therapy" or, if provided by physicians, "manual medicine." They apply highly trained palpation skills to diagnose muscle, fascia, and joint dysfunctions and assess spine function on a segmental level. In addition to numerous soft tissue and gentle manipulation techniques, they may apply high-velocity, low-amplitude manipulation impulses to spine segments and individual facet joints. The physiological effects of such spinal manipulations have been documented as increased facet gapping in human MRI studies and as reduced paraspinal muscle spindle afferents in animal studies. A 2011 Cochrane review of 26 RCTs for chronic low back

Table 10–2. Common herbs and supplements used for pain.

Name	Mechanism	Evidence for Efficacy In	Safety	Comments
Boswellia (*Boswellia serrate*)	Gum resin from the Indian frankincense tree contains boswellic acid and alpha and beta boswellic acid, which act as anti-inflammatory agents, primarily in the leukotriene pathway.	Osteoarthritis Ulcerative colitis	Well tolerated in trials lasting up to 90 days.	Classically used to treat pulmonary conditions, like asthma. Reduces pain by 25–50% in studies.
Bromelain (*Ananas comosus*)	Bromelain is a proteolytic enzyme in pineapple stem and fruit. Alters leukocyte migration and activation.	Osteoarthritis	Well tolerated in studies, occasional GI upset.	Found to be equivalent to diclofenac 50 mg in one study.
Cat's Claw (*Uncaria tomentosa* and *Uncaria guianensis*)	Root and bark contain alkaloids that inhibit production of prostaglandin E2 and TNF-alpha, decreasing inflammation.	Osteoarthritis Rheumatoid arthritis	Well tolerated in trials lasting up to 6 months.	Extracts that contain pentacyclic oxindole alkaloids and are free of tetracyclic oxindole alkaloids may be more effective.
Curcumin/Turmeric (*Curcuma longa, Curcuma domestica,* or *Curcuma aromatica*)	Curcuminoids from turmeric rhizome inhibit COX-2, prostaglandins, and leukotrienes, decreasing inflammation.	Osteoarthritis Rheumatoid arthritis	Well tolerated in trials lasting up to 8 months with doses up to 2.2 g/d.	Poor bioavailability unless combined with piperine or other absorption-enhancing agents. 500 mg qid turmeric equivalent to ibuprofen 400 mg in one trial.
Fish oil	Omega-3 fatty acids decrease production of prostaglandin E2, thromboxane B2, leukotrienes, and other inflammatory cytokines.	Rheumatoid arthritis Ulcerative colitis	3 g or less per day is considered safe. Decreases platelet activation, may increase bleeding risk.	May cause unpleasant taste or burping. This can be improved by keeping pills frozen.
Ginger (*Zingiber officinale*)	Ginger rhizome and root contain gingerol, gingerdione, shogaol, and sesquiterpene volatile oils. These appear to inhibit COX and lipoxygenase pathways, as well as TNF-alpha production, reducing inflammation.	Osteoarthritis	Well tolerated in long-term trials.	Also useful in treating nausea.
S-adenosylmethionine (SAM-e)	Naturally occurring molecule that is ubiquitous in human tissue. Concentrations decrease with age. Contributes to methylation in hundreds of biochemical reactions, including hormone synthesis, neurotransmitter synthesis, and nucleic acid synthesis.	Osteoarthritis Fibromyalgia	Well tolerated in studies lasting up to 2 years. May induce mania in patients with bipolar disorder.	Trials also show effectiveness in treating depression.

pain concluded that spinal manipulation is equally effective as other conventional therapies such as, exercise therapy, standard medical care, or physiotherapy. Other systematic reviews found no clear evidence of it being superior to other therapies or sham for patients with acute low back pain, while a large study in the British National Health System found effectiveness for pain, function, and costs above best primary care. Studies conducted by physical therapists in the United States found that spinal manipulation appears to be most effective in a subgroup of patients with a shorter duration of back pain (< 16 days), segmental hypomobility, and low fear-avoidance behavior. The guidelines by the American Pain Society (2007/2009), the American College of Physicians (2017), and the National Institute for Clinical Excellence in the United Kingdom (2016) recommend spinal manipulation for acute and chronic low back pain in patients who do not improve with self-care options. A large telephone survey in the United States in year 2003 reported that 27% of back and neck pain patients found conventional care "very helpful," whereas 61% felt that way with chiropractic care. High-velocity spinal manipulation at the upper cervical spine, however, is a procedure requiring informed patient consent due to a small but undeniable stroke risk from vertebral artery dissection.

C. Massage Therapy

Massage is an ages-old therapy and uses a wide variety of techniques: compression, friction, gliding/stroking (*effleurage*), holding, kneading (*petrissage*), lifting, movement and mobilization, and vibration. Although not covered by health insurances, a 2015 Cochrane review of 25 RCTs found moderate evidence for low back pain compared with active control in short and long term, best when combined with exercise and education, but no improvement in function and no serious side effects. Effects are larger if concordant with patient expectations. In a large 2003 telephone survey, 65% of queried US back pain patients reported that massage was "very helpful" for neck and back pain. A 2004 meta-analysis of a variety of outcomes from massage therapy studies found that massage therapy provided by far the largest effect size for a reduction in trait anxiety. The effect on pain may, at least in part, be mediated by a reduction in catastrophizing, one of the key psychological factors associated with duration and intensity of chronic pain. On a cellular and tissue level, massage has been studied for its effect on muscular pain caused by exhaustive muscular activity, which may be applicable to specific occupational settings: massage was found to improve mitochondrial biogenesis signaling and to decrease cellular stress from myofiber injury by mitigating the production of pro-inflammatory TNF-α + IL-6 and heat shock protein 27 phosphorylation.

▶ Mind-Body Therapies

Mind-body therapies are predicated on the understanding that mental processes impact the physical body and vice-versa. Because the mind-body distinction is so clearly blurred in chronic pain, these therapies have been accepted into the mainstream of chronic pain treatment and are therefore discussed above in the section on psychologically based therapies.

▶ Herbs and Supplements

In general, botanical therapies and nutritional supplements have not been studied as extensively as pharmacologic therapies for pain. On the other hand, many patients prefer these forms of treatment, not only because they may notice fewer side effects but because they tend to be less pathologizing for patients. Patients who take medications often see the medications as a sign of weakness or failure, whereas patients taking herbs and supplements seem to relate to them more as sources of strength and symbols of self-efficacy. So, despite having less clarity about efficacy, many patients and providers prefer these therapeutic options. Common herbs and supplements used for pain are listed in Table 10–2.

▶ Nutrition

Many diets are purported to have a positive impact on pain, but few have been studied sufficiently to recommend to patients. Elimination diets, in which common allergens are systematically eliminated and correlated with changes in clinical status, are frequently used for pain but not well studied. One dietary pattern supported by research is the anti-inflammatory diet. This diet appears to be useful and may be tried in inflammatory pain conditions such as rheumatoid arthritis and possibly osteoarthritis, particularly in patients motivated to make lifestyle changes. It is characterized by high vegetable, whole grain, fish, and polyunsaturated fat intake, low refined grain intake, and little to no meat or dairy.

MULTIMODAL APPROACH

Each of the above therapeutic categories addresses a different aspect of the human pain experience. Practitioners can be most effective when they design a treatment plan to impact each of those areas, particularly in cases where the physical source of pain cannot be determined or removed. This multimodal approach to pain often involves the engagement of an interdisciplinary team that either sees patients together or discusses cases regularly to generate a shared care plan. Regardless of the model, occupational medicine specialists, with their unique focus on patient function, are key members of the team.

REFERNCES

Cleeland CS, Ryan KM: Pain assessment: global use of the brief pain inventory. Ann Acad Med Singapore 1994;23(2):129-138 [PMID: 8080219].

Devan H, Hale L, Hempel D, Saipe B, Perry MA: What works and does not work in a self-management intervention for people with chronic pain? Qualitative systematic review and meta-synthesis. Phys Ther 2018 May 1;98(5):381-397 [PMID: 29669089].

Dowell D, Haegerich TM, Chou R: CDC Guideline for prescribing opioids for chronic pain—United States, 2016. MMWR Recomm Rep 2016;65(1):1-49 [PMID: 26987082].

Kean J et al: Comparative responsiveness of the PROMIS pain interference short forms, Brief Pain Inventory, PEG, and SF-36 Bodily Pain subscale. Med Care 2016;54(4):414-421 [PMID: 26807536].

Krebs EE et al: Effect of opioid vs nonopioid medications on pain-related function in patients with chronic back pain or hip or knee osteoarthritis pain: The SPACE Randomized Clinical Trial. JAMA 2018;319(9):872-882 [PMID: 29509867].

Qaseem A, Wilt TJ, McLean RM, Forciea MA, Clinical Guidelines Committee of the American College of Physicians: Noninvasive treatments for acute, subacute, and chronic low back pain: a clinical practice guideline from the american college of physicians. Ann Intern Med 2017 Apr 4;166(7):514-530 [PMID: 28192789].

Vlaeyen JWS, Crombez G: Behavioral conceptualization and treatment of chronic pain. Annu Rev Clin Psychol 2020;16:187-212 [PMID: 31821023].

■ SELF-ASSESSMENT QUESTIONS

Select the one correct answer for each question.

Question 1: Pain
a. regulation is neurologically distinct from emotion regulation
b. erases the felt aspects of emotions
c. includes a strong behavioral drive toward homeostasis
d. is unlike suffering from unpleasant emotions

Question 2: Chronic pain
a. is associated with an increase in brain matter density
b. is associated with an increase in negative neural connectivity of insula to prefrontal and thalamic regions
c. does not impair cognitive control
d. circuits develop a hypersensitive state, with pain itself being a pain predictive conditioning cue

Question 3: Opioid pain medications
a. are particularly effective for chronic pain
b. are both rewarding and behaviorally reinforcing
c. never become difficult for patients to control
d. neurologically lead to a transition from striatal to prefrontal cortical control over drug

Question 4: Depression
a. is more common in chronic pain patients than in healthy controls
b. is frequently diagnosed and overtreated in pain patients

c. is typically an antecedent of chronic pain
d. is unrelated to pain chronification

Question 5: Pharmacologic treatments for chronic pain
a. generally reduce pain scores by 80–100%
b. are usually sufficient on their own
c. are usually most effective when combined with other treatment strategies
d. rarely have side effects

Question 6: Cognitive behavioral therapy (CBT)
a. is the same as self-management support programs
b. alters patients' behaviors whether productive or destructive
c. helps patients identify destructive thought patterns and learn to generate more constructive thought patterns
d. restructures the patient's relationship with coworkers

Question 7: Pacing is
a. a technique for preventing patients from being overactive or underactive
b. a technique for teaching patients to remain constantly active without pause
c. a technique for getting things done more quickly
d. a technique for explaining to other people what it feels like to have chronic pain

Eye Injuries

Yang Hu, MD, PhD

The personal tragedy and economic loss associated with impaired vision or even blindness as a result of occupational eye injuries can be prevented by identifying workers at risk and instituting appropriate safety programs. Proper maintenance of tools and equipment by the employer and effective use of protective devices, such as safety glasses or face shields, by the employee will reduce the number of injuries, such as ocular contusions, trauma as a consequence of penetrating and nonpenetrating foreign bodies, conjunctival and corneal abrasions, lid lacerations, and optic nerve damage.

Recognition of the toxic effects of chemical agents and protection from those that may be splashed into the eyes are vital for prevention of visual damage. The ready availability of facilities for cleansing and irrigation of the face and eyes in the workplace is of the utmost importance because initial steps for treatment of chemical burns—especially those caused by strong alkalis and acids—must be carried out immediately by the employee, fellow workers, or anyone else near at hand. There is no time to wait for specialized medical care, so employee education programs for emergency care of chemical burns are essential.

The risks of ocular damage for x-ray technicians, glassblowers, welders, and other workers exposed to ionizing, infrared, and ultraviolet radiation have long been known, but damage caused by exposure to excessive amounts of visible light has been recognized only recently. Wearing protective lenses that filter the most offending wavelengths of visible light may become commonplace in the future.

ANATOMY & PHYSIOLOGY

A brief review of ocular anatomy and function will help in understanding the mechanisms of several kinds of eye injuries and how they affect the visual system (Figure 11–1). The orbit, eyelid, and conjunctiva are protective mechanisms for the eye. The orbit and its bony rim offer excellent mechanical protection from injuries, with the exception of those coming from the direct anterior or temporal directions. The eyelid and conjunctiva are essential for normal maintenance of the smooth, moist, clear anterior surface of the cornea, which, in turn, is essential for clear vision. The normal blinking mechanism depends on the third cranial nerve to open the lids and the seventh cranial nerve to close them. Moistening of the conjunctiva by lacrimal fluid depends in part on activation of the reflex arc between the sensory fifth innervation of the anterior eye and the parasympathetic secretomotor fibers that accompany the seventh cranial nerve along the petrous temporal bone into the middle fossa and then through the orbit to the lacrimal gland. Moistening of the corneal epithelium is aided by mucus from the goblet cells of the conjunctiva, particularly those on the tarsus of the upper lid. Reflex tear production by the lacrimal gland helps to dilute and wash away irritating substances that find their way into the conjunctival sac. The rich blood supply of the conjunctiva and lid also helps in resisting and limiting infections of the anterior eye.

Internal structures of the eye can be conveniently divided into anterior and posterior segments. The anterior segment includes the cornea, anterior chamber, iris, lens, and ciliary body. These structures comprise the essential optical elements of the eye. The regular pattern of the collagen fibers and posterior endothelial layer of the cornea maintain its optical clarity. Because the cornea and lens are avascular, they require a specialized source of nutrition, which is provided by aqueous humor. The ciliary body produces aqueous humor at a nearly constant rate, bathing the lens and posterior surface of the cornea and then draining near the base of the cornea through the structures associated with the Schlemm canal. A normal rate of production and drainage of aqueous humor maintains the intraocular pressure at between 10 and 21 mm Hg. Injuries causing sustained elevation of pressure can lead to significant glaucomatous visual field loss. The iris and its pupil adjust the amount of light entering the eye. Contraction of the ciliary muscle changes the shape of the lens, thereby allowing for accommodation (adjustment of focusing for seeing at different distances).

The posterior segment of the eye is the light-sensing portion of the visual system and contains the retina and its

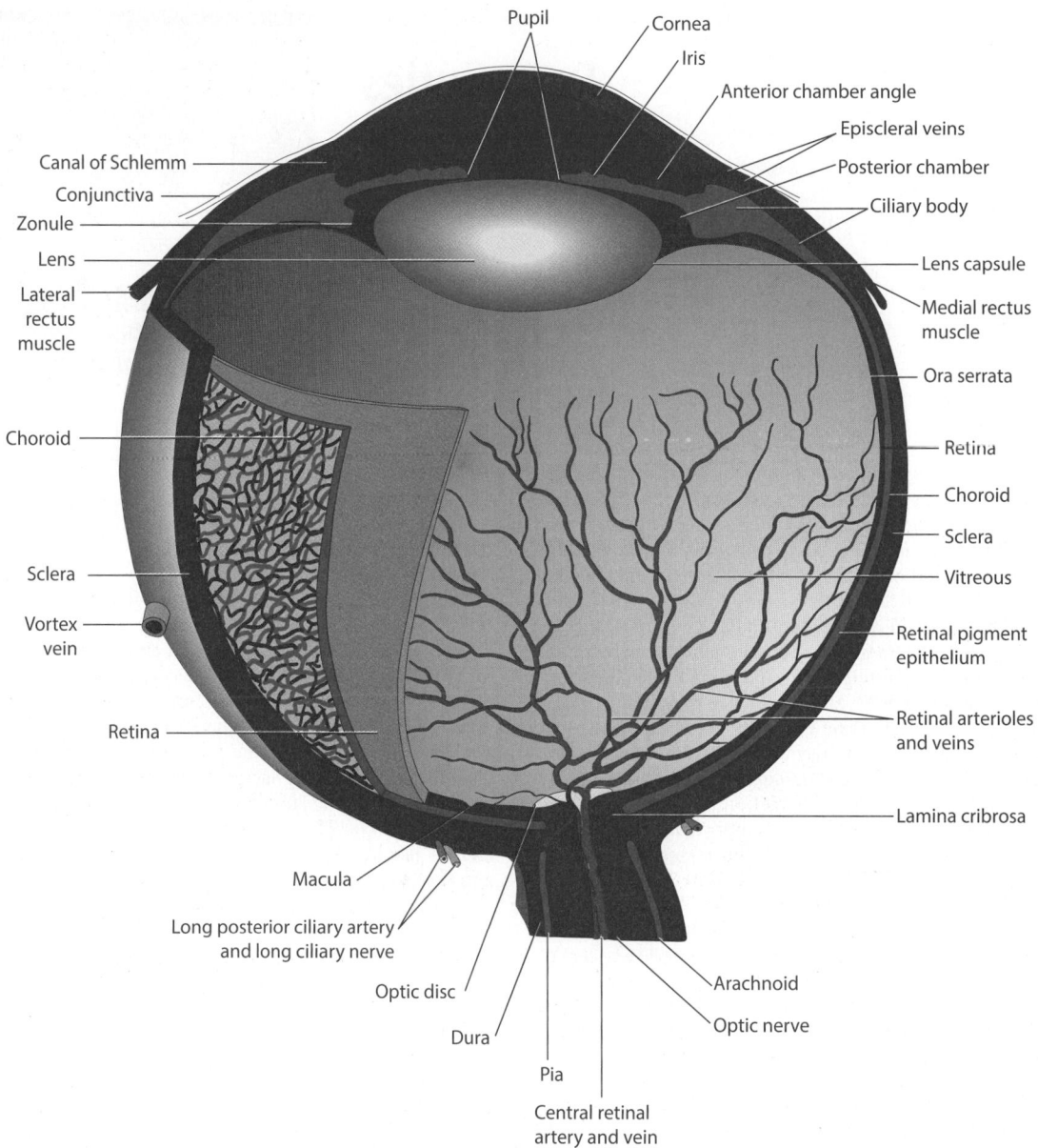

▲ Figure 11–1. View of the inferior half of the right eye.

supporting vascular layer, the choroid. The retina has more than 1 million axons that arise from the retinal ganglion cells and collect in the optic disc to form the optic nerve, which transmits visual information to the posterior visual system. These axons are not capable of healing with restoration of visual function following injuries such as penetrating wounds of the orbit or posterior orbital fractures involving the optic canal. Depending on the severity of the injury, the nerve fibers

may disappear partially or completely due to degeneration, resulting in either partial or complete atrophy of the optic disc (optic nerve head). The optic chiasm, optic tracts, and visual radiations to the cortex usually are not involved directly in eye injuries except those involving the bones of the head and the intracranial structures in traumatic brain injury.

Visual acuity depends on the optical clarity of the cornea, lens, and vitreous and proper functioning of the fovea, which is the avascular center of the retinal macula and is composed entirely of specialized cones that are color-sensitive and capable of resolving the finest images. If this small area (< 0.5 mm in diameter) is damaged, no adjacent portion of the retina is capable of assuming the fine function that provides maximum visual acuity.

Eye injuries causing retinal detachment or vitreous hemorrhage can lead to loss of peripheral vision, and injuries of the extraocular muscles or their nerves can produce diplopia (double vision).

HISTORY & EYE EXAMINATION

Caution: For chemical burns (see the section "Chemical Burns of the Eye"), emergency treatment should be started immediately, and the history and examination of the patient can proceed in due course. In cases of suspected ruptured or lacerated globe (see following discussion), care must be taken to prevent further damage to the eye during transport to the hospital and initial evaluation.

▶ History

The occupational medical history should include a variety of questions not always considered pertinent to general histories. In addition, the worker should be asked about vision before and after the injury and whether any visual loss was sudden or gradual. Sudden loss of vision without obvious injury may be caused by central retinal artery occlusion or ischemic damage to the optic nerve, occasionally caused by giant cell arteritis. These problems require emergency treatment. Progressive loss of vision following facial bone fractures or head injuries is sometimes a result of optic nerve damage, which may respond to surgery if recognized in time.

In cases of mechanical injury, the worker should be asked about previous tetanus inoculations and about the nature of the forces involved during the injury. Was the eye struck with a small, rapidly moving object that may have penetrated the globe, as sometimes occurs when a steel hammer strikes a steel tool? Or was the eye hit by a large, slowly moving object that may have caused a contusion injury or rupture of the globe? If the presence of a foreign body is suspected, the worker should be asked about the type of material that might be involved (a magnetic metal such as iron or steel, a nonmagnetic metal such as aluminum or copper, or an organic material such as wood) because this information is helpful for determining the method of treatment and for prognosis. Soluble metallic salts from iron- or copper-containing foreign bodies can cause irreversible toxic damage to the retina, best prevented by their prompt removal. Less-soluble materials, such as aluminum, plastic, or glass, are associated with a better prognosis. Organic foreign bodies, such as pieces of wood or splinters of plant material, may introduce an intraocular infection that frequently is difficult to treat and has a very poor prognosis.

If a chemical burn is present or suspected, the type of chemical (alkali or acid) will influence how quickly and deeply it penetrates the eye. If eye injuries are thought to be caused by long-term exposure to chemicals, the various substances to which the worker is exposed should be identified and a material safety data sheet (MSDS) obtained for each. The worker also should be asked about exposure to aerosols, surfactants, detergents, dust, and smoke, all of which can damage the corneal epithelium.

▶ Examination

Even if an injury is thought to have affected only one eye, both eyes should be examined carefully. If swelling prevents easy opening of the eyes for inspection, a sterile topical anesthetic can be instilled through nearly closed eyelids by applying the drops along the lid fissure. After a few minutes, smooth sterile retractors may be used carefully to lift the lids for eye examination.

A. External Eye Examination

1. Eyelids—Note symmetry of the lids of both eyes. Look for lacerations that cross the lid margins and for perforating wounds through the skin of the lid above or below the lid margin. Except in the case of a suspected ruptured or lacerated globe, the lid can be everted to search for foreign bodies on the upper tarsus. To evert the lid, the patient is asked to look down while the physician pulls gently on the lashes and applies mild pressure on the upper surface of the lid.

2. Orbits—Palpate the orbital rims, and note discontinuities and crepitus caused by subcutaneous air from fractures of the paranasal sinuses. In orbital fractures, injury to the inferior or superior orbital nerves as they pass through the floor or roof of the orbit can cause decreased sensibility of the lids and face.

3. Conjunctiva—To examine the conjunctiva, evert the lids by applying gentle pressure over the superior orbital rim of the upper lid or over the malar eminence of the lower lid, thereby avoiding direct pressure on the globe. Look for foreign bodies, hemorrhage, laceration, and inflammation.

Inflammation caused by trauma usually produces a watery discharge (tears), in contrast to the purulent mucoid discharge of bacterial conjunctivitis. Viral or chlamydial conjunctivitis is characterized by lymph follicles in the inferior fornix of the conjunctival sac along with a watery discharge. Preauricular lymph nodes are also frequently present.

4. Corneas—With a bright light, look at the light reflection on the normally smooth corneal surface. Irregularities indicate disruptions of the corneal epithelium. Because the cornea is normally clear and lustrous, the surface texture of the iris is seen easily and clearly. A corneal wound with incarceration of the iris also may be indicated by asymmetry of the pupil. A fluorescein paper strip moistened with sterile saline or a topical anesthetic can be used to stain the tears on the surface of the cornea. The stain diffuses into any area of disrupted epithelium and stains it bright green. The color is enhanced with a blue light. Details of the cornea and the anterior eye are much more easily examined with magnification such as a 2× to 4× loupe or (and preferably) with a slit lamp and microscope, if one is available.

5. Anterior chambers—The anterior chambers should appear deep and clear. Hyphema (hemorrhage into the anterior chamber) is almost always a sign of significant injury. Hypopyon (purulent material in the anterior chamber) is characterized by a white or gray layer of inflammatory cells at the chamber bottom. Hypopyon usually is caused by an infection following a penetrating injury or a bacterial or fungal corneal ulcer.

6. Pupils—The pupils should appear round, black, and equal in size. Pupillary reactions to light should be noted carefully. Normally, both pupils constrict and dilate equally and simultaneously when one pupil is stimulated by light. While the illuminated pupil is demonstrating the direct-light response, the unilluminated pupil is showing the consensual-light response. The direct-light responses of the two eyes can be compared by moving a flashlight back and forth between the eyes and pausing a few seconds at each eye to observe the pupil. Normally, each pupil constricts when illuminated; failure of one pupil to constrict but to dilate instead indicates the presence of an afferent pupillary defect (Marcus Gunn pupil), which may be the result of an optic nerve injury or extensive retinal damage on that side.

B. Test of Ocular Motility

If there are no severe eye injuries, the ocular movements may be tested safely by comparing the excursions in all directions to make sure that they are the same in both eyes. Limitation of upward or downward gaze occurs frequently in orbital floor fractures and may be the result of accompanying edema or mechanical restriction of the ocular muscles. It also can result from direct trauma to a muscle when a penetrating injury of the orbit occurs.

C. Ophthalmoscopic Examination

1. Red reflex—The presence of a good bright-red reflex demonstrates normal optical clarity of the eye. A direct ophthalmoscope with a good bright light is used to observe the red reflex (the red glow reflected from the fundus). Examination should take place in a darkened room with the instrument set at 0 or +1, and the eyes should be observed at arm's length, approximately 2 ft (60 cm), so that the reflex in both of them can be seen at the same time and compared. An opacity in the cornea, anterior chamber, lens, or vitreous or a gross change in the color of the retina will appear as a dark form against a red background or as a dull or absent red reflex.

2. Optic discs—The examiner should be as close to the patient as possible to maximize the relative size of the pupil. The optic discs should be examined for the presence of papilledema. Optic discs usually are well vascularized and have a good pink color. When nerve fibers in the optic nerve die as the result of various injuries, the blood supply to the disc

decreases in proportion to the loss of fibers. The disc will show a faint pallor if only a few fibers are missing, or it may appear completely white as a result of optic atrophy following total destruction of the nerve.

3. Optic cups—The width of each optic cup is usually one-third or less the diameter of the whole optic disc. If it is as large as half the diameter, or if the optic cups are not similar in both eyes, there is an increased risk for glaucoma. Therefore, estimating the cup size is useful for screening patients for glaucoma.

4. Retinal vessels—The vessels should be examined along the upper and lower arcades proceeding from the optic disc, and the presence of hemorrhages, exudates, and other alterations in the appearance of the retina should be noted.

5. Maculae and foveae—Each macula should be checked for alterations in its usual relatively featureless appearance. Its center, the fovea, always can be located 2.5-disc diameters temporal to the optic disc. Its concave center usually shows a small, bright foveal light reflex.

D. Measurement of Intraocular Pressure

If a lacerated or ruptured globe is suspected, intraocular pressure should not be measured. In other injuries, pressure can be measured with a Schiotz tonometer or with an applanation tonometer, if one is available on a slit lamp. If a tonometer is not available, a general impression of extremely high or low intraocular pressure can be obtained by gently palpating each globe in turn with one finger of each hand through the closed upper eyelid. Comparison of the firmness of the two eyes is occasionally useful when the intraocular pressure is extremely high, as in angle-closure glaucoma.

Angle-closure glaucoma accounts for only approximately 5% of all glaucoma; it usually presents with acute aching pain in the involved eye with moderate redness of the globe and blurred vision, sometimes described as colored halos around bright lights. It occurs when the iris root touches the back of the cornea, blocking aqueous outflow and causing intraocular pressure to rise very rapidly, thus leading to the symptoms. Angle-closure glaucoma can occur only in eyes with anatomically shallow anterior chambers and narrow chamber angles. An attack of angle-closure glaucoma requires prompt treatment. The first approach is to lower the pressure medically with topical miotics such as pilocarpine 1–4% every 15 minutes for 1–2 hours. The production of aqueous humor is reduced with a topical ophthalmic β-adrenergic blocker and a carbonic anhydrase inhibitor. Intraocular pressure can be lowered quickly by increasing the osmolarity of the blood that moves water out of the vitreous humor, thus reducing the ocular volume and the intraocular pressure. Intravenous urea or mannitol infusions are effective, but oral ingestion of glycerin is as effective, safer, and more easily available. Subsequent attacks are prevented by making an opening in the peripheral iris (iridectomy), which passes aqueous humor directly from the posterior chamber to the anterior chamber, keeping the filtration angle open. The iridectomy usually is done with a laser.

Open-angle glaucoma accounts for most cases of glaucomatous visual loss (90%). Its onset is insidious, there is no pain, and visual symptoms are noticed only after severe irreversible loss of visual field has occurred. Therefore, it becomes the physician's responsibility to see changes in the optic cup. Asymmetric cups or cups as large as one-half the disc diameter are suspicious. Such changes are an indication to request visual fields. Early lowering of intraocular pressure is the only way to prevent loss of visual field. All adults should be encouraged to have their intraocular pressures measured every 1 or 2 years.

The remaining 5% of cases of glaucoma have a variety of causes. Contusion injuries to the eye can tear the iris root and the ciliary body's attachment to the sclera, damaging the filtration angle, reducing aqueous outflow, and raising pressure. This is called angle-recession glaucoma. Blood in the anterior chamber (hyphema) and inflammatory cells in cases of chronic inflammation, such as uveitis, can block aqueous outflow channels, causing secondary glaucoma.

Although many investigators discuss enhancing blood flow and neuroprotection as potential therapies, the only treatment of open-angle and secondary glaucoma proven effective is lowering of the intraocular pressure. This can be done by medically reducing the production of aqueous humor with a topical β-adrenergic blocker, a systemic carbonic anhydrase inhibitor, or a sympathomimetic drug. Parasympathomimetics, sympathomimetics, and prostaglandin analogues increase the outflow of aqueous humor. If these measures fail to lower the pressure adequately, a surgical procedure can be used to increase the drainage of aqueous humor into the subconjunctival space.

E. Test of Visual Acuity

Visual acuity always should be tested and the results recorded before treatment is instituted. This is important both from the point of view of good care and for medicolegal reasons because patients do not always remember the amount of visual loss that occurred at the time of a severe injury. Visual acuity should be measured with a Snellen chart, if possible, or with a near-acuity card and recorded appropriately. Each eye should be tested separately, first without correction (glasses or contact lenses) and then with correction; each acuity measurement should be recorded for the right eye followed by the left. If a near-acuity card is used, it is important to record the distance at which the measurements were made and whether they were made with or without the patient's glasses. If visual acuity is poor and a refractive error is suspected, the chart or card can be read through a pinhole as a substitute for corrective lenses; an improvement in acuity will confirm the presence of a refractive error. If acuity is less than 20/200, the greatest distance at which fingers can be counted should be noted for each eye. If the patient cannot see the fingers well enough to count them, the greatest distance at which hand movements can be seen should be recorded. If vision is poorer than this, light perception can be tested with a bright flashlight held as close to the eye as possible, and the ability to perceive light in each of the four quadrants is recorded. If there is no light perception, it should be recorded as such. Visual acuity measured with a Snellen chart is based on a visual angle of 1 minute of arc; this is considered the best resolving power of the eye and is the standard used to design all types of test charts. The 20/20 letters are formed of black lines separated by white spaces, each 1 minute of arc wide; the whole letter is 5 minutes of arc high, measuring 8.7 mm (Figure 11–2). When letters of this size are read accurately at a distance of 20 ft (6 m), 20/20 vision is determined. Other letters on a chart increase in multiples of this standard dimension. The 20/200 letter is 10 times larger or 87-mm high and would appear the same size as a 20/20 letter when seen at a distance of 200 ft. Metric visual acuity charts use 6 m as the standard test distance; therefore, 6/6 = 20/20. The peak of the light-sensitivity curve of the eye is at a wavelength of about 555 nm. This means that our best vision is in yellow-green light.

There are two techniques for objectively estimating visual acuity—optokinetic nystagmus and visual-evoked response—that may be useful in certain situations, particularly when the

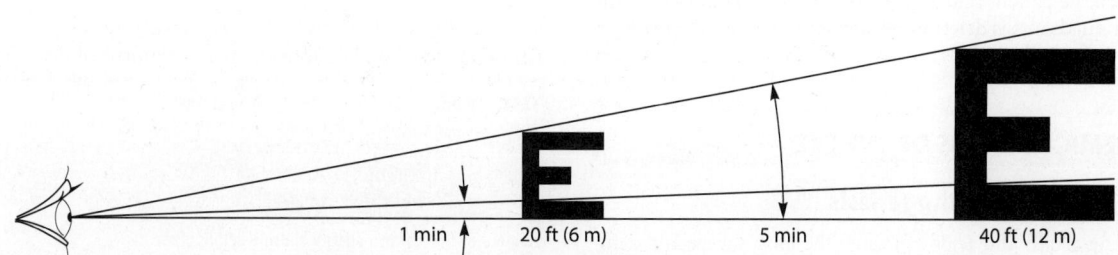

▲ **Figure 11–2.** Measurement of visual acuity. Visual acuity measurements are based on a visual angle of 1 min of arc subtending each part of a test letter. Each letter is made up of five equally sized black or white parts; therefore, the whole letter subtends a visual angle of 5 min of arc. The 20/20 letters are 8.7-mm high; the 20/40 letters are twice as large, or 17.4-mm high. This drawing is not to scale.

patient is unable or unwilling to respond to the usual subjective measures of visual acuity. Optokinetic nystagmus is a visually stimulated response to relatively large targets. These eye movements are observed in the intact visual system by passing an alternating series of dark and light stripes of equal width before the patient's eyes. Involuntary nystagmus is produced—slow following movement in the direction of movement of the stripes alternating with a quick recovery movement. The stimulus is usually presented as a series of vertical stripes 1–2 cm in width on a handheld drum 10–15 cm in diameter. The drum is held 20–30 cm from the patient and turned slowly while observing the patient's eyes to see the induced nystagmus. The stripes also can be presented on a 50-cm-long cloth strip with the stripes running across the 10–12-cm width. Normally, the nystagmus can be induced in any direction, and its rate will vary with the speed of the stimulus.

The visually evoked response is an electroencephalographic recording over the visual cortex (occipital lobe) in response to visual stimuli. The stimulus can be a simple light flash giving an on-off response, or an estimate of visual acuity can be made by presenting an alternating pattern of dark and light squares in a checkerboard pattern on a television screen. The squares can be made progressively smaller until the response is no longer recorded, and the size of the smallest squares eliciting a cortical recording can be related to standard visual acuity measurements. The responses are involuntary and cannot be controlled by the subject; acuity measurements in the range of 20/400 to 20/20 have been recorded even in infants younger than 1 year of age. This technique usually is available through neuro-ophthalmologic or neurologic consultation. It can be particularly valuable when evaluating patients with compensation or forensic problems.

F. Test of Visual Fields

Visual fields should be tested, especially in patients with suspected head injury or a significant decrease in visual acuity. Each eye is tested separately by confrontation. The patient is asked to look at the examiner's eye while the examiner's hand moves toward the center of the visual field. The point at which the patient can accurately count fingers in each of the four quadrants is determined, and the results in the two eyes are compared carefully.

CHEMICAL BURNS OF THE EYE

▶ Etiology & Pathogenesis

Strong alkalis and acids can cause the most severe and damaging chemical injuries to the eye and eyelids. Alkali burns are commonly caused by sodium and potassium hydroxide used as cleaning agents, by calcium hydroxide used in mason's mortar and plaster, and by anhydrous ammonia used in fertilizer. Battery acids and the strong acids used to

clean metal in the electroplating industry are also common causes of severe eye injury.

Alkalis affect the lipid in cell membranes and thereby reduce the normal barriers to diffusion. This allows the chemical to penetrate rapidly the interior of the eye. Because alkalis are not neutralized quickly by tissue, their destructive action can continue for hours if they are not diluted and removed immediately by irrigation of the eye. In contrast, acids tend to denature protein in tissues to form physical barriers that limits the deeper penetration of acids.

The corneal endothelium, which is essential for corneal clarity and good vision, is particularly vulnerable to chemical insult. There is often severe damage within the anterior chamber, including the aqueous outflow pathways, leading to glaucoma. Obliteration of the blood vessels of the conjunctiva and sclera can cause severe ischemia of the anterior eye, including the periphery of the cornea and the underlying ciliary body and iris. Ischemia, as well as the associated reduction in blood supply, is one of the major causes of the poor prognosis in patients with severe chemical burns.

▶ Clinical Findings

The skin on the face and eyelids shows edema and erythema, sometimes associated with sloughing of the surface. Eye examination may require use of a topical anesthetic unless nerve damage is severe enough to cause anesthesia. The conjunctiva may be mildly hyperemic, show small hemorrhages, or be blanched and have the appearance of white marble. Testing the pH of the conjunctival surface with indicator paper will help to confirm the presence of acid (low pH) or alkali (high pH) injuries. The severity of injury (Table 11–1) usually is judged by the degree of corneal opacity using the normal clarity of the pupil as a guide. The cornea may appear gray or cloudy because of epithelial and stromal edema. If the cornea is not cloudy, the anterior chamber can be seen clearly. In some cases, the iris and pupil appear hazy and indistinct. Visual acuity is decreased in proportion to the severity of corneal damage. Injuries of the nasopharynx and upper respiratory passages frequently are found in association with aspiration of the chemical irritant.

Table 11–1. Classifications of chemical burns of the eye.

Classification	Clinical Findings
Mild	Erosion of the corneal epithelium Faint haziness of the cornea No ischemic necrosis of the conjunctiva or sclera
Moderate	Corneal opacity blurring details of the iris Minimal ischemic necrosis of the conjunctiva and sclera
Severe	Corneal opacity blurring the pupillary outline Severe ischemic necrosis and blanching of the conjunctiva and sclera

Prevention

Chemical burns can be prevented by safety measures such as keeping chemicals in unbreakable containers and providing splash-protection shields and eyeglasses to employees who must handle chemicals. Workers at risk should be taught emergency treatment measures for themselves and their fellow workers.

Treatment

Emergency treatment (Table 11–2) should be started in the workplace by the patient or anyone immediately available. Any source of water (drinking fountain, hose, etc.) is adequate and should be used immediately to wash the eyes with copious amounts of water until the patient can be taken to an emergency facility. At least 1 L of saline or other isotonic solution then should be used to irrigate each eye carefully, with the lids held open to thoroughly cleanse the conjunctival sac. Use of a sterile topical anesthetic may be necessary.

Moist cotton-tipped applicators should be used to sweep the conjunctival surface free of particulate matter, such as the granules found in drainpipe cleaners and plaster. The pH of the conjunctival surface should be tested with pH test paper strips or urine pH test strips and irrigation repeated until the pH approaches the normal level of 7. As a general rule, there is no practical limit to the amount of irrigation that may be helpful. If there is any doubt about its efficacy, irrigation may be repeated for several hours while waiting for ophthalmologic consultation.

During irrigation, the gray color or cloudiness of the cornea may appear to clear, giving a false impression of improved clinical status. The change is usually a result of sloughing of the damaged corneal epithelium, which reveals the clearer corneal stroma underneath.

Diphoterine is a commercial rinsing solution used extensively by European paramedics and firefighters to decontaminate chemicals on the skin or in the eye. Although its use is not yet approved in the United States, Diphoterine is safe and effective.

After irrigation is completed, cycloplegic drops (eg, cyclopentolate or scopolamine) may be instilled to dilate the pupil and thus prevent posterior synechiae (adhesions between iris and lens). Antibiotic drops should be instilled before the eye is patched. The patch prevents blinking and should provide some comfort. The patient should be referred to an ophthalmologist.

Specific ophthalmologic treatment may include the use of topical corticosteroids and antibiotics to reduce the severe inflammatory response that occurs shortly after injury. These medications—particularly the corticosteroids—must be used with caution because they enhance the possibility of secondary infection and discourage the formation of new vessels in ischemic areas. Irrigation of the anterior chamber with saline solution may help to restore the pH to more normal levels. After the initial reaction subsides and the conjunctiva and cornea have epithelialized, the severity of the injury can be judged. A scarred cornea can be replaced by a corneal transplant, and a damaged lens (cataract) can be removed surgically and replaced with a clear synthetic lens. Glaucoma as a consequence of scarring of aqueous outflow pathways may be controlled medically—and if not, a surgical fistulization procedure may be done.

Prognosis

Emergency treatment of chemical burns usually is followed by a period of weeks or months of effort to rehabilitate the damaged ocular tissues. The degree of blanching or ischemia of the conjunctiva is an important factor influencing the final outcome. Ischemic damage, even in the presence of apparent healing, makes ultimate restoration of vision difficult. The survival of a corneal transplant depends on normal function of structures in the anterior eye. The survival of the cornea and the anterior segment of the eye are directly related to the degree of damage to the corneal endothelium, aqueous drainage pathways, and ciliary body. If the ciliary body fails to produce enough aqueous humor, the entire eye becomes soft and ultimately atrophies. In patients with severe burns, deep penetration and extensive destruction of ocular tissues can lead to perforation of the globe, infection, and loss of the eye. Milder burns in which chemical penetration is shallower may heal with little scarring.

THERMAL BURNS OF THE EYE & EYELID

Thermal burns of the eyelids and upper face may involve the eyes. However, in cases of flash burn caused by a sudden gas explosion, most individuals forcibly close their eyes, and this reflex lid closure usually protects the ocular surface. Direct contact with molten metal or glass can cause severe injury to the lids and even to the open eye. Thermal injury occurs rapidly at the time of contact. Tissue destruction is not progressive, as is the case with some chemical burns.

Table 11–2. Emergency treatment of chemical burns of the eye.

(1) **In the workplace:** Wash the eyes with copious amounts of water until the patient can be taken to an emergency facility.
(2) **In the emergency facility:**
  (a) Irrigate each eye with at least 1 L of saline or other isotonic solution, with the lids open to flush the conjunctival sac.
  (b) Use sterile topical anesthetic as necessary.
  (c) Remove particulate matter with cotton-tipped applicators.
  (d) Test the pH of the conjunctival surface, and continue irrigation until the pH approaches neutral.
  (e) Remove loose or damaged epithelium from the cornea and conjunctiva.
  (f) Dilate the pupil with cyclopentolate or scopolamine.
  (g) Give topical antibiotic drops, patch the eyes, and refer the patient to an ophthalmologist.

Eye examination may require topical anesthesia and careful use of lid retractors. Irrigation may be necessary to remove particulate matter, especially in injuries caused by explosions.

Depending on their severity, thermal burns of the eye structures are treated in the same manner as burns occurring elsewhere on the body. Extensive loss of lid skin can lead to exposure and drying of the cornea. This can be prevented by covering the eye with a transparent plastic sheet and sealing it to the surrounding skin with a sterile antibiotic ointment, thus producing a humidity chamber over the eye. Healing of lid skin frequently is followed by scarring, contraction, and distortion of the lids, which result in some degree of exposure of the globe. Plastic surgery with skin grafting may be necessary to restore lid function.

MECHANICAL INJURIES OF THE EYE & EYELID

Mechanical injuries range from superficial abrasions to complete disruption of the globe depending on the nature of the force striking the eye. Small, sharp, fast-moving objects can penetrate or lacerate the globe, whereas larger objects may exert enough compressive force to cause contusion injury or to rupture the eyeball.

▶ Laceration of the Eyelid

Lid lacerations result from two common mechanisms: (1) contact with sharp, fast-moving objects such as glass or metal parts that cut the skin and subcutaneous tissues (partial-thickness lacerations) or involve the posterior layers, the tarsus, and the conjunctiva (full-thickness lacerations) and (2) avulsion injuries that are caused by blunt trauma (eg, a blow to the malar eminence) and cause abrupt traction of the lid and tear it from its attachment to the medial canthal ligament. The type and extent of injury determine the method of treatment.

Partial-thickness lacerations can be closed by direct suturing with generally good results. Full-thickness lacerations require meticulous repair in two layers by an ophthalmic or oculofacial plastic surgeon to accurately restore the continuity of the lid margin. If notching of the margin occurs with healing, the cornea may not be moistened adequately by tears and protected from abrasions and other trauma. Deep stab wounds above the upper lid may sever the levator muscle of the lid. The cut end of the levator is easier to retrieve and repair if surgery is performed immediately after injury. Inadequate repair can result in chronic ptosis. Severe damage to the upper lid and blinking mechanism also can place the patient at risk for superficial corneal injuries.

In avulsion injuries, lid structures that have pulled away from the globe should be examined carefully and placed as close to their anatomic positions as possible to protect the eye while the patient is awaiting treatment by an ophthalmic surgeon. Retention of avulsed lid structures is important. They frequently can be repaired and usually heal well because of their rich blood supply. It is difficult to substitute skin grafts or skin flaps for the normal lid structures, particularly the tarsal and conjunctival structures that are essential for normal functioning of the lid. Avulsion of the medial canthal ligament sometimes disrupts the lacrimal drainage system, and failure to repair it will result in epiphora (the overflow of tears).

▶ Injuries to the Iris

Injuries to the iris can be caused indirectly by contusion and directly by perforating or penetrating injuries of the eye.

Contusion of the globe transmits force to the iris by the rapid displacement of aqueous humor. Because water is incompressible and the eye is essentially inelastic, these forces can be very large and destructive.

Iridoplegia is caused by damage to the pupillary sphincter. The pupil may react to light either directly or consensually and only slightly or not at all. The iris root, where it attaches to the ciliary body, may be torn, producing an iridodialysis. Sometimes the ciliary body with the iris root intact is torn away from its scleral attachment, producing an angle recession that can damage the aqueous outflow, causing a form of glaucoma.

Penetrating injuries, foreign bodies, stab wounds, corneal lacerations, and ruptured globes all may perforate, tear, or disrupt the iris. Iris tissue frequently herniates through corneal or scleral wounds.

Iris injuries usually do not require treatment other than incidental repair of the associated major injuries. Except for an increase in the amount of light entering an eye, it may have quite useful vision without an iris or with an iris with multiple holes. An eye with more than one pupil still sees only one image.

▶ Injuries of the Retina

Retinal injuries are caused by both blunt trauma (contusion) and penetrating wounds. When the eye is struck in a contusion injury, the force is transmitted by the fluid contents throughout the interior of the globe. Posteriorly, the retina may become edematous in a discrete area, frequently including the macula—a condition called commotio retinae or Berlin edema. Vision is reduced but may improve to nearly normal when the edema clears. This process may require several weeks to a month to complete. Contusion injuries also cause forceful displacement of the vitreous, resulting in traction at its anterior attachment on the surface of the retina at the posterior edge of the ciliary body. This may disinsert the retina from the ciliary body or tear a hole in the peripheral retina. Hemorrhage may result, clouding the vitreous for a time.

Retinal tears or holes frequently cause retinal detachments, which require prompt surgical repair. Visual prognosis depends on macular involvement. If the macula is intact, vision is usually good; if the macula is detached for even a few days, the prognosis is apt to be poor. Penetrating injuries cause direct perforations and tears in the retina, causing hemorrhage and detachments. Treatment of retinal detachments requires localization and closure of the tears or holes. This is done by creating an adhesion and scar between the retina and the choroid surrounding the hole. A freezing probe placed on the scleral surface over the hole will cause an inflammatory reaction in the choroid that will adhere to the retina. Sometimes it is necessary to bring the scleral, choroidal, and retinal surfaces together. Usually this is done by placing an encircling band of silicone rubber around the entire globe; it also may be done by pushing them together from the inside by injecting a gas bubble into the vitreous space.

▶ Ruptured or Lacerated Globe

If a ruptured or lacerated globe is present or suspected, placing a metal shield or other protective covering (eg, the bottom half of a paper cup) over the injured eye will prevent external pressure from causing further damage during transport to the hospital. Patching the other eye will reduce ocular movements and thus help to prevent further trauma to the injured eye.

Visual acuity should be measured and recorded. Severe injuries almost always are associated with some degree of visual loss, lid swelling, orbital swelling, exophthalmos, and hemorrhage. If lid swelling is extreme, it may be necessary to use a sterile topical anesthetic and lid retractors to lift the lids away from the globe during initial examination.

If the cornea is clear and the pupil is round and reacts to light, the globe probably is intact. Global rupture usually is characterized by the presence of brownish or grayish tissue beneath the conjunctiva (subconjunctival hemorrhage), which is caused by exposure or herniation of uveal tissue, an irregular or disrupted corneal surface, or the presence of blood or gross alteration in the appearance of the iris and pupil. Pupillary light reflexes may be abnormal. The pupil pulled or peaked toward one side of the cornea usually indicates that the iris has herniated through a laceration in that direction.

Ophthalmoscopic examination may be difficult because of corneal irregularities and hemorrhage in the anterior chamber and vitreous. If the fundus can be examined and the disc and vessels appear relatively normal, gross disruption of the globe is unlikely. A bright red reflex usually indicates that the interior of the globe is intact. Intraocular pressure should not be measured if a ruptured or lacerated globe is suspected. A radiograph for detection of any radiopaque material in the region of the globe is an essential part of the initial examination.

Definitive examination and treatment should be performed by an ophthalmic surgeon. Until a surgeon is available, both eyes should be covered again, with a sterile eye pad used on the injured eye to minimize contamination. The patient should be supported with parenteral fluids and be considered a candidate for general anesthesia. The repair of a ruptured globe or corneal laceration usually is done under general anesthesia. A local anesthetic is not considered safe because the distortion from its injection might cause additional damage.

The eye is examined safely under anesthesia, usually with an operating microscope, and the repair is carried out by suturing the torn sclera or lacerated cornea. Exposed intraocular structures such as the iris or ciliary body may be replaced in the eye or excised depending on their condition. When the repair is complete, the eye is filled with saline or an electrolyte solution that simulates aqueous humor. Antibiotics are injected subconjunctivally after the globe is closed and are continued intravenously for 4–5 days to prevent infection that may have been introduced by the injury.

A ruptured globe has a grave prognosis for restoration of vision. Corneal lacerations have a better prognosis because their surgical repair usually is accomplished easily. If scarring occurs, corneal transplant can be performed.

▶ Contusion Injuries

Blunt trauma to the eye causes various contusion injuries ranging in severity from ecchymosis of the eyelids (black eye) to major intraocular damage. Compression injuries of the anterior eye are characterized by corneal edema, anterior chamber hemorrhage, and increased intraocular pressure. These symptoms usually resolve without treatment. In some cases, however, return of normal intraocular pressure is followed several weeks or months later by another increase, which indicates the presence of angle-recession glaucoma. This is caused by a tear in the attachment of the iris and ciliary body from the internal surface of the sclera at the anterior chamber angle, damaging the aqueous outflow pathway. Patients with compression injuries always should receive follow-up care at the hands of an ophthalmologist so that angle-recession glaucoma can be detected and treated to prevent progressive damage to the optic nerve. Treatment usually begins with twice-daily drops of an ophthalmic β-blocker.

Hyphema (hemorrhage into the anterior chamber) frequently clears spontaneously, but secondary hemorrhage occurs after several hours or days in up to one-third of patients as a result of lysis of the thrombus in the injured vessels of the iris or ciliary body. Secondary hemorrhage frequently continues until the anterior chamber is completely filled with blood, during which time the intraocular pressure may rise to 50–60 mm Hg (normal 12–20 mm Hg). Lysis and reabsorption of this blood clot may take many days and cause damage to the aqueous filtration pathways and subsequent glaucoma. Breakdown products of blood also can diffuse into the cornea, stain it, and cause long-term reduction of vision. If reabsorption of the blood clot is prolonged, it sometimes can be aspirated successfully. If not, the anterior chamber is opened, and the clot is removed directly. Secondary hemorrhages may require surgical treatment. The prognosis for good vision in patients with secondary hemorrhage is poor.

The prevention of secondary hemorrhages is difficult. Bed rest with binocular patching has been a standard treatment for many years. More recent experience comparing patients treated with bed rest and others allowed normal activity showed no significant difference in the incidence of secondary hemorrhages.

Aminocaproic acid has been used to retard fibrinolysis in the injured vessels to prevent secondary hemorrhages to the benefit of many patients. This treatment slows the lysis of the primary hyphema but, when given for 5–7 days, does reduce the occurrence of secondary hemorrhages. There are significant side effects, so use of aminocaproic acid must be considered carefully and monitored.

Retinal edema, particularly in the macula, causes acute reduction of vision. Vision usually improves with clearance of edema in a few days to several weeks. Clearance is not always complete, and there may be permanent damage to the macula. In ruptures of the choroid, blood spreads beneath the retina at the time of injury, and reabsorption of blood will reveal a crescent-shaped scar concentric with the optic disk. There is no treatment. Other contusion injuries include dislocation of the lens (partial or complete), traumatic cataracts, and tears in the region of the anterior attachment of the retina to the ciliary body, which lead to vitreous hemorrhages and detachment of the retina.

A damaged lens—either dislocated or cataractous—may reduce vision or may be displaced anteriorly, causing increased intraocular pressure by closing the aqueous filtration angle. In either case, the lens is removed by using one of the cataract surgery techniques. Vitreous hemorrhages are removed with a suction-cutting vitrectomy instrument. Following this procedure, the retinal detachment is repaired by creating an adhesive scar between the choroid and retina, usually by freezing through the scleral surface (cryotherapy) over the area of the retinal tear or hole. The sclera then may be buckled inward to push the adhesion against the retina. This is usually done by compressing the globe with an encircling band of silicone rubber. Sometimes, an intraocular gas bubble is used to push the retina, choroid, and sclera into contact.

► Intraocular Foreign Bodies

An intraocular foreign body should be suspected on the basis of the occupational history, particularly if the worker complains of an irritating sensation in the eye and no superficial foreign body is found. For example, when steel tools are used to hammer other steel objects, the hammered steelwork hardens to a glassy surface from which small, sharp chips can fly and penetrate the globe with a minimum of discomfort at the moment of impact. Vision may be nearly normal if the entry wound is small. In cases such as this, in which a radiopaque foreign body is suspected, a radiograph should be taken. Ultrasonography usually will demonstrate nonradiopaque objects (eg, glass and plastic). If a foreign body is found, referral to an ophthalmologist for further evaluation and early treatment is essential.

Failure to remove iron or copper foreign bodies can cause severe impairment or loss of vision owing to their toxic effects on ocular tissue. A retained iron or copper foreign body may dissolve away in several months to a year, but the damage done to the retina by the soluble metallic salts is irreversible, and marked visual loss—even blindness—results. The prognosis for these foreign bodies is good if they are removed before they have time to dissolve. Inert materials such as glass

or plastic may cause mechanical damage to the eye, but in the absence of a local toxic reaction, the long-term prognosis is better. It is not necessary to remove every foreign body made of inert material; some of them may be left in place depending on their position in the globe and their effect on visual function. Iron-containing magnetic foreign bodies usually are removed with an ophthalmic magnet—sometimes through the entry wound or through a surgical incision made as close as possible to the foreign body. Nonmagnetic foreign bodies are removed with grasping instruments specially designed for ophthalmic microsurgery. Penetrating wounds caused by potentially contaminated objects such as agricultural implements or by wood fragments thrown from woodworking machinery can introduce severe intraocular infections that lead to complete disruption and loss of the globe; therefore, microbiologic studies and treatment with appropriate systemic and local antibiotics are required.

► Injuries to the Orbit & Optic Nerve

Orbital floor ("blowout") fractures frequently are associated with herniation of intraorbital contents into the fracture line. Usually there is severe edema within the orbit that restricts eye movements for 7–10 days. If restriction continues, surgical repair of the fracture may be indicated to free the entrapped extraocular muscles.

Facial bone and orbital fractures that extend to the posterior orbit may involve the optic canal, with damage to the optic nerve indicated by the presence of an afferent pupillary defect. Initial and later evaluations of the patient should include documentation of visual acuity. If there is progressive loss of vision, surgical decompression of the optic nerve in the canal may preserve or, occasionally, even improve the remaining vision.

Orbital injuries may cause severe hemorrhage, marked exophthalmos of the globe, and a dramatic and abrupt increase in intraocular pressure owing to compression. Although this increased pressure usually is relieved by the normal dissipation of interstitial fluid in a short period of time, it occasionally results in occlusion of the central retinal artery or vein. Pressure sometimes can be reduced by the application of gentle external massage to the globe through the closed lids. Surgical lysis of the lateral canthus of the lids may be required.

Penetrating wounds can damage the optic nerve directly by advancing through the funnel-shaped orbit to reach its apex, where the nerve and its blood supply are trapped by the optic canal. Contusion of the nerve causes severe visual impairment and sometimes is treated with large doses of systemic corticosteroids in a manner similar to treatment of spinal cord injuries.

► Injuries of the Corneal Epithelium (Abrasions & Superficial Foreign Bodies)

Abrasions of the corneal epithelium can be caused by superficial mechanical trauma (eg, prolonged wearing of contact lenses); by the presence of a foreign body; or by exposure to ultraviolet radiation, chemicals, aerosols, dust, smoke, and other irritants. The occupational medical history should be taken, as described in Chapter 2.

Photokeratoconjunctivitis (welder's flash) is a specific ocular injury caused by unprotected exposure to ultraviolet radiation with wavelengths shorter than 300 nm (actinic rays). This radiation is generated by the welder's arc and damages the exposed corneal and conjunctival epithelium. Injuries are caused both by direct observation of the arc and in persons nearby who often are not wearing protective filters.

In the first few hours after exposure, there may be only mild discomfort and slight conjunctival redness. After a latent period of several hours—even as long as 6–8 hours—the injured epithelial cells slough, causing an acute onset of severe pain sometimes said to be "as though someone had thrown hot sand in my eyes." Marked tearing, photophobia, and blepharospasm (tightly closed lids) are usual.

Examination requires a sterile topical anesthetic, which may be introduced through nearly closed eyelids by placing several drops along the lid margins. When the eyes open, more anesthetic may be instilled, along with fluorescein from a sterile paper strip. The fluorescein will diffuse over the cornea where the epithelium has sloughed, staining it bright green—best observed with a blue light. Epithelial loss is confined to the area exposed in the lid opening.

Treatment consists of instillation of an antibiotic ointment and patching the eye or eyes to prevent lid movement or blinking. The epithelium will not heal rapidly and in some cases not at all if it is frequently wiped and disturbed by blinking. It will require 12–24 hours for healing to occur; in some cases, several days may be necessary. The eyes should be examined daily. Anesthetic drops and fluorescein help in following the progress of reepithelialization. Continue to patch with antibiotic ointment until healing has occurred. Corneal epithelium heals without scarring. Antibiotic solutions or ointments containing corticosteroids sometimes are recommended for the treatment of welder's flash burns. The steroids may speed clearing of the associated hyperemia and edema, but they increase the incidence of secondary bacterial, viral, and fungal infections. If steroids are used, frequent examination (every 12–24 hours) is essential to detect early signs of infection until healing occurs. In addition, prolonged use of topical steroids (10–14 days or more), even in low doses, can raise intraocular pressure and, in time, can cause significant glaucomatous field loss. This unpredictable response occurs in approximately 10% of the population. It is therefore probably best to avoid the routine or frequent use of topical corticosteroids in the treatment of corneal and conjunctival injuries and infections.

The patient should not be given anesthetic drops or ointment to use at home. Anesthetics slow and may even prevent epithelial healing, and when used in these circumstances, they have led to severe scarring of the cornea and even the loss of an eye.

These injuries are easily prevented by wearing adequate protective filters in the face masks for the welder and goggles or ultraviolet filter glasses by visitors and workers in nearby areas where the welding flash can be seen.

Symptoms and signs of corneal abrasions include severe ocular pain, tearing, and blurring of vision. Inspection of the anterior eye with a flashlight usually shows irregular light reflections on the corneal surface in the area of the abraded epithelium. Use of sterile topical anesthetic and fluorescein paper strips is helpful for further examination. The fluorescein dye diffuses into the area of disrupted epithelium, stains it bright green, and can be observed easily with a blue light. If further evaluation reveals normal pupillary reactions, a bright red reflex, and no disruption of the anterior segment, the injury usually is confined to the anterior external layer of the cornea.

Small foreign bodies on the surface of the cornea or conjunctiva may be seen directly or detected by evidence of damaged epithelium from the fluorescein stain. Foreign bodies usually can be removed with a cotton-tipped applicator, but a sharp instrument is helpful occasionally. The side bevel of a disposable hypodermic needle can be used to gently detach foreign bodies that are firmly attached to the corneal surface. Rust deposited in the anterior layers of the cornea frequently can be removed by the same gentle scraping maneuver. If all the foreign body or rust is not removed easily, it usually can be left to slough or absorb by itself without causing damage. After foreign bodies are removed, treatment is the same as for abrasions.

Abrasions are treated by applying a sterile ophthalmic antibiotic ointment effective against both gram-positive and gram-negative organisms (eg, gentamicin, tobramycin, or a mixture containing bacitracin, polymyxin, and neomycin) and covering the affected eye with a patch dressing to keep the lids closed. Corneal epithelium usually heals promptly if the surface of the cornea is allowed to rest without blinking the lid. The initial process of healing is one in which the normal epithelial cells slide from the edge of the wound over the smooth surface of the cornea to fill the gap. The eyes should be inspected in 12–24 hours to determine if healing has occurred and to rule out corneal infection, which appears as a white or gray haze in the area of the wound. If the abrasion is not healed completely, a second application of the ointment and patch dressing for an additional 12–24 hours may be required. This process should be continued until the epithelial defect is healed. Scarring usually does not occur, and vision is restored to normal.

Caution: After the initial examination with topical anesthetic, sharp pain may return until the epithelium begins to heal. Under no circumstances should the patient be supplied with anesthetic drops or ointment to use during the healing process because topical anesthetics will delay healing and place the patient at risk for severe corneal infection and scarring. Antibiotic mixtures containing corticosteroids should not be used for treatment because they provide inadequate protection against bacterial infection and enhance the growth of viral and fungal pathogens.

Abrasions caused by fat-soluble petroleum products splashed into the eyes are treated initially by copious irrigation with water or saline solution to remove any remaining material. Staining with fluorescein will demonstrate the amount of epithelial loss, which may vary from a few punctate areas to complete denudation of the cornea. In either case, treatment is the same as outlined above. If the abraded area is large, the corneal stroma may appear slightly gray owing to some degree of edema. This clears rapidly with healing of the epithelium.

Exposure to aerosols (eg, paint sprays), detergents, surfactants, dust, smoke, and vapors can produce both acute and chronic symptoms of abrasion. Acute symptoms almost invariably include marked tearing and blepharospasm, which act to protect the eyes and wash away the offending material. Treatment for acute symptoms is as for other abrasions (see above). Chronic exposure to low-level irritants causes fatigue of the lacrimal reflex and subsequent sensations of dryness and burning of the eyes. Some degree of redness is common. Irrigation with saline solution prevents most of these chronic symptoms. Adequate ventilation and avoidance of irritants in the workplace are obviously the best preventive measures.

Exposure to some chemical substances causes a delayed loss of corneal epithelium. For example, formaldehyde fumes cause diffuse damage to epithelial cells, leading to their accelerated sloughing with normal blinking. Fortunately, the abrasion will heal without scarring when the fumes are avoided subsequently. The long list of other substances that produce this effect includes butylamine, diethylamine, hydrogen sulfide, methyl silicate, mustard gas, osmium tetroxide, podophyllum resin, and sulfur.

INDIRECT INJURIES TO THE EYE

In massive crush injuries, compression of the abdominal and chest vessels can cause sudden vascular engorgement of the retina. This leads to marked edema and diffuse hemorrhages in the fundus and can result in permanent ocular damage. Purtscher retinopathy is one form of this condition. There is no treatment. The prognosis for vision depends on the amount of damage done to the macula or optic nerve. Slow improvement in vision occurs as hemorrhages absorb for periods of up to several months.

In fractures of the long bones, fat emboli can migrate to the retina and produce small embolic changes that have the appearance of cotton-wool spots and sometimes are associated with flame-shaped hemorrhages in the fundus. Fat emboli, thrombi from heart valve disease and endocarditis, and emboli from a variety of sources occasionally obstruct branches of the retinal artery and cause infarction of a segment of the retina. Cholesterol crystals shed from atheromatous plaques in the carotid arteries also may migrate to the retina and appear as glistening intra-arterial bodies. In intravenous drug abuse, the injected drugs frequently contain inert substances such as talc, which may be seen in the retina as small white deposits. The prognosis for each of these conditions depends entirely on their location and whether or not the macula is involved. There is no ocular treatment. Clearing of the effects of these emboli—hemorrhages and edema—requires several weeks to a month. Cholesterol crystal emboli are an indication to investigate the patency of the carotid arteries.

Rarely, a septic embolus from a distant systemic infection causes endophthalmitis. Endophthalmitis generally has a poor prognosis. Specific diagnosis requires aspiration of vitreous fluid and sometimes aqueous humor for the isolation of organisms. Periocular injection of antibiotics adjacent to the scleral surface, occasionally intravitreal injection of appropriate doses of antibiotics, and intravenous antibiotics are the usual methods of treatment. The poor prognosis is a result of delay in diagnosis while the infection advances and of the unpredictable and sometimes poor ocular penetration of antibiotics.

SYMPATHETIC OPHTHALMIA

If the uveal tract (ie, the iris, ciliary body, or choroid) of one eye is injured, the uninjured (sympathizing) eye may show inflammation. This rare disorder is thought to be an autoimmune inflammatory response and can be prevented by prompt, adequate treatment of the initial injury to minimize continuing trauma to the damaged uveal tissue. Sympathetic ophthalmia can cause complete loss of vision in both eyes if unrecognized and untreated early in its course. As soon as inflammation is seen in the sympathizing eye, treatment of both eyes with local corticosteroids (topical and periocular injections) and mydriatics should be started. Large doses of systemic corticosteroids are also used frequently.

OCCLUSION OF THE CENTRAL RETINAL ARTERY

Occlusion of the central retinal artery is characterized by sudden painless loss of vision and is considered an ocular emergency. Permanent loss of vision will result if the retina is deprived of blood for 30–60 minutes; consequently, arterial circulation must be restored as soon as possible.

Diagnosis is based on the history and eye examination. Occlusion usually is seen in older patients with arteriosclerosis or following embolism from the great vessels. It also can be caused by pressure from an unusually tight dressing over the eye, particularly when there is orbital edema or hemorrhage. If the visual loss is incomplete, the patient may be able to detect some light. Ophthalmic examination reveals a bloodless retina with thin and thready arteries. Early findings include a faint retinal edema that appears as a grayish or white discoloration and is particularly noticeable around the macula, allowing the normal red color of the choroid in the fovea to show through as a cherry-red spot. Later, red cells in the blood column of the arteries may separate into segments and appear as "boxcars." The veins also appear thinner than normal. The optic disc retains its normal pink color for several weeks, but the retinal edema becomes more apparent.

Although central retinal artery occlusions usually are not associated with increased intraocular pressures, the most effective treatment is immediate reduction of the normal intraocular pressure in an attempt to dislodge the embolus or thrombus thought to be obstructing the artery at a restricted area of the vessel as it passes through the scleral shell just posterior to the optic disc. The pressure can be reduced by using two fingers to alternately massage and press the globe through the closed lids. This maneuver should be repeated four or five times over 10–15 minutes to accelerate the expression of aqueous humor and applies intermittent pressure on the artery. The patient's use of a rebreathing bag will increase the amount of carbon dioxide in the cerebral and ocular blood vessels, sometimes effecting vascular dilation.

If these maneuvers fail, paracentesis of the anterior chamber may be indicated. After a topical anesthetic is given, the conjunctiva is grasped with fine-tooth forceps. An incision is made through the clear cornea at the periphery of the anterior chamber, with the sharp scalpel blade held in the plane of the iris so as not to touch either the iris or the lens. The blade then is turned slightly to allow some of the aqueous humor to escape abruptly. This lowers the intraocular pressure and sometimes restores circulation to the retina.

▶ Anterior Ischemic Optic Neuropathy

This condition is characterized by an acute, painless loss of vision in individuals 50–70 years of age. The ischemia of the optic nerve is in or just behind the disc. The disc appears swollen or edematous at first, clearing with time and leaving various amounts of optic atrophy and usually a severe loss of vision. The same process in the 70- to 80-year-old age group may be a result of giant cell arteritis, frequently associated with temporal arteritis. Systemic steroids sometimes are helpful in the latter group to prevent involvement of the second eye.

OCCLUSION OF THE CENTRAL RETINAL VEIN

Occlusion of the central retinal vein produces painless visual loss and is seen most commonly in older patients with diabetes, hypertension, or other vascular occlusive diseases. Findings include a swollen optic disc, distended and tortuous retinal veins, and an edematous retina with flame-shaped hemorrhages.

There is no effective emergency treatment, although anticoagulants have been tried occasionally. An ophthalmologist should follow these patients. The prognosis for improvement of vision is slightly better for patients with an occluded retinal vein than it is for those patients with an occluded retinal artery.

EYE INJURIES CAUSED BY RADIATION EXPOSURE

This section describes the electromagnetic spectrum and discusses methods to prevent occupational exposure to radiation.

▶ Injuries Caused by Ionizing Radiation

X-rays, beta rays, and other radiation sources in adequate doses can cause ocular injury. The eyelid is particularly vulnerable to x-ray damage because of the thinness of its skin. Loss of lashes and scarring can lead to inversion or eversion (entropion or ectropion) of the lid margins and prevent adequate lid closure. Scarring of the conjunctiva can impair the production of mucus and the function of the lacrimal gland ducts, thereby causing dryness of the eyes. X-ray radiation in a dose of 500–800 R directed toward the lens surface can cause cataracts, sometimes with a delay of several months to a year before the opacities appear. Treatment for these injuries is the appropriate oculoplastic repair of lid deformities and scarring. Deficiencies of tears and mucus can be improved by the topical use of artificial tears and protection from evaporation by wearing protective glasses with side shields that seal to the face. Radiation cataracts can be removed surgically by the appropriate standard technique.

▶ Injuries Caused by Ultraviolet Radiation

Ultraviolet radiation of wavelengths shorter than 300 nm (actinic rays) can damage the corneal epithelium. This is most commonly the result of exposure to the sun at high altitudes and in areas where shorter wavelengths are readily reflected from bright surfaces such as snow, water, and sand. Exposure to radiation generated by a welding arc can cause welder's flash burn, a form of keratitis. After a latent period of several hours, the injured epithelial cells soften and slough, causing sudden onset of pain. Treatment of these injuries consists of applying antibiotic ointment and patches until the epithelial cells have had an opportunity to heal (see the section "Injuries of the Corneal Epithelium [Abrasions & Superficial Foreign Bodies]").

Wavelengths of 300–400 nm are transmitted through the cornea, and approximately 80% are absorbed by the lens, where they may cause cataractous changes. Accidental exposure to an inadequately shielded dental instrument used to accelerate the hardening of plastic fillings has caused significant lens opacities in dental personnel. Epidemiologic studies suggest that exposure to solar radiation in these wavelengths near the equator is correlated with an increased incidence of cataracts. They also indicate that workers exposed to bright sunlight in occupations such as farming, truck driving, and construction works appear to have a higher incidence of cataracts than do those who work primarily indoors. Experimental studies show that these wavelengths cause changes in the lens protein that lead to cataract formation in animals.

▶ Cataract

Any opacity in the lens is called a cataract. Some degree of opacity is present in almost all lenses, and the significance of the changes depends solely on their effect on vision. Peripheral opacities, for example, that do not interfere with vision are of no clinical significance.

The lens is composed of lens protein arranged in an ordered pattern of cytoplasmic fibers produced by the lens epithelium. These cells continue to produce new fibers at a slow rate throughout life. The lens thus slowly increases in volume—mainly in thickness—pushing the iris forward.

Changes in the chemistry and hydration of the lens protein create various types of cataracts. These changes may be induced by a variety of agents, including near-ultraviolet radiation of 300–400 nm. These wavelengths are absorbed by the central lens fibers, causing the brownish discoloration of lenticular nuclear sclerosis. Ocular inflammation and corticosteroids, both topical and systemic, produce typical posterior subcapsular cataracts.

Types of Cataracts

A. Age-Related Cataracts

Age-related (senile) cataract is the most common type seen. Some degree of opacity is almost universal. The progress of change and the related reduction in vision is usually quite slow. Nuclear sclerosis—an increasing density in the central mass of protein—causes a myopic change that can be corrected by changing glasses for some years—in many instances restoring vision to near normal.

B. Congenital Cataracts

These can be unilateral or bilateral, and many are thought to be of genetic origin. Some are a result of maternal rubella during the first trimester of pregnancy. If the opacity prevents a clear view of the ocular fundus, surgical removal at an early age—even 2 months—is indicated to aid in the development of useful vision.

C. Traumatic Cataracts

Contusion injuries can cause opacities that may appear right away or may develop slowly over weeks or even months. Penetrating wounds can tear the lens capsule, allowing aqueous humor to soften lens protein, usually creating major opacities. These cataracts almost always need to be removed acutely—in many cases at the time of wound repair.

D. Secondary Cataracts

These changes result from inflammatory processes in the eye (uveitis) and usually begin by producing opacities just inside the posterior lens capsule. Similar changes occur in association with retinitis pigmentosa, glaucoma, and rarely, retinal detachments.

E. Cataracts Associated With Systemic Diseases

These are usually bilateral and may appear in patients with myotonia dystrophica, hypoparathyroidism, diabetes mellitus, and Down syndrome, as well as in many other less common conditions.

F. Toxic Cataracts

Lens opacities are reported following exposure to or ingestion of numerous chemicals. They are described at some length in Grant's Toxicology of the Eye. The most common cause at present is the use of corticosteroids, either topical or systemic.

Treatment

There is no effective medical treatment for cataract. Surgical removal usually results in significant improvement of vision in approximately 90% of patients. The results depend on whether other ocular changes are present, such as macular scars or optic nerve changes. Indications for surgery depend almost entirely on the needs of the individual patient to improve vision. Minimally invasive, small incision phacoemulsification with quick post-op recovery has become the standard of care in cataract surgery all over the world.

Prognosis

The results of cataract surgery generally are excellent. Significant visual improvement is reported in nearly 90% of patients following extraction of age-related cataracts. The reduced expectations in eyes with injuries are a result of unpredictable intraocular complications such as retinal scarring and macular damage.

Injuries Caused by Visible Radiation (Light)

Visible light has a spectrum of 400–750 nm. If the wavelengths of this spectrum penetrate fully to the retina, they can cause thermal, mechanical, or photic injuries. Thermal injuries are produced by light intense enough to increase the temperature in the retina by 10–20°C (18–36°F). Lasers used in therapy can cause this type of injury. The light is absorbed by the retinal pigment epithelium, where its energy is converted to heat, and the heat causes photocoagulation of retinal tissue. Mechanical injuries can be produced by exposure to laser energy from a Q-switched or mode-locked laser, which produces sonic shock waves that disrupt retinal tissue.

Photic injuries are caused by prolonged exposure to intense light, which produces varying degrees of cellular damage in the retinal macula without a significant increase in the temperature of the tissue (usually no more than 1–2°C [1.8–3.6°F]). Recent studies show that photic injuries are not burns in the literal sense but are damage from the light itself. Sun gazing is the most common cause of this type of injury, but prolonged unprotected exposure to a welding arc also can damage the retinal macula. When the initial retinal edema clears, there is usually some scarring that leads to a permanent decrease in visual acuity. The intensity of light, length of exposure, and age of the exposed individual are all important factors. The older the individual, the more sensitive the retina appears to be to photic injuries. Anyone who has had cataract surgery is much more vulnerable because filtration of light by the lens is impaired. In photic injuries caused by exposure to welding sources or other excessively bright light, treatment with systemic corticosteroids may be tried. A large initial dose of prednisone (60–100 mg) is tapered rapidly over a period of 10–14 days. This may reduce the acute edema or inflammatory response, but it is not always effective.

Wavelengths of 500–750 nm are most useful for vision and appear not to cause photic damage to the retina at exposures most commonly encountered. However, repeated exposure to bright sunlight by working outdoors for 3–4 hours each day can cause prolongation of the dark adaptation response, thereby reducing night vision.

▶ Injuries Caused by Infrared Radiation

Wavelengths greater than 750 nm in the infrared spectrum can produce lens changes. Glassblower cataract is an example of a heat injury that damages the anterior lens capsule. Denser cataractous changes can occur in unprotected workers who observe glowing masses of glass or iron for many hours a day.

EFFECTS OF VIDEO-DISPLAY TERMINAL USE

In recent years, employees who spend 6–8 hours a day looking at video-display terminals have complained of eyestrain, headache, and general fatigue. The brightness of the light from such terminals is not great enough to produce any ocular injury. Posture, accommodative fatigue, and the early changes of presbyopia may contribute to feelings of eyestrain and physical stress. Measures to alleviate these problems associated with video-display terminal use are discussed in Chapter 6.

REFERENCES

Hall AH, Mathieu L, Maibach HI: Acute chemical skin injuries in the United States: a review. Crit Rev Toxicol 2018;48(7):540-554 [PMID: 30226392].

Lewis CJ, Al-Mousawi A, Jha A, Allison KP: Is it time for a change in the approach to chemical burns? The role of Diphoterine® in the management of cutaneous and ocular chemical injuries. J Plast Reconstr Aesthet Surg 2017;70(5):563-567 [PMID: 28330646].

Liu CC, Tong JM, Li PS, Li KK: Epidemiology and clinical outcome of intraocular foreign bodies in Hong Kong: a 13-year review. Int Ophthalmol 2017;37(1):55-61 [PMID: 27043444].

Loporchio D, Mukkamala L, Gorukanti K, Zarbin M, Langer P, Bhagat N: Intraocular foreign bodies: a review. Surv Ophthalmol 2016;61(5):582-596 [PMID: 26994871].

Lynn DD, Zukin LM, Dellavalle R: The safety and efficacy of Diphoterine for ocular and cutaneous burns in humans. Cutan Ocul Toxicol 2017;36(2):185-192 [PMID: 27486965].

Mwangi N, Mutie DM: Emergency management: penetrating eye injuries and intraocular foreign bodies. Community Eye Health 2018;31(103):70-71 [PMID: 30487690].

Tarff A, Behrens A: Ocular emergencies: red eye. Med Clin North Am 2017;101(3):615-639 [PMID: 28372717].

Zakrzewski H, Chung H, Sanders E, Hanson C, Ford B: Evaluation of occupational ocular trauma: are we doing enough to promote eye safety in the workplace? Can J Ophthalmol 2017;52(4):338-342 [PMID: 28774513].

■ SELF-ASSESSMENT QUESTIONS

Select the one correct answer for each question.

Question 1: Open-angle glaucoma
  a. accounts for most cases of glaucomatous visual loss (90%)
  b. is painful at onset
  c. distorts vision in its early stages
  d. results in smaller optic cups

Question 2: Visual fields should be tested
  a. by licensed ophthalmic technicians
  b. primarily in a hospital setting
  c. in patients with suspected head injury
  d. to confirm the diagnosis of macular degeneration

Question 3: Strong alkalis and acids
  a. are neutralized in the eye before they cause injury
  b. can cause the most severe and damaging chemical injuries to the eye and eyelids
  c. are exposure hazards in only a few industrial settings
  d. will not cause injuries away from work

Question 4: Iridoplegia
  a. is caused by damage to the pupillary sphincter
  b. predictably affects how the pupil reacts to light
  c. is not associated with injury to the iris root
  d. is unrelated to any form of glaucoma

Question 5: Hyphema with secondary hemorrhage
  a. clears spontaneously
  b. may cause an increase in intraocular pressure
  c. requires opening of the anterior chamber
  d. has a uniformly good prognosis

Question 6: Photokeratoconjunctivitis (welder's flash)
  a. is caused by unprotected exposure to ultraviolet radiation with wavelengths longer than 300 nm
  b. may be caused by the actinic rays of sunlight
  c. damages the exposed corneal and conjunctival epithelium
  d. does not affect persons passing nearby

Question 7: Sympathetic ophthalmia
  a. is a common disorder associated with injury to one eye
  b. is not likely to be an autoimmune inflammatory response
  c. cannot be prevented by prompt treatment
  d. can cause complete loss of vision in both eyes if unrecognized and untreated early in its course

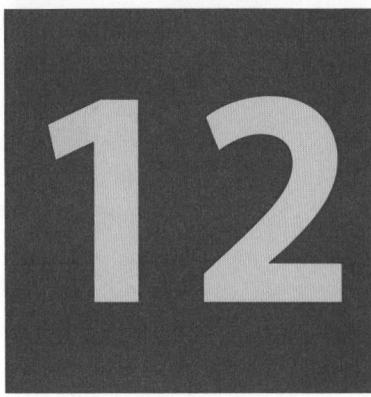

Hearing Loss

Robert Dobie, MD

Occupational hearing loss may be partial or (rarely) total, unilateral or bilateral, and conductive, sensorineural, or mixed (conductive and sensorineural). Conductive hearing loss involves the external or middle ear and impairs the passage of sound to the inner ear; sensorineural hearing loss (SNHL) results from dysfunction of the inner ear, auditory nerve, or brain. In the workplace, conductive and mixed hearing loss can be caused by blunt or penetrating head injuries, explosions, and thermal injuries such as slag burns sustained when a piece of welder's slag penetrates the eardrum. SNHL usually results from damage to the cochlea, especially loss of hair cells from the organ of Corti. Among the causes of occupational SNHL are continuous exposure to noise in excess of 85 dBA, blunt head injury, and exposure to ototoxic substances.

PHYSIOLOGY OF HEARING

Sound waves consist of alternating periods of compression and rarefaction within a medium such as air. The stronger the pressure variation, the louder the sound. Measurement of hearing in terms of sound pressure in micropascals (μPa) is cumbersome because of the enormous dynamic range of normal hearing (for the frequencies humans hear best, pressures between 20 and 20,000,000 μPa can be heard and tolerated). For this reason, the logarithmic decibel (dB) scale is used, compressing a million-fold pressure variation into a range of 120 dB. Since humans hear some frequencies better than others, audiometers are calibrated in "hearing level" (HL), a scale that defines 0 dB HL—at each frequency—as the faintest sound that the average healthy young person can detect.

Sound frequency (the number of waves passing a fixed point each second, measured in hertz [Hz]) correlates with pitch. The normal human ear can detect sounds across the frequency range from approximately 20 to 20,000 Hz. The most important range for human speech communication is between 500 and 3000 Hz.

When sound traveling in air strikes water, almost all of it is reflected, because air and water have very different acoustic impedances. To allow efficient transmission of air-conducted sound into the fluid-filled inner ear, the impedance-matching middle ear has evolved; when the ear canal is open, and the tympanic membrane and the three ossicles (malleus, incus, and stapes) are working properly, the inner ear can respond to sounds that are up to 60 dB less intense than would otherwise be the case.

The transduction of mechanical vibrations to nerve impulses by the inner hair cells takes place in the inner ear (cochlea) at the organ of Corti. The hair cells of the organ of Corti rest on the basilar membrane, and the stereocilia of the three rows of outer hair cells oscillate against the tectorial membrane. A shearing action between the stereocilia and the tectorial membrane, caused by the traveling wave motion of the basilar membrane, results in release of neurotransmitters by a single row of inner hair cells to the auditory nerve fibers that innervate them.

As the wave travels from base (high frequency) to apex (low frequency) along the basilar membrane, it reaches a peak amplitude that correlates directly with the frequency of the sound. Each point along the basilar membrane is frequency specific (tonotopically organized). The electromotility of the outer hair cells enhances the frequency tuning of the traveling wave.

EVALUATION OF HEARING

▶ Clinical Observation

The simplest form of hearing evaluation occurs during medical history taking in the examination room without any sophisticated equipment. Can the patient converse adequately face-to-face at a normal distance (about 1 m)? At lesser or greater distances? When the examiner is speaking normally, loudly, or (in cases of very severe hearing loss) shouting? When the examiner's back is turned and visual cues are lost? During handwashing, with the interfering noise of running water? While no substitute for audiometry, simple gross observations of this type should correlate with—and can serve to validate or invalidate—the results of formal hearing tests.

"Whispered-voice" tests are still used in some contexts (eg, they are permitted as a substitute for audiometry for commercial drivers' licenses).

▶ Tuning Fork Tests

Tuning fork tests should be performed with a 512-Hz tuning fork because lower frequencies may elicit a tactile response.

A. Rinne Test

In cases where the patient hears air conduction (tuning fork placed by the opening of the ear canal) better than via bone conduction (tuning fork placed on the mastoid bone), a SNHL or normal hearing is usually indicated in the test ear. When bone conduction is louder than air conduction, a conductive hearing loss is usually present (a severe unilateral sensorineural loss may show the same pattern unless masking is used to exclude the better ear).

B. Weber Test

When the tuning fork is placed on the forehead or front teeth, sound should lateralize toward the ear with a conductive loss and away from the ear with a sensorineural loss (in cases of unilateral or asymmetric hearing loss).

▶ Pure-Tone Audiometry

In a clinical audiogram, sensitivity to pure tones is measured at 250, 500, 1000, 2000, 3000, 4000, 6000, and 8000 Hz for air conduction (head phones) and, if necessary, bone conduction (bone oscillator). The threshold of hearing (the softest tone that is audible) can be measured by adjusting tone intensity either manually, or automatically under computer control; the latter is common in occupational hearing conservation programs (HCPs). Thresholds are expressed in decibels, with the normal range (for young adults) at each frequency from 0 to 20 dB HL. Because loud sounds may stimulate the opposite ear, masking that ear with competing noise is necessary when asymmetry exists. When both air and bone conduction are decreased, an SNHL exists. Conductive losses are indicated by an "air-bone gap," in which the air-conduction threshold exceeds the bone-conduction threshold. Results may be presented numerically or shown graphically (Figures 12–1 to 12–5).

▶ Bekesy (Self-Recording) Audiometry

Pure-tone thresholds also may be measured by Bekesy audiometry in which the patient uses self-directed techniques that involve pressing and releasing a signal button. This procedure used to be widespread in occupational HCPs.

▶ Speech Audiometry

Two routine tests are performed to assess speech reception and comprehension, which are the most important aspects of audition.

A. Speech Reception Threshold

The speech reception threshold (SRT) is the intensity (in decibels) at which the listener is able to repeat 50% of balanced two-syllable words known as *spondee words* (eg, **baseball, playground,** and **airplane**). The threshold is usually in close agreement (within 6–10 dB) with an average of the pure-tone thresholds for frequencies between 500 and 2000 Hz. The normal range for young adults is between 0 and 20 dB, with thresholds of 25–40 dB termed *mild hearing loss,* 40–55 dB termed *moderate,* 55–70 termed moderately severe, 70–90 dB termed *severe,* and greater than 90 dB termed *profound hearing loss.*

B. Word Recognition Score

In the word recognition score (WRS), also referred to as *speech discrimination score,* monosyllabic words that are phonetically balanced are presented at intensities usually well above the speech reception threshold (SRT plus 30–40 dB) in order to test speech comprehension. Results are expressed as a percentage of words repeated correctly. The normal range of WRSs for young adults is 88–100%. Word lists are available for most languages. Severe depression of the WRS usually indicates socially significant disability, but WRSs display high test-retest variability.

▶ Impedance (Immittance) Audiometry

The mechanical aspects of the middle ear sound transformer system can be assessed by tympanometry and acoustic reflex testing.

A. Tympanometry

Tympanometry employs an acoustic probe to measure the impedance of the eardrum and ossicular chain. Reduced middle ear compliance usually indicates a partial vacuum owing to auditory tube dysfunction, whereas noncompliance suggests either a tympanic membrane perforation or middle ear effusion. An increase in compliance suggests either laxity of the tympanic membrane or disruption of the ossicular chain.

B. Acoustic Reflex Testing

Contraction of the middle ear muscles in response to a loud noise results in a measurable rise of middle ear impedance. Interpretation of acoustic reflex testing also may yield information regarding the integrity of the auditory portion of the central nervous system. It is also an indirect measurement of recruitment (abnormal growth of loudness) that frequently accompanies SNHL.

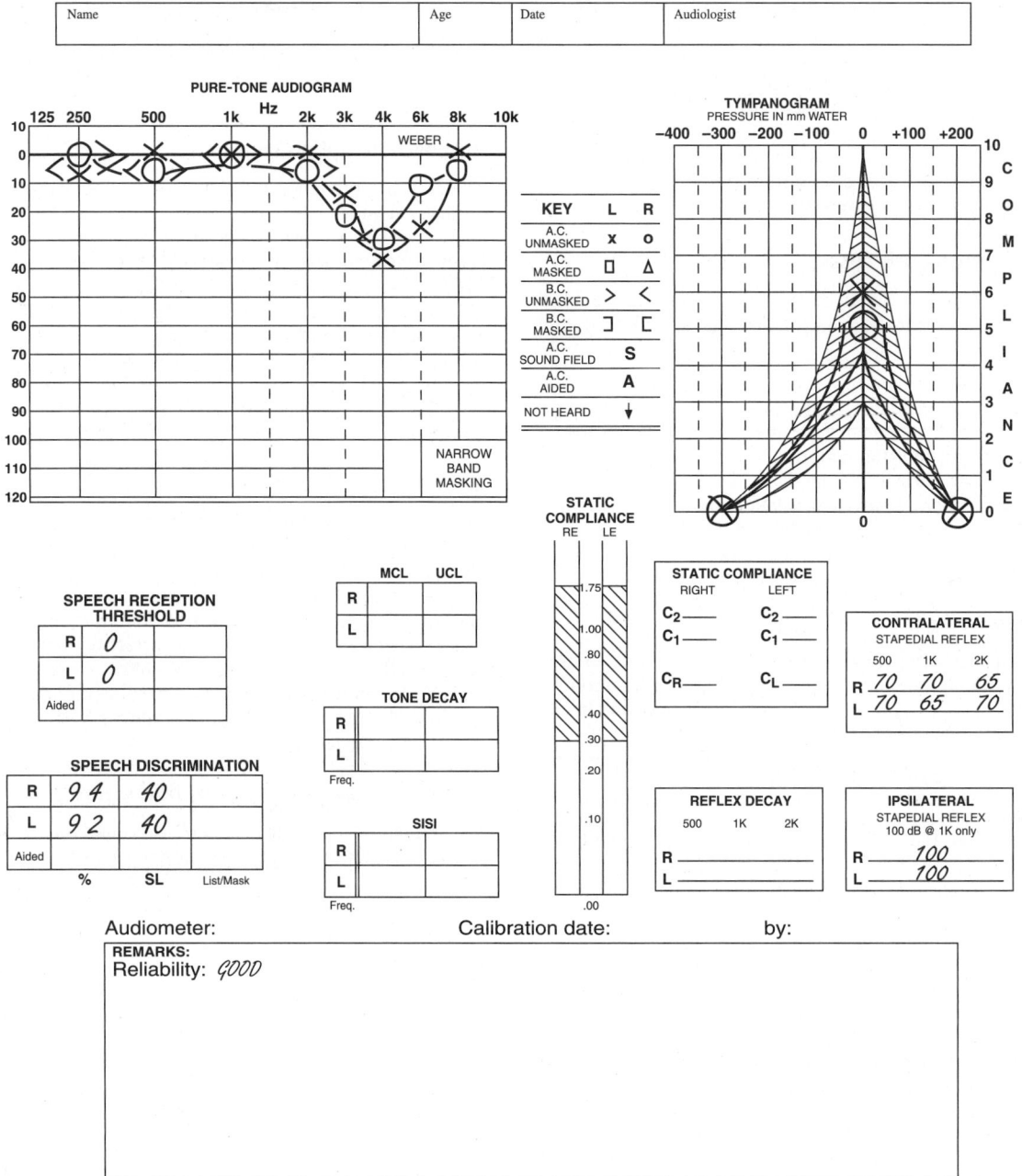

▲ Figure 12–1. Normal to mild noise-induced hearing loss. The audiogram shows typical bilateral high-frequency sensorineural hearing loss, which is most severe at 4000 Hz. Note the normal speech discrimination score.

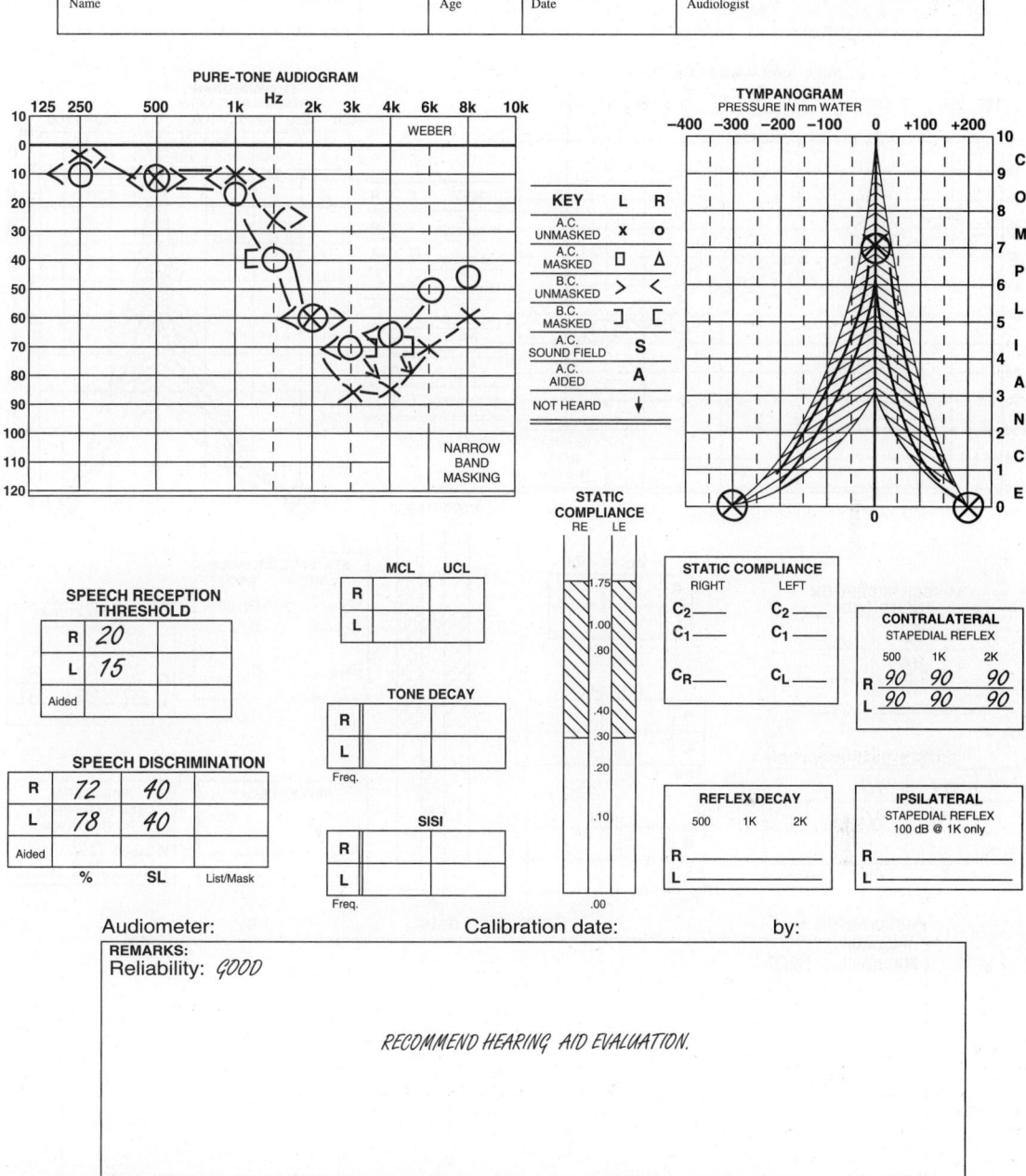

▲ **Figure 12–2.** Normal to severe noise-induced hearing loss plus age-related hearing loss. The audiogram shows moderate to severe high-frequency sensorineural hearing loss but preservation of the lower tones. Note the moderate decrease in the speech discrimination score.

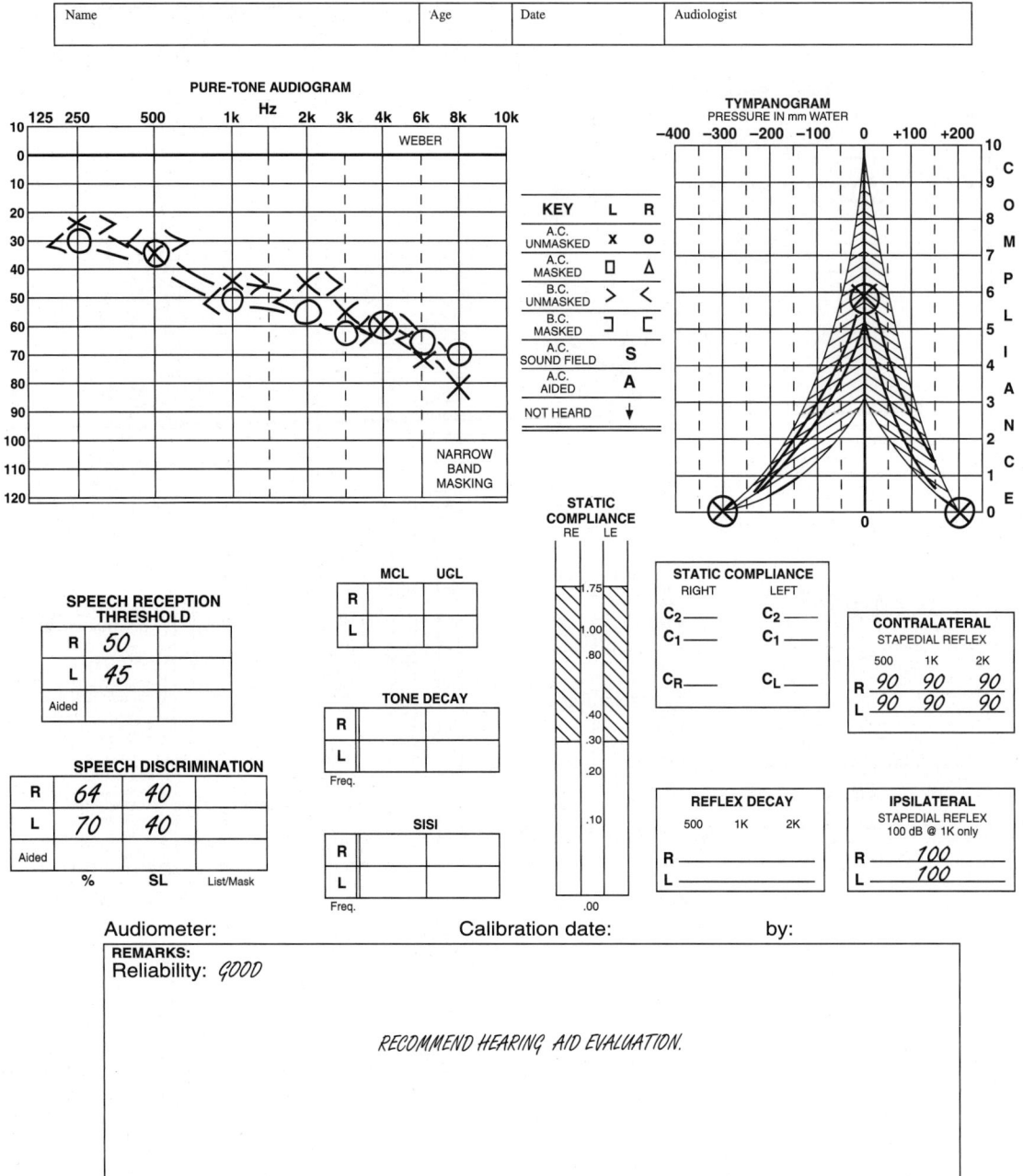

Name		Age	Date	Audiologist

PURE-TONE AUDIOGRAM

TYMPANOGRAM
PRESSURE IN mm WATER

WEBER

KEY	L	R
A.C. UNMASKED	X	o
A.C. MASKED	☐	Δ
B.C. UNMASKED	>	<
B.C. MASKED	⊐	⊏
A.C. SOUND FIELD	S	
A.C. AIDED	A	
NOT HEARD	↓	

NARROW BAND MASKING

SPEECH RECEPTION THRESHOLD

R	50	
L	45	
Aided		

	MCL	UCL
R		
L		

TONE DECAY

R		
L		
Freq.		

SPEECH DISCRIMINATION

R	64	40	
L	70	40	
Aided			
	%	SL	List/Mask

SISI

R		
L		
Freq.		

STATIC COMPLIANCE
RE   LE

STATIC COMPLIANCE

	RIGHT		LEFT	
C_2	—	C_2	—	
C_1	—	C_1	—	
C_R	—	C_L	—	

CONTRALATERAL
STAPEDIAL REFLEX

	500	1K	2K
R	90	90	90
L	90	90	90

REFLEX DECAY

	500	1K	2K
R			
L			

IPSILATERAL
STAPEDIAL REFLEX
100 dB @ 1K only

R	100
L	100

Audiometer: Calibration date: by:

REMARKS:
Reliability: GOOD

RECOMMEND HEARING AID EVALUATION.

▲ **Figure 12–3.** Presbycusis. The audiogram shows moderate to severe gently sloping sensorineural hearing loss. Note that the hearing threshold at 4000 Hz is better than at 8000 Hz, a pattern suggestive, but not diagnostic, of an aging change rather than exposure to noise.

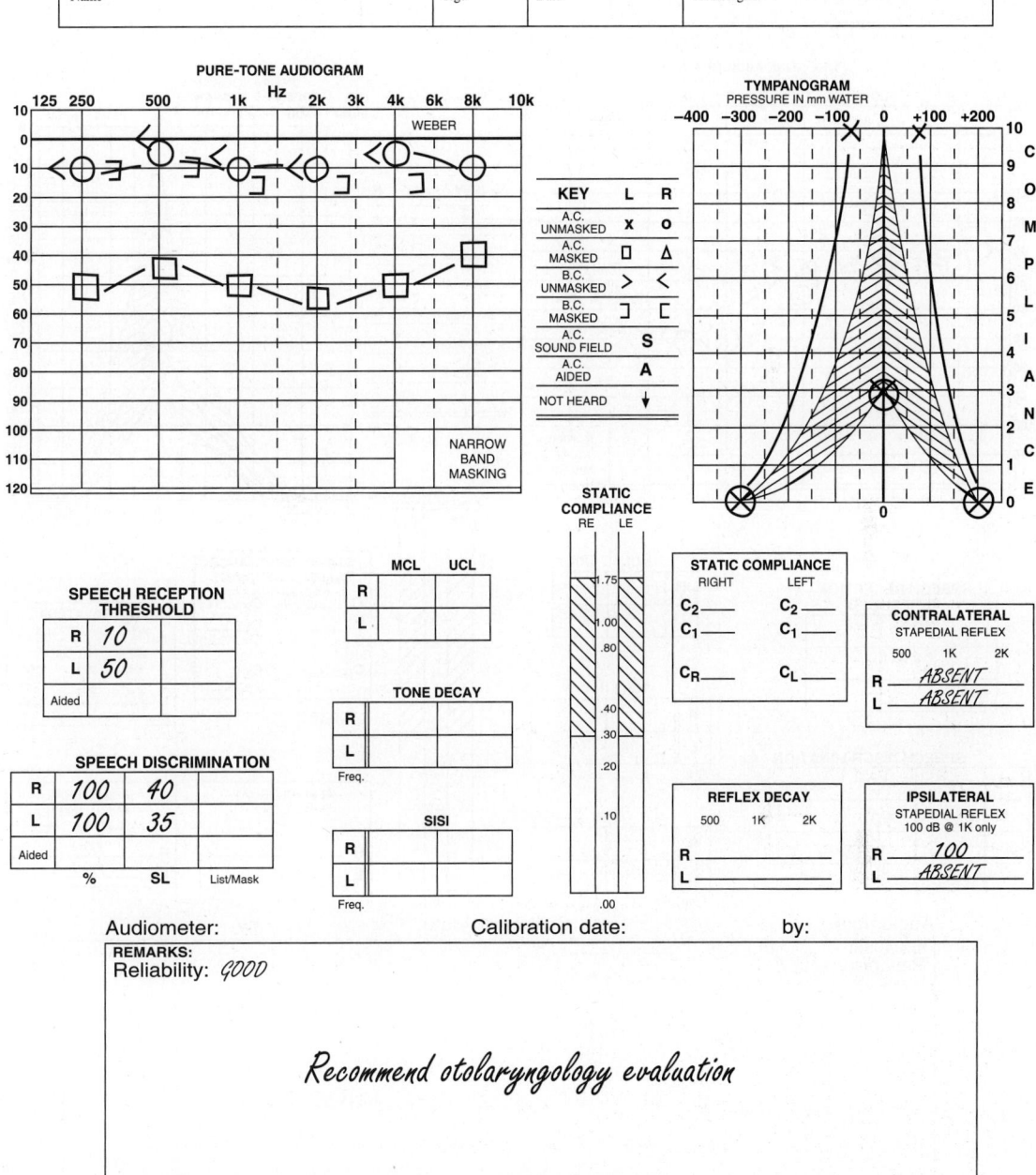

Name	Age	Date	Audiologist

PURE-TONE AUDIOGRAM

TYMPANOGRAM
PRESSURE IN mm WATER

WEBER

KEY	L	R
A.C. UNMASKED	X	O
A.C. MASKED	□	Δ
B.C. UNMASKED	>	<
B.C. MASKED	]	[
A.C. SOUND FIELD	S	
A.C. AIDED	A	
NOT HEARD	↓	

NARROW BAND MASKING

STATIC COMPLIANCE
RE   LE

SPEECH RECEPTION THRESHOLD

	MCL	UCL
R		
L		

STATIC COMPLIANCE

	RIGHT		LEFT
	C_2 ——		C_2 ——
	C_1 ——		C_1 ——
	C_R ——		C_L ——

R	*10*	
L	*50*	
Aided		

TONE DECAY

R		
L		
Freq.		

CONTRALATERAL
STAPEDIAL REFLEX

	500	1K	2K
R		*ABSENT*	
L		*ABSENT*	

SPEECH DISCRIMINATION

R	*100*	*40*
L	*100*	*35*
Aided		
	%	SL	List/Mask

SISI

R		
L		
Freq.		

REFLEX DECAY

	500	1K	2K
R		——	
L		——	

IPSILATERAL
STAPEDIAL REFLEX
100 dB @ 1K only

R	*100*	
L	*ABSENT*	

Audiometer: Calibration date: by:

REMARKS:
Reliability: *GOOD*

Recommend otolaryngology evaluation

▲ **Figure 12–4.** Moderate conductive hearing loss. The audiogram shows a disparity between the thresholds of bone conduction and air conduction. This "air-bone gap" represents the degree of hearing impairment caused by dysfunction of the external or middle ear. Tympanogram shows an increase in left middle ear compliance. The audiogram is typical of a left ossicular chain disruption.

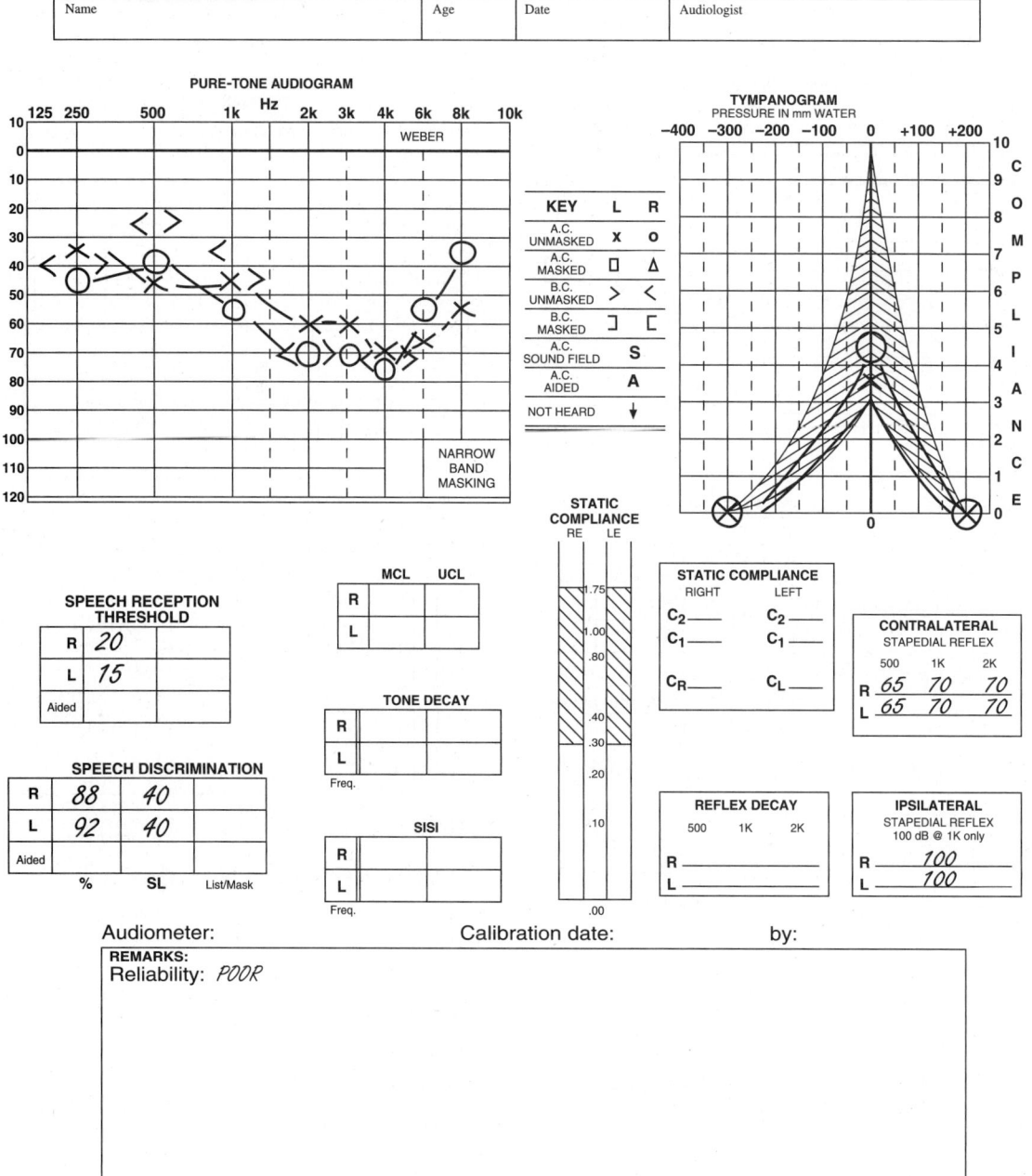

Name		Age	Date	Audiologist

PURE-TONE AUDIOGRAM

TYMPANOGRAM
PRESSURE IN mm WATER

KEY	L	R
A.C. UNMASKED	X	o
A.C. MASKED	□	Δ
B.C. UNMASKED	>	<
B.C. MASKED	]	[
A.C. SOUND FIELD	S	
A.C. AIDED	A	
NOT HEARD	↓	

NARROW BAND MASKING

STATIC COMPLIANCE
RE   LE

MCL   UCL

R		
L		

SPEECH RECEPTION THRESHOLD

R	20	
L	15	
Aided		

TONE DECAY

R		
L		
Freq.		

SPEECH DISCRIMINATION

R	88	40	
L	92	40	
Aided			
	%	SL	List/Mask

SISI

R		
L		
Freq.		

STATIC COMPLIANCE

	RIGHT	LEFT
C₂	C_2——	C_2——
C₁	C_1——	C_1——
	C_R——	C_L——

CONTRALATERAL
STAPEDIAL REFLEX

	500	1K	2K
R	65	70	70
L	65	70	70

REFLEX DECAY

	500	1K	2K
R	——————		
L	——————		

IPSILATERAL
STAPEDIAL REFLEX
100 dB @ 1K only

R	100
L	100

Audiometer: Calibration date: by:

REMARKS:
Reliability: *POOR*

▲ **Figure 12–5.** Nonorganic hearing loss. The audiogram shows pure-tone thresholds that are significantly worse than the speech reception thresholds recorded on the same data.

Evoked-Response Audiometry (Brain Stem Audiometry)

In patients who demonstrate unilateral or asymmetric SNHL, retrocochlear lesions (lesions of the eighth cranial nerve, brain stem, or cortex) must be ruled out. Evoked potentials, which typically are elicited in response to clicking noises and recorded via scalp electrodes, provide information about the location of sensorineural lesions. For individuals with normal hearing, as well as most patients with cochlear hearing losses, a series of five electroencephalographic waves may be detected, representing the central auditory system from the eighth cranial nerve (wave I) to the inferior colliculus (wave V). Any significant delay or even a complete absence of response may indicate a cerebellopontine angle tumor (eg, acoustic neuroma) or a lesion of the brain stem. More definitive diagnosis of retrocochlear lesions requires computed tomographic (CT) scanning or magnetic resonance imaging (MRI).

Stenger Test

This test is useful for detecting feigned unilateral hearing loss. The Stenger principle states that when tones of the same frequency but of different intensities are presented to both ears simultaneously, only the louder tone will be heard. When the louder tone is presented to the ear with a feigned hearing loss, the patient stops responding because the patient perceives that all the sound is coming from that side. Patients with true unilateral loss indicate that they continue to hear the sound in the opposite ear.

Otoacoustic Emissions

Otoacoustic emissions (OAEs) are a recent addition to objective hearing testing. OAEs are produced when the cochlea receives an external sound stimulus, and the mechanical properties of the outer hair cells act in a manner in which a measurable sound is produced and transmitted laterally through the middle ear to be recorded in the external auditory canal. There are two types of evoked OAEs used clinically today. They are transient-evoked otoacoustic emissions (TEOAEs) and distortion-product otoacoustic emissions (DPOAEs). Individuals with hearing better than 35 dB (TEOAEs) and 50 dB (DPOAEs) will usually produce OAEs, unless there is middle ear pathology. If an individual generates OAEs but does not admit to hearing, the middle ear and cochlea are assumed to be functional, and thus a nonorganic or retrocochlear origin must be assumed. OAEs are useful in forensic examination because OAEs are rapid (30 seconds to 3 minutes), reproducible, frequency specific (1000–10,000 Hz), and sensitive to outer hair cell dysfunction, such as the damage caused by noise. OAEs may someday prove useful in HCPs, but have not been shown to be more effective than pure-tone audiometry, and cannot detect worsening hearing in people with even mild hearing loss who have already lost their OAEs.

Fitness for Work

The hearing in noise test (HINT) has been proposed as a direct measure of functional speech perception in noise, for use in screening applicants for hearing-critical jobs. The HINT measures speech intelligibility in quiet and in spectrally matched noise at suprathreshold levels using sentence materials. The testing is done in quiet and in three background-noise environments (noise front, noise right, and noise left). The noise level is fixed at 65 dBA while the sentence (signal) level is varied; the signal-to-noise ratio (SNR) is the difference in decibels between the sentence level and the noise level at which performance is 50% correct. Young adults can usually repeat the sentences even when the noise is louder than the sentences, while people with hearing loss often require the sentences to be considerably louder than the noise. For the quiet test condition, ability to repeat 50% of sentences at a level of 28 dBA is proposed as the passing criterion. In noise, the SNRs are used to determine a percentile score based on norms for normal listeners. Some governmental employers use a fifth percentile criterion (95% of young normal listeners perform better than the subject) as a barely passing score. Tests like this are attractive because they use more realistic speech than conventional speech tests (sentences rather than isolated words) and incorporate background noise, which is important in some jobs. However, they cannot claim to simulate any specific occupational hearing situation (many jobs have unique vocabularies and types of noise) and have not been shown to correlate with or to predict job performance. There is no simple way to estimate fitness to work from hearing tests.

DIFFERENTIAL DIAGNOSIS OF SENSORINEURAL HEARING LOSS

Nonoccupational Hearing Loss

In attempting to determine the extent of occupational hearing loss in a subject, the following nonoccupational hearing-loss disorders must be considered.

A. Age-Related Hearing Loss

Age-related hearing loss (ARHL) is a slow and progressive deterioration of hearing that is associated with aging and not attributable to other causes (see Figure 12–3). It is often referred to as *presbycusis* and is associated with a variety of inner ear pathologies, including atrophy of the inner and outer hair cells, stria vascularis, and spiral ganglion in the cochlea. Other features that occur histologically include atrophy or degeneration of central auditory pathways and possibly mechanical changes in the cochlear duct affecting movement of the basement membrane. Usually the hearing loss is a gradual, more or less symmetric, progressive, high-frequency sensorineural loss associated with gradually deteriorating speech discrimination. In the US population, age is by far the most important predictor of hearing loss; the odds of having significant hearing impairment increase about threefold with every decade from age 25 to 65. The severity of ARHL at any given age is highly variable, depending in part on independent risk factors such as male sex, white race, lower socioeconomic status, heavy smoking, diabetes, and noise exposure (occupational and nonoccupational). ARHL has a large genetic component; heritability is close to 50%.

B. Hereditary Hearing Impairment

In developed countries, congenital and early-onset deafness has an important genetic origin, and at least 60% of the cases are inherited. Hereditary hearing impairment (HHI) can be conductive, mixed, or sensorineural impairment, and the pattern of inheritance can be dominant, recessive, X-linked, or mitochondrial. HHI may be accompanied by a positive family history, consanguinity, and/or physical findings consistent with a hereditary syndrome known to include hearing loss. Currently, more than 100 genes are involved in the different types of inherited deafness (syndromic and nonsyndromic). HHI is usually detected in early childhood, particularly if it is associated with syndromes (eg, autosomal-recessive Usher syndrome, autosomal-dominant branchio-oto-renal syndrome, or X-linked mixed hearing loss with stapes gusher). Autosomal-recessive nonsyndromic HHI accounts for 80% of nonsyndromic early-onset hearing loss. A single-gene locus, *DFNB1*, accounts for a high proportion of the recessive cases, with variability depending on the population. The gene involved in this type of deafness is *GJB2*, which encodes the gap-junction protein connexin 26. Connexins are transmembrane proteins that form channels that allow rapid transport of ions or small molecules between cells. Autosomal-dominant nonsyndromic HHI usually presents in early or middle adulthood and often is progressive. Genetic screening is available clinically for several nonsyndromic and syndromic mutations.

C. Metabolic Disorders

Progressive hearing loss may be related to diabetes mellitus, heavy smoking, severe thyroid dysfunction, renal failure, autoimmune disease, and perhaps hyperlipidemia. In diabetes mellitus, the pathology is varied, involving primary neuropathy and/or small-vessels disease. Other metabolic disorders may involve pathology in the stria vascularis, which is important in maintaining the ion balance and the electrical potentials within the cochlea.

D. Idiopathic Sudden Sensorineural Hearing Loss

This is differentiated by its sudden onset, usually developing within 24 hours, in the absence of precipitating factors. The hearing loss is almost always unilateral. The hearing-loss pattern in idiopathic sudden sensorineural hearing loss (ISSNHL) is variable. The degree of hearing loss is unpredictable, ranging from mild to profound; partial or total spontaneous recovery is typical. Vertigo is present in some cases of ISSNHL and suggests a worse prognosis.

The etiology of ISSNHL is unknown; viral cause, vascular insult, and inner ear membrane rupture (Reissner membrane, tectorial membrane) have been postulated. This disorder warrants a thorough evaluation in order to rule out any other known pathology.

The treatment of ISSNHL is debatable. The most common therapies are observation versus steroids (oral or intratympanic). Vasodilators, anticoagulants, and diuretics also have been used in the treatment of some ISSNHL.

E. Infectious Origin

This includes bacterial or viral infections, including meningitis and encephalitis, that may cause hearing loss. Spirochete infections such as congenital or acquired syphilis and Lyme disease can result in hearing loss and vestibular dysfunction. The congenital syphilis sufferer may develop symptoms in infancy or later in life that also may be associated with vestibular symptoms similar to Ménière syndrome; the hearing loss can be unilateral but usually is bilateral. Late syphilis may present a slowly progressive SNHL and also may exhibit associated vestibular problems.

Mumps may cause a rather severe, most typically unilateral SNHL. Other childhood viral exanthems also can cause SNHL. Congenital hearing loss also can be caused by rubella virus and cytomegalovirus.

F. Central Nervous System Disease

Cerebellopontine angle tumors, especially vestibular schwannoma (acoustic neuroma), may present with progressive SNHL that is unilateral. This is in contrast to noise-induced hearing loss and ARHL, which are usually symmetric. Patients with unilateral or asymmetric SNHL require further investigation to rule out these tumors. This investigation may require detailed audiometric studies and CT scan or MRI. Demyelinating diseases (eg, multiple sclerosis) may present a sudden unilateral hearing loss that typically recovers to some degree.

G. Ménière Disease (Endolymphatic Hydrops)

Ménière disease and its variants generally present a fluctuating low-frequency or flat unilateral SNHL, fullness or pressure in the affected ear, tinnitus, and episodic disabling vertigo. In the early stages, the hearing loss usually affects the low frequencies, but over time it may progress to a flat severe hearing loss. Although the etiology is unknown, histopathology reveals a hydropic dilatation of the endolymphatic chambers of the cochlea and membranous labyrinth.

H. Nonorganic Hearing Loss

Functional hearing loss for purposes of secondary gain is quite frequent. This may be seen in people with normal hearing and in those who embellish an existing organic hearing loss. With skillful audiometric techniques, it is usually possible to distinguish organic from nonorganic hearing loss, but this may require referral to an audiologic center with considerable experience with this problem.

There are various indications of nonorganic hearing loss. Poor correlation between the SRTs and the average of the air conduction thresholds at 500, 1000, and 2000 Hz is the most common indication of functionality (see Figure 12–5). The SRTs are generally within 6 dB of the average of the "speech frequencies." Excessive test-retest variability is also suggestive. In cases of suspected unilateral functional hearing loss, the Stenger test is useful. Evoked-response audiometry, otoacoustic emissions tests, or both also may be useful for objectively establishing hearing thresholds in patients unable or unwilling to cooperate with conventional testing.

NOISE-INDUCED HEARING LOSS

▶ Etiology & Pathogenesis

Noise-induced hearing loss (NIHL) is a complex disorder probably caused by an interaction between genetic and environmental factors. NIHL results mechanically from trauma to the sensory epithelium of the cochlea and metabolically from the generation of reactive oxygen species. The sensory epithelium of the cochlea consists of one row of stereociliated inner hair cells and three rows of stereociliated outer hair cells supported by supporting cells (Hansen and Deiter cells). The most obvious injury is to the stereocilia of the inner and outer hair cells (the electromechanical transducers of sound energy), which may become distorted or even disrupted under acoustically generated shearing forces of the tectorial membrane. All structures of the organ of Corti, however, can be affected. Vascular, chemical, and metabolic changes occurring in the sensory cells cause loss of stereocilia stiffness possibly as the result of contraction of the rootlet structures that anchor the stereocilia to the cuticular plate at the top of the hair cell.

Initially the vascular, chemical, and metabolic changes are potentially reversible, and given time, the hearing will recover. This is known as a *temporary threshold shift* (TTS). TTS can last for several hours. However, when there is permanent loss of stereocilia with apparent fracture of the rootlet structures and destruction of the sensory cells, which are replaced by nonfunctioning scar tissue, an audiogram will show *permanent threshold shift* (PTS). The outer hair cells, which are important in tuning, generally are affected before the inner hair cells. A retrograde degeneration of cochlear nerve fibers occurs progressing centrally. Noise can involve other structures in the cochlea, including vascular change in the area of the metabolically active stria vascularis. Because TTS may mimic PTS, individuals should be given audiometric tests after a recovery period of 12–24 hours following exposure to hazardous levels of noise. PTS may be caused by a brief exposure to extremely high-intensity sounds, but it is caused more commonly by prolonged repetitive exposure to lower levels of hazardous noise.

Susceptibility to NIHL is rather variable. While some individuals are able to tolerate high noise exposures for

Table 12–1. Relative intensity of common noises.

	Noise Level (dBA)
Recreational noise	
Normal conversation	50–60
Lawnmower	100
Motorcycle	110
Snowmobile	110
Firecrackers	150
Hunting weapons	160
Industry noise (average of many jobs)	
Printing and publishing	90
Truck transportation	90
Canning food products	100
Farm equipment	100
Textile mill	100
Lumber and wood products	100
Petroleum refining	110
Metal products	100
Mining, underground	110
Heavy equipment	110
Metal-tool operations	110
Military flight line	120

prolonged periods of time with minimal hearing loss, others who are subjected to the same environment can develop considerable hearing loss. Risk of permanent hearing impairment is related to the duration and intensity of exposure (Table 12–1) and probably to genetic susceptibility.

Generally, prolonged exposure to sounds louder than 85 dBA (ie, an 85-dB noise level determined by using the A scale) is potentially injurious. Although there has been no recent nationwide noise exposure survey, it is still true that millions of workers in the United States are exposed to hazardous noise that could result in hearing loss. Continuous exposure to hazardous levels of noise tends to have its maximum effect in the high-frequency regions of the cochlea. NIHL is usually most severe around 4000 Hz, with downward extension toward the "speech frequencies" (500–3000 Hz) occurring only after prolonged or severe exposure. Interestingly, this tendency of NIHL to preferentially affect the high-frequency regions of the cochlea remains true regardless of the frequency of the injurious noise and may be related to the resonance of the ear canal.

The inner ear is partially protected from the effects of continuous noise by the acoustic reflex. This reflex, which is triggered when the ear is subjected to noise louder than 90 dB, causes the middle ear muscles (the stapedius and tensor tympani) to contract, thereby stiffening the conductive system and reducing the amount of sound that enters the inner ear (this occurs only from frequencies below about 2 kHz). Because this protective reflex is neurally mediated, it is delayed in onset for a period ranging from 25 to 150 ms, depending on the intensity of the sound. Therefore, the biologic effect of impulse noise is not as dampened as the effect of continuous noise.

▶ Acoustic Trauma

While most NIHL is a result of long-term exposure, acoustic trauma, defined as a PTS from a single exposure, may result from a brief exposure to extremely loud noise. In some cases, this may follow intense impulse noises; in other cases, it may follow a single explosion. Blast injuries from explosions can result in pressures that injure middle ear structures such as the tympanic membrane. Blast injuries not only generate impulse noise but also may injure the ear through generation of overpressures and even hot combustion products that can disrupt the tympanic membrane. Although it is less common, an acute decrease in hearing also may occur following single periods of exposure to continuous noise. For example, several hours of unprotected exposure to a jet turbine producing sounds in the 120–140 dB range may result in permanent cochlear damage.

▶ Clinical Findings in NIHL and ARHL

Patients with NIHL and/or ARHL frequently complain of gradual deterioration in hearing. The most common complaint is difficulty in comprehending speech, especially in the presence of competing background noise. Because these patients have a high-frequency bias to their hearing loss, they hear vowel sounds better than consonant sounds. This leads to a distortion of speech sounds when they are listening to people with higher-pitched voices (eg, women and children). Background noise, which is usually low frequency in bias, masks the better-preserved portion of the hearing spectrum and further exacerbates the problems with speech comprehension.

All types of hearing loss are frequently accompanied by tinnitus. Most often patients describe a high-frequency tonal sound (ringing), but the sound is sometimes lower in tone (buzzing, blowing, or hissing) or even nontonal (popping or clicking). This sensation may be intermittent or continuous and may be exacerbated by further exposure to noise. Tinnitus is usually most bothersome to patients when there is little ambient noise present. Therefore, some patients may complain of inability to fall asleep or to concentrate when in a very quiet room.

On tuning fork examination, the patient hears air conduction better than bone conduction, which indicates a SNHL. Audiometric examination usually reveals a bilateral, predominantly high-frequency SNHL in both NIHL and ARHL; in NIHL there is usually a maximum drop of the pure-tone thresholds occurring at or around 4000 Hz on the pure-tone audiogram (see Figures 12–1 and 12–2).

The 4000-Hz notch, which frequently develops relatively early in the worker's exposure to hazardous noise, generally will widen as further exposure continues; thus, lower and higher frequencies become affected somewhat later if the exposure continues. Because the most important thresholds for comprehension of human speech are between 500 and 3000 Hz, significant conversational difficulties do not begin until frequencies of 3000 Hz and below are affected. The speech discrimination score is normal in the early stages of NIHL but may deteriorate as the loss becomes more severe. Because of great variability, the diagnosis of NIHL cannot always be eliminated or established by the shape of the audiogram.

Although the hearing loss in NIHL is bilateral, asymmetry can exist, particularly when the source of the noise is lateralized (eg, rifle or shotgun firing). Tinnitus (ringing or buzzing) may or may not be present. Tinnitus is a subjective complaint, and measurements of tinnitus are based on the patient's ability to match the ringing in loudness and frequency. Often the tinnitus pitch is close to the frequency of the maximum hearing loss seen on the audiogram and is about 5 dB above that threshold in loudness. Tinnitus frequently is blocked out by ambient noise. Tinnitus in the absence of hearing loss is probably not related to noise exposure.

Individuals who have acoustic trauma can present with a variety of audiometric patterns. These patients frequently experience tinnitus, and a few will have symptoms of hyperacusis and, occasionally, vertigo.

▶ Prevention

The Occupational Safety and Health Administration (OSHA) regulates exposure to noise at or above an 8-hour time-weighted average (TWA) of 85 dBA, the approximate biologic threshold above which permanent shifts in hearing are possible. Above 85-dBA TWA, OSHA requires enrolment in a HCP.

A HCP is the recognized method of preventing NIHL in the occupational environment. While there is a tendency to think of "hearing conservation" as the provision of audiometric tests and hearing protection, much more is required. An effective HCP integrates the following program elements:

1. Noise monitoring
2. Engineering controls
3. Administrative controls
4. Worker education
5. Selection and use of hearing-protection devices (HPDs)
6. Periodic audiometric evaluations

Record keeping is also important, and OSHA requires that NIHL be recorded on the OSHA 300 Log of Injuries and Illnesses. If an employee's audiogram reveals a work-related standard threshold shift (10-dB shifts in hearing acuity) in one or both ears, and the employee's total hearing level is 25 dB or more above audiometric zero (averaged at 2000, 3000, and 4000 Hz) in the same ear(s) as the STS, then the employer must record the case in Section M(5) of the OSHA 300 Log. For the purposes of injury and illness recording, this sometimes may be referred to as a *recordable threshold shift.* It should be noted that prior to recording a hearing loss, employers may seek the advice of a physician or other licensed health care professional to determine if the loss is work related, make adjustments for presbycusis, and perform additional hearing tests to verify the persistence of the hearing loss. HCP elements are outlined briefly below.

A. Noise Monitoring

If there is reason to believe that worker noise exposure will equal or exceed a TWA of 85 dBA, then noise monitoring is required. A sampling strategy must be designed to identify all workers who need to be included in the HCP. If there is a change in production, process, equipment, or controls that would affect workers' exposures, noise monitoring tests should be repeated.

B. Engineering Controls

The information collected during noise monitoring (particularly octave-band analysis, which indicates the sound level at selected frequencies) may be used to design engineering noise controls. Designers conceptualize possible engineering solutions in terms of the source (what is generating the noise), the path (the route[s] the generated noise may travel), and the receivers (the workers exposed to the noise). The noise controls may involve the use of enclosures (to isolate sources or receivers), barriers (to reduce acoustic energy along the path), or distance (to increase the path and ultimately reduce the acoustic energy at the receiver) to reduce worker noise exposure. In general, engineering controls are preferred but are not always feasible because of their costs and limits in technology.

C. Administrative Controls

Administrative controls include (1) reducing the amount of time a given worker might be exposed to a noise source in order to prevent the TWA noise exposure from reaching 85 dBA and (2) establishing purchasing guidelines to prevent introduction of equipment that would increase worker noise dose. While simple in principle, the implementation of administrative controls requires management's commitment and constant supervision, particularly in the absence of engineering or personal-protection controls. In general, administrative controls are used as an adjunct to existing HCP noise-control strategies rather than as the exclusive approach for controlling noise exposure.

D. Worker Education

Workers and management must understand the potentially harmful effects of noise in order to satisfy OSHA and, most important, to ensure that the HCP is successful in preventing NIHL. A good worker education program describes (1) program objectives, (2) existing noise hazards, (3) how hearing loss occurs, (4) purpose of audiometric testing, and (5) what workers can do to protect themselves. In addition, roles and responsibilities of the employer and the workers should be stated clearly. Training is required to be provided annually to all workers included in the HCP. Opportunities for maintaining awareness occur during periodic safety meetings, as well as during audiometric testing appointments when testing results are explained.

E. Hearing Protection Devices

Hearing protection devices (HPDs) are available in a variety of types from a number of manufacturers. There are three basic types of HPDs: (1) ear plugs, or *aurals* (premolded, formable, and custom-molded), (2) canal caps, or *semiaurals* (with a band that compresses each end against the entrance of the ear canal), and (3) ear muffs, or *circumaurals* (which surround the ear). Each of these types of devices has advantages and disadvantages that vary according to worker activity, equipment and facility noise characteristics, and the work environment (Figure 12–6). Selection of appropriate HPDs

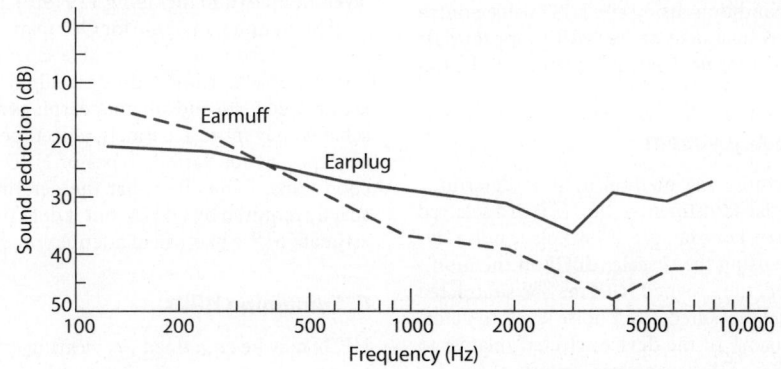

▲ **Figure 12–6.** Comparison of the attenuation properties of a molded-type earplug and an earmuff protector. Note that the earplug offers greater attenuation of the lower frequencies, whereas the earmuff is better at the higher frequencies.

should ideally include input from the industrial hygienist, the audiologist, the occupational medicine physician, and of course, the workers who will use these devices. Although the HCP is triggered by the presence of noise levels equal to or greater than an 8-hour TWA of 85 dBA, HPDs must attenuate worker exposure to an 8-hour TWA at or below 90 dBA, the OSHA 8-hour permissible exposure level (PEL) for noise.

It is important to note that—where hazardous noise levels are present—HPDs must attenuate exposure to an 8-hour TWA of 85 dBA or below for employees who have experienced a standard threshold shift. This requirement also applies to employees who have not yet had baseline audiograms. In general, the use of HPDs by employees exposed to TWA noise levels of 85 dBA or greater is recommended.

F. Audiometric Evaluations

Audiometric testing provides the only quantitative means of assessing the overall effectiveness of a hearing-conservation program. A properly managed audiometric testing program supervised by a certified audiologist or physician who is trained and experienced in occupational hearing conservation will detect changes in response to environmental noise that otherwise might be overlooked. Results of audiometric testing must be shared with employees to ensure effectiveness. The overall results or trends noted in an audiometric testing program can be used to fine-tune the HCP, that is, to determine which types of HPDs to offer to employees or to identify where additional employee training is needed.

▶ Noise Reduction Ratings & Selection of Hearing-Protection Devices

All HPDs sold in the United States are assigned a standardized value known as the *noise reduction rating* (NRR). Manufacturers of HPDs are required by the Environmental Protection Agency to have their products tested in order to obtain an NRR prior to placing them on the market. NRRs (listed in decibels) are based on laboratory attenuation data achieved under ideal conditions. Actual noise reduction achieved under field conditions using any HPD will be much lower than the NRR. Adjustment of the NRR is appropriate before a device is chosen for field use, as explained in the following discussion.

A. Weighting-Scale Adjustment

Depending on the monitoring method used to determine noise exposure, an initial adjustment to the NRR of a selected device may be necessary. For example, if workplace noise levels are determined by using the C scale (dBC) on the monitoring instrumentation, the assigned NRR may be subtracted directly from the actual measured TWA noise levels to determine the legal "adequacy" of the device selected relative to the regulatory 90-dBA TWA exposure criterion (or for employees who either [1] have standard threshold shifts or [2] have not yet had baseline audiograms, the 85-dBA TWA exposure criterion).

If workplace noise levels are determined by using the A scale (dBA) on the monitoring instrumentation, the assigned NRR should be reduced by 7 dB before being subtracted from the actual measured TWA noise levels to determine the legal "adequacy" of the device selected relative to the 90-dBA TWA exposure criterion (or for employees who either [1] have standard threshold shifts or [2] have not yet had baseline audiograms, the 85-dBA TWA exposure criterion).

The A-scale adjustment is necessary because this scale approximates the response of the human ear to speech frequencies and discounts much of the acoustic energy from the low and high frequencies that are present in the work environment. Because the C scale is essentially flat (unweighted) across the audible frequency spectrum, all the acoustic energy present is integrated into the measurement, and no adjustment is necessary.

B. Derating

The effectiveness of HPDs depends on whether they are used properly. NRRs are obtained in the laboratory under ideal conditions and reflect the attenuation that would be achieved or exceeded by 98% of subjects in this "best-case" situation. To predict the NRR of HPDs during actual use more accurately (and conservatively), the product's NRR should be derated. In auditing HCPs, OSHA derates the assigned NRR (after weighting-scale adjustment, if necessary) by one-half (50%) for *all* types of HPDs to determine the "relative performance." As a typical example, if a device has an NRR of 29 and workplace noise measurements were made using the A scale, then OSHA's predicted field attenuation of the device would be (29 − 7)/2 = 11 dB. Such a device would be expected to provide protection (per the legal OSHA 90-dBA PEL) where 8-hour TWA noise levels of up to 101 (90 + 11) dBA are present. As a worse-case example, failure to make an adjustment for A-scale noise measurements, along with a failure to apply a 50% derating, could lead an uninformed evaluator to falsely believe that this same HPD would provide protection in environments with 8-hour TWA noise levels of up to and including 119 (90 + 29) dBA.

The National Institute for Occupational Safety and Health (NIOSH) recommends a variable scheme for derating NRRs. For example, earmuffs are derated 25%, formable earplugs are derated 50%, and all other earplugs are derated 70%. This scheme may more accurately reflect the attenuation that can be expected for various types of HPDs under "real world" conditions. Remember that the derating of an HPD is not strictly required by OSHA, but it does provide a conservative estimate of the likely field attenuation that will be provided.

C. Combining HPDs

HPDs may be combined (ie, wearing earplugs and earmuffs) to provide more protection in high-noise environments. However, the NRRs of the combined devices are not added together to determine the total noise reduction. Under such circumstances, OSHA advises its inspectors that 5 dB is to be added after the weighting-scale adjustment is applied to the device with the *higher* NRR (again, OSHA does not require the 50% derating described earlier). This is a conservative approach to determining combined attenuation, and actual field attenuation (and protection) probably is higher. As a practical matter, double protection may be inadequate when TWA noise exposures exceed 105 dBA.

D. HPD Provision Versus HPD Enforcement

When 8-hour TWA noise levels are equal to or greater than 85 dBA (a 50% noise dose) but less than 90 dBA (a 100% noise dose), HPDs *must* be made available to the exposed workers. For 8-hour TWA noise dose levels at or above 90 dBA, however, HPDs must be provided to workers, *and* their proper use must be enforced by the employer (exceptions: [1] employees with standard threshold shifts must be provided with HPDs when the 8-hour TWA noise levels are equal to or greater than 85 dBA, and [2] employees who have not yet had baseline audiometric tests must be provided with HPDs). A suitable variety of HPDs must be provided. The weighting-scale adjustment of the NRR must be applied, and it is advisable to apply a derating scheme that will adjust the NRR to ensure adequate protection of the worker.

▶ Treatment

There is no medical or surgical treatment available to reverse the effects of NIHL. After the diagnosis has been established by otologic examination and performance of an audiometric test battery, the physician should counsel the patient on the likely consequences of continued exposure to excessive noise and should recommend techniques for avoidance of further noise-induced damage. Hearing amplification is reserved for patients with socially impaired hearing.

Hearing aids must be fitted carefully to optimally meet the needs of the individual with regard to frequency bias and gain. In bilateral hearing losses, bilateral amplification usually provides more satisfactory rehabilitation. Whether or not to try hearing amplification is the patient's decision. A reasonable criterion for referral to a professional for hearing aid evaluation is an SRT greater than 25 dB or a speech discrimination score of less than 80% when words are presented at a normal conversation level of 50 dB HL. In patients with high-frequency hearing loss and relatively normal low-frequency hearing, hearing aids generally are most helpful in those who have a significant hearing loss at 2000 Hz on the pure-tone audiogram. A borderline candidate may be an individual with normal hearing through 1500 Hz, a mild loss at 2000 Hz, and a moderate or greater loss at 3000 Hz and above.

Earlier hearing aids used analog circuitry, which had limited ability to match a patient's audiometric configuration and to compensate for recruitment. Almost all current hearing aids use digital circuitry, which modifies incoming sound to enhance speech and reduce ambient background noise. This noise suppression allows greater gain before producing audible feedback (suppression). Digital hearing aids also

allow for multiple and directional microphones. Programmable hearing aids can retain various programs to allow the user to adjust to various noise environments.

Hearing aids are also differentiated by style. The largest and most powerful and adjustable is the behind-the-ear (BTE) aid. There is also an in-the-ear (ITE) aid, an in-the-canal (ITC) aid, and a completely in-the-canal (CIC) aid. The CIC is the smallest but is harder to adjust and is the least powerful.

Before purchasing a hearing aid, the patient should have a hearing aid evaluation and a trial period with the patient wearing the hearing aids in various circumstances. A patient's willingness to wear a hearing aid will depend on many factors, including cosmetic considerations and concerns about the ability to insert the hearing aid and to manipulate its controls. Numerous other clever instruments, known as *assistive listening devices*, are available to enhance comprehension in small or large groups (eg, at business meetings or conventions), with telephone use, and with various audio or visual media, such as television. Most of these devices work by wireless transmission of FM signals or infrared light beams. Aural rehabilitation classes designed to enhance the patient's ability to comprehend speech also may be helpful and usually are available in urban areas.

There is no cure for tinnitus resulting from NIHL or any other cause, although numerous amelioration measures are available. In the absence of further inner ear injury, tinnitus may diminish gradually, usually over a course of weeks to months. A subtle degree of tinnitus often persists and is especially obvious when the patient is in a quiet room. For the few patients who find this to be extremely troublesome, sound therapy, in which music or other sounds are presented, is often helpful. In patients with significant hearing loss, the most successful treatment may be appropriate hearing amplification. Modified hearing aids (tinnitus maskers) designed to produce masking noises generally have been of limited success. Use of biofeedback or counseling (eg, cognitive-behavioral therapy) has helped some patients suppress their tinnitus. Sound therapy and counseling are often combined in programs such as "tinnitus retraining therapy." Psychiatric referral to manage associated depression sometimes is necessary.

▶ Prognosis

Hearing in patients with NIHL will stabilize if the patient is removed from the noxious stimulus. If it does not stabilize, hearing will continue to deteriorate, ultimately resulting in severe high-frequency hearing impairment. Although adequate hearing protection is essential and always should be recommended, other factors also may play a role in the patient's prognosis. ARHL will add to the noise-induced loss as the patient grows older.

▶ Future Therapies

In the mammalian auditory system, hair cell loss resulting from aging, ototoxic drugs, infections, noise, and other causes is irreversible and leads to permanent SNHL. To restore hearing, it is necessary to generate new functional hair cells. The advent of new approaches such as gene therapy, neural stem cell and embryonic stem cell transplantation, and genomics may lead to methods for inducing hair cell regeneration and repair in the mammalian cochlear and vestibular systems.

HEARING LOSS CAUSED BY PHYSICAL TRAUMA

▶ Etiology & Pathogenesis

A broad spectrum of injuries may cause trauma to the ears. Blunt head injury is by far the most common cause of traumatic hearing loss. A blow to the head creates a pressure wave in the skull that is transmitted through bone in a manner similar to the way a pressure wave in air is carried by the conducting mechanism of the ear. The cochlear injury observed following blunt head trauma closely resembles both histologically and audiologically that which is induced by high-intensity acoustic trauma. Motor vehicle accidents are the major cause of blunt head trauma and account for about 50% of temporal bone injuries. Penetrating injuries of the temporal bone are relatively rare, accounting for fewer than 10% of cases. Other occupational causes of ear injury include falls, explosions, and burns from caustic chemicals, open flames, or welder's slag that enters the ear canal.

▶ Examination & Treatment

In the conscious patient, hearing should be assessed immediately with a 512-Hz tuning fork. Even in an ear severely traumatized and filled with blood, sound will lateralize toward a conductive hearing loss and away from a sensorineural one. Complete audiometric examinations (see the section "Evaluation of Hearing") can be performed after the patient has been stabilized. Patients also should be checked for signs of vestibular injury (nystagmus) and facial nerve trauma (paralysis).

A. Injuries Causing Conductive Hearing Loss

1. Blunt head trauma with or without temporal bone fracture may cause hematotympanum—a collection of blood in the middle ear. If this is the sole injury, hearing usually recovers over several weeks. Blunt head trauma on rare occasion may result in separation of the bones of the middle ear (ossicular chain disruption).

2. Burns sustained when a piece of welder's slag penetrates the eardrum often heal poorly, and chronic infection often results.

3. Barotrauma can result in a conductive hearing loss with fluid or blood behind the tympanic membrane. This is generally transitory and resolves in a few days to a few weeks.

4. Traumatic membrane perforations usually heal spontaneously if secondary infection does not develop (patients should be instructed not to get the ear wet during the healing period), although hearing loss may persist.

Conductive hearing loss that persists more than 3 months after injury is usually the result of a tympanic membrane perforation or disruption of the ossicular chain (see Figure 12–4). These lesions are suitable for surgical repair, usually on a delayed basis. Repair is by grafting the tympanic membrane or by reconstructing the ossicular chain with homograft or prosthetic materials or both.

B. Injuries Causing Sensorineural Hearing Loss

Trauma to the inner ear results most commonly from blunt head injury. Labyrinthine concussion frequently occurs with transient vertigo, potentially permanent hearing loss, and tinnitus. Treatment is expectant, with vestibular suppressants such as meclizine offering symptomatic relief of vertigo.

Trauma also may cause rupture of the round or oval window membranes, which can lead to leakage of inner ear fluids into the middle ear (perilymph fistula). Most perilymphatic fistulas heal spontaneously. Persistent perilymphatic leakage is difficult to diagnose and requires surgical treatment, with autogenous material used to repair the defect. Most patients with surgically confirmed fistulas suffer recurrent episodes of vertigo and hearing loss, often temporally related to vigorous physical exercise.

C. Injuries Causing Mixed Conductive and Sensorineural Hearing Loss

Temporal bone injuries sometimes involve both the middle and inner ear, resulting in mixed, conductive, and SNHL. Fractures of the temporal bone tend to occur along lines that connect points of weakness in the skull base. Clinically, these fractures may be divided into two patterns: longitudinal and transverse. Longitudinal fractures are much more common (80% of cases) and usually result from a blow to the lateral aspect of the head. They frequently involve the structures of the middle ear but characteristically spare the inner ear, resulting in a conductive or mixed hearing loss. Transverse fractures are less common (20% of cases) and usually result from a severe occipital blow. Serious intracranial injury frequently accompanies transverse fractures. Typically, they traverse the inner ear and cause total SNHL and labyrinthine death. Fractures through the inner ear often are accompanied by severe vertigo that lasts for weeks or even months.

Temporal bone fractures are recognized clinically by the presence of blood, cerebrospinal fluid, or both in the ear canal or by the presence of blood in the middle ear behind an intact tympanic membrane. The ear canal should be cleaned carefully, using sterile suction to assess the integrity of the tympanic membrane. Under no circumstances should a recently traumatized ear be irrigated. Battle sign (ecchymosis over the mastoid region) is seen occasionally. Definitive diagnosis requires high-resolution CT scanning to demonstrate the fracture lines.

OTOTOXIC HEARING LOSS

▶ Etiology & Pathogenesis

Ototoxic hearing loss is the result of exposure to chemical substances that injure the cochlea. Most ototoxins injure hair cells either directly or through disruption of cochlear homeostatic mechanisms. In the vast majority of cases, ototoxic hearing loss stems from the use of medications such as aminoglycoside antibiotics (eg, neomycin), platinum-containing antineoplastic agents (eg, cisplatin), loop diuretics (eg, furosemide), and salicylates (eg, aspirin). The latter two classes of drugs cause only temporary hearing loss that resolves when the drug is stopped.

In industries with noisy work environments, workers who are being treated with potentially ototoxic medications may be at increased risk for hearing loss because the combination of some ototoxic drug treatments and noise trauma can lead to a greater degree of hearing loss than either would produce by itself. Aspirin, however, is probably not associated with an increased likelihood of NIHL.

Hearing loss also may result from exposure to ototoxic substances in the workplace. Heavy metals, including arsenic, cobalt, lead, lithium, mercury, and thorium, have been reported to have ototoxic potential. Other chemicals that may be ototoxic include cyanide, benzene, aniline dyes, iodine, chlorophenothane, dimethyl sulfoxide, dinitrophenol, propylene glycol, methylmercury, potassium bromate, carbon disulfide, carbon monoxide, carbon tetrachloride, and industrial solvents such as styrene and toluene.

▶ Prevention

Medicinal ototoxins should be administered in the lowest dose compatible with therapeutic efficacy. Serum peak and trough levels of aminoglycosides should be monitored to reduce the risk of excessive dosages. Simultaneous administration of multiple ototoxic drugs should be avoided when possible to minimize synergistic effects. Persons with preexisting sensory hearing loss and compromised renal or hepatic function are at substantially increased risk. Identification of those at heightened risk of ototoxic hearing loss is important to avoid this complication. Audiometric evaluation is appropriate to identify and monitor ototoxic exposure.

MEDICOLEGAL ISSUES

▶ Calculation of Binaural Hearing Impairment

Only one method for calculating the severity of hearing loss is in widespread use. The current method developed by the American Academy of Otolaryngology and Head and Neck Surgery (AAO-HNS) is as follows: (1) The average hearing threshold level at 500, 1000, 2000, and 3000 Hz is calculated for each ear. (2) The percentage of the impairment for each ear (the monaural loss) is calculated by multiplying the amount by which the preceding average exceeds 25 dBA (low fence) by 1.5, up to a maximum of 100%, which is reached at 92 dBA (high fence). (3) The hearing handicap (binaural assessment) then should be calculated by multiplying the smaller percentage (better ear) by 5, adding this figure to the larger percentage (poorer ear), and dividing the total by 6.

The American Medical Association (AMA) Guide to the Evaluation of Permanent Impairment (6th edition) describes identical calculations for rating a "binaural hearing impairment" (BHI) percentage as the AAO-HNS. In addition, the AMA Guides allow adding up to 5% for tinnitus if the tinnitus impacts the ability to perform activities of daily living. The AMA method of estimating BHI has been validated against patient's self-report of hearing disability and is used in most state and federal workers compensation programs.

For the preceding calculations to be valid, the audiometer employed must be checked daily and calibrated periodically by an independent agency. The booth used for testing must meet the standards of background noise levels established by the American National Standards Institute (ANSI) in 1977.

A note of caution is needed regarding the calculation of percentage of hearing loss based on older audiograms. Different standards for the measurement of hearing were in use prior to establishment of the current standard by the ANSI in 1969. From 1964 to 1969, the standard of the International Standards Organization (ISO) was widely used; this is essentially the same as the current ANSI standard, and no conversion is needed. However, from 1951 to 1964, and in some cases up through 1969, the standard of the American Standards Association (ASA) was used, and audiograms obtained in this period require conversion for use in the preceding formula. To convert an audiogram from the ASA to the ANSI standard, add 14 dB at 500 Hz, 10 dB at 1000 Hz, 8.5 dB at 2000 Hz, 8.5 dB at 3000 Hz, 6 dB at 4000 Hz, and 9.5 dB at 6000 Hz. In cases where the 3000-Hz threshold was not measured, the average of 2000 and 4000 Hz may be substituted.

▶ Assessment of Impairment

As indicated previously, the normal range of SRT is between 0 and 20 dB, with losses of 25–40 dB termed *mild,* 40–55 dB termed *moderate,* 55–70 dB termed *moderately severe,* 70–90 dB termed *severe,* and greater than 90 dB termed *profound.* Of course, the extent of disability suffered by the patient depends on many psychological, social, and work-related factors. Assessment of an individual's fitness to work requires knowledge about the various duties performed by that individual. Some typical work-related issues for consideration include the amount of communication with coworkers and others that is required on the job, the type of communication (eg, in person or via the telephone), and the need to hear alerting signals or emergency warning alarms.

To meet the Social Security Administration's guidelines for total disability as a result of hearing impairment, an individual must have either (1) an average hearing threshold of 90 dB or greater for the better hearing ear, based on both air and bone conduction at 500, 1000, and 2000 Hz or (2) a speech discrimination score of 40% or less in the better-hearing ear. In both cases, hearing must not be restorable by hearing amplification devices.

▶ Compensation for Occupational Hearing Loss

There is no national surveillance or injury reporting system for hearing loss. As such, comprehensive data on the economic impact of hearing loss are not available. The U.S. Department of Labor (DOL) reports that the average settlement a government worker receives for hearing loss is about $6000. This is considerably larger than the average settlement received by workers under state workers' compensation programs. The DOL treats aggravated or accelerated hearing losses in the same manner as losses entirely precipitated or proximally caused by the patient's employment. In other words, the amount of preemployment hearing loss is not subtracted when the percentage of loss is calculated. In contrast, local and state government regulations frequently take into account the level of preexisting hearing loss and some use formulas to correct for the anticipated progression of ARHL when calculating compensation awards.

The relationship between NIHL and ARHL is complex. Many studies have tried to address the issue of the aging worker who has been exposed to hazardous noise for a long period of time. The most widely held opinion is that ARHL and NIHL are essentially additive.

REFERENCES

Kerr MJ, Neitzel RL, Hong O, Sataloff RT: Historical review of efforts to reduce noise-induced hearing loss in the United States. Am J Ind Med 2017;60(6):569-577 [PMID: 28514024].

Le TN, Straatman LV, Lea J, Westerberg B: Current insights in noise-induced hearing loss: a literature review of the underlying mechanism, pathophysiology, asymmetry, and management options. J Otolaryngol Head Neck Surg 2017;46(1):41 [PMID: 28535812].

Mirza R, Kirchner DB, Dobie RA, Crawford J; ACOEM Task Force on Occupational Hearing Loss: Occupational noise-induced hearing loss. J Occup Environ Med 2018;60(9):e498-e501 [PMID: 30095587].

Sayler SK, Roberts BJ, Manning MA, Sun K, Neitzel RL: Patterns and trends in OSHA occupational noise exposure measurements from 1979 to 2013. Occup Environ Med 2019;76(2):118-124 [PMID: 30482879].

Sturman CJ, Frampton CM, Ten Cate WJF: Hearing loss asymmetry due to chronic occupational noise exposure. Otol Neurotol 2018;39(8):e627-e634 [PMID: 30113556].

■ SELF-ASSESSMENT QUESTIONS

Select the one correct answer for each question.

Question 1: In a clinical audiogram
  a. sensitivity to pure tones is measured for air conduction using a bone oscillator
  b. thresholds are expressed in decibels, with the normal range (for young adults) at each frequency from 0 to 40 dB HL
  c. when either air or bone conduction is decreased, a sensorineural hearing loss exists
  d. conductive losses are indicated by an "air-bone gap," in which the air-conduction threshold exceeds the bone-conduction threshold

Question 2: Speech reception threshold (SRT)
  a. is the intensity (in decibels) at which the listener is able to repeat all of balanced two-syllable words known as *spondee words*
  b. is usually not in close agreement with an average of the pure-tone thresholds for frequencies between 500 and 2000 Hz
  c. has a normal range for young adults between 0 and 20 dB
  d. of greater than 50 dB is termed *profound hearing loss*

Question 3: The hearing in noise test (HINT)
  a. measures speech intelligibility but does not incorporate background noise
  b. uses more realistic speech than conventional speech tests (sentences rather than isolated words)
  c. is not used to test government employees
  d. simulates specific occupational hearing situations

Question 4: Age-related hearing loss (ARHL)
  a. is a rapid and progressive deterioration of hearing associated with aging
  b. should be distinguished from what is called presbycusis
  c. is seldom associated with other inner ear pathologies
  d. has a large genetic component; heritability is close to 50%

Question 5: Idiopathic sudden sensorineural hearing loss (ISSHL)

a. usually develops within 24 hours, in the absence of precipitating factors
b. is almost always bilateral
c. seldom has partial or total spontaneous recovery
d. when accompanied by vertigo, has a better prognosis

Question 6: Noise-induced hearing loss (NIHL)

a. results mechanically from trauma to the sensory epithelium of the cochlea and metabolically from the generation of reactive oxygen species
b. is not related to the duration and intensity of exposure
c. is first measured around 500–3000 Hz
d. is usually most severe around 8000 Hz

Question 7: The acoustic reflex

a. fully protects the inner ear from the effects of continuous noise
b. is triggered when the ear is subjected to noise louder than 30 dB
c. increases the amount of sound that enters the inner ear
d. is delayed in onset depending on the intensity of the sound

Question 8: The Occupational Safety and Health Administration (OSHA)

a. regulates exposure to noise at or above an 8-hour time-weighted average (TWA) of 85 dBA
b. requires enrolment in a hearing conservation program for noise above 50-dBA TWA
c. has no jurisdiction over private company employees
d. provides a national surveillance reporting system for hearing loss

Question 9: Hearing protective devices

a. must be made available to the exposed workers when 8-hour TWA noise levels are equal to or greater than 85 dBA (a 50% noise dose) but below 90 dBA (a 100% noise dose)
b. must be provided by OSHA or state agencies to all exposed workers
c. must be provided to employees with any standard threshold shifts
d. must be provided to employees who have not yet had baseline audiometric tests

Question 10: Ototoxic hearing loss

a. is the result of exposure to chemical substances that injure the cochlea
b. does not result from the use of medications
c. does not result from exposure to heavy metals
d. is readily reversible with chelating agents

Injuries Caused by Physical Hazards

James P. Seward, MD, MPP, MMM

Joshua Potocko, MD, MPH

HYPOTHERMIA (COLD INJURY)

Cold injuries are classified as systemic or localized and as freezing (eg, frostbite) or nonfreezing (eg, immersion foot). Factors influencing the risk for these injuries include the atmospheric or water temperature, humidity, wind velocity, duration of exposure, type of protective equipment or clothing, type of work being performed and associated energy expenditure, and age and health status of the worker. Wet conditions, especially immersion, substantially increase the risk of hypothermia.

Workers at risk include both indoor and outdoor workers exposed to cold, such as meat packers and others who work inside freezers, construction workers, cold-room personnel, fishermen, woodsmen, divers, mail carriers, firefighters, utility repair workers, search and rescue staff, and road maintenance workers. The risk of hypothermia increases with age and also is increased if the individual is intoxicated with drugs or alcohol; is receiving medications such as barbiturates, antipsychotics; smokes; or has adrenal insufficiency, diabetes, myxedema, neurologic disease (affecting hypothalamic or pituitary function or causing peripheral sensory impairment), peripheral vascular disease, or cardiovascular disease (CVD) (causing diminished cardiac output).

1. Systemic Hypothermia

▶ Pathogenesis

Systemic hypothermia is reduction in the body's core temperature below 35°C (95°F). When the body is exposed to cold environments, it has two types of normal physiologic reactions: (1) constriction of superficial blood vessels in the skin and subcutaneous tissue, resulting in heat conservation, and (2) increase in metabolic heat production through voluntary movement and by shivering. In cases of systemic hypothermia, cellular and physiologic functions are diminished. Oxygen consumption is decreased by approximately 7%/°C, myocardial repolarization is slowed, and ventricular fibrillation is a major hazard.

▶ Clinical Findings

The medical history should address the circumstances under which the patient was found, the probable duration of exposure, associated injuries or frostbite, preexisting medical conditions, alcohol or drug use, and recent changes in the level of consciousness. Because body heat is lost more quickly when a person is wet, immersed in water, or exhausted, these factors should be considered.

The onset of hypothermia often is insidious, without any specific characteristics. With profound hypothermia, there is often diminished memory, a decrease in or absence of shivering, and combativeness. Initial findings may include drowsiness, slurred speech, irritability, impaired coordination, general weakness and lethargy, recent diuresis, and puffy and cool skin and face.

Physical examination often reveals diminished neurologic reflexes, slow mental and muscular reactions, weak or nonpalpable pulse, arrhythmia, low blood pressure, and increased blood viscosity. Shivering and peripheral vasoconstriction are present with the core temperature at 35°C (95°F). Heart rate, respiratory rate, and blood pressure decrease with reduced temperature. With mild hypothermia (33–35°C [91.4–95°F]), there is extensive shivering, which decreases as temperature drops below 33°C (91.4°F), wherein joint and muscle stiffness becomes more predominant.

Core temperature should be taken with a thermometer or thermocouple capable of measuring temperatures as low as 28°C (82.4°F); esophageal (especially in the intubated patient) or deep rectal measurement (15 cm) is best. The temperature may range from 25 to 35°C (77–95°F). Below 35°C (95°F), consciousness becomes dulled, causing disorientation, irrational thinking, forgetfulness, and hallucinations. Below 30°C (86°F), semiconsciousness and confusion may occur. Nerve conduction is slowed, although the central nervous system (CNS) is protected from ischemic damage.

The respiratory rate falls to 7–12 breaths/min, and gastrointestinal motility slows or ceases. There may be hemoconcentration as a result of diuresis and loss of plasma volume. The latter occurs because of subcutaneous edema, which is accompanied by an elevation in corticosteroid levels. Loss of consciousness seldom occurs at temperatures above 28°C (82.4°F).

Evaluation should include a complete blood count; measurement of blood glucose, renal and liver function tests, electrolytes, amylase, and alcohol and drug levels; urinalysis; urine volume; coagulation screen; sputum and blood cultures; thyroid function tests; arterial blood gas measurements with pH corrected for temperature (add 0.0147 pH unit for each degree <37°C [98.6°F]); chest radiograph; and electrocardiograph (ECG). There may be evidence of metabolic acidosis, hypovolemia, elevation or depression of the blood glucose level, and renal failure. The ECG may show a pathognomonic J wave at the QRS-ST junction.

Prevention

The risk of hypothermia is directly related to the wind chill index (WCI), which assesses the effects of both ambient temperature and wind velocity, as well as the activity performed. Cold stress prevention needs to take into account the environmental factors (eg, temperature, moisture, wind); the metabolic heat generation of the activity; the insulating factor of protective clothing, the duration of exposure, and other factors (Figure 13–1).

The WCI can be calculated from T and V, where T is the air temperature in Celsius (°C) and V is the wind speed at 10 meters height in kilometers per hour.

$$WCI = 13.12 + 0.6215T - 11.37V^{0.16} + 0.3965T \times V^{0.16}$$

Figure 13–2 shows the WCIs and indicates the length of exposure at a given level before frostbite is likely to occur. For the WCI, ambient temperature is measured with a dry bulb thermometer; wind velocity is measured with a standard wind gauge. Work and break schedules should take these parameters into account. Under high-risk weather conditions, workers should be under constant protective observation.

Hypothermia can be prevented by wearing clothing specially designed to resist wind and rain but that also allows water vapor generated by perspiration to escape. Overheating when strenuous work is required in extreme cold can be prevented by wearing a number of thin layers of clothing that can be removed or donned as necessary. Wet garments should be replaced as soon as possible with dry ones, and constrictive garments should not be worn.

Jobs should be designed so that workers remain relatively active when exposed to cold environments and provided with dry, wind-protected, heated shelters for tasks involving stationary work positions. Outdoor workers should have heated rest facilities and hot food and hot drinks available. Workers should be trained to "keep warm, keep moving, and keep dry."

Workers exposed to the cold should be physically fit, without underlying vascular, metabolic, or neurologic diseases that place them at increased risk for hypothermia. They should be cautioned to avoid smoking and drug or alcohol use. New workers should be introduced into the work schedule slowly and instructed in the use of protective clothing, recognition of impending frostbite and early signs and symptoms of hypothermia, proper warming procedures, and first-aid treatment.

Treatment & Prognosis

In cases of mild hypothermia (rectal temperatures >33°C [91.4°F]) in patients who are young and otherwise healthy should be treated by rewarming in a warm bed or bath or with warm packs and blankets and with oral rehydration with warmed fluids (caffeine-free and nonalcoholic). Mildly hypothermic elderly or debilitated patients should be treated conservatively, using an electric blanket heated to 37°C (98.6°F). Treatment should increase in aggressiveness with decreasing core temperature, which in severe cases may call for both selected internal and external techniques (Figure 13–3).

Cardiac rhythm and rate should be monitored. Because the risk of death from ventricular fibrillation is high with severe hypothermia (<32°C [89.6°F]), treatment methods that may trigger fibrillation (eg, central catheters, cannulas, or tubes) should be avoided unless their use is essential. However, patients who are comatose or have respiratory failure should be intubated. If cardiopulmonary resuscitation (CPR) is instituted, it should be continued until the patient has been rewarmed to at least 36°C (96.8°F). Evaluation for and treatment of localized areas of trauma and frostbite should be undertaken.

Measures should be instituted to correct acid-base deficiencies, normalize the serum potassium and blood glucose levels, increase the blood volume, maintain cardiac output and blood pressure, and provide adequate ventilation. Adequate cardiovascular support, acid-base balance, arterial oxygenation, and intravascular volume should be established as quickly as possible to minimize the risk of organ infarction during rewarming. Oxygen administration should begin prior to rewarming. Because most arrhythmias revert spontaneously to normal sinus rhythm as the patient rewarms, it is usually unnecessary to give antiarrhythmic agents unless there is a preexisting cardiac condition. Ventricular arrhythmias, however, should be treated as they are treated in a euthermic patient. Blood volume expansion with 5% dextrose–normal saline solution is recommended. Potassium-containing expanders should be avoided until the serum potassium levels are stable. If myxedema is an underlying factor or if drug intoxication is present, appropriate treatment should be given. Localized areas of frostbite should be evaluated and managed as outlined in the section "Hypothermia of the Extremities."

Use of steroids or antibiotics is not recommended unless otherwise clinically indicated. Core temperature should be monitored frequently during and after initial rewarming because of the potential for delayed, repeat hypothermia.

Active internal rewarming for severe hypothermia is more effective than external rewarming.

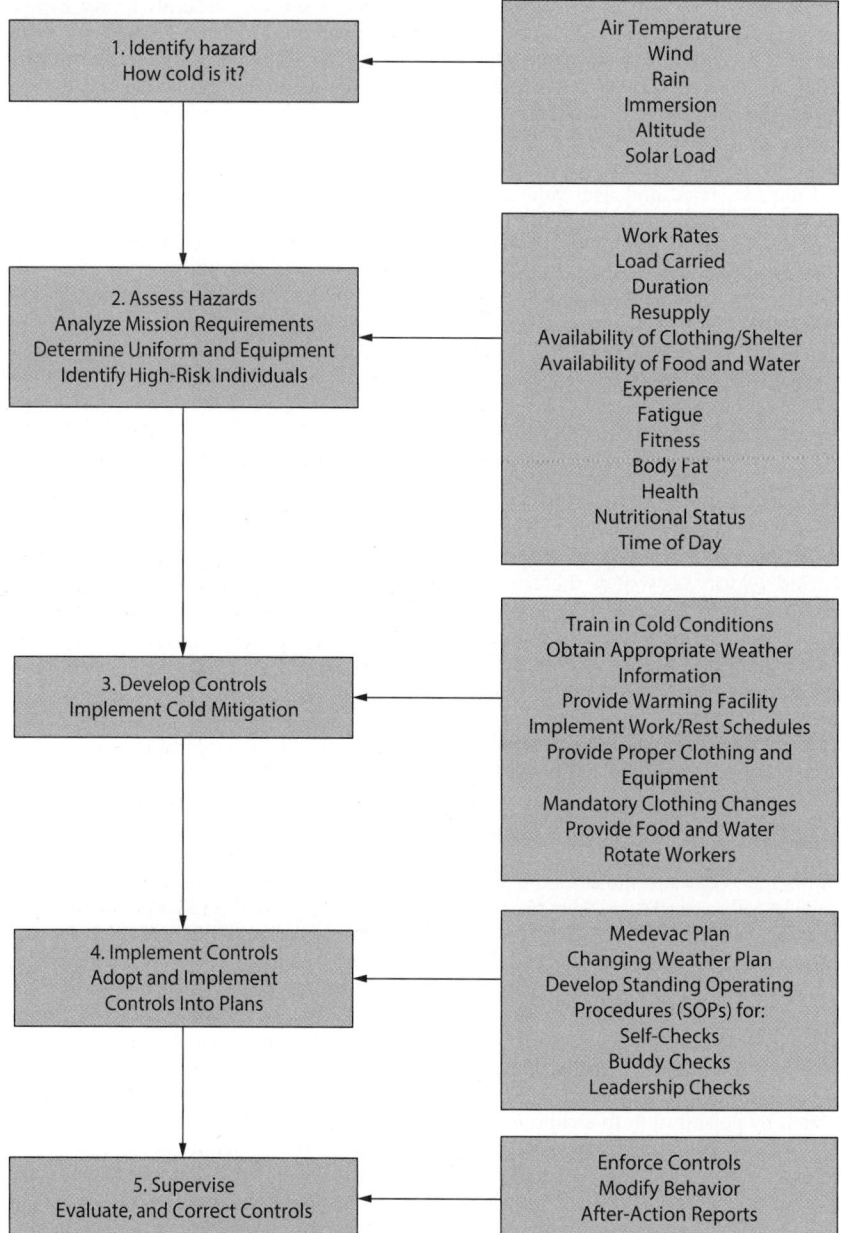

▲ **Figure 13–1.** Approach to prevention of cold-weather injuries.

A. Active External Rewarming Methods

Although relatively simple and generally available, active external warming methods may cause marked peripheral dilatation that predisposes to ventricular fibrillation and hypovolemic shock. Either heated blankets or warm baths may be used for active external rewarming. Rewarming in a warm bath is most effective and performed in a tub of stirred water at 40–42°C (104–107.6°F), with a rate of rewarming of about 1–2°C (1.8–3.6°F) per hour. It is easier, however, to monitor the patient and to carry out diagnostic and therapeutic procedures when heated blankets are used for active rewarming. Forced-air rewarming (38–43°C [100.4–109.4°F]) is

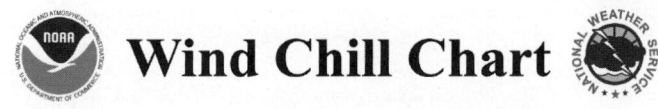

Wind Chill Chart

Temperature (°F)																	
Calm	35	30	25	20	15	10	5	0	–5	–10	–15	–20	–25	–30	–35	–40	–45
5	36	31	25	19	13	7	1	–5	–11	–16	–22	–28	–34	–40	–46	–52	–57	–63
10	34	27	21	15	9	3	–4	–10	–16	–22	–28	–35	–41	–47	–53	–59	–66	–72
15	32	25	19	13	6	0	–7	–13	–19	–26	–32	–39	–45	–51	–58	–64	–71	–77
20	30	24	17	11	4	–2	–9	–15	–22	–29	–35	–42	–48	–55	–61	–68	–74	–81
25	29	23	16	9	3	–4	–11	–17	–24	–31	–37	–44	–51	–58	–64	–71	–78	–84
30	28	22	15	8	1	–5	–12	–19	–26	–33	–39	–46	–53	–60	–67	–73	–80	–87
35	28	21	14	7	0	–7	–14	–21	–27	–34	–41	–48	–55	–62	–69	–76	–82	–89
40	27	20	13	6	–1	–8	–15	–22	–29	–36	–43	–50	–57	–64	–71	–78	–84	–91
45	26	19	12	5	–2	–9	–16	–23	–30	–37	–44	–51	–58	–65	–72	–79	–86	–93
50	26	19	12	4	–3	–10	–17	–24	–31	–38	–45	–52	–60	–67	–74	–81	–88	–95
55	25	18	11	4	–3	–11	–18	–25	–32	–39	–46	–54	–61	–68	–75	–82	–89	–97
60	25	17	10	3	–4	–11	–19	–26	–33	–40	–48	–55	–62	–69	–76	–84	–91	–98

Wind (mph)

Frostbite Times   ■ 30 minutes   ■ 10 minutes   ■ 5 minutes

$$\text{Wind Chill (°F)} = 35.74 + 0.6215T - 35.75(V^{0.16}) + 0.4275T(V^{0.16})$$
Where, T = Air Temperature (°F) V = Wind Speed (mph)

Effective 11/01/01

▲ **Figure 13–2.** Wind chill chart with time to frostbite.

recommended when extracorporeal rewarming is not available; heated blankets are recommended for transport.

B. Active Internal (Core) Rewarming Methods

Internal rewarming is essential for patients with severe hypothermia; extracorporeal blood rewarming (venoarterial extracorporeal membrane oxygenation [via the femoral artery and vein] or cardiopulmonary bypass) is the treatment of choice. If extracorporeal rewarming is not feasible, thoracic and bladder lavages are therapeutic options. Also, repeated peritoneal dialysis may be employed with 2 L of warm (43°C [109.4°F]), potassium-free dialysate solution exchanged at intervals of 10–12 minutes until the core temperature is raised to about 35°C (95°F). Parenteral fluids (5% dextrose in normal saline) should be warmed to 100–108°F before administration. Heated, humidified air warmed to 42°C (107.6°F) should be administered through a facemask or endotracheal tube. Warm colonic and gastrointestinal irrigations are of less value.

Passive rewarming (insulation from cold) is of value only for mildly hypothermic patients or as first-aid management on the scene. Hypothermia victims without vital signs should not be pronounced dead until they have been rewarmed to a

core temperature of 36°C (96.8°F) and are found to be unresponsive to continued CPR at that temperature. A key determinant of CNS effects from hypothermia will be whether brain hypoxia takes place before protective brain cooling.

Prognosis is directly related to the severity of metabolic acidosis; with low pH (6.6), elevated $Paco_2$, and/or significantly elevated serum potassium the prognosis is poor. The prognosis is good for otherwise healthy patients but worsens with the presence of underlying predisposing problems or a delay in treatment.

2. Hypothermia of the Extremities: Nonfreezing Cold Injury & Frostbite

Nonfreezing injury: Immersion foot (trench foot) is caused by a combination of cold temperature and exposure to water at temperatures from somewhat below freezing to 15°C. Immersion foot and pernio (chilblains) are nonfreezing injuries, whereas frostbite is a freezing injury. Nonfreezing injuries are a result of prolonged immersion with peripheral vasoconstriction, accompanied by local anesthesia and loss of proprioception. Predisposing factors for nonfreezing injuries include constricting boots

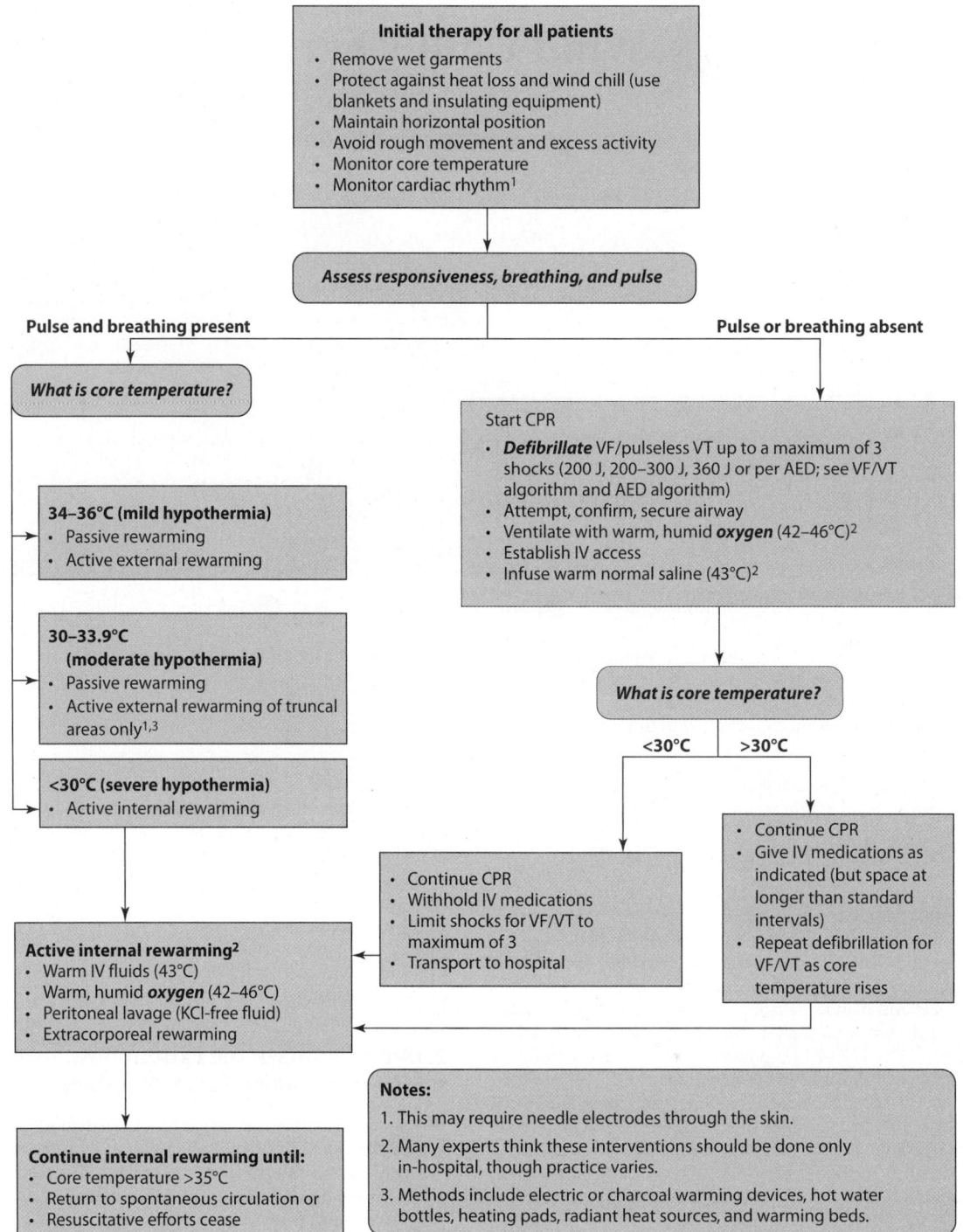

Initial therapy for all patients
- Remove wet garments
- Protect against heat loss and wind chill (use blankets and insulating equipment)
- Maintain horizontal position
- Avoid rough movement and excess activity
- Monitor core temperature
- Monitor cardiac rhythm[1]

Assess responsiveness, breathing, and pulse

Pulse and breathing present

What is core temperature?

34–36°C (mild hypothermia)
- Passive rewarming
- Active external rewarming

30–33.9°C (moderate hypothermia)
- Passive rewarming
- Active external rewarming of truncal areas only[1,3]

<30°C (severe hypothermia)
- Active internal rewarming

Active internal rewarming[2]
- Warm IV fluids (43°C)
- Warm, humid *oxygen* (42–46°C)
- Peritoneal lavage (KCl-free fluid)
- Extracorporeal rewarming

Continue internal rewarming until:
- Core temperature >35°C
- Return to spontaneous circulation or
- Resuscitative efforts cease

Pulse or breathing absent

Start CPR
- ***Defibrillate*** VF/pulseless VT up to a maximum of 3 shocks (200 J, 200–300 J, 360 J or per AED; see VF/VT algorithm and AED algorithm)
- Attempt, confirm, secure airway
- Ventilate with warm, humid *oxygen* (42–46°C)[2]
- Establish IV access
- Infuse warm normal saline (43°C)[2]

What is core temperature?

<30°C

- Continue CPR
- Withhold IV medications
- Limit shocks for VF/VT to maximum of 3
- Transport to hospital

>30°C

- Continue CPR
- Give IV medications as indicated (but space at longer than standard intervals)
- Repeat defibrillation for VF/VT as core temperature rises

Notes:
1. This may require needle electrodes through the skin.
2. Many experts think these interventions should be done only in-hospital, though practice varies.
3. Methods include electric or charcoal warming devices, hot water bottles, heating pads, radiant heat sources, and warming beds.

▲ **Figure 13–3.** Hypothermia treatment algorithm. AED = automated external defibrillator; CPR = cardiopulmonary resuscitation; IV = intravenous; J = joules; VF = ventricular fibrillation; VT = ventricular tachycardia.

and clothing, immobility, vascular compromise, and possibly tobacco use.

Frostbite: The cheeks, nose, earlobes, fingers, toes, hands, and feet are the parts of the body most likely to develop ice crystals within the tissue, resulting in localized hypothermic injury. As skin temperature falls below 25°C (77°F), tissue metabolism slows, although oxygen demand increases if work continues. There may be tissue damage at 15°C (59°F) as a consequence of ischemia and thrombosis and at –3°C (26.6°F) as a consequence of actual freezing of the tissue. Risk factors for frostbite are environmental conditions that increase heat loss or ability to generate heat. Peripheral vascular disease, diabetes, alcohol use, and dehydration increase risk.

▶ Clinical Findings

A. Pernio (Chilblains)

Pernio, also called Chilblains, consists of painful, erythematous, pruritic skin lesions caused by inflammation as a result of exposure to cold or dampness with cold. With prolonged exposure, this condition can progress to chronic pernio or "blue toes," characterized by erythematous, edematous, and ulcerating lesions of the acral parts of the toes. Scarring, fibrosis, and atrophy can follow. The emergence of skin lesions may become a chronic problem in cold conditions.

B. Immersion Foot

There are three clinical stages of recovery after removal from the cold: an ischemic stage, a hyperemic stage, and a post-hyperemic recovery stage. Initially, feet are cold, numb, swollen, and waxy white or cyanotic. Between 2 and 3 days following removal from the cold, hyperemia occurs, along with intense pain, additional swelling, redness, heat, blistering, hemorrhage, lymphangitis, ecchymoses, and, in some cases, sequelae such as cellulitis, gangrene, or thrombophlebitis. After 10–30 days, intense paresthesias sometimes occur and are accompanied by cold sensitivity and hyperhidrosis, which may persist for years. Tropical immersion foot occurring at higher temperatures is similar but usually has less intense symptoms with faster recovery.

C. Frostbite

In frostbite, freezing of superficial tissues (skin, subcutaneous) usually causes symptoms of numbness, prickling, and itching; skin is gray-white, waxy or hard. In severe cases, there may be paresthesias and stiffness, as well as injury to deeper tissues—bone, muscle, and nerve. Skin is often white and edematous. Deep frostbite may be followed by ulceration, necrosis, or gangrene.

▶ Prevention

Keep skin dry and wear moisture-resistant hats, facemasks, earmuffs, scarves, gloves, mittens, socks, and boots. Wet or constrictive socks should be replaced as soon as possible to prevent immersion foot. Pocket hand warmers may be used to warm extremities. Gloves that prevent against contact freezing on metal or other hard objects should be used. See Figure 13–2 for wind chill factors and exposure times that create a risk of frostbite. Additional prevention guidelines are the same as for systemic hypothermia (see previously).

▶ Treatment

A. Chilblains (Pernio) and Immersion Foot

Treatment is intended to improve capillary circulation and includes elevating the extremities, gradually rewarming them by exposure to air at room temperature and protecting pressure sites from trauma. Massage, ice, heat, and immersion should be avoided. Antibiotics are given if infection develops. Amitriptyline (50–100 mg at bedtime) has been used for pain. Tetanus prophylaxis is recommended. For pernio, topical steroids have been used with some success, and nifedipine may be useful for its vasodilatory properties in resistant cases, although supporting evidence is limited.

B. Frostbite

At the site of exposure, extremities can be rewarmed by removing wet gloves, socks, and shoes; drying the extremities and covering them again with dry clothing; and either elevating them or placing them next to a warmer part of the body (eg, placing the hands in the armpits). *Caution:* Rewarming should not be attempted if refreezing is likely prior to definitive therapy.

In cases of severe frostbite, hospitalization is recommended until the extent of tissue damage has been determined. The patient should be evaluated and treated, if necessary, for systemic hypothermia (see the section "Systemic Hypothermia").

Rapid rewarming of the frostbitten parts of the body can be accomplished by placing them in a moving water bath heated to 40–42°C (104–107.6°F) and leaving them there until thawing is complete but no longer (often 30 minutes). Dry heat is not recommended, and external heat should be discontinued once normal temperature has been reached. The patient should remain in bed with the affected parts elevated and uncovered at room temperature. Frostbitten parts should not be exercised, rubbed, or exposed to pressure. Dressings and bandages should not be applied. Whirlpool therapy at 37–40°C (98.6–104°F) twice daily for 15–30 minutes for 3 or more weeks helps to cleanse the skin and debrides superficial tissue.

In cases of severe frostbite injury with victims who are at risk for amputation, there is often associated thrombosis, and consideration may be given to antithrombolytic therapy with tissue plasminogen activator and heparin (or subcutaneous low-molecular-weight heparin). Imaging of cyanotic areas after rewarming by technetium scan or computed tomography (CT) angiography can help to guide treatment decisions.

Aseptic wound care is important for frostbite-damaged skin with use of nonadherent dressings and measures to avoid of tissue injury. Tetanus antitoxin or a tetanus toxoid booster may be indicated. While prophylactic antibiotics are controversial with limited supporting evidence, the skin should be monitored closely for infection and antibiotics initiated at the early signs of infection.

Surgery generally should be avoided and amputation not considered until it is certain that the tissue is devitalized. Gangrenous and necrotic tissue should be managed by surgical specialists.

Physical therapy can be instituted as healing progresses. The patient should be instructed to avoid exposure to the cold for several months and be advised of future hypersusceptibility to frostbite.

DISORDERS CAUSED BY HEAT

Five medical disorders can result from excessive exposure to hot environments: heat stroke, heat exhaustion, heat cramps, heat syncope, and skin disorders. Among the many types of workers at risk are steel workers, oven and furnace operators, glassblowers, farm workers, ranchers, fishermen, and construction workers. Heat-related illnesses have been increasing and can be expected to continue to rise with temperature spikes related to climate change.

A stable internal body temperature requires maintenance of a balance between heat production and loss, which the hypothalamus regulates by triggering changes in thirst, muscle tone, vascular tone, and sweat gland function. Production and evaporation of sweat are a major mechanism of heat removal (however, sweating causes loss of body water and sodium). The transfer of heat from the skin to surrounding air or liquid (convection) or between two solids in direct contact (conduction) also may occur, but this decreases in efficiency as ambient temperature increases. The passive transfer of heat via IR rays from a warmer to a cooler object (radiation) accounts for 65% of body heat loss under normal conditions. Radiant heat loss also decreases as ambient temperature increases up to 37.2°C (99°F), at which point heat transfer reverses. At normal temperatures, evaporation accounts for approximately 20% of body heat loss, but at excessive temperatures, it becomes the most important means for heat dissipation. It, too, is limited as humidity increases and is ineffective at 95% relative humidity. Another important physiologic response is the ability of the body to redirect blood flow from the internal organs to the skin to allow for heat dissipation.

The gradual, controlled exposure to heated environments of increasing intensity and duration (acclimatization) allows the body to adjust to heat by beginning to sweat at lower body temperatures, increasing the quantity of sweat produced, reducing the salt content of sweat, and increasing the plasma volume, cardiac output, and stroke volume while the heart rate decreases.

Health conditions that inhibit sweat production or evaporation and increase susceptibility to heat injury include obesity; skin disease; decreased cutaneous blood flow; dehydration; hypotension; cardiac disease resulting in reduced cardiac output; and the use of alcohol or medications that inhibit sweating, reduce cutaneous blood flow, or cause dehydration (eg, atropine, antipsychotics, tricyclic antidepressants, diuretics, laxatives, anticholinergics, antihistamines, monoamine oxidase inhibitors, vasoconstrictors, and beta blockers). The use of drugs that increase muscle activity and thereby increase the generation of body heat (eg, phencyclidine [PCP], lysergic acid diethylamide [LSD], amphetamines, cocaine, and lithium carbonate) is also a concern. Infections, cancer, malnutrition, thyroid dysfunction, and other debilitating medical conditions can reduce the effectiveness of the sweating mechanism and circulatory response to heat. Age and sex also affect susceptibility to heat injury. Older people do not acclimatize as easily because of their reduced sweating efficiency, and women generally generate more internal heat than men when performing the same task.

1. Heat Stroke

Heat stroke is a life-threatening medical emergency caused by thermal regulatory failure manifested by cerebral dysfunction with altered mental status, hyperpyrexia, abnormal vital signs, and, usually, hot, dry skin. Heat stroke should be diagnosed based on a clinical picture in which there are CNS signs and elevated core temperature above 40°C. It occurs in one of two forms: *classic* or *exertional*. The classic form occurs under conditions of extreme heat among those with compromised heat-dissipation capability (elderly individuals, infants, and chronically ill or debilitated patients). Exertional heat stroke results from strenuous exertion in hot environments, often in unacclimatized individuals. Morbidity or mortality can result from cerebral, cardiovascular, hepatic, or renal damage.

▶ Clinical Findings

Thermal regulatory failure is characterized by dizziness, weakness, nausea, vomiting, confusion, delirium, and visual disturbances; changes in mental status are its hallmark. Convulsions, collapse, or unconsciousness may occur. The skin is hot and initially covered with perspiration; later it dries. Blood pressure may initially be slightly elevated but later becomes hypotensive. Core temperatures usually exceed 40°C (104°F). As with heat exhaustion, hyperventilation can occur and lead to respiratory alkalosis and compensatory metabolic acidosis. There also may be liver damage, abnormal bleeding, renal failure, or arrhythmias.

Laboratory evaluation may reveal an increase in leukocytes because of dehydration; decreased serum potassium, calcium, and phosphorus levels; increased blood urea nitrogen and creatinine levels; hemoconcentration; decreased blood coagulation; and concentrated urine with proteinuria, tubular casts, and myoglobinuria. Thrombocytopenia, increased bleeding and clotting times, fibrinolysis, and consumptive coagulopathy may be present. Myocardial, liver, or renal damage may be reflected in laboratory tests (Table 13–1).

Table 13–1. Accidental hyperthermia—clinical differential.

	Heat Cramps	Heat Exhaustion	Heat Stroke
Pathophysiology	Salt deficiency	Volume/electrolyte depletion	Thermoregulatory failure
Symptoms	Painful muscle cramps/ spasm Weakness Nausea Vomiting	Weakness Headache Syncope Nausea Vomiting Intense thirst (water depletion) Fatigue Muscle cramps (salt depletion) Malaise	Irritability Confusion Prodromal heat exhaustion Collapse Severe/sustained physical exertion (exertional heat stroke) Irrational behavior
Objective findings	Euthermia	Core temperature usually ≤38°C (100.4°F) Profuse sweating Orthostatic vital signs Tachycardia Hyperventilation	Core temperature usually ≥40°C (104°F) Altered mental status—bizarre behavior Hot dry skin (classic heat stroke) Moist skin (exertional heat stroke) Coma Hypotension/shock Seizure Tachycardia Cyanosis Rales
Laboratory	Possible elevated creatine phosphokinase (CPK), creatinuria	Oliguria	Hyperuricemia CPK elevation Disseminated intravascular coagulation Respiratory alkalosis Hypokalemia Thrombocytopenia Myoglobinuria Hypoglycemia Transaminase elevation

▶ Prevention

The American Conference of Governmental Industrial Hygienists (ACGIH) review has developed an index of threshold limit values (TLVs) for exposure to heat in occupational settings. The values (wet-bulb globe temperature [WBGT]) are based on the following formula that includes the natural wet-bulb temperature T_{nwb}, the shielded dry-bulb temperature T_{db}, and black-globe temperature T_g, which are measurements that account for effects caused by solar radiant heat, air velocity, relative humidity, and ambient temperature. With direct exposure to sunlight:

$$WBGT = 0.7T_{nwb} + 0.2T_g + 0.1T_{db}$$

Without direct exposure to sunlight:

$$WBGT = 0.7T_{nwb} + 0.3T_g$$

Exposure limits take into account the type of work-rest regimen and the workload, including body position, movement, acclimatization, and limb use. These determine the heat load or metabolic rate, which is then related to the index to arrive at a recommended exposure standard for workers in a particular situation. The ACGIH has developed criteria for work-rest cycles based on the WBGT in order to limit the risk of heat-related illness. A guide and an example of the application of WBGT values to work-rest cycles can be found in the OSHA technical manual (https://www.osha.gov/dts/osta/ otm/otm_iii/otm_iii_4.html#heat_hazardassessment). A more condensed approach to the application of WBGT readings can be found in the Army Public Health Center Fact Sheet 12-005-0316 (https://phc.amedd.army.mil/phc%20resource%20library/heatillness_fs_12-005-0316.pdf).

In the absence of WBGT data, heat-index guidelines developed by the National Weather Service predict exposure risks according to ambient temperature and humidity (Figure 13–4). The standards are based on the assumption that workers are acclimatized and physically fit, are wearing appropriate clothing, and are supplied with adequate water and food. If these conditions are not met or the work environment poses special challenges, two International

Temperature (F) Versus Relative Humidity (%)

°F	90%	80%	70%	60%	50%	40%
80	85	84	82	81	80	79
85	101	96	92	90	86	84
90	121	113	105	99	94	90
95		133	122	113	105	98
100			142	129	118	109
105				148	133	121
110						135

HI[a]	Possible Heat Disorder
80°F–90°F	Fatigue possible with prolonged exposure and physical activity.
90°F–105°F	Sunstroke, heat cramps, and heat exhaustion possible.
105°F–130°F	Sunstroke, heat cramps, and heat exhaustion likely, and heat stroke possible.
≥130°F or greater	Heat stroke highly likely with continued exposure.

[a]The **Heat index** (HI) is the temperature the body feels when heat and humidity are combined. The chart shows the HI that corresponds to the actual air temperature and relative humidity. (This chart is based on shady, light wind conditions. **Exposure to direct sunlight can increase the HI by up to 15°F.**)

(Due to the nature of the heat index calculation, the values in the tables have an error +/– 1.3°F.)

▲ **Figure 13–4.** Temperature index chart.

Standards, ISO 7933 and ISO 9886, offer means to monitor the physiologic strain on workers in order to provide safe work tasks. Occupational heat exposure can be minimized with engineering controls such as air conditioning/cooling, fans, hot-air venting, reflective shielding, and spot cooling. Administrative controls such as limiting exposure duration may be necessary. Special cooled suits have been designed for hot environments.

In occupations in which workers are exposed to excessive heat, medical evaluation is recommended to identify individuals at increased risk for heat disorders caused by preexisting medical conditions or use of medications. Exposed workers should be trained to recognize early signs and symptoms of heat disorders and should be advised of the importance of proper attire, nutrition, and fluid intake. Employers should provide cool drinking water or electrolyte-carbohydrate solutions and should ensure that there are shaded rest areas close to the work site. Any advantage of sports drinks and other hypotonic electrolyte solutions over the use of water to prevent heat-illness has not been proven in the working population. However, apart from the carbohydrate load that accompanies many of the commercial products, there is little likelihood of harm. Salt tablets are not recommended because their use may exacerbate or cause electrolyte imbalance. Organized athletic events should be managed with attention to thermoregulation; the WBGT index should be monitored, water consumption should be encouraged, and medical care should be immediately accessible.

▶ **Treatment**

Treatment is aimed at rapid (within 1 hour) reduction of the core temperature and control of secondary effects. Evaporative cooling provides rapid and effective lowering of temperature and is accomplished easily in most emergency settings. Until medical care becomes available, the patient should be moved to a shady, cool place. Clothing should be removed, and the entire body should be sprayed with cool water (15°C [59°F]); cooled or ambient air should be blown across the patient at high velocity (100 ft/min). The patient should be placed in the lateral recumbent position or supported in the hands-to-knees position to expose more skin surface to the air.

The cooling process should continue in the hospital with use of wet sheets accompanied by fanning. Immersion in an iced-water or cool water bath is effective for rapid cooling down to 39°C (102.2°F) (then stop immersion), but it has a greater potential for complications of hypotension and shivering and may impede other interventions. Other treatment alternatives include ice packs (groin, axilla, and neck) and iced gastric lavage, although these are much less effective than evaporative cooling. Treatment should continue until the core temperature drops to 39°C (102.2°F). Because of the risks of hypoxia and aspiration, intubation should be considered for the unconscious patient and 100% oxygen administered until the patient is cooled. The core temperature should continue to be monitored, although it usually remains stable after it has returned to normal. Chlorpromazine, 25–50 mg intravenously, or diazepam, 5–10 mg intravenously, can be used to control shivering and thus prevent an increase in heat. Antipyretics are contraindicated (Figure 13–5).

Patients should be monitored for hypovolemic and cardiogenic shock, either or both of which may occur. Attention should be paid to maintaining a patent airway, providing oxygen, correcting fluid and electrolyte imbalances, and supporting vital processes. Central venous or pulmonary artery wedge pressure should be assessed and intravenous fluids administered if indicated. If hypovolemic shock is suspected, 500–1000 mL of 5% dextrose in normal or half-normal saline solution may be given intravenously without overloading the circulation. Other medications appropriate for cardiovascular support should be considered.

Fluid output should be monitored with an indwelling urinary catheter, and fluid administration should maintain a urine output of more than 50 mL/h. The patient should be monitored for complications, including renal failure (caused by dehydration and rhabdomyolysis), hepatic failure, or cardiac failure, respiratory distress, hypotension, electrolyte imbalance (hypokalemia), and coagulopathy. Elevated creatine phosphokinase (CPK), elevated liver enzymes, and metabolic acidosis are predictors of multiorgan dysfunction.

Because hypersensitivity to heat continues in some patients for prolonged periods following heat stroke, they should be advised to avoid re-exposure to heat for at least 4 weeks.

2. Heat Exhaustion

In individuals performing strenuous work, prolonged exposure to heat and insufficient water intake can cause heat exhaustion, dehydration, and sodium depletion or isotonic fluid loss with accompanying cardiovascular changes. Symptoms and signs may include intense thirst, weakness, nausea, fatigue, headache, confusion, a possible elevation of core (rectal) temperature, increased pulse rate, and moist skin. Symptoms associated with both heat syncope and heat cramps (see next) also may be present. Hyperventilation sometimes occurs secondary to heat exhaustion and can lead to respiratory alkalosis. Progression to heat stroke is indicated by a rise in temperature or a decrease in sweating.

Treatment consists of placing the patient in a cool and shaded environment and providing hydration (1–2 L over 2–4 hours) and salt replenishment—orally if the patient is able to swallow. Physiologic saline or isotonic glucose solution should be administered intravenously in more severe cases. At least 24 hours' rest is recommended.

3. Heat Cramps

Heat cramps usually affect the larger skeletal muscles during or after activity in the heat. A mechanism may be hyperexcitability of the nerve terminals caused by sodium loss, hypotonic fluid replacement, and extracellular fluid volume contraction. They are usually characterized by slow and painful muscle contractions and severe muscle spasms that last from 1 to 3 minutes and involve the muscles employed in strenuous work.

The skin is moist and cool, and the involved muscle groups feel hard. The temperature may be normal or slightly increased, and blood tests may show low sodium levels and hemoconcentration. Because the thirst mechanism is intact, blood volume is not diminished significantly.

The patient should be moved to a cool environment and given a balanced salt solution or an oral saline solution consisting of 4 tsp of salt per gallon of water. Salt tablets are not recommended. Rest for 1–3 days with continued salt supplementation in the diet may be necessary before returning to work.

4. Heat Syncope

In heat syncope, sudden unconsciousness results from volume depletion and cutaneous vasodilatation with consequent systemic and cerebral hypotension. Episodes occur typically following strenuous work of at least 2 hours.

The skin is cool and moist and the pulse weak. Systolic blood pressure is usually below 100 mm Hg. Treatment consists of recumbency, cooling, and rehydration. Preexisting medical conditions should be monitored and treated if necessary.

5. Skin Disorders Caused by Heat

Miliaria (heat rash) is caused by sweat retention resulting from obstruction of the sweat gland duct. In working populations, miliaria is most likely to occur with strenuous activity under hot and humid conditions. Skin occlusion with constrictive clothing or equipment may be a precipitating factor. There are three forms (listed here in increasing order of severity and depth of occurrence within the sweat gland): miliaria crystallina, miliaria rubra, and miliaria profunda. As the site of duct obstruction becomes deeper in the skin, the severity increases and presentation varies (eg, vesicles, inflammation, erythematous papules), and the condition can lead to local destruction of the sweat glands.

Erythema *ab igne* ("from fire") is characterized by the appearance of hyperkeratotic nodules following direct contact with heat that is insufficient to cause a burn. Intertrigo results from excessive sweating and often is seen in obese individuals. Skin in the body folds (eg, the groin and axillae) is erythematous and macerated. Heat urticaria (cholinergic urticaria) can be localized or generalized and is characterized by the presence of wheals with surrounding erythema ("hives").

Treatment for these disorders consists of reduction or removal of heat exposure, reduction of sweating, and control of symptoms. Antihistamines may help to relieve pruritus in patients with urticaria. Corticosteroids are not beneficial.

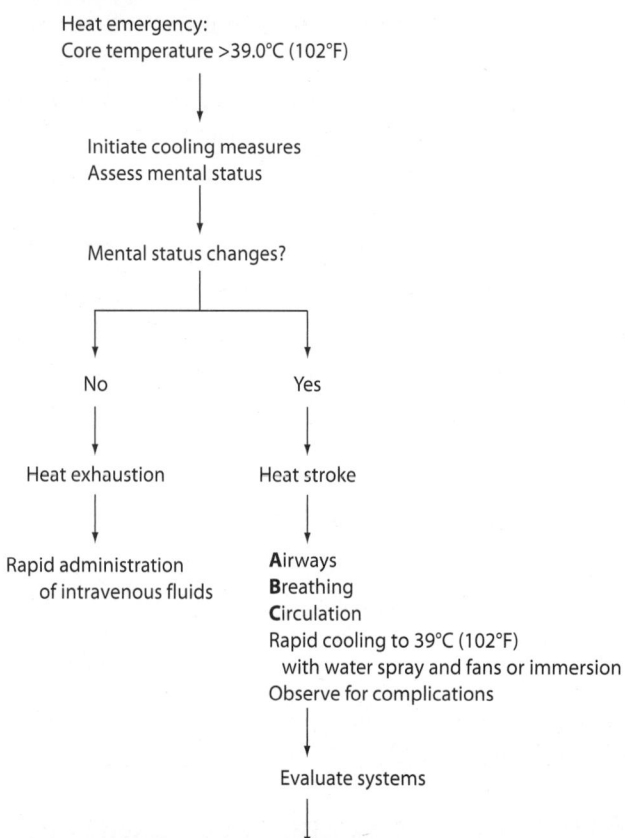

Heat emergency:
Core temperature >39.0°C (102°F)

Initiate cooling measures
Assess mental status

Mental status changes?

No — Heat exhaustion — Rapid administration of intravenous fluids

Yes — Heat stroke —

Airways
Breathing
Circulation
Rapid cooling to 39°C (102°F)
  with water spray and fans or immersion
Observe for complications

Evaluate systems

Systems	Signs	Measures
Neurologic	Persistent coma Seizures Focal deficit	CT scan of the head Lumbar puncture Intubation Ventilatory support
Cardiovascular	Hypotension Congestive heart failure	Central line PA pressure line Fluids, medication as indicated
Hematologic	Petechiae Purpura Epistaxis Hematemesis	Monitor clotting studies Platelet and factor replacement DIC: administer heparin

Renal	Oliguria
	Anuria
		High creatine kinase level
		  and myoglobinuria: maintain
		  high urine output;
		  consider dialysis

Pulmonary	Decreasing P_{O_2} Increasing airway resistance	Consider ARDS PEEP support on ventilator

▲ **Figure 13–5.** Heat illness treatment algorithm.

ELECTRICAL INJURIES

Electrical accidents comprise up to 7% of all traumatic fatal industrial injuries, mostly from very high voltages (>600 V). Electrical power-line installers and repairmen, electricians, operators of high-power electric equipment, and maintenance personnel are at greatest risk for electric shock.

The severity of the shock is related to the intensity of current (I) through the body, which, in turn, is related both to voltage (V) and resistance (R) as given by Ohm's law:

$$I = V/R$$

The severity of electrical burns is related to the amount of energy delivered, which is a function of the amount of current, the time of exposure, and the tissue resistance. Physical contact with an energized electric circuit provides a pathway for electricity to traverse the body as it seeks a ground. Resistance to electrical current is reduced by skin moisture, as well as moisture on contacting surfaces (eg, floors). Other factors influencing the type and severity of electrical injury include current type (alternating or direct current), duration of contact, area of contact, and pathway of the current through the body.

Electricity from alternating currents is more dangerous than that from direct currents. The alternating currents may cause muscle tetanization, but the direct currents do not.

Most tissue damage is related to the heat-produced conversion of the electric energy. Tissue resistance is largely reduced by the water content of the tissue, and that increases current flow and likelihood of injury. The vascular system and muscles are good conductors of electricity, whereas the bones, peripheral nerves, and dry skin have higher resistance.

A sudden exposure to intense electrical energy can cause not only tissue destruction and necrosis from heat and burning but also depolarization of electrically sensitive tissues such as nerve and heart. Alternating currents with voltages and frequencies as low as domestic circuits (100 V and 60 Hz) can produce ventricular fibrillation. High voltages (>1000 V) can cause respiratory paralysis. Most shocks involving sources exceeding 10,000 V are of such magnitude that the electrical force knocks the victim away from the power source, which reduces the electrical injury potential but often causes blunt trauma and burns.

A tetanizing effect on voluntary muscles is greatest at frequencies between 15 and 150 Hz. Most household current is in the 50- to 60-Hz range and can readily produce this effect. Current flow in amperes is the most important predictor of harm. A current flow above 10 mA is the approximate let-go threshold for electricity in the 50- to 60-Hz range. Alternating current above 20 mA can cause sustained contraction of chest respiratory muscles. Alternating currents above 40 mA can induce ventricular fibrillation with a shock duration more than 3 seconds, and higher current flows require correspondingly less time.

Direct current is more likely to cause asystole. Sustained grasp of the conductor does not usually occur at high voltages because the circuit usually arcs before contact with the victim, who is thrown back instead.

Lightning injuries, which are more like a form of direct current, differ from AC high-voltage electric shock injuries in that lightning usually involves higher voltage, briefer duration of contact, cardiorespiratory arrest with asystole rather than ventricular fibrillation, and high risk of nervous system injury. Most survivors of lightning strikes have some sequelae from blunt trauma or neurologic damage.

An arc injury can occur when a current from a voltage source jumps to the skin, causing burns but often not completing a circuit through the body.

▶ Clinical Findings

Exposure to electric current can cause shock, flash burns, flame burns, or direct tissue necrosis. Skin burns are common and can be partial or full thickness. Surface wounds covering heat-induced tissue necrosis are usually round or oval and well demarcated, and they may have a relatively innocuous yellow-brown appearance. A search must be made for both the entry and exit wounds to determine the electrical pathway through the body. Depending on the contact site and the pathway, there may be damage to nerves, muscles, or major organs such as the heart, brain, eye, kidney, and gastrointestinal tract. Arm-to-arm conduction is a high-risk concern for the heart.

In all cases, an ECG with a rhythm strip and a urine dipstick for blood and protein should be obtained, and the respiratory rhythm and rate should be checked. If organ, muscle, or nerve damage is suspected, appropriate diagnostic tests should be ordered such as urine myoglobin; renal failure can be a consequence. CPK should be monitored for at least 24 hours if muscle symptoms occur or muscle injury is otherwise suspected. With muscle injury, the CPK level can be elevated significantly (>1000 U/L), but the MB fraction will be below 3% if there is no cardiac muscle injury. Troponins may assist in making the determination of cardiac injury. Occult fractures may occur following muscle tetany or blunt trauma. Patients should be observed for several days because some develop posttraumatic myositis with rhabdomyolysis.

Electrical injury causes increased vascular permeability, which may result in reduced intravascular volume and fluid extravasation in the area of internal injury. Electrolytes, hematocrit, plasma volume, renal function studies, and urine output should be monitored closely.

Acute- and delayed-onset central and peripheral nervous system complications, including seizures, coma, respiratory center arrest, mental status changes, and localized paresis, and spinal cord injuries are potential sequelae of electrical shock. Cardiac complications usually consist of rhythm and conduction abnormalities with rare infarction. Vascular injury including small and large vein thromboses can also occur.

Prevention

Electrical injuries can be prevented in industrial settings by making sure that electrical workers are properly qualified and trained to follow safety procedures involving the installation, grounding, and disconnection of power sources. Locking out and tagging out electrical shutoff switches along with verification of the lack of voltage are effective work practices for preventing electrical injuries. Particular attention should be given to work requiring equipment manipulation during "live" operation. Nonconducting tools and clothing and other appropriate personal protective equipment should be used whenever possible. Barricades and warning signs should be placed around high-voltage areas, and procedures to exclude other employees from these areas should be strictly enforced.

Workers should be instructed in the proper measures to free a victim from contact with electric current. The rescuer must be protected during this procedure. If possible, the power should be turned off. If not, a nonconducting object such as a rope, a broom or other wooden instrument, or an article of clothing can be used to pull the victim away from the current and protect the rescuer from injury.

Avoidance of lightning strikes includes seeking shelter; if caught outdoors, finding a low area, such as a gulley, away from tall trees; and avoiding metal equipment, objects, and tools.

Treatment

Prior to CPR, first aid, or treatment, the patient must be separated from the "live" electric current. If necessary, CPR (including automated external defibrillator [AED] use) should be instituted until medical help arrives. Because the victim may have suffered spinal injury, extreme care must be taken during handling or transport.

If major electrical injuries are suspected, the patient should be hospitalized and observed for secondary organ damage, impaired renal function, hemorrhage, acidosis, and myoglobinuria. Indications for hospitalization include significant arrhythmia or ECG changes, large burns, loss of consciousness, neurologic findings, pulmonary or cardiac symptoms, or evidence of significant deep-tissue/organ damage. A tetanus booster or antitoxin should be administered if indicated.

Superficial tissue damage and burns should be addressed. If major soft-tissue damage is suspected, surgical exploration, fasciotomy, or both must be considered. Gross myoglobinuria may indicate a compartment syndrome and the need for fasciotomy.

Lactated Ringer solution should be administered intravenously at a rate sufficient to maintain urine output at between 50 and 100 mL/h. Continuous monitoring and prompt correction of acid-base or electrolyte imbalance are necessary if rhabdomyolysis occurs.

NONIONIZING RADIATION INJURIES

1. Injuries Caused by Radiofrequency & Microwave Radiation

Exposure

Injuries can be caused by the thermal effects of acute exposure to high levels of radiofrequency (RF) and microwave radiation. As with other thermal injuries, these injuries are characterized by protein denaturation and tissue necrosis at the site of tissue heating, with an accompanying inflammatory reaction and subsequent scar formation. Nonthermal effects of low-level exposure have been demonstrated in some laboratory studies, but their significance in humans is not clear.

RF radiation and microwave radiation consist of energy in wave form traveling in free space at the speed of light. The radiation is defined in terms of frequency and intensity, with the frequency portion of the electromagnetic (EMF) spectrum extending from 0 kHz to 1000 GHz (1 Hz equals 1 wave or cycle per second [cps]). Microwaves occupy only the portion of this frequency spectrum between 300 MHz and 300 GHz (Figure 13–6). Within this microwave range, cellular telephones tend to operate in the 700–900 MHz or 1700–2100 MHz windows.

RF radiation has insufficient energy to cause molecular ionization; therefore, it lacks the fundamental property of ionizing radiation which leads to carcinogenicity. However, it does cause vibration and rotation of molecules, particularly molecules that have an asymmetric charge distribution or are polar in structure, such as water. The radiation is composed of separate electric and magnetic field vectors each perpendicular to the other and both perpendicular to the direction of the resulting electromagnetic wave (Figure 13–7). The electric field component is measured in volts per meter, the magnetic component in amperes per meter, and the resulting power density in watts per square meter. The power density in W/m^2 is the key measure determining the hazard of the electromagnetic field.

Absorption of RF radiation depends partly on the orientation of the body in relation to the direction of the electromagnetic wave. Radiation at frequencies below 15 MHz and above 25 GHz is poorly absorbed by human tissues and unlikely to cause significant thermal damage, while the 80- to 100-MHz range has been shown to maximize absorption via resonance. At these frequencies, the specific absorption rate (SAR) is highest, meaning energy is absorbed by tissues at the fastest rate, measured in W/kg. As a result, regulations often focus on limiting exposures in this range. Factors affecting conduction of RF radiation within the body include the thickness, distribution, and water content of the various tissues. As the water content increases, energy absorption and thermal effects increase. RF radiation can be modulated according to amplitude (AM) and frequency (FM) and can be generated in pulsed or continuous form. Pulsed waves are considered more dangerous.

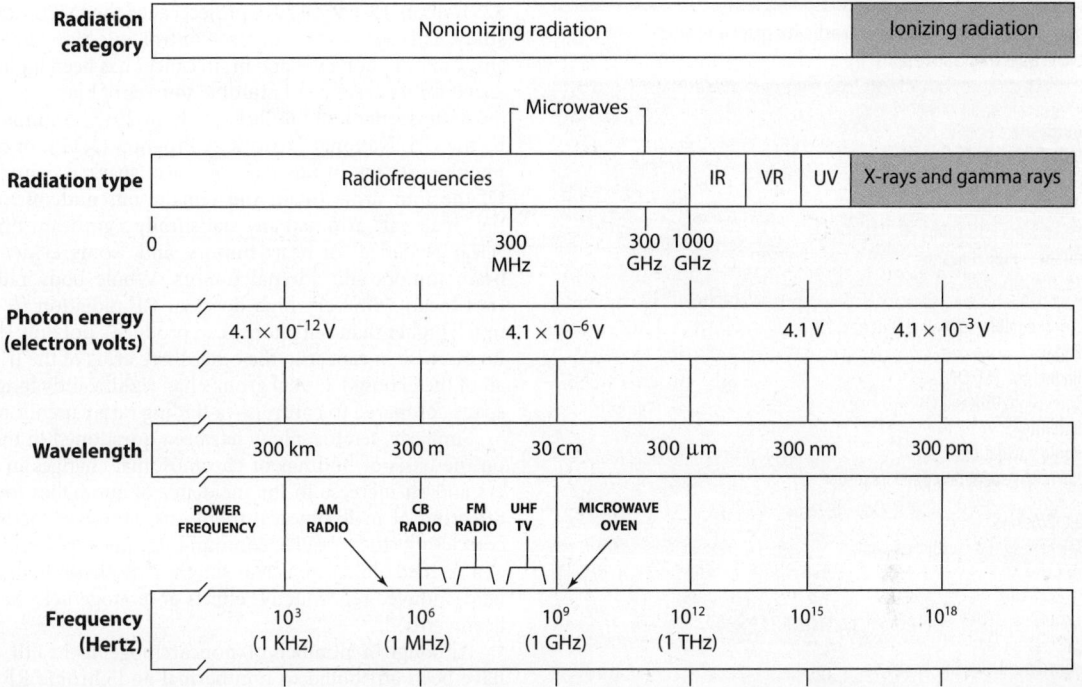

▲ **Figure 13–6.** The electromagnetic radiation spectrum. GHz = gigahertz; IR = infrared radiation; kHz = kilohertz; MHz = megahertz; THz = terahertz; UV = ultraviolet light; VR = visible radiation (light).

The risk of thermal injury increases with higher intensities of radiation and closer proximity to the radiation source. Other factors that affect human susceptibility to RF radiation injury include environmental humidity and temperature, grounding, reflecting medium, increased temperature sensitivity of tissues (eg, the testes), a lack of anatomic barriers to external radiation (eg, the eye), as well as reduced heat dissipation ability due to vascular anatomy.

Occupational exposures are likely in any workplace where employees are near equipment that generates RF

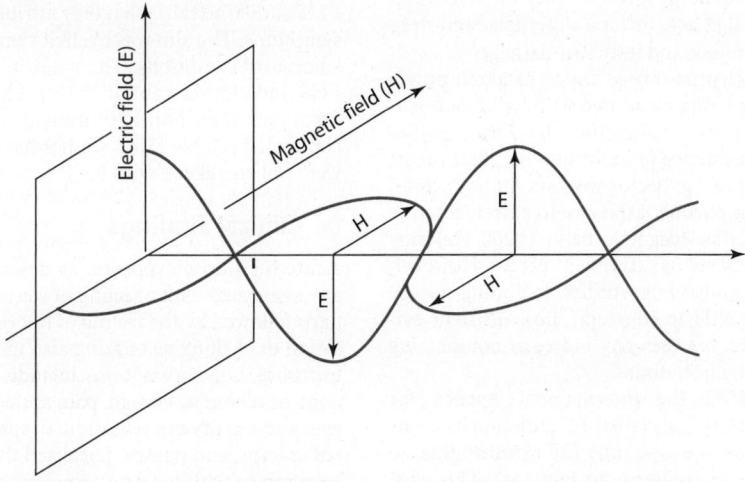

▲ **Figure 13–7.** Electric field (E) and magnetic field (H) components of radiofrequency radiation.

Table 13–2. Occupational radiofrequency and microwave exposures.

Sealing and heating equipment
Automotive trades
Furniture and woodworking
Glass-fiber production
Paper production
Plastics manufacturing and fabrication
Rubber product heating
Textile manufacturing
Electrical equipment maintenance
Radar
Radio: AM, FM, CB
Television: UHF and VHF
Satellite
Radio navigation
Microwave generators and heat sources
RF applications
Microwave tube testing and aging
RF laser
RF welding
Medical diathermy and healing promotion
Power transmission line workers

radiation, particularly equipment for dielectric heating (used in sealing of plastics and drying of wood), physiotherapy, radio communications, and maintenance of antennae and high-power electrical equipment (Table 13–2). Injuries have been documented for acute exposure to energy levels exceeding 10 mW/cm². In most cases, the levels were greater than 100 mW/cm². Most studies of RF radiation effects in animals and other biologic test systems have not demonstrated thermally induced effects at energy levels below 10 mW/cm². In animal studies, thermal effects include superficial and deep tissue destruction, cataracts, and testicular damage.

In the late 1970s scientists raised concerns about power and transmission lines being associated with childhood leukemia and brain cancer. In addition, there have been studies linking an increased incidence of brain tumors, male breast cancer, or leukemia in energy sector workers. In both cases, the prime concern was chronic exposure to extremely low-frequency (ELF) radiation magnetic fields (<200 Hz) surrounding high-voltage systems carrying a current. However, multiple more recent and robust studies, including pooled analyses, have led the NIH to conclude "no consistent evidence for an association between any source of nonionizing radiation and cancer has been found."

Nonetheless, in 2011 the International Agency for Research on Cancer (IARC) classified RF radiation as a category 2B carcinogen for the first time (2B signifies that an exposure is "possibly" carcinogenic to humans). This conclusion was almost entirely based on select findings within a

$25 million, 13-nation 2010 project called the INTERPHONE study. This age-restricted, case-control, questionnaire-based study of cell phone use and brain cancer has been highly criticized for its design and multiple sources of bias.

A subsequent $30 million study in 2017, commissioned by the U.S. National Toxicology Program (NTP), of cellular phone radiation in rats and mice also sparked controversy. Of the four arms (male and female, rats and mice), only the "male rat" arm had any statistically significant findings: "clear evidence" of heart tumors, and "some evidence" of brain tumors and adrenal tumors. Whole body radiation (not local) with very high doses of RF radiation (6 W/kg, much higher than cell phones can produce), not only showed no increase in cancer in the other three arms of the trial, but all of the exposed animal groups had significantly longer life spans compared to controls—a finding rarely mentioned.

Similarly, teratogenicity has been questioned in the past, on the basis of findings of chromosomal changes in workers and an increase in the incidence of anomalies found in offspring of male physical therapists. However, because of conflicting study results, confounding exposures, and a lack of a verified biologic mechanism, the hypotheses of magnetic field–induced reproductive effects or teratogenicity have not been verified.

Although a number of noncarcinogenic health effects have been attributed to nonthermal and chronic RF exposures (including microwave and ELF radiation), current data do not support an association with cardiovascular, neurologic, or reproductive outcomes. Patient advocacy groups have claimed there should be a new clinical syndrome caused by RF exposure labeled "electromagnetic hypersensitivity" (EHS), characterized by nonspecific, intermittent symptoms that may involve any body part or system. Alleged sources include power lines, Wi-Fi routers, and household appliances. The World Health Organization (WHO) has investigated these concerns, noting: "A number of studies have been conducted where EHS individuals were exposed to EMF similar to those that they attributed to the cause of their symptoms. The aim was to elicit symptoms under controlled laboratory conditions. The majority of studies indicate that EHS individuals cannot detect EMF exposure any more accurately than non-EHS individuals. Well controlled and conducted double-blind studies have shown that symptoms were not correlated with EMF exposure."

▶ **Clinical Findings**

Acute high-dose exposure, as described previously, is usually associated with a feeling of warmth on the exposed body part, followed by the feeling of hot or burning skin. The sensation of clicking or buzzing also may be present during the exposure. Other symptoms include irritability, headache or light-headedness, vertigo, pain at the site of exposure, watery eyes and a gritty eye sensation, dysphagia, anorexia, abdominal cramps, and nausea. Localized thermally induced masses may appear within days of exposure and consist of interstitial edema and coagulation necrosis.

The exposed skin has a sunburned appearance, with erythema and slight induration. There may be vesiculation or bullae. Blood pressure may be increased, and CPK levels may be elevated. Hematologic values, electroencephalographic and brain scan findings, sedimentation rate, and electrolyte values usually are within normal limits.

Beyond the immediately evident thermal injury, no further structural injury would be anticipated. Symptoms of posttraumatic stress disorder have occurred, with emotional lability and insomnia persisting for as long as 1 year.

▶ Prevention

Exposure assessment should include the following factors: the distance between the power source and exposed workers, the peak power density at the time of exposure, the frequency and type of radiation wave (pulsed or continuous), and the duration of exposure (in minutes). Metal barriers around the energy source can be used to contain RF radiation. Intensity is proportional to $1/d^2$, where d is distance from the source. Accordingly, there is a rapid decrease in power density over distance, and specification of a "Personnel not allowed" area can provide an effective barrier. Procedures to de-energize equipment are recommended when employees are working close to exposed sources. Protective clothing generally is ineffective. Periodic environmental RF radiation measurements for equipment exposures are essential.

▶ Treatment & Prognosis

Treatment is the same as for other thermal injuries. Thermal injuries usually heal without problems. If hypertension develops, it usually will resolve following a short course of antihypertensive therapy. Posttraumatic stress disorder and other psychological sequelae generally are responsive to short-term therapy.

2. Injuries Caused by Infrared Radiation

Infrared (IR) radiation covers the portion of the electromagnetic spectrum between visible and RF radiation (see Figure 13–6). It has wavelengths between 760 nm and 1 mm and is composed of three spectral bands—IR-A ("near"), IR-B ("middle"), and IR-C ("far")—that begin at 750, 1400, and 3000 nm, respectively. IR radiation is given off by any object having a temperature greater than absolute zero. Occupational exposures—in addition to sunlight—include processes in which thermal energy from IR radiation is used, such as heating and dehydrating processes, welding, glassmaking, and the drying and baking of coatings on consumer products. In addition, workers near molten metals and glass may be exposed to high levels of IR radiation. In recent years, the use of IR lasers, such as neodymium-doped yttrium aluminum garnet (nd:YAG) and high-intensity light sources, such as xenon-arc searchlights, has increased the potential for accidental high-power exposure to IR radiation.

Acute, high-intensity exposure to IR wavelengths shorter than 3000 nm (IR A and B) has potential to cause thermal damage to the cornea, iris, or lens. Wavelengths in this range cause molecular excitation and vibration, resulting in heat that is absorbed by tissues. The cornea may be thermally damaged by IR exposures, and energy absorbed from surrounding structures at different wavelengths is postulated to contribute to corneal damage. Such exposure is also capable of producing cataracts, a problem noted in glassblowers and in steel furnace workers. IR-A (near infrared) wavelengths can be focused on the retina, causing chorioretinal damage and blindspots from thermal injury, although photochemical injury may also occur from wavelengths in the visible spectrum. Thermal injury to the skin can also occur, but it is usually self-limited by withdrawal from the pain and results in an acute skin burn with increased pigmentation.

Prevention of injuries can be achieved by shielding heat sources, using protective eye and skin wear, and monitoring exposure levels. The ACGIH has developed a TLV formula for limiting exposure to the energy from IR radiation in the wavelength spectrum of 770–3000 nm.

3. Injuries Caused by Visible Radiation

Chorioretinal injury: Visible radiation (light) covers the portion of the electromagnetic spectrum between IR and ultraviolet (UV) radiation (see Figure 13–6) and the wavelengths between 400 and 760 nm. The eye is the most sensitive target organ, with damage resulting from structural, thermal, or photochemical light-induced reactions. Workers at risk are those with prolonged or repeated exposure to intense light sources, including sunlight, high-intensity lamps, lasers, flashbulbs, spotlights, and welding arcs and fluorescent and other sources of high-intensity blue light. It has been well documented that intense exposures to visible light spectrum from directly observing solar eclipses or from intense human-made sources can result in chorioretinal injury.

The retina is the usual site of injury and is most sensitive to the wavelengths of 440–500 nm, which cause a destructive photochemical reaction. Absorption of energy by the choroid and retina is greatest in the 500- to 700-nm range. Blue light (400–500 nm) is responsible for solar retinitis (eclipse blindness) and can also cause subclinical changes with chronic exposure. It may contribute to retinal aging and to senile macular degeneration, which can result in central visual field acuity loss. Because the lens partially filters out wavelengths between 320 and 500 nm, it provides some protection of the retina from blue light. Individuals with aphakia (absence of the lens), who are more susceptible to retinal damage, should be cautioned against looking into the midday sun and other intense light sources and should be urged to wear spectacle filters when working in bright environments. Short bursts of high-intensity light can cause flash blindness in which the temporary visual loss and afterimage are a result of bleaching of visual pigments. As the light intensity and exposure duration increase, the afterimage persists longer. With mild to moderate exposures, symptoms of flash blindness resolve quickly.

Measures to prevent injury include interlocks, filters and warnings on intense light sources, special filtration of blue-light wavelengths, proper illumination of the workplace to reduce glare, and use of goggles or face shields by welders and other exposed workers. Workers with aphakia or a history of light sensitivity who are at-risk for exposure may need special protections and medical surveillance to detect changes in visual acuity or early signs of ocular damage. The ACGIH has a TLV to protect against the effects of chronic blue light exposure.

Other problems related to visible light: Insufficient lighting or reflected light (glare) can cause asthenopia (eyestrain), visual fatigue, headache, and eye irritation. These problems are more likely to occur in people older than 40 years. Symptoms are transient, and there is no indication that repeated episodes lead to ocular damage.

Contrast from surrounding light sources on areas of lesser intensity has led to complaints of asthenopia associated with video-display terminal use. This usually can be corrected by decreasing surrounding light intensities, using antiglare filters, and adjusting the contrast of the characters on the screen.

4. Injuries Caused by Ultraviolet Radiation

UV radiation covers the portion of the electromagnetic spectrum between visible radiation and ionizing radiation (see Figure 13–6) and has wavelengths between 100 and 400 nm. The wavelengths are divided into three spectral bands—A, B, and C—with the A and B bands representing the longer wavelengths and producing the greatest biologic effects (Table 13–3). Wavelengths shorter than 200 nm are absorbed over extremely short distances in air, preventing health effects. Wavelengths of 200–290 nm are absorbed primarily in the stratum corneum of the skin or the cornea of the eye, whereas the longer wavelengths can affect the dermis, lens, iris, or retina.

Because UV radiation has relatively poor penetration, the only organs it affects are the eye and skin. Eye injury is caused by thermal action from pulsed or brief high-power exposures, and skin damage is caused more commonly by photochemical reactions (including toxic and hypersensitivity reactions) from brief high-power or extended low-power exposures. The thermal effects of protein coagulation and tissue necrosis are rapid in onset. The effects of chronic exposure include accelerated aging of the skin, characterized by loss of elasticity, hyperpigmentation, wrinkling, and telangiectasia.

UV injuries occur in occupations involving drying and curing processes, arc welding, or use of lasers or germicidal UV lights (Table 13–4), but by far the greatest proportion

Table 13–4. Workers potentially exposed to ultraviolet radiation.

Natural sunlight	
Agricultural workers	Oil field workers
Brick masons	Open pit miners
Ranchers	Outdoor maintenance workers
Construction workers	Pipeline workers
Farmers	Police officers
Fishermen	Postal carriers
Gardeners	Railroad workers
Groundskeepers	Road workers
Horticultural workers	Sailors
Landscapers	Ski instructors
Lifeguards	Sports professionals
Lumberjacks	Surveyors
Military personnel	Other outdoor workers
Arc welding/torch cutting	
Welders	
Pipeline workers	
Pipecutters	
Maintenance workers	
Germicidal ultraviolet	
Physicians	
Nurses	
Laboratory technicians	
Bacteriology laboratory personnel	
Barbers	
Cosmetologists	
Kitchen workers	
Dentists/dental technicians	
Laser	
Laboratory workers	
Drying and curing processes	
Printers	
Lithographers	
Painters	
Wood curers	
Plastics workers	

Table 13–3. Ultraviolet light spectrum: ultraviolet A (UVA) and ultraviolet B (UVB) comparison.

	UVA	UVB
Wavelength	315–400 nm	280–315 nm
Penetration Physical Biological	Air, water, glass, quartz, through eye to retina	Air, quartz Anterior chamber only
Health effects	Skin and eye injury require greater energy than UVB	Skin erythema at 280–315 nm Peak carcinogenicity at 280–320 nm Peak photokeratitis sensitivity at 270 nm Cataract
Proportion of natural background UV	97%	3%

of injuries result from occupations that expose workers to natural sunlight during the peak time of UV energy dissemination, 10 AM to 3 PM. Factors affecting the severity of injury include exposure duration, radiation intensity, distance from the radiation source, altitude, and orientation of the exposed individual relative to the source and its wave-propagation plane. UV reflections from water and snow or their surrounding surfaces may increase exposure intensity.

▶ Clinical Findings & Treatment

A. Photokeratoconjunctivitis (Welder's Flash)

Ocular exposure to UV wavelengths shorter than 315 nm (especially wavelengths of 270 nm, to which the eye is most sensitive) can cause photo keratoconjunctivitis. Symptoms occur 6–12 hours after exposure and include severe pain, photophobia, a sensation of a foreign body or sand in the eyes, and tearing. After a latency period that varies inversely with the severity of the exposure, conjunctivitis appears, sometimes accompanied by erythema and swelling of the eyelids and facial skin. Fluorescein examination may reveal diffuse punctate staining of both corneas.

Treatment consists of providing symptomatic relief, which may include ice packs, systemic analgesics, eye patches, and mild sedation. Local anesthetics should not be used because of the risk of further injury to the anesthetized eye. Symptoms usually resolve within 48 hours. Permanent sequelae are rare, and the eye does not develop tolerance to repeated exposure (Table 13–5).

B. Cataracts

Cataractogenesis (cortical) is attributed to both photochemical and thermal effects of intense exposure to UV wavelengths of 295–320 nm and usually appears within 24 hours. Cataract formation following repeated exposures to UV wavelengths longer than 324 nm has been reported but is not well documented. Treatment is by corrective surgery.

Table 13–5. Eye injuries caused by ultraviolet light.

Location	UV Effect
Conjunctiva	Conjunctivitis
Sclera	Hyperemia
Cornea	Keratitis
Cataracts	Lens
Aqueous	Toxic photochemicals
Vitreous	Degradation in aphakics
Retina	Chromophore damage in aphakics

Intraocular lenses implanted after cataract removal often provide UV filtration to protect the retina.

C. Other Eye Injuries

The cornea and lens protect the retina from the effects of UV wavelengths shorter than 300 nm, but damage to the iris and retina is possible if individuals with aphakia are exposed to these wavelengths. In others, damage is possible with exposure to longer wavelengths or to high-power UV lasers. Treatment is supportive. Two lesions of the bulbar conjunctiva have been associated with repeated exposures to UV radiation: pterygium (a benign hyperplasia) and epidermoid carcinoma.

D. Erythema

Absorbed UV radiation reacts with photoactive substances present in the skin and 2–24 hours later causes erythema (sunburn), the most common acute UV effect. Erythema is most severe following exposure to wavelengths of 290–320 nm and may be accompanied by edema, blistering, desquamation, chills, fever, nausea, and, rarely, circulatory collapse.

Treatment of acute sunburn and any blistering that occurs is supportive and symptomatic and may include topical and mild systemic analgesics. Most symptoms subside within 48 hours. The resulting scaling, darkening of the skin (caused by increased melanin production), and thickening of the stratum corneum provide increased protection against subsequent exposures.

E. Photosensitivity Reactions

Two types of acute photosensitivity reactions of the skin can occur following exposure to UV radiation: phototoxic (nonallergic) and photoallergic reactions. Phototoxic reactions are much more common and frequently occur in association with use of medications such as griseofulvin, tetracycline, sulfonamides, thiazides, and preparations containing coal tar or psoralens. Phototoxicity may exaggerate or aggravate the effects of some systemic diseases, including lupus erythematosus, dermatomyositis, congenital erythropoietic porphyria, porphyria cutanea tarda symptomatica, pellagra, actinic reticuloid, herpes simplex, and pemphigus foliaceus. Photosensitivity reactions may be characterized by blisters, bullae, and other skin manifestations.

Exposure to UV wavelengths above 320 nm after skin contact with furocoumarin-producing plants such as celery can cause phytophotodermatitis. A mild phototoxic reaction causes pigmentary changes along the pattern of points of contact, whereas bullae may result from a more severe inflammatory reaction. Photoallergic reactions to UV radiation occur in association with bacteriostatic agents and perfume ingredients, which cause skin irritation, erythema, and blistering. Treatment of photosensitivity reactions depends on the particular underlying or associative cause and ranges from symptomatic care in mild cases to hospitalization and use of systemic corticosteroids in cases of severe reactions.

F. Premalignant and Malignant Skin Lesions

Premalignant lesions associated with chronic exposure to UV radiation include actinic keratosis, keratoacanthoma, and Hutchinson melanosis. Malignant lesions associated with exposure are basal cell carcinoma (the most common), squamous cell carcinoma, and malignant melanoma. Hazardous UV wavelengths are thought to be between 256 and 320 nm. UV radiation also promotes carcinogenesis following exposure to some chemicals, including those found in tar and pitch. Increased risk for premalignant and malignant lesions occurs in fair-skinned individuals and in those who have repeated sunburns or tan poorly. Patients with a history of xeroderma pigmentosum are at greater risk for malignant melanoma.

Patients should be referred to a dermatologist for definitive diagnosis and treatment. Premalignant lesions may be treated by removal or use of topical medication. Treatment of malignant lesions may involve simple excision, radiation, or major surgery.

▶ Prevention

Exposure guidelines are based on wavelength and irradiance. Exposed individuals should be counseled concerning photosensitizing agents. Welders should be required to wear goggles or face shields to protect their eyes. Outdoor workers should be instructed to wear wide-brim hats, sunglasses, protective clothing, and to use broad-spectrum sunscreen with an SPF of 15 or higher. Persons at increased risk due to skin type, family history, preexisting medical conditions, or excessive exposure should be examined periodically for the presence of premalignant or malignant lesions.

IONIZING RADIATION INJURIES

Ionizing radiation can cause both acute injuries in which the tissue *damage* increases with dose and chronic health effects such as cancer for which the *risk* increases with exposure. The acute radiation syndrome (ARS) is a well-understood and catastrophic tissue effect of ionizing radiation that follows a brief but massive exposure. Researchers have also documented chronic effects of radiation, most notably cancer, the risk of which can result either from brief high-dose exposure or excessive cumulative exposures. More than 200 significant radiation incidents have occurred since 1940 as a result of exposure to radioisotopes, x-ray generators and accelerators, radar generators, and similar sources of ionizing radiation. Workers at risk, based on their history of exposures and resulting injury, include radiologists and x-ray technologists, uranium miners, nuclear power plant operators, laboratory workers, military personnel, and many others. Radioactive sources or x-ray generating devices are found in a wide range of occupational settings.

Ionizing radiation is emitted from radioactive atomic structures as high-energy electromagnetic x-rays or gamma rays or as energized particles (alpha, beta, proton, and neutron particles) that impart energy through collision with other structures. The different forms of ionizing radiation vary by natural source, energy, frequency, and penetrability, but they all share the ability to ionize incident materials. X-rays and gamma rays exist at the highest energies and frequencies of the electromagnetic spectrum (see Figure 13–6). Dislocation of an electron from an incident atom and the resulting biomolecular chemical reactions and instability can cause tissue damage.

External biologic exposure to x-rays, gamma rays, and proton and neutron radiation results in high absorption, whereas beta particles penetrate skin poorly and alpha particles do not penetrate at all. Internal exposure to alpha or beta particles by radioisotope inhalation, implantation, or ingestion can result in serious acute or delayed injury. If radioactive surface contamination is suspected, contamination control procedures should be followed scrupulously during all phases of patient management.

As an emergency resource, the Oak Ridge Institute for Science and Education maintains the Radiation Emergency Assistance Center/Training Site (REAC/TS) with 24-hour phone access to consultation regarding medical and health physics problems associated with radiation accidents (1-865-576-1005).

A few definitions will help the reader to understand the terminology used in classifying the health effects of radiation:

- *Tissue effects (also called deterministic effects)*: injury as a result of cellular damage that occurs at a threshold dose and increases in severity with additional dose in all exposed individuals (eg, radiation skin burns and ARS)
- *Stochastic effects*: effects, such as cancer, that increase in probability but not severity with higher dose and that are assumed to have no threshold for risk.

The way in which dose to an individual is expressed depends, in part, on what kind of health effect that is being assessed. Some units of measurement for exposure and other related quantities that will be used in this section include (Table 13–6):

- *Absorbed dose*: The energy imparted by ionizing radiation to a given mass of tissue in J/kg. This is expressed in grays (Gy) in the international system (SI) units. The rad is the older name in CGS units for this measure that is still commonly found in older US publications and is gradually being replaced. Absorbed dose is used most commonly for characterizing adverse tissue effects.
- *Equivalent dose*: This is the absorbed dose adjusted by a weighting factor for the type of radiation to correct for different biological effectiveness between different radiation sources and particles. For example, alpha particles are given a weighting factor of 20. The name for equivalent dose in the SI system is sievert (Sv). The rem is the older

Table 13–6. Radiation units used in this chapter.

Parameter	SI Units[a]	CGS Units[b]	Conversion
Activity = rate of decay (disintegrations per second)	becquerel (Bq)	curie	1 Ci = 3.7 × 1010 Bq 1 Bq = 2.703 × 10^{-11} Ci
Absorbed dose = quantity of radiation energy absorbed per unit of mass joules/kg (used for tissue effects)	gray (Gy) joules (J)/kg	rad	1 Gy = 1 J/kg 1 Gy = 100 rads 1 rad = 0.01 Gy
Equivalent dose = absorbed dose × weighting factor for type of radiation (used for stochastic effects)	sievert (Sv)	rem	1 Sv = 100 rem 1 rem = 0.01 Sv

[a]SI = International System of Units.
[b]CGS = centigram-gram-second system of units now being replaced by SI units.

name for this measure in CGS units that is still commonly found in older US publications and is gradually being replaced. Both external and internal sources are considered when calculating equivalent dose. This measure is used in reference to stochastic effects, such as cancer risk. A related term is *effective dose* that adds a tissue-weighting factor for different body parts and organs. It is also expressed in sieverts. This measure allows for comparison of the stochastic risks from different exposure situations and types.

- *Becquerel (Bq)*: The becquerel is a measure of the activity of a radionuclide and represents one nuclear transformation/second. The term corresponds to curies in the CGS system. Measurements of the amount of radon/radon progeny in the air are made in becquerels or picocuries (pCi.).

1. Background Radiation

The general public is exposed to both natural background radiation and radiation from medical and other human-generated sources. Natural background radiation averages about 3.2 mSv/y in the United States and varies somewhat by location and altitude, although the largest contributor is radon decay products. Medical radiation has been a growing exposure source as a result of increased use of imaging technologies, such as CT and now accounts for approximately 3 mSv/person/y averaged across the US population.

2. Tissue Effects: Acute Radiation Syndrome

ARS is a consequence of brief but intense whole body (trunk, head) exposure to ionizing radiation. The radiation disrupts chemical bonds, which causes molecular excitation and free-radical formation. Highly reactive free radicals react with other essential molecules such as nucleic acids and enzymes; in turn, this disrupts cellular function. The clinical presentation and severity of illness are determined by the dosage, body part(s) exposed, and duration of exposure. Tissues with the most rapid cellular turnover are the most radiosensitive:

reproductive, hematopoietic, and gastrointestinal tissues. Table 13–7 summarizes the clinical effects seen with the ARS.

▶ Clinical Findings

In ARS many organs can be affected, although the predominant findings are in the hematologic, gastrointestinal, and central nervous systems with increasing exposure. ARS is an example of tissue effects (also called deterministic effects) in which specific clinical effects are almost certain to occur in a dose-dependent manner. Exposure effects on these organ systems constitute sub-syndromes that may be seen in the ARS victim. The hematologic syndrome is commonly seen at threshold absorbed doses above 1 Gy and is characterized by early onset of lymphocytopenia followed by declines in granulocytes and other blood cell lines. Individuals who become severely neutropenic need to be managed to support bone marrow and to avoid infection. At absorbed doses above 6 Gy, the gastrointestinal syndrome becomes a clinical concern with potential for severe nausea, vomiting, diarrhea, GI bleeding, malabsorption, electrolyte imbalances, and infection. A neurologic syndrome may manifest at absorbed doses above 8 Gy with neurovascular signs including severe headache, confusion, hypotension, fever, diminishing consciousness, and death. The magnitude of exposure can often be assessed by the latency period from exposure to onset of nausea and vomiting with short latency of under 1 hour usually indicating a high dose in the 6 Gy range.

Assuming sufficient exposure to cause ARS, patients may pass through four phases: prodrome, latent phase, illness, and recovery. Prodromal symptoms and signs may include anorexia, nausea, vomiting, diarrhea, and fever. The prodrome is sometimes followed by a period of relative well-being prior to the onset of illness. In cases of exposure to higher doses of radiation, the latent period is shortened or eliminated. In the illness phase, the patient exhibits the findings consistent with the sub-syndromes described previously and commensurate with the dose received. With good supportive care about half of the patients exposed at the 6 Gy dose can be expected to survive beyond 2 months. Radiation

Table 13–7. Acute radiation syndrome clinical spectrum.

Dose in grays (Gy)	<2 Gy	2–6 Gy	6–8 Gy	8–10 Gy	>10 Gy
Time to vomiting	None expected at lower levels	4.5 h at 2 Gy	1 h at 6 Gy	2/3 h at 8 Gy	½ h at 10 Gy
Clinical syndrome	Subclinical hematologic	hematologic	Gastrointestinal (Pulmonary)	Neurologic Vascular	Neurologic Vascular
Clinical findings	Early declines in total lymphocytes and possibly other cell lines later	Bone marrow suppression Infection	Diarrhea Hematochezia Electrolyte imbalance Malabsorption Infection	Headache Confusion Fever Prostration Vascular instability	Convulsions Headache Confusion Fever Prostration Vascular instability
Key therapies	Decontamination and observation	Colony-stimulating factors Observation and Rx for Infection	Supportive Antibiotics	Supportive	Supportive Palliative
Mortality	No fatalities expected	Most Survive	Up to 50% exposed at 6 Gy survive with supportive care	Most die	Essentially 100% mortality

effects on other organs often complicate the clinical course and contribute to morbidity. Delayed effects following high-dose may include endarteritis obliterans, dry-eye syndrome, myelopathy, pericarditis, hepatitis, nephritis, coronary artery disease, intestinal stenosis, pulmonary fibrosis, and cataracts.

Reproductive effects. Absorbed doses to the testes as low as 0.15 Gy, may cause transient male reproductive system effects, including oligospermia. Doses in the 3- to 4-Gy range may lead to sterility in males. The ovarian dose to create sterility in women is in the range of 2–3 Gy. Fetal and embryo toxicity or death also can occur. Fetal growth retardation has been demonstrated with doses above 0.5 Gy. Radiation exposure to the fetus can also cause dose-dependent mental retardation, microcephaly, and increased risk of leukemia and solid tumors. By contrast, gonadal radiation has not been demonstrated to cause heritable genetic defects in humans, although animal models indicate that possibility.

▶ **Treatment**

The ARS patient should be decontaminated as necessary; hospitalized at tertiary care center; and receive consultation from hematology and infectious disease, as well as radiation exposure experts at REAC/TS. Serial complete blood counts with differentials and total lymphocyte counts every 6 hours for the first 2 days should be performed to monitor lymphocyte populations—a sensitive prognostic indicator of exposure. Vital signs; fluid and electrolyte balance; and hematopoietic, gastrointestinal, and CNS functions should be monitored closely. Consultation with a health physicist should be expedited to attempt to assess the radiation dose.

Key medical interventions are aimed at controlling nausea and vomiting, supporting hematopoiesis, controlling diarrhea, and preventing and treating infection. Ondansetron is

often effective for vomiting. Loperamide may be beneficial for diarrhea. Patients with marrow-threatening exposures should receive colony-stimulating factors (CSFs). Neutropenic patients are at risk for reactivation of viral infections, such as herpes, and prophylactic treatment should be considered. Careful monitoring for bacterial infection should also be maintained. Bone marrow transplants have been used with questionable success in combating intractable hemorrhage and infection and promoting survival.

3. Tissue Effects: Acute Localized Radiation Injuries

Industrial and medical radioactive sources are a relatively common cause of exposures causing local injury. Localized exposure of skin to ionizing radiation can result in dose-dependent adverse tissue effects including hair loss at 2–4 weeks (absorbed doses above 3 Gy), erythema (doses above 6 Gy), dry desquamation (10–15 Gy), wet desquamation (15–25 Gy), and necrosis. Surgical consultation should be obtained early in the course. Other key considerations are careful wound management, treatment of pain, and prevention of infections. To conserve joint motion and prevent contractures, splinting and physical therapy may be required during convalescence. Injuries should be followed closely because the extent of tissue damage often is not readily apparent. Subsequent fibrosis, ulceration, infection, necrosis, or gangrene may occur and require grafting. Radiodermatitis is a chronic tissue effect that often occurs as a consequence of ionizing radiation therapy. The skin is dry, smooth, shiny, thin, pruritic, and sensitive, and there are signs of telangiectasia, atrophy, and diffuse pigmentation. The nails are brittle and striated.

4. Other Tissue (Deterministic) Effects of Radiation

An increased risk of cataracts has been found in atomic bomb survivors and in employed populations such as those working with medical fluoroscopy. The typical lesion is a posterior subcapsular cataract, although other types of cataract have also been noted. The National Council on Radiation Protection has lowered its recommendation for ocular (lens) exposure to 50 mGy/y of absorbed dose in view of the concern that cataracts may develop at lesser doses than previously recognized.

It has been established that atomic bomb survivors and others with relatively high-dose external radiation exposure have an elevated risk of CVD. Recent studies of workers exposed to relatively low dose radiation (<0.1 Gy/y) in nuclear power-related industries have also shown an increased risk of CVD.

5. External and Internal Radionuclide Contamination

Skin contamination with radionuclides is rarely life-threatening. Immediate decontamination measures consist of gently scrubbing the skin with soap and warm water and, if necessary, cutting the hair. Hair clippings, material removed by scrubbing, swabs of the nares and mouth, clothing, and personal effects should be saved for radioactivity analysis and dosage calculation.

Inadvertent internal contamination with radioactive materials is less common than external exposure but may occur by inhalation, transdermal implantation, or ingestion at worksites where radionuclides are used. The health effects in these situations depend on the distribution kinetics of the radionuclide within the body to its target organ(s) (eg, radioiodine I-131 to the thyroid and strontium-90 to bone). For contaminated open wounds, irrigation should be performed and gentle surgical debridement considered. Depending on the type of radionuclide involved, administration of a chelating agent may be indicated. For plutonium and some other alpha emitters, diethylene-triamine-pentaacetic acid (DTPA) is effective and can be administered systemically, as well as in the wound irrigation solution. Agents that block uptake into target organs may also be considered, as in the case of iodine tablets for radioiodines. To assist with dose measurement, urine and feces for the first 24 hours (or longer) should be collected in consultation with a health physicist with experience in internal dosimetry. The reader is directed to other sources for a full description of the specialized management of internal contamination situations.

6. Stochastic Effects of Radiation

The principal stochastic effect of ionizing radiation that has been demonstrated in humans is a dose-related increase in the risk of cancer. Based on the International Commission on Radiological Protection's (ICRP) findings, there is approximately a 5% risk of a fatal cancer or other life-impairing health detriment per 1 Sv equivalent dose of whole body exposure to ionizing radiation. The effects of exposure are expected to be cumulative. However, there are uncertainties in making projections with low-dose numbers and adding doses over time. The age of the exposed individual, dose level and rate, and other individual characteristics are significant factors. The weight of scientific evidence points to a linear no-threshold model for cancer from ionizing radiation exposure. Human epidemiology has established that doses above 0.1 Sv cause an increase in cancer risk in an exposed population, and more recent studies point to an increased risk in the 0.05- to 0.1-Sv range. The Japanese Atomic Bomb Long Term Survivors Study has shown an increased risk of leukemia, developing 2 years after exposure and peaking at 8 years; it also has established an elevated risk for many solid tumors, beginning at 10 years after exposure and persisting over the survivors' lifetimes.

In addition, there are many corroborating findings of increased cancer risk from studies of medical radiation, occupationally exposed groups, and accidental exposures. Uranium miners have increased rates of lung cancer related to inhalation of alpha-emitting radon progeny (decay products). Radon progeny are also a significant contributor to lung cancer from contaminated dwellings. Findings from large cohorts of workers involved in nuclear industries indicted dose-related increases in leukemia, lymphoma, and solid cancers. Radiology technicians exposed to fluoroscopy and radiologists (the latter group historically) show increases in some cancers. Children exposed to radioiodine after the Chernobyl meltdown have had elevated rates of papillary cancer of the thyroid.

7. Stochastic Risks: Heritable Genetic Defects

Heritable genetic defects have not yet been demonstrated in humans as a result of ionizing radiation exposure. There has been careful study of offspring of survivors of the Japanese Atomic Bombs to assess this issue. Animal models have shown that heritable genetic abnormalities can occur, and this possibility requires ongoing research in humans.

Both tissue effects to the human fetus (as discussed previously) and stochastic risks in the form of increased cancer risk have been shown from ionizing radiation exposure to the embryo.

▶ Prevention

The prevention and control of radiation exposure in the occupational setting is based on three general principles as set out by the National Commission on Radiologic Protection and Measurement (NCRP):

- *Justification*: Decisions to permit an individual to be exposed require a solid rationale of overall benefit over harm.

- *Optimization*: The number of individuals exposed and the extent of exposure should be minimized by the best protective measures available under the circumstances. The principle "as low as reasonably achievable" applies.

- *Dose limits*: Exposures should not exceed numerical dose limits as recommended for occupational and nonoccupational exposures. Table 13–8 lists the recommended external exposure limits. Exposure limits apply to different human tissues and to the fetus. Exposures should be optimized below these levels whenever possible.

Occupational exposure to ionizing radiation must be monitored. The monitoring technology varies with the type of radiation and the target site. Personal exposure measurement devices include film badges (x-rays, gamma, and beta), thermoluminescent dosimeters (x-ray, gamma, beta, and neutron), and ionization dosimeters. For internal contamination, a scintillation counter can be used to measure some radioisotopes in urine specimens or in tissue from target organs. Environment- or area-monitoring devices include the Geiger-Müller counter, ionization chamber, and scintillation detector.

Ionizing radiation exposures can be prevented by limiting the amount of radioactive material used, shielding, reducing

exposure time, and increasing distance from the source. The use of lead or other high-density material that can shield the worker from the source is a common technique.

LASER INJURIES

The energy of the laser source is transformed through atomic excitation into a coherent, collimated, monochromatic beam of radiation. Lasers operate at one wavelength, usually in the UV, visible, or IR portion of the electromagnetic spectrum. They may emit radiation in continuous or pulsed waves.

The list of industrial laser applications that may result in human exposures is a long one and is growing. Familiar uses of low-power lasers using visible light include bar code scanning, laser pointers, and laser leveling. Moderate-power lasers can perform material cutting, soldering, and brazing operations. Medical applications include skin treatment, tattoo removal, and retinal surgery. Intense laser sources are used to cut hard metals and diamonds.

Lasers have been categorized by their ability to cause injury in the ANSI standard Z136.1. The basic categories are classes 1, 1M, 2M, 3R, 3B, and 4. These categories are based on the maximum power that the laser can generate at its wavelength over a given amount of time as measured in a standardized way. The maximum permissible exposure (MPE) indicates the highest energy density of a laser that is safe. Laser classifications provide some indication of relative hazard, but many other variables in the laser environment and application contribute to the overall risk. Laser safety officers are specially trained in the more sophisticated risk analysis, and should be consulted both in the prevention of and response to laser injuries.

Class 1 lasers are generally regarded as safe, although there is some risk of energy concentration through optical equipment with 1M lasers. Class 2 laser beams are not expected to ever cause injuries due to the blink reflex, again barring optical concentration of the 2M beam. Class 3 lasers have the potential to injure the eye, but not the skin. From a practical perspective, class 3R lasers are considered safe when handled carefully with restricted beam exposure; however, class 3B lasers can exceed the MPE and cause retinal injury both from direct eye exposure and potentially from non-diffuse reflections. One should be aware that not every laser is classified correctly: some green lasers labeled class 1 have been found to exceed the power level of that classification.

The nature, mechanism, and location in the eye of laser injuries depend primarily on the wavelength and power of the laser. Infrared lasers in the IR-B and IR-C wavelengths may cause thermal corneal injury as well as burns to lids and adjacent structures. UV lasers also may damage the cornea but the mechanism is photochemical denaturation. Visible and near-infrared laser radiation (IR-A) passes to the retina where it can produce injury by thermal, photochemical, or other energetic mechanisms. Permanent injuries have not been associated with repeated low-intensity exposures. Eye symptoms of accidental high-intensity laser exposure include photophobia or a sudden visual flash followed by scotoma or shadow of unusual size and color. Visual acuity or fields may

Table 13–8. External radiation exposure limits.

Occupational Exposure	Radiation Limit
*Stochastic Risks**	
Adults> 18 y	50 mSv)/y
	not to exceed 10 mSv times age in years
Individuals <18 y	Not to exceed 1 mSv/y
Embryo or fetus of pregnant worker (in declared pregnancy)	Not to exceed 0.5 mSv/mo equivalent dose to embryo/fetus
Radon in workplace	Include exposure in occupational limits if activity in air >300 Bq/m³ after radon mitigation
Tissue Effects	
Skin and extremities	Should not exceed 500 mGy/y averaged over most highly exposed 10 cm² of surface area
Lens of eye	Should not exceed 50 mGy/y
Public Exposure	
Stochastic Risks[a]	
Stable Source subject to advance control	Should not exceed 1 mSv/y
Radioactive material not previously subject to control	Should not exceed 20 mSv in first year, optimize protection in subsequent years
Radon in dwellings	Mitigate if activity >300 Bq/m³ in air
Tissue Effects	
Skin, extremities	Same as for occupational
Lens of eye	Should not Exceed 15 mGy/y

[a]Doses for stochastic risks are effective doses.
Source: Adapted from NCRP 180 (2018).

be reduced. Retinal changes, including edema, coagulation, hemorrhage, can occur, and the vitreous can be opacified. Prompt treatment for laser eye injuries by an ophthalmologist is important and often includes corticosteroids.

To prevent injuries, proper engineering and administrative controls are key considerations, and personal protective equipment, typically safety eye protection matched to the laser wavelength, must be used. A qualified laser safety officer should review controls, especially for class 3b and 4 lasers. Engineering controls may include enclosures and interlocks. The establishment of limited access areas is an important consideration.

Individuals working in proximity to high-power lasers should be instructed in proper operating procedures and provided with protective eyewear designed for the specific wavelength of the laser. In some cases, the eyewear does not by itself offer sufficient protection owing to possible laser reflections, or ultrashort laser pulses. Other devices, including door interlocks, barriers, and where possible, remote viewing equipment, should be considered. Skin protection is also important when high-power lasers are used. If feasible, systems should be designed with the beam line totally enclosed.

Preplacement examinations should be considered for individuals who will work with class 3B and 4 lasers and should consist of, at a minimum, the medical history, tests for visual acuity (near and far), refractive errors, visual fields, and inspection of the outer eye and skin. Baseline retinal photographs can be useful in evaluating patients after they have experienced a laser flash sensation. Skin exams should be considered for individuals with regular exposure to UV lasers. Routine periodic eye examinations are not recommended. Evaluation of workers following laser exposures should include an assessment of exposure intensity, wavelength, duration, viewing angle, and ANSI laser hazard classification. Medical evaluation, usually by an ophthalmologist, is recommended to assess the eye and surrounding skin, cornea, retina, and other ophthalmic structures.

ATMOSPHERIC PRESSURE DISORDERS (DYSBARISM)

Sudden shift to an environment of lower ambient pressure, as occurs with rapid ascension to the surface from deep-sea diving or with loss of cabin pressure while flying at high altitudes, causes decompression sickness (DCS); in its most severe form, DCS can be rapidly incapacitating or lethal. Acute pulmonary injuries are not uncommon with rapid ascent from diving, and may be difficult to differentiate from DCS. Compression sickness can also occur following movement to an environment of higher ambient pressure, but the most likely injury is localized barotrauma, as opposed to any systemic effects.

1. Decompression Sickness (Caisson Disease)

DCS results from mechanical and physiologic effects of expanding gases and bubbles in blood and tissue. When the body is exposed to an environment of higher than atmospheric gas pressure, as in tunneling or diving, it absorbs more of the inhaled gases than it does at sea level. Aided by its fat solubility, nitrogen concentrations increase in tissues, particularly those of the nervous system, bone marrow, and fat. Because the blood supply is poor in bone marrow and fat, nitrogen enters and leaves these tissues more slowly than oxygen or carbon dioxide does. As the surrounding pressure decreases (decompression), nitrogen expands and will form gas bubbles if there is insufficient time for its dissolution from tissues. Because oxygen and carbon dioxide have greater fluid solubility and move more easily between tissue compartments, their tendency for bubble formation is reduced. Remaining nitrogen gas bubbles are more destructive, especially in less elastic structures or tissues (eg, joints and CNS). Most cases of DCS have occurred after rapid ascension from sea depths in excess of 9 m (29.5 ft) or after sudden cabin pressure loss at altitudes in excess of 7000 m (22,966 ft).

▶ Clinical Findings

A complete evaluation of the systems affected—as determined by the history and physical examination—should be performed with appropriate x-rays and other diagnostic procedures. Anyone exhibiting signs or symptoms of DCS within 48 hours of a high-pressure exposure should be given a compression test in which 100% oxygen at 3 atmospheres (atm) pressure is administered for 20 minutes in a hyperbaric chamber. The U.S. Navy reports that 42 percent of cases present within 1 hour, and 98 percent of cases present within 24 hours.

The most common DCS classification scheme differentiates two types of DCS, as described next. The type and severity of symptoms will depend on the age, weight/body fat, smoking status and physical condition of the patient, the degree of physical exertion, the depth or altitude before decompression, duration of compression, and rate and duration of decompression.

A. Type I Decompression Sickness

This type, which has the best prognosis, affects the joints skin, or lymphatics. Acute pain, usually around a frequently used joint, may be incapacitating and cause the patient to assume a stooped posture (the "bends"). Patients may erroneously attribute musculoskeletal pain to acute trauma, overuse injury, or arthritis; the clinician must consider Type I DCS in their evaluation. Pain may begin immediately after decompression or up to 12 hours later and sometimes is accompanied by urticarial and bluish red mottling and itching of the skin ("diver's lice"). A more severe mottling with a marbled, raised appearance, known as cutis marmorata can sometimes signal later development of Type II DCS illness. Lymphatic obstruction can result in swelling and pain, especially distal to areas of anatomic lymph node concentration.

B. Type II Decompression Sickness

Type II DCS is more severe than Type I, and almost always includes neurologic symptoms. Symptoms and signs of central and peripheral nerve damage may include vertigo, "pins-and-needles" paresthesias, hypoesthesia, ataxic gait, hyperreflexia, Babinski sign, paralysis or weakness of the limbs, headache, seizures, vomiting, visual loss or visual field defects, incontinence, impaired speech, tremor, and coma. Pulmonary manifestations (the "chokes") may include substernal pain, chest tightness, severe coughing, dyspnea, pulmonary edema, and shallow respirations. Cardiovascular findings include arrhythmia and hypertension. Hypotensive shock due to central and peripheral nerve dysfunction occurs in the most severe cases.

Type 2 DCS, which is probably caused by gas bubbles in the CNS and spinal cord, may have significant sequelae, such as vascular obstruction and tissue infarction (which sometimes are accompanied by hemoconcentration, changes in osmotic pressure or lipid emboli, hemorrhagic infarcts of the lungs, ulcers of the colon, multifocal degeneration of white matter, and hypercoagulation of blood). Patients with any concern for any severity of type 2 DCS should be referred to a tertiary medical center, with hyperbaric capabilities.

C. Pulmonary Overinflation Syndromes (POIS)

POIS is characterized by the presence of pulmonary barotrauma-induced pneumothorax, mediastinal pneumomediastinum, or arterial gas embolism (AGE). AGE can mimic cardiopulmonary symptoms of Type II DCS, but both are treated emergently with compression and oxygen; AGE is also the second leading cause of death in divers (drowning is first). The primary mechanism for POIS is a diver who fails to adequately exhale while ascending, such as a diver who panics and swims rapidly to the surface. Ischemic stroke caused by AGE usually causes a more sudden and severe neurologic deficit than Type II DCS without AGE.

D. Other Conditions

A localized decompression-related illness is aseptic necrosis of bone, also known as dysbaric osteonecrosis (DON). This condition frequently involves the head or shaft of the humerus and less often involves either end of the femur or the tibial head. DON usually occurs 6–60 months following decompression and is asymptomatic unless there is joint involvement, which can cause permanent impairment. Radiographic examination may show bone sclerosis and mottling. Lesions are often symmetric. DON may be the result of nitrogen bubbles obstructing the capillaries and has been reported in up to 50% of technical divers and diving fishermen, although disability occurs in fewer than 3%.

An increased incidence of memory deficits, retrograde amnesia, emotional instability, and other neurologic and psychiatric symptoms has been observed in divers with a history of multiple episodes of any type of DCS.

▶ Prevention

Divers, underwater workers, and pilots should be screened to make that sure they are in good physical condition— not overweight and with no other conditions imposing an increased risk for dysbarism, such as vascular disorders,

hypercoagulopathy, obstructive airways disease, pneumothorax, sinusitis, otitis media, dehydration, substance abuse, or recent bone fractures. Workers should receive training and education in proper compression and decompression procedures and in recognizing the symptoms and signs of DCS.

▶ Treatment

A. Types I and II Decompression Sickness

The patient should be placed in a supine position. For immediate first aid, 100% oxygen should be administered, and aspirin may be given for analgesia. The patient should be transported rapidly to an emergency facility that has a hyperbaric chamber for recompression and decompression. Information about the nearest facility and advice about recompression can be obtained 24 hours a day by calling the National Divers Alert Network (DAN) at +1-919-684-8111.

In the hyperbaric chamber, the patient is placed in an atmosphere of raised pressure. The pressure then is reduced at a slow rate, with decompression pressures and schedules determined on the basis of the duration and pressure exposure of the inciting incident. Compression protocols vary by provider; the U.S. Navy treatment schedules are commonly followed in the United States. Breathing 100% oxygen by mask, alternating with breathing normal air should shorten the period of decompression. Some centers use oxygen-helium mixtures as an alternative to protocols requiring 100% oxygen in an effort to speed decompression without causing oxygen toxicity.

Corticosteroids, diuretics, or both can be used for cerebral or spinal edema. Volume depletion should be corrected with oral or parenteral fluids (normal saline or lactated Ringer solution). In severe cases, anticoagulation with heparin or plasma volume expansion with low-molecular-weight dextran 40 is effective. Diazepam is used for treatment of agitated or delirious states and oxygen toxicity if oxygen is administered during treatment.

In cases of type 2 sickness, decompression may take several days. Careful monitoring should be maintained to guard against oxygen toxicity of the lungs and CNS.

B. Stroke-like symptoms: Type II DCS and AGE

Type II DCS or AGE-induced neurologic injury often results in activation of a stroke code, however, unlike other ischemic strokes, medication-induced or catheter-based reperfusion strategies are not indicated. Recompression therapy with hyperbaric oxygen is the only reliable treatment, with some patients being able to make a full recovery, especially when treatment is initiated early.

2. Compression Sickness

When atmospheric pressure is increased, internal gases become compressed, usually with little effect. The common form of compression sickness is otic barotrauma, or barotitis. This can occur with descent of an aircraft from a high altitude, under water during diving descent, or during hyperbaric oxygen therapy, any of which causes a relative vacuum in the middle ear space if the auditory tube is already obstructed because of allergies or upper respiratory tract infection. Symptoms may include pain, fullness, dizziness, nausea, and vertigo. In more severe cases, the tympanic membrane may appear inflamed and retracted or ruptured.

Barotitis can be prevented in people at risk by avoiding high-pressure exposures or, for short exposures, by using oral and topical decongestants and descending slowly where practical. Barotitis is usually self-limiting but can be treated with pain control, decongestant nose drops, a nasal vasoconstrictor inhaler, or use of a Valsalva maneuver.

DISORDERS CAUSED BY VIBRATION

Vibration occurs when mechanical energy from an oscillating source is transmitted to another structure. Every structure has its own natural vibration level, including the human body as a whole and each of its parts. When vibration of the same frequency is applied, resonance (amplification) of that vibration occurs, often with adverse effects. For example, at a frequency of 5 Hz, whole-body resonance occurs, and the body acts in concert with externally generated vibration and amplifies that effect. In the occupational setting, vibration-related health concerns can be divided into two major categories—whole-body vibration (WBV) and hand-arm vibration. With a few exceptions, such as jackhammer use, they tend to occur separately.

1. Effects of Whole-Body Vibration

Truck and bus drivers, heavy-equipment operators, miners, and others exposed to long-term WBV have been reported to have a higher incidence of musculoskeletal, neurologic, circulatory, and digestive system disorders than does the general population. Low back pain, intervertebral disk damage, and spinal degeneration are found frequently. European studies have found associated bony abnormalities (intervertebral osteochondrosis and calcification of intervertebral disks) and adverse reproductive effects (spontaneous abortion, congenital malformations, and menstrual changes). "Vibration sickness," characterized by gastrointestinal problems, decreased visual acuity, labyrinthine disorders, and intense musculoskeletal pain, also has been reported in these workers. Despite these reports, a relationship between exposure intensity or quantity and the disorders found in occupationally exposed groups has not been clearly defined. Although many questions remain unanswered regarding the effects of long-term WBV exposure, neurologic and spinal effects appear likely.

The primary focus of research on WBV has been on the spine. Given the difficulty of studying vibration in isolation in workers with multiple risk factors (eg, lifting, prolonged sitting), the research is inconclusive but suggestive of a relationship between WBV and low back pain. There is evidence for increased mechanical stresses on the spine from WBV; enhanced strain due to harmonic resonance (especially around 5 Hz); and muscular fatigue. While contracting to cushion the force of vibration, the spinal musculature may not be able to adapt to the vibratory frequency, as a result contracting out of phase and increasing stress on the spine. Research on cadaver spine segments has shown that vibration can cause annual tears in the lumbar discs. In addition, many occupations settings with WBV (eg, tractors, train locomotives) are also subject also unpredictable erratic jolts that increase spinal loads.

The measurement of WBV exposure depends on factors such as the amplitude, acceleration, duration, and direction (in three planes) of the vibrating force. Several standards have been developed for measuring and controlling WBV, including The International Standards Organization (ISO) 2631 (2010), the ACGIH TLV's (2018), and the European Union Physical Agents Directive (2002). These standards provide methods to quantify and monitor vibration. Employers should try to appropriately control WBV exposures of their employees by limiting the duration of exposure. Equipment that separates workers from vibration, seating and engineering designs that reduce vibrations, and mechanisms that reduce jolts and impacts are appropriate protections. In addition, provision of rest breaks when transitioning from an activity involving WBV will allow for muscular recovery.

2. Vibration-Induced White-Finger Disease (Hand-Arm Vibration Syndrome)

Vibration-induced white-finger disease (hand-arm vibration syndrome [HAVS]) is an occupational injury caused by segmental vibration of the hands. In the United States, more than 1 million workers are estimated to have significant exposure to vibration from hand tools such as power saws, grinders, sanders, pneumatic drills, jackhammers, and other equipment used in construction, foundry work, machining, and mining. Although segmental vibration injury can occur with frequencies ranging from 5 to 1500 Hz, it usually occurs with frequencies of 125–300 Hz. Other factors affecting risk include the amplitude and acceleration of the equipment used and the duration of use.

HAVS is characterized by spasms of the digital arteries (Raynaud phenomenon) caused by vibration-induced damage of the peripheral nerve and vascular tissue, subcutaneous tissue, bones, and joints of the hands and fingers. The pathologic process also may involve arterial muscle wall hypertrophy; demyelinating peripheral neuropathy; excess connective-tissue deposition in perivascular, perineural, and subcutaneous tissues; and microvascular occlusion.

▶ Clinical Findings

Attacks of cold-induced vasospasm can last from 15 minutes to hours and are more likely to occur with exposure to the cold and with strenuous physical exertion. They are usually easily reversible if the individual is removed from vibration exposure. Early symptoms consist of tingling followed by numbness of the fingers. The fingers later begin to turn white in a cold environment or when cold objects are touched. Intermittent blanching often starts with the tip of one finger but extends progressively to other fingertips and eventually to the tips and bases of all fingers on the exposed hands. With increasing severity of disease, blanching or cyanosis of the fingers may extend into the summer season. Return of blood circulation (reactive hyperemia, or "red flush") following each episode is accompanied by redness and swelling, acute pain, throbbing, and paresthesias.

In more advanced cases, there may be degeneration of bone and cartilage, with resulting joint stiffness, restriction of motion, and arthralgia. Manual dexterity may decrease and clumsiness increase. With greater intensities of vibration, the period between exposure to vibration and the appearance of "white finger" is shorter. Diagnostic staging of HAVS is based on the Stockholm Workshop Scale from 0-SN to 3-SN based on vascular and neurologic symptoms and signs.

Diagnosis is based on exposure history and response to cold. Specific diagnostic tests can include finger systolic pressure response to cold stress, finger temperature response to cold, ultrasonic measurements of blood flow, thermography, and tests neurologic function (nerve conduction, two-point discrimination, vibration threshold, hot/cold perception). Nailfold capillary microscopy can be done to distinguish primary Raynaud disease.

▶ Differential Diagnosis

The diagnosis of HAVS is based on the occupational history of vibration exposures, the association of these exposures with episodes of Raynaud phenomenon (digital vasospasms), and exclusion of idiopathic Raynaud disease and other causes of Raynaud phenomenon, including trauma of the fingers and hands, frostbite, occlusive vascular disease, connective-tissue disorders, neurogenic disorders, drug intoxication, and exposure to vinyl chloride monomer. Carpal tunnel may coexist with HAVS and some symptoms may overlap.

▶ Prevention

Segmental vibration can be prevented by using ergonomically-designed tools with good grips, wearing gloves to minimize vibration and keep the hands warm, following a work-rest schedule that prevents long periods of exposure to vibration, and gripping the tool as lightly as safety allows. Workers should be instructed about the early symptoms and signs of HAVS and advised of factors that may place them at higher risk, such as the use of vasoactive drugs and cigarette smoking. Exposure limits developed by the ACGIH rely on measurements of the acceleration of the tool in each of three directional axes.

▶ Treatment

In most cases, symptoms and signs disappear in the early phase of the disease when the worker is removed from exposure to vibration. Other measures include avoidance of cold exposure (whole body and digits), smoking cessation, and avoidance of sympathomimetic drugs. More severe cases may require pharmacologic treatment with a calcium channel blocker (eg, nifedipine) for vasodilation. Other potential therapies include topical nitrates, phosphodiesterase 5 inhibitors. Chemical or surgical sympathectomy may be considered for more unresponsive cases.

HIGH-PRESSURE INJECTION INJURIES

Use of pressurized tools and systems in manufacturing and service industries occasionally results in severe injection injury. These puncture wounds fall into two broad categories: those caused by spontaneous leak or rupture of high-pressure hoses, and those caused by a sprayer or gun designed to eject material from a nozzle. Common types of materials injected include diesel fuel, oil, hydraulic fluid, paint and paint thinner, and to a lesser extent, air and water. The nondominant hand is the most common injury location, often during nozzle cleaning or troubleshooting, but other sites such as face, neck, leg, and foot have been reported.

▶ Pathogenesis

The type and amount of material injected, the anatomic location, and the velocity of injection determine the extent of injury. Hydrocarbons such as paint thinners and diesel fuel result in a high amputation rate (well over 50%), whereas air and water injections rarely result in amputation. The nondominant index finger is the most commonly injured body part, followed by the long finger. Materials from higher velocity injections travel along tendon sheaths or fascial planes, leading to widespread damage and diffuse foreign-body deposition compared to other types of puncture wounds. Injections over 1000 psi have been found to double the amputation rate compared to those less than 1000 psi.

Pathologic response occurs in three stages. The first stage involves acute inflammation associated with vascular compromise from tissue distension. Gangrene and/or infection often complicate the first stage. The second stage involves chemically induced inflammation and foreign-body granuloma formation. The late stage involves tissue fibrosis and breakdown of skin overlying granulomas, resulting in ulceration and subcutaneous sinus formation.

▶ Clinical Findings

With the initial event, the patient may feel a momentary stinging sensation; numbness and swelling are the initial symptoms. In fact, the initial appearance of the injury often does not reflect the severity of the injury, extending the time to appropriate treatment and resulting in worse outcomes. Most injuries appear similar to other benign puncture wounds, from which some of the injected material may be oozing. Pressure exerted around the puncture may increase the amount of oozing. There is no reliable method at the job site to determine whether the wound contains more widely dispersed material. However, there are fluorescent dyes available for oil and hydraulic system leak detection. These are also advertised as potentially useful for injection injury evaluation at remote work sites, by indicating whether there is a necessity for urgent medical transport.

Within a few hours, throbbing pain and pallor or cyanosis may develop. The pain sometimes is described as a burning sensation. Patients who do not seek immediate evaluation may present hours to several days later with leukocytosis and evidence of lymphangitis. Laboratory tests include radiography for evidence of radiopaque materials such as metals, cement, gypsum, and metallic paints. CT scanning has been used to demonstrate localized edema, gas pockets, and globe distortion involved in orbital injection injuries.

▶ Treatment

The goal of treatment is preservation of neurovascular structures. Aggressive decompression, debridement, and irrigation are recommended. Incision and debridement of devitalized tissues and removal of as much of the injected material should be done as soon as possible. Open debridement of all contaminated structures including tendon sheaths is recommended. Amputation may be required and is most frequent in injections involving paint or solvents. Pulsed-lavage irrigation, drainage, and open packing techniques have been used successfully. Delayed wound closure or closure by secondary intention is recommended.

Broad-spectrum antibiotic and tetanus prophylaxis, if indicated, should be provided. Early range-of-motion and intense physical therapy should be provided; twice-daily hand soaks in povidone-iodine and daily whirlpool treatments have been used successfully.

Initially, analgesics will be required, but local anesthesia, digital ring blocks, and Bier blocks should be avoided because of the risk of further vascular compromise. This results in nearly every serious case being admitted and taken to the operating room for general anesthesia. The value of steroid or dextran use has not been demonstrated for injection injuries, with the possible exception of steroids for high-pressure orbital injections, for which surgical debridement is more difficult or may not be appropriate.

▶ Sequelae & Prevention

Generally, high-pressure injection injuries occur in the workplace, with over 70% associated with a Workers' Compensation claim. Permanent deficits are virtually inevitable, including pain, range-of-motion limitation, loss of grip strength, paresthesias, hypersensitivity, and temperature intolerance. Average return to work takes longer than 7 months, with fewer than half of patients able to return to their previous job.

Various preventive approaches have been attempted, including adequate worker training and supervision, inspecting and replacing high-pressure lines more frequently, and mechanical solutions such as hydraulic line protective sleeves. However, safety gloves, including those with Kevlar and other specialized materials, have been unable to prevent or mitigate these injuries. As of 2015 a new glove was brought to market by a hydraulic servicing company. One manufacturer has developed a puncture-resistant glove that has been tested under ANSI Standards up to 10,500 psi in a UK safety lab; however, the performance of this glove under workplace conditions does not yet appear to have been carefully studied.

REFERENCES

Clark AT, Wolf S: Electrical injury. JAMA 2017;318(12):1198 [PMID: 28973623].

Johanning E: Whole-body vibration-related health disorders in occupational medicine—an international comparison. Ergonomics 2015;58(7): 1239-1252 [PMID: 25655650].

National Commission on Radiologic Protection and Measurement: Management of Exposure to Ionizing Radiation: Radiation Protection Guidance for the United States (2018). NCRP Report no. 180. https://ncrponline.org/shop/reports/report-no-180.

Ozasa K, Grant E, Kodama K: Japanese Legacy Cohorts: the life span study atomic bomb survivor cohort and survivors' offspring. J Epidemiol 2018;28(4):162-169 [PMID: 29553058].

Radiation Emergency Assistance Center/Training Site (REAC/TS): The Medical Aspects of Radiation Incidents. https://orise .orau.gov/reacts/.

U.S. Navy Diving Manual Revision 7 SS521-AG-PRO-010 0910-LP-115-1921 (PDF). Washington, DC.: US Naval Sea Systems Command.

Zafren K: Out-of-hospital evaluation and treatment of accidental hypothermia. Emerg Med Clin North Am 2017;35(2):261-279 [PMID: 28411927].

■ SELF-ASSESSMENT QUESTIONS

Select the one correct answer for each question.

Question 1: Systemic hypothermia
  a. is reduction of the body's core temperature below 35°C (95°F)
  b. onset is reliably symptomatic
  c. may result in hemoconcentration as a result of internal bleeding
  d. loss of consciousness is irreversible

Question 2: Heat stroke
  a. presents with increased alertness
  b. presents with cold, dry skin
  c. stabilizes as the core (rectal) temperature approaches 41.1°C (106°F)
  d. may cause cerebral, cardiovascular, hepatic, or renal damage

Question 3: Electrical injuries
  a. comprise up to 15% of all fatal industrial accidents
  b. from alternating currents are less dangerous than those from direct currents
  c. can cause not only tissue destruction and necrosis from heat and burning but also depolarization of electrically sensitive tissues such as nerve and heart
  d. involving currents exceeding 10,000 V freeze the worker to the source

Question 4: Acute radiation syndrome
  a. largely spares tissues with the most rapid cellular turnover
  b. primarily affects reproductive, hematopoietic, and renal tissues
  c. from doses exceeding 1000 cGy are uniformly lethal
  d. patients with significant exposure show an early spike in total lymphocyte count

Question 5: Decompression sickness (Caisson disease)
  a. results from mechanical and physiologic effects of toxic gases
  b. reflects nitrogen concentration in the nervous system, bone marrow, and liver
  c. symptoms are related to oxygen and carbon dioxide bubble formation
  d. occurs after rapid ascension from sea depths in excess of 9 m (29.5 ft) or after sudden cabin pressure loss at altitudes in excess of 7000 m (22,966 ft)

Question 6: Laser eye injuries
  a. only occur when looking directly into a laser beam
  b. are not related to the laser's power
  c. only occur with visible light lasers
  d. are much more likely when exposed to class 3b or stronger lasers

Question 7: High-pressure injection injuries
  a. should be treated conservatively and allowed to drain spontaneously
  b. usually occur in the dominant hand
  c. often require urgent debridement with delayed closure
  d. rarely result in amputation

Medical Toxicology

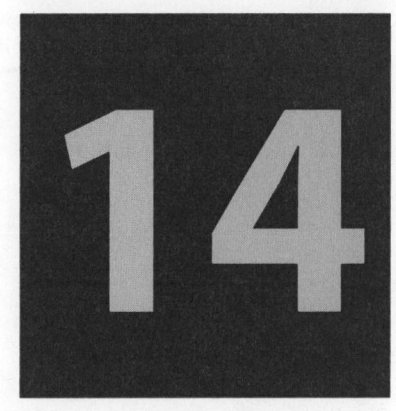

Timur S. Durrani, MD, MPH, MBA
Kent R. Olson, MD

Medical toxicology is a subspecialty focusing on the diagnosis, management, and prevention of poisoning and other adverse health effects due to drugs, occupational and environmental toxic substances, and biological agents. In the adult population all substances are potentially toxic; it is the dose that makes the poison. Many activities, including occupations and hobbies, can result in exposure to toxic substances. Although occupational exposure to toxic substances is considered to be underreported, it is estimated that 5% of all poison control consultations are occupationally related, suggesting a high rate of chemical exposure in the workplace. Table 14–1 lists selected activities and potential toxic exposures. Historically, many populations have also been recognized to be at risk for toxic environmental exposure (Table 14–2).

Toxicity does not necessarily equate with hazard. An extremely toxic chemical that is in a sealed container on a shelf has inherent toxicity but presents little or no hazard. However, when the chemical is removed from the shelf and used by a worker without appropriate protection, the hazard may become significant. The manner of use affects how hazardous the substance will be in the workplace.

TOXIC AGENTS & THEIR EFFECTS

▶ Classification of Toxic Agents

Toxic agents can be classified by their:

A. Physical State

A metal such as lead may be harmless in solid form, moderately toxic as a dust, and extremely toxic as a fume.

B. Chemical Structure

Chemical structure can determine toxicity. Often, one but not another isomer of a compound possesses toxicity. For example, aromatic amines are carcinogenic when substituted in other than the para-positions. The stability of a substance and the presence of impurities, contaminants, or additives can also affect toxicity.

C. Size

Nanoparticles are engineered structures that are less than 100 nm in size. These structures have demonstrated unique physical and chemical properties, which may be independent of the dose. Their small size and unique shape may facilitate absorption, theoretically allowing them direct access to the central nervous system via the olfactory nerve or causing increased fibrosis in the lung similar to asbestos. Due to their unique properties, these materials may display altered biological activity, which may result in positive health effects (eg, antioxidant effects, improved absorption for drug delivery), negative health effects (eg, unexpected toxicity, oxidative stress), or mixed effects. These materials are used in a number of products including computers, food storage containers, clothing, cosmetics, and medications. There is little known about their human toxicity. The measurement of dose and of levels in biological tissues may be difficult for some nanostructures.

D. Medium or Solution

The medium in which a toxic substance is found in part determines the population exposed and thus to some extent the hazard. Some toxic substances occur in a specific medium—for example, oxides of nitrogen in air (from vehicular exhaust), trihalomethanes in water (from chlorination), and nitrosamines in food (from nitrites). Often, the active chemical in a commercial product is dissolved in a liquid solvent because it is insoluble in water; the solvent may have potential toxicity independent of the active ingredient.

E. Site of Injury

Toxic agents can be described in terms of their effects on target organs (hepatotoxins, nephrotoxins, etc).

Table 14–1. Selected job processes at high risk for specific toxic exposures.

Job Process	Exposure
Aerospace and other specialty metal work	Beryllium
Artificial nail application	Methacrylate
Artificial nail removal	Acetonitrile, nitroethane
Artificial leather making, fabric coating	Dimethylformamide
Auto body painting	Isocyanates
Battery recycling	Lead and cadmium fumes and dust
Bathtub refinishing	Methylene chloride
Carburetor cleaning (car repair)	Methylene chloride
Cement manufacture	Sulfur dioxide
Commercial refrigeration	Ammonia, sulfur dioxide
Concrete application	Chromic acid
Custodial work	Chlorine (hypochlorite + acid mixes)
Dry cleaning	Chlorinated hydrocarbon solvents
Epoxy glue and coatings use	Trimellitic anhydride
Explosives work	Nitrate oxidants
Fermentation operation	Carbon dioxide
Firefighting	Carbon monoxide, cyanide, acrolein
Fumigation	Methyl bromide, methyl iodide, Vikane (sulfuryl fluoride), phosphine
Furniture stripping	Methylene chloride
Furniture and wood floor finishing	Isocyanates
Gas-shielded welding	Nitrogen dioxide
Gold refining	Mercury vapor
Hospital sterilizer work	Ethylene oxide, glutaraldehyde
Indoor forklift or compressor operation	Carbon monoxide
Manure pit operation	Hydrogen sulfide
Metal blade specialty cutting	Tungsten carbide-cobalt
Metal degreasing	Chlorinated hydrocarbon solvents
Metal plating	Cyanide, acid mists
Microelectronics chip etching	Hydrofluoric acid
Microelectronic chip doping	Arsine gas, diborane gas

(continued)

Table 14–1. Selected job processes at high risk for specific toxic exposures. (Continued)

Job Process	Exposure
Paint stripping	Methylene chloride
Paper pulp work	Chlorine, chlorine dioxide, ozone
Pool and hot tub disinfection	Chlorine, bromine
Pottery glazing and glassmaking	Lead dust
Radiator repair	Lead fumes
Rayon manufacturing	Carbon disulfide
Rubber cement glue use	*n*-Hexane, other solvents
Rocket and jet fuel work	Hydrazine, monomethylhydrazine
Sandblasting, concrete finishing	Silica dust
Sewage work	Hydrogen sulfide
Silo work with fresh silage	Nitrogen dioxide
Sheet metal flame cutting or brazing	Cadmium fumes
Structural paint refurbishing	Lead fumes and dust
Tobacco harvesting	Nicotine
Water treatment or purification	Chlorine, ozone
Welding galvanized steel	Zinc oxide fumes
Welding solvent-contaminated metal	Phosgene

Table 14–2. Examples of toxic exposures affecting public health.

Toxin	Incident
Lead	Widespread pediatric lead poisoning in Zamfara, Nigeria, due to unsafe mining practices
Arsenic	Estimated 70 million people exposed to arsenic due to well water contamination surrounding the Ganges delta in Bangladesh
Nitrates	Methemoglobinemia in infants due to nitrates in well water
Hydrogen sulfide	Frequent cause of multiple deaths in enclosed sewers or manure pits
Methyl isocyanate	3800 deaths in Bhopal India, due to accidental release in a pesticide plant
Methylene chloride	Widely used solvent in paint stripping, degreasing, decaffeination; recently recognized cause of death in bathtub refinishers
Methyl mercury	Minamata bay (Japan, 1950s); contaminated grain in Iraq (1972)

F. Mechanism of Action

Simple asphyxiants (inert gases, such as carbon dioxide) act by displacing oxygen in tissue without causing other toxic effects. In contrast, chemical asphyxiants such as carbon monoxide actively interfere with the delivery or utilization of oxygen by combining with hemoglobin to form carboxyhemoglobin, which decreases the oxygen-carrying capacity of the blood and inhibits release of oxygen to tissues.

G. Clinical Effects

1. Onset of effects—Toxic effects can be immediate, as occurs with some irritants that cause direct damage to tissues at the point of initial contact, usually resulting in inflammation; or delayed, as with chemical carcinogens.

2. Reversibility of effects—Whether or not the toxic effects of a substance are reversible depends on the capacity of damaged cells to regenerate or recover. For instance, brain and other nervous system cells have little capacity to regenerate, whereas liver and muscle cells are more likely to regenerate or recover after injury.

▶ Factors Affecting Clinical Response to a Toxic Agent

The following factors affect the dose-response relationship and the clinical response of humans to a toxic agent:

A. Duration, Frequency, and Route of Exposure

The severity of injury is related to the duration, frequency, and route of exposure. For example, ethylene glycol is toxic when ingested but poses little threat in the workplace except when sprayed or heated.

B. Environmental Factors

Toxicity is affected by atmospheric pressure, temperature, and humidity. For example, a concentration of carbon monoxide that has little effect at sea level can cause impairment of work capacity at an altitude of 5000 ft. Chemicals are more readily absorbed through skin that is injured or wet with perspiration and has increased blood flow in response to heat and humidity.

C. Individual Factors

Individual factors that determine "susceptibility" include racial and genetic background, age and maturity, gender, body weight, nutrition, lifestyle, immunologic and hormonal status, and presence of disease or stress. These factors are not independent of one another. For instance, genetic factors determine many of the other factors, and poor nutrition can affect immunologic status.

1. While much concern about the effect of age on individual susceptibility has focused on the fetus, the elderly also metabolize many chemicals less efficiently. As the work force ages, this may become an increasing concern.

2. The effect of nutritional deficiency on susceptibility to toxic agents has been of concern in developed countries primarily during war or famine, but it is relevant in developing countries as they industrialize. While toxicologic studies in animals readily demonstrate the effects of nutritional deficiency on susceptibility, the results of these studies are difficult to extrapolate to humans. There is controversy about the role of genetic factors and the development and use of genetic screening tests to identify individuals with increased susceptibility to toxic agents in the workplace. It is questioned whether such tests are accurate and whether job discrimination could result from their use as preemployment screening. Examples of genetic traits that might increase the risk of toxicity from exposure to chemicals or radiation glucose-6-phosphate dehydrogenase (G6PD) deficiency, sickle cell anemia, and α_1-antitrypsin deficiency.

G6PD deficiency is an X-linked recessive disorder that primarily affects African American males and persons of Mediterranean descent. Affected individuals are susceptible to hemolysis from many drugs. Some chemicals—notably naphthalene and arsine—can cause hemolysis following overexposure. There is no evidence that G6PD-affected workers exposed to these chemicals are at increased risk. Screening for G6PD deficiency is not supported by solid evidence of its utility.

Similarly, there is no evidence that any of the 7–13% of African Americans with sickle cell trait are at increased risk of hypoxia when working as airplane pilots or of hemolysis when working with hemolytic agents, despite the fact that these "risks" have been cited to justify screening of individuals for these occupations.

Severe α_1-antitrypsin deficiency, when present in the rare homozygous genotype, can lead to early emphysema in the absence of environmental agents. The more common heterozygous genotype, which affects 4–9% of the US population, may in combination with other factors place affected individuals at increased risk of developing emphysema from exposure to environmental agents.

TOXICOKINETICS & TOXICODYNAMICS

Toxicokinetics is the study of the movement of toxic substances within the body (ie, their absorption, distribution, metabolism, and excretion) and the relationship between the dose that enters the body and the level of toxic substance found in the blood or other biological sample. Toxicodynamics is the study of the relationship between the dose that enters the body and the measured response. *Simply put, toxicokinetics is the study of the effect of the body on the substance, and toxicodynamics is the study of the effects of the substance on the body.* The magnitude of a toxic response is usually related to the concentration of the toxic substance at its site of action.

Bioavailability

The bioavailability of a toxic substance indicates the extent to which the agent reaches its site of action. In some instances, an agent will be inactivated before it reaches the site of action. For example, when cyanide is taken orally, it is absorbed and passes to the liver, where the enzyme rhodanese may detoxify a portion of the ingested cyanide. On the other hand, if the cyanide in the form of gaseous hydrocyanic acid (HCN) is absorbed through the pulmonary circulation, it goes directly to the brain, where it may cause damage due to hypoxia.

Cell Membrane Permeability & Cellular Barriers & Cell Signaling

Absorption, distribution, metabolism, and excretion, all involve passage of toxic agents across cell membranes. Permeability is dependent on a toxic substance's molecular size and shape, degree of ionization, and relative lipid solubility. The distribution of some toxic agents is altered by unique cellular barriers, for example, the blood-brain barrier, the blood-testis barrier, and the placenta, which may exclude toxic substances.

Bone is an important deep reservoir for many heavy metals (especially lead) and for radioactive materials, and the effects of these materials can persist long after they have left the circulation. This storage property can be used in determining previous exposure and toxic burden. *Substances rely on many different cell signaling pathways to induce toxicity. These pathways include G-protein–coupled receptors (for muscarinic receptors that are susceptible to organophosphate agonism), ligand gated ion channels (used by nicotine), and intracellular enzymes such as soluble guanylate cyclase (used by nitrovasodilators such as nitrate).*

Absorption

The rate of absorption is dependent on the concentration and solubility of the toxic agent. Absorption is enhanced at sites that have increased blood flow or large absorptive surfaces such as the adult lung and gastrointestinal tract.

A. Gastrointestinal Absorption

The amount of absorption through the gastrointestinal tract is usually proportionate to the gastrointestinal surface area and its blood flow and depends on the physical state of the agent. Most toxic substances are absorbed in the small intestine. Therefore, agents that accelerate gastric emptying will increase the absorption rate, while factors that delay gastric emptying will decrease it. Some toxic substances may be affected by gastric juice; for example, the acidity of the stomach may release cyanide products and form hydrogen cyanide gas, which is even more toxic than the cyanide salt.

B. Pulmonary Absorption

The most common route of occupational exposure is pulmonary absorption. Gaseous and volatile toxic substances may be inhaled and absorbed through the pulmonary epithelium and mucous membranes in the respiratory tract. Access to the circulation is rapid because the surface area of the lungs is large and the blood flow is great. The nasal hair, the cough reflex, and the mucociliary barrier help prevent dust particles and fumes from reaching the lung.

The solubility of gases affects their absorption. Highly water-soluble gases such as ammonia and sulfur dioxide are absorbed in the upper airways and cause marked irritation there. This serves as a warning and may help limit the injury to the lung because the victim leaves the site of exposure. In contrast, noxious gases of lower water solubility such as nitrogen dioxide and phosgene, which have few early warning properties, can reach the bronchioles and alveoli and cause delayed injury (Table 14–3).

Table 14–3. Irritant gases.

Low Water Solubility (poor warning properties)	High Water Solubility (good warning properties)
Ozone	Ammonia
Phosgene	Chloramine
Nitrogen dioxide	Sulfur dioxide
Nitric oxide	Nitric acid

C. Percutaneous Absorption

Many toxic substances can pass through intact or broken skin. The amount of skin absorption is generally proportionate to the surface area of contact and to the lipid solubility of the toxic agent. The epidermis acts as a lipid barrier, and the stratum corneum provides a protective barrier against noxious agents. The dermis, however, is freely permeable to many toxic substances. Absorption is enhanced by toxic agents that increase the blood flow to the skin. It is also enhanced by use of occlusive skin coverings (eg, including clothing and industrial gloves) and topical application of fat-solubilizing vehicles. Hydrated skin is more permeable than dry skin. The thick skin on the palms of the hands and the soles of the feet is more resistant to absorption than is the thin skin on the face, neck, and scrotum. Burns, abrasions, dermatitis, and other injuries to the skin may alter its protective properties and allow absorption of larger quantities of the toxic substance.

The pH of the substance can affect the degree of tissue injury and ultimate skin. Highly acidic substances can cause an immediate coagulation-type necrosis that creates an eschar, which tends to self-limit further damage. In contrast, highly alkaline substances cause a liquefactive necrosis with saponification and continued penetration into deeper tissues, resulting in extensive damage.

D. Ocular Absorption

The eye is also a ready site of absorption. When chemicals enter the body through the conjunctiva, they bypass hepatic first-pass elimination and may cause systemic toxicity. Early decontamination of the eye may thus prevent systemic as well as local damage.

▶ Distribution of Toxins in the Body

After absorption, toxic substances are transported to various regions of the body. Some are removed by the lymph, and some insoluble compounds are transported through tissues such as the lung via cells such as macrophages. Most toxic substances enter the bloodstream and are distributed into interstitial and cellular fluids. The pattern of distribution depends on the physiologic and physicochemical properties of the material. The initial phase of distribution usually reflects the cardiac output and regional blood flow. Agents that penetrate membranes poorly are restricted in their distribution, and their potential sites of action are therefore limited. The blood-brain and blood-testis barriers limit the distribution of water-soluble but not lipid-soluble chemicals to these organs. Distribution may also be limited by the binding of toxic substances to plasma proteins. Toxic agents can accumulate in higher concentration in some tissues as a result of pH gradients, binding to special cellular proteins, or partitioning into lipids. Some agents accumulate in tissue reservoirs, and this may serve to prolong the toxic action, for example, lead may be stored for years in bone and may be released later. Some properties allow for substances to be removed by extracorporeal means such as dialysis. Substances with a small volume of distribution, low molecular weight, high water solubility, and low protein binding are more likely to be removed by dialysis.

▶ Metabolism

Before a toxic substance can be excreted, it may require metabolic conversion (biotransformation), for example, to a more water-soluble substance that can be eliminated in the urine. The most common site for biotransformation is the liver, but it can also occur in plasma, lung, or other tissue. Biotransformation may result in either a decrease (detoxification or inactivation) or an increase (activation) in the toxicity of a compound. Differences in the metabolism of toxic substances account for much of the observed differences between individuals and between animal species.

Biotransformation occurs in the liver by hydrolysis, oxidation, reduction, and conjugation. Microsomal cytochrome P450 metabolizing enzymes play a key role in the process by primarily catalyzing the oxidation of toxic substances. The activity of the CYP450 enzyme system can be increased (induced) by many environmental and pharmacologic agents. Individual differences in microsomal enzyme activity and susceptibility to induction are genetically determined and account for the marked variability in bioavailability of many toxic substances. Other factors that regulate key liver enzyme systems are hormones (which account for some gender-dependent differences) and disease states (eg, the presence of hepatitis, cirrhosis, or heart failure). Because the activity of many hepatic metabolizing systems is low in neonates—particularly premature neonates—they may be much more susceptible to toxic substances that are inactivated by liver metabolism. Inefficient metabolizing systems, an altered blood-brain barrier, and inadequate mechanisms of excretion combine to make the fetus and neonate more sensitive to the toxic effects of many agents.

▶ Excretion

A. Pathways and Mechanisms of Excretion

Toxic substances are excreted either unchanged or as metabolites. Excretory organs other than the lungs eliminate polar (water-soluble) compounds more efficiently than they eliminate nonpolar (lipid-soluble) compounds. The kidney is the primary organ of elimination for most polar compounds and metabolites. Excretion of toxic substances in the urine involves glomerular filtration, active secretion, and passive tubular reabsorption. Alkalization or acidification of the urine may dramatically change excretion of some agents. When tubular urine is more alkaline, weak acids are excreted more rapidly because they are ionized and passive tubular reabsorption is decreased. In contrast, when tubular urine is made more acid, excretion of weak acid is reduced.

Many toxic substances metabolized by the liver are excreted first in the bile and later eliminated in the stool. After biliary excretion, some substances are efficiently reabsorbed into the blood, a process known as enterohepatic recirculation. This recirculation can be a cause of repeat exposure and injury. This process can be interrupted by the use of binding agents, such as activated charcoal given in multiple doses. Toxic substances can also be excreted in sweat, saliva, and breast milk, and there may be some minor removal in hair or skin.

B. Clearance

Clearance is the rate at which a toxic agent is excreted, divided by the average concentration of the agent in the plasma. Most toxic substances are eliminated as a function of concentration; that is, a constant fraction of the toxic material is eliminated per unit of time, a process known as "first-order" elimination. If the point of saturation is reached, the body will no longer be able to eliminate a constant fraction of the material but will instead eliminate a constant amount per unit of time, a process known as "zero-order" elimination. Under these circumstances, the clearance becomes quite variable. Note that clearance is a measure not of how many *milligrams* of toxin is being removed but rather of the *volume* of fluid that is freed of the toxic agent per unit of time.

C. Volume of Distribution

The volume of distribution is calculated by dividing the amount of the toxic substance in the body (eg, a known dose) by the concentration measured in the blood. This number is not necessarily a physiologic volume; it is an "apparent" volume that reflects the degree of distribution of the toxic agent in tissues. The volume of distribution for most toxic agents depends on its size, pH, protein binding, partition coefficients, and regional differences in blood flow and binding to special tissues.

D. Half-Time and Half-Life

The time it takes for the plasma concentration of a substance to be reduced by 50% is the half-time. For substances that are eliminated according to first-order kinetics, the time it takes to eliminate 50% of the substance is called the half-life. For a substance eliminated by first-order kinetics, about 90% of the amount in the body will be eliminated in 3.5 half-lives after the end of the period of exposure.

TESTS OF TOXIC EFFECTS

Much of our information about the toxic effects of different agents comes from studying various strains and species of animals. Toxic substances frequently cause effects in animals, some immediately after administration and others after a prolonged period. Acute effects are sometimes qualitatively quite different from chronic effects. For example, the acute effect of benzene is central nervous system depression, while its chronic effects are aplastic anemia and leukemia.

Although tests in animals are the most common methods of identifying agents that cause toxicity, the results are difficult to extrapolate to humans, given the disparity among life spans (18–24 months for rodents vs 75 years for humans). In addition, different strains and species of animals may show both qualitative and quantitative differences in the pattern or intensity of response to a toxic agent. Even with the best statistical approaches and the best evidence of toxic responses in animals, there is no certain way of estimating the incidence of toxicity or determining the type of response to a toxic substance in a human population. Furthermore, there is no absolute certainty that safety factors for exposure to a toxic substance based on studies in animals would be valid for humans.

► Tests for Acute, Subacute, & Chronic Toxic Effects

Tests for acute effects are usually performed when there are no data available on the potential toxicity of a single exposure or a few exposures to a specific agent. An appropriate route of administration is chosen, and a specific end point (eg, death of the laboratory animal) is selected. The signs and symptoms before death are observed, and the animal is later examined for gross and histologic damage to tissues. In some cases, topical application of an agent is used to test for skin or eye injury.

Tests for subacute or sublethal effects of a specific agent are usually performed during a period of 21–90 days in animals, with the route of administration chosen on the basis of anticipated human exposure. Two different species of rodents are usually involved in each test.

Tests for chronic effects are performed in animals when long-term human exposure to a specific agent is anticipated or a long latency period between exposure and toxicity is expected. Rats and mice are usually exposed from a few weeks of age until their premature death or their sacrifice at the end of the expected lifetime. Short-term tests for genotoxicity, including mutagenicity, are used to prioritize agents for long-term testing or to provide supportive data for the results of long-term testing.

► Tests for Teratogenesis & Toxic Effects on Reproductive Organs

Teratologic tests involve exposing pregnant female animals to a specific agent at a critical time during pregnancy and then examining their offspring for malformations. Usually two or three species are used for comparison and controls. In reproductive studies, male and female animals are exposed to an agent and subsequently observed for reproductive failure or success. In cases of successful reproduction, the first- and second-generation offspring are also observed for their ability to reproduce. In cases of unsuccessful reproduction, male animals are often tested for sperm motility, count, and morphology.

TOXICOLOGIC RISK ASSESSMENT

► Steps in Risk Assessment

Risk assessment is the characterization of the potential adverse health effects of human exposure to hazardous substances. It can be divided into the following steps:

Step 1. Hazard identification—(a) Description of the population exposed to a substance (population at risk). (b) Determination of the adverse health effects that would be caused by that substance (eg, cancer and birth defects).

Step 2. Dose-response assessment—(a) Collection of epidemiologic and experimental dose-response data on the effects of the substance. (b) Identification of a "critical" dose-response relationship (discussed in detail below). (c) Quantitative expression of the dose-response relationship by mathematical extrapolation from high doses in animals to low doses in humans.

Step 3. Exposure assessment—Estimation of past, present, and future exposure levels of the population at risk and of actual doses received.

Step 4. Risk characterization—Estimation of the incidence of adverse health effects in the population predicted from the dose-response assessment (step 2) as applied to the exposure assessment (step 3).

► Uncertainties Inherent in Risk Assessment

There are a number of uncertainties inherent in risk assessment for toxic substances: (1) Human data are frequently lacking or are limited due to inability to detect low-incidence effects. Epidemiologic studies do not demonstrate causation or provide quantitative dose-response data, nor do they account for mixed and multiple exposures, a sufficient latency period for effects to be expressed, and differences between the populations studied. (2) Animal data are often of uncertain relevance to humans. A rational choice of the most appropriate species may not be possible. Toxicokinetic and toxicodynamic data are usually lacking. The route, frequency, and duration of exposure may be different from those of the human population. The doses are usually much higher, and the animals studied are genetically homogeneous and free of exposure to other toxic substances. (3) The mechanisms of action for effects are poorly understood. (4) The exposure of the population at risk may not be quantified, and calculation of doses may not be possible.

Because of these uncertainties, the practice of quantitative risk assessment is sometimes criticized for being "unscientific." However, since human exposure to toxic substances may result in medical and public health risks, risk assessment often provides the only basis for decisions on how to manage potential risks. Methods for estimation of health risk assessment are discussed in Chapter 55.

DOSE-RESPONSE CURVES

A dose-response relationship exists when changes in dose are followed by consistent changes in response, as shown in dose-response curves. A variety of toxicologic phenomena can be demonstrated by these curves. Figure 14–1 shows the intensity of the response to various doses in an individual. Line L depicts a linear response, where there is a linear relationship between dose and toxicity. Line T depicts a threshold response, where a toxic response is not elicited until a dose above a particular threshold is met. Line H depicts hormesis, a theoretical

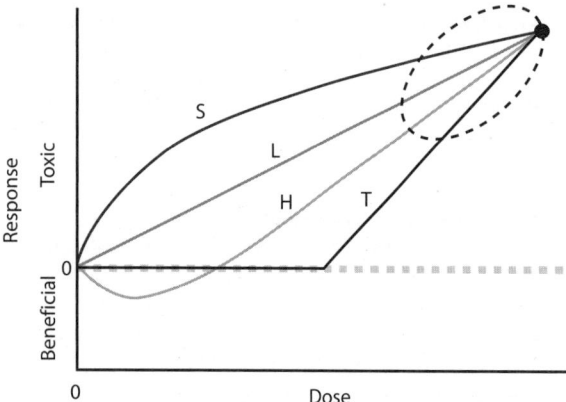

▲ **Figure 14–1.** In this figure, dose-response curves are abbreviated as follows: H = hormetic (biphasic); L = linear (no threshold); S = supralinear; T = threshold. The dose-response curves show the range of possible dose response relationships in an individual.

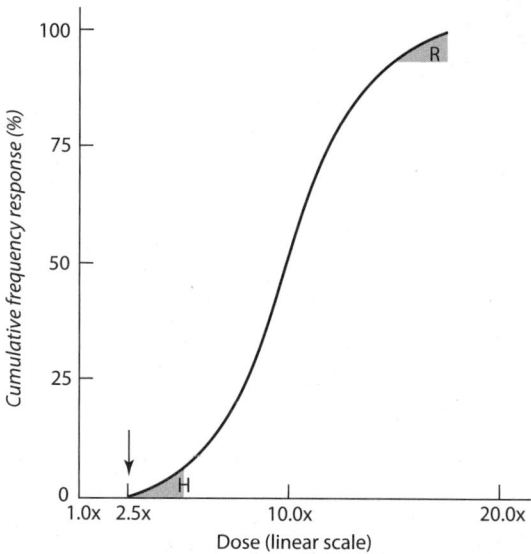

▲ **Figure 14–2.** The existence of a threshold in this dose response curve is indicated by the arrow. Doses below this point do not produce a response. Individuals who exhibit the response at doses well below the average or the mean are considered hypersusceptible (H), whereas those who respond only to doses well above the average or the mean are considered resistant (R).

dose-response, where a minimal dose results in a protective response, such as increasing detoxification ability, but at a higher dose, results in a toxic response, where by the organ can no longer detoxify and is subsequently harmed. Line S depicts a supralinear dose response, where toxicity is increased in relation to dose, particularly at the lower spectrum.

The frequency of a response in a population can be related to dose as a frequency distribution (as in Figure 14–2) or as a cumulative frequency (as in Figures 14–3 and 14–4).

In Figure 14–2, the existence of a threshold is indicated by the arrow at the point where the curve intersects the dose coordinate. Doses below this point do not produce a response. Individuals who exhibit the response at doses well below the average or the mean are considered hypersusceptible (H in Figure 14–2), while those who respond only to doses well above the average or the mean are considered resistant (R in Figure 14–2).

In Figure 14–3, cumulative frequency curves are used to compare two doses of the same toxic substance to the dose that is lethal to 50% of the population (LD50) and the dose that has an effect on 50% (ED50). The ED50 may, for example, represent an effect that is not harmful, such as odor. The ratio between comparable points on the curves (ie, the ratio of LD50 to ED50) will then represent the margin of safety for odor as a warning against a toxic or lethal effect.

In Figure 14–4, cumulative frequency curves are used to compare the doses at which the same toxic effect is elicited

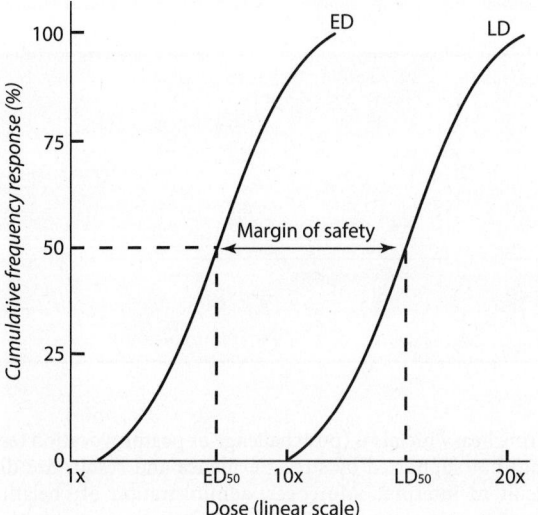

▲ **Figure 14–3.** Dose-response curves comparing two doses of the same toxic substance. ED = effective dose; LD = lethal dose. The area between the ED and LD is the margin of safety.

by three different toxic substances (A, B, and C). Substance A is clearly the most toxic, because at every dose level a greater percentage of the population exhibits the response to A than to B or C. The LD50, the ED10, and the threshold for A are all lower than the corresponding values for B and C. The comparison between B and C is less clear and demonstrates the need to consider the entire dose-response curves rather than individual points when comparing toxicities. Because the LD50 of B is lower than that of C, at this dose B is more toxic than C. However, because the ED10 of C is lower than that of B, at the lower dose C is more toxic than B. The shape of a dose-response curve is important for assessing the hazard of a toxic substance. A substance that has a low threshold and shallow dose-response curve (such as C) may be more hazardous at low doses, while a substance that has a steep dose-response curve (such as B) may be more hazardous as the dose increases. Adequate assessment of the hazard of a toxic substance requires evaluation of dose-response data over a wide range of doses.

DIAGNOSIS OF TOXIC EFFECTS

In general, the manifestations of acute toxicity due to high-dose exposures will be more overt than those due to chronic toxicity or toxicity associated with low-dose exposures.

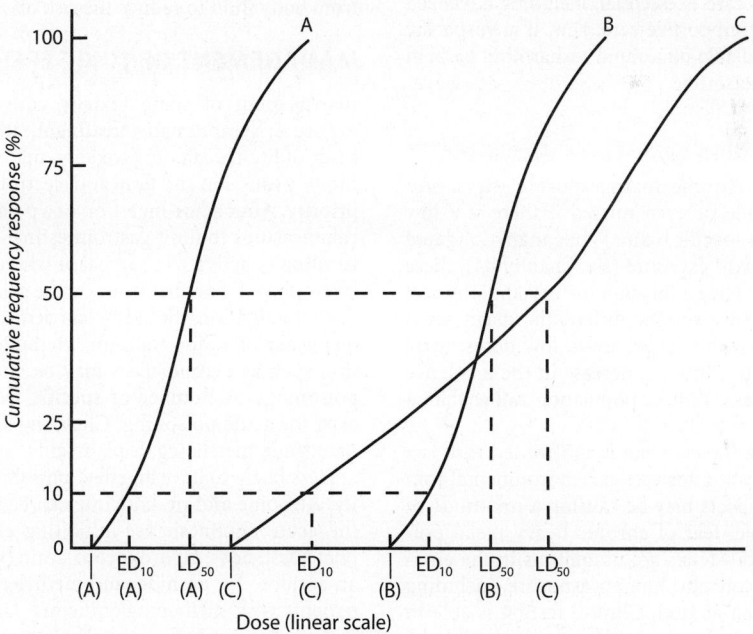

▲ **Figure 14–4.** Dose-response curves comparing the doses at which the same toxic effect is elicited by three different toxic substances (A, B, and C).

Table 14–4. Occupational/environmental toxic syndromes.

	Blood Pressure	Pulse Rate	Pupil Size	Sweating	Peristalsis
Sympathomimetic (cocaine or amphetamine intoxication)	+	+	+	+	−
Sympatholytic (opiate, ethanol, or benzodiazepine intoxication)	−	−	−−	−	−
Nicotinic (tobacco plant harvesting)	+	+	±	+	+
	−	−−	−−	+	+
Mixed cholinergic (organophosphate or carbamate pesticide exposure)	±	±	−−	+	+
Antimuscarinic (anticholinergic state, eg, from antihistamines)	±	+	+	−−	−−

Table 14-4 lists selected occupational exposures and their symptoms and signs.

ACUTE EXPOSURE

Recognition of symptoms consistent with toxic exposure is key to evaluating and ultimately ordering tests to confirm acute exposure. Vital signs including blood pressure and pulse rate as well as examination of the pupils, skin, and bowel sounds can assist in the diagnosis (see Table 14–4, Toxidromes). For example, a worker who becomes ill after harvesting tobacco may present with an increased blood pressure, heart rate, pupil size, and sweating, due to the toxic effects of nicotine absorbed across the skin. In the setting of an acute poisoning, access to adequate emergency care is essential, including advanced cardiac and respiratory supportive care. Few, if any, specific toxicologic tests are available on a rapid turnaround basis in the setting of an acute poisoning.

CHRONIC EXPOSURE

In cases of suspected chronic toxin exposure, signs and symptoms may be subtle or even missed if there is a low index of suspicion for a specific toxin. While many validated tests are available for toxin exposure (see Chapter 44), these tests are best employed after a through history and physical has been performed, and a specific differential diagnosis is being explored. With chronic exposure to low doses, toxic agents are more likely to cause an increase in the incidence of disorders already present in the population rather than a novel disorder.

A common scenario the clinician is confronted with is a patient who requests testing for various environmental toxins that the patient suspects may be causing a multitude of symptoms. For example, fear of chronic heavy metal poisoning is often invoked. Metals are ubiquitous in the environment, resulting in constant human exposure, including nonessential metals such as lead. Clinical testing is able to detect very low levels of heavy metals, at concentrations lower than those associated with known toxic effects. The practice of administering a chelating agent then testing for

urine heavy metals is (postchallenge or postprovocation testing) not supported by strong evidence and results are difficult to interpret. Moreover, administration of chelating agents can increase the elimination of some essential minerals such as iron, copper, and zinc.

Hair analysis has been used to determine exposure to heavy metals including arsenic, methyl mercury, and selenium and drugs of abuse including amphetamines. However, the results of hair testing are difficult to interpret as hair samples are subject to external contamination.

Trace metals analysis can be technically difficult, as specimens are easily contaminated during the collection process, including needles and vacutainers used in collection. Special care should be used in collection and testing of trace metals from body fluid to reduce the risk of contamination.

MANAGEMENT OF TOXIC EFFECTS

Management of acute toxicity consists of removal from exposure, symptomatic treatment, and supportive care. In cases of life-threatening toxicity, maintenance of cardiopulmonary function and fluid and electrolyte balance are of high priority. After acute ingestion of a poisonous drug or chemical, measures to limit gastrointestinal absorption by administration of activated charcoal or whole bowel irrigation may be employed. For chemicals on the skin or in the eye, topical decontamination should be carried out, usually with copious water or saline solution. Methods to enhance elimination such as hemodialysis may be effective for a few acute poisonings. A number of specific treatments or antidotes exist for acute poisoning. Chelating agents may help eliminate some metals (eg, lead, arsenic, and mercury), but they are less likely to have an effect on subacute or chronic toxicity. Atropine and pralidoxime can be lifesaving in reversing the acute cholinesterase-inhibiting effects of organophosphate pesticides. Hydroxocobalamin (vitamin B_{12a}) is used as an antidote for cyanide, and methylene blue can be used in patients with methemoglobinemia. Use of oxygen counters the effect and enhances the elimination of carbon monoxide. Table 14–5 lists several common antidotes used in occupational and environmental toxic exposures.

Table 14–5. Common antidotes used in occupational and environmental exposure.

Toxin/Exposure	Antidote
Methemoglobinemia	Methylene blue
Hydrogen cyanide	Hydroxocobalamin; sodium thiosulfate/sodium nitrite
Carbon monoxide	Oxygen
Animal or insect envenomations	Specific antivenom
Anticholinergics	Physostigmine
Organophosphates	Atropine, pralidoxime
Lead	EDTA, dimercaprol, succimer
Arsenic	Dimercaprol, succimer
Mercury	Dimercaprol, succimer

▶ **Carcinogens**

The International Agency for Research on Cancer (IARC) rates the carcinogenic potential of chemical agents for humans. The agency currently rates over 100 chemical agents as "known" carcinogens. These ratings are based primarily on human and animal data.

Although substances are implicated in the abnormal development of the fetus, less than 10% of birth defects can be attributed to exposure to a toxic substance. The human fetus is most susceptible to teratogenic agents in first 3–8 weeks of gestation. Known workplace teratogens include antineoplastic agents, carbon monoxide, mercury, lead, and tobacco smoke.

RESOURCES

American Associations of Poison Control Centers: www.aapcc.org
American College of Medical Toxicology: Toxicology Reference Data. https://www.acmt.net/resources_tex.html
International Agency for Research on Cancer: www.iarc.fr

■ SELF-ASSESSMENT QUESTIONS

Select the one correct answer for each question.

Question 1: Nanoparticles
   a. are engineered structures that are less than 100 nm in size
   b. have no chemical properties
   c. are blocked from the central nervous system
   d. are easily measured in biological tissues

Question 2: Toxicity
   a. affects all ages to the same degree
   b. is independent of racial and genetic background
   c. has no important genetic factors
   d. is affected by atmospheric pressure, temperature, and humidity

Question 3: G6PD deficiency
   a. primarily affects white males and persons of Mediterranean descent
   b. is an X-linked recessive disorder
   c. prevents hemolysis from many drugs
   d. screening is supported by solid evidence

Question 4: Biotransformation
   a. occurs in the liver by hydrolysis, oxidation, reduction, and conjugation
   b. is independent of microsomal cytochrome P450
   c. can be arrested by many environmental and pharmacologic agents
   d. is accelerated in neonates

Question 5: Clearance
   a. is the rate at which a toxic agent is excreted, multiplied by the average concentration of the agent in the plasma
   b. is a function of concentration in the urine, unrelated to dose
   c. is a measure of how many milligrams of toxin is being removed
   d. is a measure of the volume of fluid that is freed of the toxic agent per unit of time

Question 6: Hair analysis
   a. is used only for evaluating heavy metal exposures
   b. is the preferred method for evaluating toxic exposures
   c. requires little training in collection and analysis
   d. results are difficult to interpret as hair samples are subject to external contamination

Question 7: Management of acute toxicity
   a. consists of removal from exposure, symptomatic treatment, and supportive care
   b. first identifies the exact toxin so the appropriate antidote can be given
   c. follows contact with public health authorities
   d. focuses on preventing damage to the central nervous system

Clinical Immunology

Karin A. Pacheco, MD, MSPH

The immune system lies at the intersection of the external environment and internal host organ systems and modulates these interactions to protect the host from damage and disease. Although much of the response is organized to protect against infectious diseases, some responses are also directed against environmental irritants and agents that can perturb host homeostatic processes. In some cases, an unchecked or dysfunctional immune response in reaction to certain occupational exposures plays an important role in causing occupational diseases. This chapter will review the basic components and functions of the immune system and then discuss in more depth common occupational diseases driven by innate and adaptive immune responses.

OVERVIEW OF THE IMMUNE RESPONSE

The basic function of the immune system is to protect the host from invasion or damage by foreign organisms, first by distinguishing "self" from "nonself" antigens, then by elaborating a protective response, and finally by turning off the response once the danger threat has been neutralized. In most cases, such a response is beneficial. The exposures that turn on the immune response are carefully defined, and the response is orchestrated along set pathways. In some settings, however, where the immune response is directed against either irrelevant or self-antigens, or is overly aggressive or not downregulated, the system can trigger tissue damage and disease in the host.

Immune responses can be broadly categorized into innate versus adaptive immunity. Broadly speaking, the innate response is designed for rapid pattern recognition and neutralization, whereas the adaptive response is more targeted and specific, and takes time to be elaborated.

As a general principle, consider the immune system to function similarly to the Marvel comics character Daredevil. While technically blind, the system is constantly sampling the environment by shape, size, pattern, ion fluxes, pH changes, and other signals to distinguish self from nonself, and friend from enemy, to initiate the most appropriate and best response.

INNATE IMMUNITY

Most living organisms, from bacteria and plants to humans, possess a rapid innate system of immune responses based on basic pattern recognition that automatically triggers defensive responses. Innate immunity is present from birth, and, importantly, does not require previous antigenic exposure for the response. Four main components are considered to constitute the innate immune system.

1. **Physical obstacles**, including the intact skin and mucosal barriers of the gastro-intestinal and respiratory tracts, serve as the first line of defense. Colonization with beneficial bacteria, viruses, and fungi that constitute the normal human microbiome serve to limit availability of these potential ecological niches for growth of harmful organisms.

2. **Phagocytic barriers** mediated by neutrophils, macrophages, and natural killer cells (NK cells) serve as the next level of protection. **Neutrophils** are the most abundant of circulating white blood cells and are rapidly recruited to the sites of infection and inflammation by a gradient of chemotactic factors such as n-formyl bacterial peptides, complement derived C5a, LTB4, G-CSF and GM-CSF, IL-8, and certain antimicrobial peptides. The diffusion gradient left by these factors serves as a trail to guide incoming neutrophils to the site of action. **Monocytes** derive from bone marrow precursors and differentiate into effector macrophages after conditioning by specific tissue environments. Examples include interstitial and alveolar macrophages of the lung, Kuepfer cells in the liver, osteoclasts in bone, and microglia in brain and retina. Each resident, tissue-specific macrophage type can further differentiate into proinflammatory, microbicidal M1 macrophages, or anti-inflammatory M2 macrophages. **NK T cells** are T cells dedicated to the

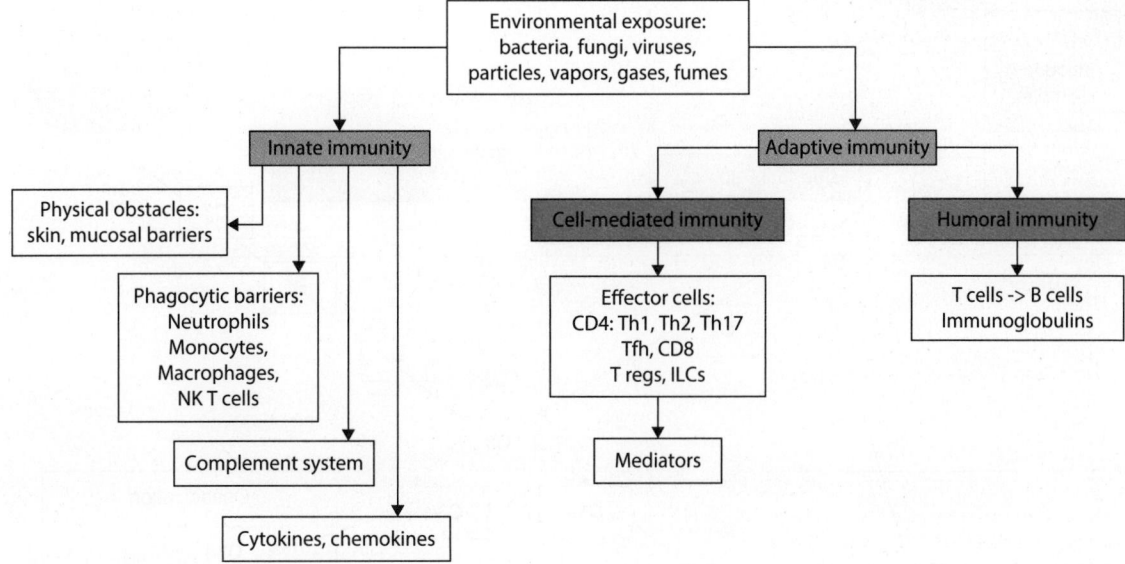

▲ **Figure 15–1.** Overview of the Immune System.

innate immune system and respond to precise molecular patterns. They do not express T-cell receptors specific for antigen, or surface immunoglobulins (Ig), and distinguish invaders from self by recognizing and binding to Major Histocompatibility Complex (MHC) Class I receptors. Viruses and tumor cells, because they downregulate their MHC Class I surface molecules, become more susceptible to recognition by NK T cells which then bind and release their granules containing perforins and granzymes.

3. The **complement system components** recognize and bind bacterial cell surface constituents (the alternative pathway), mannose binding protein attached to pathogen surfaces (the lectin pathway), or antibody bound to pathogen surface antigens (the classical pathway related to adaptive immunity). Complement binding creates pores in the target cells leading to their destruction or apoptosis.

4. **Cytokines and chemokines** produced by neutrophils, macrophages, and NK T cells lay down a trail to the site of action and initiate and mediate inflammatory reactions designed to clear the pathogens. A number of cytokines are produced by cells specific to the innate immune system (Table 15–1).

PATTERN RECOGNITION RECEPTORS

The key to the specificity of the innate immune response lies in pattern recognition receptors (PRRs) that are targeted to critical and distinguishing microbial surface proteins. PRRs can be secreted and circulating molecules, as well as stationary receptors present on effector cell surfaces or in their cytoplasm.

Secreted and Circulating PRRs

Some PRRs are released directly into the circulation and function to coat microbial pathogens for binding, ingestion, and killing by phagocytic cells. These include antimicrobial/ host defense peptides, collectins, lectins, and pentraxins.

1. **Host defense peptides** respond to bacterial invaders and manage the normal host bacterial load and diversity of the microbiome. **Defensins** are secreted primarily by neutrophils and epithelial cells and bind specifically to the negatively charged phospholipids present in bacterial outer membranes, but are not attracted to animal cell membranes, which contain cholesterol. Binding leads to pore formation, loss of membrane integrity, and bacterial cell death. **Beta defensins** constitute a large gene family, including **human alpha defensins 1–4** contained in the azurophilic neutrophil granules, and **human beta defensins 1–6** expressed on all epithelial cell surfaces and induced by inflammatory cytokines released from damaged epithelium. **Cathelicidins** are another group of cationic antimicrobial peptides stored in the secretory granules of neutrophils and macrophages, and also released by epithelial cells, with activity against bacteria, enveloped viruses, and fungi. They neutralize lipopolysaccharide (LPS) from gram-negative bacteria and are important in wound healing, angiogenesis, and clearing apoptotic cells. One role of vitamin D in immunity is to induce the expression of specific cathelicidin LL-37. Interestingly, organisms of the normal microbiome are relatively resistant to the effects of host defense peptides.

2. **Collectins** contain a tail characteristic of collagen molecules, and a lectin or carbohydrate-binding domain at

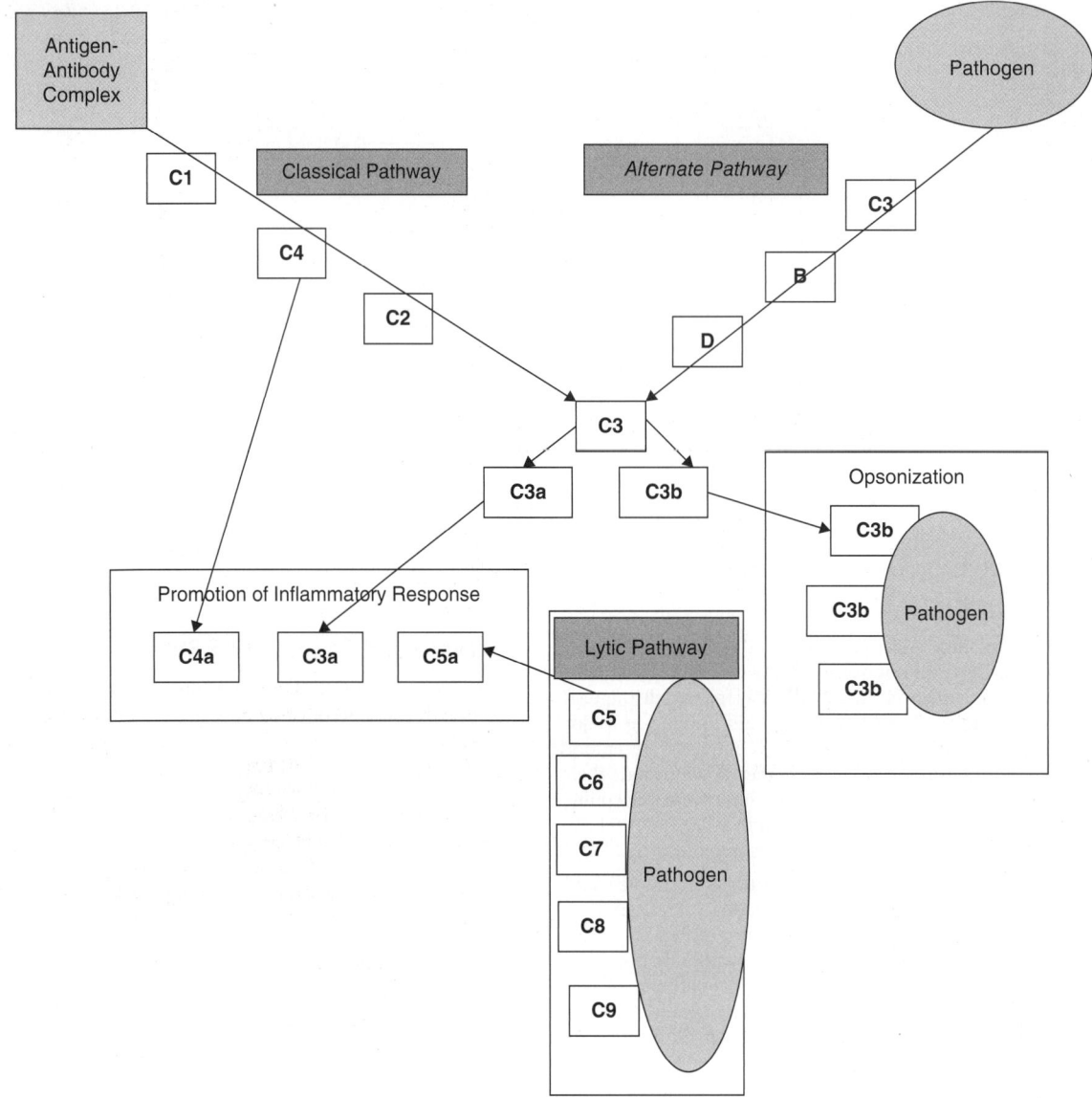

▲ **Figure 15–2.** Complement pathways.

the head; the two regions joined by a neck region. Collectins bind to carbohydrates in microbial cell walls and label the cell for destruction or promote uptake of apoptotic cells. Examples include the first component of complement, **C1q**, and **pulmonary surfactant proteins A and D** that bind to oligosaccharides on microbial cell membranes to mark and opsonize them for destruction.

3. **Lectins** are ubiquitous proteins that bind to specific carbohydrate structures on pathogen cell surfaces to identify

them for complement-mediated destruction or disrupt cell membranes and kill these directly. Subtypes include **Galectins**, that recognize the β-galactoside carbohydrate structure, **Ficolins** that bind N-acetyl glucosamine, and the **annexin family**, defined by calcium-dependent membrane phospholipid binding proteins. In cancer biology, aberrant expression of carbohydrate residues by tumor cells evades lectin binding and cell destruction.

4. **Pentraxins** are acute phase reactants secreted in response to toll-like receptor (TLR) binding or proinflammatory

Table 15–1. Cytokines of the innate immune system.

Cytokine	Cellular Source	Function
TNF-α	Macrophages and T cells	Activates endothelial cells and neutrophils Induces fever and synthesis of acute phase proteins
Type I Interferons (IFN-α, IFN-β)	Macrophages and fibroblasts	Activate NK cells Induce expression of MHC-I
IL-1	Macrophages and endothelial cells	Activates endothelial cells and neutrophils Induces fever and synthesis of acute phase proteins
IL-6	Macrophages, endothelial and T cells	Induces synthesis of acute phase proteins Induces proliferation of B cells and antibody production
IL-10	Macrophages and Th2 cells	Induces proliferation of B cells Inhibits proinflammatory cytokine production and MHC-II expression
IL-12	Macrophages and dendritic cells	Activates NK and T cells Induces synthesis of IFN-γ Increases cytolytic activity Induces differentiation of T cells toward Th1 cells
IL-15	Macrophages	Induces NK and T-cell proliferation
IL-18	Macrophages	Activates NK and T cells Induces IFN-g synthesis
Chemokines	Macrophages, endothelial and T cells	Induce chemotaxis and cell activation

Source: From Chapter 2, Innate immune system Beatriz Aristizábal and Ángel González. *Autoimmunity: From Bench to Bedside* [Internet]. Anaya JM, Shoenfeld Y, Rojas-Villarraga A, et al, eds. Bogota (Colombia): El Rosario University Press; 2013 Jul 18. © 2013 Universidad del Rosario. NCBI Bookshelf. A service of the National Library of Medicine, National Institutes of Health.

cytokines TNF-α or IL-1β. **C-reactive protein** (CRP) and **serum amyloid P** are short pentraxins, and **Pentraxin 3** (PTX3) is a member of the long pentraxins. PTX3 binds strongly to *Aspergillus fumigatus, Pseudomonas aeruginosa*, and C1q and launches the classical pathway of complement activation and pathogen destruction. PTX3 also plays a key role in initiating and driving the development of cardiovascular disease (CVD), thus highlighting the association of CVD with inflammation.

C-reactive protein was initially identified as an opsonin for strep pneumoniae. Its inflammatory activity is also measurable in sterile settings and levels can be increased in cardiac, autoimmune, and other inflammatory conditions.

Membrane-bound PRRs

Membrane-bound PRRs are constitutively expressed on many innate immune cells, as well as on antigen presenting cells including macrophages, dendritic cells, monocytes, and B cells. They recognize conserved pathogen-associated molecular patterns (PAMPs) which are uniquely associated with the pathogen and fundamental to its survival such that it cannot be easily mutated to evade host PRRs. The major classes of PRRs include TLRs, RIG-1-like receptors (RLRs), NOD-like receptors (NLRs), and C-type lectins (Table 15–2).

TLRs are the most important and ubiquitous PRRs. TLRs 1–2, 4–6, and 11 localize to the plasma membrane, and bind circulating host-derived damage-associated molecular patterns or DAMPs. Specific TLRs (3, 7, 8, 9, and 10) are internal and reside in endolysosomes containing host enzymes that break down bacterial and viral invaders. These TLRs recognize foreign nucleic acid taken up into endolysosomes and stimulate the production of antiviral cytokines IFN-α, IFN-β, and IFN-γ. The class shares an Myd88 signaling pathway that induces NF-Kappa-B and AP-1 (activating protein-1), which then induce production of proinflammatory cytokines IL-1β, TNF, and IL-6.

RIG-1-like receptors (RLRs) are intracellular RNA helicases found in most tissues. They detect short pieces of single- or double-stranded RNA viruses that have invaded the host cell to trigger downstream type 1 interferon production that initiates antiviral defences. The RLR family includes RIG-I (retinoic acid-inducible gene I), MDA5 (melanoma differentiation associated factor 5), and LGP2 (laboratory of

Table 15–2. Pattern recognition receptors and their ligands.

PRRs	Localization	Ligand	Origin of the Ligand
Toll-like Receptors (TLRs)			
TLR1	Plasma membrane	Triacyl lipoprotein	Bacteria
TLR2	Plasma membrane	Lipoprotein	Bacteria, viruses, parasites, self
TLR3	Endolysosome	dsRNA	Virus
TLR4	Plasma membrane	LPS	Bacteria, viruses, self
TLR5	Plasma membrane	Flagellin	Bacteria
TLR6	Plasma membrane	Diacyl lipoprotein	Bacteria, viruses
TLR7 (human TLR8)	Endolysosome	ssRNA	Virus, bacteria, self
TLR9	Endolysosome	CpG-DNA	Virus, bacteria, protozoa, self
TLR10	Endolysosome	Unknown	Unknown
TLR11	Plasma membrane	Profilin-like molecule	Protozoa
RIG-I-like Receptors or Retinoic Acid-Inducible Gene-I-like Receptors (RLRs)			
RIG-I	Cytoplasm	short dsRNA, 5′triphosphate dsRNA	RNA viruses, DNA virus
MDA5	Cytoplasm	Long dsRNA	RNA viruses (Picornaviridae)
LGP2	Cytoplasm	Unknown	RNA viruses
NOD-like Receptors, or Nucleotide-Binding Oligomerization Domain-like Receptors (NLRs)			
NOD1	Cytoplasm	iE-DAP	Bacteria
NOD2	Cytoplasm	MDP	Bacteria
C-Type Lectin Receptors (CLRs)			
Dectin-1	Plasma membrane	β-Glucan	Fungi
Dectin-2	Plasma membrane	β-Glucan	Fungi
MINCLE	Plasma membrane	SAP130	Self, fungi

Source: From Takeuchi O, Akira S. PRRs and inflammation. Cell 2010;140:805-820.

genetics and physiology 2). Dysregulated RLR expression is associated with the development of autoimmune diseases.

NLRs, or NOD-like (nucleotide-binding and oligo-merization domain) receptors, recognize both structural motifs of bacterial peptidoglycans (PAMPs) and host DAMPs. NLRs are highly conserved throughout both plant and animal evolution, and in humans are found in lymphocytes, macrophages, dendritic cells, and epithelial cells. Their binding activates an NF-κ-B cascade also leading to the production of proinflammatory mediators. Mammalian NLRs are divided into four families (A, B, C, and P) based on variation in the N-terminal domain. After the NLR binds a ligand, the auto-inhibitory leucine

rich repeat (LRR) changes conformation to expose the N-terminal domain which forms a complex with limited numbers of repeating units. These NLR platforms recruit and activate the inflammatory protease caspase-1 and are referred to as **inflammasomes**. Caspase-1 is required to process inflammatory cytokines IL-1β and IL-18 and leads to an inflammatory form of cell death termed pyroptosis. Given the importance of NLRs, genetic variants have been implicated in a number of human diseases.

The **AIM-2** inflammasome binds dsDNA from viruses and bacteria, and engages ASC (apoptosis-associated speck-like protein containing CARD [caspase activation and recruitment domain]) to form a caspase-1 activating inflammasome in dendritic cells and macrophages. It is essential in the response to *Francisella tularensis,* vaccinia virus, and *Listeria monocytogenes.* **DAI (DNA-dependent activator of IFN regulatory factors)**, functions as a dsDNA sensor that dimerizes using DNA as a scaffold, causing activation of type I IFN genes. Other surface PRRs include the **macrophage scavenger receptor** which binds bacterial cell walls, the **macrophage mannose receptor** which recognizes fungal carbohydrates with terminal mannan, **Dectin-1** which recognizes fungal membrane beta-glucan, and the **formyl peptide receptor** specific for bacterial membrane n-formyl methionine. These serve to opsonize bacteria and/or fungi for lysis.

RAGE (receptor for advanced glycation end-products) belongs to the immunoglobulin superfamily and is encoded by a gene located in the MHC class II region on human chromosome 6. It is expressed by immune cells and binds many of their secreted products that act as DAMPs. Binding activates NFκB, which translocates to the nucleus and turns on innate and adaptive cytokine genes, antiapoptotic genes such as Bcl proteins, the MAP kinase signaling pathway inducing cell proliferation, and TGF-β signaling cascades of the Ras homolog family and Rho-associated kinase, which set in motion stable actin filament formation and subsequent cell migration. Conversely, soluble RAGE molecules bind to DAMPs to prevent cell activation. Abnormal RAGE signaling pathways are associated with several human diseases, including diabetes, cancers, and CVDs, and hence blockade of the RAGE pathways is being investigated as treatment.

Pathogen recognition receptors are keyed to conserved **PAMPs** that are distinct from the host. Typical PAMPs include LPS, peptidoglycan, lipoteichoic acids, mannans, unmethylated microbial DNA, viral RNA, and polysaccharides and proteins specific to pathogens but not the host.

Some PRRs also recognize host-derived danger signals known as **DAMPs (danger or damage associated molecular patterns)**. These are host derived macromolecules released by damaged tissues that trigger a noninfectious, sterile, inflammatory response (Table 15–3). For example, ATP is one of the oldest and best-conserved DAMPs that activates PRRs, NLRP3, and the inflammasome in both plants and animals. Other DAMPs include heat shock proteins (HSP), mRNA, ssRNA, hyaluronic acid, and heparin sulfate. DAMPs may also trigger systemic inflammatory responses and persistent tissue damage and remodeling in myocardial infarctions, type 2 diabetes, Alzheimer disease, as well as malignant and infectious diseases.

THE INFLAMMASOME

Inflammasomes are large, three-dimensional, multimolecular structures that assemble in response to signals from cellular damage or microbial invasion, that is, triggering by DAMPs or PAMPs to elicit inflammation. The classic or canonical inflammasome complex consists of three main components: (1) a cytosolic sensor protein such as an NLR or ALR protein, (2) a central adaptor protein ASC, and (3) an effector protein caspase procaspase-1. ASC orchestrates the activity of the inflammasome with an N-terminal pyrin domain (PYD) that binds to the sensor, and a c-terminal CARD that binds to the caspase procaspase-1.

> **Importance for Occupational Medicine**
> The inflammasome is the innate immune basis for the fibrotic responses that characterize silicosis and asbestosis.

Assembly of the inflammasome is triggered by activation of the sensor, that then recruits the ASC component which serves as a scaffold for the procaspase-1. When assembled, procaspase-1 undergoes auto proteolysis to active caspase-1 which cleaves the pyroptosis effector molecule GSDMD as well as pro-IL-1β and pro-IL-18 to generate active cytokines which initiate a protective cascade. IL-1 and IL-18 are different from other cytokines whose expression is induced by specific inflammatory signals. Instead, IL-1 and IL-18 are constitutively expressed in a "pro" form and can be quickly activated when needed by the assembly of the inflammasome.

The sensor can be activated by four different methods: (1) traditional binding of microbial products, such as NLRC4 to flagellin or bacterial secretory proteins, (2) reactivity to microbial proteases, such as murine NLRP1b and anthrax lethal factor, (3) reactivity to changes in cellular signaling cascades, such as PYRIN-Rho GTPase, and (4) sensing of the loss of integrity of the host membrane, such as potassium efflux.

Once assembled the inflammasome functions as a structure for caspase activation. Activated caspase-1 not only cleaves pro-IL1-β and pro-IL-18 into active moieties, it also can induce pyroptosis, a proinflammatory form of lytic cell death, by cleavage and activation of the pore-forming gasdermin gene family. These proteins bind to acidic phospholipids such as phosphoinositides found on the inner leaflet of mammalian plasma membranes to form pores leading to cell death. Such pores will also cause potassium efflux, the major trigger of NLRP3 inflammasome assembly. In contrast, necroptosis, a programmed form of necrotic cell death, is triggered by ligand binding of cytosolic death domains of the TNF superfamily receptors (including TNFR1, CD95, TRAIL-R1, and TRAIL-R2). Whereas pyroptosis triggers a primary cellular response after sensing damaging messages such as pathogen ligands, DAMPs, and altered host metabolites, necroptosis is considered a backup cell death defense mechanism that comes into play when apoptosis is blocked during pathogen infection.

NLRP3 INFLAMMASOME

The NLRP3 is among the best characterized inflammasome and one of the most relevant to occupational lung diseases. It is expressed in granulocytes, monocytes, macrophages,

Table 15–3. Danger-associated molecular patterns (DAMPs) and their receptors.

Origin		Major DAMPs	Receptors
Extracellular matrix		LMW hyaluronan	TL42, TLR4, NLRP3
		Heparan sulfate	TLR4
		Fibronectin (EDA domain) (extra-domain A)	TLR4
		Fibrinogen	TLR4
		Tenascin C	TLR4
Intracellar compartments	Plasma membrane	Syndecans	TLR4
		Glypicans	TLR4
	Cytosol	Uric acid	NLRP3, P2X7
		S100 proteins	TLR2, TLR4, RAGE
		Heat shock proteins	TLR2, TLR4, CD91
		ATP	P2X7, P2Y2
		F-actin	DNGR-1
		Cyclophilin A	CD147
		Amyloid β	TLR2, NLRP1, NLRP3, CD36, RAGE
	Nuclear	DNA	TLR9, AIM2
		Histones	TLR2, TLR4
		RNA	TLR3, TLR7, TLR8, RIG-I, MDA5
		HMGB1 (high mobility group box protein 1)	TLR2, TLR4, RAGE
		HMGN1 (high mobility group nucleosome binding domain 1)	TLR4
		IL-1α	IL-1R
		IL-33	ST2
	Mitochondria	mtDNA	TLR9
		TFAM (transcription factor A, mitochondrial)	RAGE
		Formyl peptide	FPR1
		mROS (mitochondrial reactive oxygen species)	NLRP3
	ER (Endoplasmic Reticulum)	Calreticulin	CD91
	Granules	Defensins	TLR4
		Cathelicidin (LL37)	P2X7, FPR2
		EDN (eosinophil-derived neurotoxin)	TLR2
		Granulysin	TLR4

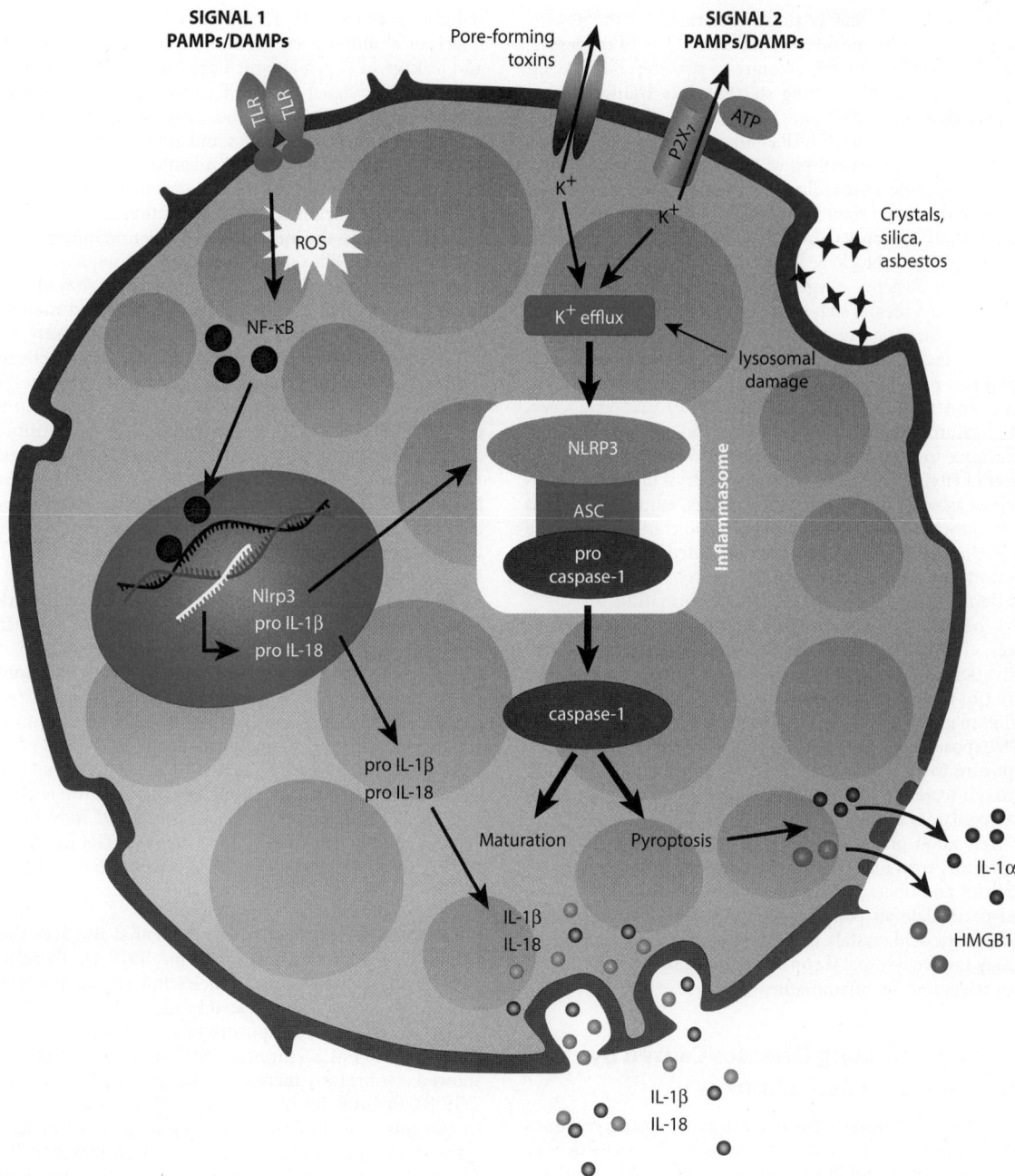

▲ **Figure 15–3.** Structure of the inflammasome.

and dendritic cells and is similarly formed by the assembly of NLRP3 with the adaptor protein ASC and caspase-1. The NLRP3 inflammasome requires a two-step mechanism to be activated. The priming step involves transcriptional upregulation of NLRP3 and pro-IL-1β by TLR signaling. Then assembly of the NLRP3 inflammasome is triggered by sensing potassium efflux, which is the pathogenic effect of a pathogen-derived molecule and an indirect measure of cell viability, rather than by recognizing the pathogen itself. Other NLRP3 agonists damage cellular integrity by high osmotic pressure, blockage of glycolysis, and oxidative phosphorylation. Reactive oxygen species can prime the inflammasome but a second step is still needed to activate it.

Many other triggers serve to assemble the NLRP3 inflammasome, including interaction with nucleic acids, muramyl dipeptide, pore-forming toxins such as pneumolysin, nigericin, and maitotoxin, extracellular ATP, uric acid crystals, hyaluronan and heparin sulfate, and amyloid-β fibrils. Relevance to occupational medicine includes the triggering effect of environmental large inorganic crystalline structures such as asbestos and silica, nanoparticles, adjuvants such as aluminum hydroxide (alum), and ultraviolet irradiation. The NLRP3 inflammasome can also be activated by irritants such as trinitro phenyl chloride, trinitro chlorobenzene, and dinitro fluorobenzene which cause contact dermatitis.

Whereas many of the NLRP3 triggers involve acute exposures, chronic exposures may down regulate inflammasome activation. For example, whereas acute, short-term LPS exposure (up to 4 hours), followed by ATP, activates the NLRP3 inflammasome in macrophages, prolonged (12–24 hours) LPS exposure has the opposite effect. In this setting, longer exposure to LPS reduces NLRP3 inflammasome activation through secretion of IL-10 and caspase-8 activation, a negative regulatory element.

Activation of the NLRP3 inflammasome in cells of the respiratory tract manages the response to a variety of inhaled particles and fibers including asbestos, silica, nanoparticles, and particulate air pollution. Ingestion of diverse particles such as uric acid crystals, alum, hydroxyapatite, and amyloid B may induce lysosomal rupture and release of cathepsin B, thus triggering an inflammatory cascade.

Occupational Lung Diseases Caused by Inflammasome Activation

1. Silica and asbestos—The innate immune system responds to disruption by particulates such as silica and asbestos with an inflammatory and fibrotic reaction. The NALP3 inflammasome is a key factor in the pathway of IL-1β secretion stimulated by asbestos and silica particulates, where inflammasome activation manages the balance between tissue repair and inflammation induced by inhalation of these particles. NALP3 $^{-/-}$ (knock-out) mice exposed to asbestos particles by inhalation showed decreased recruitment of lymphocytes, eosinophils, and neutrophils to the lungs and

reduced secretion of IL-1β. Uptake of silica crystals, asbestos fibers, or aluminum salts leads to lysosomal destabilization and leakage of enzymes which are interpreted as an endogenous danger signal and lead to the secondary activation of the NALP3 inflammasome. Indeed, the inflammatory response to inhalation of silica and asbestos, and subsequent development of fibrosis, is dependent on the NALP3 inflammasome and abrogated in NALP3 deficient species.

Inflammasome priming and activation are speculated to play a key role in the initial lung and pleural injury induced by asbestos and silica particles, as well subsequent development of fibrosis. The NRLP3 inflammasome may also contribute to the development of lung cancer and malignant mesothelioma seen with these exposures. Conversely, some data suggest that inhibition of the inflammasome activation pathway and/or inflammasome produced cytokines can diminish the fibrotic response in both *in vitro* and *in vivo* disease model. For example, treatment with the antifibrotic drug pirfenidone in mice with acute lung injury induced by LPS, was able to reduce lung inflammation and fibrosis by blocking NLRP3 inflammasome activation. This indirectly suggests that pirfenidone may be beneficial in treating lung fibrosis because it targets the major pathway: persistent NLRP3 activation.

Because the severity of silicosis varies among workers with similar dust exposures, genetic variants of key factors in the process, including NALP3, caspase-1, and IL-1β, may play a role in the magnitude of the outcome. A case control study of 179 workers with silicosis and 201 workers without silicosis from a large cohort working in an iron mine in China examined the interactions of genetic variants of these three factors on susceptibility to silicosis. After adjusting for age, smoking status, and cumulative dust exposure, subjects with the T allele of Ex4-849 C -> T versus CC in Nalp3, and the GA genotype of Ex2+37 G -> A versus GG in caspase-1 had significantly increased risks of silicosis, 2.40 (1.12–5.12) and 3.62 (1.63–8.02) respectively.

2. Particulates—Fine particulate matter has also been shown to activate the NLRP3 inflammasome. THP-1 cells cultured with PM 2.5 will ingest the particles and activate the NLRP3 inflammasome as demonstrated by markedly elevated secretion of IL-1β. *In vivo* exposure of mice to increasing concentrations of PM 2.5 through oropharyngeal aspiration also showed significantly increased concentrations of IL-1β and TGF-β1 in bronchoalveolar lavage (BAL) fluid compared to controls. Trichrome-stained lung tissue after 21 days of exposure to fine particulates revealed increased collagen deposition around small airways suggesting a potential pathway of lung inflammation and fibrosis.

3. Cigarette and other smoke—Development of chronic airway inflammation in chronic obstructive pulmonary disease (COPD) is thought to be caused by inhalation of noxious particles, most commonly cigarette smoke although other particulate exposures behave similarly. Their effect is to trigger sustained activation of NLRP3. Cigarette smoke exposure can activate TLR4 and also cause epithelial cell injury resulting in release of DAMPs from lung tissue. These will activate the NLRP3 inflammasome leading to release of IL-1β, with higher serum levels shown to correlate with increased severity of COPD, and suggesting that COPD is a state of chronic inflammation. Increased levels of mRNA from NLRP3, caspase-1, ASC, IL-18, and IL-1 β have been found in bronchial biopsies of COPD patients with acute exacerbations compared to smokers without exacerbations and those with stable COPD. Levels of IL-1 β and IL-18 in both serum and BAL fluid supernatants, an indirect measure of NLRP3 inflammasome activation, were significantly higher in the same COPD patients with acute exacerbations.

4. Asthma—A subset of patients with severe, predominantly neutrophilic asthma have markers of inflammasome activation in their airways, presumed important in the pathogenesis of this subset of the disease. Sputum from these patients demonstrates significantly higher levels of extracellular DNA (eDNA) released from neutrophils, and neutrophil extracellular traps (NETs) derived from eDNA and known to activate inflammasomes, compared to others with severe asthma but without the neutrophilic signature. Sputum levels of NLRP3, along with other markers of inflammasome activation, including caspase-1 and IL-1β, are also significantly increased in these patients.

Interestingly, the link between silicosis and autoimmune disease may lie in the crossover effect of inflammasome activation. Priming of inflammasomes is increased in autoimmune disease either due to genetic polymorphisms or the chronic proinflammatory cellular environment including cellular debris released from damaged cells. NLRP1, NLRP3, and AIM2 inflammasomes are all known to be activated in autoimmune diseases and play key roles in tissue injury and organ damage. For example, IL-1β and IL-18 levels in BAL fluid and in BAL fluid macrophage cultures were significantly elevated in rheumatoid arthritis (RA) patients with interstitial lung disease (UIP) consistent with chronic inflammasome activation. Although data are incomplete and somewhat conflicting, NLRP3 inflammasome activation has also been linked to systemic lupus erythematosus (SLE), RA, systemic sclerosis (SSC), and inflammatory bowel disease (IBD). This mechanism may explain the association between silicosis and the development of autoimmune diseases such as RA, SLE, and SSC.

The Adaptive Immune Response Requires Activation by Innate Immune Triggers

Found in lymph nodes, skin, and mucosal surfaces, dendritic cells and other antigen presenting cells (APCs) link innate with adaptive immunity. They are the crossover cells that express pathogen recognition receptors activated by PAMPs and DAMPs, and, in response to activation, release inflammatory cytokines, express costimulatory molecules such as CD80 (B7-1) and CD86 (B7-2), and process and present antigen to initiate the more targeted adaptive immune response. They regulate adaptive immunity by determining the appropriate effector class of response: whether an antigen should initiate a cell-mediated response or an antibody-mediated response. Dendritic cells are the only APCs able to present antigen and activate naïve T cells, and as such, are essential for initiating a primary adaptive immune response. In addition, mast cells and basophils express TLRs and contain preformed granules containing vasoactive substances, histamine, cytokines, and chemokines that direct immune traffic to the site of inflammation and modulate dendritic cell activation, antigen presentation, and expression of costimulatory molecules necessary to engage and activate specific T cells. Basophils also produce IL-4 necessary for TH2 differentiation and responses to parasites and allergens.

In addition, inflammasomes and IL-1 family cytokines are instrumental in T-cell activation and memory cell formation. IL-1α or cleaved IL1β bind to IL1-R, trigger a short-lived release of IL-2, and upregulate IL-2R surface expression to expand naïve and memory T cells and prolong T cell help to B cells for antibody production. Inflammasomes and their IL-1 family cytokines initiate adaptive immune responses to infection and vaccination, as well as in autoimmunity including multiple sclerosis (MS), RA, SLE, and cancer.

Interestingly, NLRP3 is also expressed in T cells, but rather than being cytosolic, is localized to the nucleus. Here, it lacks the ability to form inflammasomes, but specifically controls TH2 cell differentiation. NLRP3 interacts with transcription factor IRF4 (interferon regulatory factor 4) and then binds to the promoter regions of TH2 cytokine genes to induce their expression. In contrast, NLRP12 is a negative regulator of cell inflammation by dampening NF-Kβ and Extracellular signal-regulated kinase (ERK) activation. It downregulates osteoclastogenesis, impairs neutrophil migration, and negatively regulates T cell IL-4 production. There is also evidence that, in turn, the adaptive immune system exerts control on inflammasome signaling. CD4 T cells constitutively express pro-IL-1β, and if activated, can release active IL-1β which may serve as an autocrine survival signal for pathogenic T cells.

Hence, although the innate and the adaptive immune system are often considered separately, the two responses orchestrate together for maximum speed, efficiency, and precision in host protection.

ADAPTIVE IMMUNITY

The adaptive immune response is also characterized by pattern recognition, similar to innate immunity, but of greater specificity for individual foreign (and occasionally self) antigens. Whereas innate immunity systems are found throughout the animal kingdom and in many plants, the adaptive component of the immune system is present only in higher animals. Compared to innate immunity, the adaptive immune system is capable of developing far more specific responses to foreign antigens, with the potential for immune memory and thus faster protective responses with each subsequent encounter with the antigen. Different from the innate response, the primary adaptive responses occur distant from the site of antigen encounter, in regional lymph nodes, rather than in the directly affected tissue. The cost to this system of immunity is time—initial responses generally require 10–14 days to be fully expressed—and known as latency. With immune memory, however, subsequent responses can develop in hours to days, rather than weeks, and is the basis for vaccine success. Such a system also requires regulatory procedures to suppress immune responses to self-antigens and to dampen and turn off the adaptive response when it is no longer needed. Decreased function of the regulatory system underlies the development of autoimmunity, allergy, and persistent inflammatory states. Conversely, excessive downregulation of the adaptive immune system can be permissive for the development of cancer.

> **Importance of occupational medicine:**
> The time, a minimum of 1–2 weeks and usually months to years, to develop a specific adaptive immune response is the source of **latency** observed for immune occupational diseases such as asthma, sinusitis, or Hypersensitivity Pneumonitis (HP).

The essence of the adaptive response is the unsystematic generation of T cells and B cells with a vast, but random array of multiple possible antigen specificities that are subsequently whittled down to the most specific responses. Hence, the repertoire of adaptive responses is tremendously diverse, with an estimated 10^9 antigenic specificities that can be elaborated to match the enormous array of external antigens. Adaptive immunity is not an efficient system, as it is on the development of so many random antigen specificities, many of which will be irrelevant and subsequently deleted. However, it is an effective system, in that it is capable of recognizing and responding to almost all potentially dangerous antigens and invaders, and can do so with memory.

MHC I versus II

The key receptors that present antigens to adaptive immune cells and trigger immune activation are the major histocompatibility complex or MHC. The general function of the MHC is to bind peptide fragments derived from pathogens and foreign antigens and to display these on the cell surface for recognition and subsequent activation of selected T cells.

The MHC class I is a glycoprotein cluster present on the surface of nearly all nucleated cells, consisting of an alpha chain with three domains (α1, α2, and α3) associated with β2-microglobulin. Differences in the sequence of the peptide-binding groove of the receptor mean that different MHC I

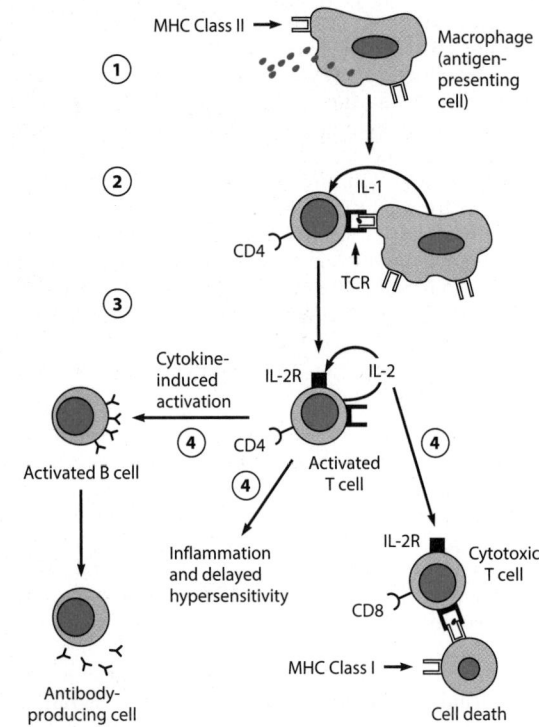

▲ **Figure 15–4.** The normal MHCII immune response.

molecules bind many different peptides, although limited to short peptides 8–10 amino acids in length. Hence, a single MHC I gene is able to bind the same short peptide derived from many different larger foreign proteins. The *human* MHC I gene cluster is located on chromosome 6, and codes for three different alpha chains: human leukocyte antigens (HLA) A, B, and C gene products that are highly polymorphic. Peptides presented by MHC I are typically viral proteins taken up by phagocytosis/endocytosis or forced entry by the virus, broken down into short fragments, loaded onto an MHC I complex in the endoplasmic reticulum, and then transported back to the cell surface. MHC I receptors then present these short peptide antigens to cytotoxic CD8+ T cells.

In contrast, MHC class II receptors are limited to a few types of APCs, including macrophages, dendritic cells, B cells, and activated endothelial cells. Genes coding for MHC II receptors are adjacent to those for MHC I on chromosome 6 and include HLA-DR, HLA-DP, and HLA-DQ. MHC II also consists of two, alpha and beta, peptide chains. Extracellular pathogens such as bacteria are taken up by these APCs, processed into peptides, and then loaded in the endoplasmic reticulum onto the MHC II peptide-binding groove by displacing the invariant chain peptide. Translocated to the cell surface, MHC II plus antigen interacts with CD4+ T helper cells to activate them.

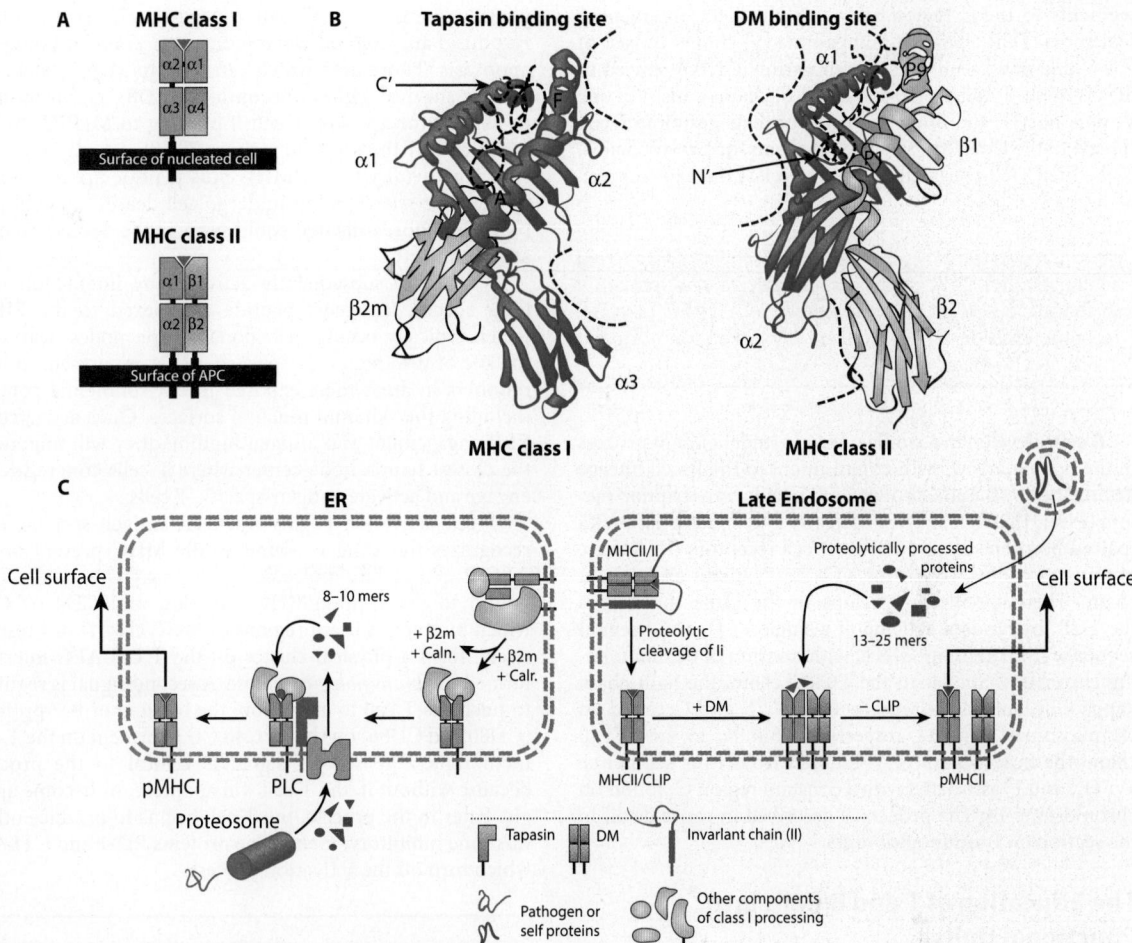

▲ **Figure 15–5.** Structural characteristics of MHC class I and MHC class II proteins and their compartment-dependent loading with processed peptides. **A.** Domain topology of a pMHC class I and pMHC class II complex. **B.** Structure of HLA-A68 in complex with an HIV-derived peptide (PDB: 4HWZ, left) and HLA-DR1 in complex with a hemagglutinin-derived peptide (1DLH, right). Indicated are the supposed interaction sites of MHC class I with tapasin and of MHC class II with DM as dashed gray lines. The peptide is shown in yellow with its N and C-terminus marked and relevant pockets are labeled green. **C.** Simplified illustration of MHC class I (left) and II (right) processing and peptide-editing pathways. Caln., calnexin; Calr., calreticulin; CLIP, class II-associated invariant chain peptide; ER, endoplasmic reticulum; PLC, peptide loading complex. (Used with permission from Wieczorek M et al: Major Histocompatibility Complex (MHC) Class I and HMC Class II Proteins: Conformational Plasticity in Antigen Presentation. 2017;8:292, Fig. 3)

CELLULAR (T CELL) AND HUMORAL (B CELL) ADAPTIVE IMMUNITY

The fundamental nature of adaptive immunity is based on a highly regulated interplay between T cells and B cells. The two share a similar method of developing antigen-specific receptors that are likely developed from a common ancestor. The contribution of cytokines and signals derived from other antigen presenting and accessory cells helps direct the response.

Overview

T cells develop in the fetal thymus from common lymphoid progenitor cells coming from bone marrow or fetal liver and commit to the T-cell lineage when stimulated by IL-7. Their germline (undifferentiated) DNA contains multiple variable (V region), diversity (D region), and joining (J region) sequences upstream of the C or constant region. Cells initially develop TCR antigen specificity independent of antigen by a random splicing of one variant from each of these segments to the C region and excision of the intervening sequences. TCR alpha (α) and gamma (γ) chains consist of one V and one J sequence of their germline DNA spliced to the C region. TCR beta (β) and delta (δ) chains consist of one V, plus one D, and one J sequence of their germline DNA spliced to the C region. The two αβ chains, or two γδ chains, of the final TCR are assembled at the cell surface in complex with CD3.

> These excised TCR segments circularize and remain in the nucleus as an episome known as a TREC (T-cell receptor excision circle) and are a marker for normal T cell development.

B cells develop in a similar, antigen-independent process in the bone marrow, with commitment to the B-cell lineage determined by the effects of several specific transcription factors (PU.1, IKAROS, E2A, EBF [early B-cell factor 1], PAX5 [paired box gene 5], and IRF8). B-cell receptors (BCRs) are immunoglobulins, consisting of a heavy chain and a light chain. Their specificity develops in the same manner as the TCR, by random splicing of a single V, D, and J region sequence from germline DNA, with excision of the intervening chromatin. Similar to the TCR α chain, the light chain kappa κ or lambda λ assembles from V_l, J_l, and C_l found on chromosomes 2 and 22, respectively. Similar to the TCR β chain, the heavy chain is assembled from four segments: V_h, D_h, and J_h associated with a constant region C_h found on chromosome 14. The process is described in more detail in the section on **Immunoglobulins.**

The Education of T and B Cells Into Functional Units

T cells

Similar to almost all other human systems, the immune system is quite plastic in infancy and requires education by interaction with the environment to mature. Once early T cells express productive, but random, TCRs, either an αβ or γδ TCR on their surface, they are double positive for CD4 and CD8 and still reside in the thymic cortex. They then undergo positive and negative selection, passing through the thymic medulla, to weed out those receptors which cannot stimulate a productive immune response and those receptors which bind to self-peptides and might cause autoimmunity. Given the important role of the TCR in facilitating antigen recognition and cellular killing, it is vitally important that the TCRs produced by somatic recombination (1) are capable of binding MHC complexes and (2) will not recognize their own (host) cells, which express MHC proteins that may be bound to normal, self-peptides. T cells, then, must walk a very fine line between recognition of that which is foreign and harmful, and that which is self and safe. T cells which are *unable to bind to MHC I or II* that is complexed with small

peptides (and hence cannot engage an effective immune response) are *eliminated via positive selection* and undergo apoptosis. Those cells which can bind to MHC I or II will receive survival signals, becoming a CD8+ cell if binding to MHC I, or a CD4+ T cell if binding to MHCII. At the other end of the spectrum, those T cells which *bind with very high avidity* to self MHC plus peptide are *eliminated by negative selection* and undergo cell death, to avoid perpetuating those cells that could support the development of autoimmunity.

T cells are subsequently activated by interaction with their specific antigenic peptide complexed to the MHC, which typically occurs in regional lymph nodes nearest to the site of the antigenic exposure. APCs are present in high numbers in areas most exposed to environmental contact, including the skin and mucosal surfaces. Once activated by PRR engagement and antigen binding, they will migrate to the closest lymph node center where T cells congregate, to engage and activate antigen-specific T cells.

T-cell activation begins when an antigen-specific TCR recognizes the antigen bound to the MHC present on an APC. T-cell surface molecules, including CD3 and the TCR bound to the peptide/MHC complex, and CD4 or CD8 which bind to invariant regions of MHC class II or I respectively, form a physical cluster on the T cell-APC interface termed the *immunologic synapse*. A second signal is required to push the T cell to activation: the binding of B-7 proteins (CD80 and CD86) on the APC to CD28 present on the T-cell membrane. The second signal is critical to the process, because without it, the T cell will apoptose, or become anergic. Later in the process, the T cell begins to produce other, this time inhibitory, membrane proteins PD-1 and CTLA-4, which turn off the activation process.

> Immune checkpoint inhibitors used in cancer therapy target PD-1 or CTLA-4. They work to bind, block, or turn off these receptors that inhibit immune responses. The result is enhanced immune function against the tumor.

T-Cell Effector Subsets

The adaptive immune process requires both actors and regulators, with a number of different T-cell effector subsets. The most common T cells are the **CD4+ αβ TCR** population; most serve a helper function and are designated **T helper cells (T_H cells)**. T_H1 cells provide primary immunity against intracellular organisms and differentiate from T_H0 cells by the secretion of **IL-12** and **IFN-γ** by the APC and the **T-bet** (T box expressed in T cells) transcription factor. T_H1 cells produce IFN-γ and TNF-α, along with the universal T-cell helper cytokine IL-2. T_H1 cells drive cell-mediated responses and activate macrophages to kill the pathogens sequestered in their phagosomes, and cytotoxic T cells and NK cells to kill bacterially and virally infected cells. **T_H2 type T cells** differentiate under the influence of **IL-4** and the transcription factor **GATA-3**. These cells produce IL-4, IL-5, IL-10, and IL-13, and provide immunity from extracellular pathogens and parasites. T_H2 T cells stimulate B cells to produce most classes of antibodies, including IgE that binds to mast cells, basophils, and eosinophils. In the absence of parasites, or adequate stimulation of the T_H1 pathway, T_H2 cells may default to allergy and hypersensitivity responses.

Follicular helper T cells (Tfh) are found in lymph nodes and the spleen. **IL-6, I-12, IL-23**, and **TGF-β** produced by dendritic and monocyte cell types triggers their differentiation from T_H0 cells. IL-6 signaling through **STAT3** is necessary for early **CXCR5** expression, considered the defining marker of Tfh cells. Interaction with antigen-specific B cells in the lymph node is essential for the development of Tfh cells, and, conversely, Tfh cells are essential for the development of memory B cells and the production of most high-affinity antibodies.

T_H17 **cells** are CD4+ T cells induced by **IL-6** and **TGF-β**, sustained by **IL-23**, and the transcription factor **RORγ τ** (retinoic acid receptor related orphan receptor γτ) plays a critical role in their differentiation. T_H17 cells produce five different IL-17 homologues, along with other potent proinflammatory cytokines that drive granulocyte recruitment and tissue damage. T_H17 cells are also active in autoimmunity, and RA, MS, IBD, and psoriasis appear to be IL-17-mediated diseases. They are also prominent in the more severe phenotypes of asthma that are characterized by neutrophilic inflammation.

Cytotoxic T Cells

CD8 T cells have been termed the foot soldiers of the immune system and are thus critical for defense against intracellular pathogens such as bacteria and viruses. For example, the mononucleosis caused by EBV infection is, in fact, hordes of CD8+ T cells released to counter the virus. CD8 T cells secrete TNF-α and IFN-γ which have antimicrobial and antitumor effects, release cytotoxic granules into the immune synapse, and express Fas ligand which binds to Fas present on target cells that activates apoptosis. They also provide critical recognition, elimination, and defense against tumor cells.

However, persistent antigen stimulation of CD8 T cells leads to expression of TOX and PD1 and promotes an exhausted or dysfunctional phenotype. This may be important to prevent overstimulation and activation-induced cell death and thus limit tissue damage. The downside to this function, however, includes decreased antitumor effector T-cell function. Building CD4 T cell help sequences into vaccine antigens, and decreasing the expression of TOX in CD8 T cells may develop more effective antipathogen and antitumor vaccines.

T-regulatory cells are critical players that turn down the immune response when the immediate threat is gone and maintain tolerance to irrelevant antigens. There are nT_{regs} **or natural** T_{regs} that develop in the thymus following positive and negative selection, and iT_{regs} **or induced**

T regulatory cells that develop from naïve CD4+ T cells in the periphery at the site of antigen exposure. Both carry a TCR specific for a single antigen. The **foxp3** (forkhead box p3) transcription factor is critical to the development of T_{reg} cells, along with interaction with costimulatory molecules CD28, CD40, CD80/86, and IL2rβ, exogenous IL-2 which they cannot synthesize themselves, and TGF-β signaling. Intranasal and oral exposure to antigen are the routes most likely to generate T regs. Dendritic cells in the gut-associated lymphoid tissue (GALT) are especially efficient at inducing T_{reg} formation, as well as dendritic cells present in tumor microenvironments. T regs suppress immune activation through cell to cell contact, along with secretion of IL-10 and TGF-β.

Innate lymphoid cells (ILCs) constitute a family of adaptable immune responder cells similar to Th cells, and include NK cells, ILC1, ILC2, ILC3, and lymphoid tissue inducer cells. Subtypes can morph into other subtypes based on their environmental triggers.

Type 2 innate lymphoid cells, or ILC2s, are the ILC most associated with allergic disease. They are derived from a common lymphoid progenitor, but do not express either TCRs or BCRs because they lack the RAG genes necessary for variability, diversity, and joining segment (VDJ) recombination. ILC2s regulate host defense against parasites, allergic inflammation in skin and lungs, adipose tissue metabolism, and tissue repair. They are found at mucosal barriers, including skin, lungs, liver, and gut, and in higher concentrations in specific allergic tissues, such as nasal polyps or atopic dermatitis lesional skin. As such, they are sentinel cells that provide the first innate immune response to infectious invaders, but are also responsible for initiating and orchestrating an adaptive immune response. Once activated, ILC2s release significant quantities of type 2 cytokines including IL-4, IL-5, IL-13, IL-9, and amphiregulin which direct Th2 cell polarization and function and also contributes to tissue repair. For example, patients with successful lung transplants for COPD or ILD had increased frequency of ILC2 cells after allograft perfusion, compared to transplanted patients with primary graft dysfunction who had significantly fewer ILC2s. ILC2s are inhibited by Type I and II interferons as well as by β2 adrenergic receptor agonists, glucocorticoids, IL-10, and TGF-β.

Cells of the Parasitic/Allergic Response

Allergic sensitization, defined as positive skin tests to seasonal or perennial allergens as the marker for specific IgE production, is so common in industrialized countries that it is easy to forget that the original purpose of the Th2 adaptive immune response was to protect against parasitic infections. The rise in prevalence of allergic diseases has continued in the industrialized world for more than 50 years with sensitization rates to one or more common allergens among school children currently approaching 40–50%. There are many suspected environmental causes of this increase, including the reduced prevalence of infectious diseases, increased

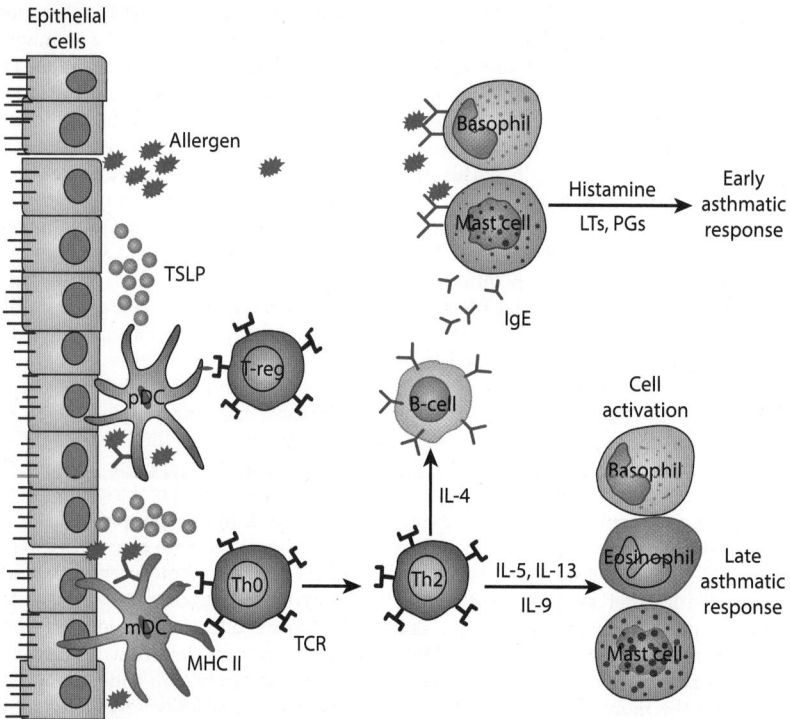

▲ **Figure 15–6.** Cells of the allergic phenotype: Origin, education, function, mediators. The role of airway epithelium, dendritic cells, and IgE in the initiation of allergic airway inflammation. IL: interleukin; LT: leukotriene; mDC: myeloid dendritic cell; MHC: major histocompatibility complex; pDC: plasmacytoid dendritic cell; PG: prostaglandin; TCR: T-cell receptor; Th: helper T-cell; Treg: regulatory T-cell; TSLP: thymic stromal lymphopoietin. (Used with permission from Gauvreau GM, El-Gammal AI, O'Byrne PM: Allergen-induced airway responses. Eur Respir J 2015;46(3):819-831.)

exposure to particulate air pollution, and changes in diet in "first world" compared to "third world" countries. The allergic response is defined as the type I immune response of the Gell & Coombs classification system, and is described in more detail in that section. Airway epithelium, dendritic cells, Th2, and T$_{reg}$ cells are critical in the induction and regulation of allergen responses in the airways, whereas mast cells, basophils, and eosinophils are responsible for the actual process of allergic inflammation.

B Cells: Active in Both Innate and Adaptive Humoral Immune Responses

B cells are the key players in the elaboration of specific antibodies of different classes. **B1a type B cells** develop only in the fetus and constitute the innate arm of the B-cell lineage. These migrate to pleural and peritoneal cavities and the gut lamina propria and provide a sentinel innate response to pathogens. They are T-cell independent and constitutively secrete only IgM, either of low affinity to self-antigens or directed toward common surface polysaccharides expressed by certain pathogens such as *Streptococcus pneumoniae*. This IgM forms the first line of defense against this group of

pathogens and is considered part of innate immunity providing an initial, rapid response. **Conventional B-cell lineages** develop later *in utero*. These cells are generated continuously in the bone marrow during adult life from pluripotent hematopoietic stem cells (pHSCs), are able to develop more diverse antigen-binding regions, and support the development of peripheral pools of B cells.

The early development of all B cells in adult life is antigen independent—The initial commitment to the B-cell lineage occurs in the bone marrow where B cells undergo random VDJ rearrangement to generate a BCR. The process is similar to the development of early T-cell antigen specificity and is also directed by the action of recombinase activating genes 1 and 2 (RAG1 and RAG2). The immature B cell then exits the bone marrow into the peripheral circulation and travels to the spleen.

Three out of five immune checkpoints in the development of B cells take place in the bone marrow. B cells with an Ig heavy chain segment unable to pair with a surrogate (nonspecific) light chain, or with a BCR that binds to self-peptides, are deleted. Only cells expressing a functional light chain capable of binding the heavy chain to form a functioning BCR, which is not autoreactive, persist. It is estimated that over 85% of newly formed B cells die at one of these checkpoints in the bone marrow.

Two types of B cells exit the bone marrow. A small percentage are **B-1b type B cells** (distinct from B-1a type B cells) that have a more limited antibody repertoire but can develop into memory cells and generate effective and long-lasting responses to *Borrelia hermsii*, *S pneumoniae*, *Salmonella enterica*, *Salmonella typhi*, and *Enterobacter cloacae* bacteria. Some human B-1b cells express low-affinity autoreactive BCRs and secrete autoantibodies, playing a role in onset or persistence of autoimmune diseases. For example, a small survey of lupus patients identified greater numbers of CD11b+ B-1b cells in patients than in unaffected controls.

The majority of B cells enter the bloodstream as conventional **B-2 type B cells** that are further educated in the spleen and lymph nodes. These are the workhorses of the adaptive immune system. After surviving negative selection in the spleen, B-2 cells then circulate to the secondary lymphoid tissues, including spleen, lymph nodes, and mucosal-associated lymphoid tissues where they will encounter antigens and differentiate into memory cells or long-lived plasma cells. The B cells with the BCRs most effective at enhanced T cell–antigen interaction will receive activation and survival signals and produce an ever more precise BCR capable of interacting with antigen and T cell in a process termed *affinity maturation*.

Response to T Independent Antigens: Type I and Type II

As another extension of the innate immune system, B cells can proliferate and produce antibody *without T cell help* in response to some plant lectins such as poke weed mitogen (PWM), a TI (T independent) type 1 antigen. B cells can also respond to TI type 2 antigens, which possess repeating molecular patterns, such as polymerized proteins or polysaccharides capable of cross-linking multiple immunoglobulin receptors. The common second signal for both T-independent type 1 and 2 antigens comes from TLR binding. Such interactions can promote immunoglobulin class switching independent of T cells and may provide a rapid immune response to bacterial polysaccharide antigens before a more specific B-cell response has been formulated.

> Response to PWM is used as a positive control to mark normal B-cell function in some immunologic assays.

B-Cell Subsets

Human marginal zone B cells are mainly involved in the immune response to bacterial LPS found in the capsules of *S pneumoniae*, *Neisseria meningitidis*, and *Haemophilus influenzae*. These B cells have high levels of TLR expression and higher basal levels of costimulatory molecules CD80 and CD86 which may explain their ability to respond rapidly to certain bacterial pathogens. **Age-associated B cells (ABCs)** are a unique B-cell subset that express the transcription factor t-bet, have high expression levels of CD11c, and progressively accumulate with age. They are poorly responsive to BCR and CD40 ligation, responding much more vigorously to TLR7 and TLR9 ligation by viral particles which enables them to rapidly differentiate into IgG2a or IgG2c secreting plasma cells. These cells appear in high frequencies in patients with autoimmune diseases. **IRA B cells** (innate response activator B cells) develop from B1a innate-like B cells responding to LPS-TLR4 binding. They secrete GM-CSF and IL-3 in response to sepsis and rapidly respond to infection with the generation of polyreactive IgM that recognize bacterial components. **NK-like B cells** demonstrate convergent phenotypes of both B cells and NK cells, expressing a fully rearranged BCR, B-cell lineage markers CD19 and MHC-II along with NK cell markers CD161 and CD335. These cells do not possess cytotoxic activity (as compared to NK cells), but efficiently secrete IL-12 and IL-18 in response to microbial infections, which then rapidly primes both NK cells and ILC1 cells to respond. Other identified, but as yet poorly characterized, innate-like B cells include **IL-17 producing B cells** that develop in response to *Trypanosoma cruzi* parasitic infection and **innate-like V_H4-34 immunoglobulin expressing B cells** found in autoimmune disorders such as SLE, as well as in chronic infectious diseases such as mononucleosis, AIDS, and hepatitis C.

Immunoglobulin Production/ Class-switching/Somatic Hypermutation

Immunoglobulins consist of two longer, inner heavy chains and two shorter, outer light chains of either kappa or lambda variety. They are identical to the BCR, but lack a transmembrane domain. The immunoglobulin molecule can be fragmented by *papain* digestion into two Fab' regions containing the variable domains that are able to bind antigen and one Fc' region containing the class specificity. In contrast, *pepsin* digestion cleaves the immunoglobulin molecule into a single $F(ab)_2$ fragment that binds and cross-links antigen and an Fc fragment.

> The ability to manipulate immunoglobulin structures and isolate the specific antigen-binding segments lies at the heart of monoclonal antibody production and the development of biologics.

The variable region, which carries the antigen-binding specificity of the molecule, is further divided into three hypervariable segments called complementarity-determining regions (CDRs), interspersed with four stable framework

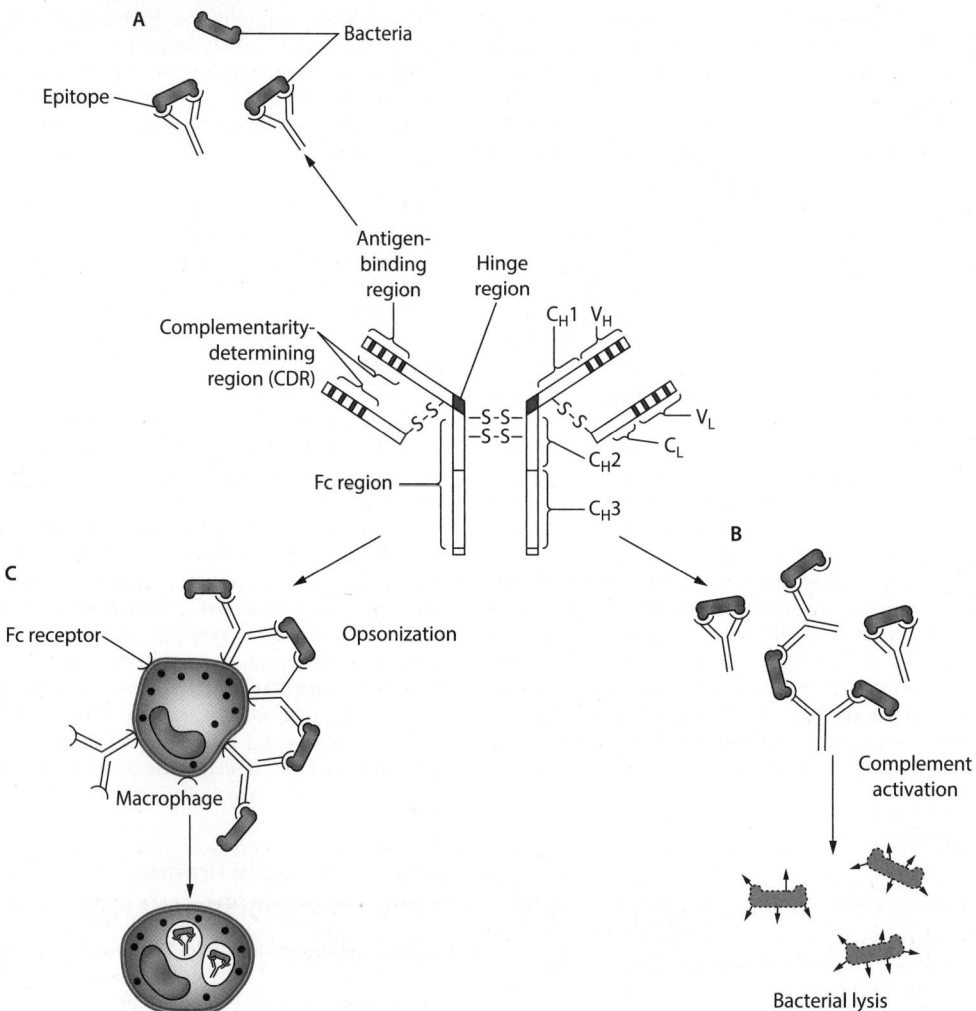

▲ **Figure 15–7.** Immunoglobulin function. Antibody has multiple functions. The prototypical antibody consists of two heavy (H) and two light (L) chains, each subdivided into constant (CL, CH) and variable (VL, VH) domains. The structure is held together by intra- and inter-chain disulfide bridges. (**A**) The complementarity-determining region (CDR) of the antigen-binding portion of the antibody engages the antigenic determinant (epitope) in a lock and key fashion. (**B**) Antigen-antibody complexes activate complement to produce split complement components that cause bacterial lysis. (**C**) The Fc portion of antibodies binds to Fc receptors on phagocytes (eg, macrophages, neutrophils) and facilitates uptake of bacteria (opsonization).

regions (FR). The extreme variability in the immunoglobulin repertoire is due to the multiple possible arrangement of different Variable$_H$ (V$_H$) gene segments with Diversity$_H$ (D$_H$) and Joining$_H$ (J$_H$) segments. More than 10^7 different VDJ segments can be generated in this way, which, adding the variability contributed by the association with the light chain, is estimated to generate more than 10^{16} different immunoglobulins.

The second phase of immunoglobulin development takes place in germinal centers and requires the presence of antigen as well as T-cell help. Follicular B cells (termed centrocytes) interact with follicular dendritic cells and follicular T helper cells presenting antigen to the T cells. If both T and B cells are able to bind to the same antigen, the B cell receives activation signals via CD40-CD40 ligand binding, migrates to the dark zone to downregulate the BCR, and rapidly divides.

After several divisions, the B cells, now termed centroblasts, express activation-induced cytidine deaminase (AID). This enzyme is able to create random mutations in the immunoglobulin genes that may enhance (or decrease) their affinity to bind the antigen in question, in a process termed *somatic hypermutation*. Recurrent cycles of somatic hypermutation result in *affinity maturation*—the development of highly precise immunoglobulins targeted to bind with high affinity to the antigen in question.

Class-Switch Recombination

At the same time, T-cell cytokines direct the process of class-switch recombination to a specific immunoglobulin subtype. Downstream of the VDJ loci of the B cell are nine functional Constant$_H$ (C$_H$) chain genes, each encoding a different immunoglobulin class. In linear order, they code for IgM, IgD, IgG$_3$, IgG$_1$, IgA$_1$, IgG$_2$, IgG$_4$, Ig$_E$, and IgA$_2$ isotypes. While the variable region confers antigen-binding specificity, it is the constant region of the immunoglobulin molecule that defines its effector functions by determining binding to the specific Fc receptor on effector cells. Despite amino acid differences between the immunoglobulin subclasses, the three or four constant regions fold into a similar structure consisting of a β-pleated sheet held together by internal disulfide bonds.

Immunoglobulins are *glycoproteins*, and the number and kind of attached sugars also affect binding to Fc receptors on effector cells. Type III immune responses, known as complement-dependent cytotoxicity, depend on binding of the Fc portion of the immunoglobulin to complement protein C1q. Specific glycosylation patterns are necessary for binding the immunoglobulin C1q–antigen complex to an effector cell that then permits complement binding and destruction of the target.

> Antibody-dependent cellular cytotoxicity (ADCC, or Type III immune reactions) is an immune process in which antibody-coated antigens bind to Fc receptors and activate NK cells or monocytes to destroy them.

Heavy Chain Isotypes

Table 15–4 gives a brief review of the structure and function of the five main immunoglobulin subclasses.

IgM

IgM is the first immunoglobulin to be expressed on B cells and associated with heterodimer CD79a and b to form the first BCR. With maturation and antigenic stimulation IgM is secreted and can be linked by disulfide bonds and a J polypeptide chain to form pentamers. IgM antibodies are often the first to appear in an infectious challenge and are of low specificity. Their benefit comes from rapid deployment early in infection, and, for this reason, detection of specific IgM antibodies signifies an acute infection. IgM binding avidity is much enhanced with the pentameric version, especially if the

Table 15–4. Characteristics of immunoglobulin isotypes and subclasses.

	Serum (%)	Structure	Complement Fixation	Opsonizing	Cross Placenta	Other Functions	Fc Receptor
IgG	75	Monomer	+	+++	+	For all IgG subclasses	FcγR
IgG$_1$	67% of IgG	Monomer	Yes	Yes	+	Secondary response	I,II,III
IgG$_2$	22% of IgG	Monomer	Yes	Yes	+	Neutralize toxins and virus	II
IgG$_3$	7% of IgG	Monomer	Yes	Yes	+		I,II,III
IgG$_4$	4% of IgG	Monomer	No	No	+		I,II
IgM	10	Pentamer	+++	+	−	Primary response	
IgA	15	Monomer, Dimer	−	−	−	Mucosal response	FcαR (CD89)
IgA$_1$		Monomer, Dimer	−	−	−		
IgA$_2$		Monomer, Dimer	−	−	−		
IgD	<0.5	Monomer	−	−	−	Homeostasis	FcδR
IgE	<0.01	Monomer	−	−	−	Allergy	FcεR I,II

Source: From Schroeder HW, Cavacini L: Structure and function of immunoglobulins. 2010;125(2 Suppl 2):S41-52.

antigen contains repeating epitopes (such as bacterial carbohydrates).

> IgM immunoglobulins are the first to appear in response to infection. Measurable IgM antibodies to a specific pathogen signals an acute infection, whereas IgG antibodies are markers of a previous infection and the presence of immune memory.

IgD

Membrane-bound IgD is the second antibody to appear in early B-cell maturation. It is expressed on the B-cell surface as it leaves the bone marrow for secondary lymphoid organs. It is produced by class switching to the D heavy chain, but is usually present with IgM, and both are specific for the same variable region. Both IgD and IgM will form a functional BCR. IgD is rarely secreted, with a short serum half-life. Certain bacterial proteins can bind to the constant region of IgD and thus stimulate and activate the B cell.

IgG

IgG is the mainstay of the immunoglobulin family and is the most common antibody type found. It has the longest half-life in serum, approximately 3 months, and includes four subclasses, numbered in their order of serum levels: from IgG_1 with the highest concentration, to IgG_4 with the lowest. Differences in the heavy chain regions of subtypes 1–4 affect immunoglobulin flexibility of the F(ab) and Fc regions, primarily at the hinge region, as well as functional affinity. The four subclasses of IgG have discrete affinity for different antigens. IgG_1 and IgG_3 antibodies are produced in response to protein antigens, have the greatest binding affinity for C1q, the first component of the complement pathway, and both bind to all three Fcγ (gamma) receptor classes I, II, and III. IgG_2 and IgG_4 antibodies are formed in response to polysaccharide antigens. IgG_2 has the weakest binding to C1q, whereas IgG_4 does not bind C1q at all. IgG_4 is able to bind to Fcγ receptors II and III, and IgG_2 only binds to Fcγ receptor II. Fcγ receptors are generally found on immune cells such as macrophages, neutrophils, eosinophils, and dendritic cells.

IgA

IgA is predominantly a mucosal antibody with much higher levels in saliva, colostrum, and breast milk than IgG. It is predominantly monomeric in serum but forms a dimer associated with a J-chain and a secretory component polypeptide chain at mucosal surfaces. Interestingly, only those B cells present in mucosal areas, such as the lamina propria of the gut, can synthesize J chains that are essential for the polymerization and secretion of IgA. There are two isoforms IgA_1 and IgA_2 that differ primarily in their hinge regions. IgA_1 has a longer hinge region that makes it more susceptible to bacterial proteases; hence IgA_2 is the predominant form in

mucosal secretions. It provides the first level of protection against bacterial and viral invaders that enter through mucosal surfaces. Its polymeric nature makes it more effective at binding specific bacterial products such as *Clostridium difficile* toxin A. Fc (α) receptors are found on myeloid cells such as neutrophils, eosinophils, monocytes, some macrophages, and some dendritic cells.

IgE

IgE is primarily a tissue-bound antibody and thus has the lowest serum concentrations and shortest serum half-life of all the immunoglobulins. It binds with high affinity to FcεR1 receptors present on basophils, eosinophils, mast cells, and Langerhans cells. Cross-linking surface-bound IgE with antigen triggers activation and degranulation of these cells. IgE binds with much lower affinity to FcεRII receptors present on B cells, NK cells, and platelets, as well as the same cast of cells listed earlier. Whereas IgE is the predominant antibody made against parasites, in the absence of parasitic infections it will default to mediating allergic and hypersensitivity reactions.

Because affinity maturation and class switch recombination take time, the peak germinal response only occurs between 10 to 14 days after the initial antigen exposure. What remains afterwards are high-affinity, somatically mutated plasma cells and memory B cells. These memory B cells can persist in the periphery without specific antigen stimulation, but can rapidly proliferate and secrete antibody with a subsequent specific antigen encounter. Affinity matured plasma cells disappear from the spleen after about 2 weeks, but may be found in the bone marrow continuing to secrete antibody for up to a year later. It is likely that plasma cells exist for much longer in survival niches in the bone marrow, estimated at up to 60 years, as well as a fewer number in the spleen.

CLASSIFICATION OF IMMUNE HYPERSENSITIVITY DISORDERS

In 1963, Philip Gell and Robin Coombs classified immune hypersensitivity diseases into four immunopathologic categories. This classification should be viewed in its historical context as an attempt to order and explain the reactions to treatment with antitoxins, blood transfusions, and impure drugs that constituted the best medical practice available at the turn of the twentieth century. Since that time, our understanding of the interactions of the immune system with the outside world has exploded in complexity and precision. However, the Gell & Coombs classification system is still a useful way to identify immune reactions, although type I allergic and type IV T-cell mediated, remain the most helpful and frequently used today.

Gell and Coombs defined four distinct types of immune reactions (types I–IV). Type I, allergic, encompass those reactions mediated by IgE antibodies, although the IgE antibody was not identified until 1966 and 1967 by Teruko and Kimishige Ishizaka and Gunnar Johansson and Hans Bennich, respectively. Type II, cytotoxic hypersensitivity reactions, describe a process in which host antibodies recognize and bind fixed cell surface or tissue antigens, activate complement, and initiate the complement cascade of destruction. Type III, antibody-antigen reactions, involve circulating host antibodies that bind circulating foreign antigens in reactions that can occur locally or systemically, again fixing complement and initiating tissue damage. Type IV reactions result from the actions of sensitized T lymphocytes (cell-mediated immune response). Each of the four mechanisms requires an initial exposure to antigen, which induces sensitization, a clinically silent primary immune response. Subsequent challenge—exposure to the same antigen—following a short lag period (usually at least 1 week) evokes the hypersensitivity response.

Type I: Anaphylactic or Immediate Hypersensitivity Reactions

Occupational Examples: Occupational Asthma, Rhinitis, Contact Urticaria, Anaphylaxis

These reactions are initiated by the interaction of antigen with specific IgE antibodies bound to mast cells and basophils with the subsequent release of inflammatory mediators. Examples of type I reactions in the practice of occupational

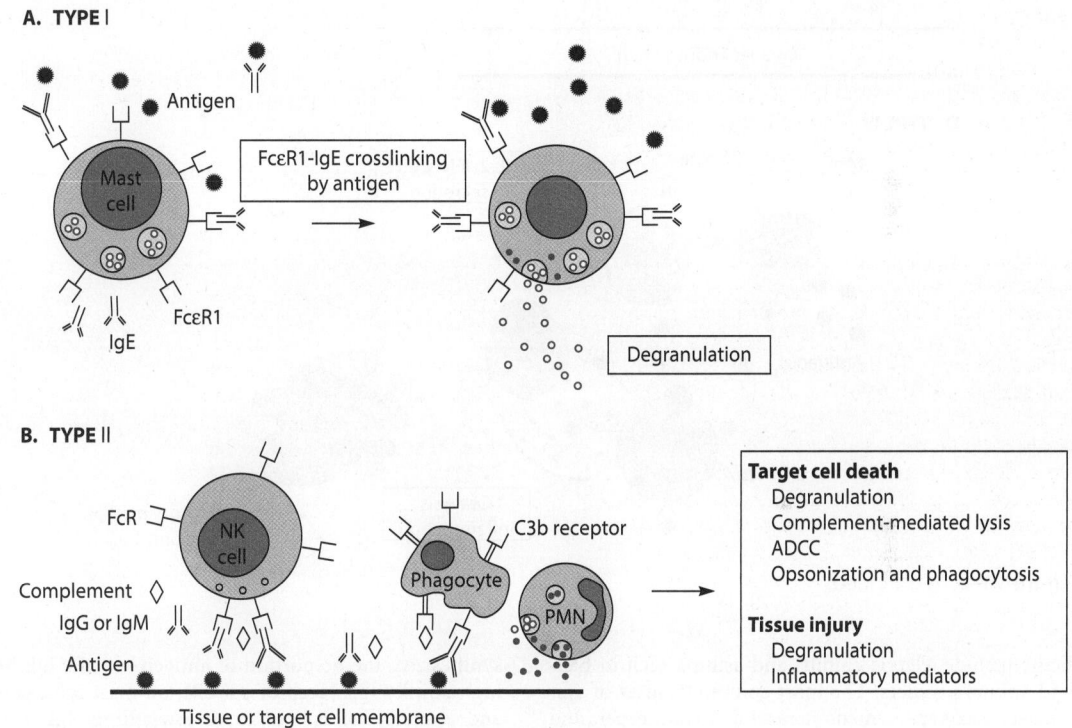

▲ **Figure 15–8.** Hypersensitivity immune responses. **A.** Type I reaction. Mast cells and basophils bind IgE via high-affinity Fc receptors (FcεR1). Antigen-binding and cross-linking of FcεR1-IgE complexes induce cellular degranulation and release of inflammatory mediators. **B.** Type II reaction. IgG or IgM antibodies against tissue or cellular antigens induce complement activation which results in cell death and tissue injury. **C.** Type III reaction. Circulating immune complexes composed of soluble antigen and IgG or IgM deposit on vascular endothelium of various tissues which activates the complement cascade. Polymorphonuclear leukocytes (PMNs) and other phagocytes are attracted to these sites of immune complex deposition via their Fc and C3b receptors and are induced to degranulate and phagocytose the complexes, resulting in local tissue injury and vasculitis. **D.** Type IV reaction. Via their T-cell receptors, helper T cells recognize target cell antigenic peptides bound to antigen-presenting cells. This T-cell recognition results in the secretion of interleukin 2, interferon-gamma, and other cytokines that are required for the activation of tissue macrophages and cytotoxic T cells. Cytotoxic T cells recognize the same antigen bound to target cells and induce lysis by perforin and other molecules secreted by cytotoxic T cells. ADCC, antibody-dependent cell-mediated cytotoxicity; APC, antigen-presenting cell; Tc, cytotoxic T cell; TCR, T-cell receptor; TH, T helper cell.

C. TYPE III

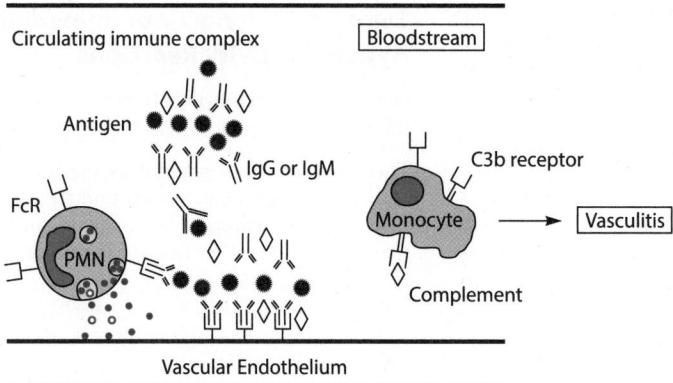

D. TYPE IV

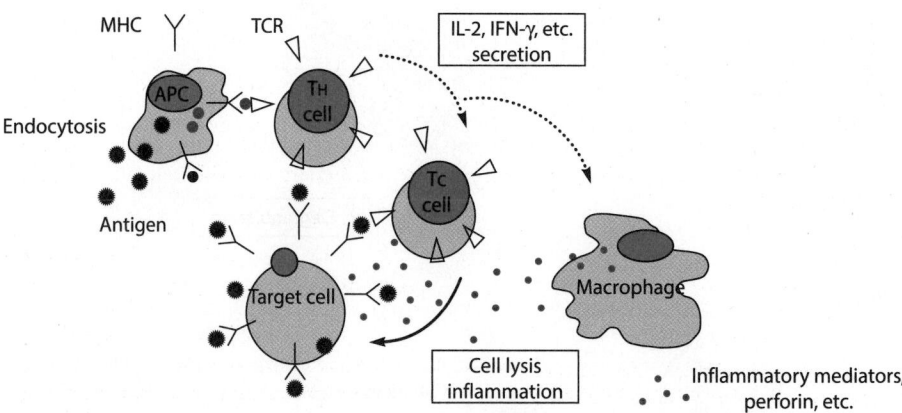

▲ **Figure 15–8.** (Continued)

medicine include allergic rhinitis and asthma seen in bakers and animal handlers. The most common causes of systemic anaphylaxis are Hymenoptera stings in beekeepers and greenhouse workers and natural rubber latex in health care workers.

A. Type 1 Reaction

Mast cells and basophils bind IgE via high-affinity Fc receptors (FcεR1). Antigen-binding and cross-linking of FcεR1-IgE complexes induce cellular degranulation and release of inflammatory mediators.

Initial exposure to antigen in a genetically predisposed host leads to the synthesis of antigen-specific IgE by mature B cells, constituting the atopic state. Indeed, a history of allergies to plant and animal allergens is a risk factor for the development of occupational allergic disease. Once

synthesized, the Fc portion of antigen-specific IgE binds to high-affinity IgE receptors, FcεRI, on mast cells, basophils, and eosinophils, as well as to low-affinity IgE receptors, FcεRII or CD23, on lymphocytes, macrophages, eosinophils, and platelets, thus priming these cells for future allergen encounters. Re-exposure to the allergen will cross-link the adjacent IgE receptors, activating enzymes leading to degranulation of allergic mediators. These include both preformed mediators from cytoplasmic granules (histamine, chemotactic factors, and enzymes) and newly generated mediators (prostaglandins, leukotrienes, and platelet-activating factor). Eosinophils contain four major proteins, including major basic protein (MBP), eosinophil cationic protein (ECP), eosinophil peroxidase (EPO), and eosinophil-derived neurotoxin (EDN). Tryptase is a serine protease primarily produced and stored in mast cells with lower concentrations in basophils. With an allergic or anaphylactic reaction, serum levels of tryptase peak in 1–2 hours after allergen exposure and can remain elevated for up to 12–24 hours depending on the reaction. To document that a clinical response was due to allergy or anaphylaxis, the serum tryptase should be measured with a few hours. Serum tryptase that is low or normal within an hour of a reaction strongly suggests that the cause was not allergic. If serum tryptase is measured several hours after the initial response, it may be low or undetectable and, in that case, is not helpful in determining if the cause was allergic. In contrast, histamine levels peak early and return to baseline within 15–30 minutes after a reaction.

The allergic response can include only an early-phase response, only a late-phase response, or a dual or biphasic response. The early response is characterized by the release of mast cell, basophil, and eosinophil mediators causing vasodilation, vascular leakiness, edema, smooth-muscle constriction, mucus hypersecretion, pruritus, and a mild cellular infiltrate. Clinically, this presents as erythema, swelling, rhinorrhea, cough, chest tightness, itching, and hives occurring within minutes of an allergen exposure. Depending on the severity of the response, effective treatment may include subcutaneous epinephrine at 1 mg/mL (1:1000), antihistamines, and/or bronchodilators. (Note that injectable solutions of epinephrine are 10-fold diluted at 0.1 mg/mL or 1:10,000.)

The **late-phase response**, characterized by mucosal edema and the influx of inflammatory cells, may either follow the early-phase response (as a dual response) or occur as an isolated event (isolated late phase). Late-phase reactions begin 2–4 hours after the initial antigen exposure, reach maximal activity at 6–12 hours, and usually resolve within 12–24 hours. The late-phase response is characterized clinically by erythema, edema, and induration at the site of the allergen exposure, heat, burning, and itching. Asthma may present as cough, shortness of breath, or a silent chest indicating little air movement. Wheezing is more common in children and less common in adults. Microscopically, there is an influx of primarily eosinophils and mononuclear cells. Eosinophils are frequently sampled from the nasal mucosa of patients with allergic rhinitis and from the sputum of asthmatics. Products of activated eosinophils such as MBP and eosinophilic cationic protein are destructive to airway epithelial tissue and are associated with airways hyperreactivity. Epithelial disruption is a feature of patients with both contact dermatitis and asthma. Immune cells infiltrating tissues in the late response may further elaborate cytokines and histamine-releasing factors that perpetuate the inflammatory response, leading to a sustained hyperresponsiveness and disruption of the target tissue in bronchi, skin, or nasal mucosa. If exposure to the inciting allergen persists, the onset and resolution of the late-phase response becomes blurred as chronic tissue inflammation develops. Late-phase reactivity has been found in many atopic disease states including allergic rhinitis and conjunctivitis, asthma, and anaphylaxis. The dual asthmatic responses seen in detergent worker's asthma, trimellitic anhydride (TMA) asthma, and baker's asthma represent clinical examples of asthmatic late-phase

responses. The late-phase response requires treatment with anti-inflammatory therapies including oral, inhaled, and topical corticosteroids, in addition to treatment with antihistamines, leukotriene inhibitors, and bronchodilators for the immediate symptoms.

The hallmark of immediate hypersensitivity reactions is the presence of allergen-specific IgE. It can be demonstrated *in vivo* by a prick or intradermal skin test to a specific antigen. Because the skin test measures tissue bound IgE, positive reactions presenting as an itchy wheal and flare (ie, a small hive) will be evident within 15 minutes. Prick skin testing is always performed with both a negative control, usually saline, and a positive control, usually histamine at 1 mg/mL. Skin testing is less sensitive but more specific than *in vitro* testing by the radioallergosorbent test (RAST) or the enzyme-linked immunosorbent assay (ELISA). In many cases, however, commercially available skin testing extracts are not available. Testing can be performed to a home-made "puddle" extract, but should be performed by someone trained in that procedure to avoid potentially harmful or caustic effects.

Type II: Cytotoxic Reactions

Occupational Examples: Transfusion Reactions, TMA Pulmonary Disease-Anemia Syndrome

A. Type II Reaction

IgG or IgM antibodies against tissue or cellular antigens induce complement activation which results in cell death and tissue injury.

In type II reactions, the target antigen is a cell surface protein or antigenic substance that binds covalently to a cell surface protein. Antibody then attaches to the cell surface-bound antigen labelling it for demolition. The antibody-antigen complex can facilitate phagocytosis or fix complement to initiate the terminal complement sequence leading to cell lysis. In transfusion reactions, the antigen is a protein on the cell membrane of the incompatible erythrocyte. IgG then binds to the protein and marks the cell for destruction. The direct Coombs test measures IgG antibody bound to the surface of red blood cells (RBCs) and leukocytes, and is used to diagnose autoimmune hemolytic anemia. Here, the patient's RBCs are washed to remove unbound antibodies and then incubated with antihuman IgG (the Coombs reagent); if the RBCs agglutinate, the test indicates IgG bound to the RBC surface. The indirect Coombs test measures circulating anti-RBC antibodies in the serum and is used in cases of Rh or ABO incompatibility, or prior to a transfusion. In this test, the patient's serum is incubated with foreign RBCs of known antigenicity and then antihuman IgG (the Coombs reagent) is added; if the RBCs agglutinate, it indicates the presence of circulating anti-RBC antibodies in the patient. In some type II hypersensitivity disorders, a LMW chemical such as TMA acts as a hapten and attaches to a host cell surface protein that acts as a carrier, forming a complete antigen. In workers repeatedly exposed to high concentrations of volatile TMA, the chemical can combine with an erythrocyte membrane protein or pulmonary basement cell membrane protein that then stimulates the formation of anti-TMA-conjugate IgG or IgM antibodies. Clinically, affected workers present with cough, hemoptysis, dyspnea, pulmonary infiltrates, restrictive lung function, hypoxemia, and anemia: the pulmonary disease-anemia syndrome. Rat models of TMA-induced pulmonary disease-anemia demonstrate elevated antibody titers that correlate with intra-alveolar hemorrhage, alveolar septal inflammatory nodules, and endothelial and epithelial cell injury.

Type III: Immune Complex Reaction

Occupational Examples: Local Arthus Reaction, Serum Sickness

A. Type III reaction

Circulating immune complexes composed of soluble antigen and IgG or IgM deposit on vascular endothelium of various tissues, which activates the complement cascade. Neutrophils and other phagocytes are attracted to these sites of immune complex deposition via their Fc and C3b receptors and are induced to degranulate and phagocytose the complexes, resulting in local tissue injury and vasculitis.

Type III reactions depend on the union of soluble antigen with soluble IgG or IgM antibody and subsequent activation of the complement sequence with end-organ tissue damage. When the immune complex is formed locally, such as in the skin, the type III reaction is termed an Arthus reaction; in the second subtype, serum sickness, circulating complexes are deposited in renal glomeruli or pulmonary basement membranes.

Arthus reactions are the result of local antigen deposition to which circulating antibodies adhere *in situ*, causing induration and erythema at the injection site in 2 hours, which peaks at 6 hours and resolves in 12–24 hours. In some instances necrosis may develop. The process involves localized immune complexes that activate the complement cascade forming opsonins that enhance phagocytosis by neutrophils and generate C3a, C4a, and C5a anaphylatoxins leading to vasodilatation and increased vascular permeability. This facilitates the diffusion of other mediators and effector cells to the reaction site and stimulates the release of lysosomal enzymes, platelet-activating factor (PAF), and thromboxane that activate and aggregate platelets leading to thrombus formation.

In serum sickness, or "immune complex disease," circulating antigen and IgG antibodies combine forming immune complexes and microprecipitates. These are filtered from the circulation at the postcapillary venule in tissues such as skin, kidney, joints, and lungs. Classic serum sickness occurs 7–14 days after injection of a foreign serum or administration of a drug and resolves within a few weeks of discontinuation of the drug. Clinical manifestations of serum sickness include morbilliform rash, urticaria, arthritis, pleuritis, pericarditis, fever, and nephritis. It was a common complication of early treatment with equine-based antitoxins or treatment with rabbit antithymocyte globulin in early kidney transplant patients, for example. Although patients may appear very ill in the acute presentation, the disease is self-limited and the prognosis is excellent once the offending drug is discontinued.

Type IV: Cellular Immunity

Occupational Examples: Contact Dermatitis, Hypersensitivity Pneumonitis

Type IV **delayed hypersensitivity reactions** are not mediated by antibody; instead, they are mediated primarily by T lymphocytes (cell-mediated immunity). In contrast to type I reactions, which often occur within minutes of antigen challenge dose, type IV reactions require 24–72 hours to appear. Classic examples of type IV immune reactions are the tuberculin skin test reactions and contact dermatitis, such as the poison ivy response.

A. Type IV Reaction

Via their TRCs, helper T cells recognize target cell antigenic peptides bound to antigen-presenting cells. This T-cell recognition results in the secretion of IL-2, interferon-gamma, and other cytokines that are required for the activation of tissue macrophages and cytotoxic T cells. Cytotoxic T cells recognize the same antigen bound to target cells and induce lysis by perforins and other molecules secreted by cytotoxic T cells.

In the case of skin contact with allergen, the process is initiated by uptake of the allergen by Langerhans or dendritic cells which migrate to regional lymph nodes where they present the allergen/antigen to circulating T cells. Those that recognize the antigen will migrate back into the site of exposure and secrete cytokines that attract and activate other inflammatory cells causing a contact dermatitis. Type IV delayed hypersensitivity responses are mediated by T cells through three different pathways. When type 1 helper (Th1) T cells recognize antigen they release γ-interferon that activates macrophages and causes tissue injury. The prototype example is the positive tuberculin test presenting as local tissue induration and erythema. In a Th2-mediated response, Th2 cells release cytokines that recruit and activate eosinophils that degranulate and cause itching as well as tissue injury. A common example is the reaction to poison ivy or to nickel, characterized by erythema, pruritus, induration, vesicles, weeping, and blistering if severe. T_H17 cells produce IL-17 family cytokines that amplify the Th2 response. In the third pathway, damage is caused directly by cytotoxic T cells.

The antigen specificity of contact dermatitis is established by patch testing. This is a process of placing a solution of the antigen in either petrolatum or saline onto the skin for 48 hours, to allow sufficient time for uptake of the antigen. The patch sites are re-examined after 72–96 hours for erythema, induration, vesicles, and itching. Generally speaking, skin reactions that are present at 48 hours on the removal of the patch and then fade, is more than likely an irritant response. Reactions that gradually increase in size and severity after the patch is removed are more likely representative of true sensitization. The prolonged nature of the test over several days recapitulates the lag time in type IV hypersensitivity reactions: It takes time to take up the antigen, migrate to the regional lymph node, and then persuade antigen-specific T cells to migrate back into the site of the patch test to initiate a reaction. Patch testing is also limited by a narrow selection of commercially available extracts as there are many occupational exposures with no testing material available. Although sometimes patch testing with the suspected material is possible, it is *very important* to make sure the material is not toxic or caustic or harmful and is best left to an allergist or dermatologist. In addition, the practitioner is constantly grappling with the question as to whether the skin reaction is due to specific sensitization to an allergen or is an irritant response to the material's qualities or concentration. Although occupational dermatitis is one of the most common work-related conditions, 80% are due to an irritant reaction. Of these, wet work involving frequent hand washing with soap, is the most common.

In some autoimmune diseases, effector T cells have been shown to specifically recognize self-antigens and cause tissue damage internally, either by direct cytotoxicity or by inflammatory responses mediated by activated macrophages. For example, in type 1 insulin-dependent diabetes mellitus, T cells orchestrate destruction of B cells of the pancreatic islets. In MS, IFN-γ–producing T cells specific for myelin basic proteins have been implicated as the cause of tissue damage.

Hypersensitivity pneumonitis (HP), also called extrinsic allergic alveolitis, is considered an example of both type III and type IV immune responses. It is an inflammatory lung disease caused by an immune response to repeated exposure to inhaled organic dusts, or, rarely, to certain chemicals. Prevalence estimates are low depending on the population, generally from 4% to 15% of all interstitial lung disease (ILD) cases. Although the disease has been characterized as either acute/subacute or chronic, in many cases the symptoms come on insidiously or are misdiagnosed as recurrent episodes of pneumonia. The clinical presentation of the sudden onset of fever, chills, cough, myalgias, and shortness of breath, associated with exposure to a bioaerosol in the previous 24–48 hours, is considered characteristic of acute HP. The chronic form presents with worsening dyspnea over time, with a chronic cough, fatigue, and weight loss, but is easily missed by both physician and patient due to the subtle presentation at first. Chronic HP is often only picked up on a chest x-ray showing an upper lung predominant or diffuse interstitial infiltrate associated with reduced lung volumes, decreased FVC, and decreased diffusion capacity. In both acute and chronic cases, it is important to ask about

exposures, current or previous, to home floods or leaks, visible mold or moldy odors, the presence of a hot tub, sauna, humidifier or swamp cooler, or birds in the home, either as pets or an infestation. Many professions where HP is a concern involve exposure to a bioaerosol, either due to mold or birds, or to a chemical used in the workplace. Although there are many specific and esoteric exposure related examples of HP, such as Alternaria species in wood pulp causing woodworker's lung or *Aspergillus clavatus* in moldy grains causing malt worker's lung, it is not necessary to memorize these lists. In general, exposure to stored or germinated plant materials such as with mushroom growing or beer making, animal infestations such as birds or bats, or to standing water such as in humidifiers, storage ponds, hot tubs, or metal working fluids, are potential reservoirs of bioaerosols that could cause HP.

HP is considered an example of a type III immune response due to the presence of specific antibodies to the causative agent. The presence of such antibodies has, in the past, been tested in an Ouchterlony double diffusion test, where the suspected antigen is added to serum antibodies from the patient. If the patient has made antibodies to the suspected agent, such as *A fumigatus*, a line of precipitation will form where the two components meet, bind, and form a lattice resulting in a precipitin line. Although specific precipitins to the bioaerosol are considered a core part of the diagnosis, these are often unhelpful except in the case of bird antigens. This is in part due to the fact that there are so many subspecies of mold, or multiple molds in one exposure that the proper antigen is not used in the test. So negative precipitins do not rule out the diagnosis, and positive precipitins indicate exposure but not disease. In general, we advise against checking mold precipitins because they are often negative and usually simply involve a guess as to the actual exposure.

The diagnosis is made on the basis of transbronchial lung biopsies showing granulomas, usually poorly formed, and, on occasion, an organizing pneumonia. The BAL fluid usually contains an elevated lymphocyte count, although there are no set standards. Acute HP may also contain elevated neutrophil counts. A decreased CD4/CD8 ratio is not always present and not always helpful, and an elevated CD4 count does not rule out the diagnosis. We generally interpret the BAL cell count in context with the biopsy results, the clinical presentation, and a suspected exposure to establish the diagnosis. One set of suggested criteria to establish the diagnosis identified six important predictors is as follows: (1) exposure to a known causative antigen, (2) presence of precipitins to the suspected causative antigen, (3) recurrent respiratory and systemic symptoms, (4) inspiratory crackles detected by physical examination, (5) symptoms occurring 4–8 hours after exposure, and (6) weight loss. An EAACI position paper on occupational HP categorized the principal agents into the following groups (Table 15-5): (1) bacteria (eg, *Thermophilic actinomycetes*, *Klebsiella*, *Bacillus subtilis*, *Mycobacterium avium*), (2) fungi (eg, *Aspergillus*, *Penicillium*), (3) enzymes (eg, phytase, subtilisin), (4) animal and insect proteins (eg, avian serum and feathers), (7) plant proteins (eg, soy, malt,

Table 15–5. Principal agents causing occupational hypersensitivity pneumonitis.

Categories	Agents	Examples of Jobs and Occupational Exposures
Bacteria	*Thermophilic actinomycetes*	Farmers; bagasse workers; mushroom workers, potato riddlers (sizers/graders), compost workers, HVAC workers
	Lichtheimia corymbifera	Farmers
	Acinetobacter, Ochrobactrum	Metal working fluids
	Streptomyces albus	Compost workers
	Klebsiella oxytoca	Humidifiers
	Bacillus subtilis enzymes	Detergent industry
	Mycobacterium avium complex and other nontuberculous mycobacteria	Spa workers/hot tubs, steam rooms
	Mycobacterium immunogenum	Metal working fluids, machine operators
Fungi	*Alternaria alternata*	Humidifiers, wood workers
	Aspergillus spp.	Stucco workers, tobacco growers, malt workers
	Trichosporon cutaneum	Summer-type HP
	Penicillium glabrum	Cork workers
	Penicillium roqueforti	Cheese workers
	Penicillium verrucosum	Food processors
	Penicillium camemberti	Food processors
	Penicillium citreonigrum	Peat moss processing workers
	Cryptostroma corticale	Maple bark strippers, florists
	Botrytis cinerea	Wine makers
	Mucor stolonifer	Paprika slicers
	Rhodotorula	Humidifiers
	Mushrooms: *Shiitake, Bunashimeji, Pleurotus, Pholiota, Shimeji, Agaricus*	Mushroom growers
Enzymes	Phytase, subtilisin	Animal feeding, cleaners
Animal & insect proteins	Avian serum and feather proteins	Bird breeders
	Rat serum proteins	Laboratory workers
	Pearl	Pearl industry
	Mollusk shell	Nacre industry
	Silk	Textile workers
	Carmine	Food and cosmetic industry
	Sitophilus granarius	Farmers

(continued)

Table 15–5. Principal agents causing occupational hypersensitivity pneumonitis. (Continued)

Categories	Agents	Examples of Jobs and Occupational Exposures
Plant proteins	Tiger nut	Food processors
	Legumes (eg, soy)	Food processors
	Malt	Food processors
	Alginate	Seaweed workers
	Woods: ramin, pine	Wood workers
	Esparto dust	Stucco workers
Low molecular weight chemicals	Diisocyanates	Chemical and polyurethane industry, painters
	Acid anhydrides	Plastic workers, aircraft industry
	Triglycidyl isocyanurate	Painters (powder paint)
	Pharmaceutical agents: penicillins, cephalosporins	Pharmaceutical industry
	Dimethyl phthalate and styrene	Yacht manufacturing
Metals	Cobalt	Hard-metal workers
	Zinc	Smelters
	Zirconium	Ceramic workers

Source: From Quirce S: Occupational HP: an EAACI position paper. Allergy. 2/23/2016; https://doi.org/10.1111/all.12866.

woods), (8) LMW chemicals (diisocyanates, acid anhydrides, phthalates), and (9) metals (cobalt, zinc, and zirconium).

NONSPECIFIC ACTIVATION OF INFLAMMATORY REACTIONS

A number of plant- and chemical-derived substances can activate cells and mediators of inflammation **without** triggering a specific immune response characterized by explicit recognition of antigen. Triggers include plant-derived lectins such as concanavalin A from the jack bean, phytohemagglutinins from the red kidney bean, and pokeweed mitogen from the American pokeweed. Their nonspecific effect of activation of the immune system is why one of these is often used as the positive control in an immunologic assay. Other examples include gram-negative polysaccharides, pneumococcal polysaccharides, fungal by-products, trypsin, papain, silica, zinc oxide, and asbestos, for example, that can nonspecifically activate lymphocytes, macrophages, mast cells, basophils, and, in some cases, the complement system through their physicochemical properties, interaction with toll receptors, ability to split complement, and the like. Such triggers are sometimes able to initiate an inflammatory process that then opens the door for specific immune responses to associated antigens. **Organic dust toxic syndrome** is a short-lived constellation of symptoms triggered by exposure to dust from hay, grain, fuel chips, straw, and livestock. Organic dust includes molds, pollens, bacteria, pesticides, chemicals, feed and bedding particles, and animal particles including hair, feathers, and droppings; their toxic constituents include endotoxin, mycotoxins, and volatile organic compounds. The clinical presentation occurs reasonably rapidly, usually within 4–12 hours of exposure, with the onset of fever and chills, chest discomfort, shortness of breath, dry cough, body and muscle aching, weakness, headache, and fatigue. Chest x-rays are often normal and symptoms resolve without sequelae after 2–12 days. Other, nonimmune, toxic syndromes caused by inhalation of agricultural dusts and gases may cause bronchitis, silo filler's disease, an acute toxic inflammation of the lung caused by exposure to nitrogen oxides in freshly filled silos, and death by asphyxiation (suffocation) from inhalation of toxic gases in manure pits, for example.

Occupational exposure to some organic acids, such as plicatic acid (red cedar) and abietic acid (colophony or resin), can cause airway epithelial cell desquamation, activation of complement, induction of bronchial hyperreactivity, and stimulation of afferent C fibers, without a specific immune response, and hence, without latency. These agents can induce asthma and airways inflammation through toxic injury and neurogenic mechanisms. In the clinical reactions to toxic agents, the severity of response is more often related to the magnitude and nature of the exposure, rather than individual susceptibility or reactivity.

Reactive airways dysfunction syndrome (RADS) is a syndrome characterized by the acute emergence of bronchial hyperreactivity and symptoms of asthma, after an acute exposure to high levels of respiratory irritants, usually toxic chemicals, smoke, or particulates. Symptoms develop within the first 24 hours of exposure, and in contrast to the hypersensitivity syndromes, there is no latency period. By definition, there is an absence of preexisting pulmonary disease in affected workers, and despite the lack of re-exposure to the specific agent, asthma symptoms and bronchial hyperreactivity may persist due to damage to the airways. The pathogenesis is believed to involve respiratory epithelial injury with subsequent neurogenic inflammation and airway remodeling. A well-described example of RADS occurred in 2001 during rescue efforts in the New York City terrorist attacks. Emergency and recovery workers, fire fighters, and police officers were exposed to a highly complex mixture of smoke, particulate matter, and pollutants, and many of the most highly exposed developed asthma that did not resolve. The asthma caused by RADS is thought to persist due to continuing airway damage that heals with scarring, as compared to immunologically mediated asthma that can sometimes resolve out of exposure to the inciting allergen.

Pneumoconiosis

The pneumoconioses refer to dust-related lung diseases, fibrotic changes caused by the chronic inhalation of fine powdered chemicals and particulates. The primary types of pneumoconiosis include coal workers' pneumoconiosis due to inhalation of coal dust, silicosis due to silica dust from rock and sand, and asbestosis due to inhalation of asbestos fibers. These are diseases of latency, with onset of cough and dyspnea after a minimum of 10 and usually more years of exposure. Unlike biological agents, these dusts cannot be broken down and eliminated by the immune system and instead persist in the lungs. The immune system attempts to isolate the particles of coal, silica, or asbestos by forming coal macules, silicotic nodules, and asbestos bodies—fibers of asbestos coated with an iron-rich material derived from ferritin and hemosiderin and formed by macrophages that have phagocytosed and attempted to digest the fibers. Asbestos and silica particles also prime and activate inflammasomes that may play a key role in the initial lung and pleural injury, as well the subsequent development of fibrosis. Hence, although these particles do not elicit an immune response specific to a surface marker, they do engage the immune system nonspecifically as foreign particles that are sequestered and as activators of inflammasomes that initiate the fibrotic process. Fibrosis develops over years, in part driven by high levels of exposure and in part by the persistence of inhaled particles that cannot be broken down or removed. There does appear to be a genetic component

as to who will develop more severe disease, and that risk is related to variants of specific inflammasome components. The disease presents as the insidious onset of dyspnea and cough that is often mistakenly attributed to an infection. Treatment is primarily supportive, and there is no cure for any of these diseases.

Chronic or classic silicosis may take years to develop and demonstrates predominantly upper lobe silicotic nodules and eggshell calcification of the hilar lymph nodes. Acute high-level exposure can cause acute silicosis presenting as a pulmonary alveolar proteinosis in response to the high particulate load. Accelerated silicosis develops over 3–10 years in response to a higher level of exposure as well. Common occupations include hard rock miners, granite cutters and polishers, sandblasters, stone workers, glass makers, foundry and quarry workers, and construction workers. Engineered stone fabrication workers making stone counter tops are the newest occupation reported at risk of developing silicosis and accelerated silicosis. Silicosis increases susceptibility to tuberculosis, as well as to immune-mediated diseases such as systemic sclerosis, RA, and SLE.

Asbestos workers are at risk of developing asbestosis over many years of working with asbestos fibers. Occupations at risk include auto mechanics working with brakes from older cars, blacksmiths, carpenters, boilermakers, cement plant workers, chemical plant workers, engineers, HVAC mechanics, and electricians, to name a few. Prolonged asbestos exposure can also cause pleural plaques, felt to originate from asbestos fibers migrating to the periphery of the lungs and then encapsulated in fibrotic material, and rounded atelectasis, caused by entrapment of the subpleural lung at the site of pleural effusion or thickening, with a rounded appearance of chest radiographs. Benign pleural effusions are similarly caused by migration of asbestos fibers to the periphery of the lung, and mesothelioma, a malignant disease of the pleura exclusively caused by asbestos fibers. Asbestos exposure is also a risk factor for peritoneal and GI cancers and alone or in conjunction with cigarette smoking is a cause of lung cancer.

Coal workers, principally underground coal miners, who inhale dust from high carbon coal such as anthracite and bituminous, and rarely graphite, can develop simple coal workers' pneumoconiosis or black lung disease. The chest x-ray will show small, 1–5 mm round nodular opacities occasionally with small central calcifications and favoring the upper lungs. Higher intensity exposure can lead to progressive massive fibrosis, presenting on chest x-ray as upper lung predominant coal macules that coalesce to form fibrotic masses that may be associated with surrounding emphysema. Coal miners with black lung disease are at increased risk of tuberculosis and the development of RA known as Caplan syndrome.

Biological Effects of Diesel Exhaust Particles

A growing body of evidence has documented proinflammatory effects of diesel exhaust particles (DEP) on airway epithelial cells and immune cells, with intriguing data suggesting that DEP, when present with specific allergen, can potentiate allergic responses with increased IgE production. *In vitro* studies of DEP demonstrate they exert an adjuvant effect, increasing IL-4 production by cultured B cells, as well as specific IgE production. Animal models show enhanced airways hyperresponsiveness with eosinophilia and goblet cell hyperplasia, histological hallmarks of allergy, and asthma. While the pathophysiologic mechanisms are still under investigation, numerous epidemiologic studies have shown associations between proximity to car traffic and incidence of cough, asthmatic exacerbations, bronchitis, and allergic sensitization.

COMMON-IMMUNE MEDIATED OCCUPATIONAL DISEASES

The most common immune hypersensitivity occupational disorders include allergic asthma or rhinoconjunctivitis, HP, and allergic contact dermatitis (ACD). The reactions are dependent on the host, and the exposure, including the duration, the degree and type of sensitization, and the antigen.

Allergic asthma and allergic rhinitis occur when sensitized workers inhale specific antigen. **Occupational asthma** is probably one of the most common of the immunologically mediated occupational disorders, although knowledge of its incidence is limited by failure to make the association with occupation, underreporting, selection bias, and differences in the distribution of different industries in different countries. The population attributable risk of asthma due to occupation, based on a meta-analysis of 21 studies from around the world, found a range from 4% to 58%, with a median value of 15%. Variable airflow limitation, bronchial hyperresponsiveness, or both, as a result of conditions in a particular work environment, mark occupational asthma. Histamine and arachidonic acid metabolites contribute to acute bronchoconstriction but chronic airways obstruction also develops as a consequence of edema of bronchial mucosa, hyperplasia of bronchial smooth muscle, hypersecretion of mucus, and airway-remodeling with sub–basement membrane thickening. Both occupational asthma and work-aggravated asthma are associated with wheezing, chest tightness, dyspnea, cough, or some combination of these symptoms. Bronchial hyperreactivity is a hallmark of asthma and is characterized by a heightened sensitivity to allergenic triggers in the case of immune-mediated asthma, and nonallergenic stimuli such as methacholine used in a challenge to establish the diagnosis. Common nonspecific triggers for asthma include inhalation of cold, dry air, exercise, and exposure to respiratory irritants like exhaust fumes, smoke, particulate matter, and strong odors.

Sensitization may result from a broad array of natural or synthesized chemicals that may appear in a diverse range of materials and processes. The list of documented causal agents has expanded rapidly over the past 5–10 years and now numbers more than 250 (Table 15-6).

In general, atopic patients are predisposed to sensitization to large-molecular-weight inhalants (proteins) such as animal proteins, pollens, plant proteins, enzymes, mold spores, and house dust. Exposure to **high-molecular-weight**

(HMW) antigens generally induces classic type I, IgE-mediated hypersensitivity reactions. In contrast, there is no atopic predisposition to sensitization by low-molecular-weight (LMW) chemicals such as toluene diisocyanate (TDI), TMA, or epoxy resins. Some **low-molecular-weight compounds**, such as anhydrides and isocyanates, act as haptens and may induce specific IgE antibodies by combining with a cell surface or carrier protein to form a new antigen.

Several clinical patterns have been observed after respiratory exposure to inhalants including (1) acute bronchospasm with rapid resolution after removal of exposure; (2) late onset with the development of symptoms 4–6 hours after the exposure (often after a worker has returned home); or (3) acute onset of continuous asthma symptoms without remission between early- and late-phase responses. In general, IgE-mediated reactions occur as isolated early-phase events or biphasic reactions, whereas IgE-independent reactions often occur as isolated late-phase, or atypical, asthmatic reactions.

Surveys among workers in high-risk occupations suggest that the etiologic agent or exposure is the most important risk factor for the development of occupational asthma. The incidence of allergic rhinitis or allergic asthma in workers with exposure to animal proteins is estimated to be between 20% and 30%. The prevalence of occupational asthma in workers exposed to anhydrides is estimated to be 20%, as compared to the National Health Interview Survey estimation of 5% prevalence of asthma in the general adult population in 1994.

A personal or family history of atopy and concurrent smoking are independent risk factors for IgE-mediated occupational asthma but do not appear to influence IgE-independent processes. Patients may develop occupational asthma early in the course of antigen exposure or may develop symptoms after 10 years of exposure.

Pathologic airway changes characterized by inflammatory cell infiltrates (primarily eosinophils), edema, hypertrophy of smooth muscle, subepithelial fibrosis, and obstruction of the airway lumen by exudate or mucus are similar for all patients with asthma, occupational or environmental.

In principle, any agent that causes occupational asthma can also cause **allergic rhinitis** or allergic conjunctivitis. The sneezing, rhinorrhea, and nasal pruritus seen in allergic rhinitis are the result of tissue effects from early-phase mediators causing increased vascular permeability, tissue edema, stimulation of efferent C fibers, and mucus glandular secretions. Chronic nasal obstruction appears to be caused by the late-phase reaction with cellular recruitment of mononuclear cells, eosinophils, and production of other inflammatory mediators. A phenomenon of priming has been observed, where frequent or chronic exposure to an allergen will lower the threshold for elicitation of symptoms caused by the accumulation of inflammatory cells in the affected tissues. Recent studies estimate the cumulative prevalence of allergic rhinitis to be 20% in the general US population. Occupational rhinitis can develop through both allergic and irritant mechanisms and may exist alone or be superimposed on allergic rhinitis caused by environmental pollens, dust mite, animal dander, or molds. Many patients with allergic rhinitis will

Table 15–6. Materials causally linked to rhinitis and asthma in the workplace.

	Allergen	Occupational Exposure
Plant material	Aromatic herbs, spices	Food industry workers
	Carob bean flour	Food industry workers
	Coffee beans, green	Coffee roasters
	Colophony (abietic acid)	Solder workers
	Cotton	Cotton workers
	Fibers (jute, linen)	Fiber processors
	Flowers (chrysanthemum, carnation, sunflower)	Florists
	Fodder	Dairy farmers
	Grain dust (wheat, buckwheat, soy bean)	Bakers, millers
	Henna	Hairdressers
	Hops	Brewers
	Latex	Health care workers, laboratory workers, latex processing workers, housekeepers
	Obeche (African maple)	Sauna builders
	Pentadecylcatechol (Poison oak)	Poison oak
	Sesame, fennel, anise seeds	Food industry workers
	Rose hips	Health food workers
	Tobacco	Tobacco workers
	Vegetables (garlic dust, artichokes, beans, cabbage)	Food industry workers
	Vegetable gums (Arabic, guar)	Carpet manufacturers, food industry, hairdressers, pharmaceutical workers, printers
	Wood dusts (ash, cedar, mahogany, oak, zebrawood)	Construction workers, carpenters, sawmill workers, craftsmen
Animal and insect products	Animal dander	Veterinarians, farmers, zoo handlers
	Animal urinary proteins	Laboratory animal workers (rodents)
	Casein	Food industry workers, tanners
	Crustaceans	Food processors
	Egg	Food processors
	Feathers, droppings	Bird breeders, farmers
	Food mites	Food handlers (especially handling cheese, poultry, chorizo, salty ham)
	Grasshoppers, midges	Fish feeders, laboratory workers
	Grain weevils	Grain handlers
	Lactalbumin (cow's milk, egg proteins)	Bakers, confectioners, food processors
	Live fish bait	Anglers
	Red spider mites	Nursery workers

(continued)

Table 15–6. Materials causally linked to rhinitis and asthma in the workplace. (Continued)

	Allergen	Occupational Exposure
	Silk worms	Silk workers
	Storage mites	Grain workers, bakers
Fungi and mold	Aspergillus sp, Penicillium sp, T actinomyces,	Farmers, gardeners, laboratory workers, librarians, loggers, mushroom workers, refuse collection workers, vintners
Chemicals	Anhydrides (acid, phtalic, trimetallic)	Plastic manufacturers
	Diacrylates	Auto body workers
	Diisocyanates	Polyurethane plastic and foam workers, spray painters
	Drugs (antibiotics, opiates, psyllium)	Pharmaceutical workers
	Dyes	Carmine extractors, hairdressers, photographers, textile workers
	Epoxy resins	Epoxy manufacturers
	Ethylene dioxide	Healthcare workers
	Formaldehyde	Hospital workers, manufacturers, morticians
	Glutaraldehyde	Hospital workers, paper industry workers
	Metabisulfite	Agricultural workers
	Persulfates (permanent wave solution)	Beauticians
	Reactive dyes	Dye manufacturers
	Sulfites	Food processors
Enzymes	β-Amylase	Bakers
	Bacterial enzymes (alcalase, proteases, peptidase)	Detergent, pharmaceutical workers
	Lactase	Pharmaceutical workers
	Lysozyme	Food, pharmaceutical industry workers
	Pectinase, glucanase	Fruit processors
	Papain	Pharmaceutical workers
	Pepsin	Food industry (cheese), pharmaceutical workers
	Trypsin	Food, laboratory, plastic manufacturing workers
Metals	Aluminum	Solder workers
	Chromium	Cement workers, tanners
	Cobalt	Hard metal workers
	Nickel	Metal workers
	Platinum salts	Catalyst manufacturers
	Stainless steel vapor	Welders
Pharmaceuticals	Antibiotics	Health care providers
	Corticotropin-releasing hormone	Pharmaceutical workers
	Psyllium	Health care providers

also suffer from concomitant **allergic conjunctivitis** manifest by conjunctival injection, eye pruritus, discharge, or discomfort. Although a non–life-threatening disorder, allergic rhinoconjunctivitis has a measurable impact on quality of life. In some surveys, the impact of rhinoconjunctivitis surpasses that of asthma because of its effect on physical, social, emotional functioning and well-being, at home, school, and work. Furthermore, uncontrolled rhinitis may lead to complications such as bacterial sinusitis, cough, and asthma.

HP is a parenchymal pulmonary disease resulting from sensitization and subsequent exposure to a variety of inhaled organic dusts and related occupational antigens. Bacterial products, small amounts of serum present in the excreta of animals, T actinomycetes (eg, *Micropolyspora faeni, Tectibacter vulgaris,* and *Thermoactinomyces sacchari*), fungi, and vegetable proteins have all caused HP (Table 15-5).

Examples include pigeon breeder's disease, farmer's lung, humidifier lung, malt worker's lung, mushroom worker's lung, and bagassosis from processing sugarcane. Chemicals demonstrated to induce HP include the diisocyanates found in most polyurethane paints, foams, and coatings, and the epoxy resins found in most plastics. HP caused by plastics appears to have a more insidious course than does the classic farmer's lung. Prolonged treatment with systemic steroids may be required to clear inflammation and improve the ventilatory impairment. The incidence varies with the type and frequency of antigen exposure and is not age dependent. Sensitization is favored by the alveolar deposition of particulate antigen less than 5 μm in diameter.

With short-term high-level exposure to antigen the acute disease is characterized by fever, cough, dyspnea, and myalgias which occur 4–12 hours after heavy exposure and remit within hours to days. The subacute or chronic form of the disease is associated with long-term, low-level antigen exposure and induces an insidious onset of cough and dyspnea and eventually an irreversible restrictive ventilatory impairment.

There is evidence both to support and reject the concept that HP is a type III reaction. Up to 90% of patients have antigen-specific precipitins in their serum. However, 50% of similarly exposed asymptomatic subjects also have precipitins to the same antigens which suggests that the precipitins may merely be markers of antigen exposure. In patients, the presence of specific precipitins can only be interpreted as a sign of exposure, not disease. Evidence suggests that a type IV or cell-mediated immune reaction to inhaled antigen may play a more predominant role in the development of HP. Histopathologic study of the lesions reveals an infiltrate with neutrophils, lymphocytes, and macrophages. Noncaseating granulomas, giant cells, and fibrosis may be present. Granuloma formation favors the diagnosis of cell-mediated immune reaction; however, this may also be induced by non-phagocytosed antigen-antibody complexes. The lymphocytes of sensitized patients release cytokines when exposed to the specific antigen. Experimentally, lesions resembling alveolitis can be induced by first sensitizing rabbits using methods favoring a cell-mediated immune response and then challenging with inhaled antigen. Furthermore, when rabbits are passively sensitized by lymphocytes from sensitized rabbits and then challenged, typical lesions consistent with alveolitis develop. These studies favor a type IV response. It is possible that nonimmune activation of effector mechanisms of hypersensitivity may also be operative.

Although previously a diagnosis of HP required finding specific IgG antibodies (precipitins) against the offending agents, that is no longer the case. Bird precipitins are a reasonable marker of exposure and the elaboration of a specific immune response, but in many cases, there are no appropriate testing reagents. Testing for precipitins to fungi is generally not helpful, in part because of the plethora of fungal species, subspecies, and mixtures that may not be adequately represented in a commercially available test. Efforts now focus on finding an intense alveolar lymphocytosis on bronchoalveolar lavage. Lavage fluid in HP can be marked by increased numbers of CD8+ T cells, although not always depending on the timing of antigen exposure and the state of the disease. In contrast, CD4+ T cells typically predominate in sarcoidosis and neutrophils in idiopathic pulmonary fibrosis. Radiographic imaging and pulmonary function testing can establish interstitial involvement but BAL and transbronchial lung biopsies may sometimes be necessary.

ACD is a type IV, delayed hypersensitivity disorder, caused by a variety of agents in the occupational setting including latex, nickel, formaldehyde, potassium dichromate, thiurams, epoxy resins, mercaptos, parabens, quaternium-15, ethylenediamine, and cobalt. Rhus or poison ivy, oak, and sumac ACD is caused by cutaneous exposure to oils from the toxicodendron plants (Table 15-7). Acutely,

Table 15–7. Occupational agents causing allergic contact dermatitis.

Acrylates
Aldehydes
Anhydrides
Ammonium persulfate
Aromatic amines
Aromatic nitros
Carbamates
Disinfectants
Enzymes
Epoxy resins
Fungicides
Herbicides
Isocyanates
Lanolin
Metals
Phenols
Phthalates
Plant extracts
Pharmaceutical agents
Preservatives
Rubber additives
Solvents

the dermatitis is characterized by intense pruritus and local erythema and induration with vesicle formation, exudation, and crusting in more advanced stages. Chronic ACD may be associated with fissuring, lichenification, or dyspigmentation. The face and hands are disproportionately affected because of their higher likelihood of exposure. Indeed, the appearance may resemble other forms of dermatitis, such as atopic dermatitis or irritant dermatitis.

Note that irritant dermatitis is four times more common than ACD. In contrast to agents causing ACD, irritant reactions are not characterized by a sensitization phase and do not result in an antigen-mediated inflammatory response. Their appearance is often similar to ACD but they are more frequently characterized by burning and pain, and less frequently characterized by intense pruritus. Wet work, involving skin contact with water, surfactants, and solvents are common causes of irritant contact dermatitis.

OCCUPATIONS AND EXPOSURES THAT CAN CAUSE OCCUPATIONAL IMMUNE DISEASES

Antigens inducing occupational immune hypersensitivity disorders may be of animal, vegetable, or chemical origin. Immune hypersensitivity reactions occur when a sensitized worker encounters antigens in the work environment.

Animal Products

Occupational exposure to animal products may cause a type I immediate response manifested by symptoms of acute or chronic asthma and rhinitis. Animal danders and excreta, insects, shellfish, and animal enzymes induce IgE antibodies and type I reactions. Cat and dog hair, dander, saliva, and urine may induce occupational allergies in veterinarians and animal handlers. Allergens found in the urine, saliva, and pelt from mice, rats, rabbits, and guinea pigs may sensitize laboratory workers and cause respiratory allergy. Of the 5641 workers who were exposed to animals at 137 laboratory animal facilities in Japan, approximately 25% had one or more allergic symptoms related to laboratory animals, most commonly rhinitis. Approximately 70% of workers developed symptoms during their first 3 years of exposure. The presence of atopy, the number of animal species handled, and the time spent in handling correlated significantly with the development of allergy. Cow epithelial and urinary proteins have been demonstrated to cause asthma and rhinitis in farmers, as demonstrated by immunologic tests and bronchial or nasal provocation. Insects including the red spider mite and other arthropods have induced occupational allergic disease in technicians and pest control workers.

In today's laundry detergents, enzymes such as proteases and amylases are some of the active ingredients. In the United States, about 50% of liquid detergents, 25% of powder detergents, and almost all powdered bleach additives now contain enzymes to help break down stains that are otherwise hard to remove with conventional surfactants alone.

For example, amylase catalyzes the breakdown of starch-based stains to smaller oligosaccharides and dextrins that are soluble and released from the fabric surface. The action of proteases is similar to that of amylase, except that a large protein molecule is hydrolyzed. During the process of hydrolysis, the peptide bonds are broken down, releasing smaller polypeptides (<100 aa) and individual amino acid units. Currently, these enzymes are manufactured commercially in large quantities through fermentation by common soil bacteria B subtilis or B licheniformis. When detergents containing enzymes were first manufactured in Great Britain, the manufacturing facilities noted extremely high rates of asthma and rhinosinusitis. The issue of worker exposure was solved by encapsulating the enzymes, although occupational asthma to bacterial enzymes has still been diagnosed in workers exposed to encapsulated enzymes. More recently bacterial enzymes used to sterilize medical scopes have been reported to cause occupational asthma in nurses and technicians.

Vegetable Products

Castor bean, soy bean, and green coffee bean dust are potent antigens for some people, inducing a type I immediate hypersensitivity response manifested as rhinitis and asthma. There are reports of patients living near castor bean processing plants who have developed severe asthma secondary to wind shifts resulting in inhalation of minute amounts of this dust. The inhalation of soybean dust released during the unloading of soybeans into a silo caused outbreaks of asthma in Spain. Installing filters on silos to prevent airborne dissemination of allergenic soybean dust eliminated these outbreaks. It is estimated that 10% of workers handling green coffee beans develop IgE-mediated symptoms, especially rhinoconjunctivitis. The antigenicity of the green coffee bean is destroyed by roasting. Workers who have an adverse immune response to green coffee dust are able to handle the roasted beans without difficulty.

A common problem and public health threat in the 1990s and early 2000s was hypersensitivity to natural rubber latex antigens derived from the commercial rubber tree Hevea brasiliensis. Between 1989 and 1993, the U.S. Food and Drug Administration (FDA) received more than 1100 reports of injury and 15 deaths associated with latex allergy. Latex is a complex plant product, the essential functional unit of which is the rubber particle, a spherical droplet of polyisoprene coated with a layer of protein, lipid, and phospholipid. Approximately 250 Hevea polypeptides have been identified, of which a few have been found to be the most highly sensitizing. These include Hev b 1.2, 2, 3, 4, 5, 6.02, 7.01, and 13. Hev b1, the rubber elongation factor, and Hev b3 require direct mucosal contact to sensitize, and hence are the most allergenic for spina bifida patients and others with frequent mucosal contact with rubber products such as foley catheters. Hev b5 and Hev b 6.01/6.02 are proteins released from dipped products, such as latex gloves and are the major allergens that sensitize health care workers. Type I, immediate hypersensitivity reactions to latex, may range from mild to life-threatening and include systemic urticaria, rhinitis, conjunctivitis, bronchospasm, and anaphylaxis and may occur following cutaneous, mucosal, or parenteral contact. Aerosol transmission of antigens is a commonly reported route of exposure. Workers at risk of latex allergy include health care workers and rubber industry workers. Since latex can be ubiquitous in certain settings, and the incidence latex hypersensitivity may approach 1% in the general public, it can be difficult to establish the source and onset of sensitization. Furthermore, up to 3000-fold differences in allergen content have been noted when various brands of natural latex gloves were examined. So the risk of sensitization in the same setting, for example, ER, diagnostic lab, etc., may differ based on the brand of gloves used.

Risk factors for sensitization include increased exposure and atopy. Studies looking at nurses and surgeons have estimated the prevalence of latex hypersensitivity to range between 5% and 17%. The growing numbers of affected workers has been blamed on changes in latex processing and the increased number of exposed individuals because of body fluid exposure precautions in the last two decades. In 1998, Germany banned the use of powdered latex gloves and the incidence of occupational latex allergy has decreased by 80%, demonstrating the impact of exposure reduction measures. ACD may also be caused by latex exposure, although these type IV, delayed hypersensitivity reactions are caused by rubber additives, such as thiurams, carbamates, benzothiazoles, thioureas, and amines. These chemical components are added to the plant-derived latex extracts during the manufacturing process as antioxidants, accelerating agents, or dyes. A curious condition, "latex fruit syndrome," has also been seen in up to 52% of latex allergic patients. Because of immunologic cross-reactivity between latex allergens and those found in avocado, banana, chestnut, kiwi, peach, tomato, potato, and bell pepper, ingestion, particularly of fresh fruits, by latex allergic individuals can cause a systemic allergic reaction.

Five percent of workers in the western US red cedar lumber industry develop asthma after a latent period of exposure that averages about 3–4 years. They exhibit bronchospasm to inhalation challenge with plicatic acid, a LMW derivative of red cedar. Skin testing and RAST demonstrate IgE sensitivity in approximately 50% of affected workers, but positive results are also found in unaffected workers and hence are more indicative of sensitization. Atopy does not predispose workers to sensitization, although it is possible that some cases are caused by IgE-mediated processes. Other wood dusts may also cause occupational asthma, including oak, mahogany, zebrawood, and ash, but many sawmill workers also have significant exposure to molds as well.

Colophony, a pine resin by-product (rosin) that is used as solder flux, causes both immediate and dual respiratory reactions in sensitized workers. The reaction is probably an IgE-mediated hypersensitivity to the allergen, abietic acid.

In the United States, the most common agent causing occupational dermatitis is the oil from plants of the genus *Rhus* (poison oak, poison ivy, and poison sumac). Poison oak is found west of the Rocky Mountains; poison ivy and poison sumac are found to the east. The active allergen is located in the oily sap, urushiol, a LMW substance that binds to a skin protein and forms a complete antigen. Studies reveal that more than 90% of subjects are sensitized on exposure to these antigens. A subject will develop a type IV ACD reaction 24–72 hours after exposure.

Respiratory symptoms secondary to exposure to flour dust occur in bakers. Potential allergens can be from cereal grain and also from mold spore contaminants, storage mites, egg proteins, or enzymes used in cooking and fermentation. The mean annual incidence of occupational respiratory diseases among bakery workers over a 10-year period in Finland was reported to be 374 per 100,000 workers, compared with a rate of 31 per 100,000 workers in general. Affected workers may exhibit (1) an immediate or (2) an immediate followed by a late-onset reaction; both are probably IgE mediated. There is a direct relation between duration of exposure and the percentage of bakers who exhibit skin test reactivity.

Chemical Agents

Workers in industrial plants may be exposed to a wide variety of chemical agents. Two that have been extensively studied are the isocyanates and anhydrides. In contrast to biological allergens, which are HMW sensitizers, these agents are LMW and must haptenate before becoming immunogenic. **Isocyanates** are used in the manufacture of pesticides, polyurethane foams, synthetic varnishes, spray foam insulation, truck-bed liners, and two-part car paints. There are many case reports of asthma related to TDI. These occur with equal frequency in atopic and nonatopic workers. The mechanism of developing disease has not been elucidated, but several different pathways explain the pathogenesis, include the following:

1. *RADS due to acute high dose exposure.* In this case, there is no latency period, but asthma develops soon after a sudden, high concentration exposure.

2. *Direct pharmacologic action. In vitro* studies demonstrate that TDI can act as a weak beta-adrenergic blocking agent and may also stimulate neuroimmune mechanisms, enhancing substance P and neuropeptide-mediated actions.

3. *Airway epithelial cell and innate immune responses.* These may mediate cytokine release, oxidative stress reactions, and inflammation, independent of IgE. Isocyanate exposure has also been associated with increased chemoattractant release and monocytic and neutrophilic cell accumulation.

4. *Immune hypersensitivity response.* This form of isocyanate-induced asthma presents with the insidious onset of symptoms after a latency period of weeks to months, peripheral eosinophilia, and the induction of symptoms in sensitized workers on re-exposure to minute quantities of the material. RAST and skin testing with a LMW isocyanate conjugate with human serum albumin (HSA)

have demonstrated specific IgE antibodies, and in some cases, IgG antibodies; however, because the antibodies can be demonstrated in affected and nonaffected workers, they may better correlate with exposure and not with clinical disease. The ability to mount an immunologic response against isocyanates appears to be genetically determined, as certain HLA genes have been linked to disease susceptibility.

TMA is used to manufacture plastics, epoxy resins, and paints. TMA dust or fumes have been associated with four different clinical syndromes:

1. The *TMA immediate-type reaction* is caused by IgE antibodies to trimellitic-human serum albumin (TM-HSA) conjugates. The reaction requires a latent period of exposure before the onset of clinical disease which is characterized by allergic-type symptoms of rhinitis, conjunctivitis, or asthma. Interestingly, affected workers have no atopic predisposition, despite this being a type I reaction.

2. The *late-reacting systemic syndrome ("TMA flu")* is characterized by cough, occasional wheezing, dyspnea, and systemic symptoms of malaise, chills, myalgia, and arthralgia. These reactions occur 4–6 hours after exposure to TMA and are a type III disorder in which IgG antibodies to TM-HSA form immune complexes with TMA protein conjugates. Consistent with a specific immune response, repeated exposure and a latent period of weeks to months are required before symptoms develop.

3. The *pulmonary disease–anemia syndrome* develops after repeated high-dose exposure to the volatile fumes of TMA sprayed on heated metal surfaces to prevent corrosion. This is a type II cytotoxic reaction in which IgG antibodies to TM-HSA and to a trimellitic-erythrocyte conjugate develop and are directed toward TMA bound to erythrocytes and the pulmonary basement membrane. The clinical outcome is a Coombs-positive hemolytic anemia and respiratory failure.

4. An *irritant respiratory syndrome*, characterized by cough and dyspnea and consistent with RADS may occur with a first high-dose exposure to TMA powder and fumes. This is not caused by immune sensitization to TMA conjugates.

Hexahydrophthalic anhydride (HHPA) is a component of some epoxy resin systems. A high fraction of HHPA-exposed workers displays nasal symptoms and some of them have serum IgE antibodies specific to HHPA. Eleven subjects, who were IgE sensitized against an HHPA-HSA conjugate and who reported work-related nasal symptoms, responded to an HHPA-HSA nasal provocation with a significant increase of nasal symptoms and a decrease of nasal inspiratory peak flow. Symptoms were associated with significant increases in eosinophil and neutrophil counts and in levels of tryptase and albumin in nasal lavage fluid. Nine subjects who were not sensitized but complained of work-related symptoms, and 11 subjects who were not sensitized and had no symptoms, displayed no changes in any of these parameters following challenge. Another study reported that risk factors for the development of immunologically mediated respiratory disease caused by HHPA in 57 exposed workers included exposure level and the development of specific IgE or IgG antibodies.

Reactive metallic compounds are found in a wide range of industrial settings. Metallic salts are an important cause of immune hypersensitivity. After poison oak, nickel is the most common cause of contact dermatitis, a type IV reaction. There are also reports of asthma secondary to inhalation of fumes of nickel and platinum salts. These salts act as haptens and bind to serum proteins, creating a new antigen that induces the production of specific IgE. Subsequent exposure may then trigger bronchial asthma. Challenge studies with bronchial provocation by offending metallic substances have demonstrated bronchospasm and bronchial hyperreactivity after exposure to platinum salts, nickel sulfate, cobalt chloride, and vanadium. IgE-mediated hypersensitivity has been found with some but not all of these metallic compounds. Notably, this process is distinct from a type IV immune reaction leading to a contact dermatitis to the metals.

DIAGNOSIS OF HYPERSENSITIVITY DISEASES IN OCCUPATIONAL MEDICINE

From the standpoint of both the patient and the employer, it is important to establish an early diagnosis. Many obstructive pulmonary problems that are reversible with proper early management can become fixed disabilities with prolonged exposure to causative agents. The diagnosis of occupational hypersensitivity diseases should include both making the clinical diagnosis and establishing the relationship with the workplace. Requirements for establishing the relationship to work are generally more stringent for medical diagnoses than for field epidemiologic surveys. Occupational hypersensitivity illnesses should be suspected in a person exposed at work to agents known to cause disease, although the failure to identify a known agent does not rule out the disorder.

▶ History & Physical Examination

The initial workup should include a detailed history and physical examination and, when indicated, a chest film, pulmonary function tests (PFTs), and a blood count.

Note the type of symptoms, aggravating and relieving factors, and the timing of onset after starting the current job to address the issue of latency. Also record their temporal relationship with the work environment and the effects of vacation and weekends. A history of improvement of symptoms during weekends and holidays and a worsening on return to work suggests but does not confirm occupational hypersensitivity disease. Late-onset respiratory reactions may not occur until a patient has returned home from work. Be sure to detail past and current exposures because early exposure to an agent may have induced sensitization that then manifests as asthma in the next job. Ask about a personal or family history of atopy (hay fever, allergic asthma, or atopic dermatitis) as a risk factor for sensitization to HMW allergens. With the presence of bronchospasm, it is important to review current medications, including beta-blockers, aspirin, and nonsteroidal anti-inflammatory drugs, all of which may induce bronchial asthma; angiotensin-converting enzyme inhibitors may cause cough. Ask about the home environment including any changes that have occurred, the presence of pets and molds, any recent moves, hobbies, and the use of tobacco by the patient or others in the household. Finally, elicit a detailed occupational history, including information regarding present and past employment and a detailed history of specific job duties and work processes for both the patient and coworkers. Assess the frequency and intensity of exposures and peak concentrations of potential agents. Also review safety data sheets for chemicals in the workplace, industrial hygiene data, and employee health records.

At times it is helpful—with the employer's permission—to visit the work site to get a better idea of the work processes and potential exposures.

Focus the physical examination on evaluation of the skin and the upper and lower respiratory tracts, but a full examination should be performed to identify signs of systemic or other medical illness. Look for evidence of atopic disease, including the presence of allergic facies or allergic shiners, cobblestoning of the conjunctiva, pale and swollen mucous membranes, posterior pharyngeal lymphoid plaques, expiratory wheezing, cough, rhonchi, or a silent chest indicating more severe asthma. Examine the skin of the face, "V" of the neck, forearms, and hands for signs of a contact or atopic dermatitis. Listen for dry crackles or rales and look for cyanosis, clubbing, and an increased anteroposterior diameter of the chest.

▶ Laboratory Investigation

The diagnosis of occupational disease should be confirmed by objective data. A complete blood count demonstrating evidence of eosinophilia may aid in the diagnosis of atopy. The presence of serum eosinophilia suggests a diagnosis of allergic disease, whereas eosinophils in sputum or nasal secretions is consistent with asthma and allergic rhinitis, respectively. However, neither is required to make a diagnosis of allergic disease. Total serum IgE level is often elevated in atopic patients, although this test is neither sensitive nor specific for establishing the diagnosis of atopy.

Baseline posteroanterior and lateral radiographs of the chest should be obtained in patients with pulmonary problems, noting increased anteroposterior chest diameter, flattening of the diaphragms, infiltrates, enlarged lymph nodes, evidence of bronchiectasis, hyperinflation, and/or diffuse micronodularity.

Pulmonary function studies before and after bronchodilator should be obtained in the case of respiratory symptoms;

at a minimum, they should include forced expiratory volume in 1 second (FEV_1), forced vital capacity (FVC), forced expiratory flow (FEF) between 25% and 75% of FVC, and peak expiratory flow rate (PEFR). A significant response to bronchodilator is considered to include both a greater than or equal to 12% improvement in the FEV_1 after albuterol, as well as greater than or equal to 200 mL improvement in airflow. Complete PFTs including lung volumes and diffusion capacity (DL_{CO}) are necessary to establish a restrictive component of lung disease. Measurements of blood gases may prove helpful to establish hypoxemia, hypo- or hyperventilation.

Measurement of bronchial hyperresponsiveness to pharmacologic agents such as methacholine or histamine is important in the diagnosis of asthma, especially when a bronchodilator response is not evident on spirometry or cough is the only marker of lung disease. It is important to note that, in otherwise healthy individuals, PFTs may be completely normal but a methacholine challenge can be positive for asthma.

In a methacholine challenge test, the subject inhales increasing doses of methacholine and performs spirometry after inhaling each one. If bronchial hyperreactivity is present, the FEV_1 will decline by a minimum of 20% at low doses of methacholine. Asthmatics are up to 1000 times more sensitive than normal individuals to methacholine bronchoprovocation challenge. The absence of bronchial hyperresponsiveness, that is a positive methacholine challenge, after a person has worked for 2 weeks under normal working conditions virtually rules out the diagnosis of occupational asthma. Once bronchial hyperresponsiveness has been established, further testing is required to demonstrate the relationship of asthma to the workplace. Note that demonstration of sensitization to an antigen at work implicated in triggering symptoms, along with pharmacologically induced bronchial hyperresponsiveness, that is, a positive methacholine challenge, have an 80% likelihood of demonstrating asthma to the antigen in a laboratory challenge.

More recently, measurements of FE_{NO} (fractional exhaled nitric oxide) have been utilized in bronchial asthma to quantify airway inflammation. Rapid, reproducible, and simple to measure FE_{NO} is a noninvasive biomarker that may be an adjunct to measurements of airflow and elevated levels associated with allergic sensitization.

▶ Immunologic Tests

Based on the initial evaluation, specific immunologic tests may be obtained to confirm the diagnosis, including immediate allergy skin tests, patch tests, *in vitro* tests for IgE antibodies, Ouchterlony gel diffusion tests, and provocative challenge with specific antigens.

A. Skin Tests

Epicutaneous (prick) and intradermal skin tests are helpful in establishing IgE-mediated sensitization to a number of inhalant protein antigens, including mold spores, house dust mites, animal danders, feathers, pollens, and extracts of suspected HMW antigens in the work environment, although many standardized occupational allergens are not commercially available at present. Skin tests are *in vivo*, rapid, cost-effective, and more sensitive and more specific than currently available *in vitro* allergen-specific IgE assays. Testing can be accomplished in 30–60 minutes at experienced centers. A positive skin test is marked by a pruritic wheal-and-flare reaction, which peaks at 20 minutes, confirming the presence of antigen-specific IgE bound to skin mast cells. The initial wheal-and-flare reaction may be followed in 4–6 hours by an IgE-mediated late-phase reaction evidenced by erythema, induration, pruritus, and tenderness at the skin test site. LMW materials usually do not give a positive immediate skin test response unless they are linked to a protein carrier such as HSA.

B. Patch Testing

Patch tests are useful in evaluating skin contact sensitization (type IV delayed hypersensitivity). The test employs antigen-impregnated patches applied to the skin. The patches are removed after 48 hours, and the test sites are evaluated, although this reading is considered preliminary. A positive reaction consists of erythema, induration, and, in some cases, vesiculation. A follow-up reading is usually done 24–48 hours after the first reading, allowing the technician to discriminate between true delayed hypersensitivity and irritant reactions that typically have faded by the time of the second reading. A standardized antigen patch test kit, the T.R.U.E. Test, may be purchased from SmartPractice (Phoenix, AZ). Other antigens, including sets organized by job or profession, may be obtained from a number of different companies, including SmartPractice Dermatology and Dormer/Chemotechnique. Suspected materials from the work environment may be used, although testing should be performed by an experienced allergist or dermatologist, as some materials are too toxic or irritating to be used.

C. In Vitro Antibody Tests

RAST and ELISA are *in vitro* immunoassays that are used to detect circulating antigen-specific IgE antibodies. In these tests, inert particles coated with antigen are incubated with the patient's serum. If a specific antibody is present, it binds to the specific particle-bound antigen. The complex is then washed, incubated with radiolabeled or enzyme-labeled anti-IgE, and washed again. The amount of anti-IgE measured by radioactivity or enzyme activity indirectly measures the amount of bound antigen-specific IgE from the patient. Such *in vitro* tests may be valuable in cases when appropriate skin testing reagents are unavailable or in patients with severe dermatographism on treatment with long-acting antihistamines or tricyclic antidepressants that would suppress prick skin testing or with an increased risk of systemic anaphylaxis. AlaSTAT (Diagnostic Products Corporation), Immuno-CAP (Pharmacia-UpJohn), and HY-TEC EIA (Hycor) are serologically tested, FDA-approved kits for use in the diagnosis of latex allergy in the United States.

D. Ouchterlony Gel Diffusion Test

This semiquantitative test is used to demonstrate IgG precipitating antibody to a specific antigen. Suspected antigens and the patient's serum are placed in separate wells cut into a gel-coated plate. The antigen and serum diffuse toward one another. If sufficient antibody specific to the antigen is present, precipitin lines, composed of antigen-antibody complexes, form at an intermediate point between the two wells. Detection of serum precipitins can confirm a type III hypersensitivity reaction. Commercially available precipitating antibodies specific for avian proteins can be found in some cases of HP.

E. Inhalation Challenge Tests

These tests are conducted by exposing the worker to the suspected antigen. *Caution:* Inhalation challenge studies are not without risk. The measurable endpoints are typically a 20% deterioration in airflow. Sensitized patients are susceptible to late-onset asthmatic reactions that may develop up to 12 hours after the initial challenge. These reactions are often refractory to bronchodilator treatment. The severity of the underlying lung disease or the inability to stop corticosteroids, antihistamines, and/or bronchodilators prior to the test may be contraindications for these procedures.

The challenge may be performed in the work environment or in a hospital laboratory situation. The patient probably should be hospitalized and observed for 12–24 hours after a laboratory challenge.

1. Workplace challenge—A workplace challenge may be indicated to establish the association between workplace exposure levels and respiratory responses. The patient is instructed to use a hand-held peak-flow meter to monitor and record PEFR four times a day for 2 weeks while at work and for an additional 2 weeks while away from work. The general timing should include a measurement at home upon arising, a measurement during the first half of the work shift, a measurement in the second half of the work shift, and a final measurement sometime after work. There is good correlation with results from specific inhalation challenges; however, peak-flow diaries can be subject to patient bias and effort. Combining measurement of peak flow with serial measurements of bronchial hyperresponsiveness (eg, methacholine challenge) does not appear to improve sensitivity or specificity. The use of computerized peak-flow meters may improve accuracy and record patient effort. If initial peak-flow monitoring is suggestive of occupational asthma, a technician may be sent to the workplace to monitor hourly spirometry during the workday.

2. Laboratory inhalation challenge—When there is uncertainty regarding the etiologic relevance of a specific occupational agent and respiratory hazard, an inhalation challenge may be performed in a clinic or hospital setting. This can be obtained in three ways:

1. After the worker's condition is stabilized off work, baseline spirometry is obtained; the worker is placed in a closed environment and asked to transfer suspected antigen dust, mixed in lactose powder, back and forth between two trays. If possible, testing should also include a placebo transfer, using lactose powder alone. Spirometry should be obtained every 30–60 minutes over the following 6–8 hours to assess for a late asthmatic response.

2. In another variation in a hospital setting, the subject is exposed to various volatile agents (eg, solder, varnish) by actually working with the materials. Spirometry is obtained immediately before and for at least 6–8 hours after exposure.

3. Aerosol inhalation challenge involves the administration of gradually increasing amounts of aerosolized suspected material while spirometry is similarly monitored. A 20% or greater fall in FEV_1 is considered a positive response. False-negative inhalation challenge test results may occur if the incorrect agent or dose is used or if the patient has had an extended absence from work and has lost bronchial hyperresponsiveness.

▶ Treatment

The diagnosis of occupational hypersensitivity disease has considerable economic implications for the worker and the worker's family, the employers, and government agencies. Although pharmacotherapy can help manage symptoms, it is environmental avoidance measures that are the cornerstone of any treatment plan. However, safe or threshold levels of exposure are not well known or clearly defined for many agents. Complete removal of the worker from the workplace environment may be ideal but may place considerable economic hardships on all involved. An attempt may be made to retrain workers for other roles within the same company or with another employer, to reduce exposure by improving ventilation or providing a respirator, or to make changes in the workplace to abide by existing laws. Public health agencies should be enlisted to begin surveillance programs when index cases have been identified. Patients who return to the same workplace require close medical monitoring and follow-up. Even after removal from the workplace, many patients may continue to have chronic airway disease and require the use of medications. Experience with western red cedar (plicatic acid), TDI, and other LMW substances reveals that at least half of the patients will continue to have persistent, even worsening asthma despite removal from exposure. Duration of symptoms greater than 6 months before removal and severity of asthma are strong risk factors for progressive disease even after removal from the workplace. Workers may be impaired or even disabled from occupational asthma and they should be evaluated for appropriate compensation.

REFERENCES

Baur X et al: Immunological methods for diagnosis and monitoring of IgE-mediated allergy caused by industrial sensitizing agents (IMExAllergy). Allergy 2019;74(10):1885-1897 [PMID: 30953599].

Caillaud D, Leynaert B, Keirsbulck M, Nadif R, mould ANSES working group: Indoor mould exposure, asthma and rhinitis: findings from systematic reviews and recent longitudinal studies. Eur Respir Rev 2018;27(148):170137 [PMID: 29769295].

Pacheco KA: Occupational dermatitis: how to identify the exposures, make the diagnosis, and treat the disease. Ann Allergy Asthma Immunol 2018;120(6):583-591 [PMID: 29698693].

Quirce S et al: Occupational hypersensitivity pneumonitis: an EAACI position paper. Allergy 2016;71(6):765-779 [PMID: 26913451].

Rachiotis G, Savani R, Brant A, MacNeill SJ, Newman Taylor A, Cullinan P. Outcome of occupational asthma after cessation of exposure: a systematic review. Thorax 2007;62:147-52. Epub 2006 Oct 13.

Raulf M, Quirce S, Vandenplas O: Addressing molecular diagnosis of occupational allergies. Curr Allergy Asthma Rep 2018;18(1):6 [PMID: 29445888].

■ SELF-ASSESSMENT QUESTIONS

Select the one correct answer for each question.

Question 1: Lymphocytes are
   a. about 70–80% B cells
   b. about 10–15% T cells
   c. responsible for the initial specific recognition of antigen
   d. distinguished visually from each other under the microscope

Question 2: Cytotoxic or "killer" T cells are
   a. generated after immature T cells interact with foreign antigens
   b. responsible for defense against intracellular pathogens
   c. unable to cause programmed cell death
   d. do not secrete TNF

Question 3: Macrophages
  a. become monocytes after they are recruited to sites of inflammation
  b. are unable to synthesize proinflammatory mediators
  c. are involved in the ingestion, processing, and presentation of antigens for interaction with lymphocytes
  d. inhibit production of bacterial endotoxin

Question 4: Eosinophils
  a. play both a proactive and a modulating role in inflammation
  b. are attracted to the site of the antigen-antibody reactions by temperature change
  c. play no role in the defense against parasites
  d. primarily release prostaglandins

Question 5: Type I anaphylactic or immediate hypersensitivity reactions
  a. are initiated by the interaction of antigen with specific IgE antibodies
  b. have no subsequent release of inflammatory mediators
  c. have a destructive role in inflammation
  d. are unrelated to proinflammatory mediators

Question 6: Reactive airways dysfunction syndrome (RADS)
  a. symptoms develop slowly
  b. is characterized by symptoms of asthma

  c. has a long latency period
  d. occurs in the presence of preexisting pulmonary disease

Question 7: Allergic contact dermatitis (ACD)
  a. usually involves skin covered by clothing
  b. is not caused by exposure to latex
  c. predominantly results from solvent exposure
  d. is a type IV, delayed hypersensitivity disorder

Question 8: Trimellitic anhydride (TMA) flu
  a. is characterized by cough, occasional wheezing, and dyspnea
  b. is a type IV disorder
  c. occurs after low-dose exposure to TMA fumes
  d. occurs immediately following exposure to TMA fumes

Question 9: Patch testing
  a. is useful in evaluating irritant contact dermatitis
  b. is useful in evaluating skin contact sensitivity
  c. is read after 24 hours
  d. follow-up reading is done 1 week after the first reading

Question 10: Inhalation challenge tests
  a. expose the worker to the suspected antigen
  b. entail no significant risk
  c. should not be performed in the work environment
  d. do not require omitting corticosteroids, antihistamine, and bronchodilators prior to the test

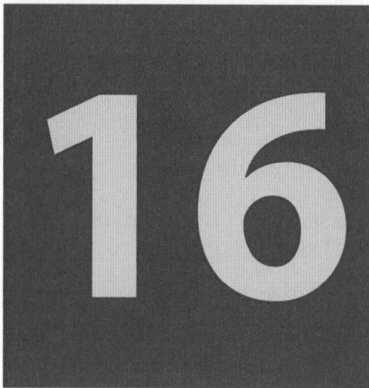

Occupational Infections

Timur S. Durrani, MD, MPH, MBA

Lisa Winston, MD

Occupational infections are human diseases caused by work-associated exposure to microbial agents, including bacteria, viruses, fungi, and parasites. Occupational infection can occur following contact with infected persons or surfaces, as in the case of health care workers; with infected animal or human tissue, secretions, or excretions, as with laboratory workers; with asymptomatic or unknown contagious humans, as happens during business travel; or with infected animals, as in agriculture. See Table 16–1 for work-related pathogens by specific job title.

The etiology, pathogenesis, clinical findings, diagnosis, and treatment of occupational, nonoccupational, and bioterrorism infections are essentially the same except for practical differences related to identification of the source of exposure, epidemiologic control, and prevention. This chapter focuses on the occupational aspects of microbial exposures and relevant strategies for prevention. This chapter highlights viral hemorrhagic fevers (VHFs), coronaviruses, influenza, tuberculosis, hepatitis B and C, human immunodeficiency virus (HIV), and travel-related infections as examples of different types of exposures.

VHFs, coronaviruses, influenza, and tuberculosis can be spread by the aerosol route. Aerosol transmittable diseases require precautions in health care facilities to reduce the risk of spreading infection. Aerosol transmission can occur by droplet or airborne particles. Droplets are larger and can be propelled up to 6 ft and deposited on the mouth, nose, and eyes. Droplets also can contaminate surfaces where some pathogens can survive on certain surfaces for up to several days, allowing the surface to be a fomite which can transmit infection. Airborne particles in the respirable size containing infectious agents can remain infective over time and distance. Microorganisms carried in this manner may be dispersed over long distances by air currents and may also be inhaled by susceptible individuals who have not had face-to-face contact with (or have been in the same room with) the infectious individual.

The Centers for Disease Control and Prevention (CDC) recommends airborne precautions for the management of hospitalized patients with the organisms listed in Table 16–2. These precautions include basic hygiene measures incorporating respiratory hygiene/cough etiquette, use of personal protective equipment (PPE), in particular fit-tested National Institute of Occupational Health and Safety (NIOSH)-approved N95 or higher-level respirators, use of negative pressure airborne infection isolation rooms (AIIR), and procedural protocols for the use of ventilators, nebulizers, endotracheal intubation, and other droplet- and aerosol-generating devices and procedures.

EMERGING INFECTIOUS DISEASES

▶ Viral Hemorrhagic Fevers

Viral hemorrhagic fevers (VHFs) refer to a group of illnesses that are caused by five families of viruses: *Arenaviridae*, *Bunyaviridae*, *Filoviridae*, *Flaviviridae*, and *Paramyxoviridae*. Three genera of *Filoviridae* have been identified: Cuevavirus, Marburgvirus, and Ebolavirus. In general, the term "viral hemorrhagic fever" is used to describe a severe syndrome in which multiple organ systems in the body are affected. Characteristically, the overall vascular system is damaged, and the body's ability to regulate itself is impaired. These symptoms are often accompanied by hemorrhage (bleeding); however, the bleeding is itself rarely life threatening. While some types of hemorrhagic fever viruses can cause relatively mild illnesses, many of these viruses cause severe, life-threatening disease.

On March 23, 2014, the World Health Organization (WHO) reported cases of Ebola virus disease (EVD) in the forested rural region of southeastern Guinea. The identification of these early cases marked the beginning of the West Africa Ebola epidemic, the largest in history. Two and a half years after the first case was discovered, the outbreak ended after more than 28,600 cases and 11,325 deaths. On September 30, 2014, the CDC confirmed the first travel-associated case of EVD diagnosed in the United States in a man who traveled from West Africa to Dallas, Texas. The patient

Table 16–1. Work-related pathogens by specific job title or broader occupational groups.

Occupation	Pathogen
Abattoir workers	*Brucella* spp, (swine) influenza virus, *Campylobacter* spp, *Coxiella burnetii*, *Escherichia coli*, hepatitis E virus, *Leptospira hardjo*, *Leptospira pomona*, *Toxocara canis*, *Erysipelothrix rhusiopathiae*
Archaeologists	Coccidioidomycosis, histoplasmosis
Armed forces	*Leishmania* spp, *Acinetobacter*, *Coccidioides immitis*, and rabies
Childcare providers	*Cryptosporidium parvum*, cytomegalovirus, *Giardia lamblia*, hepatitis A virus, parvovirus, varicella zoster virus
Divers	*Blastomyces dermatitidis*, *Pseudomonas aeruginosa*
Farm workers, animal handlers	(Methicillin resistant) *Staphylococcus aureus*, (swine and avian) influenza virus, *Borrelia burgdorferi*, *Brucella* spp, *Campylobacter* spp, *Chlamydophila psittaci*, *Clostridium tetani*, *C burnetii*, hepatitis E virus, *Leptospira icterohaemorrhagiae*, *Mycobacterium bovis*, *Streptococcus suis*, *Strongyloides stercoralis*, *T canis*, *Toxoplasma gondii*, West Nile virus
Farm workers, crop harvesters	*B burgdorferi*, *C tetani*, *C burnetii*, *E coli*, *Leishmania* spp, *S stercoralis*, *T canis*
Fishermen, fishmongers	*Anisakis simplex*, *E rhusiopathiae*, and *Mycobacterium marinum*.
Forestry workers	*Anaplasma phagocytophilum*, *B burgdorferi*, *C burnetii*, hantavirus, *Rickettsia conorii*, *Rickettsia helvetica*, tick-borne encephalitis virus, *T gondii*
Funeral service workers	*Mycobacterium tuberculosis*
Gardeners	*Francisella tularensis*, *Sporothrix schenckii*
Health care workers	(Methicillin resistant) *S aureus*, *Bordetella pertussis*, cytomegalovirus, hepatitis B virus, hepatitis C virus, human herpes virus, human immunodeficiency virus (HIV), human parvovirus, influenza virus, measles virus, mumps virus,, *M tuberculosis*, rubella virus, severe acute respiratory syndrome (SARS) coronavirus, *Streptococcus pyogenes*, vancomycin-resistant enterococci, varicella zoster virus, scabies
Hunter, trapper	*B burgdorferi*, *Brucella* spp, *Echinococcus granulosus*, *Echinococcus multilocularis*, *Ehrlichia chaffeensis*, *F tularensis*, hantavirus, *L icterohaemorrhagiae*, *Leptospira interrogans*, *T canis*
Clinical laboratory workers	*C immitis*, *Brucella* spp, *Neisseria meningitidis*, *Francisella tularensis*. Note: Researchers who work with a variety of live organisms may be at risk.
Prison guards	*M tuberculosis*, methicillin-resistant *S aureus*
Sex workers (also adult movie actors)	*Chlamydia trachomatis*, hepatitis A, hepatitis B virus, hepatitis C virus, herpes simplex virus, HIV, human papilloma virus, human T-lymphotropic virus, *Neisseria gonorrhoeae*, *Treponema pallidum*, *Trichomonas vaginalis*
Teachers, primary	Influenza, rhinovirus, parainfluenza virus, human metapneumovirus, respiratory syncytial virus, adenovirus, coronaviruses, other respiratory viruses, measles, and mumps
Domestic animal care workers	(Methicillin resistant) *S aureus*, (swine) influenza virus, *Bartonella henselae*, *Brucella* spp, *Campylobacter* spp, *C psittaci*, *C tetani*, *C burnetii*, hepatitis E virus, monkey pox virus, *Pasteurella multocida*, *Salmonella* spp, *T canis*, *T gondii*
Waste collectors	*Brucella* spp, hepatitis A virus, hepatitis B virus, hepatitis C virus, *T gondii*

(the index case) died on October 8, 2014. Two health care workers who cared for him in Dallas tested positive for EVD. Both recovered. In total, 11 people were treated for Ebola in the United States during the 2014–2016 epidemic.

▶ Response in Health Care Facilities

As part of the response to the Ebola outbreak in West Africa, US hospitals were asked by public health officials to evaluate their capacity to serve as assessment hospitals versus definitive treatment facilities. The CDC recommended that assessment hospitals should be able to provide up to 96 hours of evaluation and care for patients under investigation for Ebola until the diagnosis was either confirmed or ruled out and until discharge or transfer was completed. The CDC has provided guidance on infection control measures, including the use of PPE such as gowns, masks, gloves, goggles, face shields, respirators, and booties as well as the use of

Table 16–2. Pathogens requiring airborne precautions

Diseases/pathogens requiring airborne precautions
Aerosolizable spore-containing powder or other substance that is capable of causing serious human disease, eg, Anthrax/*Bacillus anthracis*
Avian influenza/avian influenza A viruses (strains capable of causing serious disease in humans)
Varicella disease (chickenpox, shingles)/varicella zoster and herpes zoster viruses, disseminated disease in any patient. Localized disease in immunocompromised patient until disseminated infection ruled out
Measles (rubeola)/measles virus
Monkeypox/monkeypox virus
Novel or unknown pathogens
Severe acute respiratory syndrome (SARS)
Smallpox (variola)/variola virus
Tuberculosis (TB)/*Mycobacterium tuberculosis*—Extrapulmonary, draining lesion; pulmonary or laryngeal disease, confirmed; pulmonary or laryngeal disease, suspected

EPA-registered hospital disinfectants with a label claim for use against nonenveloped viruses for disinfection. Several vaccines against Ebola are currently being tested and have been used as part of ring vaccination strategies in the Ebola outbreak in the Democratic Republic of Congo 2017–2019.

▶ Coronaviruses

Middle East respiratory syndrome (MERS) and severe acute respiratory syndrome (SARS) are respiratory viruses and part of the Coronavirus family. Coronaviruses are transmitted primarily by respiratory droplets from coughing and sneezing. In 2003, the SARS epidemic evoked a global public health emergency response as the disease, in the absence of control measures, spread rapidly worldwide. SARS was clearly an occupational health hazard because health care workers who cared for patients accounted for a large proportion of all cases (>50% in some settings). Health care workers were not only affected but also propagated the outbreaks in hospitals and in the community. Other groups who were at risk included workers at live animal markets, laboratory workers, traveling workers, and flight attendants.

MERS is a viral respiratory illness first reported in Saudi Arabia in 2012. Symptoms include fever, cough, and shortness of breath. Most people who have been confirmed to have MERS infection developed severe acute respiratory illness. The overall case fatality rate is estimated to be about 35%, with mortality greater than 60% for those who require mechanical ventilation. All MERS cases to date have been linked directly or indirectly to countries in or near the Arabian Peninsula. The 2015 MERS outbreak in South Korea linked to a returning traveler provided a poignant example of transmission in the hospital setting both to health care workers and other patients in the absence of meticulous infection control measures.

SARS-CoV- 2 is the virus that causes Coronavirus Disease 2019 (COVID-19). COVID-19 cases were initially reported in Wuhan, China in December of 2019 as a pneumonia of unknown cause. By January 21, 2020, COVID-19 cases were reported in Thailand, Japan, the Republic of Korea and the United States; as of early 2021 over 90 million cases were reported worldwide, with close to 2 million deaths. Thousands of workplace outbreaks have occurred throughout the world, making SARS-CoV-2 the most significant occupational infectious disease in modern history. Essential or "front line" workers such as health care workers, food production, construction and agricultural workers are at higher risk of infection due to exposure to patients, clients, customers or co-workers. SARS-CoV-2 infection has occurred at higher rates among Latino and African-American individuals who work as front line workers, have disparate access to prompt health care, and have a greater prevalence of comorbidities that increase risk of hospitalization and death. In communities with high rates of transmission it may be difficult to distinguish work-related and community infection.

Transmission of severe acute respiratory syndrome SARS-CoV-2 occurs primarily through respiratory transmission, via particles of different sizes. Droplets are larger particles created by sneezing and coughing that can be propelled by force into the face (nose, mouth, and eyes). This type of transmission requires being relatively close (within 0.5 meters) to and facing an infectious source. Transmission can also occur through smaller particles that can remain suspended in the air for long periods of time and can be inhaled at short to medium distances. More than 50% of infection occurs without symptoms, making prevention of widespread community and workplace transmission through case-contact tracing extremely challenging. Many countries have implemented public health measures for control including shelter in place, business and school closures and mass testing for infection. The SARS-CoV-2 pandemic has resulted in a global economic dislocation and recession, with enormous impact on poverty rates in many countries.

As with all occupational exposures, reducing SARS-CoV-2 transmission relies on the hierarchy of controls, to include administrative measures (social distancing, face coverings, limited indoor gatherings), adequate ventilation, and the use of personal protective equipment. Personal protective equipment should include eye protection, a fit-tested respirator, and gown and gloves for workers with high risk of exposure. In addition, rapid and accessible testing for SARS-CoV-2 is essential for symptomatic workers, case contact investigation and ongoing surveillance among high risk workers. Quarantine of workers exposed to a positive case must be implemented to prevent ongoing workplace transmission, with return to work after at least 7 days if asymptomatic and with a negative SARS-CoV-2 molecular test. Individuals with SARS-CoV-2 infection - or if exposed and symptomatic - can return to work 10 days after symptoms first develop, and at least 24 hours have passed since last fever without the use of fever-reducing medications and symptoms have improved. As of January 2021, development and duration of immunity to SARS-CoV-2 after infection is several months but is under investigation. Highly effective vaccines for SARS-CoV-2 have been approved for immunization in late 2020. Increasing evidence is emerging that systemic, respiratory and neuropsychological symptoms of SARS-CoV-2 infection may be prolonged for several months.

▶ Occupational Issues With Emerging Infections

When infections arise that threaten workers, some health care workers may be placed on "working quarantine" (allowed to travel only between home and health care facility) to ensure sufficient staffing levels. Other measures may be warranted, including closure of businesses and cancelation of public gatherings. The International Labor Office (ILO) documented a working paper on practical and administrative responses to SARS in the workplace in relation to preexisting ILO standards.

INFLUENZA

Influenza (commonly called flu) is a respiratory infection caused by several types of viruses.

Seasonal influenza is the term used to refer to outbreaks that occur annually, mainly in the late fall and winter. Pandemic influenza refers to particular novel strains of influenza A that spread rapidly from person to person to create a worldwide epidemic (pandemic).

Influenza viruses are classified as types A, B, and C. Influenza A viruses are divided into subtypes based on two proteins on the surface of the virus: hemagglutinin (H; 15 subtypes: H1–H15) and neuraminidase (N; 9 subtypes: N1–N9). Wild birds are the primary natural reservoir for all subtypes of influenza A viruses, and while shedding the viruses, they usually remain healthy hosts. When domesticated birds (eg, chickens, ducks, and turkeys) become infected, the infection often spreads quickly and widely and may lead to an avian influenza outbreak in poultry. If the virus is of a highly pathogenic type, the epidemic is highly lethal. Viruses can be transmitted from farm to farm by contaminated equipment, vehicles, feed, cages, or clothing. Thus, the standard control measures in poultry are quarantine and depopulation (or culling) and surveillance around affected flocks. Although the risk of infection to humans from avian influenza is generally low, people should avoid contact with infected birds or contaminated surfaces and should be careful when handling and cooking poultry.

Influenza A viruses are genetically labile and well adapted to escape host defenses. Consequently, small changes constantly occur in the antigenic composition (*antigenic drift*). Alternatively, an abrupt major change (*antigenic shift*) may occur if two different viruses infect the same host and mix together; for viruses that may impact humans, mixing is thought to occur most commonly in pigs. The new virus may acquire genes from human, avian, and swine origins, and a minority of viruses will have receptors that enable efficient person-to-person spread.

In the twentieth century, four influenza pandemics have occurred, caused by newly circulating influenza A viruses. The great influenza pandemic of 1918–1919 ("Spanish flu" [A(H1N1)]) caused an estimated 40–50 million deaths worldwide and was followed by pandemics in 1957–1958 ("Asian flu" [A(H2N2)]) and 1968–1969 ("Hong Kong flu" [A(H3N2)]). Although the origin of the 1918–1919 pandemic virus is not entirely clear, the latter two pandemics were caused by viruses containing a combination of genes from a human influenza virus and an avian influenza virus. Influenza pandemics may occur when new virus subtypes emerge and are readily transmitted from person to person. Influenza pandemics are distinct from the seasonal influenza outbreaks that occur yearly in temperate regions and are caused by type A or B influenza viruses (type C causes mild respiratory illness and does not cause epidemics). The pandemic of 2009 was caused by a novel H1N1 influenza A strain with both swine and avian genetic elements. An outbreak of human infections with a new avian influenza A (H7N9) virus was first reported in China in 2013, and sporadic human infections with H5N1, which gained attention in 2003, continue to occur.

While each workplace is unique, and workers' risk for occupational exposure to influenza can vary widely depending on the nature of their jobs, the CDC encourages workplaces to promote influenza vaccination among workers, to encourage proper hand and respiratory hygiene practices, and to educate workers on influenza signs and symptoms. Influenza vaccination of health care and other workers has been shown to decrease absenteeism. Because health care workers and first responders will be at high risk of infection in a pandemic situation, preparedness strategies with a strong occupational health component are warranted, including education regarding respiratory etiquette in the workplace and staying home when ill.

Guidance for screening, prevention, and treatment of influenza are updated regularly.

INFECTIONS CAUSED BY THE WORKERS ENVIRONMENT

Workers can be exposed to a variety of infectious agents when they come in contact with other humans, animals, insects, or environmental agents such as soil or contaminated air.

▶ Histoplasmosis

Histoplasmosis is an infectious disease caused by inhaling the spores of a fungus called *Histoplasma capsulatum*. *H capsulatum* is a dimorphic fungus. It is a mold (mycelial phase) in soil at ambient temperatures, and after being inhaled by humans or animals, it produces a yeast phase when spores undergo genetic, biochemical, and physical alterations. Although the fungus has a worldwide distribution, the proportion of people infected by *H capsulatum* is higher in certain areas, including US central and eastern states, especially along the Ohio and Mississippi River valleys. Histoplasmosis primarily affects the lungs. The vast majority of infected people are asymptomatic, or they experience symptoms so mild they do not seek medical attention. If symptoms do occur, they will usually start within 3–17 days after exposure, with an average of 10 days. Histoplasmosis can appear as a mild, influenza-like respiratory illness and has a combination of symptoms, including malaise (a general ill feeling), fever, chest pain, dry or nonproductive cough, headache, loss of appetite, shortness of breath, joint and muscle pains, chills, and hoarseness.

Diagnosis of acute illness can be made by detecting *H capsulatum* polysaccharide antigen (HPA) levels in a patient's urine, serum, and other body fluids or by culturing the organism from infected sites. HPA is detected in body fluid samples of most patients with disseminated infection and in the urine and serum of 25–50% of those with less severe infections.

Anyone working at a job or present near activities where material contaminated with *H capsulatum* becomes airborne can develop histoplasmosis if enough spores are inhaled. To reduce worker risk of contracting *H capsulatum*, NIOSH recommends posting health risk warnings, controlling aerosolized dust, and the use of PPE such as NIOSH-approved respirators.

▶ Coccidioidomycosis

Coccidioidomycosis, also known as Valley fever, is a recognized occupational illness that has been reported in workers engaged in soil-disrupting activities, including agricultural and construction workers, military personnel, anthropologists, and archaeologists working in endemic areas. In nonendemic areas, work-related cases of disease have been reported in various occupations, including laboratory personnel; precautions must be taken to prevent transmission of Coccidioides when it is grown in clinical or research laboratories.

Coccidioidomycosis is caused by the inhalation of airborne fungal spores following soil disruption from either of the two soil-dwelling *Coccidioides* species: *C immitis* and *C. posadasii*. The fungus is endemic to certain semiarid areas of California, Arizona, New Mexico, Nevada, and Texas, and to some parts of Central and South Americas. Coccidioidomycosis can be a severe illness and result in disability due to pulmonary involvement and disseminated disease; however, most infections are asymptomatic. Influenza-like illness is the most common clinical presentation, but a delay in diagnosis can result in disseminated disease. Infection generally imparts immunity to reinfection, although cases of reinfection have been reported. Groups at increased risk for developing disseminated disease are African Americans and Asians, people of Filipino descent, pregnant women during their third trimester, and immunocompromised patients.

Prevention of occupationally acquired coccidioidomycosis requires a multidisciplinary approach, including engineering controls such as continuous soil wetting of disturbed soil and washing all equipment prior to removal from the worksite; administrative controls such as increasing training on prevention, signs, and symptoms of infection; and use of PPE such as NIOSH-approved respiratory protection with particulate filters rated as N95, N99, N100, P100, or HEPA and requiring a change of clothing at the worksite.

Most patients with coccidioidomycosis, including those with meningitis, are treated with fluconazole. Some patients, including those with meningitis, require lifelong therapy to prevent relapses. Amphotericin preparations are used for severe disease.

▶ *Legionella*

Legionnaires' disease and Pontiac fever are collectively known as legionellosis, a disease caused by *Legionella* bacteria. Legionnaires disease is a serious, potentially deadly, lung infection and Pontiac fever is a less serious infection with milder symptoms. *Legionella* is transmitted via inhalation of aerosolized water containing the bacteria. Occupational *Legionella* infection has been reported primarily in industrial settings, office buildings, and hospitals but has also been reported among street cleaning workers, car washing workers, water treatment plant workers, and aboard ships. Preventing worker exposures and legionellosis cases depend on implementing an effective water management program. These programs focus on identifying areas where *Legionella* could grow and implementing control measures.

▶ Hantavirus

Hantavirus of the bunyavirus family of viruses is a negative-sense, single-stranded RNA virus. Animal laboratory workers and persons working in rodent-infested buildings are at increased risk for coming in contact with dried droppings, urine, or saliva of mice and rats that carry Hantavirus and developing Hantavirus pulmonary syndrome (HPS). The disease begins as an influenza-like illness characterized by fever, chills, and muscle aches, but it can rapidly progress to life-threatening respiratory failure.

Prevention of exposure should rely on sealing holes in workplace structures to prevent entry of rodents, placing traps to reduce rodent population, and placing food in sealed containers to eliminate nesting sites. If rodent excreta are found, the CDC recommends cleaning with wetting agents and disinfectants prior to creating aerosolized dust.

Prevention of occupational exposure to Hantavirus should include minimization of airborne dust, particularly when cleaning rodent droppings. Workers involved in general cleanup activities where there is not heavy accumulation of droppings should wear disposable protective clothing and gloves (neoprene, nitrile, or latex-free), rubber boots, and a disposable N95 respirator. For cleaning up rodent contaminated areas with heavy accumulations of droppings, it is necessary to use powered air-purifying (PARP) or air-supplied respirators with P100 filters and eye or face protection to avoid contact with any aerosols. Dead mice, nests, and droppings should be soaked thoroughly with a 1:10 solution of sodium hypochlorite. The contaminated material should be placed in a plastic bag and sealed for disposal. All reusable respirator surfaces, gloves, rubber boots, and goggles should be disinfected with bleach solution. All disposable protective clothing, gloves, and respirators should be placed in plastic bags and sealed for disposal. Hands should be washed thoroughly after removing the gloves. Biosafety level 2 (BSL-2) facilities and BSL-2 practices are recommended for laboratory handling of sera and tissues from persons potentially infected with the agents of HPS.

There is no specific treatment or cure for hantavirus infection. Treatment of patients with HPS remains supportive in nature. Patients should receive appropriate antibiotic therapy while awaiting confirmation of a diagnosis of HPS. Care during the initial stages of the disease should include antipyretics and analgesia as needed. If there is a high degree of suspicion of HPS, patients should be immediately transferred to an emergency department or intensive care unit (ICU) for close monitoring and care.

▶ Tick-Borne Illnesses

Outdoor workers are at risk of exposure to tick-borne diseases if they work at sites with ticks. Worksites with woods, bushes, high grass, or leaf litter are likely to have more ticks. Outdoor workers in most regions of the United States should be especially careful to protect themselves in the spring, summer, and fall when ticks are most active. Ticks may be active all year in some regions with warmer weather. Workers at risk for tick-borne diseases include construction workers, painters, roofers, pavers, laborers, mechanics, landscapers, forestry workers, brush clearers, land surveyors, farmers, railroad workers, oil field workers, utility line workers, park or wildlife management workers, entomologists, and wildlife biologists. Other diseases transmitted by ticks include Lyme disease, babesiosis, ehrlichiosis, anaplasmosis, Rocky Mountain spotted fever, tick-borne relapsing fever, tularemia, and Q fever.

Prevention of tick-borne diseases includes wearing light-colored clothing, including long-sleeved shirts and long pants tucked into boots or socks, use of insect repellents containing 20–30% DEET on exposed skin and application of permethrin to pants, socks, and shoes, which typically stays effective through several washings. Workers should be advised to check their skin and clothes for ticks every day. The immature forms of these ticks are small and may be hard to see. Workers should also be advised to shower or bathe as soon as possible after working outdoors in order to wash off and check for ticks, particularly in the hair, underarms, and groin. Any ticks discovered should be removed immediately using fine-tipped tweezers and the area cleansed with soap and water. Removing infected ticks within 24 hours prevents infection with the Lyme disease bacterium. Work clothes may be dried in a hot dryer after washing to kill any ticks present.

In the United States, ticks are usually more active in the months of April through October and peak in the summer months of June through August. The time of year when ticks are active may vary with the geographic region and climate. Common symptoms of infections with tick-borne diseases include body/muscle aches, fever, headaches, fatigue, joint pain, or rash. Tick-borne diseases are suspected based on symptoms and the possibility that the worker has been exposed to infected ticks. Tick-borne diseases caused by bacteria can be treated with antibiotics, most commonly doxycycline.

INFECTIONS CAUSED BY EXPOSURE TO INFECTED HUMANS OR THEIR TISSUES

Health care and clinical laboratory workers may be at increased risk of infection by organisms whose natural hosts are humans, such as hepatitis viruses, HIV, and *Mycobacterium tuberculosis*. Some infections may be transmitted through close personal contact with infected patients. Infections caused by many viruses, bacteria, fungi, and parasites pathogenic for humans can result from direct contact with the organism in culture or in human tissue. Tuberculosis is an example of an occupational infection resulting from repeated close contact with infected patients, and hepatitis B exemplifies a serious and previously frequent infection resulting from manipulation of infected human blood and inoculation by infectious virus particles.

▶ Varicella

Varicella (chickenpox) is caused by varicella-zoster virus (VZV), a DNA virus that is a member of the herpesvirus group. After the primary infection, VZV remains in the sensory nerve ganglia as a latent infection. Primary infection with VZV causes varicella. Reactivation of latent infection causes herpes zoster (shingles).

Varicella is highly contagious. It can be spread from person to person by direct contact, inhalation of aerosols from vesicular fluid of skin lesions of acute varicella or zoster, and through infected respiratory secretions that also may be aerosolized. Localized zoster can be transmitted to persons without immunity resulting in primary varicella but only with close contact. A person with varicella is contagious beginning 1–2 days before rash onset until all the chickenpox lesions have crusted. The Advisory Committee on Immunization Practices (ACIP) recommends that healthy people who do not have evidence of immunity to varicella should get vaccinated against this disease. Varicella vaccination is important for health care professionals, people who care for or are around immunocompromised people, teachers, child care workers, staff in nursing homes and residential settings, staff of correctional institutions, military personnel, and international travelers.

▶ Methicillin-Resistant *Staphylococcus aureus*

Custodial populations have increased rates of methicillin-resistant *S* (MRSA). Correctional staff (officers and staff working in jails or prisons) may be at increased risk of exposure to MRSA. There is variability in studies as to whether health care workers are more likely to be colonized with MRSA than the local population. Other locations where risk of MRSA exposure may be increased include schools (including athletic departments), dormitories, military barracks, households of persons with MRSA, and daycare centers. Factors that increase risk of transmission of MRSA include crowding, frequent skin-to-skin contact, compromised skin, and contaminated items (such as towels or used bandages). MRSA is transmitted most frequently by direct skin-to-skin contact or contact with shared items or surfaces that have been contaminated. MRSA infections can vary from simple skin abscesses to life-threatening systemic infections.

Environmental measures in settings with increased risk of transmission should include daily use of commercially available cleaners or detergents on high-touch surfaces (eg, doorknobs, counters, bedside tables, bedrails bathtubs, toilet seats) that may come in contact with skin. In health care settings, contact isolation, with use of gowns and gloves for health care workers and private rooms for patients, can be considered, particularly if spread is confirmed or suspected despite the use of standard precautions.

Simple abscesses or boils traditionally have been managed with incision and drainage alone; newer data suggest benefit from the addition of antibiotics for 5–10 days to decrease risk for complications and recurrence. Oral antibiotic options for treating skin and soft-tissue infections in patients with community-associated MRSA include clindamycin and trimethoprim/sulfamethoxazole.

Decolonization may be considered if a worker develops a recurrent infection despite good personal hygiene and wound care or if other household members develop infections. Strategies include nasal decolonization with mupirocin twice per day for 5–10 days, or nasal decolonization with mupirocin twice per day for 5–10 days plus topical body decolonization with a skin antiseptic solution (eg, chlorhexidine), or dilute bleach baths for 5–14 days. Decolonization typically results in short-term eradication of MRSA, and repeated courses of decolonization treatment may be needed in those at high risk for infection.

TUBERCULOSIS

M tuberculosis can cause disseminated disease but most frequently causes pulmonary infections. The bacilli are transmitted by the airborne route and, depending on host factors, may lead to latent tuberculosis infection (LTBI) or tuberculosis disease (TB). People who are ill with TB of the lungs or upper airways are infectious, whereas people with LTBI are not.

Globally, the WHO estimates that TB caused 10 million incident cases and 1.6 million deaths in 2017. Geographically, the burden of TB is highest in Asia and Africa. India and China combined have almost 40% of the world's TB cases; the South-East Asia and Western Pacific Regions of which they are a part account for more than 60%. The African region has approximately one-quarter of the world's cases and the highest rates of cases and deaths relative to population. There has been major progress in reducing TB cases and deaths in the past two decades, with TB incidence falling globally for several years at an annual rate of 2%, and the TB mortality rate falling by 3% per year.

Work environments with concern for TB transmission include most health care settings (especially hospitals, long-term care facilities, and dialysis centers), refugee/immigration centers, homeless shelters, substance abuse treatment centers, and correctional institutions.

Tubercle bacilli may be present in sputum, gastric fluid, cerebrospinal fluid, urine, and other tissues. Infectious patients disseminate the organism when coughing, sneezing, or talking by expelling small infectious droplets that may remain suspended in the air for several hours and then be inhaled by susceptible persons. After an incubation period of 4–12 weeks, infection usually remains subclinical and dormant without development of active disease, but the Mantoux tuberculin skin test (TST) will become positive. The risk of developing active tuberculosis is highest in the first 2 years following infection. However, the organism may be activated at any time, resulting in pulmonary or systemic disease. The risk of development of clinical disease following infection is higher in those younger than 5 years, in states of undernutrition, in certain immunopathologic states (eg, in persons with HIV), with certain genetic predisposition (persons with HLA-Bw15 histocompatibility antigen), and in persons with some coexisting diseases (silicosis, end-stage renal disease, leukemia, lymphoma, upper gastrointestinal tract carcinoma, diabetes).

▶ Tuberculin Skin Test

TST is a chemical fractionation product of tubercle bacilli culture filtrate. Intradermal injection of 5 tuberculin units of TST in a patient with LTBI or active tuberculous infection results in a delayed hypersensitivity reaction manifested by induration at the site of injection within 48–72 hours. A minimum of 5 mm of induration is required for a test to be positive or reactive in close contacts of infectious patients, those with fibrotic changes on chest radiograph consistent with prior TB, organ transplant recipients, persons with human immunodeficiency infection (HIV) infection, and persons with other types of significant immunosuppression. A reaction of 10 mm or more is considered positive in high-risk occupational groups (including employees in prisons or jails, health care facilities, or mycobacterial laboratories), injection drug users, persons who have immigrated in the past 5 years from countries with high TB prevalence, children younger than 5 years, those with the coexisting diseases mentioned previously, and children exposed to adults at high risk for developing active TB. In persons with none of the previously mentioned risk factors, induration of 15 mm or more is required for a positive reaction. The TST test may be negative in the presence of overwhelming tuberculosis, measles, Hodgkin disease, sarcoidosis, or immunosuppressive states. If the initial test is negative in individuals with suspected reduced immune response or in those who will be screened annually because of occupational or other risk, it should be repeated.

▶ "Two-Step" Method

Some people infected with *M tuberculosis* may have a negative reaction to the TST if many years have passed since they became infected. They may have a positive reaction to a subsequent TST because the initial test stimulates their ability to react to the test. This is commonly referred to as the "booster phenomenon" and may incorrectly be interpreted as a skin test conversion (going from negative to positive). For this reason, the "two-step method" is recommended at the time of initial testing for individuals who may be tested periodically (eg, health care workers). If the first TST result in the two-step baseline testing is positive, consider the person infected and evaluate and treat the person accordingly. If the first test result is negative, the TST should be repeated in 1–3 weeks. If the second test result is positive, consider the person infected and evaluate and treat the person accordingly; if both steps are negative, consider the person uninfected and classify the TST as negative at baseline testing.

TST skin testing is an accepted method for screening high-risk populations for TB infection. Persons having a reactive test are at risk of developing active clinical infection at any time (lifelong) following the primary infection owing to reactivation as long as viable tubercle bacilli remain in the body.

▶ Blood Tests for TB Infection

Interferon-gamma release assays (IGRAs) are whole-blood tests that can aid in diagnosing *M tuberculosis* infection. They do not differentiate LTBI from active tuberculosis disease. The advantages of the IGRAs, when compared to TSTs, include requiring only a single patient visit to conduct the test, results can be available within 24 hours, there is no "booster phenomenon" measured by subsequent tests, and prior bacille Calmette-Guérin (BCG) vaccination does not cause a false-positive IGRA result. Disadvantages include a higher false-positive rate than TSTs in relatively low-risk, serially tested workers, such as US health care workers. Newly positive test results in health care workers without recent TB exposure are usually just above the threshold for positivity and are often negative on repeat testing. Additional disadvantages include the requirement that samples be processed within a specified time (8–30 hours) after collection while white blood cells are still viable and that errors in collecting or transporting blood specimens or in running and interpreting the assay can decrease the accuracy of IGRAs. Cost of the IGRA may be above or below administration of the TST, depending on local health care labor costs and lost productivity of the tested worker.

▶ TB Control & Treatment

In 2016, the American Thoracic Society, Infectious Diseases Society of America, and the CDC published clinical practice guidelines on the diagnosis of tuberculosis in adults and children. They identify three risk groups for screening of LTBI: those at high risk of infection with a high risk of progressing to active TB, those with a high risk of infection and low to intermediate risk of progressing to active TB, and those with a low risk of infection. Decisions to test workers should rely on a risk assessment; however, some workers, regardless of

risk of infection, are mandated by law or their employers to undergo LTBI screening.

Serial testing (biennially or more frequently) can identify recently infected individuals whose tests have become reactive (*converters*) within the past 2 years.

Occupational candidates who should be given high priority for LTBI treatment include employees of high-risk congregate settings including correctional facilities, nursing homes, homeless shelters, hospitals, other health care facilities, and mycobacteriology laboratory personnel. The CDC-recommended treatment regimens for LTBI are isoniazid (INH) plus rifapentine dosed weekly for 12 doses, rifampin dosed daily for 4 months, or INH dosed daily for 6 or 9 months. All the regimens have advantages and disadvantages; people are more likely to complete treatment with the shorter regimens. Treatment must be modified if the person with LTBI is a contact of an individual with drug-resistant TB disease. Consultation with a TB expert is advised if the known source of TB infection has drug-resistant TB.

Bacilli in the lungs may develop resistance to anti-TB medicines when the patient fails to complete standard treatment regimens or is given the wrong treatment regimen. A particularly dangerous form of drug-resistant TB is multidrug-resistant TB (MDR-TB), which is defined as disease caused by TB bacilli resistant to at least INH and rifampin. Some countries have high rates of MDR-TB, which threaten TB control efforts. For cost-effective control of TB, the WHO and other international organizations advocate a comprehensive strategy centered on direct observed therapy (DOT). Health and community workers or trained volunteers observe patients swallowing the full course of the correct dosage of anti-TB medicines. The goals of DOT are to facilitate completion of treatment and to prevent the development of drug resistance.

Persons not known to have a previously positive skin test who have substantial contact with a person with infectious TB should be skin tested immediately and then retested 8–12 weeks after the infectious contact. If conversion occurs, physical examination and chest radiography should occur to rule out acute clinical infection before beginning therapy for LTBI.

Attenuated tubercle bacilli—particularly BCG—is used in many countries as a vaccine. However, BCG has variable efficacy in preventing the adult forms of TB and interferes with skin testing for latent TB infection. Thus, it is not recommended routine for use in the United States.

HEPATITIS A

Hepatitis A causes an acute viral hepatitis that is usually symptomatic in adults. Symptoms include nausea, anorexia, fever, malaise, and abdominal pain; patients often have jaundice on physical examination and elevated serum aminotransferase levels and bilirubin levels on laboratory testing. Hepatitis A does not result in chronic infection but can cause severe disease, including liver failure and death. Because the clinical characteristics are similar for all types of acute viral hepatitis, hepatitis A diagnosis must be confirmed by a positive serologic test for immunoglobulin M (IgM) antibody to hepatitis A virus, or the case must meet the clinical case definition and occur in a person who has an epidemiologic link with a person who has laboratory-confirmed hepatitis A during the 15–50 days before the onset of symptoms.

Hepatitis A is generally not considered an occupationally transmitted infection. It is spread person-to-person through the fecal-oral route or consumption of contaminated food or water. It can also spread from close personal contact with an infected person such as through sex or caring for someone who is ill. However, with recent outbreaks in the United States among persons who are homeless and/or use drugs, vaccinating people who work with these populations is now recommended by many public health departments.

HEPATITIS B

Prior to the introduction of the hepatitis B vaccine in 1981, hepatitis B was a frequent occupational infection among health care workers in the United States, with laboratory and public safety workers also at risk. Hepatitis B virus (HBV) can cause fulminant hepatitis and also can lead to chronic carrier states in up to 10% of persons following acute infection. Chronic carriers suffer higher rates of cirrhosis and liver failure as well as liver cancer.

Blood contains the highest titers of virus in infected individuals, with lower levels in various other body fluids, including cerebrospinal, synovial, pleural, peritoneal, pericardial, and amniotic fluids, as well as semen and vaginal secretions. Viral titers in urine, feces, tears, and saliva are low enough that these are not felt to be routes of transmission except in cases of human bites that involve some blood transmission. Sexual and maternal-child transmissions are the most common modes of HBV transmission in the general population.

The risk for transmission of HBV through needlestick injuries is approximately 30% when the source patient has high level of replicating HBV. HBV can remain viable for at least 1 month on dried surfaces at room temperature. This poses additional opportunities to acquire occupational HBV infections when individuals with open cuts or abraded skin or mucous membranes contact contaminated surfaces. Historically, most occupational infections have had no clear percutaneous injury leading to HBV transmission.

Prescreening serologic testing prior to vaccination generally is not recommended because the prevalence of HBV infection in the United States is low. Some groups have instituted prescreening of all potential vaccine recipients with hepatitis B core antibodies when a high percentage of potential vaccines come from endemic countries. Positive core antibodies indicate past or present HBV infections and should prompt testing for surface antigen to identify chronic carriers and for surface antibodies to identify those with resolved past infections.

Since 1991, it has been recommended to vaccinate newborn infants at birth. That same year, the Bloodborne Pathogens Act was passed, mandating employer-funded vaccination for at-risk health care workers. Since that time, a dramatic reduction in occupational HBV transmission has occurred. However, there are still some workers who have not completed or have refused vaccination and remain vulnerable to infection. Some people who are vaccinated do not develop protective antibodies and remain susceptible to infection.

Known exposures to HBV-infected blood or blood products in those who were not vaccinated require the use of hepatitis B immune globulin (HBIG), which can be given as a single dose if hepatitis B vaccination is administered concomitantly. For those who were vaccinated and did not develop antibodies, two doses of HBIG 1 month apart are needed.

The usual schedule for HBV vaccination for health care workers, public safety workers, and other workers at risk for exposure to blood or body fluids is two doses separated by no less than 4 weeks, followed by a third dose 4–6 months after the second dose. Those who have received only one or two doses do not need to restart the series: they only need to complete the doses they did not receive (as with most other vaccines requiring multiple dosing). A new, adjuvanted hepatitis B vaccine (Heplisav-B) is now available and requires only two doses given at least one month apart.

The current recommendations are to check for hepatitis B surface antibodies 4–8 weeks following the vaccine series. In the United States, those who test positive (surface antibody level >10 mIU/mL) are considered to have lifelong immunity, even if the antibody level later wanes. In persons who test negative for surface antibodies, one additional dose of vaccine will induce antibody protection in 15–25% of nonresponders and three additional doses (for a total of six doses) will induce antibodies in 30–50% of nonresponders. With traditional vaccine, additional doses can be given following the 0-, 1-, and 6-month schedule or using an abbreviated schedule. Use of the newer adjuvanted hepatitis B vaccine can also be considered, as seroconversion rates with this vaccine appear to be higher after the primary vaccine series. However, data are not yet available for vaccine nonresponders.

See Table 16–3 on interpretation of hepatitis B serologic test results.

HEPATITIS C

Hepatitis C is a viral infection of the liver caused by the hepatitis C virus (HCV). In the United States, HCV is most frequently associated with a history of blood transfusion (prior to the introduction of enzyme immunoassay [EIA] in the late 1980s), injection drug use, and, less commonly, sexual exposure, especially in those with multiple partners. Some people with HCV infection do not have clearly identifiable risk factors. Worldwide, there are six major genotypes of HCV, with type 1 the most frequent in the United States.

Transmission occurs rarely in health care settings as a result of exposure to the blood of a person infected with HCV. The current estimate for transmission of HCV following a needlestick injury from a positive carrier of HCV is approximately 1.8%. Transmission following mucous membrane exposure is very rare, with no apparent transfer following exposures to intact skin.

Table 16–3. Interpretation of hepatitis B serologic test results.

Test	Result	Interpretation
HBsAg anti-HBc anti-HBs	Negative Negative Negative	Susceptible
HBsAg anti-HBc anti-HBs	Negative Positive Positive	Immune due to natural infection
HBsAg anti-HBc anti-HBs	Negative Negative Positive	Immune due to hepatitis B vaccination
HBsAg anti-HBc anti-HBs IgM anti-HBc	Positive Positive Negative Positive	Acutely infected
HBsAg anti-HBc anti-HBs IgM anti-HBc	Positive Positive Negative Negative	Chronically infected
HBsAg anti-HBc anti-HBs IgM anti-HBc	Negative Positive Negative	Interpretation unclear; four possibilities: 1. Resolved infection (most common) 2. False-positive anti-HBc, thus susceptible 3. "Low level" chronic infection 4. Resolving acute infection

With EIA testing, antibodies against HCV can be detected in many people by 4–10 weeks after infection and in more than 97% of those who are infected by 6 months after exposure. Antibodies against HCV indicate exposure to the virus and are used for diagnostic purposes, but they do not correlate with clearance of the virus. Approximately 75–85% of those infected with HCV develop chronic infection. Those with chronic infection have about a 20% chance of developing cirrhosis and, particularly in those with cirrhosis, an increased risk for developing hepatocellular carcinomas. Positive EIA tests usually warrant confirmatory testing with highly sensitive polymerase chain reaction (PCR) assays for HCV RNA. The presence of HCV RNA indicates current infection.

Major advances in the treatment of those with chronic HCV infection have occurred recently with the use of anti-HCV direct-acting antiviral (DAA) agents. Regardless of genotype, most persons with HCV infection can now be cured with 8–12 weeks of oral therapy. Those who have a sustained virologic response with no detectable virus at 12 weeks after the completion of therapy are considered cured, as late relapses are uncommon.

Following exposures to known HCV-positive blood or blood products, HCV RNA testing is often considered 2–4 weeks after exposure as a sensitive diagnostic tool to detect early disease.

While postexposure prophylaxis is not indicated after exposure, early HCV treatment can be offered.

HUMAN IMMUNODEFICIENCY VIRUS

Approximately 37 million people are now living with HIV, with the African continent suffering the greatest impact. With the availability of effective antiretroviral therapy, the mortality rate has declined, but many people worldwide still do not have access to therapy. For those who receive continuous treatment, life expectancy is long, and infection with HIV can be managed as a chronic illness.

HIV transmission occurs via blood and sexual contact. In the United States, occupationally acquired infection has been a rare (albeit serious) occurrence. The body fluids other than blood that are considered to confer risk for HIV transmission include semen and vaginal secretions and cerebrospinal, synovial, pleural, peritoneal, pericardial, and amniotic fluids. Nasal secretions, saliva, sputum, sweat, tears, urine, and vomitus are not considered potentially infectious unless they are visibly bloody.

The established rate of transmission following an HIV exposure from a needlestick injury is approximately 0.3%, making it approximately ten fold less transmissible than HCV and 100-fold less transmissible than HBV. Moreover, the incidence of occupational HIV transmission appears to have declined substantially in recent years. There are several factors that may account for this decrease, including the widespread use of antiretroviral agents in persons living with HIV, leading to lower viral loads, as well as broad use of effective antiretroviral treatment following HIV exposures.

After contact with blood or a potentially infectious body fluid following a needlestick or splash to mucous membranes, postexposure prophylaxis may be warranted if the source of the exposure is known to have HIV or, when unknown and the exposure is concerning, until HIV testing of the source can be performed. In almost all cases in which postexposure prophylaxis is indicated, a three-drug regimen is used for 28 days. The most common regimens prescribed are a combination of tenofovir disoproxil fumarate and emtricitabine (co-formulated as Truvada) plus an integrase inhibitor (either raltegravir twice daily or dolutegravir once daily). Caution is indicated with dolutegravir in early pregnancy and in persons who may become pregnant due to concern for increased risk of neural tube defects. The most worrisome exposures involve either larger amounts of blood or higher concentrations of virus, including needlesticks with large-bore needles, deep punctures, and sticks with visible blood on devices or needles that were used in arteries or veins or exposure to persons with a high viral load or to concentrated virus in the laboratory.

Baseline HIV testing of the exposed person should be performed at the time of the exposure, with follow-up testing at 6 weeks and 3–4 months. Prolonged testing up to 12 months is only suggested if the exposed person contracts HCV as a result of the exposure or if the exposed individual has preexisting HCV infection.

Response to potential exposures should be considered urgent, as potential exposure can provoke considerable anxiety and, when indicated, postexposure prophylaxis should be started as quickly as possible.

Preexposure prophylaxis (PrEP) is recommended for people at very high risk for HIV to decrease the chance of infection. The current regimen used for PrEP is a combination of tenofovir disoproxil fumarate and emtricitabine (Truvada), which is usually taken once daily. PrEP is highly effective for preventing HIV if used as prescribed, but it is much less effective when not taken consistently. PrEP should be recommended for sex workers, as well as appropriate immunizations and PPE, such as barrier devices to limit body fluid contact.

TRAVEL

With the expansion of global commerce, international business travel has become increasingly common. Travel to developing areas of the world warrants special considerations because there are many vaccine-or medication-preventable diseases that can have significant morbidity and mortality in healthy adults. Control of most of these diseases does not appear imminent, and it has been hypothesized that certain infectious diseases such as malaria, dengue fever, and cholera will become even more prevalent with climate change. Illnesses contracted during travel that are specific to the destination, such as malaria or hepatitis A, are covered under workers' compensation. Serious travel-related infections are an important threat to workers' health, but even milder, self-limited illnesses significantly impede productivity.

Few vaccinations are currently required for entry into some countries. However, vaccines are frequently recommended, depending on the destination, length of stay, and activities that are planned. Those who are working with refugees or performing disaster relief may be at particular risk. The most commonly administered travel vaccines include hepatitis A (for those who are not immune) and typhoid, which are indicated for travel to most parts of the developing world. Vaccines indicated for certain destinations include cholera, polio, Japanese encephalitis, and quadrivalent meningococcal vaccine. Rabies vaccine is important if occupational duties may bring workers into contact with dogs, bats, or other mammals. Hepatitis B vaccination is recommended for those who might be exposed to blood or body fluids. Risk likely increases with increased duration of travel, which may not be continuous. Pretravel screening is important for all family members who are traveling when preparing for long-term foreign assignments.

Updated guidelines for determining which vaccines would be appropriate for a particular country can be found on the CDC's Travelers, Health Web site (https://wwwnc.cdc.gov/travel) or by referring to the CDC's *Health Information for International Travel* (also known as the "Yellow Book"). Further information regarding immunization of military personnel can be obtained at the US Military Health System web site (https://www.health.mil/Military-Health-Topics/Health-Readiness/Immunization-Healthcare.

REQUIRED TRAVEL VACCINATIONS

▶ Yellow Fever

Yellow fever is an acute viral hemorrhagic disease transmitted by mosquitoes that occurs in tropical and subtropical areas of Africa, South America, and parts of Panama. Yellow fever vaccination may be required when entering a country (even if only in transit) when travel has occurred through another country where yellow fever is known or thought to be present. Recent deaths due to yellow fever have occurred in unimmunized travelers to Brazil, which is experiencing a yellow fever outbreak that includes regions where yellow fever was not previously found.

Vaccination must be obtained from a certified yellow fever vaccination center, where the International Certificate of Vaccination (or "yellow card") is stamped and signed. These centers can be located by checking the CDC web site (http://wwwnc.cdc.gov/travel/yellow-fever-vaccination-clinics/search). The Certificate of Vaccination must be presented at customs in order to enter and is valid 10 days following vaccination. For most people, a single dose of vaccine provides lifelong protection, and a booster dose is not needed. However, a booster dose can be considered in travelers going to areas with ongoing outbreaks if more than 10 years has elapsed since the last dose, and some countries may require vaccination within 10 years.

Since yellow fever vaccine is a live-virus vaccination, it should not be given to immunosuppressed individuals and is relatively contraindicated in pregnancy (although it can be given if travel to high-risk areas is unavoidable). It is contraindicated in those with severe allergies to eggs or when a severe allergic reaction has occurred with previous doses. There have been rare cases of yellow fever vaccine–associated neurotropic disease (YEL-AND), primarily in children but also in a few adults. Rare cases of vaccine-associated viscerotropic disease (YEL-AVD) with febrile multiorgan-system failure also have been reported in first-time vaccines and seem to occur more frequently in those older than 60 years. Thymic disorders associated with immune dysfunction (eg, myasthenia gravis) appear to be a risk factor for severe complications of yellow fever vaccine and are a contraindication to vaccination.

Other live-virus vaccines (eg, MMR and varicella) must be given simultaneously or be separated by at least 4 weeks.

▶ Travel Prophylaxis

A. Malaria

Malaria is a significant protozoal disease transmitted by infected female *Anopheles* mosquitoes, which bite between dusk and dawn. Those who are infected multiple times develop a partial immunity, which provides protection from severe disease. Persons traveling from nonendemic countries such as the United States have a greater chance for developing severe illness. Symptoms may develop months after returning from regions with malaria, and the diagnosis may be missed. There are four types of malaria generally recognized to infect humans: *Plasmodium falciparum*, *P vivax*, *P ovale*, and *P malariae*. *P falciparum* is the most serious form and has developed resistance in many areas of the world. *P knowlesi*, which infects macaques, is now appreciated as a cause of human infections in Southeast Asia. Other animal species may rarely infect humans.

In areas where *P falciparum* remains susceptible (areas in Central America and the Middle East), chloroquine can be used for malaria prophylaxis. This medication is taken weekly beginning 1 week before travel, weekly during travel, and for 4 weeks after leaving the malarious area.

In areas with chloroquine resistance (Asia, Southeast Asia, India, Africa, and South America), other forms of malaria prophylaxis must be used. These include mefloquine, doxycycline, and atovaquone-proguanil. Mefloquine has been associated with bad dreams, anxiety, depression, psychosis, a lowered seizure threshold, and cardiac conduction abnormalities. This drug is taken once a week in a schedule similar to chloroquine. Doxycycline, as a form of tetracycline, has been associated with photosensitivity, gastrointestinal disorders, rash, and diarrhea. This is taken once a day starting 1–2 days before travel, during travel, and continued for 4 weeks after leaving the malarious area. Atovaquone-proguanil has relatively few adverse effects that include abdominal pain, nausea, vomiting, diarrhea, headache, elevated transaminases, and pruritus. This medication is taken daily starting 1–2 days before travel, during travel, and continued for 7 days after leaving the malarious region.

Since antimalarial medications are highly but not completely protective, additional measures to reduce mosquito bites are important and also help to protect against other mosquito-borne diseases. These should include the use of an effective DEET or picaridin-containing repellent on exposed skin (avoiding the eyes and mouth), use of mosquito netting if sleeping in unscreened areas, treatment of clothing and mosquito netting with permethrin, and avoidance of outdoor activity when mosquitoes are biting.

B. Traveler's Diarrhea

Traveler's diarrhea (TD) is common with travel to the developing world. This problem affects up to 30–70% of travelers during the first 2 weeks of travel and is usually caused by an infection. Enterotoxigenic *Escherichia coli* (ETEC) is thought to be the most common cause; other bacterial agents include *Campylobacter*, *Salmonella*, *Shigella*, enteroaggregative *E coli*, and other agents. Viral agents include norovirus (which has affected many cruise ships) as well as rotaviruses. Protozoal infections are less likely and often lead to more chronic diarrheal states.

Eating piping-hot foods, avoiding foods handled by hand and not thoroughly cooked, and avoiding contaminated water (including ice) may be useful in preventing TD, but adherence to these measures is difficult. Treatment with a fluoroquinolone antibiotics (given either as a single dose or as a 3-day course) or rifaximin (a nonabsorbable antibiotic given three times daily for 3 days) can be used to shorten the course of diarrhea. Fluoroquinolones have a number of potentially serious side effects. An alternative to fluoroquinolones is azithromycin, particularly for Southeast Asia where fluoroquinolone resistance is common. Loperamide can be used as symptomatic treatment so long as fever and bloody diarrhea are absent.

INFECTIONS TRANSMITTED FROM ANIMALS TO HUMANS: ZOONOSES

Zoonoses are defined as diseases that are naturally transmissible from vertebrate animals to humans. Occupations involving contact with infected animals and/or their infected secretions or tissues or contact with arthropod vectors that transmit diseases from infected animals can result in work-related zoonotic disease.

Nipah Virus

Nipah virus was initially isolated and identified in 1999 during an outbreak of encephalitis and respiratory illness among pig farmers and people with close contact with pigs in Sungai Nipah, Malaysia. It can be transmitted from person to person, requiring standard infection control precautions. The diagnosis is confirmed with laboratory testing. The drug ribavirin has been shown to be effective against the viruses in vitro, but human investigations to date have been inconclusive and the clinical usefulness of ribavirin remains uncertain.

Rabies

Rabies is a preventable viral disease of mammals most often transmitted through the bite of a rabid animal. In the United States, the vast majority of rabies cases reported each year occur in wild animals like raccoons, skunks, bats, and foxes. Human rabies in the United States is rare and most commonly occurs as a result of bat exposure. Worldwide, dog bites cause most cases of human rabies.

▶ Prevention

Preexposure vaccination should be offered to persons in high-risk groups, such as veterinarians and their staff, animal handlers, rabies researchers, and certain laboratory workers. Preexposure vaccination also should be considered for persons whose activities bring them into frequent contact with rabies virus or potentially rabid bats, raccoons, skunks, cats, dogs, or other species at risk for having rabies. In addition, some international travelers might be candidates for preexposure vaccination if they are likely to come in contact with animals in areas where dog or other animal rabies is enzootic and immediate access to appropriate medical care, including rabies vaccine and immune globulin, might be limited. Routine PrEP for the general US population or routine travelers to areas where rabies is not enzootic is not recommended.

▶ Pathogenesis & Clinical Findings

Patient history is important to identify a possible exposure to rabies and other encephalitides; however, rabies should never be ruled out based solely on the absence of definite exposure history. The rabies virus infects the central nervous system, ultimately causing disease in the central nervous system and death. The early symptoms of rabies in people are similar to that of many other illnesses, including fever, headache, and general weakness, or discomfort. Death usually occurs within days of the onset of these symptoms.

▶ Diagnosis & Treatment

Diagnosis of rabies in animals requires examination of brain tissue after the animal has been euthanized. After a bite from a healthy-appearing dog or cat, the animal can be quarantined for 10 days. If the dog or cat has not developed symptoms in that time period, rabies in the animal is ruled out. For diagnosis of rabies in humans, several laboratory tests are required. Postexposure antirabies vaccination should always include administration of both passive antibody and vaccine in those who have not received preexposure vaccination. The combination of human rabies immune globulin (HRIG) and vaccine is recommended for both bite and nonbite exposures, regardless of the interval between exposure and initiation of treatment.

BRUCELLOSIS

Brucellosis is an infectious disease caused by the bacteria of the genus *Brucella*. Different species infect different animal hosts: *B abortus*, cattle; *B melitensis*, goats and sheep; *B suis*, swine; and *B canis*, dogs. Currently, US cattle herds are nearly free of *B abortus* infection. The risk of contracting brucellosis through occupational exposure to livestock in the United States or consumption of domestically produced, properly pasteurized dairy products is minimal. The majority of US cases of brucellosis occur among returned travelers or recent immigrants from endemic areas.

▶ Pathogenesis & Clinical Findings

Occupational brucellosis occurs as a result of mucous membrane or skin contact with infected animal tissues. Aborted placental and fetal membrane tissues from cattle, swine, sheep, and goats are well-documented sources of human exposure. The incubation period is 1–6 weeks. The onset is usually insidious, with fever, sweats, malaise, aches, and weakness. The fever may have a characteristic pattern, often rising in the afternoon and falling during the night (*undulant fever*). The infection is systemic and may result in gastric, intestinal, neurologic, hepatic, or musculoskeletal involvement.

▶ Diagnosis & Treatment

Brucellosis is diagnosed by finding *Brucella* organisms in samples of blood or bone marrow or by detecting antibodies.

Most infections are treated with a combination of doxycycline plus either streptomycin or rifampin. Prolonged treatment often is necessary.

▶ Prevention

Identification and treatment or slaughter of infected animals combined with effective immunization of susceptible animals can eliminate disease in livestock populations. Personal hygiene and protective precautions should be observed in handling potentially infected animal tissues or secretions, particularly those resulting from abortion. Antibiotic postexposure prophylaxis may be recommended in certain circumstances, such as inadvertent exposure to *Brucella* cultures in the laboratory.

Q FEVER

Q fever is a zoonosis caused by *Coxiella burnetii*, an intracellular bacterium that infects mononuclear phagocytes but can infect other cell types as well. Infection in humans usually occurs by inhalation of bacteria from air that is contaminated by excreta of infected animals.

Q fever is an occupational disease in persons whose work involves contact with animals, such as slaughterhouse workers, veterinarians, and farmers, although infection is not limited to these groups. Q fever outbreaks have been reported among workers in animal research facilities, military units, and, rarely, hospitals and diagnostic laboratories. Urban outbreaks and cases with no known exposure or close proximity to livestock have been reported. Cases of acute Q fever were reported in US military personnel who were deployed to Iraq in the 2000s. Investigations of these cases linked illness to tick bites, sleeping in barns, and living near helicopter zones with environmental exposure resulting from helicopter-generated aerosols.

Acute Q fever symptoms vary, and the condition typically is characterized by a nonspecific febrile illness, hepatitis, or pneumonia. Asymptomatic infections followed by seroconversion have been reported in up to 60% of cases identified during outbreak investigations. Onset of symptoms usually occurs within 2–3 weeks of exposure, and symptomatic patients might be ill for weeks or months if untreated. Chronic Q fever can manifest within a few months or several years after acute infection and can follow symptomatic or asymptomatic infections. Chronic disease is rare and typically is characterized by endocarditis in patients with preexisting risk factors such as valvular or vascular defects. Unlike acute Q fever which has a low mortality rate, chronic Q fever endocarditis is fatal if untreated. Routine blood cultures are negative in patients with chronic Q fever endocarditis. Diagnosis of chronic Q fever endocarditis can be difficult because vegetative lesions may not be visualized by echocardiography.

▶ Diagnosis

A. Acute Clinical Features

A prolonged fever greater than 10 days with a normal leukocyte count, thrombocytopenia, and increased liver enzymes is suggestive of acute Q fever infection in the appropriate epidemiological setting.

Women infected with Q fever during pregnancy are at increased risk for miscarriage and preterm delivery.

B. Chronic Clinical Features

Conditions that increase the risk for development of chronic Q fever include preexisting valvular heart disease, vascular grafts, or arterial aneurysms. Infection during pregnancy and immunosuppression (eg, from chemotherapy) are both conditions that have been linked to chronic Q fever development.

C. Laboratory Analysis

PCR of whole blood or serum provides rapid results and can be used to diagnose acute Q fever in approximately the first 2 weeks after symptom onset, especially if obtained before antibiotic administration. A fourfold increase in phase II immunoglobulin G (IgG) antibody titer by immunofluorescent assay (IFA) of paired acute and convalescent specimens is the diagnostic gold standard to confirm diagnosis of acute Q fever. A negative acute titer does not rule out Q fever because an IFA is negative during the first stages of acute illness. Most patients seroconvert by the third week of illness. A single convalescent sample can be tested using IFA in patients past the acute stage of illness; however, a demonstrated fourfold rise between acute and convalescent samples has much higher sensitivity and specificity than a single elevated, convalescent titer. Diagnosis of chronic Q fever is made by an increased phase I IgG antibody ($\geq$1:1024) and an identifiable persistent infection (eg, endocarditis). PCR, immunohistochemistry, or culture of affected tissue can provide definitive confirmation of infection by *C burnetii*.

▶ Treatment & Management

Because of the delay in seroconversion that is often necessary to confirm diagnosis, antibiotic treatment should never be withheld pending laboratory tests or discontinued on the basis of a negative acute specimen. In contrast, treatment of chronic Q fever should be initiated only after diagnostic confirmation. Treatment for acute or chronic Q fever should only be given in clinically compatible cases and not based on elevated serologic titers alone. Doxycycline is the drug of choice, and 2 weeks of treatment is recommended for adults with acute disease. Women who are pregnant when acute Q fever is diagnosed should be treated with a prolonged course of trimethoprim/sulfamethoxazole, which is often given until the eighth month of pregnancy. Serologic monitoring is recommended following acute Q fever infection to assess possible progression to chronic infection. The recommended schedule for monitoring is based on the patient's risk for chronic infection.

▶ Prevention

Educational efforts should particularly target groups vulnerable to development of chronic Q fever, such as workers who have preexisting valvulopathy, a prosthetic heart valve, a vascular prosthesis, an aneurysm, are pregnant or might become pregnant, or are immunosuppressed, because these employees have a higher risk for a severe outcome or death if infected. Although protection for at-risk workers can be provided by Q fever vaccination, a licensed vaccine is not available in the United States.

▶ Management of Occupational Exposure

The majority of occupationally related Q fever outbreaks in the United States have occurred among biomedical research facility workers exposed to infected pregnant ewes. Workplaces with employees at high risk for *C burnetii* exposure (eg, laboratories that experiment with *C burnetii* and animal research facilities) should institute a Q fever medical surveillance and health education monitoring program. Engineering controls, administrative controls, and use of PPE are recommended when appropriate. The use of standard precautions by health care providers is sufficient to prevent Q fever transmission during routine care. Additional precautions should be used during aerosol-generating procedures. The use of postexposure prophylaxis is not recommended for workers after a known or potential exposure; any acute febrile illness that occurs within 6 weeks of exposure warrants immediate treatment and medical evaluation.

B VIRUS

B virus infection is caused by Macacine herpesvirus 1, an alpha-herpesvirus closely related to herpes simplex virus. B virus is also commonly referred to as herpes B, monkey B virus, herpesvirus simiae, and herpesvirus B.

The virus is commonly found among macaque monkeys, including rhesus macaques, pig-tailed macaques, and cynomolgus monkeys, any of which can harbor latent B virus infection and appear to be natural hosts for the virus. Monkeys infected with B virus usually have no or only mild symptoms. In addition, rabbits, guinea pigs, and mice can be experimentally infected with B virus.

Infection with B virus is extremely rare in humans; however, when it does occur, the infection can result in severe neurologic sequelae or fatal encephalomyelitis if the patient is not treated soon after exposure.

Initial treatment of workers exposed to B virus infection should include cleaning of the exposed area by thoroughly washing and scrubbing the area or wound with soap, concentrated solution of detergent, povidone-iodine, or chlorhexidine and water, and irrigating the washed area with running water for 15–20 minutes. A specimen for testing should not be obtained from the wound area prior to washing the site because it could force virus more deeply into the wound, reducing the effectiveness of the cleansing protocol. After the site is cleaned, a serum specimen should be obtained from the patient to provide a baseline antibody level. Consideration should be given to prophylaxis with valacyclovir 1 g three times daily × 14 days or acyclovir 800 mg 5 times/day for 14 days.

The affected worker should be counseled to seek immediate care if skin lesions, influenza-like symptoms or neurologic symptoms develop.

OCCUPATIONAL IMMUNIZATION & BIOLOGIC SURVEILLANCE

As discussed previously, workers with specific risk factors should be considered for appropriate immunization, prophylaxis, and surveillance, if available. For example, vaccination with a quadrivalent meningococcal vaccine (protects against serotypes A, C, Y, and W135) and a serogroup B meningococcal vaccine is recommended for those who may be exposed to meningococcus in clinical microbiology laboratories. Since adenovirus can spread rapidly and cause significant disease in military recruits, adenovirus vaccine is recommended for certain military personnel.

Serologic testing for evidence of subclinical infection may be helpful in selected circumstances.

▶ Exposure Evaluation

Serologic or other clinical microbiologic tests can be used to investigate human or animal sources of infectious agents. Environmental exposure evaluation associated with sources such as contaminated ventilation systems or water requires special techniques. However, technologies exist for collection and measurement of certain environmental organisms. A knowledgeable industrial hygienist can select the appropriate instrumentation and sampling strategy based on factors such as the suspected organism, air velocity, sampler efficiency, anticipated concentration, particle size, sampler physical requirements, and the study objective.

REFERENCES

Alwan NA, Burgess RA, Ashworth S, et al: Scientific consensus on the COVID-19 pandemic: we need to act now. Lancet. 2020;396(10260):e71-e72. Erratum in: Lancet. 2020;396(10261):1490. [PMID: 33069277].

Centers for Disease Control and Prevention: Infection Control in Healthcare Personnel—Infrastructure and Routine Practices for Occupational Infection Prevention and Control Services (2019). https://www.cdc.gov/infectioncontrol/pdf/guidelines/infection-control-HCP-H.pdf.

Freedman M, Jackson BR, McCotter O, Benedict K: Coccidioidomycosis outbreaks, United States and worldwide, 1940-2015. Emerg Infect Dis 2018;24(3):417-423 [PMID: 29460741].

Kuhar DT, Henderson DK, Struble KA, et al: Updated US Public Health Service guidelines for the management of occupational exposures to human immunodeficiency virus and recommendations for postexposure prophylaxis. Infect Control Hosp Epidemiol 2013;34(9):875-892. Erratum in: Infect Control Hosp Epidemiol 2013;34(11):1238 [PMID: 23917901].

Larremore DB, Wilder B, Lester E, et al: Test sensitivity is secondary to frequency and turnaround time for COVID-19 screening. Sci Adv. 2020 Nov 20:eabd5393. Epub ahead of print. [PMID: 33219112].

Milton DK: A Rosetta Stone for Understanding Infectious Drops and Aerosols. J Pediatric Infect Dis Soc. 2020;9(4):413-415. [PMID: 32706376].

Paltiel AD, Schwartz JL, Zheng A, Walensky RP: Clinical outcomes of a COVID-19 vaccine: Implementation over efficacy. Health Aff (Millwood). 2021;40(1):42-52. [PMID: 33211536].

Principe L, Tomao P, Visca P: Legionellosis in the occupational setting. Environ Res 2017;152:485-495 [PMID: 27717486].

Su CP, de Perio MA, Cummings KJ, McCague AB, Luckhaupt SE, Sweeney MH: Case investigations of infectious diseases occurring in workplaces, United States, 2006-2015. Emerg Infect Dis 2019;25(3):397-405 [PMID: 30789129].

■ SELF-ASSESSMENT QUESTIONS

Select the one correct answer for each question.

Question 1: Hepatitis A
  a. is a viral hepatitis transmitted through the fecal-oral route
  b. is rarely encountered by travelers
  c. always causes pronounced acute symptoms in children
  d. has been eradicated in the United States

Question 2: Positive hepatitis B core antibodies
  a. indicate past or present HBV infections
  b. do not prompt testing for HBV surface antigens
  c. result from percutaneous injury
  d. indicate susceptibility to HBV infection

Question 3: Hepatitis C
  a. is a bacterial infection of the liver caused by the hepatitis C virus
  b. causes chronic infection in a minority of those who are infected
  c. is infrequently associated with a history of blood transfusion
  d. is transmitted rarely following mucous membrane exposure, with no apparent transfer following exposures to intact skin

Question 4: Tuberculin skin test
  a. is recommended on a monthly basis for occupational high-risk workers
  b. is reliably positive even in the presence of overwhelming tuberculosis
  c. is reliably positive even in the presence of measles, Hodgkin disease, sarcoidosis, or immunosuppressive states
  d. is considered positive in high-risk occupational groups with a reaction of 10 mm or more

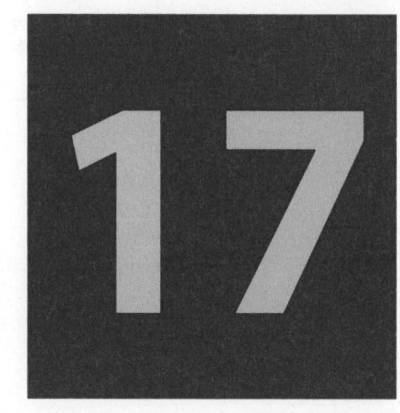

Occupational Skin Disorders

Howard I. Maibach, MD
Becky S. Li, MD
John H. Cary, MD

Although human skin can withstand many assaults of a hostile environment, it is the most commonly injured organ in industry. Skin disorders comprise more than 35% of all occupationally related diseases, affecting annually approximately one worker per thousand. Reporting remains highly incomplete, however, and the hardship and financial loss to workers and employers alike are substantial. Most occupational skin disease results from contact with chemicals, of which there are more than 90,000 in the environment today. Under certain conditions, all of them can irritate the skin, and approximately 2000 substances are now recognized as contact allergens. In addition, workers bring to their work preexisting diseases, which can be aggravated by their work.

Contact dermatitis (CD) of the hands is the most common occupational skin disease and atopy is often an important cofactor. CD can be subdivided into irritant contact dermatitis (ICD) and allergic contact dermatitis (ACD) (Figure 17–1).

GENERAL APPROACH TO DIAGNOSIS & TREATMENT OF OCCUPATIONAL SKIN DISORDERS

The workup and diagnosis of patients with work-related skin disease requires much more time than does a general dermatologic workup. Making a premature diagnosis before studying all the evidence should be resisted because an incorrect diagnosis can have long-lasting and severely detrimental effects. Review of the medical records, patch testing, fungal and bacterial cultures, biopsy, and plant visits often are necessary to reach a correct diagnosis. While an endogenous or constitutional eczema or dermatitis may be the primary cause, detailed analysis of

work-relate risk factors should be undertaken where appropriate. Atopic eczema, although inherited, often has onset for the first time in adult life when precipitated by work activities, and aggravation often is considered work-related. Many other constitutional diseases can be considered similarly.

Table 17–1 outlines a typical evaluation of a work-related illness. The following headings can serve as a form for recording the results of the workup. The text under each heading details the information that should be gathered and recorded.

▶ History of Injury/Problem & Current Complaints

Learn exactly which anatomic skin site was first affected. With a diagnosis of CD, the eruption should begin at the site of contact with the offending agents. Spreading then occurs, especially in the case of allergic sensitization. The date of the initial appearance of the dermatitis is important because often a change in workplace ergonomics, contact with new substances, or increased contact with long-used substances can precipitate dermatitis. Itching is important because ICD, and especially ACD, is almost always pruritic. If improvement occurs away from work and aggravation regularly takes place on resumption of the same work, a work relationship is almost always found. Over-the-counter medicines and home

Photographs of the occupational dermatoses discussed in this chapter can be found at: NIOSH Occupational Dermatoses: https://www.cdc.gov/niosh/topics/skin/occderm-slides/ocderm.html

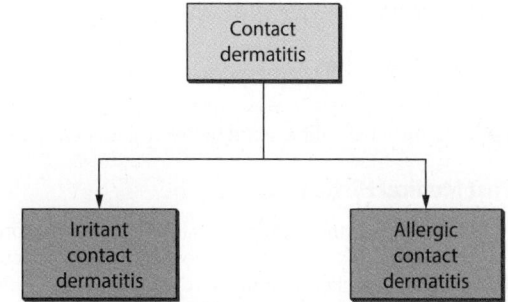

▲ **Figure 17–1.** Types of contact dermatitis.

Table 17–1. Outline for dermatologic examinations for workers' compensation patients.

History
Job description
Current treatment
Present complaints
Medical history
Family history
Social history
Personal data
Medical record review
Physical examination
Diagnosis
Support for diagnosis
Discussion
Disability status
Factors of disability
Subjective
Objective
Apportionment
Future medical care
Vocational rehabilitation
Work restrictions

remedies often contain contact allergens that sometimes can be the sole cause.

A. Occupational History

A description of the job as provided by the patient is often more accurate than the official job title. Often the worker has performed the same job for a long period of time before onset of dermatitis. This suggests a new process or contactant introduced into the workplace or home environment.

B. Prior Employment

The nature of previous jobs and dermatitis, as well as previous exposure to irritants and potential sensitizers, is important.

C. Nonwork Activities

The 40-hour workweek leaves sufficient opportunity for other part-time jobs, hobbies, and house and garden work.

D. Past Medical History

Although 15–20% of the population has a family or personal history of atopy, it is an often-overlooked cause of recurrent dermatitis, especially among hairdressers, kitchen helpers, medical and dental personnel, and automobile repair workers. Even persons with mild atopy may develop major

work-related hand dermatitis at the time of first employment, following repeated contact with irritants. Psoriasis also can be precipitated by trauma, especially repeated intense friction and pressure on the hands.

E. Family History

A family history of atopy is most important. Psoriasis (type 1) also may be a relevant family condition.

F. Hobbies/Habits

Hobbies and off-work activities should be explored during the history taking, including habitual traumatic activities such as picking and digging the skin, especially with wooden or metal articles used for scratching and rubbing.

G. Review of Systems

A general review of body systems should be done.

▶ Review of Medical Records

The medical records must be examined thoroughly to supplement the history as provided by the patient.

▶ Examination

Examination should not be limited to the part affected because the presence of dermatitis elsewhere and other skin conditions can change an initial impression. This is especially true when psoriasis, tinea infections, and lichen planus are found.

A. Special Investigations

Patch testing is the most important special investigation and should include not only suspected specific allergens but also a standard series of common allergens.

B. Diagnosis

The specific diagnosis should be recorded with an opinion regarding a work relationship.

C. Summary

This should be a brief summary of the findings with an explanation of the conclusions. Nonmedical terms should be used as much as possible.

1. Temporary and total disability—The disability status, total or partial, is described here. In most cases of hand dermatitis, the disability is temporary, but total disability is also possible.

2. Permanent and stationary (P&S) status—Once the dermatitis has reached a plateau and no further improvement is anticipated, P&S status is reported. This does not mean, however, that treatment should not continue should the condition warrant or a recurrence cause a worsening of symptoms.

3. Objective findings—A brief review of the objective findings is recorded here.

4. Subjective findings—A review of the patient's complaints and a description of any impairment are provided here.

5. Work restrictions—Work restrictions, if any, can be recorded here.

6. Loss of preinjury capacity—For purposes of permanent disability rating, one should describe any loss of preinjury capacity, such as may occur with contact allergy.

7. Causation and apportionment—If any aspect of the impairment is related to a previous employment or any pre-existing disability, this is explained here, estimating the percentage of impairment associated with each.

8. Future medical treatment—An estimation of the type and duration of future medical treatment is given here.

9. Vocational rehabilitation—Once a P&S state is reached, vocational rehabilitation must be considered. It is important to offer guidance to vocational rehabilitation personnel in job selection for disabled workers.

10. Patch testing—The most important diagnostic test for occupational skin disease is the patch test. Since irritant and allergic dermatitis can be similar clinically, differentiation can be done only by patch testing, which not only will reveal the specific cause of a work-related dermatitis but also when negative after testing all possible allergens in the patient's work will effectively rule out ACD as a cause. Unfortunately, the test is often performed inadequately or incompletely, if at all. Patch testing should be done by experienced physicians according to accepted methods with nonirritating concentrations of test substances, preferably chemicals obtained commercially from manufacturers of patch test materials. Table 17–2 lists and describes common contact allergens.

11. Additional diagnostic tests—Fungal, bacterial, and viral smears and cultures, biopsies and photopatch testing. The prick testing, if contact urticaria is suspected, sometimes is required. Plant visits are an essential and integral part of the evaluation, often providing information vastly different from that learned during the patient's evaluation.

▶ Prevention

Prevention of occupational skin disorder is highly important as it reduces the risk of progression to more severe skin diseases such as hand eczema, disfigurement, and even skin cancers. This requires close cooperation between the employee, employers, company physicians, dermatologists, and other relevant stakeholders such as workers unions.

In general, prevention of occupational skin disorders can be subdivided into three categories: primary, secondary, and tertiary preventions.

A. Primary Prevention

This involves identifying, avoiding, and/or replacing any potentially harmful substances. This should include providing employees with information on the involved chemical

Table 17–2. Allergens tested in various standard series: Main uses (European, International, British).

1.	Potassium dichromate 0.5% petro-latum (pet)	Tanning leather, cement
2.	4-Phenylenediamine base 1% pet	Azo dye intermediate, hair dye
3.	Thiuram mix 1% pet	Rubber accelerator, fungicides
4.	Neomycin sulfate 20% pet	Antibiotic in creams
5.	Cobalt(II) chloride hexahydrate 1% pet	Metal
6.	Benzocaine 5% pet	Local anesthetic in creams
7.	Nickel sulfate hexahydrate 5% pet	Metal
8.	Clioquinol 5% pet	Synthetic anti-infective agent
9.	Colophony 20% pet	Pine resin, adhesives, printing ink
10.	Paraben mix 16% pet	Preservatives in creams
11.	*N*-Isopropyl-*N*-phenyl-4-phenylenediamine (IPPD)	Black rubber chemical
12.	Wool alcohols 30% pet	Ointment base in creams
13.	Mercapto mix 2% pet	Rubber additives
14.	Epoxy resin 1% pet	Resin in adhesives, paint, insulation
15.	Balsam of Peru 25% pet	Fragrance and flavoring agent
16.	4-*tert*-Butylphenoformaldehyde resin (PTBP) 1% pet	Resin in adhesives
17.	2-Mercaptobenzothiazole 2% pet	Rubber chemical
18.	Formaldehyde 1% aqueous (aq)	Disinfectants, cosmetic preservatives
19.	Fragrance mix 8% pet	Fragrances
20.	Sesquiterpene lactone mix 0.1% pet	Plants
21.	Quaternium 15 1% pet	Formaldehyde releaser
22.	Primin 0.01% pet	Main allergen in primula dermatitis
23.	5-Chloro-2-methyl-4-isothiazolin-3-one 0.01% aq	Preservative in oils and creams
24.	Budesonide 0.01% pet	Nonhalogenated steroid
25.	Tixocortol-21-pivalate 0.1% pet	Topical steroids (hydrocortisone)

substances and putting in place risk reduction strategies at organizational level.

B. Secondary Prevention

Employers should make available skin protective measure. Employees should ensure individual skin protection by wearing of protective gloves, application of protective skin ointments before working, adequate skin cleansing, and skin care measures to support regeneration following work. A careful analysis of the harmful effects to the skin at the workplace is necessary for the appropriate choice of suitable skin protective measures.

C. Tertiary Prevention

Individuals with patients with severe skin diseases suspected to be of occupational origin may benefit from an inpatient/outpatient prevention program. In general, this is most applicable to clinically severe and/or chronic occupational disease for which outpatient methods of secondary prevention have been inadequate.

► Treatment

In many occupations, avoidance of irritants and allergens is not always possible. Prophylactic measures are necessary in industry to avoid the risk of developing ICD and ACD. The specific treatment of occupational skin disease depends on the cause and does not differ from treatment of nonoccupational skin disease. Protective measures include moisturizers, barrier creams, and appropriate gloves and clothing. In many cases, a specific cause is not found, and recurrences may continue to affect the patient; hence, treatment with topical or oral corticosteroids often continues for prolonged period of time, leading to atrophy of skin and systemic complications. Although recovery may occur rapidly following treatment, the skin retains a nonspecific hypersensitivity for several weeks, and hence work should not be resumed too early.

CONTACT DERMATITIS

Irritant Contact Dermatitis

ESSENTIALS OF DIAGNOSIS

Acute and subacute effects

▶ Single exposure to a strong irritant is sufficient
▶ Usually hands involved
▶ Raw appearance and erythema of the affected body part
▶ Demarcated areas from the normal skin
▶ Cracking/chapping of the affected body part
▶ Fissuring
▶ Bleeding

▶ Pustular skin changes
▶ Itching/burning with or without visible skin changes

Chronic effects

▶ Repeated exposures required
▶ Skin dryness
▶ Hyperkeratosis
▶ Skin itching (less than in ACD)
▶ Skin wrinkling
▶ Development of ACD

► General Considerations

ICD is a spectrum of disease processes with a complex pathophysiology, a varied natural history, and divergent clinical appearance. This contrasts with ACD, in which a specific chemical is the central cause. Many factors can induce irritant reactions, either in isolation or in combination. These include the intrinsic nature of the substance (ie, pH, solubility, physical state, and concentration), environmental factors (ie, molecular weight, partition coefficient, temperature, humidity, and pressure), predisposing individual characteristics (ie, age, gender, ethnicity, concurrent and preexisting skin disease, and the skin region exposed), and genetic factors such as filaggrin (FLG) gene mutation. ICD is a common form of occupational skin disease and, in the United States, accounts for nearly 80% of all occupational dermatitis.

There are at least 14 biological entities within the irritant dermatitis syndrome.

Acute irritation/corrosion refers to a single exposure of a material that is so irritant that damage is seen within hours to a day or so. Typically, this is caused by exposure to strong acids and bases (Table 17–3). Many other chemicals produce similar exaggerated effects. The likelihood of a mixture producing such acute irritation frequently can be estimated by high concentrations of chemicals with extremes of pH.

Table 17–3. Examples of contact irritants and allergens.

Irritants
Soaps/detergents
Water
Acids/alkalis
Organic solvents
Metalworking fluids
Allergens
Chromate
Epoxy resins
Biocides
Fragrances
Formaldehyde
Rubber chemicals
Methacrylates

Irritant reaction refers to a slowly developing redness and chapping of the skin that, with prompt cessation, usually leads to prompt amelioration without therapy. The prototypic situation is the hairdresser trainee who becomes the shampoo person, washing heads many times a day for weeks and months. The erythema and chapping frequently start on the dorsal hand. When discontinued, resolution is rapid. Many (but not all) moisturizers will inhibit the response. Some individuals will go on, with repeated exposure, to a cumulative irritant dermatitis, which may become severe.

Delayed acute irritant dermatitis refers to acute (primary) irritant dermatitis that develops within hours to a day or so. Another form exists in which a single exposure produces irritation as late as 2 and 3 days. This form of irritant dermatitis can be confused with ACD responses.

Subjective/sensory irritation is a form of irritation that consists of burn, sting, itch, and other discomfort but without visible signs. The same symptoms can occur with visible dermatitis, but this is not then called subjective/sensory irritation. The syndrome is readily confused with low-dose chemicals that also produce burn, sting, and itch but which, with higher doses, will produce contact urticaria. This must be ruled out in order for the symptoms to be defined as subjective/sensory irritation. Although visible damage does not occur, some individuals are highly annoyed by the symptoms. A classic chemical class that induces this is the pyrethroids.

Suberythematous irritation is defined as skin discomfort in which there is no visible erythema, induration, or scaling. However, careful examination of the skin with a stratum corneum assay (squamometry) reveals changes in the protein conformation of the stratum corneum. This nonvisible clinical problem is well worth noting by the occupational health care professional because it can be the first sign of early clinical (visible) irritant dermatitis.

Cumulative irritation is often confused with ACD. This biological entity refers to the fact that some chemicals (frequently at appropriately low doses) may not produce irritation on multiple exposures until weeks, months, or years of exposure. It is essential, when a visible dermatitis develops after a prolonged period of time, to exclude ACD with appropriate diagnostic patch testing. If the worker is patch-test-negative, the clinical dermatitis then may be cumulative irritation. Discontinuing the irritant and allowing healing eventually may allow the chemical to be used without clinical intolerance.

Traumative irritant dermatitis refers to an uncommon and little understood clinical phenomenon where a small area of dermatitis heals and then exacerbates. The subsequent dermatitis may be long lasting (weeks to years). Triggering factors include acute irritant dermatitis, occasionally ACD, and trauma such as cuts.

Pustular and acneiform irritant dermatitis occurs in individuals who develop, on exposure to irritants such as oils, greases, and tars, acne-like lesions such as comedones (Tables 17–4 and 17–5). They also develop pustules, which the individual frequently identifies, if on the face, as acne.

Table 17–4. Examples of acne in the workplace.

Type	Occupation
Cosmetic acne	Actors, models, cosmetologists
Acne mechanica	Auto and truck mechanics, athletes, telephone operators
Ultraviolet acne	Models, lifeguards
Oil acne	Machinists, auto mechanics, fry cooks, roofers, petroleum refinery workers, rubber workers, highway pavers

Exsiccation eczematoid dermatitis refers to a chronic low-humidity dermatitis leading to an eczematous morphology. The trigger is low humidity and often frequent changes of air. This is nonimmunologic, and management consists of raising the relative humidity.

Friction occurs in many industries with repetitive exposures of the skin leading to friction. Friction has been studied extensively and can be measured readily with bioengineering instruments. This form of irritation is not chemically induced.

Nonimmunologic contact urticaria (NICU) is a common event but fortunately is typically of minimal clinical significance. An appropriate dose of a chemical such as sorbic acid or dimethyl sulfoxide (DMSO) will produce at low doses burn, sting, and itch. At higher doses, they will produce erythema, and at still higher doses will produce a frank wheal. Involution is rapid.

Airborne irritant dermatitis refers to irritation (with appropriate negative patch tests and a photopatch test) in a photoexposed area.

Photoirritation (phototoxicity) refers to chemical irritation that requires typically ultraviolet light A (UVA) to elicit it. It would not occur in the dark. The prototype chemical that has been most studied is bergapten. Predictive tests to identify chemicals that produce photoirritation are well developed and highly predictive. Management generally requires removing the chemical from the environment.

Tandem irritant dermatitis refers to cases when one irritant may not produce clinical disease, but two irritants may do so. This is not a common phenomenon, and some combinations do not produce tandem irritation.

Table 17–5. Chloracne-producing chemicals.

Polyhalogenated naphthalenes
Polyhalogenated biphenyls
Polyhalogenated dibenzofurans
Contaminants of polychlorophenol compounds: herbicide 4, 5-T
Contaminants of 3,4-dichloroaniline and related herbicides
Dichlorodiphenyltrichloroethane (DDT) (crude trichlorobenzene)

Other general clinical patterns include repeated rubbing and friction in many individuals producing a thickened, sharply demarcated, scaly plaque resembling psoriasis known as *lichen simplex*. Excessive sweating, especially under occlusion, and ultraviolet (UV) and infrared radiation may cause miliaria. Irritation also may result in hyperpigmentation or hypopigmentation, alopecia, urticaria, and granulomas.

▶ Mechanisms of Action

ICD is a nonimmunogenic skin reaction to toxic substances either in low or high concentrations. Any substance (including water after long-term exposure) has a potential to cause skin irritation. Skin exposure to irritating toxic substances in minor concentrations over a long period is a predisposing factor, as are atopic skin diathesis and hyperhidrosis.

The exact mechanisms of ICD are not fully elucidated. Currently, either alone or in combination, two mechanisms have been proposed: damage to the barrier function of the stratum corneum of the skin, and/or the direct effect of the irritant on the skin cells.

ICD results from the denaturation and delipidation of the lipid-rich stratum corneum leading to altered barrier function and transepidermal water loss. This may result in the further penetration of and damage to the deeper epidermal layer containing living keratinocytes.

ICD mechanism is best illustrated by surfactants and emulsifiers (Figure 17–2). Surfactants have hydrophilic and hydrophobic tails; hence, they can reduce the surface tension of and form micelles in solution. They cause cytoplasm release of pro-inflammatory cytokines such as IL-1α which further expresses IL-6, IL-8, phospholipase A_2 (PLA$_2$), and tumor necrosis factor-α (TNF-α). The process is then followed by the morphologic changes and clinical manifestations of ICD.

▶ Clinical Findings

A. Symptoms and Signs

Clinical features vary and depend on many factors. These include the skin integrity, physical and chemical properties of the substance involved, duration of exposure, surface area of the exposed skin and the location. The commonest predisposing factor to ICD in workplace is atopy, occurring in 15–20% of the population. Dry skin and advancing age are also important predisposing factors. ICD in workplace manifests as erythema, edema, and scaling. It usually involves the hands and results from exposures to irritants. Symptoms appear at work, some improvements occur over the weekend and holidays with complete resolution only after a prolonged leave of absence or change of job.

Anatomic differences in exposure site are important. Irritation usually is greater in areas where the skin is thin, such as dorsa of the hands, between the fingers, volar forearms, inner thighs, and dorsum of the feet. Irritant dermatitis from airborne substances such as dusts and volatile chemicals develops most commonly on regions most heavily exposed, such as the face, hands, and arms.

B. Special Tests

The diagnosis of ICD is often confirmed by exclusion of ACD. Patch testing is necessary to rule out ACD, but it

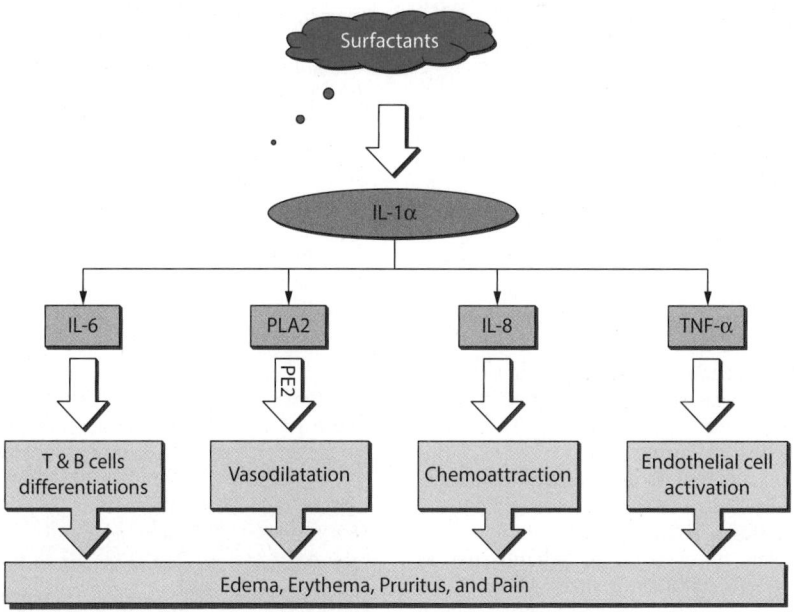

▲ **Figure 17–2.** Pathophysiology of irritant contact dermatitis.

Table 17–6. Causes of phototoxic (photoirritant) reactions.

Coal tars
Furocoumarins: Psoralen; 8-methoxypsoralen; 4,5,8-trimethylpsoralen
Aminobenzoic acid derivative: Amyl-ortho-dimethylaminobenzoic acid
Dyes: Disperse blue 35
Drugs: Sulfonamides; phenothiazines; tetracyclines; thiazides

should be emphasized that testing should be avoided with irritants unless in nonirritant concentrations.

▶ Specific Types of Cutaneous Irritation

A. Phototoxic (Photoirritation) Reactions

A nonimmunologic phototoxic eruption may result from contact with certain chemicals, such as the juice of a plant, with simultaneous exposure to natural or artificial light. Vesicle and bullae formation are characteristic, with sunburn-like erythema, followed by hyperpigmentation. Pseudoporphyria, photo-onycholysis, slate-gray hyperpigmentation, and lichenoid eruptions are less frequent. The degree of phototoxicity is correlated to the dose or concentration of the phototoxic substance and the amount of UV exposure. The most common causes are the polycyclic aromatic hydrocarbons in tar and furocoumarins (psoralens) found in certain plants (Table 17–6). Numerous systemic drugs also can cause these reactions. The exact mechanism of photoirritation has not been fully elucidated; ultraviolet absorption (usually UVA spectrum), tissue damage from reactive oxygen species (ROS) generation, photodynamic lipid peroxidation and DNA cleavage have been considered to play major roles in the process. Avoiding the offending substance(s) is curative.

B. Cement Burns

Severe burns can result from contact with wet cement because of its high alkalinity resulting from the presence of calcium oxide and hydroxide. The burns usually result from workers kneeling in wet cement or spilling it into their boots or gloves. Workers frequently delay removing contaminated boots and gloves in order to finish a job before the concrete hardens. Initially, there is burning and erythema, with ulceration delayed for several hours and followed by deep necrosis. Healing is slow, requiring several weeks and leaving disfiguring scars.

The loss of work in these cases is extensive, lasting many weeks. There are numerous cosmetic and functional residual problems. The importance of taking precautionary measures by cement users cannot be overemphasized.

C. Fiberglass Dermatitis

Commercially produced since the 1930s, fiberglass is available in two forms: wool fiberglass and textile fiberglass. The former is used chiefly for insulation, acoustic panels, and ceiling boards in construction. Textile fiberglass is made into yarns or processed into short fibers for reinforcement of plastics, rubber, and paper. Binders are used on wool fiberglass, such as thermosetting phenol formaldehyde-type resins. The sizing agent for textile fiberglass varies, but once the sizing agent is cured, the risk of ACD is diminished. Almost all fiberglass manufactured has a diameter of more than 4.5 μm, which can readily penetrate stratum corneum and cause irritation.

Contact with fiberglass produces irritation, with itching and prickling of the skin, especially in skin folds and areas where clothing rubs. A maculopapular rash may be present, usually obscured by excoriations. When widespread, the rash can be diagnosed incorrectly as scabies. Application of a piece of cellophane tape to the skin and then to a microscopic slide will disclose the uniform, rodlike fibers of glass (readily visualized with polarization).

The symptoms usually subside after a few days. Allergic sensitization has not been proven, and many workers develop "hardening" and thus are able to return to work and continue without recurrence.

D. Pigmentary Changes

Chemical agents may induce either increased or decreased pigmentation or sometimes both in the same patient. *Melanosis* denotes hyperpigmentation, whereas *leukoderma* refers to loss of pigment. Inflammation usually precedes the color change. Repeated trauma, friction, chemical and thermal burns, and exposure to UV light can increase pigmentation, especially in dark-skinned persons. Coal tar, pitch, asphalt, creosote, and other tar and petroleum derivatives can induce skin darkening. Psoralens, found in certain plants, induce phytophotodermatitis with contact followed by sun exposure, which can cause hyperpigmentation.

Occupational leukoderma resembles idiopathic vitiligo, and differentiation can be difficult. However, to be considered work-induced, the initial site of leukoderma, usually the hands and forearms, should be the site of repeated contact with a known depigmenting chemical (Table 17–7). With continued contact, depigmentation may spread to distant body sites not in direct contact with the chemical.

Table 17–7. Chemicals causing leukoderma.

Hydroquinone
Monobenzyl ether of hydroquinone
Monomethyl ether of hydroquinone
para-Tertiary-butylphenol
para-Tertiary-butylcatechol
para-Tertiary-amylphenol
para-Isopropyl catechol

Chemical leukoderma is reversible if exposure is discontinued soon after onset. If continued exposure occurs, it may be permanent. Topical and oral psoralen and ultraviolet A (PUVA) therapy has been used to induce repigmentation, but acral lesions, especially on the hands, often are refractory to treatment.

▶ Differential Diagnosis

- ACD
- Atopic dermatitis\endogenous eczema
- Lichen simplex chronicus
- Pompholyx
- Palmoplantar pustulosis
- Phytophotodermatitis
- Id reaction
- Dermatitis artefacta—self-induced lesions that are seen occasionally and can be recognized by their bizarre shapes and locations with an inconsistent and suspicious history of occurrence.
- Scabies
- Drug eruptions
- Porphyria cutanea tarda
- Pseudoporphyria
- Bullous diseases of dialysis

ALLERGIC CONTACT DERMATITIS

ESSENTIALS OF DIAGNOSIS

- ▶ Once allergic sensitization has occurred, the dermatitis begins within 24 hours to several days after contact.
- ▶ Pruritus—very prominent feature.
- ▶ Erythema—usually rapid.
- ▶ Papule formation.
- ▶ Vesicles.
- ▶ Blistering.

▶ General Considerations

Although reportedly occurring less often than ICD, ACD is of great importance because ordinary protective measures can be ineffective, and many workers have to change jobs or learn a new trade. By contrast, workers with irritant dermatitis often can return to work, provided they use adequate personal protective measures, such as gloves, and if the workplace is made less hazardous.

ACD is an immunologic reaction classified as a delayed type IV or cell-mediated hypersensitivity. This distinguishes it from type I reactions, which are immediate and antibody mediated.

A. Mechanisms of Action

Development of ACD results from a complex interplay of inherited risk factors such as polymorphism (genetic variations) and acquired risk factors like include atopic dermatitis, ICD, and venous stasis. The mechanisms are not fully understood.

Langerhans cells (LCs), epidermal and dermal dendritic cells (DCs) play vital roles in the sensitization and elicitation of ACD. During sensitization, the potential allergens react with DCs via interaction with neighboring keratinocytes, migration to the local draining lymph nodes and the priming of naive T cells. These processes are mediated by inflammatory cytokines, chemokines, and adhesion molecules. When skin is in contact with the same allergens, the allergen-specific effector T cells are then recruited resulting in elicitation. Following their recruitment, these T cells are then activated by antigen-presenting skin cells, including LCs, dermal DCs, and most likely keratinocytes.

Cytotoxic effector T cells in the dermoepidermal junction will attack (causing cell death) among others, keratinocytes at the suprabasal layer. The interaction of DCs, keratinocytes and the loss of regulatory T (Treg) cell–mediated inhibition will result in the subsequent activation of skin-specific effector cells, that is, cytotoxic T (CD8+ Tc1) cells and T helper (Th) cells 1 and 17 (Figure 17–3).

Lymphocyte-mediated immune mechanisms in contact allergy include a sensitization phase. The contact allergen interacts with DCs in the skin via "pattern recognition receptors" such as toll-like receptors (TLRs). Subsequently naive T helper (Th) cells are polarized upon specific recognition of the haptenated allergen by the major histocompatibility complex (MHC), costimulatory signals and cytokines such as IL-12, IL-4, IL-1b, and IL-6. This process is followed by the elicitation phase where hapten-specific cytotoxic CD8 T lymphocytes (CTLs) release inflammatory cytokines and induce disease-specific local skin lesions following reexposure of the skin to the same contact allergen.

Occasionally a more acute dermatitis can occur on reexposure to the allergen or with aggravation by contact with irritating substances. There is considerable variation in the intensity of reaction depending on the body area affected. The mucous membranes usually are not affected, and the hair-bearing scalp usually is much less involved than the adjacent skin. The palms and soles may be less affected than the dorsal and interdigital areas. The eyelids and periorbital skin are especially sensitive, whereas involvement of the vault of the axillae is rare. It is important to consider and address the perception of patients regarding their symptom as this is beneficial in relieving the symptoms on the long term.

Examples of occupational contact allergens include epoxy resins, biocides, chromate, and formaldehyde (see Table 17–3).

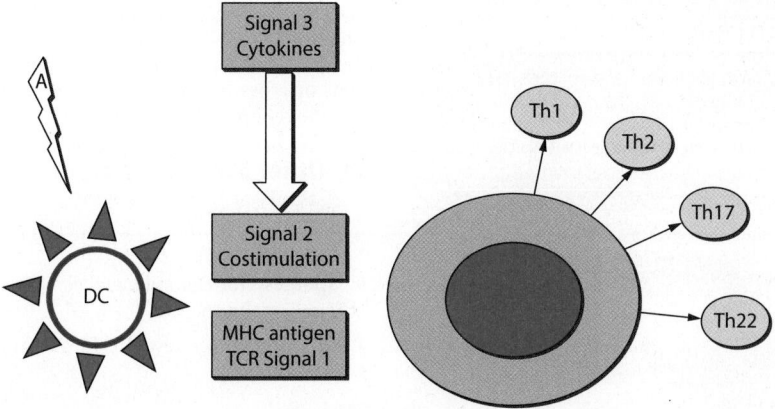

▲ **Figure 17–3.** Pathophysiology of allergic contact dermatitis.

▶ Clinical Findings

A. Symptoms and Signs

Although most contact allergens produce sensitization in only a small percentage of exposed persons, great variation exists among individuals depending on numerous factors such as the nature of the allergen itself. The allergen in poison ivy or poison oak will sensitize nearly 70% of exposed persons, whereas *p*-phenylenediamine, the allergen in permanent hair dyes, sensitizes a relatively small percentage of persons who repeatedly contact with it.

Sensitization requires at least 4 days to develop. Many workers, however, contact an allergen repeatedly in their work for months and even years before developing clinical sensitivity. The precipitating cause of sensitization can be a minor episode of irritant dermatitis or even increased frequency of contact with greater pressure and sweating at the site. After poison oak, nickel is the most common cause of CD.

The dermatitis originates at the site of contact with the allergen, but new lesions may appear at distant, seemingly unrelated sites, usually because of inadvertent transfer of the allergen by the hands.

A subacute and chronic stage can evolve. It is characterized by skin thickening, dryness, and fissuring.

B. Patch Testing

The key to diagnosis of ACD is diagnostic patch testing. The opportunity to select the site of application and the ability to use only a minute concentration of test substance, confining it to a small area, are important features. The organ tested is the same as that affected by the disease and the same mechanism for production of the disease is used; hence, the patch test remains one of the most direct and valuable of all methods of medical testing.

Standardized procedures in patch testing are important, especially the concentration of the allergen and the type and characteristics of the vehicle. During recent decades, attempts to standardize patch testing have occurred.

Two methods are currently in use worldwide. The older method is the Finn chamber, which employs an aluminum cup, 8 mm in diameter, fixed to a strip of Scanpor tape, a finely meshed paper tape with a polyacrylate adhesive. The allergens are applied to the cups, covering more than half the diameter of each cup, and fixed to the skin with Scanpor tape.

A newer method, the T.R.U.E. (thin layer rapid use epicutaneous) test, manufactured in Denmark, is a convenient, ready-to-use strip of tape on which a measured amount of allergen is incorporated in a thin hydrophilic gel film printed on a polyester patch measuring 9 × 9 mm. The patches contain 35 different allergens, are mounted on strips of acrylic tape protected by a plastic sheet, and are packaged in airtight envelopes. The thin sheet of plastic is removed, and the strips are placed on the skin. On contact with skin moisture, the dry film dissolves into the gel, and the allergen is released onto the skin. This method permits rapid application and avoids the hazard of mistakes in preparation of the application. The T.R.U.E. test system was not designed for occupational use and is now out of date in terms of current knowledge.

The upper back is the favored site for patch testing. Any hair must be removed using an electric rather than a safety razor to minimize damage to the keratin layer. The patches remain on the skin for 48 hours and then removed, and the sites are identified with a fluorescent-inked pen. Reading is done at 72 or 96 hours after application and occasionally at 1 week. When a fluorescent pen has been used to delineate the allergens, a hand-held black light will identify the sites. A single reading at 48 hours misses approximately 35% of positive results. Table 17–8 lists patch test interpretation codes.

Clinical interpretation is the most difficult aspect of patch testing. Irritant reactions show varied patterns such as fine wrinkling, erythematous follicular papules, petechiae, pustules, and sometimes large bullae. A classic positive patch test reaction consists of erythema, mild edema, and small, closely set vesicles.

Table 17–8. Patch test interpretation codes.

1	+	=	Weak reaction, nonvesicular, erythema, mild infiltration
2	+	=	Strong reaction, erythema, edema, vesicles
3	+	=	Extreme reaction, spreading, bullous, ulcerative
4		=	Doubtful, faint erythema only
5		=	Irritant reaction
6		=	Negative
7		=	Excited skin reaction
8		=	Not tested

Table 17–2 describes the allergens present in the T.R.U.E. test and additional allergens for detecting vehicle and preservative allergy. Table 17–9 lists other additional occupational series available for patch testing.

Adverse reactions can rarely occur. The most common are increased pigmentation at the site of a positive reaction, persistence of a reaction (especially with a positive reaction to gold), mild flare of the original dermatitis with brisk reactions, the development of psoriasis in a positive test site (rare), active sensitization (very rare), and anaphylactoid reactions (exceedingly rare).

Keep in mind that the test is a template of allergic contact sensitization developed over a person's lifetime. Therefore, clinical relevance of each positive reaction must be determined. This can be accomplished only with extensive knowledge of commercial and industrial materials and their ingredients. Information can be obtained from numerous

Table 17–9. Additional occupational series for patch testing.

Hairdressing
Bakery
Dental
Epoxy
Fragrance
Isocyanate
Oils and cooling fluid
Methacrylates: dental, nails, printers
Photographic chemicals
Plant
Plastics and glues
Rubber additives
Textile colors and finish

sources, including standard textbooks, manufacturers, and material safety data sheets. A review of the patient's clinical history, a workplace visit, chemical analysis of other allergens or cross-reacting substances, and further patch testing may be required.

▶ **Other Special Tests**

- Photopatch test
- Prick test
- Spot test, for example, nickel, epoxy resin, formaldehyde, isothiazolinone, etc.
- Provocative use test (PUT) or a repeat open application test (ROAT)

SPECIFIC TYPES OF ALLERGIC CONTACT DERMATITIS

Epoxy Resin Dermatitis

Epoxy resins are used commonly as adhesives and can be found in paints, cement, and electrical insulation. Most epoxy resins are based on diglycidyl ether of bisphenol A. Epichlorohydrin combined with bisphenol A produces an epoxy resin of varying molecular weights from 340 to larger polymers, which are less sensitizing.

However, there are other potential allergens, including pigments, fillers, reactive diluents, and solvents, that are mixed with a curing or hardening agent to polymerize the resin. Once hardened, the sensitizing potential is reduced.

Patch testing to epoxy resins must be thorough because there may be unknown compounds, and testing with the patient's own resins is essential. Irritant reactions and sensitization on patch testing may occur, particularly to the amine epoxy hardeners. Facial dermatitis may suggest allergy to hardener rather than to the epoxy resin itself, because the latter has low volatility. Detection of epoxy resin can be undertaken by a spot test with sulfuric acid or thin-layer chromatography.

Epoxy resin dermatitis can be prevented with exclusion or low concentrations of molecular weight 340 and 624 epoxy oligomers, high-molecular-weight (>1000) reactive diluents, and hardeners that exclude aliphatic amines.

Photoallergic Reactions

Photoallergic reactions are immunologically based. They are less common than phototoxic reactions and develop only in individuals previously sensitized by simultaneous exposure to a photosensitizing chemical and appropriate UV radiation. The biological process is similar to ACD, except that UV converts the chemical to a complete allergen. The radiation is usually in the UVA spectrum, although it may extend into the UVB.

Photoallergic reactions appear suddenly with an acute eczematous eruption, later becoming lichenoid and

Table 17–10. Causes of photoallergic reactions.

Halogenated salicylanilides
Tetrachlorosalicylanilide
3,4,5-tribromosalicylanilide
4,5-dibromosalicylanilide
Phenothiazines: Chlorpromazine, promethazine
Fragrances: Musk ambrette
Optical brighteners (stilbenes)
Sunscreens: PABA esters, benzophenone 3, butyl methoxydibenzoylmethane
Compositae plants

thickened, on the face, neck, dorsum of the hands, and exposed arms, often extending to other areas. The diagnosis is suggested by the distribution and character of the eruption, but confirmation requires careful questioning and photopatch testing. Sparing of skin under the chin and upper eyelids is strongly suggestive of a photo eruption. Table 17–10 lists some causes of photoallergic reaction.

Operational Definition of Occupational ACD

There are eight steps in the full assessment (or operational definition) of occupational ACD to be considered:

1. Relevant clinical history
2. Appropriate morphology
3. Positive diagnostic patch test with appropriate vehicle and concentration
4. Repeat patch test, when appropriate, to exclude "excited skin syndrome" and "angry back"
5. Perform serial dilution (when necessary)
6. Reviewing controls for non irritating concentrations and perform special test for uncommonly utilized allergens
7. Perform a PUT or ROAT
8. Clearing

The assessment begins with a comprehensive personal history, which includes dermatologic history of atopy or psoriasis, occupational history, and history of allergen exposure. A time relationship between exposure and onset of dermatitis should also be noted. Other factors required are a consistent morphology of ACD and positive diagnostic testing (patch testing) with appropriate vehicle and concentration. The diagnostic process is bidirectional; hence, patch test results will guide further questioning and investigation. Clinical relevance needs to be defined, with an allergen being clinically relevant if: (1) an exposure is established and (2) dermatitis occurred secondary to that exposure. This may sometimes require a PUT or ROAT with the suspected allergens.

Serial dilutions of the chemicals tested may be needed to confirm initial findings and suspicions. Control subject testing is essential to confirm nonirritating concentrations. Finally, clearing of the dermatitis once the allergen is removed or exposure is reduced significantly provides further information regarding the relevance of the allergen.

▶ Differential Diagnosis

- ICD
- Atopic dermatitis, psoriasis
- Pustular eruptions of the palms and soles (palmoplantar pustulosis)
- Herpes simplex and zoster
- Idiopathic vesicular reactions secondary to *Trichophyton* infections of the feet
- Dyshidrotic and nummular eczemas
- Drug eruptions

▶ Prevention Contact Dermatitis

In addition to the aforementioned treatment strategies, other measures to lower the incidence of CD in the workplace include

- Identification of potential irritants and allergens in the workplace
- Chemical substitution or removal to prevent recurrence
- Personal protective measures
- Personal and environmental hygiene
- Education to promote awareness of potential irritants and allergens both at work and at home
- Preemployment and periodic health screening and
- Engineering controls with automated, closed systems

▶ Treatment of Contact Dermatitis

Treatment of CD depends on the stage of the disease. Acute vesicular eruptions are treated with wet dressings for the first 24–36 hours using Burow's solution or potassium permanganate $KMNO_4$ solutions, followed by a topical corticosteroid; only the most potent topical corticoids (classes 1 and 2) are effective in the acute phase. In addition, based on current evidence, cold compresses have been shown to decrease inflammation in CD.

A. Corticosteroids

When the eruption begins to dry, corticosteroid creams can be used, accompanied by oral sedating antihistamines for itching. Oral antibiotic therapy is indicated only when secondary infection is suspected. Topical antibiotic and antihistamine preparations should be avoided, however, because of risk of sensitization. High-potency topical corticosteroids decrease mild to moderate, but not severe, ACD. Topical corticosteroids are possibly not significantly effective with some irritants such as sodium lauryl sulphate. There are no controlled studies, but oral corticosteroids are effective in severe ACD.

B. Skin Cleaners

These should be readily available and designed for the use intended, for example, heavy-duty cleansers for mechanics and others working with grease and oils and mild bar or liquid soaps for workers in less dirty occupations. Industrial cleansers often contain harsh abrasives and potentially allergenic antibacterial agents.

Waterless hand cleaners remove industrial dirt without water and can be of value in work sites without convenient washing facilities. Most are based on relatively nonirritating detergents and are removed from the skin with towels, waste papers, or rags. When used repeatedly, rags may contain a large number of irritants from the work site.

C. Protective Clothing and Gloves

Protective clothing is available for most work situations and exposures. It must be selected with specific consideration of the type of work and exposure and must be inspected regularly for holes and tears. Remember that certain allergens, such as methyl and ethyl methacrylate, glyceryl monothioglycolate, and paraphenylenediamine, pass readily through many rubber gloves. Workers may wear gloves to protect an active dermatitis, but the occlusion can aggravate an existing eruption, and contact with rubber can lead to allergic sensitization to ingredients of the gloves.

D. Barrier Creams

Barrier creams are popularly termed "invisible gloves." Although the benefit of this physical barrier to penetration is debated widely, barrier creams have reduced ACD and ICD in both experimental and clinical studies. Barrier creams should be applied to intact skin only and prior to contact with irritants, including application after breaks. High frequency of application with adequate amounts is essential. Barrier creams may induce ICD or ACD caused by various preservatives, lanolin, and fragrances. Workers should not become lax in other protective measures because of this "invisible glove" provides a sense of false security.

E. Emollients

Emollients and moisturizers are designed to increase the water content of the skin and can be used on irritated skin. They play an important role in treating and preventing ICD, but further assessment is required in both animal and human models in the workplace.

Regular prophylactic skin cream application is widely acknowledged to be an effective prevention strategy against occupational CD. However, compliance and prevention remain low. To address low compliance rates, Hines and associates proposed three moments for skin cream application in the work place to drive down rates of occupational ICD. These are (1) before starting the work period, (2) after washing hands during work, and (3) after work. Combining these recommendations with implementation strategies from principles of organizational change management may prove useful.

▶ Complications of Contact Dermatitis

A. Disease Complications

- Lichen simplex chronicus
- Contractures, for example, severe hydrofluoric acid burns
- Loss of job/income
- Career change
- Psychosocial problems

B. Treatment Complications

- Topical corticosteroids
- Atrophy
- Hypopigmentation
- Systemic corticosteroids

May cause several side effects such as acne, osteoporosis, weight gain, hypertension, etc. Bone protection measures such as intake of bisphosphonates is recommended in any patients especially elderly taking corticoids for more than 2 months.

Also, prolonged use absorption of topical corticoids may result in systemic effects.

Other systemic medications: Cyclosporine, azathioprine, mycophenolate mofetil, and methotrexate may cause wide range of side effects and need to be closely monitored.

▶ Prognosis

ACD may wax and wane despite treatment especially if the allergens are not identified or the skin protective measures are not strictly adhered to. ACD to chromium (less common than ICD) appears to be persistent in the affected individuals despite appropriate treatment and rigorous skin protection. Lichen simplex chronicus is sequelae of repeated scratching in the affected body parts. Unchanged work practices, age more than 45 years, food-related occupations, respiratory atopy, and male sex are considered to be the risk factors for continuing occupational CD. Discontinuation of the causative agents' exposure leads to clinical improvement and healing. A change in work activities, modification of work environment, and the presence of easily avoidable work-related allergies are associated with a good prognosis.

CONTACT URTICARIA

▶ General Considerations

Contact urticaria develops within minutes to an hour following contact with a substance. Interest in and knowledge of this reaction have increased greatly during the past 25 years, particularly with natural rubber latex allergy.

▶ Types

A. Nonimmunologic (Nonallergic) Contact Urticaria

With sufficient provocation, nearly all exposed individuals will develop a reaction. Previous sensitization is not necessary. Gardeners may develop reactions from contact with nettles and other plants, caterpillar hair, moths, and other insects; cooks from cinnamic acid and aldehyde, sodium benzoate, sorbic acid, fruits, vegetables, fish, and meat; and medical personnel from alcohols, balsam of Peru, and DMSO.

B. Immunologic (Allergic) Contact Urticaria

Immunologic (allergic) contact urticaria is caused most commonly by latex in natural rubber, especially gloves, which is a problem for medical and dental personnel, kitchen and dairy workers, pharmacists, semiconductor workers, and others who must wear gloves throughout the workday. The reactions range from mild erythema with itching at the site of contact to severe anaphylactic reactions, sometimes resulting in death. They are immunoglobulin E (IgE)–mediated type I immediate hypersensitivity reactions and appear to be more common in atopics. The cause is natural latex from the sap of the tree *Hevea brasiliensis*, a *cis*-1,4-polyisoprene, the precursor of the rubber molecule. It is estimated that there are 50 or 60 different proteins in latex that provoke the allergic response.

▶ Clinical Findings

Signs and symptoms:

- Onset within minutes of contact and when mild, disappear without treatment within 2–3 hours
- Itching
- Redness
- Wheal-and-flare reaction

Severe reactions progress rapidly and include generalized urticaria, swelling of the face and lips, asthma, collapse, and death.

Natural rubber latex gloves most commonly cause these reactions, but condoms, urinary catheters, elastic bandages, adhesive tapes, wound drains, dental dams, hemodialysis equipment, balloons, pacifiers, barium enema tips, and many other latex-based rubber products are implicated. Cross-reactions can occur to foods such as avocados, water chestnuts, kiwi, papaya, and bananas, provoking reactions in sensitive persons.

Dermatographism, a common form of urticaria, occurs when the skin becomes raised and inflamed when stroked, scratched, or rubbed. Airborne contamination by rubber glove powder also may induce symptoms in very sensitive patients.

A. Prick and Open Testing

Open testing on intact skin and skin prick testing are the most common diagnostic methods for this condition. A standardized test material should be used, and testing should be performed only if resuscitation measures are readily available. "Use tests" with a glove or a single finger of a glove should be performed with special care in patients who have a history of anaphylaxis or when the results of skin prick test or the latex radioallergosorbent test (RAST; Pharmacia, Sweden) are positive. Note that the RAST is only 60–65% sensitive.

The Food and Drug Administration (FDA) prohibits the labeling of latex-containing medical products as "hypoallergenic" and requires the statement: "This product contains natural rubber latex" on all latex-containing products that are directly or indirectly in contact with the body.

▶ Differential Diagnosis

- Acquired angioedema
- ACD
- ICD
- Other forms of urticaria: cholinergic, pressure, vasculitic, and solar

▶ Prognosis

The long-term prognosis is generally good if proper precautions are taken and by avoiding the causative and precipitating factors. These can be achieved through continuous education of the individuals and organizations involved.

Generally, fewer compounds produce immune mediated contact urticaria compared to the non immune mediated type. In an occupational setting, if these compounds are not rigorously sought early, it may lead to eczematous skin changes resulting from the ACD. This in turn may cause debilitating chronic hand dermatitis. It is advisable to perform extensive patch testing as the allergen(s) may be missed using the standard battery.

Extracutaneous manifestations of contact urticaria include rhinitis, conjunctivitis, dyspnea, and anaphylaxis.

OCCUPATIONAL ACNE

Oil Acne (Folliculitis)

Oil acne, or oil folliculitis, is a common condition resulting from heavy exposure to oil, especially under oil-soaked clothing. The arms and thighs usually are affected with numerous, often black comedones, pustules, furuncles, and sometimes carbuncles. This condition was once very common, especially in oil fields and refineries, but with improved engineering and less heavy contact with oils, it is seen much less often today. Many cases are never reported because most workers know that with better hygiene the condition improves. The most common sources are insoluble cutting oils in machinists and greases and lubricating oils in mechanics. Melanosis and photosensitivity also occur. Workers handling heavy tar distillates and coal tar pitch, roofers, oil well drillers, coke oven workers, petroleum refiners, rubber workers, textile mill workers, and road pavers are affected commonly.

Another form of environmental acne is acne cosmetica, occurring in actors and cosmetologists. Acne mechanica secondary to local pressure, friction, rubbing, squeezing, and stretching can occur in the wearers of heavy clothing and helmets. Tropical acne is common in hot, moist climates. During World War II, thousands of military personnel were evacuated from the South Pacific because of this condition. The so-called McDonald acne results from contact with the grease and fat of frying hamburgers (see Table 17–4). Nonoccupational sources of environmental acne also should be considered, including acne from medications such as corticosteroids, testosterone, progesterone, isoniazid, iodides, and bromides.

Treatment of oil folliculitis consists of oil-impervious aprons and environmental measures to limit exposure. Gloves usually cannot be worn by machinists and mechanics because of the danger of catching them in the machinery. Modernization of cutting machines with automation and special guards decreases skin contact.

Chloracne

Chloracne is a rare condition with multiple closed comedones and pale-yellow cysts on the skin from cutaneous and systemic exposure to certain halogenated chemicals (see Table 17–5). Body areas affected are the cheeks, forehead, and neck. The shoulders, chest, back, buttocks, and abdomen also may be involved. The genitalia are especially affected, whereas the nose often is spared, except in systemic exposure. In addition, there may be hypertrichosis, hyperpigmentation, and increased skin fragility suggesting porphyria cutanea tarda. Conjunctivitis, swelling, and discharge from swollen meibomian glands of the eyelids can be seen, as well as a brownish pigmentation of the nails. Peripheral neuritis and hepatotoxicity may occur, suggesting systemic toxicity.

Although treatment of chloracne is often unsatisfactory, oral antibiotics, oral isotretinoin, acne surgery, and occasionally dermabrasion may be helpful. The majority of cases clear within 1–2 years following cessation of exposure.

OCCUPATIONAL SKIN CANCER

Approximately 400,000 new cases of nonmelanoma skin cancer occur in the United States each year, comprising approximately 30–40% of all cancers reported annually. Malignant melanoma accounts for another 18,000 cases. The exact number of skin cancers induced by the workplace is disputed, but most observers agree that it is a significant proportion. The most common causes of skin cancers in the work environment are UV light, polycyclic aromatic hydrocarbons, arsenic, ionizing radiation, and trauma.

Ultraviolet Light

Sunlight is the most common cause of skin cancer, but workers seldom consider sunlight from the workplace as contributing to their actinically damaged skin and skin cancer. The most common skin cancers are squamous cell and basal cell carcinomas. These are related to prolonged exposure to sunlight but also may be initiated by tar and oils, mechanical trauma, and burns. The primary carcinogenic action spectrum of sunlight is in the UVB range (290–320 nm), but UVC (100–290 nm) and UVA (320–400 nm) rays also are photocarcinogenic. UVA rays accelerate UVB-induced malignancy, and even though UVC rays are not present in sunlight, there is exposure from welding arcs and germicidal lamps.

The evidence for the skin carcinogenicity of UVB and UVA is overwhelming. Such cancers occur much more frequently in outdoor workers and in persons with fair skin and light hair and eye color and in those who tan poorly and burn easily. In fact, there is a specific compensation scheme in the United Kingdom for war veterans who served in tropical countries and later developed skin cancers. Other professionals who are at risk of developing skin cancers as a result of chronic sun exposure include builders, farmers, horticulturists, etc. In addition to the time spent in sunlight, the UV radiation received by an outdoor worker depends on the latitude, season, time of day, altitude, and weather.

The exposure of UVB and UVA is not only limited to natural sunshine but also includes man-made sources like tanning beds. In fact, artificial tanning even raises the risk of melanoma, the deadliest skin cancer. With such alarming data, several nations have passed strong antitanning legislation. In 2009, Brazil imposed a total ban of tanning devices for cosmetic purposes for the entire population. In 2012, New South Wales (Australia) projected a total ban by 2014. France, Germany, Austria, and the United Kingdom banned under-18 indoor tanning, and South Australia banned artificial tanning for those younger than 18 and for anyone with type I skin.

Other artificial sources of carcinogenic UV radiation include welding arcs; germicidal lamps; devices for curing and drying printing ink, plastics, and paint; UV lasers; mercury vapor lamps; and medical UV therapy machines. Radiometers are available that can measure the amount of UV radiation a worker is receiving.

Epidemiologic studies in countries where there is a large blond, fair-skinned population, as in Australia, show a higher incidence of melanomas of the head, face, and neck in outdoor workers, which contrasts with office workers, who have melanomas more commonly on the covered parts of the trunk and limbs. Lentigo maligna is almost always present on exposed, sun-damaged skin and becomes invasive after a variable period of time. Persons with xeroderma pigmentosa, a hereditary disease, are extremely sensitive to the carcinogenic effects of sunlight. A frequent cause of death in these individuals is malignant melanoma, often occurring at a young age.

Polycyclic Aromatic Hydrocarbons

For 250 years, coal tar products and certain petroleum oils were considered potential causes of cutaneous cancers in individuals who work in certain industries. In the twentieth century, the relationship became firmly established not only from experimental animal studies but also from numerous epidemiologic surveys. Polycyclic aromatic hydrocarbons, such as those found in soot and carbon black, coal tar, pitch and tarry products, creosote oil, and certain oils, account for the majority of cutaneous tumors. Photosensitization develops initially, with recurring erythema and intense burning of the exposed skin. After repeated episodes, poikilodermatous changes appear, especially on the exposed skin of the face, neck, and hands. Keratotic papillomas (tar warts) then develop, which later may become squamous cell carcinomas, basal cell carcinomas, and keratoacanthomas. Polycyclic aromatic hydrocarbons and UVB appear to act synergistically to induce malignant change.

Arsenic

Since the late 1940s, epidemiologic studies have strongly linked inorganic arsenic exposure to squamous cell cancers of skin and lungs. Arsenic keratoses, characteristic of chronic arsenicalism, are multiple yellow, punctate keratoses distributed symmetrically on the palms and soles. Squamous cell carcinomas and multiple lesions of intraepidermal squamous cell carcinoma (Bowen disease) may develop from these keratoses. Basal cell carcinomas also occur from arsenic exposure, and they are often multiple, superficial, and pigmented.

Occupational arsenic exposure occurs in ceramic enamel workers, copper smelters, fireworks makers, gold refiners, hide preservers, carpenters (removing old wallpaper), semiconductor workers, and taxidermists. Arsenic is rarely used as an insecticide today but is still employed as a rodenticide.

OTHER CAUSES OF OCCUPATIONAL SKIN DISORDERS

Biological Causes

▶ Bacterial Diseases

A. Staphylococcal and Streptococcal Infections

Infection of minor lacerations, abrasions, burns, and puncture wounds accounts for most staphylococcal and streptococcal infections. A work relationship is not always easy to establish, however, and many cases are unreported. Nevertheless, these infections are common in certain occupations, especially agricultural and construction workers, butchers, meat packers, and slaughterhouse workers. The history should clarify whether a work relationship is likely, although frequently in workers' compensation cases the patient's statements must be accepted as valid.

Furunculosis is common among automobile and truck repair persons, especially in dirty jobs, such as tire repair.

Paronychia may be seen in occupations such as nurses, hairdressers, and manicurists.

Atopic dermatitis patients are especially likely to experience skin colonization with staphylococci. In a high percentage of atopics, *Staphylococcus aureus* can be cultured from their eczematous skin, which often has been made worse by heavy and prolonged application of corticosteroid creams and ointments. Prophylactic oral antibiotics should be part of the long-term treatment of these patients. Employment of persons with active atopic dermatitis in food service industries and hospital patient care may need to be restricted.

B. Cutaneous Mycobacterial Infections

A classic example of tuberculosis of the skin acquired through inoculation of *Mycobacterium tuberculosis hominis* is seen in pathologists (*prosector's wart*) and morgue attendants (*necrogenic wart* or *anatomic tubercle*). Surgeons are also at risk for such granulomatous infections. Veterinarians, farmers, and butchers may acquire infection with *M tuberculosis* var. *bovis,* which at one time was a common cause of disease in livestock in the United States, but bovine tuberculosis has declined since the mid-1930s. In some countries, however, the disease is still common. In the United States and other parts of the world, as a result of population movement and the increasing prevalence of human immunodeficiency virus (HIV) infection, the incidence of infection with human strains of tuberculosis has increased greatly. Between 1985 and 1991, 39,000 more cases occurred in the United States than expected, and drug resistance, especially in those with HIV infection, has seriously compounded the problem.

The typical skin lesions are slowly progressive, warty, hyperkeratotic plaques, which, if left untreated, eventually regress after many months or years, leaving disfiguring scars. Demonstration of organisms either directly or from cultures is often difficult.

C. Atypical Mycobacterial Infections

Atypical mycobacterial infections are caused most commonly by infection with *M marinum*. This infection usually is acquired from exposure to infected fish, especially in aquariums and fish tanks by persons who clean these tanks. Swimming pools have become contaminated with this organism, and pool attendants and cleaners are also at risk. Treatment with rifampicin or ethambutol is usually effective.

As in other mycobacterial skin infections, the clinical picture consists of granulomatous papules and nodules that ulcerate and exude a clear, thin serum. Sometimes a pattern resembling sporotrichosis develops, with nodules and papules ascending the arm (or leg) along the course of regional lymphatics. Persons with AIDS are at special risk for developing these infections. Other atypical mycobacteria include *M ulcerans, M fortuitum, M avium, M intracellulare, M kansasii,* and *M chelonae.*

▶ Viral Diseases

A. Herpes Simplex

Herpes simplex is the most frequent viral infection of occupational origin, affecting dentists and dental assistants, physicians and nurses, and respiratory technicians. This is caused by the herpes simplex virus (HSV). Transmission is by contaminated saliva or pharyngeal or laryngotracheal secretions. Wearing disposable gloves, masks, and safety glasses reduces the risk of infection in these workers.

B. Viral Warts

Meat handlers, especially butchers and slaughterhouse workers, are at greatest risk for development of the common wart, caused by the human papilloma virus (HPV), of which there are at least 35 types. These warts are most numerous on the hands and fingers of these workers, and minor cuts and abrasions inoculate the virus. Molluscum contagiosum occurs in wrestlers, boxers, and other sportsmen.

C. Orf

Endemic in sheep and goats, orf is caused by infection with a parapoxvirus, usually involving the mouth and nose of infected animals. Mostly farmers and veterinarians are affected with this relatively mild, self-limited disease. Only one or two lesions may be present, almost always on fingers, and are associated with mild fever, lymphangitis, and regional lymphadenopathy. An erythema multiforme–like rash occurs 10–14 days after onset. Treatment is symptomatic, with antibiotics given only for complications such as secondary infection.

▶ Fungal Infections

A. *Candida*

Infection with *Candida*, mainly *Candida albicans*, is the most common occupationally related fungal disease. The organism is ubiquitous, and proliferation is favored by moisture, occlusion, and irritation. Most occupationally acquired candidal infections are on the hands, especially in the paronychial areas and interdigital spaces. Occupations in which prolonged wearing of rubber gloves is required, such as dentistry, medicine, and technical work in clean rooms in the semiconductor industry, show the highest incidence of this condition. Diabetics and neutropenic, immunocompromised patients are especially at risk.

B. Dermatophytes

Dermatophytic infections are common. *Trichophyton verrucosum* is an animal fungus that readily infects farmers and cattle tenders. The lesions are often quite inflammatory and may resemble pyoderma. Farmers, milkers, cattle tenders, veterinarians, and tannery workers, especially hide sorters, are at risk. *T rubrum* and *T mentagrophytes* are examples of fungi that cause tinea infections in the general population, especially tinea manuum and tinea pedis. *Microsporum canis* frequently infects small animals and causes infection in pet shop workers, veterinarians, and personnel in contact with laboratory animals. *M gypseum* is a rare fungus found in soil, causing occasional infection in agricultural workers.

Physicians are often requested to decide whether a *Trichophyton* infection is work-related, especially *T rubrum* and *T mentagrophytes* infections of the hands and nails. Onychomycosis is extremely common, and most of those affected do not seek medical attention. Workers engaged in repetitive hand activities, especially where there is sweating and pressure or repetitive nail trauma in the case of onychomycosis, may believe their work to be the primary cause of the infection. Each case must be studied individually, but most often the work cannot be considered a primary cause.

▶ Parasitic Diseases

A. Protozoa

1. Cutaneous leishmaniasis—Most parasitic diseases, such as amoebiasis, giardiasis, and malaria, present with general rather than cutaneous health problems. An exception is cutaneous leishmaniasis, caused by *Leishmania tropica* (Oriental sore, bouton d'orient) found in the Middle East, and *L braziliensis* (American leishmaniasis, uta) found in Central and South America. The disease is transmitted by sandflies that thrive in warm climates and is endemic in persons working in tropical forests in southeastern Mexico, Colombia, and Venezuela. The disease manifests as cutaneous ulcers with metastatic mucocutaneous lesions known as *espundia*. Pentavalent antimonials, such as sodium stibogluconate, are the treatment of choice. Pentamidine and liposomal or conventional amphotericin are alternatives.

2. Helminths—Penetration of the cercariae of schistosomes into the papillary dermis induces a highly pruritic papular eruption termed *swimmer's itch*. Urticaria may accompany the rash and be widespread. Migratory birds usually are the definitive hosts, with saltwater molluscs serving as intermediate hosts. The condition lasts for 2–3 weeks, often with secondary infection of excoriated lesions. Skin divers, lifeguards, dock workers, and workers who maintain lakes and ponds may be affected. Treatment is symptomatic.

Larva migrans (creeping eruption) occurs in subtropical and tropical regions where people work on moist soil infected with hookworm larvae. Dogs, cats, cattle, and human feces carry the larvae, and humans are the final host. A threadlike, red or flesh-colored, circuitous, slightly raised line occurs often on the feet, legs, back, or buttocks caused by movement of the larva in the epidermis. Humans are infected with the larvae of *Ancylostoma braziliense* and *Necator americanus*, the ova of which are deposited in the soil. Topical application of 10% suspension of thiabendazole to affected areas four times daily for 7–10 days is usually curative. Agricultural workers, lifeguards, shoreline fishermen, ditch diggers, and sewer workers are at greatest risk.

Other nematode diseases that are occasionally occupational include trichinosis, dracunculosis, filariasis, loiasis, enterobiasis, strongyloidiasis, and toxocariasis.

3. Scabies—Epidemics of scabies have occurred in nursing homes, hospitals, and residential facilities for the aged. The disease is highly contagious and spreads rapidly, especially in the immunosuppressed. It is often initiated by an infected employee who transmits the mite to patients. They then spread the disease to other personnel. The scabicide of choice is permethrin, but treatment of the more severe types of scabies (eg, crusted scabies) can be difficult and may require repeated treatments with other scabicides such as lindane, permethrin, precipitated sulfur, and oral ivermectin.

4. Lyme disease—Lyme disease is an important inflammatory disease that follows tick-induced erythema chronicum migrans (ECM) weeks or months after inoculation. ECM begins with a small erythematous macule, usually on an extremity, that enlarges with central clearing. The lesion sometimes reaches a diameter of 50 cm, and smaller satellite lesions often are present. In nearly half the patients, a type of arthritis occurs within weeks or months of the ECM, and there may be associated neurologic abnormalities, as well as myocardial conduction alterations, serum cryoprecipitates, elevated serum immunoglobulin M (IgM) levels, and an increased sedimentation rate. Elevated serum IgM and later IgG appear within weeks of infection with circulating cryoprecipitates and other immune complexes. ECM is an important diagnostic marker for this disease. The ticks *Ixodes dammini, I pacificus* (in the United States), and *I ricinus* (in Europe) transmit the spirochete *Borrelia burgdorferi* that is responsible for the disease. In some cases, localized scleroderma appears to be linked to *Borrelia* infection. Tick bites are common in outdoor workers, loggers, wilderness construction workers, guides, and ranchers. Other major tick-borne diseases in the United States are relapsing fever, tularemia, Rocky Mountain spotted fever, ehrlichiosis, Colorado tick fever, babesiosis, and tick paralysis.

Physical Causes

▶ Mechanical Trauma

Intermittent friction of low intensity will induce lichenification (thickening) of the skin. With greater pressure, corns and calluses appear. After minor trauma, calluses frequently develop painful fissures, which may become infected. After years of repeated frictional hand trauma during work, permanent calluses may result, leading to disability and early retirement. With increasing automation, less frequent manual operation of tools, and better protective clothing, occupational marks are less frequent and have almost disappeared from many industries.

▶ Heat

A. Burns

Burns arising from the occupation are common and exhibit characteristic occupational patterns. The resulting scarring and pigmentary changes are of chief concern to dermatologists, who rarely treat acute burns. Hypopigmentation is especially susceptible to actinic damage, and scars and the hyperpigmentation often are disfiguring.

B. Miliaria

Miliaria is caused by sweat retention and often is seen in the work environment. The eruption can be extensive, accompanied by burning and itching. The most superficial form, miliaria crystallina, is caused by poral closure and rupture of the ducts within the upper level of the epidermis. The condition commonly occurs on the palms and in intertriginous areas, with asymptomatic desquamation of the surface. When the closure occurs deeper in the epidermis, vesiculation with marked pruritus results. Miliaria rubra, or prickly heat, is the type most likely to be confused with CD. If poral obstruction extends deeper in the epidermis and into the upper dermis, the condition is known as *miliaria profunda,* resulting in deep-seated, asymptomatic vesicles. This condition is caused by prolonged exposure to a hot environment and often follows an extended period of miliaria rubra. Heat exhaustion and collapse may be sequelae.

C. Intertrigo

A macerated, erythematous eruption in body folds, intertrigo results from excessive sweating, especially in obese workers. Secondary bacterial and candidal infections are common. The interdigital space between the third and fourth fingers is a common site in workers whose hands are continuously wet, especially from rubber gloves. Medical and dental personnel, bartenders, cannery workers, cooks, swimming instructors, and housekeepers are especially predisposed to this condition.

Overheating, especially in conjunction with physical exercise, may result in heat-induced urticaria and, rarely, in anaphylaxis. Acne vulgaris and rosacea are aggravated by prolonged exposure to heat, especially from ovens, steam, open furnaces, and heat torches. Herpes simplex may be triggered by intense heat, especially with sunburn and UVB exposure.

▶ Cold

A. Chilblains (Perniosis)

This mild form of cold injury, although an abnormal reaction to cold, is less common in very cold climates where homes are usually well heated and warm clothing is worn. The northern United States and Europe are areas where this condition is seen frequently. The lesions are reddish blue, swollen, boggy discolorations with bullae and ulcerations. The fingers, toes, heels, lower legs, nose, and ears are especially affected. Genetic factors with vasomotor instability often are found to be important background features. Treatment is symptomatic with calcium channel blockers such as nifedipine.

▶ Vibration Syndrome

Vibrations of handheld tools and Raynaud phenomenon have been known to be associated since the early twentieth century.

Popular names include *dead fingers* and *white fingers*; clinically, the condition is a type of Raynaud phenomenon. Operation of heavy vibrating tools such as jackhammers, especially in cold weather, produces vasospasm of the digital arteries, causing episodic pallor, cyanosis, and erythema of the fingers. Chain saws, handheld grinders, riveting hammers, and other pneumatic tools also are associated with this condition. Tingling and numbness, blanching of the tips of one or more fingers, and clumsiness of the fingers and hands occur. The symptoms may be indistinguishable from other forms of Raynaud phenomenon, but asymmetry usually is observed. Occupational disability seldom results and most workers continue at their jobs. Vibration frequencies between 30 and 300 Hz are most likely to be responsible.

▶ Ionizing Radiation

Numerous industrial processes use ionizing radiation, including the curing of plastics, sterilization of food and drugs, testing of metals and other materials, medical and dental radiography, therapy with radioisotopes, and operation of high-powered electronic equipment. Exposure is much less now than it was several decades ago mainly as a consequence of better construction and shielding of the radiographic equipment. Measurements of radiation emissions from video display terminals have consistently shown nondetectable or background levels.

Occupational exposure to ionizing radiation may be acute or chronic and usually is localized. Acute radiodermatitis often results from a single accidental exposure to around 1000 R and presents with rapid onset of erythema, edema, and blanching of the skin, reaching a peak at about 48 hours. Anorexia, nausea, vomiting, and other systemic symptoms also occur. There follows a latent period of apparent recovery lasting a few days, after which the skin again becomes erythematous, with purplish ecchymotic areas that become vesicular and bullous. Pain is intense, usually requiring narcotics. A repair stage follows, and as reepithelialization takes place, the skin becomes atrophic, hairless, and lacks functioning sebaceous glands. With large single doses, ulceration usually follows but often is delayed for 2–3 months. Healing is very slow, and an atrophic, disfiguring scar is left.

Chronic radiodermatitis results from exposures to smaller doses of ionizing radiation (300–800 R) received daily or weekly over a long period of time to a total dose of 5000–6000 R. The skin becomes red and eczematous with burning and hyperesthesia. Often the epidermis sloughs, and regrowth occurs slowly over a period of 4–6 weeks. Hair is also lost, often permanently, and the sebaceous glands cease activity. The skin becomes hypopigmented and atrophic with multiple telangiectasias.

REFERENCES

Elmas ÖF, Akdeniz N, Atasoy M, Karadag AS.Clin. Contact dermatitis: A great imitator. Dermatol. 2020 Mar-Apr;38(2):176-192. PMID: 32513398 Review.

Holness DL: Occupational dermatosis. Curr Allergy Asthma Rep 2019;19(9):42 [PMID: 31352594].

Lampel HP, Powell HB: Occupational and hand dermatitis: a practical approach. Clin Rev Allergy Immunol 2019;56(1):60-71 [PMID: 30171459].

Nassau S, Fonacier L. Allergic Contact Dermatitis. Med Clin North Am. 2020 Jan;104(1):61-76. PMID: 31757238.

Pacheco KA: Occupational dermatitis: how to identify the exposures, make the diagnosis, and treat the disease. Ann Allergy Asthma Immunol 2018;120(6):583-591 [PMID: 29698693].

Papadatou Z, Williams H, Cooper K: Effectiveness of interventions for preventing occupational irritant hand dermatitis: a quantitative systematic review. JBI Database Syst Rev Implement Rep 2018;16(6):1398-1417 [PMID: 29894409].

■ SELF-ASSESSMENT QUESTIONS

Select the one correct answer for each question.

Question 1: Irritant contact dermatitis (ICD)
  a. accounts for nearly 80% of all occupational dermatitis
  b. is caused by a single chemical
  c. is unrelated to environmental factors
  d. is not affected by ethnicity

Question 2: ICD
  a. is an immunogenic skin reaction to toxic substances
  b. is caused by a limited number of substances
  c. has no predisposing factors
  d. is caused by skin exposure to irritating toxic substances

Question 3: Phototoxic (Photoirritation) reactions
  a. may result from exposure to natural or artificial light alone
  b. can be caused by numerous systemic drugs
  c. is unrelated to the dose or concentration of phototoxic substance
  d. may be followed by loss of pigmentation

Question 4: Occupational leukoderma
  a. results in hyperpigmentation
  b. occurs without inflammation
  c. usually involves the hands and forearms
  d. remains localized

Question 5: Allergic contact dermatitis (ACD)
a. is controlled by ordinary protective measures
b. seldom requires job change
c. does not prevent immediate return to work
d. is an immunologic reaction classified as a delayed type IV

Question 6: ACD
a. is less severe when following reexposure to the allergen
b. can evolve into subacute but not chronic stages
c. produces considerable variation in the intensity of reaction depending on the body area affected
d. usually affects the mucous membranes

Question 7: ACD
a. sensitization requires at least 4 days to develop
b. eventually affects all workers exposed to allergens
c. is unrelated to irritant dermatitis
d. is unrelated to epoxy resins, biocides, chromate, and formaldehyde

Question 8: Patch testing
a. is the key to diagnosis of ACD
b. allows the use of a large concentration of test substance
c. tests a more resistant organ than that affected by the disease
d. tests a different mechanism than that which causes the disease

Question 9: Photoallergic reactions
a. are more common than phototoxic reactions
b. are immunologically based
c. appear slowly with an acute eczematous eruption
d. appear only on the face, neck, and dorsum of the hands

Question 10: Nonimmunologic (nonallergic) contact urticaria
a. affects only a few exposed individuals
b. requires no previous sensitization
c. spares gardeners
d. spares cooks and other food handlers

Question 11: Immunologic (allergic) contact urticaria
a. is caused most commonly by latex in natural rubber, but not rubber gloves
b. is limited to mild erythema with itching at the site of contact

c. reactions are IgE-mediated type I
d. is less common in atopics

Question 12: Chloracne
a. is a common occupational skin disorder
b. especially affects the nose
c. spares the conjunctivae
d. may lead to peripheral neuritis and hepatotoxicity, suggesting systemic toxicity

Question 13: Atopic dermatitis
a. protects workers from skin colonization with staphylococci
b. produces immunity through development of eczematous skin
c. requires prophylactic oral antibiotics
d. may restrict employment in food service industries and hospital patient care

Question 14: Atypical mycobacterial infections
a. are caused most commonly by infection with *Mycobacterium chelonae*
b. are acquired from exposure to infected fowl
c. are usually effectively treated with rifampicin or ethambutol
d. are not predisposed in persons with AIDS

Question 15: In the management of contact dermatitis (CD)
a. avoidance and protective measures remain the best approach
b. highly potent steroids are always required
c. water-based cleaners are recommended as skin cleansers
d. alcohol-based cleaners are recommended as skin cleansers

Question 16: Prevention of occupational skin disorders
a. is not necessary because the long-term outcome is always the same once exposure has occurred
b. should be limited to the affected employees to prevent stigmatization
c. requires close cooperation between the employee, employers, company physicians, dermatologists, and other relevant stakeholders such as workers unions
d. does not involve giving employees information on the involved chemical substances

Upper Respiratory Tract Disorders

Dennis J. Shusterman, MD, MPH

The upper airway contributes to respiratory function by providing air conditioning, filtering, and sensory monitoring of the ambient environment. These same structures are vulnerable to the effects of inhaled irritants and allergens. A growing body of evidence links the development of rhinitis with that of asthma, making the prevention (and early recognition) of upper airway inflammation a priority.

FUNCTIONAL ANATOMY OF THE UPPER AIRWAY

Anatomy of the Upper Airway

The upper airway extends from the nares to the larynx (Figure 18–1). The surface area of the upper airway is increased by the presence of the nasal turbinates, which enhance the nose's air conditioning and filtering ability. The anterior nasal cavity is lined with a squamous epithelium; posterior to the tip of the inferior turbinate, it transitions to a ciliated epithelium, complete with secretory cells, submucous glands, and venous capacitance vessels. The nasal vasculature responds to a variety of humoral and neural factors which, by changing the nasal mucosal thickness, affect upper airway patency. These stimuli also affect glandular secretion, giving rise to the two main symptoms associated with nasal disease: rhinorrhea and airflow obstruction. An area at the superior margin of each nasal cavity is dedicated to the olfactory (cranial nerve I) neuroepithelium, the only portion of the central nervous system (CNS) exposed directly to the environment, and the only portion of the CNS which continuously regenerates throughout one's lifespan. The entire nasal and oral cavities (as well as the cornea and conjunctivae) are also innervated by the trigeminal nerve (cranial nerve V), which gives rise to sensations of temperature, mechanical stimulation, and chemical irritation (Figure 18–2).

Functions of the Upper Airway

The upper respiratory tract performs several essential physiologic functions. These include air conditioning, filtering,

microbial defense, sensation, and phonation (Table 18–1). During the fraction of a second that inspired air travels through the upper airway, its temperature is adjusted to near body temperature, and its relative humidity regulated between 75% and 80%. These physical alterations to inspired air help minimize thermal and osmotic stresses on the tracheobronchial tree. The major fraction of particulate matter larger than 1 μm in diameter is deposited in the upper airway (Figure 18–3). The majority of impacted material—captured in the mucous blanket—is transported posteriorly via ciliary action until it empties into the nasopharynx and then is swallowed (a smaller fraction being transported anteriorly to the nasal vestibule). The high surface area of the turbinates and the high water content of nasal mucus further provide a "scrubbing" mechanism for water-soluble air pollutants (Figure 18–4). Thus, depending on the concentration and duration of exposure, water-soluble gases and vapors may have their initial (or principal) irritative effect on the mucous membranes of the nose, throat, and eye.

The sensory functions of the upper airway are twofold: olfaction and irritant perception. Odor perception, mediated by the olfactory nerve, contributes to quality of life—allowing one to appreciate fragrances, as well as augmenting the primary tastes in the appreciation of food. In addition, olfaction has a safety function. Individuals lacking odor perception (anosmics) cannot distinguish fresh from spoiled food, tell that a gas pilot light has gone out in their kitchen, or sense that a respirator filter cartridge has become saturated with an odorous vapor against which they are to be protected. Upper respiratory tract irritation (conveyed by the trigeminal nerve) can be protective, in that nose and throat (as well as eye) irritation triggers escape behavior during an industrial mishap, at times before chemical injury to the lung can occur. With lower-level exposures, trigeminal (eye, nose, and throat) irritation (collectively referred to as "sensory irritation") may be the primary health endpoint of concern, and indeed is a major symptom complex in nonspecific building-related illness (so-called "sick building syndrome").

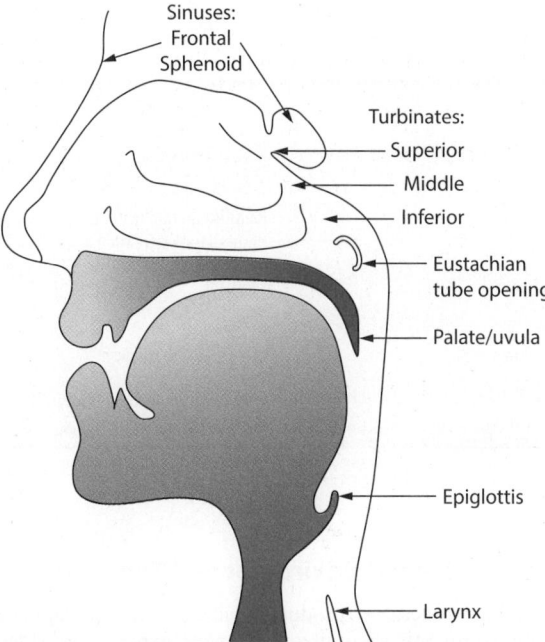

▲ **Figure 18–1.** Anatomy of the upper airway.

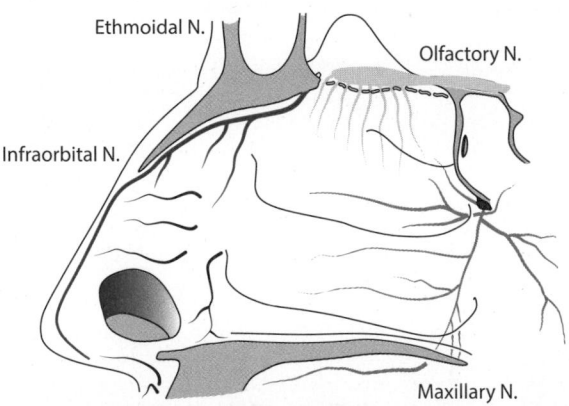

▲ **Figure 18–2.** Innervation of the nasal cavity. The olfactory epithelium connects, via perforations in the cribriform plate, with the olfactory bulbs. The ethmoid and infraorbital nerves arise from the ophthalmic (first) division of the trigeminal nerve; the maxillary nerve constitutes the second division of the trigeminal.

Table 18–1. Functions of the upper airway.

General	Specific
Air conditioning	Heating Humidification
Air filtration	Microbes (inactivation) Particulates (mucociliary clearance) Gases and vapors (scrubbing)
Sensation	Olfaction (odor perception) Chemesthesis (irritant perception)
Communication	Hearing (pressure regulation of the middle ear) Speech

OCCUPATIONAL & ENVIRONMENTAL CONDITIONS OF THE UPPER AIRWAY

A variety of exposure-related health effects involve the upper airway. Structures potentially affected include the nasal cavity, paranasal sinuses, sensory nerves, Eustachian tubes/middle ear, and larynx (Table 18–2).

Occupational & Environmental Allergic Rhinitis

ESSENTIALS OF DIAGNOSIS

▶ Rhinorrhea, nasal airflow obstruction, nasal pruritus, and sneezing.

▶ Symptoms may occur seasonally ("intermittent") or perennially ("persistent").

▶ Common aeroallergens encountered in the general environment include pollens, mold spores, and animal-related allergens.

▶ Allergens responsible for occupational allergic rhinitis are identical to those producing occupational asthma, and include both high- and low-molecular-weight substances.

▶ Diagnosis involves confirmatory allergy testing (either epicutaneous skin prick testing or *in vitro* measurement of antigen-specific IgE).

▶ General Considerations

It has been estimated that, worldwide, 20% of the population suffers from allergic rhinitis, and another 5% suffers from various forms of nonallergic rhinitis. As a result of exposure to common aeroallergens, individuals may experience: (1) seasonal pollinosis; (2) perennial allergy to common indoor allergens (eg, dust mite, molds, or pet allergens); or

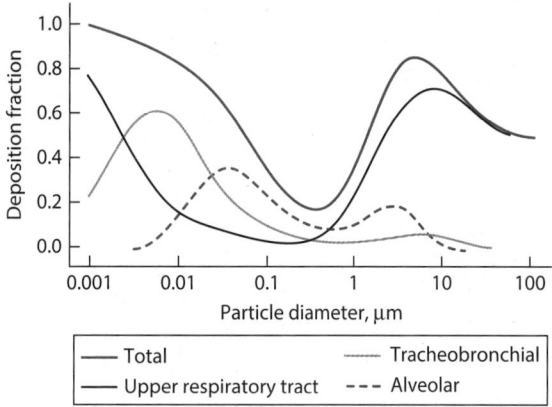

▲ **Figure 18–3.** Fractional deposition of particulate matter in the upper respiratory tract, tracheobronchial tree, and alveoli, by particle diameter.

Table 18–2. Upper airway health effects associated with occupational and environmental agents.

Structure	Conditions
Sensory apparatus	Olfactory dysfunction Sensory irritation
Nasal cavity	Rhinitis (allergic/irritant) Nasal septal perforation
Paranasal sinuses	Sinusitis Sinonasal cancer
Middle ear	Otitis media in children
Larynx	Overuse dysphonia Vocal cord dysfunction

(3) a mixed pattern. Both conditions produce symptoms of nasal pruritus, sneezing, rhinorrhea, and nasal congestion. Patients with perennial allergic rhinitis frequently adapt to their symptoms (particularly congestion) to the degree that additional prompting may be necessary to elicit a complete history (a useful screening question for dust mite allergy being "do you often wake up with a stuffy nose?"). The terms "seasonal" and "perennial" allergic rhinitis are increasingly being replaced by the terms "intermittent" and "persistent" allergic rhinitis. Seasonal allergens vary geographically, and some areas have already shown pollen changes as a result of long-term climate change. Dust mites require a minimum of approximately 40% relative humidity to survive, and therefore are rarely found in far northern latitudes.

Occupational & Environmental Exposure

Workplace allergens producing allergic rhinitis may be either commonly encountered allergens, exposure to which may be incidental to the work environment (eg, grass pollen exposure in a landscaping gardener), or unusual agents encountered only in industrial environments (eg, trimellitic anhydride exposure in a plastics worker). As is the case with asthma, work-related allergic rhinitis may either be work-induced ("occupational") or work-exacerbated. Table 18–3 lists representative agents producing occupational allergic rhinitis; the reader will recognize that these same agents can produce occupational asthma (and, indeed, many sensitized individuals suffer from both conditions). Figure 18–5 depicts

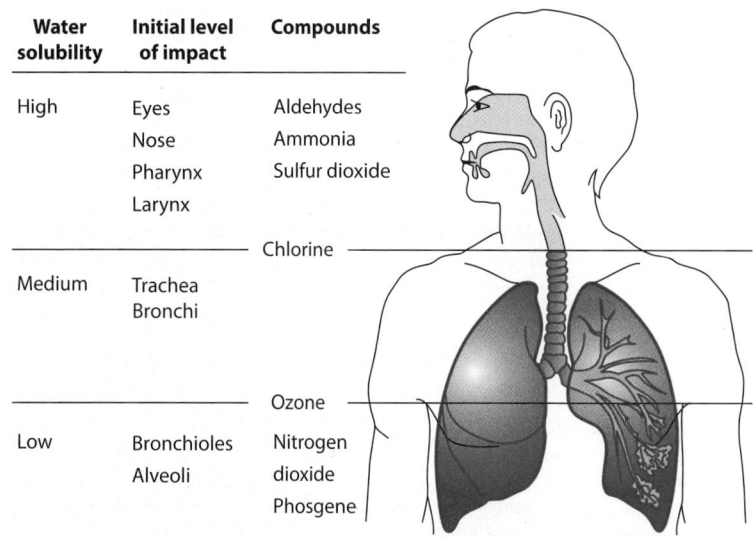

Water solubility	Initial level of impact	Compounds
High	Eyes Nose Pharynx Larynx	Aldehydes Ammonia Sulfur dioxide
		Chlorine
Medium	Trachea Bronchi	
		Ozone
Low	Bronchioles Alveoli	Nitrogen dioxide Phosgene

▲ **Figure 18–4.** Water solubility and site of initial impact of airborne irritants. Highly water-soluble pollutants dissolve quickly in mucous membrane water, and alert the individual to the presence of the pollutant via trigeminal irritation.

Table 18-3. Some agents associated with occupational allergic rhinitis.

General Class	Specific Agent	Occupation Affected
High molecular weight	Baking flour; α-amylase Animal proteins (urinary, salivary) Proteolytic enzymes Mold spores Insect antigens Natural rubber latex	Bakers Laboratory animal handlers Veterinary personnel Detergent manufacturers Librarians; composters Flood control workers Pharmaceutical workers (too restrictive) Health care personnel Food service workers Florists
Low molecular weight	Trimellitic anhydride (epoxy component) Diisocyanates (polyure-thane component) Plicatic acid (from Western Red Cedar) Abietic acid/colophony (from rosin core solder)	Fabricators (various) Auto body painters Boatbuilders Shipping clerks Sawyers Solderers (electronics)

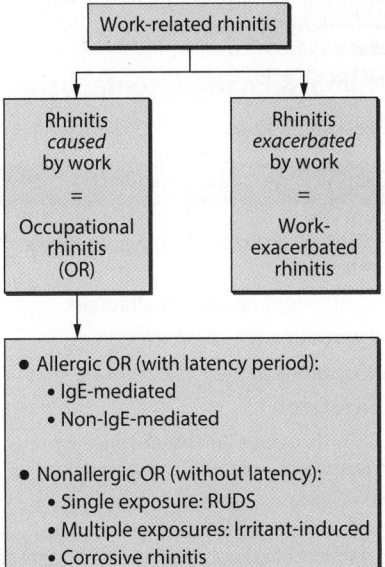

▲ **Figure 18–5.** Classification of occupational rhinitis, analogous to that for occupational asthma, as proposed by the European Academy of Allergy and Clinical Immunology.

a classification of work-related rhinitis, analogous to that of work-related asthma.

▶ **Metabolism & Mechanisms of Action**

In sensitized individuals, specific antigen can initiate mast cell degranulation in the nasal mucosa, resulting in immediate release of such preformed mediators as histamine, heparin, tryptase, and leukocyte chemotactic factors, as well as rapidly generating lipid breakdown products, including leukotrienes and prostaglandins. A "late-phase" reaction, occurring 2–6 hours later, may release cytokines and chemokines, which in turn trigger longer-lasting symptoms and recruit additional inflammatory cells. The effects of these mediators include glandular secretion (rhinorrhea), nerve stimulation (nasal pruritus and sneezing), vasodilation (congestion), and chemotaxis (inflammation). Of importance, the mucous membranes of the nose and conjunctivae are contiguous, and are often affected by the same antigen exposures (hence the term, "rhinoconjunctivitis").

▶ **Clinical Findings**

A. Symptoms and Signs

Allergic rhinitis is typically manifest by symptoms of rhinorrhea, nasal airflow obstruction, nasal pruritus, and sneezing. Symptoms may occur seasonally ("intermittent") or perennially ("persistent"). Signs on anterior rhinoscopy include swollen, pale nasal turbinates, copious, watery secretions, and "mucus stranding" (clear strands of mucus bridging the inferior turbinate and nasal septum).

B. Laboratory Findings

- Eosinophilia on nasal cytology
- Positive epicutaneous skin prick testing[1]
- Allergen-specific IgE on *in vitro* testing (RAST or ELISA)[1]
- Increased total serum IgE (variable finding)
- Peripheral eosinophilia (variable finding)

C. Imaging Studies

Swelling of nasal turbinates may be observed on computed tomographic (CT) scanning.

D. Special Tests

- *Nasal inspiratory peak-flow measurements.* This ambulatory, self-administered test may provide objective validation of cross-shift nasal obstruction and can be employed

---

[1]If neither an *in vitro* test system nor a skin test reagent is available for a given occupational allergen, response to allergen avoidance or workplace challenge may provide the best clue to the specific diagnosis.

during adjacent periods of allergen avoidance and normal work routine to help establish an occupational etiology.

- *Sensory testing.* Qualitative and quantitative tests of olfactory function can help document the response to allergen avoidance and medical therapy.

E. Special Examinations

- *Rhinolaryngoscopy.* Flexible (fiberoptic) rhinolaryngoscopy allows the examining physician to visualize the sinus ostia, larynx, and olfactory cleft, as well as to assess for the presence of nasal polyps.

▶ Differential Diagnosis

- Irritant rhinitis
- Nonallergic rhinitis
- Viral upper respiratory tract infection

▶ Prevention

Allergen avoidance should be the key component of therapy, both to control nasal symptoms and to prevent the progression of allergic rhinitis to asthma. In terms of common environmental aeroallergens, the major exposures within the realm of control of patients (or employers) are perennial allergens encountered in the home (or office) environment.

In the industrial workplace, engineering controls or personal protective equipment may be sufficient to control antigen exposures. However, some individuals may require reassignment, particularly if chest symptoms are coincident. In some cases, substitute chemicals or processes have been effective in ameliorating the risk of occupational sensitization (not only for the "index" patient but also for coworkers). After a peak incidence of sensitization of health care workers to natural rubber latex in the mid-1990s, for example, the use of nonlatex gloves (and lower-antigen-content, nonpowdered latex gloves) resulted in a dramatic reduction of new cases.

▶ Treatment

Medical therapies for allergic rhinitis include oral medications (antihistamines and leukotriene inhibitors) and topical medications (nasal corticosteroids, cromolyn sodium, antihistamines, and cholinergic blockers). Topical saline flushes have also been employed as an adjunct to traditional medications. The use of biologics (ie, monoclonal antibodies) in occupational rhinitis and asthma is currently being explored, and their safety and efficacy are unclear.

Of the oral antihistamines, second- and third-generation drugs may enable patients to control symptoms while simultaneously staying productive and alert. These include, among others, fexofenadine, loratadine, desloratadine, cetirizine, and levocetirizine. As many as 2 weeks of therapy may be necessary before an optimal response is observed from topical anti-inflammatory medications (corticosteroids; cromolyn sodium; or the combined antihistaminic/anti-inflammatory agents, azelastine and olopatadine).

Topical nasal decongestants are to be avoided except for very brief control of acute symptoms. Continuous therapy with topical decongestants poses a risk of tachyphylaxis and rebound congestion (*rhinitis medicamentosa*). For patients complaining of prominent secretions, a trial of ipratropium bromide nasal spray (a cholinergic blocker) may be indicated.

The efficacy of desensitization therapy ("allergy shots") has been better evaluated for common aeroallergens than for specific occupational sensitizers. Patients electing to use saline flushes should either use commercial products or be cautioned regarding the hazards of microbial contamination of home preparations.

▶ Prognosis

Assuming the practicality of allergen avoidance (and absent progression to rhinosinusitis), allergic rhinitis has an excellent prognosis. Untreated occupational allergic rhinitis may progress to occupational asthma.

Limited data link allergic rhinitis to obstructive sleep apnea. High-grade nasal obstruction predisposes to oral breathing, bypassing the filtration and air-conditioning functions of the upper airway. This may be one of the mechanisms whereby rhinitis and asthma severity are linked. Nasal mucosal swelling may also occlude the ostia of the paranasal sinuses and/or middle ear (Eustachian tubes). Ostial occlusion leads to pressure imbalance, effusion, and eventually infection (sinusitis or otitis media).

Occupational & Environmental Irritant Rhinitis

ESSENTIALS OF DIAGNOSIS

- ▶ Nasal irritation, dryness, stinging, burning, rhinorrhea, nasal obstruction.
- ▶ Facial pressure and decreased olfaction.
- ▶ Mucosal erythema is a common sign.
- ▶ Punctate erosions of the nasal septum.
- ▶ Septal perforation.
- ▶ Irritant rhinitis occurs in the absence of specific sensitization (although it may occur coincident with allergic rhinitis).
- ▶ Irritant rhinitis is dose-related, often occurring in a substantial fraction of coworkers in an industrial setting.
- ▶ Cytologic changes consistent with irritant rhinitis have been documented among urban dwellers whose primary exposure is to high levels of photochemical oxidants (smog).

General Considerations

The eyes, nose, and throat are sensitive to chemical irritants (including gases, vapors, dusts, and smokes), with sensory irritation being the most commonly reported symptom complex in problematic indoor work environments. Types of chemical irritants in home or office air include (1) combustion products (from tobacco smoke and malfunctioning appliances) and (2) volatile organic compounds (VOCs; from cleaning products, office supplies and machines, building materials and furnishings, and microbial sources). Industrial environments present workers with an even wider range of airborne irritants, with the majority of permissible exposure levels (PELs) being based on the irritancy of the compound in question. Extreme forms of industrial irritant rhinitis ("corrosive rhinitis") occur in electroplaters and others exposed to chromic acid, who may develop nasal mucosal ulcerations and even septal perforation. Ambient exposure to photochemical air pollution can produce objective inflammatory changes in the upper airway, including squamous metaplasia. Representative environmental and occupational irritants appear in Tables 18–4 and 18–5, respectively.

Persistent rhinitis symptoms and signs after a one-time high-level irritant exposure has been termed *reactive upper airways dysfunction syndrome* (RUDS). This diagnosis is analogous to the lower airway condition referred to as *irritant-induced asthma* or *reactive airways dysfunction syndrome* (RADS). However, in contradistinction to irritant-induced asthma, RUDS lacks objective diagnostic criteria (ie, physiologic changes on provocation testing), making the diagnosis one based on clinical criteria alone.

Table 18–4. Environmental irritants.

Source or Class	Specific Pollutant	Comment
Combustion products	Second hand smoke (SHS) Nitrogen oxides (NOx) Sulfur oxides (SOx) Ozone + PAN (peroxyacetyl nitrite) Particulate matter	Complex mixture of vapors, gases, and particulates Unvented stoves and heaters Vehicular exhaust Oil refineries; coal- and oil-burning power plants Photochemical reaction products of NOx + VOCs from vehicular exhaust Fireplaces and wood-burning stoves; power plants
Cleaning products	Hypochlorite, ammonia Chloramines, chlorine gas	Reaction products of inappropriate mixing
Volatile organic compounds (VOCs)	Formaldehyde, glycol ethers, various others Various	Off-gassing construction materials and furnishings Stationery and art materials; polishes and waxes

Table 18–5. Selected occupational irritants.

Occupation	Irritant
Agricultural workers	Ammonia, nitrogen dioxide, hydrogen sulfide
Custodians	Ammonia, bleach (hypochlorite), chloramines
Firefighters	Smoke, hazardous materials releases
Food service workers	Cooking vapors, cigarette smoke
Health professionals	Glutaraldehyde, formaldehyde
Laboratory workers	Solvent vapors, inorganic acid vapors/mists
Military personnel	Zinc chloride smoke
Power plant and oil refinery workers	Sulfur dioxide
Printers, painters	Solvent vapors
Pulp mill workers	Chlorine, chlorine dioxide, hydrogen sulfide
Railroad personnel, miners, truck drivers	Diesel exhaust
Refrigeration workers (commercial)	Ammonia
Roofers, pavers	Asphalt vapors, PAHs
Swimming pool service workers	Chlorine, hydrogen chloride, nitrogen trichloride
Wastewater treatment workers	Chlorine, hydrogen sulfide
Welders	Metallic oxide fumes, nitrogen oxides, ozone
Woodworkers	Wood dust

Metabolism & Mechanisms of Action

"Irritation" encompasses a spectrum of effects, including (1) subjective sensory irritation, (2) stimulation of neurogenic reflexes, and (3) actual tissue damage. Neurogenic reflexes triggered by physical or chemical stimuli are also prominent in a subset of nonallergic rhinitis referred to as "idiopathic" (formerly, "vasomotor") rhinitis (see discussion below). Stimulation of trigeminal nerve afferents—which are sensitive to low pH, endogenous inflammatory mediators (such as bradykinin), and various chemical irritants—results in two major types of reflex response: (1) parasympathetic reflexes, conveyed by the facial nerve (cranial nerve VII), and (2) the axon reflex, an antidromic response involving neuropeptides released from afferent branches of the trigeminal nerve.

Two familiar examples of parasympathetic reflexes are (1) gustatory rhinitis (a copious, watery rhinorrhea that occurs with the ingestion of spicy foods) and (2) "skier's nose" (watery rhinorrhea in response to cold, dry air). Consistent with their mechanism, both of these conditions can be blocked by the topical anticholinergic agent, ipratropium bromide.

The axon reflex, through the release of substance P, also acutely triggers glandular secretion and vascular dilatation. Subacutely, substance P potentiates the response of mast cells to antigens, forming one of several known links between the allergic response and chemical irritation. In another such link, both diesel exhaust particles and second-hand tobacco smoke **enhance allergic sensitization** (act as *adjuvants*) and **intensify the allergic response** (*priming*). In return, pre-existing nasal allergies increase an individual's sensitivity to chemical irritants (*neuromodulation*). Thus, our understanding of the immunologic and neurogenic systems in the airway has come to include reciprocal modulatory effects elicited by allergens and chemical irritants.

▶ Clinical Findings

A. Symptoms and Signs

Irritant rhinitis is marked by subjective irritation (often expressed as "dryness," "stinging," or "burning"). Pruritus and sneezing are not typical symptoms. Rhinorrhea and nasal congestion (airflow obstruction) are secondary (reflex) symptoms that occur variably among individuals affected by irritant rhinitis. A sensation of facial pressure and/or decreased olfaction are also common.

On examination, mucosal erythema is a common sign. There may be punctate erosions of the nasal septum. Nasal erosions (as well as septal perforation) can occur with concentrated and protracted exposures to airborne irritants. This has been termed "corrosive rhinitis."

B. Laboratory Findings

Irritant rhinitis yields a negative allergy workup. Polymorphonuclear leukocytes (neutrophils) predominate on nasal smear.

C. Imaging Studies

If reflex congestion is present, turbinate hypertrophy may be apparent on **CT scanning**.

D. Special Tests

- *Nasal inspiratory peak-flow measurements.* If subjective congestion is prominent in response to workplace or environmental exposures, exposure-related changes in nasal patency may be documented utilizing a nasal peak inspiratory flow meter.
- *Sensory testing.* Qualitative and quantitative tests of olfactory function can help document the response to irritant avoidance and medical therapy.

E. Special Examinations

Flexible (fiberoptic) rhinolaryngoscopy allows the examining physician to visualize the sinus ostia, larynx, and olfactory cleft, as well as to assess for the presence of nasal polyps.

▶ Differential Diagnosis

- Allergic rhinitis
- Nonallergic rhinitis
- Viral upper respiratory infection

▶ Prevention

The majority of occupational permissible exposure limits have been set for the avoidance of chemical irritant effects, in particular sensory irritation. Similar logic underlies several ambient air quality standards, as well as statutory restrictions on smoking in public spaces.

High-grade nasal obstruction predisposes to oral breathing, bypassing the filtration and air-conditioning functions of the upper airway. This may be one of the mechanisms whereby rhinitis and asthma severity are linked. Nasal mucosal swelling may also occlude the ostia of the paranasal sinuses and/or middle ear (Eustachian tubes). Ostial occlusion leads to pressure imbalance, effusion, and eventually infection (sinusitis or otitis media).

▶ Treatment

- Reduction of exposure.
- Nonspecific supportive measures (eg, saline nasal lavage).
- Topical steroids (of questionable value).
- Topical cholinergic blockers (ipratropium bromide) for prominent rhinorrhea.
- In atopic patients, control of intercurrent allergic rhinitis—whether occupational or nonoccupational—may decrease reactivity to chemical irritants.

▶ Prognosis

With the exception of corrosive rhinitis with nasal septal perforation, the prognosis for irritant rhinitis after exposure reduction is excellent. However, some individuals with RUDS may show persistent nasal hyperesthesia and nasal hyperreactivity (exaggerated responsiveness to nonspecific physical and chemical stimuli), despite therapy.

Occupational & Environmental Nonallergic Rhinitis

Nonallergic rhinitis encompasses a variety of entities, including idiopathic (formerly, "vasomotor") rhinitis, endocrine rhinitis (including rhinitis of pregnancy), rhinitis medicamentosa, nonallergic rhinitis with eosinophilia ("NARES") syndrome, rhinitis of granulomatous disease (Wegener granulomatosis), immotile cilia/Kartagener syndrome, and rhinitis in cystic fibrosis. In idiopathic rhinitis (the most prevalent form of nonallergic rhinitis), the mechanism(s) underlying nasal hyperreactivity are poorly understood.

ESSENTIALS OF DIAGNOSIS

▸ Symptoms of idiopathic nonallergic rhinitis are variable, including rhinorrhea, nasal obstruction, facial pressure, and decreased olfaction.

▸ There are no characteristic physical findings in idiopathic nonallergic rhinitis.

▸ Negative allergy workup.

▸ Lack of inflammatory cells on nasal smear.

▶ General Considerations

Idiopathic (formerly, vasomotor) rhinitis, a subcategory of nonallergic rhinitis, is a term that is often used to describe increased nasal reactivity to nonspecific physical and chemical stimuli. Symptoms of rhinorrhea and/or congestion tend to predominate, with neither subjective irritation nor nasal pruritus being prominent. Relevant physical stimuli include low humidity, extremes in or rapid changes of temperature, and excessive air motion. Relevant chemical stimuli include smokes (including second-hand tobacco smoke), household cleaning products, perfumes, and industrial irritants. Possibly linked to this diagnosis are *gustatory rhinitis* (rhinorrhea in response to the ingestion of spicy foods) and *bright-light rhinitis* (self-explanatory). Roughly 40% of individuals with allergic rhinitis also complain of reactivity to nonspecific physical and chemical stimuli. Problematic occupations include outdoor work, biotechnology and food processing (cold rooms), and office work. The American Society of Heating, Refrigerating, and Air-Conditioning Engineers (ASHRAE) has promulgated guidelines for temperature and humidity control in indoor air; these parameters should be assessed as part of any "problem building" investigation.

High-grade nasal obstruction predisposes to oral breathing, bypassing the filtration and air-conditioning functions of the upper airway. This may be one of the mechanisms whereby rhinitis and asthma severity are linked. Nasal mucosal swelling may also occlude the ostia of the paranasal sinuses and/or middle ear (Eustachian tubes). Ostial occlusion leads to pressure imbalance, effusion, and eventually infection (sinusitis or otitis media).

▶ Metabolism & Mechanisms of Action

The pathogenesis of vasomotor rhinitis is unclear. In some studies, parasympathetic overactivity appears to be responsible for hypersecretion. Other studies have postulated that overexpression of irritant sensors in the nasal mucosa is the pathogenic key. Finally, researchers have identified a subset of patients with local mucosal allergy (ie, sensitized nasal mucosal mast cells in the absence of skin test reactivity or circulating antigen-specific IgE). This condition has been termed "local allergic rhinitis," requires nasal provocation testing to diagnose, and has been more extensively studied with common aeroallergens than with occupational agents.

▶ Clinical Findings

A. Symptoms and Signs

Symptoms in idiopathic rhinitis are variable. They include rhinorrhea, nasal obstruction, facial pressure, and decreased olfaction. There are no characteristic physical findings in idiopathic nonallergic rhinitis.

B. Laboratory Findings

- Negative allergy workup
- Lack of inflammatory cells on nasal smear

C. Imaging Studies

- If reflex congestion is present, turbinate hypertrophy may be apparent on **CT scanning**.

D. Special Tests

- *Nasal inspiratory peak-flow measurements.* If subjective congestion is prominent in response to workplace or environmental exposures, exposure-related changes in nasal patency may be documented utilizing a nasal peak inspiratory flow meter.

- *Nasal provocation with cold, dry air.* When exposed to cold, dry air, individuals with idiopathic rhinitis, on average, congest more than do normal controls. Because of high interindividual variability, however, this test has limits to its sensitivity and specificity.

- *Histamine challenge.* Histamine has been used, in titrated doses, to document nonspecific nasal reactivity. The concentration is increased by a fixed ratio until a predetermined increase in nasal airway resistance (NAR) is documented (analogous to the methacholine challenge test). However, there is considerable overlap in response among diagnostic groups.

- *Nasal allergen challenge.* As indicated above, some individuals with rhinitis symptoms react to local instillation of antigen in the nose, while simultaneously maintaining negative skin test reactivity and a lack of antigen-specific IgE in the serum. These individuals would be classified as having "local allergic rhinitis" rather than idiopathic nonallergic rhinitis.

E. Special Examinations

- *Rhinolaryngoscopy.* Flexible (fiberoptic) rhinolaryngoscopy allows the examining physician to visualize the sinus ostia, larynx, and olfactory cleft, as well as to assess for the presence of nasal polyps.

► Differential Diagnosis

- Allergic rhinitis
- Irritant rhinitis
- Viral upper respiratory infection

► Prevention

There is no known primary prevention for vasomotor rhinitis. Avoidance of extremes of temperature and humidity, as well as avoidance of chemical irritant exposure, may provide symptomatic relief in some individuals.

► Treatment

Approved therapies for vasomotor rhinitis include selected topical steroids (fluticasone propionate and beclomethasone dipropionate), topical antihistamines (azelastine and olopatadine), and topical cholinergic blockers (ipratropium bromide).

► Prognosis

The prognosis for resolution of vasomotor rhinitis is very guarded. Some referral centers claim long-lasting relief after capsaicin desensitization, which is considered an investigational procedure at this time.

PARANASAL SINUS DISEASE

Sinusitis

ESSENTIALS OF DIAGNOSIS

- ► Sinusitis may affect single or multiple sinuses, unilaterally or bilaterally.
- ► Sinusitis is classified as acute (up to 4 weeks duration); subacute (4–12 weeks); and chronic (>12 weeks).
- ► Primary symptoms are nasal congestion, facial pressure, purulent nasal discharge, decreased olfaction, and systemic symptoms (such as fatigue and, occasionally, fever).
- ► Findings on CT scanning may include mucoperiosteal thickening, air-fluid levels, and obstruction of the ostiomeatal complex. Nasal polyposis may be an associated finding.
- ► The role of sinusitis in the genesis of headaches is the subject of active discussion at this time.
- ► Sinusitis has been linked to asthma incidence and severity.

► General Considerations

Both allergic and irritant rhinitis can progress to *rhinosinusitis*. Epidemiologically, active smokers are at higher risk for developing acute (and chronic) sinusitis. Evidence for a link between sinusitis and second-hand tobacco smoke exposure appears to be mounting, as well. Relatively few studies have systematically examined the endpoint of sinusitis and occupational exposures. Surveys of furriers, spice workers, vegetable picklers, hemp workers, and grain and flour workers all include increased prevalence rates for sinusitis; however, these studies are based on self-report. More recently, cohort studies of World Trade Center responders have suggested increased rates of upper airway disorders, including sinusitis and vocal cord dysfunction, compared to unexposed individuals.

► Metabolism & Mechanisms of Action

Irritant- and allergen-induced nasal mucosal swelling can compromise the patency of the paranasal sinus ostia, thereby producing pressure imbalance, effusion, and impaired clearance of secretions, and leading to the development of sinusitis. Most bouts of acute sinusitis result from viral upper respiratory tract infections, and are self-limited. In acute bacterial sinusitis, the most common organisms involved include *Streptococcus pneumoniae*, *Haemophilus influenzae*, and *Moraxella catarrhalis*. Less frequently, *Staphylococcus aureus*, anaerobes, or gram-negative organisms are present. *Invasive fungal sinusitis* may be seen with immune suppression (eg, in the presence of diabetes mellitus). *Noninvasive allergic fungal sinusitis* has also been described, in which affected sinuses are colonized by one or more fungal species (such as *Schizophyllum commune*), which in turn attract eosinophils. Considerable tissue damage can occur from the inflammatory mediators released by these inflammatory cells.

Chronic rhinosinusitis, with or without polyposis, involves some component of noninfectious chronic inflammation, the mechanisms of which have yet to be fully elucidated. Inflammation in the upper and lower respiratory tracts appears to be linked, in that active sinusitis typically augments nonspecific bronchial reactivity in asthmatics. Postulated mechanisms include upregulation of neurogenic and humoral responses; loss of air conditioning and filtration functions due to chronic oral breathing; and aspiration of biochemical-mediator-laden nasal secretions into the lower respiratory tract. The model linking allergic inflammation in the upper and lower respiratory tracts has been termed the "united airway hypothesis."

► Clinical Findings

A. Symptoms and Signs

Symptoms include nasal airflow obstruction (congestion), facial pressure, impaired olfaction, and systemic symptoms of fatigue and variable fever. Signs include sinus tap tenderness (frontal/maxillary) and mucopurulent nasal secretions visible on routine examination or on flexible rhinolaryngoscopy.

B. Laboratory Findings

Abnormalities of the complete blood count (leukocytosis) and elevations of the erythrocyte sedimentation rate or C-reactive protein are both nonspecific and insensitive measures in acute or chronic sinusitis.

C. Imaging Studies

Potential findings on CT scanning include mucoperiosteal thickening, air-fluid levels, and obstruction of the ostiomeatal complex. Polyposis and bony erosions may also be found.

D. Special Tests

- *Nasal nitric oxide sampling.* Because the sinuses serve as a reservoir for nitric oxide (NO), nasal NO levels tend to be higher than levels measured in exhaled breath. However, nasal NO trends down with increasing obstruction of the ostiomeatal complex (ie, obstruction due to sinusitis and/ or nasal polyposis).

E. Special Examinations

- *Rhinolaryngoscopy.* Mucopurulent discharge per sinus ostia is a common sinusitis-related finding on rhinolaryngoscopy.

▶ Differential Diagnosis

- Viral upper respiratory tract infection
- Odontogenic (dental) pain
- Migraine headache
- Sinus neoplasm
- Nasal foreign body
- Invasive fungal sinusitis
- Allergic fungal sinusitis
- Underlying immune deficiency or mucociliary disorder (cystic fibrosis; immotile cilia syndrome)
- Underlying granulomatous process (Wegener's)

▶ Prevention

- Irritant and allergen avoidance
- Effective medical therapy for allergic rhinitis
- Nasal hygiene (saline flushes) for those working in dusty environments

▶ Treatment

Acute and uncomplicated sinusitis lasting 10 or fewer days should be treated as a self-limited condition, and presumed to be of viral origin. Acute sinusitis symptoms lasting greater than 10 days may be a candidate for antibiotic therapy. Given the potential role of β-lactamase producing organisms, recommended empiric antibiotic therapy is evolving.

Therapy for *chronic rhinosinusitis* (with or without polyps) emphasizes topical corticosteroids initially, at times augmented by oral leukotriene antagonists or biologics. When exposure controls and medical therapy fail to yield expected improvement, patients should undergo an allergy workup and otolaryngologic consultation. In some cases, *functional endoscopic sinus surgery* may be indicated to promote effective sinus drainage. Therapy for **invasive fungal sinusitis** relies heavily on systemic antifungal agents, often in conjunction with surgery. Therapy for **allergic fungal sinusitis**, on the other hand, relies on oral steroids and saline lavage, typically in a post-operative setting. Clinical trials have shown inconsistent benefit from the administration of antifungal agents in the latter condition.

▶ Prognosis

The prognosis for resolution of acute sinusitis is good. The prognosis for resolution of chronic sinusitis is variable, depending on a variety of factors (including anatomy, atopy, and inflammatory subtype).

Sinonasal Cancer

A number of occupations and imputed exposures have been linked with the development of malignant neoplasms of the paranasal sinuses. The strongest (and most consistent) findings pertain to formaldehyde-exposed workers and to leather- and woodworkers, although some studies also have found nickel- and chrome-refining and chrome-plating workers to be at risk.

Laryngeal Pathology

Symptoms referable to phonation (typically, hoarseness) can also occur in work settings. Temporary and reversible hoarseness may occur either from exposure to inhaled chemical irritants or from overuse of the voice. Although overuse is most widely recognized in lecturers and singers, it also occurs among industrial employees who need to shout in order to communicate in noisy environments. The most ominous condition heralded by hoarseness—squamous cell carcinoma of the larynx—has been associated with a number of exposures/occupations, including: polycyclic aromatic hydrocarbon exposure (cigarette smoking, metalworking fluids, work in aluminum reduction plants, use of coal as a cooking fuel indoors), as well as exposure to asbestos and personal consumption of ethanol.

Two other occupational/environmental conditions deserve mention. After significant smoke inhalation injury laryngeal strictures may occur, resulting either from the initial chemical/thermal insult or secondary to prolonged intubation. In addition, laryngeal papillomatosis has been described in a case report of a physician whose apparent exposure was human papillomavirus aerosolized during laser surgery.

A functional laryngeal condition of note is *vocal cord dysfunction* (VCD) (also referred to as "paradoxical vocal fold motion"). VCD involves episodic hoarseness, shortness of breath, stridor (often confused with wheezing), and globus (a pressure sensation in the throat or upper chest). Coughing is also common in VCD. Because of overlapping symptoms with asthma, VCD may be misdiagnosed as the latter. Predisposing conditions include postnasal drip and gastroesophageal reflux. In the occupational setting, VCD has been documented after acute irritant exposures, giving rise to the diagnosis of "irritant-associated VCD." Most recently, this condition has been documented among a subset of individuals exposed to alkaline dust as World Trade Center responders.

Diagnosis of VCD requires documentation of paradoxical vocal cord motion (adduction during inspiration as visualized during rhinolaryngoscopy). Alternatively, the finding of variable extrathoracic obstruction during the inspiratory phase of the flow-volume loop is highly suggestive for this condition. After ruling out more serious conditions (eg, neoplasms, vocal cord paralysis, and spasmodic dysphonia), treatment consists of voice rest, hydration, and biofeedback/voice training under the supervision of a qualified speech pathologist.

Otitis Media in Children

An increased incidence of otitis media with effusion has been reported among children exposed to second-hand tobacco smoke. Postulated mechanisms center on Eustachian tube dysfunction, with second-hand tobacco smoke producing ciliostasis and mucous membrane congestion, resulting in impaired pressure equalization, middle ear effusion, and reduced drainage of middle ear secretions. Because of the strength and consistency of this finding, the workup of recurrent otitis media in young children always should include questions about parental smoking.

Sensory (Olfactory) Alterations

Both temporary and long-lasting alterations in olfactory function have been reported among workers exposed to a variety of industrial chemicals. Chemically induced olfactory dysfunction may include (1) *quantitative defects*, including hyposmia (reduced odor acuity) and anosmia (absent odor perception), and (2) *qualitative defects*, including olfactory agnosia (decreased ability to identify odors) and various dysosmias (distorted odor perception). Occupational groups and exposures for which defects in odor detection or identification have been identified include alkaline battery workers and braziers (cadmium ± nickel exposure), tank cleaners (hydrocarbon exposure), paint formulators (solvent ± acrylic acid exposure), and chemical plant workers (ammonia and sulfuric acid exposures). Of note, olfactory deficits have also been identified among World Trade Center responders, compared to age-, sex-, and smoking status-matched controls. At high concentrations (levels in excess of approximately 50 ppm), hydrogen sulfide is known to produce acute and reversible olfactory fatigue.

Chemical irritants may cause hyposmia via nasal obstruction, or alternatively, may produce direct damage to the olfactory neuroepithelium. Experimentally, at least one study has shown the olfactory equivalent of a *temporary threshold shift* (reversible olfactory deficit) after several hours of controlled exposure to solvents (toluene or xylene); subjects recovered olfactory acuity within about 2 hours of cessation of exposure. Of note, no perceptual deficit was evident for a test compound unrelated to the exposure (methylphenyl carbinol). This reversible and specific phenomenon might therefore be thought of as an extension of the familiar process of *odor adaptation*, in which odors lose their intensity during continuous exposure.

Other causes of olfactory impairment not directly related to chemical exposures include head trauma, chronic nasal obstruction from rhinosinusitis, postinfectious inflammation, neurodegenerative disorders (Alzheimer and parkinsonism), endocrine disorders, hepatic and renal disease, neoplasms, various drugs, ionizing radiation, selected psychiatric conditions, and congenital defects (eg, Kallmann syndrome). Loss of olfactory and gustatory function can also occur with viral infections, such as SARS-CoV-2 (i.e., COVID-19), which can potentially be acquired occupationally.

DIAGNOSTIC TECHNIQUES

A number of diagnostic tools are useful in the study of nasal responses to environmental agents; unfortunately, they are underutilized in clinical practice. Accordingly, these have been classified here as either semiroutine or techniques used exclusively in clinical referral or research centers (Table 18–6).

Semiroutine Methods

A. Nasal Cytology

Nasal smears for cytologic analysis are used to provide information regarding the types of inflammatory cells in nasal mucus and/or the superficial mucosal layers. Samples are taken from the medial surface of the inferior turbinate using a curette, and are done under direct visualization. Typically, eosinophils predominate in allergic inflammation, whereas neutrophils predominate with viral and bacterial infections.

Table 18–6. Diagnostic tools for the upper airway.

Routine	Physical examination; insufflation tympanometry Impedance tympanometry Nasal endoscopy Allergy skin testing In vitro allergy tests (RAST or ELISA) Plain films and CT scans of the paranasal sinuses
Semiroutine	Nasal cytology Nasal peak flow measurement
Referral centers	Rhinomanometry, acoustic rhinometry Nasal mucociliary clearance tests Olfactory function tests (detection, identification)
Research centers	Nasal lavage (cell counts/biochemical mediators) Nasal mucosal blood flow measurement Negative mucosal potentials Chemosensory-evoked potentials

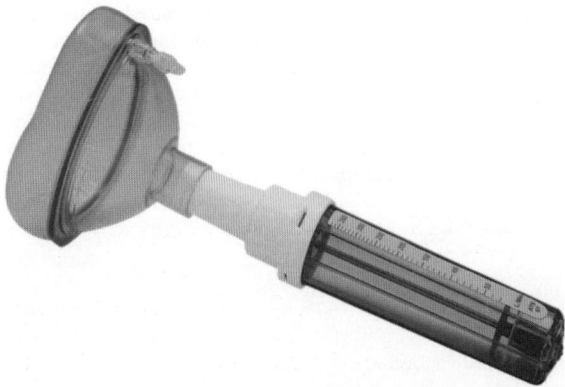

▲ **Figure 18–6.** Commercial nasal inspiratory flow meter.

Neutrophils also predominate in nasal smears taken from individuals with irritant rhinitis, whereas inflammatory cells may absent altogether in patients with nonallergic (particularly idiopathic) rhinitis.

B. Peak Nasal Flow Measurement

Nasal inspiratory peak-flow measurement is listed here as semiroutine, not because of any technical challenges involved, but because the technique and equipment are unfamiliar to many health care providers. Commercially available nasal inspiratory flow meters have become more compact and rugged than in the past (Figure 18–6). To take a measurement, the patient breathes out maximally (to residual volume), places the mask over his or her nose and mouth, and then inhales forcefully through the nose to total lung capacity. Three replicate measures are normally taken, with the highest value being taken as representative.

A diary of nasal peak-flow measurements (along with nasal symptoms) can be kept, with the patient recording peak flow before, during, and after a work shift. If possible, recordings should be taken over a full work week, along with contiguous weekends. Interpretation of these data is analogous to the process of interpreting peak expiratory flow data in the diagnosis of occupational asthma, although no consensus standards exist for "significant" work-related decrements in peak flow.

Techniques Used in Referral Centers

A. Rhinomanometry

Rhinomanometry, or the measurement of NAR, involves simultaneously measuring airflow and pressure between the nasopharynx and anterior nares. With *posterior rhinomanometry*, the individual being tested breathes nasally with an anesthesia mask applied over the nose and mouth, and with a small plastic pressure tap held between the tongue and palate. In *anterior rhinomanometry*, one nostril at a time is occluded with a pressure tap while the subject breathes slowly through the opposite nostril with a flow meter applied.

Anterior rhinomanometry is particularly useful for documenting fixed anatomic pathology that may be unilateral in distribution (eg, deviated septum or polyposis). Posterior rhinomanometry gives a more stable estimate of total NAR than does the anterior technique and is therefore of particular utility in documenting the response of the nose to challenge agents (allergens or irritants).

NAR has been used as the endpoint for various pharmacologic challenge protocols, principally to document the so-called *nonspecific nasal hyperreactivity*. This procedure requires the use of serially increasing concentrations of histamine or methacholine, with the endpoint being the concentration necessary to induce a predetermined percentage increase in NAR. Using this method, allergic rhinitics studied in and out of season show systematic differences in nonspecific nasal reactivity (greater during allergy season). Rhinomanometry can also be used as an objective endpoint after specific (nasal allergen) or nonspecific physical (cold/dry air) challenge.

B. Acoustic Rhinometry

Another technique designed to measure nasal airway patency is acoustic rhinometry (AR). The apparatus consists of a tube with an acoustic pulse generator (and microphone) at one end and a nasal adaptor at the other; the instrument alternately sends and receives sound pulses. By measuring the intensity of reflected sound waves at various time intervals from the initial pulse, an acoustic rhinometer produces a map of total nasal cross-sectional area as a function of distance from the nares. Like rhinomanometry, AR is often used to document the response to pharmacologic, irritant, cold air, or allergen challenge. The relationship between cross-sectional area and NAR, however, is a complex one, rendering the physiologic and symptomatic interpretation of AR challenging at times.

C. Sensory Testing

Olfactory sensory testing focuses on alternative endpoints: *qualitative* or *quantitative*. *Qualitative odor testing* uses panels of test odorants to assess odor identification ability. Typically, such tests are administered as a multiple-choice task in order to prevent the patient's personal experience from having undue influence on testing results. One commercially available qualitative test, the University of Pennsylvania Smell Identification Test (UPSIT), takes the form of scratch-and-sniff panels on a paper base; the test has been well standardized with extensive population norms. The advantage of this test is its portability, and the fact that results generally correlate well with quantitative endpoints.

In the clinical setting, *quantitative olfactory testing* consists of olfactory threshold testing. The simplest clinical screening test is the *alcohol sniff test*. The alcohol sniff test utilizes commonly available packaged isopropanol swabs, opened at the top and held below the breathing zone of a patient whose eyes are closed and who is breathing nasally. The swab is advanced vertically (starting at 30 cm below the nares) by 1 cm with each breath, until the patient reports perceiving an odor. With normal olfactory acuity, the patient should be able to detect an odor by the time the stimulus reaches 20 cm below the nose. More formally, odor threshold testing can be carried out utilizing a forced-choice discrimination task using a series of squeeze bottles with matching blanks. A threshold so obtained is an *odor detection threshold*. Alternate systems utilize a series of pen-like devices whose wicks are saturated with test odorants.

D. Mucociliary Clearance Tests

Mucociliary clearance tests include both invasive and noninvasive procedures. The best-standardized test is the observation of ciliary beat frequency in vitro. This method is often employed as a screening step (prior to electron microscopy) in the diagnosis of disorders involving ultrastructural abnormalities in epithelial cilia (eg, primary ciliary dyskinesia/ Kartagener syndrome). Specimens typically are obtained either by scraping or biopsy of the inferior turbinate; ciliary beat frequency is normally in the range of 9–15 Hz. In addition to frequency, trained observers can note the degree of spatial coordination of adjacent ciliary units, an important component of intact function.

The *saccharine transit time test* is the simplest measure of nasal mucociliary dysfunction. In this procedure, a small grain of saccharine is placed on the anterior portion of the inferior turbinate, and the time interval before the subject tastes the saccharine is recorded. A prolonged test—defined as greater than 30 minutes—indicates impaired mucociliary function.

Mucociliary clearance is important because of its essential function in microbial defense. Patients with impaired mucus formation (cystic fibrosis) or impaired ciliary function (primary ciliary dyskinesia) experience repeated episodes of bronchitis, otitis, and sinusitis, often with ultimate cardiopulmonary complications (bronchiectasis and cor pulmonale). Environmental factors that have been noted to impair mucociliary clearance include viral infection, antigen challenge, cigarette smoke, and sulfur dioxide exposure.

REFERENCES

Anderson JA: Work-associated irritable larynx syndrome. Curr Opin Allergy Clin Immunol 2015;15(2):150 [PMID: 25961388].

Balogun RA, Siracusa A, Shusterman D: Occupational rhinitis and occupational asthma: Association or progression? Am J Ind Med 2018;61(4):293 [PMID: 29411403].

Marcinow AM, Thompson J, Forrest LA, deSilva BW: Irritant-induced paradoxical vocal fold motion disorder: diagnosis and management. Otolaryngol Head Neck Surg. 2015;153(6):996 [PMID: 26307573].

Schwartz DA, Vinnikov D, Blanc PD: Occupation and obstructive sleep apnea: a meta-analysis. J Occup Environ Med 2017;59(6):502 [PMID: 28598928].

Shao Z, Bernstein JA: Occupational rhinitis: classification, diagnosis, and therapeutics. Curr Allergy Asthma Rep. 2019;19(12):54 [PMID: 31776689].

Shusterman D: Nonallergic rhinitis: environmental determinants. Immunol Allergy Clin North Am 2016;36(2):379 [PMID: 27083110].

Van Gerven L, Alpizar YA, Steelant B et al: Enhanced chemosensory sensitivity in patients with idiopathic rhinitis and its reversal by nasal capsaicin treatment. J Allergy Clin Immunol 2017;140(2):437-46.e2 [PMID: 28389389].

■ SELF-ASSESSMENT QUESTIONS

Select the one correct answer for each question.

Question 1: Occupational allergic rhinitis
 a. occurs on a work-exacerbated, but not work-induced, basis
 b. may be linked with occupational asthma
 c. is exclusively histamine-mediated
 d. is associated with a negative epicutaneous skin prick test in all cases

Question 2: Allergens responsible for work-related allergic rhinitis
 a. are distinct from those producing occupational asthma
 b. include only low-molecular-weight substances
 c. include only high-molecular-weight substances
 d. may include common aeroallergens, such as grass pollen

Question 3: Irritant rhinitis
 a. has no symptom overlap with allergic rhinitis
 b. is diagnosed by a positive allergy workup
 c. predisposes to oral breathing via reflex nasal congestion
 d. never occurs on the first exposure to a given irritant chemical

Question 4: Idiopathic rhinitis
 a. is a subcategory of allergic rhinitis
 b. is defined by reactivity to a single specific chemical stimulus
 c. causes rhinorrhea, with nasal pruritus being definitive
 d. is characterized by nasal hyperreactivity (rhinorrhea and/or congestion) to nonspecific physical and chemical stimuli

Question 5: Sinusitis
 a. has been linked to asthma incidence and severity
 b. may follow allergic but not irritant rhinitis
 c. spares active smokers because they develop resistance
 d. always involves bacterial infections

Occupational Lung Diseases

John R. Balmes, MD

The respiratory tract is often the site of injury from occupational exposures. The widespread use of potentially toxic materials in the environment poses a major threat to both the airways and lung parenchyma. The respiratory tract has a limited number of ways to respond to injury. Acute responses include rhinosinusitis, laryngitis, upper airway obstruction, bronchitis, bronchoconstriction, alveolitis, and pulmonary edema. Chronic responses include asthma, bronchitis, bronchiolitis, parenchymal fibrosis, pleural fibrosis, and cancer. Early recognition and appropriate treatment of occupational lung diseases by physicians can reduce both morbidity and mortality significantly and greatly affect patient outcome. This chapter focuses on common occupational lung diseases and on how to diagnose and manage them.

The site of deposition of inhaled materials depends on water solubility for gases and particle size for solids (Table 19–1). Water-soluble gases and particles with a diameter in excess of 10 μm tend to get deposited in the upper airways, whereas insoluble gases and smaller particles penetrate to the lower airways. Subsequent respiratory injury depends on both the site of toxin deposition and the type of cell/structure damaged.

EVALUATION OF PATIENTS WITH OCCUPATIONAL LUNG DISEASE

A careful evaluation can identify and diagnose occupational lung disease successfully in most cases. The following four approaches are recommended: (1) detailed history, including occupational and environmental exposures, (2) thorough physical examination, (3) appropriate imaging studies, and (4) pulmonary function testing.

▶ History

A detailed history of both the patient's complaints and environmental/occupational exposures is essential. Work practices should be explored extensively with attention to types and durations of exposures, whether appropriate environmental controls are present, and if respiratory protective gear is used. If available, safety data sheets (SDSs) should be reviewed. These documents profile the important health, safety, and toxicologic properties of the product's ingredients and under federal law must be furnished by the employer to the worker or to the worker's health care provider on request.

If available, actual industrial hygiene data on the level of exposure and the agent to which the patient was exposed should be obtained. The history should include the condition of the patient's home, any hobbies, and social habits because exposures outside the workplace that contribute to or cause the lung injury may be discovered.

▶ Physical Examination

Occupational lung diseases do not present with specific clinical findings. It is difficult, for example, to distinguish asbestosis from idiopathic pulmonary fibrosis or chronic beryllium disease from sarcoidosis. Only in the context of the exposure history will the correct diagnosis be made. A physician who suspects the presence of an occupational lung disease should, nonetheless, perform a complete physical examination rather than focus narrowly on findings suggested by the exposure history. Relevant nonoccupational disease otherwise may be missed.

The physical examination may be helpful if abnormal, but it is, in general, insensitive for detection of mild respiratory tract injury. The vital signs and the level of respiratory distress, if any, should be assessed. The presence of cyanosis and finger clubbing should be noted. Examination of the skin and eyes can yield signs of irritation and inflammation. Oropharyngeal and nasal areas should be inspected for inflammation, ulcers, and polyps. The presence of wheezing, rhonchi, or both is evidence of airways disease, and crackles are suggestive of the presence of parenchymal disease. Examination of the cardiovascular system for evidence of left ventricular failure is important when crackles are heard. The presence of isolated right ventricular failure suggests the possibility of

Table 19–1. Site of respiratory tract deposition and effect.

Water Solubility	Examples	Site of Injury
High	Ammonia, formaldehyde	Upper airway
Moderate	Chlorine, sulfur dioxide	Lower airways
Low	Nitrogen oxides, phosgene	Lung parenchyma
Particle size (aerodynamic diameter)		
>10 μm	Dust from Earth's crust	Upper airway
2.5–6 μm	Some fire smoke particles	Lower airways
<2.5 μm	Metal fumes, asbestos fibers	Lung parenchyma

cor pulmonale as a result of chronic severe lung disease with hypoxemia.

▶ Imaging Studies

A chest radiograph should be part of the workup when lung disease is suspected. However, normal radiographic findings do not exclude significant damage to the lung. Immediately after toxic inhalational injury, the chest radiograph frequently is normal. On the other hand, dramatically abnormal chest radiographs can be seen in individuals without significant lung injury who are exposed chronically to iron oxide or tin oxide. Abnormalities on the chest radiograph do not necessarily correlate with the degree of pulmonary impairment or disability. These are better assessed by pulmonary function testing and arterial blood gas determination.

With dust-exposed persons, chest films should be interpreted according to the International Labor Organization (ILO) classification for pneumoconiosis, in addition to the routine interpretation. The purpose of the ILO classification is to provide a standardized, descriptive coding system for the appearance and extent of radiographic change caused by pneumoconiosis. The classification scheme consists of a glossary of terms and a set of standard radiographs that demonstrate various degrees of pleural and parenchymal change caused by pneumoconiosis. The standard films are now available in digital format from the National Institute for Occupational Safety and Health (NIOSH). The worker's posteroanterior chest film is scored in comparison with the standard films. In the United States, a certification process for readers using the ILO classification was developed under the auspices of NIOSH. In NIOSH parlance, an "A reader" has taken the American College of Radiology (ACR) pneumoconiosis course but has not passed the certification examination. A "B reader" has taken the ACR course and passed the examination.

Computed tomographic (CT) scanning is a radiographic technique that scans axial cross sections and produces tomographic slices of the organ(s) scanned. Conventional CT scanning of the chest is better able to detect abnormalities of the pleura and the mediastinal structures than is plain chest radiography in large part because it is more sensitive to differences in density. When performed after the administration of intravenous contrast medium, CT scanning is considered to be the imaging study of choice for evaluation of the pulmonary hila.

High-resolution CT (HRCT) scanning incorporates thin collimation (1–2 mm as opposed to 10 mm in conventional CT) with high spatial-frequency reconstruction algorithms that sharpen interfaces between adjacent structures. Studies suggest that HRCT scanning is more sensitive than either conventional CT scanning or chest radiography for assessing the presence, character, and severity of a number of diffuse lung processes such as emphysema and interstitial lung disease (ILD).

▶ Pulmonary Function Testing

Pulmonary function testing is used to detect and quantify abnormal lung function. Measurement of lung volumes and diffusing capacity, gas exchange analysis, and exercise testing need to be performed in a well-equipped pulmonary function laboratory, but spirometry can and should be done in most evaluating centers. There are two different types of spirometers: volume- and flow-sensing devices. Modern computerized versions of both types of spirometers can produce exhaled volume-time and expiratory flow-volume curves. There are advantages and disadvantages to each type of spirometer. Whether a volume- or flow-sensing device is chosen, the best spirometers have comparable accuracy and precision. Performance requirements for spirometers of either type are described in an American Thoracic Society (ATS)/European Respiratory Society (ERS) statement.

The most valuable of all pulmonary function parameters are those obtained from spirometry, namely, forced expiratory volume in 1 second (FEV_1), forced vital capacity (FVC), and the FEV_1:FVC ratio. These parameters provide the best method of detecting the presence and severity of airway obstruction, as well as the most reliable assessment of overall respiratory impairment. The forced expiratory flow from 25% to 75% of vital capacity (FEF_{25-75}) and the shape of the expiratory flow-volume curve are more sensitive indicators of mild airway obstruction. A simple portable spirometer can be used to obtain the necessary measurements. Lack of patient cooperation, poor testing methods, and unreliable equipment can produce misleading results. The ATS/ERS statement contains criteria for the performance of spirometry, and NIOSH oversees courses for spirometry technicians that lead to their certification. Results of spirometry can be compared with predicted values from reference populations (adjusted for age, height, and sex) and expressed as a percentage of the predicted value. The presence of obstructive, restrictive, or mixed ventilatory impairment then can be determined from the comparison of observed with predicted values. Because the commonly used reference populations consist entirely of whites, there can be problems using predicted values to evaluate patients of nonwhite background. A NIOSH study produced separate reference-value equations for whites, African Americans, and Mexican Americans.

Another commonly used single-breath test that reflects the degree of airway obstruction is the peak expiratory flow rate (PEFR). Portable instruments such as the mini-Wright peak-flow meter can be used for its measurement. The major limitation of the PEFR is that patient self-recording of measurements usually is done, and thus there is a potential for malingering. Despite this limitation, the test is useful in detecting changes in airway obstruction over time. In addition, the use of computerized instruments, although more expensive than simple mechanical peak-flow meters, avoids the problems of patient self-recording. Serial peak-flow measurements are especially valuable in the diagnosis of occupational asthma to document delayed responses after the work shift is over.

Because FVC can be reduced as a consequence of disease processes that either restrict airflow into or obstruct airflow from the lungs, differentiation of restrictive from obstructive processes often requires measurement of static lung volumes, that is, total lung capacity (TLC), functional residual capacity (FRC), and residual volume (RV). These lung volumes are measured by inert gas dilution or body plethysmography. Restrictive lung diseases cause a reduction in TLC and other lung volumes, whereas obstructive diseases may result in hyperinflation and air trapping, that is, increased TLC and RV:TLC ratio.

The diffusing capacity of the lung for carbon monoxide (DL_{CO}) is a test of gas exchange in which the amount of inhaled carbon monoxide absorbed per unit time is measured. The DL_{CO} is closely correlated with the capacity of the lungs to absorb oxygen. A reduced DL_{CO} is a nonspecific finding; obstructive, restrictive, or vascular diseases all can cause reductions. Nevertheless, the DL_{CO} is used often in combination with other clinical evidence to support a specific diagnosis or to assess respiratory impairment.

▶ Bronchoprovocation Tests

Bronchoprovocation tests are useful in the diagnosis of occupational asthma. Pulmonary function responses to inhaled histamine and methacholine are relatively easy to measure and give an indication of the presence and degree of nonspecific hyperresponsiveness of the airways. A measure of airway obstruction, such as FEV_1, is obtained repeatedly after progressively increasing doses of histamine or methacholine so as to generate a dose-response curve. The test is usually terminated after a 20% fall in FEV_1. Patients with asthma typically respond with such a change in lung function after a relatively low cumulative dose of methacholine. Nonspecific challenge testing, as described earlier, is relatively inexpensive and can be performed on an outpatient basis. An ATS statement provides guidelines for the proper conduct of methacholine challenge.

Inhalation challenge testing with specific allergens thought to be causing occupational asthma also can be performed. Bronchoconstriction may occur early (within 30 minutes), late (in 4–8 hours), or in a dual response (Figure 19–1). The occurrence of any of these responses after inhaled allergen is specific and diagnostic of occupational asthma. Unfortunately, specific inhalation challenge tests are both expensive and potentially hazardous. These tests should be performed only at specialized centers.

TOXIC INHALATION INJURY

ESSENTIALS OF DIAGNOSIS

- ▶ Inhalational exposure to irritating agents can cause injury along the respiratory tract.
- ▶ The site of injury depends on the physical and chemical properties of the inhaled agent.
- ▶ The severity of injury depends on the intensity and duration of the exposure.
- ▶ Effects can range from transient, mild irritation of the mucous membranes of the upper airways to life-threatening pulmonary edema.

▶ General Considerations

Short-term exposures to high concentrations of noxious gases, fumes, or mists generally are a result of industrial or transportation accidents or fires. Inhalation injury from high-intensity exposures can result in severe respiratory impairment or death.

Details about the exposure in most cases should establish the causative chemical. The more serious exposures generally occur after major spills from industrial or transportation accidents or fires. Early effects depend on the level of exposure and may range from mild conjunctival and upper respiratory membrane irritation in low-dose exposures to life-threatening laryngeal or pulmonary edema in high-dose exposures.

The site of injury depends on the physical and chemical properties of the inhaled agent. The site of deposition of an inhaled gas is determined primarily by water solubility. Other important factors are the duration of exposure and the minute ventilation of the victim. The concentration of an inhaled water-soluble gas such as ammonia is greatly reduced by the time it reaches the trachea because of the efficient scrubbing mechanisms of the moist surfaces of the nose and throat. In contrast, a relatively water-insoluble gas, such as phosgene, is not well absorbed by the upper airways and thus may penetrate to the alveoli.

▶ Pathogenesis

The effects of inhalational exposure to toxic materials can range from transient, mild irritation of the mucous membranes of the upper airways to fatal adult respiratory distress syndrome (ARDS) (Table 19–2).

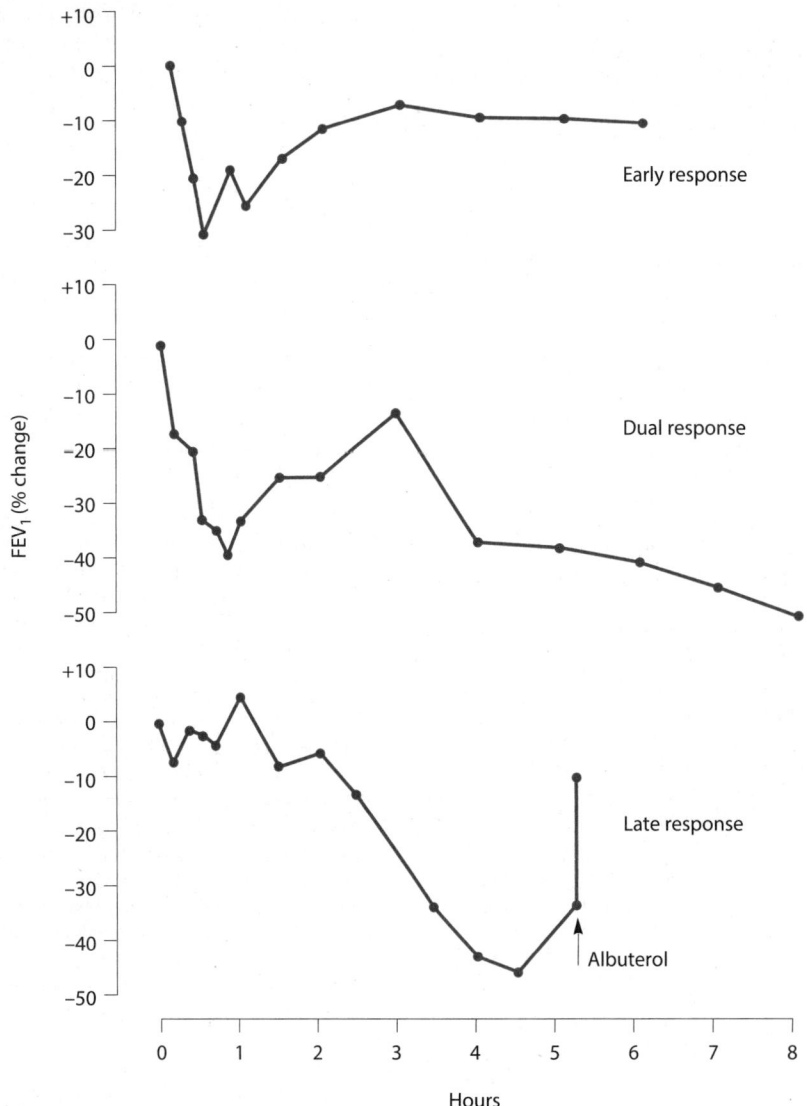

▲ **Figure 19–1.** Potential responses to inhalation of allergen in sensitized workers with asthma.

The adverse respiratory effects depend on the concentration of the substances inhaled. Low-dose exposure to a water-soluble agent such as ammonia or chlorine usually produces local irritation of conjunctival membranes and the upper airway. Moderate exposure to such an agent can result in hoarseness, cough, and bronchospasm. Acute high-level exposure can cause ARDS. Because of poor water solubility, certain agents, such as phosgene and oxides of nitrogen, are only mildly irritating to the upper respiratory tract. Once inhaled and deposited in the lower respiratory tract, however, these agents are highly irritating to the pulmonary parenchyma and may cause tissue necrosis.

▶ **Prevention**

The most effective approach to the prevention of acute lung injury from exposure to toxic agents is to substitute less toxic materials in products and processes.

▶ **Clinical Findings**

The initial focus of the physical examination must be on the airway. If the nose and throat are badly burned, or if there is hoarseness or stridor, chemical laryngitis should be suspected. The presence of early wheezing suggests that the exposure was relatively heavy. Spirometry or peak-flow

Table 19–2. Potential effects of inhaled irritants.

Site of Injury	Acute Effects	Chronic Effects
Eye, nose, sinuses, oropharynx	Irritation, inflammation	Corneal scarring, nasal polyps
Upper airway	Laryngeal edema, upper airway obstruction	Laryngeal polyps
Lower airways	Tracheobronchitis, bronchorrhea, decreased mucociliary clearance	Asthma, bronchiectasis
Lung parenchyma	Pneumonitis, pulmonary edema/adult respiratory distress syndrome	Pulmonary fibrosis, bronchiolitis obliterans

measurements may demonstrate airway obstruction relatively early after exposure.

The chest radiograph usually will be normal immediately postexposure. Chemical pneumonitis and pulmonary edema (ARDS) may develop within 4–8 hours of heavy exposure. Arterial blood gas measurements may show hypoxemia prior to radiographic evidence of parenchymal injury. Because of the relative lack of immediate signs and frequent delayed reactions to poorly water-soluble agents such as phosgene and oxides of nitrogen, patients exposed to significant concentrations of these agents should be observed for a minimum of 24 hours.

▶ **Complications**

Long-term sequelae from toxic inhalation injury include bronchiectasis, bronchiolitis obliterans, persistent asthma (see the discussion of irritant-induced asthma later in the text), and pulmonary fibrosis.

▶ **Treatment**

Management of toxic inhalation injury should include immediate decontamination of exposed cutaneous and conjunctival areas by irrigation with water. If facial cutaneous burns are noted, direct laryngoscopy or fiberoptic bronchoscopy is recommended by some to assess for the presence of laryngeal edema. If present, endotracheal intubation should be considered. However, it is by no means clear who will develop life-threatening upper airway obstruction. A conservative approach of careful clinical monitoring of the victim in an intensive-care unit may be appropriate. If bronchoscopy is performed, evidence of significant inhalation injury includes erythema, edema, ulceration, and/or hemorrhage of the airway mucosa. If particulate material was inhaled, it may be visualized on the airway mucosa.

Simple spirometry or peak expiratory flow measurements to detect early airway obstruction are often quite useful. Flow-volume loops have been used both to diagnose upper airway obstruction and as a more sensitive detector of early lower

airway obstruction and they do so better than simple spirometry or PEFRs. Supplemental oxygen should be administered if there is any sign of respiratory distress. Wheezing should be treated with an inhaled bronchodilator. Serial periodic clinical examinations, spirometry or peak-flow measurements, chest radiographs, and arterial blood gases are useful in monitoring progression of disease. There is no evidence to support the use of prophylactic antibiotics or the immediate use of corticosteroids in exposed patients.

Vigorous bronchial hygiene measures are required in those who develop severe tracheobronchitis. Drainage of mucus plugs and respiratory secretions should be encouraged by postural drainage, chest physical therapy, deep inspiratory maneuvers, and adequate hydration. If intubated, frequent suctioning of the airways should be performed to remove any adherent soot that may contain irritant and corrosive chemicals. Some authors recommend fiberoptic bronchoscopy to lavage off this adherent material.

Patients who develop pulmonary edema/ARDS require intensive-care-unit management, including mechanical ventilatory assistance. However, if such patients can be supported through the acute phase of the disease process, they may recover with no significant loss of lung function.

▶ **Prognosis**

Controversy exists, however, about the potential for long-term pulmonary sequelae after toxic inhalation injury. For example, there are well-documented reports of persisting airway obstruction, nonspecific airway hyperresponsiveness, and sequential reduction in RV following acute chlorine gas exposure. Until this controversy is resolved, it would seem prudent to follow exposed individuals with periodic clinical examinations and pulmonary function testing for the development of any persistent respiratory impairment. Although there is no controlled experimental evidence to support the practice, a trial of corticosteroids can be considered in a patient who is not recovering promptly. Such a trial may be especially beneficial in a patient with bronchiolitis obliterans following inhalation injury.

▼ **OCCUPATIONAL ASTHMA**

ESSENTIALS OF DIAGNOSIS

▶ Patients complain of dyspnea, wheezing, and/or cough that correlate with workplace exposures.

▶ Patients often report feeling better in the evenings or during weekends and vacations.

▶ Symptoms may occur 4–8 hours after exposure to the offending antigen. This may occur after the patient has left work or even at night.

▶ The suspected diagnosis should be confirmed with changes in lung function (spirometry or peak flow).

General Considerations

Asthma is characterized by airway obstruction that is reversible (but not completely so in some patients), either spontaneously or with treatment, airway inflammation, and increased airway responsiveness to a variety of stimuli. In occupational asthma, there is variable airway obstruction and/or airway hyperresponsiveness as a consequence of workplace exposure(s). Work-related variable airway obstruction can be caused by several mechanisms, including type I immune (immediate hypersensitivity) reactions, pharmacologic effects, inflammatory processes, and direct airway irritation. More than 250 agents in the workplace cause asthma, and the list is growing as new materials and processes are introduced. Work-aggravated asthma occurs when workplace exposures lead to exacerbations of preexisting nonoccupational asthma. In the United States, asthma occurs in approximately 5% of the general population. Work-related asthma (ie, both occupational asthma and work-aggravated asthma) has been estimated to be 15–20% of all adult asthma.

There are two major types of occupational asthma. Sensitizer-induced asthma is characterized by a variable time during which *sensitization* to an agent present in the work site takes place. Irritant-induced asthma occurs without a latent period after substantial exposure to an irritating dust, mist, vapor, or fume. *Reactive airways dysfunction syndrome* (RADS) is a term used to describe irritant-induced asthma caused by a short-term, high-intensity exposure. Sensitizing agents known to cause occupational asthma can be divided into high-molecular-weight (>1000 Da) and low-molecular-weight compounds (Table 19–3). High-molecular-weight compounds tend to cause occupational asthma via type I immunoglobulin E (IgE)–mediated reactions, whereas the mechanism(s) of low-molecular-weight compounds is (are) unknown. Sensitizer-induced asthma is characterized by specific responsiveness to the etiologic agent. The mechanism of irritant-induced asthma is also unknown, but there is no clinical evidence of sensitization. Irritant-induced asthma involves persistent nonspecific airway hyperresponsiveness but not specific responsiveness to an etiologic agent. While there is no doubt that irritant-induced asthma can be caused by a single intense exposure (eg, RADS), it appears that lower-level exposure over a longer duration of time (months to years) also can cause the disease.

Pathogenesis

Airway inflammation is now recognized as the paramount feature of asthma. Asthmatic airways are characterized by (1) infiltration with inflammatory cells, especially eosinophils, (2) edema, and (3) loss of epithelial integrity. Airway obstruction in asthma is believed to be the result of changes associated with airway inflammation. Airway inflammation is also believed to play an important role in the genesis of airway hyperresponsiveness.

Most of the research on mechanisms that mediate airway inflammation in asthma has focused on high-molecular-weight allergen-induced responses. In a previously sensitized individual, inhalation of a specific allergen allows interaction of the allergen with airway cells (mast cells and alveolar macrophages) that have specific antibodies (usually IgE) on the cell surface. This interaction initiates a series of redundant amplifying events that lead to airway inflammation. These events include mast-cell secretion of mediators, macrophage and lymphocyte activation, and eosinophil recruitment to the airways. The generation and release of various cytokines from alveolar macrophages, mast cells, sensitized lymphocytes, and bronchial epithelial cells are central to the inflammatory process (Figure 19–2). Cytokine networking, with both enhancing and inhibitory feedback loops, is responsible for inflammatory cell targeting to the bronchial epithelium, activation of infiltrating cells, and potential amplification of epithelial injury. Adhesion molecules also play critical roles in the amplification of the inflammatory process. The expression of various adhesion molecules is upregulated during the inflammatory cascade, and these molecules are essential for cell movement, cell attachment to the extracellular matrix and other cells, and possibly cell activation.

Table 19–3. Some agents causing occupational asthma.

Mechanism	Examples
Without "sensitization"	
Anticholinesterase effect	Organophosphate pesticide (agricultural workers)
Endotoxin effects	Cotton dust (textile workers)
Airway inflammation	Acids, ammonia, chlorine (custodial workers, paper manufacturing workers)
Airway irritation	Dusts, fumes, mists, vapors, cold (construction workers, chemical workers)
With "sensitization"	
High-molecular-weight agents IgE-mediated (complete allergens)	Animal and plant proteins (laboratory workers, bakers)
Low-molecular-weight agents IgE-mediated (haptens)	Antibiotics, metals (pharmaceutical workers, metal plating workers)
Mechanism undefined	Acid anhydrides, diisocyanates, plicatic acid (epoxy plastics and paints, polyurethane foams and paints, western red cedar products)

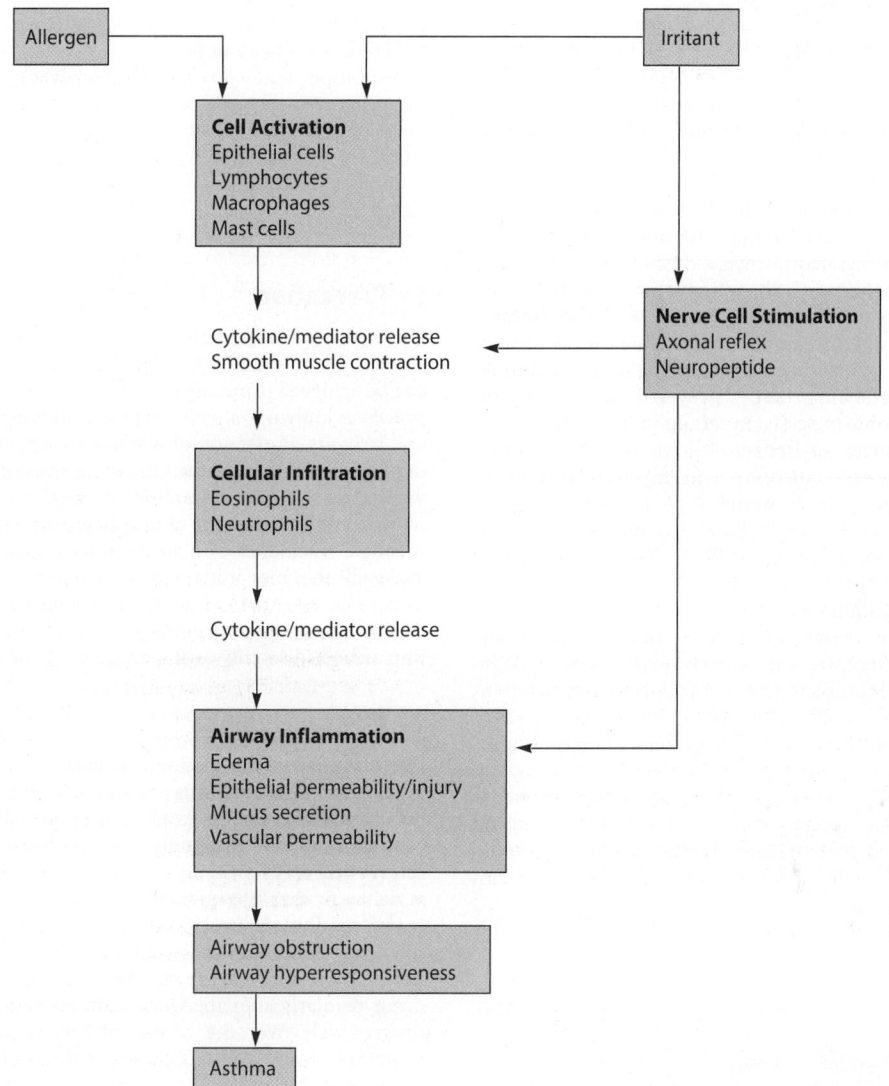

▲ **Figure 19–2.** Proposed pathways in the pathogenesis of asthma.

The mechanism of low-molecular-weight sensitizer-induced asthma is not well understood, although bronchial biopsy studies of affected workers clearly have demonstrated that airway inflammation is present.

Inhalation of the specific etiologic agent in a worker with sensitizer-induced asthma often will trigger rapid-onset but self-limited bronchoconstriction, called the *early response* (see Figure 19–1). In many sensitized workers, a delayed reaction will occur 4–8 hours later, called the *late response*. The late response is characterized by airway inflammation, persistent airway obstruction, and airway hyperresponsiveness. In some workers, there is a dual response, and in others,

only an isolated late response (see Figure 19–1). Mast-cell degranulation and release of mediators such as histamine are believed to be responsible for the early response. The role of the mast cell in the genesis of the late response is more controversial, but the release of chemoattractant substances such as leukotrienes, chemokines (eg, regulated on activation, normal T-cell expressed, and secreted [RANTES] and interleukin-8 [IL-8]) and cytokines (eg, IL-4, IL-5, and IL-13) may be involved in the influx of neutrophils and eosinophils into the airway epithelium. The eosinophil can release proteins (eg, major basic protein, eosinophilic cationic protein, eosinophil-derived neurotoxin, and enzymes), lipid mediators, and oxygen radicals that can cause epithelial injury. There is increasing evidence that lymphocytes, especially a CD4+ subset known as T-helper 2 (TH_2) cells, are involved in the release of cytokines that may activate both mast cells and eosinophils. In IgE-mediated allergic asthma, TH_2 cells may be responsible for the maintenance of chronic airway inflammation.

Although the mechanisms by which airway inflammation occurs in irritant-induced asthma are not well understood, neurogenic pathways may be involved (see Figure 19–2). The axonal reflex involving C-fiber stimulation and the release of neuropeptides have been implicated in models of irritant-induced airway inflammation. With high-level irritant exposure, direct chemical injury can lead to an inflammatory response. The important unanswered question is what causes this response to persist in certain individuals.

As the sensitizer- or irritant-induced airway inflammatory process proceeds, mucosal edema, mucus secretion, and vascular and epithelial permeability all increase, leading to a reduction of the caliber of the airway lumen and resulting airflow obstruction (Figure 19–3). The level of airway obstruction in patients with asthma is a marker of the severity of disease. With mild asthma, there may be no evidence of obstruction between acute exacerbations, but nonspecific airway hyperresponsiveness is likely to be present. With more severe asthma, there is increased airway hyperresponsiveness, and airway obstruction is present between attacks.

Two other mechanisms by which variable airway obstruction owing to workplace exposure can occur are reflex and pharmacologic bronchoconstriction. In reflex bronchoconstriction, neuroreceptors in the airway are stimulated by agents such as cold air, dusts, mists, vapors, and fumes. The reaction does not involve immunologic mechanisms

and does not lead to airway inflammation. In most cases, the patient has a history of preexisting nonoccupational asthma with nonspecific airway hyperresponsiveness so that this is the primary mechanism of work-aggravated asthma. Pharmacologic bronchoconstriction occurs when an agent in the workplace causes the direct release of mediators (eg, cotton dust in textile mills) or a direct effect on the autonomic regulation of bronchomotor tone (eg, organophosphate pesticides inhibit cholinesterase).

▶ Prevention

Prevention of further occupational asthma should be considered in all workplaces where cases are diagnosed. This can be achieved primarily through environmental control of processes known to involve exposure to potential sensitizers and irritants. Protection of workers by substitution of other materials for asthma-inducing agents, the use of appropriate ventilation systems, respiratory protective equipment, and worker education about appropriate procedures is recommended. Avoidance of high-intensity exposures from leaks and spills that may initiate the development of occupational asthma is essential. Medical surveillance for early detection of cases also can contribute to reducing the burden of impairment/disability owing to occupational asthma.

▶ Clinical Findings

The diagnosis of occupational asthma is made by confirming the diagnosis of asthma and by establishing a relationship between asthma and the work environment. The diagnosis of asthma should be made only when both intermittent respiratory symptoms and physiologic evidence of reversible or variable airways obstruction are present. The relationship between asthma and workplace exposure may fit any of the following patterns: (1) symptoms occur only at work, (2) symptoms improve on weekends or vacations, (3) symptoms occur regularly after the work shift, (4) symptoms increase progressively over the course of the workweek, and (5) symptoms improve after a change in the work environment.

At least one of the symptoms of wheezing, shortness of breath, cough, and chest tightness should occur while the worker is at or within 4–8 hours of leaving the workplace. Often the worker's symptoms improve during days off work or while away from the worker's usual job. With persistent exposure, the symptoms may become chronic and lose an obvious relationship to the workplace. Concomitant eye and upper respiratory tract symptoms also may be noted. The diagnosis of occupational asthma also should be considered when there is a history of recurrent episodes of work-related "bronchitis" characterized by cough and sputum production in an otherwise healthy individual. While high-molecular-weight sensitizers typically cause early or dual responses, the low-molecular-weight sensitizers tend to induce isolated late responses that may occur hours after the work shift is over.

The evaluation for possible occupational asthma requires a detailed history of the work environment (Figure 19–4).

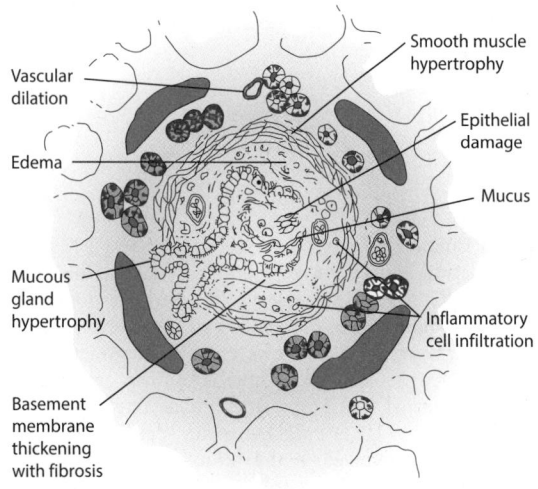

Smooth muscle hypertrophy

Vascular dilation

Epithelial damage

Edema

Mucus

Mucous gland hypertrophy

Inflammatory cell infiltration

Basement membrane thickening with fibrosis

▲ **Figure 19–3.** Morphologic changes in asthma.

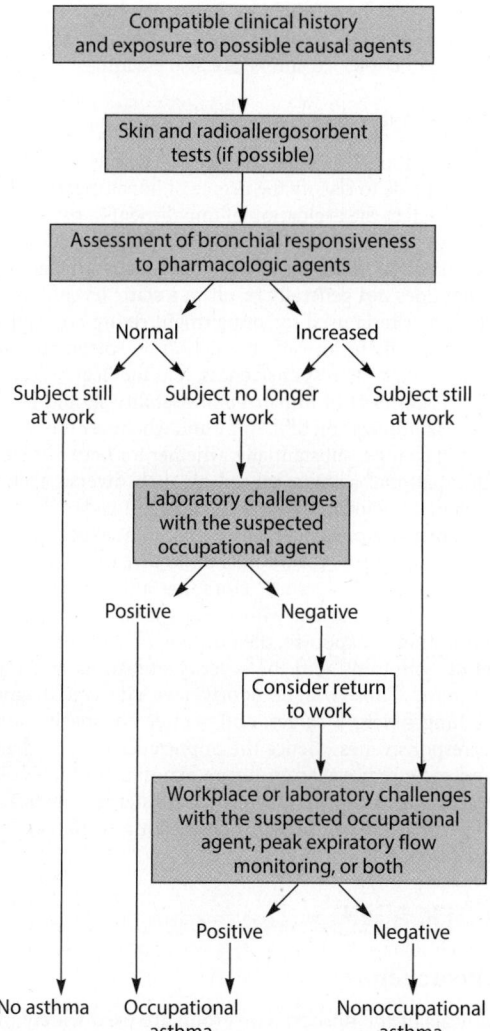

▲ **Figure 19–4.** Algorithm for the clinical investigation of occupational asthma.

than the lung parenchyma. Hyperinflation and flattening of the diaphragms, indicating air trapping, may be seen during exacerbations. Fleeting infiltrates indicating mucus plugging and bronchial wall thickening reflecting chronic inflammation also may be noted.

Spirometry for measurement of FEV_1 and FVC is the most reliable method for assessing airway obstruction. However, because asthmatic patients typically have reversible airway obstruction, they may have normal lung function during intervals between acute attacks. The response to inhaled bronchodilator administration has been used as a measure of airway hyperresponsiveness. A 12% improvement in FEV_1 of at least 200 mL after inhaled bronchodilator is how the ATS defines a significant improvement indicative of hyperresponsive airways. Across-work-shift spirometry, when available, can provide objective evidence of occupational asthma. A greater than 10% fall in FEV_1 across a work shift is suggestive of an asthmatic response.

Serial recording of PEFR over a period of weeks to months is often the best way to document the work-relatedness of asthma. The worker records his or her PEFR at least four times while awake, as well as respiratory symptoms and medication use. When interpreting the worker's log, attention should be given to any work-related pattern of change. A 20% or greater diurnal variability in PEFR is considered evidence of an asthmatic response (Figure 19–5). The major advantage of serial PEFR measurement over spirometry is the ability to detect late responses that occur after the work shift ends.

Methacholine or histamine challenge can demonstrate the presence of nonspecific airway hyperresponsiveness in a worker suspected of having occupational asthma who has normal spirometry. Such testing can be particularly valuable if it demonstrates an increase in airway responsiveness on

As noted earlier, attention should be given to the agents to which the worker is exposed, the type of ventilation in the workplace, whether respiratory protective equipment is used, and if possible, the level of exposure (ie, whether it is high or low or if accidental exposure through spills ever occurs). A helpful clue to a significant problem in a workplace is the presence of other workers with episodic respiratory symptoms.

The detection of wheezing on chest auscultation is helpful, but the physical examination is frequently normal in asthmatic patients not currently suffering from an exacerbation. Chest radiographs are normal in most individuals with asthma because the disease involves the airways rather

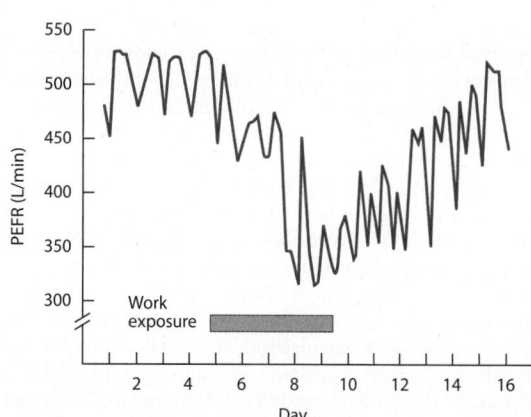

▲ **Figure 19–5.** Serial peak expiratory flow rates (PEFRs) during a 16-day period in a worker with occupational asthma before, during, and after 1 week of exposure to the inciting agent.

returning to work or a decrease when away from work. Specific inhalational challenge testing, that is, challenging the patient with the suspected agent at levels and under conditions that mimic workplace conditions, can be done for medicolegal purposes or to determine the precise etiology in a complex exposure scenario. However, specific challenge testing is time-consuming and potentially dangerous, and usually should be reserved for evaluation of patients in whom there is diagnostic uncertainty.

Allergy skin tests with common aeroallergens can be used to establish whether or not the worker is atopic. Atopy is a risk factor for high-molecular-weight sensitizer-induced asthma. When high-molecular-weight compounds are responsible for occupational asthma, skin tests with the appropriate extracts may help to identify the etiologic agent. Extracts of materials such as flour, animal proteins, and coffee will give positive skin tests in specifically sensitized individuals. Skin testing also may be helpful for a few low-molecular-weight compounds such as platinum salts. IgE antibodies assayed by the radioallergosorbent test (RAST) or by enzyme-linked immunoabsorbent assay (ELISA) may confirm exposure to allergens such as flour, animal proteins, acid anhydrides, plicatic acid, or isocyanates. However, the presence of positive skin reactions and/or specific antibodies is not always correlated with the presence of occupational asthma.

▶ Treatment

Acute asthma attacks requiring emergency management should be treated with supplemental oxygen, beta-agonists, corticosteroids, and if infection is suspected, antibiotics. Hospitalization should be considered in the more severe cases because of the potential for respiratory failure.

Once the diagnosis of occupational asthma is made, the primary intervention is to reduce or eliminate the worker's exposure to the offending agent. This may be achieved through modifications in the workplace. It may be possible to substitute the offending agent with another safer one. Improved local exhaust ventilation and enclosure of specific processes also may be helpful. With irritant-induced asthma, the use of personal protective equipment may lower exposures to levels that do not induce bronchospasm. Workers who are allowed to continue in the job should have regular follow-up visits, including monitoring of their lung function and nonspecific airway responsiveness. With sensitizer-induced asthma, however, the worker should be precluded from further exposure to the sensitizing agent. It may be necessary to completely remove the worker from the workplace because exposure to even minute quantities of the offending agent may induce bronchospasm. If a worker is required to leave the workplace (eg, a baker with flour-induced asthma), the worker should be considered 100% impaired on a permanent basis for the job that caused the illness and for other jobs with exposure to the same causative agent.

In addition to reduction or elimination of exposure to any specific offending agent, the worker also should avoid exposure to other materials/processes that may exacerbate the worker's asthma, such as irritating dusts, mists, and vapors. Cessation of smoking and avoidance of exposure to environmental tobacco smoke are also essential.

▶ Prognosis

Once occupational asthma has been diagnosed, an attempt should be made to classify the degree of impairment/disability. An approach to the evaluation of impairment in patients with asthma was developed by the ATS and has been adopted by the American Medical Association. Asthma is a dynamic disease that does not generally result in a static level of impairment. The criteria used for impairment rating are degree of postbronchodilator airway obstruction by spirometry, measurement of airway responsiveness, and medication requirements. Assessment of impairment/disability should be done only after optimization of therapy and whenever the worker's condition changes substantially, whether for better or worse.

Occupational asthma caused by such diverse agents as diisocyanates, snow crab, and western red cedar show persistence of symptoms and the presence of nonspecific airway hyperresponsiveness for periods up to 6 years after removal from the offending agent. Factors that affect the long-term prognosis of the patient with occupational asthma are the total duration of exposure, the duration of exposure after the onset of symptoms, and the severity of asthma at the time of diagnosis. Those who do poorly have a delayed diagnosis, lower lung function values, and greater nonspecific airway hyperresponsiveness, hence the importance of early diagnosis and early removal from future exposure to the etiologic agent. Treatment with inhaled corticosteroid medications has been shown to improve prognosis for sensitizer-induced occupational asthma.

SPECIFIC AGENTS

1. Diisocyanates

Chemicals of the diisocyanate group are used widely in the manufacture of polyurethane surface coatings, insulation materials, car upholstery, and furniture. The most commonly used diisocyanate is toluene diisocyanate (TDI). Because of its high vapor pressure, the less volatile agent methylene diphenyl diisocyanate (MDI) is used in some production processes. Other diisocyanates, such as hexamethylene diisocyanate (HDI), naphthalene diisocyanate (NDI), and isophorone diisocyanate (IPDI), also have commercial uses. These chemicals are all highly reactive because of the presence of –N–C–O groups, which easily react with biologic molecules and are potent irritants to the respiratory tract. Upper respiratory tract inflammation occurs in almost everyone exposed to TDI levels of 0.5 ppm or more.

Five major patterns of airway response to TDI have been described in humans: (1) occupational asthma of the sensitizer-type, which occurs in 5–10% of exposed workers weeks to months after the onset of exposure, (2) chemical bronchitis, (3) acute but asymptomatic deterioration of respiratory function during a work shift, (4) chronic deterioration of respiratory function associated with chronic exposure to low doses, and (5) persistent asthma or RADS after exposure to high doses.

2. Vegetable Dusts, Including Cotton (Byssinosis), Flax, Hemp, & Jute

Byssinosis occurs in certain workers in the cotton textile industry. The characteristic symptoms are chest tightness, cough, and dyspnea 1–2 hours after the patient returns to work after several days off. The symptoms usually resolve overnight and on subsequent days become milder until by the end of the workweek the worker may become asymptomatic. The prevalence of byssinosis is higher in workers with longer duration of exposure and with greater respirable dust exposure, such as during opening bales and carding, and lowest in those with a shorter exposure history and with lesser dust exposure. The mechanism underlying byssinosis remains unclear. Cotton-dust extracts are capable of causing direct release of histamine and contain endotoxins that can induce a number of inflammatory responses.

3. Metal Salts

Complex salts of platinum used in electroplating, platinum refinery operations, manufacture of fluorescent screens, and jewelry making are known to cause occupational asthma. Specific IgE antibodies to platinum salts conjugated to human serum albumin have been found in sensitized workers by RAST. Rhinitis and urticaria frequently accompany asthma, and this triad is sometimes called *platinosis*. Nickel, vanadium, chromium, and cobalt are other metals known to cause occupational asthma.

4. Acid Anhydrides

Epoxy resins often contain acid anhydrides as curing or hardening agents. Phthalic anhydride, trimellitic anhydride (TMA), and tetrachlorophthalic anhydride (TCPA) are several of the more commonly used acid anhydrides. Occupational asthma occurs in a small percentage of exposed workers. The serum of affected workers typically contains specific IgE antibodies against acid anhydride–protein conjugates. TMA exposure can give rise to four clinical syndromes: (1) symptoms of immediate airway irritation, (2) immediate rhinitis and asthma, (3) late asthma with systemic symptoms of fever and malaise, and (4) infiltrative lung disease (hemorrhagic alveolitis) with hemoptysis and anemia.

5. Wood Dusts

A large number of wood dusts are known to cause rhinitis and asthma. Western red cedar is the best studied. This wood contains the low-molecular-weight compound plicatic acid, which is believed to be responsible for causing asthma

through an unclear mechanism. Western red cedar asthma falls under the category of low-molecular-weight sensitizer-induced asthma and clinically is much like diisocyanate asthma. There is often a long period between onset of exposure and onset of symptoms, and asthma only develops in a small proportion of exposed subjects. A small dose of plicatic acid can induce a severe asthmatic attack in a sensitized individual, and many workers continue to have persistent asthma years after cessation of exposure.

HYPERSENSITIVITY PNEUMONITIS

ESSENTIALS OF DIAGNOSIS

▶ A link between symptoms and antigen exposure may be obtained from the work or environmental history.

▶ The antigen can be a microbial agent, animal protein, or chemical sensitizer.

▶ The clinical presentation can be acute, subacute, or chronic (insidious onset).

▶ General Considerations

Hypersensitivity pneumonitis, also known as *extrinsic allergic alveolitis*, refers to an immunologically mediated inflammatory disease of the lung parenchyma that is induced by inhalation of organic dusts that contain a variety of etiologic agents (eg, bacteria, fungi, amebae, animal proteins, and several low-molecular-weight chemicals). Although many different antigens are capable of causing hypersensitivity pneumonitis (Table 19–4), the basic clinical and pathologic findings are similar regardless of the nature of the inhaled dust. The nature of the inhaled antigen, the exposure conditions, and the nature of the host immune response all contribute to the risk for the disease. Hypersensitivity pneumonitis is characterized initially by a lymphocytic alveolitis and granulomatous pneumonitis, with improvement or complete resolution if antigen exposure is terminated early. Continued antigen exposure may lead to progressive interstitial fibrosis.

Inhalational exposure to antigen in a sensitized individual may result in either an acute or chronic presentation of hypersensitivity pneumonitis depending on the exposure conditions. The acute and more common form of presentation of hypersensitivity pneumonitis usually occurs within 4–6 hours of an intense exposure to the offending antigen. Recurrent low-level exposure to an appropriate antigen may result in the insidious onset of chronic ILD with fibrosis.

▶ Pathogenesis

The pathogenesis of hypersensitivity pneumonitis involves repeated inhalational exposure to the antigen, sensitization of the exposed individual, and immunologically mediated damage to the lung. The inflammatory response that results in hypersensitivity pneumonitis appears to involve

Table 19–4. Some agents causing hypersensitivity pneumonitis.

Antigen	Exposure	Syndrome
Bacteria		
Faenia rectivirgula	Moldy hay	Farmer's lung
Thermoactinomyces vulgaris	Moldy grain, compost	Grain worker's lung, mushroom worker's lung
Thermoactinomyces sacchari	Moldy sugar cane fiber	Bagassosis
Thermoactinomyces candidus	Heated water reservoirs	Humidifier lung
Bacillus subtilis	Detergent	Detergent worker's lung
Fungi		
Aspergillus clavatus	Moldy malt	Malt worker's lung
Penicillium casei	Moldy cheese	Cheese worker's lung
Penicillium frequentans	Moldy cork dust	Suberosis
Cryptostroma corticale	Moldy maple bark	Maple bark stripper's lung
Aureobasidium pullulans	Moldy redwood dust	Sequoiosis
Graphium spp.		
Amoebae		
Naegleria gruberi	Contaminated water	Humidifier lung
Acanthamoeba castellani		
Animal proteins		
Avian proteins	Bird droppings, feathers	Bird breeder's lung
Rodent proteins	Urine, sera, pelts	Animal handler's lung
Wheat weevil	Infested flour	Wheat weevil lung
Chemicals		
Toluene diisocyanate	Paints, coatings	Isocyanate lung
Hexamethylene diisocyanate		
Diphenylmethane diisocyanate	Polyurethane foam	
Trimellitic anhydride	Epoxy resins, paints	Trimellitic anhydride pulmonary hemorrhage-anemia syndrome

a combination of humoral, immune complex–mediated (type III), and cell-mediated (type IV) immune reactions to the inhaled antigen. In the presence of excess antigen, immune complexes may be deposited in the lungs. These complexes activate complement, leading to an influx of neutrophils. The local immune response later shifts to a T-lymphocyte-predominant alveolitis, with a differential cell count in bronchoalveolar lavage (BAL) fluid of up to 70% lymphocytes. Examination of BAL lymphocyte subpopulations in patients with hypersensitivity pneumonitis often has revealed a predominance of CD8+ suppressor/cytoxic cells. The peripheral blood and BAL T lymphocytes from patients with hypersensitivity pneumonitis will proliferate and undergo blastogenic transformation with cytokine generation when exposed in vitro to antigen. Animal models also support the role of cell-mediated immunity in the disease. Passive transfer of lymphocytes from sensitized animals to unexposed, nonsensitized animals results in a hypersensitivity pneumonitis–like disease when the latter animals subsequently are exposed to the specific antigen by inhalation. Alveolar macrophages also may play an important role in the pathogenesis of the disease by processing and presenting inhaled antigen to T-helper lymphocytes, as well as by releasing cytokines, which may help to amplify the inflammatory response.

Because only a small number of exposed persons ever develop hypersensitivity pneumonitis, the underlying mechanism of the disease may be a form of immune dysfunction in which a normal host defense response cannot be appropriately downregulated. This immune dysfunction may be, at least in part, genetically mediated. Other environmental factors also may be involved because a number of studies show that hypersensitivity pneumonitis occurs more frequently in nonsmokers than in smokers.

▶ **Prevention**

Exposure to agents capable of causing hypersensitivity pneumonitis should be avoided. Any area of a workplace or home where there is water damage involves potential risk of exposure to molds that could cause hypersensitivity pneumonitis. Such an area should be thoroughly cleaned and repaired. Moldy silage, compost, and plant material (eg, sugarcane, cork, redwood) as well as areas with heavy bird congregation should be avoided.

▶ **Clinical Findings**

Symptoms of chills, fever, malaise, myalgia, cough, headache, and dyspnea are noted commonly. Physical examination may reveal a relatively ill-appearing patient with bibasilar inspiratory crackles on chest auscultation. Frequently, acute hypersensitivity pneumonitis is misdiagnosed as an acute viral syndrome or pneumonia because it tends to closely mimic these conditions. Laboratory findings include peripheral blood leukocytosis with increased neutrophils and a relatively decreased lymphopenia. Arterial blood gas values may show hypoxemia.

Chest radiographic findings may be completely normal even in symptomatic individuals. Typically, however, the acute phase is associated with the presence of a reticulonodular pattern. Patchy densities that tend to coalesce also may be seen. These infiltrates usually are bilaterally distributed, but a more focal presentation sometimes occurs.

Pulmonary function testing may reveal a decrease in the FEV_1 and FVC with an unchanged FEV_1:FVC ratio consistent with a restrictive impairment. A decrease in the DL_{CO} reflecting impaired gas exchange also is typical of the acute presentation. The acute form generally progresses for up to 18–24 hours and then begins to resolve. Recurrence of the syndrome may be seen subsequently with reexposure to the antigen.

Progressive respiratory impairment with symptoms of dyspnea, cough, excessive fatigue, and weight loss may develop without acute episodes. Physical examination may reveal cyanosis, clubbing, and inspiratory crackles. Chest radiographic findings include diffusely increased linear markings and reduced lung size. Findings on HRCT scanning of the chest include centrilobular micronodules, ground-glass opacification, patchy airspace consolidation, and linear densities. Chest CT findings can be suggestive of the diagnosis of hypersensitivity pneumonitis but are not always pathognomonic. Pulmonary function testing usually will show a restrictive impairment with a decreased DL_{CO}, although some patients may be seen with a mixed or obstructive pattern.

The diagnosis of hypersensitivity pneumonitis should be suspected in patients with episodic respiratory symptoms and evidence of fleeting infiltrates on chest radiographs or restrictive impairment on pulmonary function testing. A careful history may elicit the onset of respiratory symptoms with exposure to the offending antigen. The temporal relationship of symptom development after exposure is crucial to the diagnosis. Additional supporting evidence is provided by the remission of symptoms and signs after cessation of exposure to the antigen and their reappearance on reexposure. The home environment also can be a source of the offending antigen. Workplace and home inspections may provide information supportive of the diagnosis (eg, evidence of mold or water damage).

Serologic studies demonstrating specific IgG precipitating antibodies by the traditional double-immunodiffusion technique will be positive in most patients with hypersensitivity pneumonitis if the correct antigen is used, although such antibodies are also detected frequently in exposed individuals who are healthy. False-positive results may be obtained with the use of more sensitive assays for IgG, such

as ELISA. False-negative results frequently are a result of the failure to test for the correct antigen. Most commercially available hypersensitivity pneumonitis panels involve only a limited number of common antigens. Inhalational challenge studies with the suspected antigen may assist in the diagnosis of hypersensitivity pneumonitis. Antigen extracts may be administered in an aerosolized form followed by serial pulmonary function testing. Specific challenge testing should be conducted only by a laboratory experienced in the technique. While such challenges provide the "gold standard" method of confirming a direct relationship between a suspected offending antigen and the disease process, workplace studies involving the actual conditions of patient exposure are safer and usually easier to conduct.

Analysis of BAL fluid obtained by fiberoptic bronchoscopy in patients with hypersensitivity pneumonitis often demonstrates an increased percentage of T lymphocytes that are primarily CD8+ suppressor cells. In sarcoidosis, another condition characterized by increased T lymphocytes in BAL, the predominant cells are of the CD4+ helper subtype.

Lung biopsy may be necessary to make the diagnosis in difficult cases, such as those with the chronic form and an insidious presentation of dyspnea. Video-assisted thoracoscopic surgery (VATS) or open lung biopsy is preferred because transbronchial biopsy may not provide adequate tissue for pathologic differentiation of hypersensitivity pneumonitis from other diseases such as sarcoidosis. In acute or early chronic (subacute) hypersensitivity pneumonitis, there is patchy infiltration of predominantly lymphocytes in a bronchocentric distribution, usually with accompanying epithelioid (ie, noncaseating) granulomas. The granulomas are likely what appear as centrilobular micronodules on HRCT scanning. In chronic hypersensitivity pneumonitis, peribronchiolar inflammation remains prominent, and bronchiolitis obliterans is common. Large histiocytes with foamy cytoplasm may be seen in the alveoli and interstitium. Interstitial fibrosis with honeycombing occurs in advanced disease, by which time granulomas no longer may be evident.

▶ Complications

The primary complication of hypersensitivity pneumonitis is the development of irreversible lung fibrosis.

▶ Treatment

The key to successful treatment of hypersensitivity pneumonitis is avoidance of the offending antigen. As described for occupational asthma, this may be achieved by product substitution or institution of effective engineering controls. Respiratory protective equipment also may be appropriate in situations where possible exposure is only occasional. If persistence of symptoms occurs despite engineering control measures and respiratory protective equipment, complete removal of the worker from exposure is necessary.

Corticosteroids remain the mainstay of treatment of patients with severe or progressive hypersensitivity pneumonitis, despite the lack of controlled data regarding the effect of these agents on the disease process. An empirical trial of prednisone (1 mg/kg/d), with monitoring of chest radiographic and pulmonary function changes 1 month after starting the trial, is a reasonable approach. Therapy should be continued until there is significant clinical improvement. If bronchospasm is present, beta-agonists should be administered. Supplemental oxygen should be given to patients with hypoxemia, and intensive-care-unit support may be needed in particularly severe acute cases.

▶ **Prognosis**

Workers with a diagnosis of hypersensitivity pneumonitis should have frequent follow-up, especially if continued exposure to antigen is possible. If further exposure to the offending agent is avoided, the prognosis is good. Significant pulmonary morbidity may occur if persistent exposure is allowed.

▼ INHALATION FEVERS

ESSENTIALS OF DIAGNOSIS

▶ Inhalational exposure to organic dusts, polymer fumes, and certain metals can cause a flu-like illness.

▶ The illness is usually self-limited.

▶ Bilateral infiltrates on chest x-ray are usually present.

▶ **General Considerations**

Inhalation fever refers to several syndromes that are characterized by short-term but debilitating flulike symptoms after exposure to organic dusts, polymer fumes, and metal fumes (Table 19–5). In addition to fever, the symptoms

Table 19–5. Some agents causing inhalation fever.

Agent	Syndrome
Metals Zinc Copper Magnesium	Metal fume fever
Teflon pyrolysis products Polytetrafluoroethylene	Polymer fume fever
Bioaerosols Contaminated water Moldy silage, compost, wood chips Sewage sludge Cotton, jute, hemp, flax dust Grain dust	Humidifier fever Organic dust toxic syndrome Mill fever Grain fever

include chills, myalgia, headache, malaise, cough, and chest discomfort.

In contrast to occupational asthma and hypersensitivity pneumonitis, which require susceptibility and/or sensitization, the attack rate for the inhalation fevers is high; that is, most people will experience symptoms as a result of high-level exposure to the etiologic agents.

SPECIFIC SYNDROMES

1. Metal Fume Fever

▶ **General Considerations**

Inhalation of certain freshly formed metal oxides can cause metal fume fever, an acute self-limiting flulike illness. The most common cause of this syndrome is the inhalation of zinc oxide, which is generated from molten bronze or welding galvanized steel. The oxides of only two other metals, copper and magnesium, have been proven to cause metal fume fever. When zinc is heated to its melting point, zinc oxide fumes are generated. The particle size of the generated fumes ranges from 0.1 to 1 μm in diameter, although aggregation with the formation of larger particles occurs readily. The underlying pathogenesis of metal fume fever is incompletely understood. However, there is evidence from controlled human exposure studies that zinc oxide fume inhalation induces a leukocyte recruitment to the lungs with an associated release of cytokines, which causes systemic symptoms.

It is estimated that more than 700,000 workers in the United States are involved in welding operations, so the potential for inhalational exposure and metal fume fever is great. The clinical syndrome begins 3–10 hours after exposure to zinc oxide. The initial symptom may be a metallic taste associated with throat irritation and followed within several hours by the onset of fever, chills, myalgia, malaise, and a nonproductive cough. Occasionally, nausea, vomiting, and headache are noted. Physical examination during the episode may reveal a febrile patient with crackles on auscultation of the chest. Laboratory evaluation frequently reveals a leukocytosis with a left shift and an elevated serum lactate dehydrogenase level. The chest radiograph, pulmonary function tests, and arterial blood gas measurements usually are normal. Transient chest radiographic infiltrates and reduced lung volumes and DL_{CO} have been reported in severe cases. Signs and symptoms generally peak at 18 hours and resolve spontaneously with complete resolution of abnormalities within 1–2 days.

Treatment of metal fume fever is entirely symptomatic. Control of elevated body temperature by antipyretics and oxygen therapy for hypoxemia may be required. There is no evidence that steroid therapy is of any benefit. Prevention relies on appropriate engineering controls and/or personal protective equipment to reduce exposure. There are no good data on the long-term sequelae of repeated exposures.

2. Polymer Fume Fever

A syndrome similar to metal fume fever may occur after inhalation of combustion products of polytetrafluoroethylene (Teflon) resins. The properties of Teflon—strength, thermal stability, and chemical inertness—make it a widely used product in the manufacture of cooking utensils, electric appliances, and insulating material. When Teflon is heated to temperatures greater than 300°C (572°F), numerous degradation products are formed that appear to cause the syndrome. Exposure to such combustion products can occur during welding of metal coated with Teflon, during the operation of molding machines, and while smoking cigarettes contaminated with the polymer.

Exposure to a high concentration of polymer fumes causes a fever to develop within several hours. Often this occurs toward the end of the work shift or in the evening after work. The symptoms, signs, and laboratory findings of polymer fume fever are essentially the same as those of metal fume fever. The syndrome is self-limiting and resolves within 12–48 hours. Exposure to very high concentrations of polymer fumes may lead to the development of severe chemical pneumonitis with pulmonary edema. In such cases, the symptoms, signs, and laboratory features are similar to pulmonary edema from other causes.

3. Organic Dust Toxic Syndrome

Inhalation of various bioaerosols contaminated with fungi, bacteria, and/or endotoxins can cause an acute febrile syndrome known as *organic dust toxic syndrome* (ODTS). Exposures to moldy silage, moldy wood chips, compost, sewage sludge, grain dust (grain fever), cotton dust (mill fever), animal confinement building environments, and contaminated humidifier mist (humidifier fever) are associated with the development of inhalation fever. The clinical syndrome of ODTS is essentially identical to that described earlier for metal or polymer fume fever. Severe pulmonary inflammatory reactions have been described with massive exposures, but these are rare.

▼ METAL-INDUCED LUNG DISEASE

ESSENTIALS OF DIAGNOSIS

▶ Inhalational exposure to several metals can cause immune-mediated ILD. The clinical presentation is similar to that of other types of ILD.

▶ General Considerations

Metal-induced ILD appears to be due to cell-mediated sensitization to the offending agent. While greater exposure is associated with increased risk, likely genetic predisposition plays an important role.

SPECIFIC METALS

1. Hard Metal

Hard metal is a cemented alloy of tungsten carbide with cobalt, although other metals such as titanium, tantalum, chromium, molybdenum, or nickel also may be added. These cemented carbides have found wide industrial use because of their properties of extreme hardness, strength, and heat resistance. Their major use is in the manufacture of cutting tools and drill-tip surfaces.

Workers exposed to hard metal are at risk for developing ILD, the so-called hard-metal disease, and occupational asthma. The putative cause of both these disease processes is cobalt. Some workers may present with features of both hard metal–induced airway and parenchymal diseases. Workers at risk for these diseases are those engaged in the manufacture of the alloy, grinders and sharpeners of hard metal tools, and diamond polishers and others who use disks containing cobalt and metal coaters who use powdered hard metal. Occupational asthma caused by cobalt in hard-metal workers is similar to that caused by other low-molecular-weight sensitizer agents.

Workers with hard-metal disease typically complain of symptoms of dyspnea on exertion, cough, sputum production, chest tightness, and fatigue. Physical examination may reveal evidence of crackles on chest auscultation, reduced chest expansion, clubbing, and in advanced cases, cyanosis. Chest radiographs may show bilateral rounded and/or irregular opacities with no pathognomonic features. Pulmonary function tests tend to show both a restrictive ventilatory impairment and a decreased DL_{CO}. The diagnosis of hard-metal disease often is made on the basis of pathologic examination of lung tissue rather than by clinical evaluation. The histologic findings are those of interstitial pneumonitis, frequently of the giant-cell type (eg, giant-cell interstitial pneumonia), and interstitial fibrosis. Characteristic multinucleated giant histiocytes may be seen in BAL fluid as well.

The primary treatment of hard-metal disease is removal of the affected worker from further exposure. Relatively rapid progression to impairment is not infrequent, and resolution after cessation of exposure may not occur. Complete removal from cobalt exposure is advisable because a case has been reported of a worker who developed rapidly fatal lung disease with continued exposure. Because hard-metal disease is often progressive, empirical therapy with corticosteroids may be required.

2. Beryllium

Beryllium is a light-weight, tensile metal that has a high melting point and good alloying properties. It has a wide range of applications in modern industrial processes. Although beryllium is no longer used in the manufacture of fluorescent light tubes, it is used commonly in the ceramics, electronics, aerospace, and nuclear weapons/power industries. Workers at risk are those involved in processes that generate airborne beryllium, including melting, casting, grinding, drilling, extracting, and smelting of beryllium. Acute beryllium-induced pneumonitis can occur after high-intensity exposure but has largely disappeared owing to improved workplace control of exposures. Chronic beryllium disease, which involves sensitization to the metal through a cell-mediated (type IV) mechanism, still occurs after lower-level exposures in susceptible workers. Beryllium can be phagocytosed by macrophages that present beryllium antigen to lymphocytes, resulting in sensitization and proliferation of beryllium-specific CD4+ T cells. Beryllium-activated T cells may release various cytokines and other inflammatory mediators, resulting in granuloma formation. Latency from time of initial beryllium exposure to the development of clinically manifest disease ranges from months to many years.

Why only a small percentage of an exposed population becomes sensitized to beryllium is not well understood. Genetic studies have found markers of risk for beryllium sensitization, especially a glutamic acid substitution in residue 69 of the beta chain of the major histocompatibility complex molecule HLA-DP.

Chronic beryllium disease is a granulomatous inflammatory disorder that is very similar to sarcoidosis. In fact, the histologic findings in chronic beryllium disease are identical to those of sarcoidosis; that is, epithelioid (noncaseating) granulomas with mononuclear cell infiltrates and varying degrees of interstitial fibrosis. Chronic beryllium disease usually affects only the lungs, but involvement of other organs may occur. Extrapulmonary involvement is less common than in sarcoidosis.

Workers with chronic beryllium disease commonly present with insidious onset of dyspnea on exertion, cough, and fatigue. Anorexia, weight loss, fever, chest pain, and arthralgias also may occur. Physical examination findings usually are confined to the lungs, with crackles being the most common, but they may be absent with mild disease.

Chest radiographic findings are ill-defined nodular or irregular opacities and hilar adenopathy. The latter is seen somewhat less frequently than in sarcoidosis and rarely occurs in the absence of parenchymal changes. The small nodular opacities sometimes are more prominent in the upper lung zones and may coalesce into more conglomerate masses. HRCT scanning is more sensitive than plain chest radiography, but histologically confirmed cases occur with normal scans.

Pulmonary function testing may be normal with mild disease, but there is usually a restrictive, obstructive, or mixed pattern of impairment and a reduced DL_{CO}. Resting arterial hypoxemia and further desaturation with exercise are common with more severe disease.

Often a meticulously obtained occupational history is required to suggest beryllium as the causative agent. Because of the similarity between chronic beryllium disease and sarcoidosis, demonstration of beryllium sensitization is necessary to confirm the diagnosis. A relatively specific blood lymphocyte proliferation test (LPT) is available in which the beryllium-specific uptake of radiolabeled DNA precursors by the patient's lymphocytes cultured in vitro is quantitated. The sensitivity of the LPT for chronic beryllium disease is greater than 90% when using peripheral blood lymphocytes and can be increased if lung lymphocytes obtained from BAL are used. The blood LPT also can be used to screen for sensitization among beryllium-exposed workers.

The current criteria for the diagnosis of chronic beryllium disease are (1) a history of beryllium exposure, (2) a positive peripheral blood or BAL LPT, and (3) the presence of epithelioid granulomas and mononuclear infiltrates, in the absence of infection, in lung tissue. This approach relies on the LPT to confirm sensitization to beryllium and transbronchial biopsy of lung tissue to confirm the presence of disease.

Because the disease process involves a type of hypersensitivity, a worker with chronic beryllium disease should be completely removed from further beryllium exposure. A trial of corticosteroids is warranted in symptomatic workers with documented pulmonary physiologic abnormalities because this may induce a remission in some. If steroid therapy is initiated, objective parameters of response such as chest radiographs and pulmonary function test results should be monitored serially in order to adjust appropriately the dose and duration of treatment. Chronic beryllium disease has the propensity to develop into chronic irreversible pulmonary fibrosis, so careful monitoring of affected workers is necessary.

3. Other Metals

Inhalation of relatively high concentrations of cadmium, chromium, or nickel fumes or mercury vapor can cause toxic pneumonitis. Occupational exposure to certain metals (eg, antimony, barium, iron, and tin) can lead to deposition of sufficient radiodense dust that chest radiographs demonstrate opacities in the absence of lung parenchymal inflammation and fibrosis. Indium-tin-oxide (ITO) is an indium compound with widespread applications, including touch screens and photovoltaic cells. Exposure of workers involved in the production, use, or reclamation of ITO can develop a potentially fatal condition characterized by pulmonary alveolar proteinosis (PAP) that may progress to fibrosis with or without emphysema.

▼ PNEUMOCONIOSES

ESSENTIALS OF DIAGNOSIS

▶ Chronic exposure, usually over years, to mineral dusts can cause fibrotic ILD.

▶ Symptoms are typically progressive dyspnea and dry cough.

▶ Diagnosis is usually made on the basis of radiographic abnormalities, which may precede lung function impairment.

▶ General Considerations

The pneumoconioses are a group of conditions resulting from the deposition of mineral dust in the lung and the subsequent fibrotic lung tissue reaction to the dust. The diagnosis is usually made based on chest imaging. Radiographically evident interstitial opacities may appear before impairment of pulmonary function or symptoms.

The risk of disease is clearly associated with level of exposure. Chronic exposure (ie, years) is required for most types of pneumoconiosis. Typically, a long latent period (>5 years) between onset of exposure and clinical manifestation of disease is also required.

SPECIFIC PNEUMOCONIOSES

1. Silicosis

Silicosis is a parenchymal lung disease that results from the inhalation of silicon dioxide, or silica, in crystalline form. Silica is a major component of rock and sand. Workers with potential for exposure are miners, sandblasters, foundry workers, tunnel drillers, quarry workers, stone carvers, ceramic workers, and silica flour production workers.

Exposure to silica can lead to one of three disease patterns: (1) chronic simple silicosis, which usually follows more than 10 years of exposure to respirable dust with less than 30% quartz, (2) subacute/accelerated silicosis, which generally follows shorter, heavier exposures (ie, 2–5 years), and (3) acute silicosis, which is seen often following intense exposure to fine dust of high silica content over a several-month period.

Chronic silicosis is characterized by the formation of silicotic nodules in the pulmonary parenchyma and the hilar lymph nodes (Figure 19–6). The lesions in the hilar lymph

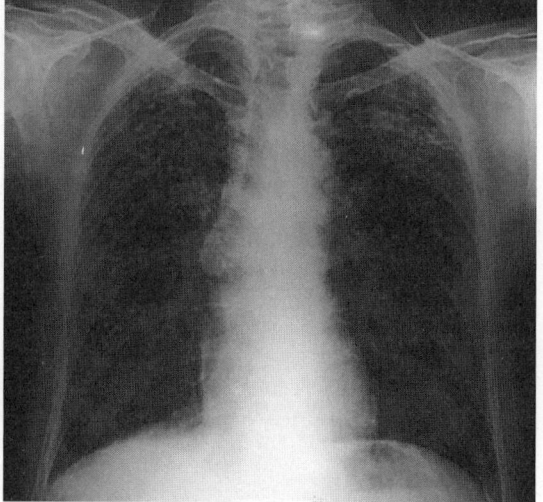

▲ **Figure 19–6.** Radiographic changes of simple silicosis.

nodes may calcify in an "egg shell" pattern that, while only occurring in a small proportion of cases, is virtually pathognomonic for silicosis. Lung parenchymal involvement tends to have a predilection for the upper lobes. The coalescence of small silicotic nodules into larger fibrotic masses, called *progressive massive fibrosis* (PMF), may complicate a minority of cases. PMF tends to occur in the upper lung fields, may obliterate blood vessels and bronchioles, causes gross distortion of lung architecture, and leads to respiratory insufficiency.

Accelerated silicosis is similar to chronic silicosis except that the time span is shorter and the complication of PMF is seen more frequently. Two modern exposure scenarios that have been associated with accelerated silicosis are "aging" of denim jeans through sandblasting and the fabrication of artificial stone countertops. Acute silicosis is a rare condition seen in workers who are exposed to very high concentrations of free silica dust with fine particle size. Such exposures occur frequently in the absence of adequate respiratory protection. The characteristic findings differ from chronic silicosis in that the lungs show consolidation without silicotic nodules, and the alveolar spaces are filled with fluid similar to that found in PAP. Acute silicosis leads to death in most cases.

Alveolar macrophages play an important role in the pathogenesis of silicosis because these cells ingest inhaled silica and then release cytokines that recruit and/or stimulate other cells. Although crystalline silica can be cytotoxic secondary to direct chemical damage to cellular membranes, the primary effect of inhaled silica on macrophages is activation. The silica-activated macrophages recruit and activate T lymphocytes, which, in turn, recruit and activate a secondary population of monocytes-macrophages. The activated macrophages produce cytokines, which stimulate fibroblasts to proliferate and produce increased amounts of collagen.

There are few symptoms and signs of chronic simple silicosis. The diagnosis usually is made by chest radiographs, which frequently reveal small round opacities (<10 mm in diameter) in both lungs, with a predilection for the upper lung zones. If an adequate occupational history is obtained from the patient along with a thorough review of the chest radiographs, the diagnosis of silicosis should not present any great difficulty. Pulmonary function testing in patients with simple silicosis is usually normal but occasionally may demonstrate evidence of a mild restrictive ventilatory defect and decreased lung compliance. In addition, a mild obstructive impairment is found occasionally in patients with simple silicosis, often as a consequence of chronic bronchitis caused by nonspecific dust effects and/or smoking. With complicated silicosis involving progressive fibrosis (nodules >10 mm in diameter), increasing dyspnea is noted, initially with exertion and then progressing to dyspnea at rest. Complicated chronic silicosis is associated with greater reductions in lung volumes, decreased diffusing capacity, and hypoxemia with exercise. PMF is the end-stage of complicated chronic silicosis.

There is an increased incidence of mycobacterial disease, both typical and atypical, in silicosis. Fungal diseases (especially cryptococcosis, blastomycosis, and coccidioidomycosis) are also seen with greater frequency. The mechanism by which the immune-inflammatory responses to inhaled silica lead to the increased incidence of mycobacterial and fungal infections is not clearly understood. Silicosis is also associated with increased risk for autoimmune diseases such as rheumatoid arthritis and systemic sclerosis.

Because no treatment for silicosis is currently known, management is directed toward the prevention of progression and the development of complications. Continued exposure should be avoided, and surveillance for tuberculosis should be instituted. Tuberculin-positive persons with silicosis have an approximately 30-fold greater risk for developing tuberculosis and should be treated for latent tuberculosis with a regimen proven to be efficacious. In acute silicosis, therapeutic whole-lung lavage has been employed to physically remove silica from the alveoli.

The prognosis for patients with chronic silicosis is good, especially if they are removed from exposure. Mortality remains high, however, in those who develop PMF.

2. Asbestosis

Asbestos is the name for the fibrous forms of a group of mineral silicates. The types of asbestos that have been used commercially are chrysotile, amosite, crocidolite, anthophyllite, tremolite, and actinolite, with chrysotile being the most commonly used. The durability, heat resistance, and ability to be woven into textiles of asbestos led to a wide variety of industrial applications. Major occupational exposures occurred with asbestos mining and milling, manufacture or installation of insulation for ships or buildings, manufacture of friction materials for brake linings and clutch facings, asbestos cement manufacture, asbestos textile manufacture, and asbestos-containing spray products for decorative, acoustical, and fireproofing purposes.

Asbestosis refers to the diffuse interstitial pulmonary fibrosis caused by inhalation of asbestos fibers. The inhaled fibers are deposited primarily at the bifurcations of conducting airways and alveoli, where they are phagocytosed by macrophages. The initial injury is characterized by damage to the alveolar epithelium, incomplete phagocytosis by and activation of alveolar and interstitial macrophages, and release of proinflammatory cytokines as well as cytotoxic oxygen radicals by activated macrophages. A peribronchiolar inflammatory response ensues involving fibroblast proliferation and stimulation, which eventually may lead to fibrosis. Many factors are felt to play a role in disease initiation and progression, including the type and size of fiber, the intensity and duration of exposure, history of cigarette smoking, and individual susceptibility. A dose-response relationship exists such that asbestosis is more common in workers with a higher exposure level. Once asbestosis begins, it may progress irrespective of removal from continued exposure. Finally, there is a considerable latency period (usually at least 20 years) between onset of exposure and development of clinically apparent disease. The diagnosis of asbestosis is made by a thorough exposure history, clinical examination,

appropriate imaging studies, and pulmonary function testing. The symptoms of asbestosis are indistinguishable from those of any other gradually progressive interstitial pulmonary fibrosing disorder, with progressive dyspnea and nonproductive cough being the most prominent. Bibasilar crackles with a "Velcro" quality can be auscultated over the posterolateral chest in the middle to late phase of inspiration. The crackles of asbestosis are unaffected by coughing.

Imaging studies that are helpful in the evaluation of asbestos-exposed patients are the chest radiograph and HRCT scan. The chest radiograph shows characteristic small, irregular or linear opacities distributed throughout the lung fields but more prominent in the lower zones. There is loss of definition of the heart border and hemidiaphragms. The most useful radiographic finding is the presence of bilateral pleural thickening, which does not occur commonly with other diseases-causing interstitial pulmonary fibroses (Figure 19–7). Diaphragmatic or pericardial calcification is almost a pathognomonic sign of asbestos exposure. The ILO classification system is often used in the United States to rate the degree of profusion of small, irregular opacities and of pleural thickening on the chest radiograph. Conventional chest CT scanning is more sensitive than chest radiography for the detection of pleural disease but not for parenchymal disease. HRCT scanning is the most sensitive imaging method for detecting early asbestosis.

Depending on the severity of disease, pulmonary function testing will show varying degrees of restrictive impairment

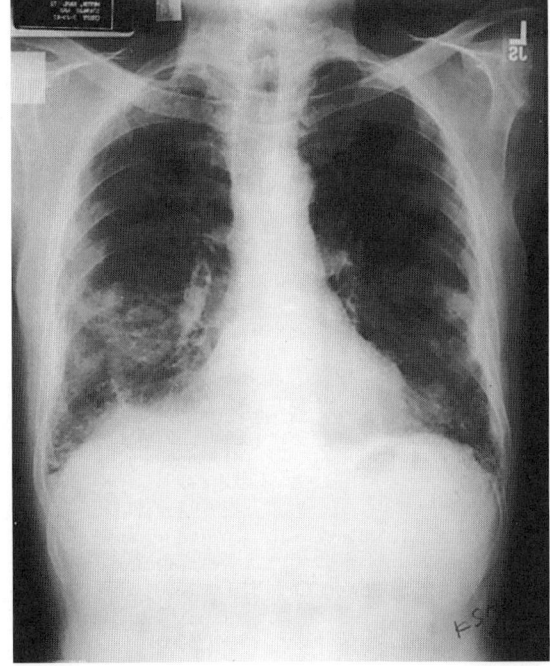

▲ **Figure 19–7.** Radiographic changes of asbestosis.

and decreased DL_{CO}. Because asbestosis begins as a peribronchiolar process, reduced flow rates at low lung volumes, indicative of small airways obstruction, may be seen.

As for silicosis, there is no known treatment for asbestosis. Fortunately, only a minority of those exposed are likely to develop radiographically evident disease, and among these, most do not develop significant respiratory impairment. Workers with asbestosis should be removed from further asbestos exposure because the risk that parenchymal scarring will progress appears to increase with cumulative asbestos exposure. Any other factors that may contribute to respiratory disease should be reduced or eliminated. This is especially true of cigarette smoking because there is some evidence that it may contribute to the initiation and progression of asbestosis.

The substitution of other fibrous materials for asbestos and the institution of strict environmental controls where it is still present have led to a dramatic reduction in occupational exposures to asbestos. Medical surveillance of all currently exposed workers in the United States is required by Occupational Safety and Health Administration (OSHA) regulation.

3. Coal Workers' Pneumoconiosis

Coal workers' pneumoconiosis is the term used to describe parenchymal lung disease caused by the inhalation of coal dust. Miners who work at the coal face in underground mining and drillers in surface mines are at greatest risk of contracting this disease. A heavy coal dust burden is required to induce coal workers' pneumoconiosis, and the condition is seen rarely in those who have spent fewer than 20 years underground. However, modern US coal industry practices have been associated with a higher rate of coal workers' pneumoconiosis, including PMF, in recent years, perhaps due to due to increased mechanization and higher silica content of coal dust.

The coal macule is the primary lesion in coal workers' pneumoconiosis. It is formed when the inhaled dust burden exceeds the amount that can be removed by alveolar macrophages and mucociliary clearance. This leads to retention of coal dust in the terminal respiratory units. Prolonged retention causes lung fibroblasts to secrete a limiting layer of reticulin around the dust collection, or macule, near the respiratory bronchiole. Progressive enlargement of the macule may weaken the bronchiole wall to create a focal area of centrilobular emphysema; coalescence of small macules into larger lesions may occur. Initially, there is a predilection for the upper lung lobes, but with progression of the disease, the lower lobes become involved. As for silicosis, coal workers' pneumoconiosis can be characterized as simple (radiographic lesions <10 mm in diameter) or complicated (lesions >10 mm in diameter). Only a small proportion of miners develop complicated or progressive fibrotic disease, but that proportion has been increasing over the last decade. PMF, identical to that described earlier for silicosis, may occur.

The symptoms of cough and sputum production are common among coal miners and often are the result of chronic bronchitis from dust inhalation rather than coal workers' pneumoconiosis. As with silicosis, simple coal workers' pneumoconiosis is often asymptomatic. The symptoms and signs associated with complicated disease are the same as those described earlier for silicosis. PMF almost invariably leads to respiratory insufficiency and death.

The chest radiograph in simple coal workers' pneumoconiosis shows the presence of small, rounded opacities in the lung parenchyma. Often seen first in the upper lung zones, these opacities may involve the lower zones in the later stage of the disease. Calcification of the hilar lymph nodes is not seen unless there is concomitant silica exposure. Complicated coal workers' pneumococcosis/PMF is diagnosed when large parenchymal opacities are present.

Caplan syndrome may occur in coal miners with rheumatoid arthritis and is characterized by the appearance of rapidly evolving rounded densities on chest radiographs. These have a propensity to cavitate and histologically are composed of layers of necrotic collagen and coal dust. The pulmonary manifestations of Caplan syndrome may precede or coincide with the onset of arthritis.

Pulmonary function findings vary with the stage of disease in a manner similar to that described for silicosis. In simple disease, there are usually no significant pulmonary function abnormalities. In complicated disease, either a restrictive or mixed restrictive and obstructive pattern may occur with a decreased diffusing capacity and abnormal arterial blood gases. It is important to remember that an obstructive ventilatory impairment in a coal miner may be a result of chronic bronchitis, coal workers' pneumoconiosis, or both.

Simple coal workers' pneumoconiosis usually follows a benign course. Unlike silicosis, no increase is seen in either pulmonary tuberculosis or fungal infections of the lung. In complicated disease, the affected worker may have mild to severe respiratory symptoms and significant impairment. In such cases, depending on the degree of impairment, the worker should be removed from continued dust exposure. In the United States, underground miners are able to participate in a federally run medical surveillance program that provides free periodic chest radiographs. If coal workers' pneumoconiosis is evident on the chest radiograph, the affected miner has the right to work in a low-dust job in the mine without loss of pay. In addition, personal dust exposure is monitored to confirm that exposures remain low.

Prevention of coal mine dust-related respiratory disease depends primarily on effective control of exposure to coal mine dust. In the United States, good progress had been made in reducing the incidence and prevalence of coal workers' pneumoconiosis since the passage in 1969 of the Coal Mine Health and Safety Act, which established programs to monitor dust levels in mines and to provide radiographic surveillance of miners. As noted above, however, the reduced incidence of coal workers' pneumoconiosis achieved in the United States appears to have abated with increased mechanization and mining of coal veins with greater surrounding silica. The latter factor in particular may be the reason for the increased incidence of PMF.

4. Other Pneumoconioses

Other mineral dusts capable of causing pulmonary parenchymal fibrosis include graphite (which causes disease similar to coal workers' pneumoconiosis), kaolin and diatomaceous earth (which cause silicosis-like disease), and talc and mica (which cause disease that has features of both silicosis and asbestosis). A metal dust that can cause pneumoconiosis is aluminum oxide, which can form fibers under certain conditions.

A new cause of ILD was reported involving a series of cases of ILD from a single nylon flock manufacturing plant. Finely cut nylon, called *flock*, is used to make fabric for upholstery, clothing, and automobiles. Nylon flock fibers are 10–15 μm in diameter, but respirable-size particles are generated during cutting operations. Lung biopsies from patients with nylon flock–related ILD have shown lymphocytic bronchiolitis and peribronchiolitis with lymphoid hyperplasia.

▼ CHRONIC OBSTRUCTIVE PULMONARY DISEASE

Chronic obstructive pulmonary disease (COPD) is typically divided into two main categories, chronic bronchitis and emphysema, although many patients with COPD have features of both. Work-related COPD is usually of the chronic bronchitis category, although cadmium and coal dust have been associated with emphysema.

CHRONIC BRONCHITIS

ESSENTIALS OF DIAGNOSIS

▶ History of chronic exposure to inhaled irritants at work is necessary for the diagnosis of occupational COPD. There may or may not be a history of coexistent cigarette smoking.

▶ Chronic cough and sputum production are required for the diagnosis of chronic bronchitis.

▶ Airflow limitation as evidenced by a decreased FEV_1:FVC ratio that does not improve with inhaled bronchodilator is another essential feature of COPD.

▶ General Considerations

Chronic bronchitis is characterized by inflammation of the bronchial tree and is manifested by persistent cough productive of sputum on most days for at least 3 months of the year for at least 2 successive years. The inhalation of irritant dusts, fumes, and gases can cause chronic simple bronchitis, that is, persistent sputum production without airflow obstruction (Table 19–6).

The diagnosis of chronic bronchitis is straightforward and based entirely on whether the worker's history is

Table 19–6. Some agents causing chronic bronchitis.

Minerals
Coal
Oil mist
Silica
Silicates
Synthetic vitreous fibers
Portland cement
Metals
Osmium
Vanadium
Welding fumes
Organic dusts
Cotton
Grain
Wood
Smoke
Tobacco smoke
Fire smoke
Engine exhaust

consistent with the definition given earlier. Once chronic bronchitis has been diagnosed, establishing a causal role for an occupational exposure is also based on the history obtained from the worker. Symptoms of cough and sputum production that are temporally associated with workplace exposure should suggest the diagnosis. Whether workers with chronic simple bronchitis are at risk for the development of chronic airflow obstruction and permanent respiratory impairment is an area of controversy that has yet to be completely resolved. The development of permanent respiratory impairment may depend on a variety of host factors such as preexisting nonspecific airway hyperresponsiveness, protease-antiprotease activity, and whether there is concomitant cigarette smoking. The population attributable risk is approximately 15% for occupational factors in the etiology of COPD. Smoking workers are at greater risk of developing respiratory symptoms with exposure to other irritants, and a work-related contribution to their symptoms should be considered.

▶ Pathogenesis

Airway inflammation and lung injury are key features of COPD. Exposure to irritating agents in the workplace is hypothesized to cause airway inflammation by activating epithelial cells and macrophages to release chemokines, prostanoids, and proinflammatory cytokines. Activated macrophages and recruited neutrophils release various proteases, including matrix metalloproteases (MMPs) that can damage lung tissue, stimulate mucus hypersecretion, and lead to airway remodeling. In addition, there is increasing evidence that CD8+ T lymphocytes are also recruited as part of the irritant-induced inflammatory response and play a role in the pathogenesis of COPD.

Prevention

Reduction of exposure to irritants in the workplace can prevent cases of chronic bronchitis through the application of the hierarchy of control strategies as described for occupational asthma. Protection of workers by substitution of nonirritating materials, the use of appropriate ventilation systems, respiratory protective equipment, and worker education about appropriate procedures is recommended.

Clinical Findings

Upper respiratory tract inflammatory symptoms, eye irritation, and an increased incidence of symptoms among coworkers all are features that support a work-related problem. Physical examination may demonstrate no evidence of pulmonary abnormality. Spirometry and expiratory flow-volume curves may or may not show evidence of airway obstruction. A nonsmoking worker exposed to high concentrations of an irritant at the workplace who has evidence of airway obstruction and no history of asthma should be suspected of having occupationally induced chronic bronchitis.

Treatment

Because chronic bronchitis often has a multifactorial etiology, a multifocal approach to management should be taken. If the worker smokes, cessation should be encouraged. Work exposure to the suspected agent should be reduced or eliminated. Pharmacologic agents of benefit are the beta$_2$-agonists, inhaled steroids, and inhaled anticholinergic agents. Periodic follow-up with particular attention to symptoms and worsening airway obstruction on serial spirometry is warranted.

Prognosis

The prognosis of workers with chronic irritant-induced bronchitis has not been well described. Some data, however, suggest that accelerated loss of ventilatory function can occur. In light of this, it may be prudent to assume that all workers with chronic work-related bronchitis are at risk of developing permanent respiratory impairment. Those with worsening symptoms or lung function abnormalities should be considered for removal from further exposure.

BRONCHIOLITIS OBLITERANS

ESSENTIALS OF DIAGNOSIS

▶ The clinical presentation is usually insidious onset of cough and dyspnea.

▶ Irreversible airflow limitation is present on pulmonary function testing.

▶ Minimal changes are found on chest radiographs.

General Considerations

When there is a history of a relevant exposure to a toxic agent, the small airways can be injured. Bronchiolitis is inflammation of the small airways, and when the inflammatory response leads to obstruction of bronchiolar lumens, the term *bronchiolitis obliterans* is used. The bronchiolar obstruction is caused by intraluminal polyps of organizing connective tissue (proliferative-type) and/or airway remodeling and smooth-muscle hypertrophy (constrictive-type). The most common occupational cause is irritant gas inhalation (eg, oxides of nitrogen, chlorine, phosgene, ozone, hydrogen sulfide, and sulfur dioxide) (see discussion of toxic gas inhalation above). Bronchiolitis obliterans also has been reported in nylon-flock workers, battery workers (exposed to thionyl chloride), and textile workers exposed to polyamide-amine dyes. In 2002, bronchiolitis obliterans was reported in a group of workers from a microwave popcorn plant exposed to diacetyl, with a high prevalence of obstructive-type spirometric abnormalities with an exposure-response relationship. Cases of bronchiolitis obliterans and airways disease (primarily obstructive, but also mixed obstructive/restrictive) have since been identified in several other food production facilities and in a coffee production facility where diacetyl was used as a flavoring. Based on the risk of serious lung disease, the NIOSH recommends that exposure to diacetyl should not exceed 5 ppb as a time-weighted average (TWA) for up to 8 h/d during a 40-hour work week, and 25 parts per billion for a 15-minute time period. NIOSH also recommends that worker exposure to a related diketone (2,3-pentanedione) be kept below 9.3 ppb as an 8-hour TWA during a 40-hour work week and 31 parts per billion during a 15-minute period.

PLEURAL DISORDERS

ESSENTIALS OF DIAGNOSIS

▶ Pleuritic pain, that is, sharp pain on inspiration, may accompany pleural disease caused by occupational exposures, but the diagnosis is usually made on the basis of chest imaging.

General Considerations

The pleura is the serous membrane that lines the lungs, mediastinum, diaphragm, and rib cage. It is divided into the *visceral pleura*, which lines the lung surface, and the *parietal pleura*, which lines the remaining structures. The primary cause of occupationally induced pleural disease is asbestos, although talc and mica can cause benign pleural disease and zeolite can cause mesothelioma.

BENIGN PLEURAL EFFUSIONS

Pleural effusions resulting from asbestos exposure may occur in up to 3% of exposed workers. The risk of developing an effusion is greater in those with heavy exposure. Benign asbestos effusions tend to develop within 5–20 years of the onset of exposure.

A pleural effusion can be attributed to asbestos if the following criteria are met: (1) a significant history of occupational exposure with an appropriate latent period since onset of exposure, (2) exclusion of other known causes of pleural effusion, and (3) a repeat evaluation of the effusion within a minimum of 2 years confirms that it is benign.

The majority of workers who have pleural effusions from asbestos exposure are asymptomatic. Physical examination in those with large effusions may show diminished rib cage expansion, dullness to percussion, and decreased breath sounds on the side of the effusion. Chest radiographs typically show small to moderately large, unilateral pleural effusions. Bilateral involvement occurs in approximately 10% of cases of benign asbestos effusions. Pleural thickening may be noted, although often the effusion is the first manifestation of asbestos-induced disease. Diffuse pleural thickening involving both pleural surfaces and obliteration of the costophrenic angle may develop in the wake of benign asbestos effusions. Thoracentesis will obtain pleural liquid that is a sterile exudate with no specific findings, although increased eosinophils are suggestive of an asbestos etiology.

It is essential to exclude other etiologies of pleural effusion, especially tuberculosis and malignancy. Regular follow-up with repeat thoracentesis if pleural fluid persists is essential. There is no known treatment. Recurrences occur, but in most cases the effusion clears spontaneously within a year without any obvious residual pleural disease.

PLEURAL PLAQUES

Pleural plaques are circumscribed areas of pleural thickening that are the most common radiographic findings as a result of chronic asbestos exposure. Plaques usually involve the parietal pleural surface and tend to occur over the central portions of the hemidiaphragm and along the inferior posterolateral aspect of the lower ribs.

Bilateral pleural plaques almost invariably are a result of past asbestos exposure, and their prevalence is related to both the intensity of exposure and the duration since onset of exposure. Workers with a greater exposure have a higher chance of developing plaques. In workers without asbestosis, plaques rarely cause signs and symptoms. The diagnosis usually is made from a routine chest radiograph. When plaques lie parallel to the beam, they appear as slightly to moderately protuberant linear or ovoid opacities along the costal or diaphragmatic margins. If calcified, they have an irregular, unevenly dense appearance. Although oblique radiographic views are recommended by some, chest CT scanning provides the most sensitive and specific technique for confirming the presence of plaques. Pathologically, the plaques are composed mainly of collagen with little accompanying inflammation. Asbestos fibers can be demonstrated in plaque tissue by electron microscopy, although this is not required for routine clinical diagnosis.

A worker with a past history of asbestos exposure and pleural plaques on chest radiograph should be evaluated for the presence of asbestosis. Even if no evidence of parenchymal disease is found, the worker should be monitored periodically for the possible development of this condition. Although workers with pleural plaques and no parenchymal disease typically do not develop respiratory impairment, there is evidence that heavily exposed workers with radiographic evidence of plaques, but no asbestosis, tend to have decreased lung function in comparison with workers with similar exposure histories whose chest radiographs are normal.

Because of the risk of development of bronchogenic carcinoma with asbestos exposure, cigarette smoking should be discouraged. The increased risk of lung cancer is not due to the plaques but to the cumulative dose of asbestos, the plaques merely acting as a marker of exposure.

Diffuse pleural thickening involving both visceral and parietal pleura also can result from past asbestos exposure. Such thickening occasionally is associated with a restrictive-type respiratory impairment even in the absence of asbestosis. Neither circumscribed plaques nor diffuse pleural thickening is believed to undergo malignant transformation to mesothelioma.

LUNG CANCER & MESOTHELIOMA

Lung cancer and mesothelioma are discussed in Chapter 17.

REFERENCES

Almberg KS: Progressive massive fibrosis resurgence identified in U.S. coal miners filing for Black Lung Benefits, 1970-2016. Ann Am Thorac Soc 2018;15:1420 [PMID: 30114941].

Balmes JR: An official American Thoracic Society statement: diagnosis and management of beryllium sensitivity and chronic beryllium disease. Am J Respir Crit Care Med 2014;190:e34 [PMID: 25398119].

Blanc PD: The occupational burden of nonmalignant respiratory diseases. An official American Thoracic Society and European Respiratory Society statement. Am J Respir Crit Care Med 2019;199:1312 [PMID: 31149852].

Choi S: Interstitial lung disorders in the indium workers of Korea: an update study for the relationship with biological exposure indices. Am J Ind Med 2015;58:61 [PMID: 25345911].

de Lange DW: Do corticosteroids have a role in preventing or reducing acute toxic lung injury caused by inhalation of chemical agents? Clin Toxicol (Phila) 2011;49:61 [PMID: 21370942].

Greenberg MI: Metal fume fever and polymer fume fever. Clin Toxicol (Phila) 2015;53:195 [PMID: 25706449].

Lacasse Y: Recent advances in hypersensitivity pneumonitis. Chest 2012;142:208 [PMID: 22796841].

Leso V: Artificial stone associated silicosis: a systematic review. Int J Environ Res Public Health 2019;16 pii: E568 [PMID: 30781462].

Marcon A: Can an airway challenge test predict respiratory diseases? A population-based international study. J Allergy Clin Immunol 2014;133:104 [PMID: 23683511].

Myers R: Asbestos-related pleural disease. Curr Opin Pulm Med 2012;18:377 [PMID: 22617814].

NIOSH: B reader program: http://www.cdc.gov/niosh/topics/chestradiography/breader.html.

Quirce S: Occupational hypersensitivity pneumonitis: an EAACI position paper. Allergy 2016;71:765 [PMID: 26913451].

Rose C: Early detection, clinical diagnosis, and management of lung disease from exposure to diacetyl. Toxicology 2017;388:9 [PMID: 28344095].

Seaton A: Farewell, king coal! Thorax 2016;71:364 [PMID: 2685636].

Vandenplas O: Diagnosing occupational asthma. Clin Exp Allergy 2017;47:6 [PMID: 27883240].

Vasakova M: Hypersensitivity pneumonitis: current concepts of pathogenesis and potential targets for treatment. Am J Respir Crit Care Med 2019 May 31 [Epub ahead of print] [PMID: 31150272].

■ SELF-ASSESSMENT QUESTIONS

Select the one correct answer for each question.

Question 1: The diffusing capacity of the lung for carbon monoxide (DL_{CO})

a. is the amount of inhaled carbon monoxide returned in exhaled air

b. is closely correlated with the capacity of the lungs to absorb oxygen

c. is increased with obstructive, restrictive, or vascular diseases

d. is often misused to assess respiratory impairment

Question 2: Bronchoprovocation tests

a. are useful in the diagnosis of occupational asthma

b. should be done in a hospital environment

c. give an indication of the presence and degree of inflammation of the airways

d. are usually terminated after a 40% fall in FEV_1

Question 3: The site of deposition of an inhaled gas

a. depends on the duration of exposure and its concentration

b. is determined primarily by water solubility

c. such as phosgene is the moist surfaces of the nose and throat

d. such as ammonia is likely the alveoli

Question 4: Occupational asthma

a. may be caused by such diverse agents as diisocyanates, snow crab, and western red cedar

b. resolves rapidly after removal from the offending agent

c. is predicted by a history of childhood asthma

d. treatment with inhaled corticosteroids does not improve prognosis

Question 5: Hypersensitivity pneumonitis

a. should be distinguished from extrinsic allergic alveolitis

b. is an immunologically mediated inflammatory disease of the airway

c. is induced by inhalation of organic dusts that contain a variety of etiologic agents

d. has different clinical and pathologic findings for each etiologic agent

Question 6: Silicosis

a. is a thoracic pleural disease

b. results from the inhalation of silicon dioxide, or silica, in crystalline form

c. is primarily the result of cytotoxic effects on lymphocytes

d. produces small round opacities (<10 mm in diameter) in both lungs, with a predilection for the lower lung zones

Question 7: Coal workers' pneumoconiosis

a. is, unlike silicosis, often asymptomatic

b. is seen often in those who have spent more than 2 years in underground mining

c. may lead to PMF, identical to that of silicosis

d. is confirmed by biopsy of the coal macule

Question 8: In reflex bronchoconstriction

a. neuroreceptors in the airway are stimulated by agents such as cold air, dusts, mists, vapors, and fumes

b. the reaction involves immunologic mechanisms and leads to airway inflammation

c. the patient has no history of preexisting nonoccupational asthma

d. there is no history of nonspecific airway hyperresponsiveness

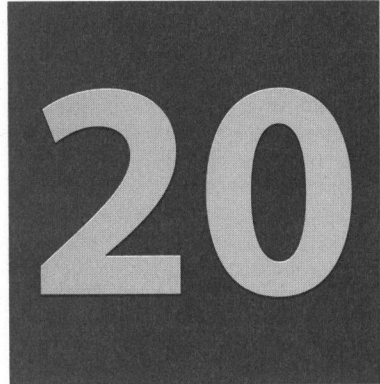

Cardiovascular Toxicology

Timur S. Durrani, MD, MPH, MBA

Neal L. Benowitz, MD

Heart disease and stroke cause the majority of deaths in the United States. The major risk factors for coronary heart disease—family history, hypertension, diabetes, lipid abnormalities, and cigarette smoking—explain only a minority of the cases. Other factors, such as stress and exposure to occupational or environmental toxic agents, are believed to contribute to the development of heart disease, although the magnitude of the risk is unknown.

CAUSATION IN TOXIC CARDIOVASCULAR DISEASE

Table 20–1 lists the types and possible toxic causes of cardiovascular disease. Massive exposure may occur (eg, in acute carbon monoxide poisoning), but toxic cardiovascular disease usually is the result of chronic low-level exposures.

Problems in establishing the cause of cardiovascular disease include the following:

- Cardiovascular disease is common even in the absence of toxic exposures.
- There is usually nothing specific, either clinically or pathologically, to point to toxic cardiovascular disease.
- It is rarely possible to document high tissue levels of suspected toxic substances.
- It is difficult to establish occupational exposure levels over the 20 or more years it may take to develop cardiovascular disease.
- Cardiovascular toxic substances are likely to interact with other risk factors in causing or manifesting cardiovascular disease.

With these limitations in mind, this chapter discusses current information concerning toxic cardiovascular disease.

EVALUATION OF PATIENTS

Evaluation of patients with suspected toxic cardiovascular disease should include the following steps:

1. Take a detailed occupational history with attention to the temporal relationship between cardiovascular symptoms and exposure to toxic substances in the workplace.

2. Attempt to document exposure to suspected toxic substances by obtaining industrial hygiene data and, if possible, monitoring worker exposure directly.

3. Evaluate other cardiovascular risk factors.

4. Perform a complete physical examination.

5. Perform appropriate diagnostic studies such as exercise stress testing and coronary angiography to establish the presence and extent of coronary artery disease; echocardiography or radionuclide angiography to establish myocardial disease and the presence of cardiomyopathy; and ambulatory electrocardiographic recordings taken on workdays and at other times to document work-related arrhythmias, paying particular attention to variations in intervals such as PR, QT, and QRS.

CARDIOVASCULAR ABNORMALITIES CAUSED BY CARBON DISULFIDE

Chronic exposure to carbon disulfide appears to accelerate atherosclerosis and/or precipitate acute coronary ischemic events. Carbon disulfide is a widely used solvent, especially in the rubber and viscose rayon industries, in the manufacture of carbon tetrachloride and ammonium salts, and as a degreasing solvent. Early epidemiologic studies indicated that there is a 2.5- to 5-fold increase in the risk of death from coronary heart disease in workers exposed to carbon disulfide. However, more recent analyses of the results of multiple studies found association between carbon disulfide exposure and circulatory disease to be weaker and inconsistent.

▶ Pathogenesis

The mechanism of accelerated atherogenesis caused by carbon disulfide has not been proved. One theory is that carbon disulfide reacts with amino- and thiol-containing

Table 20–1. Classification of cardiovascular diseases and possible toxic causes.

Condition	Toxic Agent
Cardiac arrhythmia	Arsenic Chlorofluorocarbon propellants Hydrocarbon solvents (eg, 1,1,1- 　trichloroethane and trichloroethylene) Organophosphate and carbamate insecticides
Coronary artery disease	Air pollution Carbon disulfide Carbon monoxide Lead(?)
Hypertension	Cadmium Carbon disulfide Lead
Myocardial asphyxiation	Carbon monoxide Cyanide Hydrogen sulfide
Myocardial injury	Antimony Arsenic Arsine Cobalt Lead
Nonatheromatous ischemic heart disease	Organic nitrates (eg nitroglycerin and 　ethylene glycol dinitrate)
Peripheral arterial occlusive disease	Arsenic Cadmium Lead

compounds in the body to produce thiocarbamates, which are capable of complexing trace metals and inhibiting many enzyme systems. This causes metabolic abnormalities such as disturbances of lipid metabolism and thyroid function and can lead to elevations of low-density lipoprotein/cholesterol concentrations and hypothyroidism, which are risk factors for atherosclerosis. Aldehyde dehydrogenase may be inhibited, resulting in a disulfiram-like reaction after alcohol ingestion. Other possible contributors to ischemic heart disease in workers exposed to carbon disulfide are increased vascular permeability, which may lead to greater lipid deposition; interference with normal inhibition of elastase activity, resulting in excess elastase activity with disruption of blood vessel walls and formation of aneurysms; depressed fibrinolytic activity, resulting in a greater tendency to thrombosis; and hypertension.

Pathology

The findings are those of accelerated atherosclerotic vascular disease involving the coronary, cerebral, and peripheral arteries. Renovascular hypertension also has been reported.

Clinical Findings

A. Symptoms and Signs

Acute intoxication may produce symptoms and signs of encephalopathy or polyneuropathy, including fatigue, headaches, dizziness, disorientation, paresthesias, psychosis, and delirium. In cases of chronic exposure, patients may present with hypertension or manifestations of atherosclerotic vascular disease such as angina or myocardial infarction. An early sign of chronic carbon disulfide poisoning is abnormal ocular microcirculation, characterized by microaneurysms and hemorrhages resembling those of diabetic retinopathy. Disturbed color vision may be reported. Presenile dementia, stroke, and sudden death have been reported in patients with chronic poisoning.

B. Laboratory Findings

Findings may include a decrease in serum thyroxine levels and an increase in serum cholesterol levels, particularly those of the very-low-density lipoproteins. There are no practical methods for measuring carbon disulfide levels in biologic fluids.

C. Cardiovascular Studies

Delayed filling of the retinal arteries, as measured by fluorescein angiography, may be an early sign of vascular disease. The electrocardiogram sometimes shows evidence of ischemia or previous myocardial infarction. The presence of coronary artery disease may be confirmed by exercise stress testing and coronary angiography.

Differential Diagnosis

The vascular findings in patients with chronic carbon disulfide poisoning are the same as those seen in any patient with atherosclerotic vascular disease. The most specific finding is abnormal ocular microcirculation in the absence of diabetes. The diagnosis is based on a clinical picture of premature vascular disease and a history of exposure to excessive levels of carbon disulfide for more than 5 or 10 years.

Prevention

Carbon disulfide exposure is primarily by inhalation. The Occupational Safety and Health Administration (OSHA) recommends that workplace exposure be limited to 20 ppm (parts per million) as an 8-hour time-weighted average (TWA) concentration, 30 ppm as an acceptable peak concentration for 30 minutes, and 100 ppm as a maximum peak. Periodic examination of the ocular fundi may help to detect early signs of vascular disease.

Treatment

Treatment consists of removing the worker from sources of carbon disulfide exposure and providing medical measures for atherosclerotic vascular disease.

Course & Prognosis

The course of the disease is similar to that of any atherosclerotic vascular disease. There is evidence of reversibility—at least of ocular changes—after exposure to carbon disulfide is discontinued.

CARDIOVASCULAR ABNORMALITIES CAUSED BY CARBON MONOXIDE

Excessive carbon monoxide exposure can reduce maximal exercise capacity in healthy workers; aggravate angina pectoris, intermittent claudication, and chronic obstructive lung disease; and aggravate or induce cardiac arrhythmias. Acute intoxications can cause myocardial infarction or sudden death. Chronic high-level carbon monoxide exposure may result in congestive cardiomyopathy.

Carbon monoxide is the most widely distributed of all industrial toxic agents and accounts for the greatest number of intoxications and deaths. It is formed wherever combustion engines or other types of combustion are present. Workers at high risk include forklift operators, foundry workers, miners, mechanics, garage attendants, and firefighters. Carbon monoxide poisoning also may occur with the use of faulty furnaces or heaters, particularly improperly vented kerosene or charcoal heaters. Cigarette smoking is an important source of carbon monoxide, and occupational sources may be additive to exposure from cigarettes. The solvent methylene chloride is metabolized within the body to carbon monoxide.

Pathogenesis

The affinity of carbon monoxide for hemoglobin is more than 200 times that of oxygen. The binding of carbon monoxide and hemoglobin to form carboxyhemoglobin reduces the delivery of oxygen to body tissues because the oxygen-carrying capacity of hemoglobin is decreased and because less oxygen is released to tissues at any given oxygen tension (ie, there is a shift in the oxygen dissociation curve). Thus, a carboxyhemoglobin concentration of 20% represents a greater reduction in oxygen delivery than a 20% reduction in erythrocyte count. Other heme-containing proteins (eg, myoglobin, cytochrome oxidase, and cytochrome P450) bind 10–15% of the total-body carbon monoxide, but the medical significance of their binding at usual levels of exposure to carbon monoxide is unclear.

In healthy individuals exposed to carbon monoxide, the decrease in delivery of oxygen to tissues causes the cardiac output and coronary blood flow to increase to meet the metabolic demands of the heart. Although these compensatory responses enable healthy individuals to perform at normal work levels, their maximal exercise capacity is decreased. If, on the other hand, compensatory responses are limited, as in patients with coronary artery disease, carbon monoxide exposure may cause angina or myocardial infarction (Figure 20–1). Reduced exercise thresholds for the development of angina have been reported when carboxyhemoglobin concentrations are as low as 2.7% (Table 20–2). Carbon monoxide decreases the ventricular fibrillation threshold in experimental animals and may do the same in humans. This would explain why sudden death occurs in people who have coronary artery disease and are exposed to carbon monoxide, as has been reported to occur on smoggy days in large cities. Severe carbon monoxide poisoning (carboxyhemoglobin concentrations >50%) can cause severe hypoxic injury, including cardiovascular collapse.

Chronic exposure to carbon monoxide is thought to accelerate atherogenesis. Cigarette smokers demonstrate advanced coronary and peripheral atherosclerosis, and carbon monoxide is believed to contribute. Several animal studies have tested the effects of chronic high-level carbon monoxide exposure combined with feeding of atherogenic diets; the results of some of these studies showed increased severity of atherosclerosis. Possible mechanisms include abnormal vascular permeability, increased vascular uptake of lipids, and increased platelet adhesiveness. Whether atherosclerosis is accelerated at levels of carbon monoxide commonly encountered in the workplace is unclear.

Chronic exposure to carbon monoxide results in increased red blood cell mass in response to chronic tissue hypoxia and in increased blood viscosity, which could contribute to acute cardiac events.

Pathology

Cardiac necrosis is observed often in cases of fatal carbon monoxide poisoning and presumably is due to severe hypoxia. Myocardial infarction may occur in workers who have coronary artery disease and are exposed to high levels of carbon monoxide, particularly while performing strenuous work or exercise. Cardiomyopathy with cardiac enlargement and congestive heart failure has been described in workers with chronic high-level exposure to carbon monoxide (carboxyhemoglobin concentrations >30%).

Clinical Findings

A. Symptoms and Signs

Headache is typically the first symptom of carbon monoxide poisoning and may occur at carboxyhemoglobin concentrations as low as 10%. At higher concentrations, nausea, dizziness, fatigue, and dimmed vision are reported commonly.

In patients with angina pectoris or peripheral arterial occlusive disease, carbon monoxide exposure may reduce exercise capacity to the point of angina or claudication (see Table 20–2). All workers experience a reduction in maximal exercise capacity.

Although symptoms correlate poorly to carboxyhemoglobin levels, neuropsychiatric testing may reveal findings such as increased reaction time and decreased manual dexterity may be seen at carboxyhemoglobin concentrations

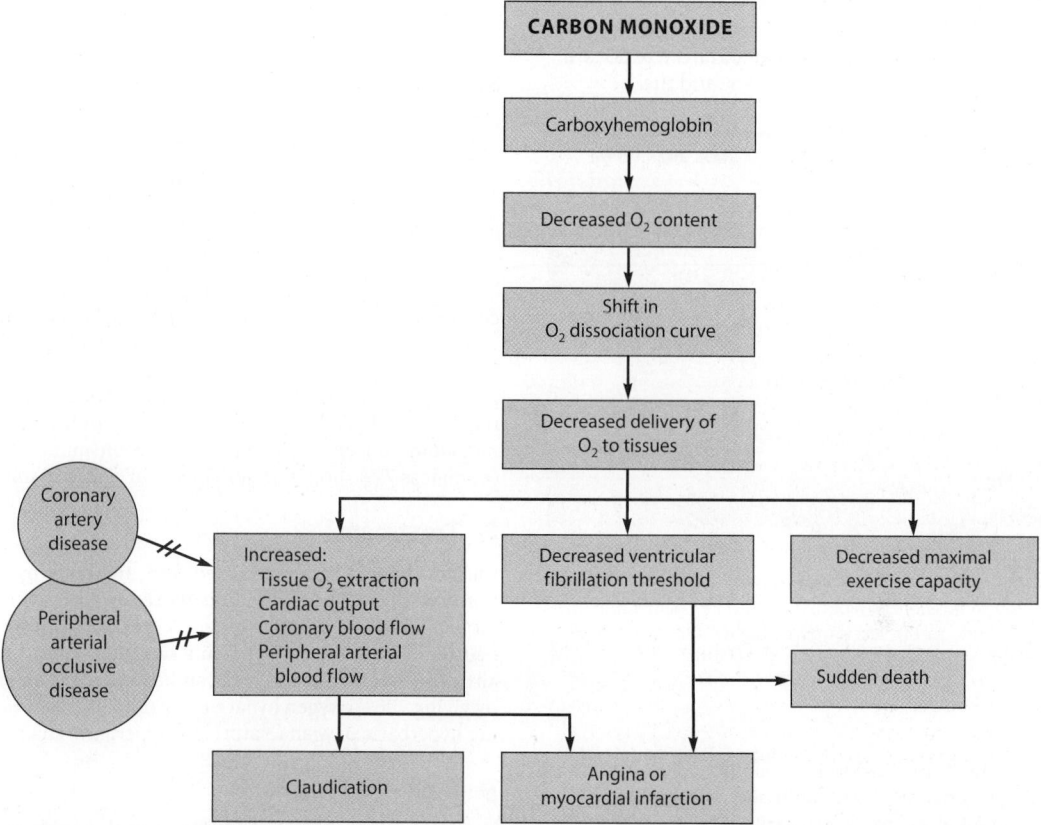

▲ **Figure 20–1.** Cardiovascular consequences of exposure to carbon monoxide. The presence of coronary artery disease or peripheral arterial occlusive disease prevents (//) the usual compensatory increase in coronary or peripheral arterial blood flow, which results in symptoms of arterial insufficiency.

between 5% and 10%. At concentrations of 25%, there may be decreased visual acuity and impaired cognitive function; at 35%, ataxia; at 50%, vomiting, tachypnea, tachycardia, and hypertension; and at higher levels, coma, convulsions, and cardiovascular and respiratory depression. Myocardial ischemia may be evident at any carboxyhemoglobin concentration in susceptible individuals.

B. Laboratory Findings

The only finding specific for carbon monoxide intoxication is elevation of the carboxyhemoglobin concentration. Table 20–3 lists normal carboxyhemoglobin concentrations and provides examples of concentrations resulting from exposure to carbon monoxide in the environment and the workplace.

Table 20–2. Effects of carbon monoxide on exercise capacity.

Group	Baseline Exercise Duration(s)	Level of Exposure to Carbon Monoxide	Increase in Concentration of Carboxyhemoglobin	Exercise Duration After Exposure(s)	Exercise Endpoint
Healthy individuals	698	100 ppm for 1 h	1.7% → 4%	662	Exhaustion
Patients with angina pectoris	224	50 ppm for 2 h	1% → 2.7%	188	Angina
Patients with intermittent claudication	174	50 ppm for 2 h	1.1% → 2.8%	144	Claudication
Patients with chronic lung disease	219	100 ppm for 1 h	1.4% → 4.1%	147	Dyspnea

Table 20–3. Normal carboxyhemoglobin concentrations and examples of concentrations resulting from exposure to carbon monoxide in the environment and the workplace.

Source of Carbon Monoxide	Carboxyhemoglobin Concentration	
	Average (%)	Range (%)
Endogenous metabolism (normal level[a])	0.5	—
Environmental exposure Air pollution	2	1.5–2.5
Cigarette smoking	6	3–15
Occupational exposure (nonsmokers) Foundry workers	4	2–9
Mechanics	5	—
Garage attendants	7	—

[a]Carbon monoxide is normally formed as a product of metabolism of hemoglobin. Endogenous levels may be higher if there is increased hemoglobin turnover.

Measurement of carboxyhemoglobin levels must be done using CO-oximetry with arterial or venous blood. The routine arterial blood gas instruments measures the partial pressure of oxygen dissolved in plasma (Po_2), but oxygen saturation is calculated from the Po_2 and is therefore unreliable in patients with CO poisoning. Conventional pulse oximetry gives falsely normal readings because it is unable to distinguish between oxyhemoglobin and carboxyhemoglobin. A newer pulse CO-oximeter can detect carboxyhemoglobin.

Although respiratory alkalosis caused by hyperventilation is observed commonly, there is respiratory failure in the most severe poisonings. When there is marked tissue hypoxia, lactic acidosis develops.

C. Cardiovascular Studies

The electrocardiograph (ECG) may show ischemic changes or myocardial infarction. Various types of arrhythmias, including atrial fibrillation and premature atrial and ventricular contractions, are observed. Abnormalities seen on the ECG usually are transient, although ST-T-wave abnormalities may persist for days or weeks.

▶ Differential Diagnosis

The most important clue to carbon monoxide poisoning is the occupational or environmental exposure history. A typical symptom, such as headache, confusion, or sudden collapse, with findings of myocardial ischemia or metabolic acidosis should suggest the diagnosis, and carboxyhemoglobin concentrations should be measured.

▶ Prevention

Levels of carbon monoxide should be monitored if there are sources of combustion such as combustion engines or furnaces in the workplace. The current ACGIH 8-hour threshold limit value is 25 ppm, which at the end of an 8-hour workday results in a carboxyhemoglobin concentration of 2–3%. This concentration is tolerated well by healthy individuals but may impair function in people with cardiovascular or chronic lung disease. Workplace monitoring is done easily with a portable carbon monoxide meter. Biologic monitoring of workers involves measuring either the carboxyhemoglobin concentration in blood or the level of expired carbon monoxide, which is directly proportional to the carboxyhemoglobin concentration. Elevated carbon monoxide levels (as high as 7%) should be anticipated in cigarette smokers.

▶ Treatment

Carbon monoxide is eliminated from the body by respiration, and the rate of elimination depends on ventilation, pulmonary blood flow, and inspired oxygen concentration. The half-life of carbon monoxide in a sedentary adult breathing air is 4–5 hours. The half-life can be reduced to 80 minutes by giving 100% oxygen by face mask or to 25 minutes by giving hyperbaric oxygen (3 atm) in a hyperbaric chamber.

▶ Course & Prognosis

Recovery usually is complete after mild to moderate carbon monoxide intoxication in the absence of a cardiac complication such as myocardial infarction.

CARDIOVASCULAR ABNORMALITIES CAUSED BY ORGANIC NITRATES

In the 1950s, an epidemic of sudden death in young munitions workers who hand-packed cartridges of explosives were observed. It was discovered subsequently that abrupt withdrawal from excessive exposure to organic nitrates, particularly nitroglycerin and ethylene glycol dinitrate, may result in myocardial ischemia even in the absence of coronary artery disease. Occupations in which workers may be exposed to organic nitrates include explosives manufacturing, construction work involving blasting, weapons handling in the armed forces, and pharmaceutical manufacturing of nitrates.

▶ Pathogenesis

Nitrates directly dilate blood vessels, including those of the coronary circulation. With prolonged exposure (usually 1–4 years), compensatory vasoconstriction develops that is believed to be mediated by sympathetic neural responses, activation of the rennin-angiotensin system, or both. When

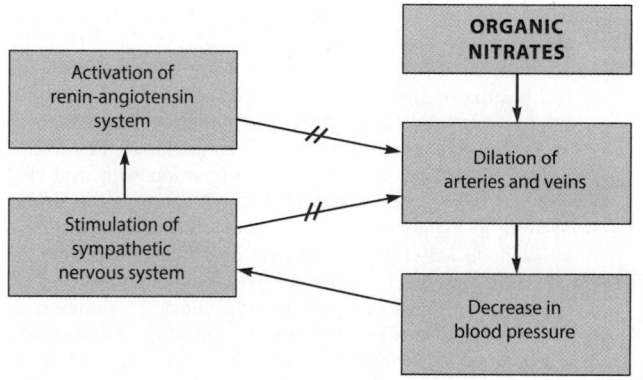

▲ **Figure 20–2.** Mechanism of vasospasm after withdrawal from chronic exposure to nitrates. Vasoconstrictor forces antagonize (//) nitrate-induced vasodilation. Withdrawal from exposure to nitrates results in unopposed vasoconstriction and in coronary vasospasm.

exposure to nitrates is stopped, the compensatory vasoconstriction becomes unopposed (Figure 20–2). Coronary vasospasm with angina, myocardial infarction, or sudden death may result. Chest pain occurring during nitrate withdrawal has been termed Monday morning angina because it typically occurs 2–3 days after the last day of nitrate exposure. Case-control studies suggest a 2.5- to 4-fold increase in the risk of cardiovascular death in workers handling explosives.

▶ Pathology

In patients who have died following withdrawal from nitrates, there is often no or minimal coronary atherosclerosis. In one patient, coronary vasospasm was observed during angiography, and the spasm was reversed promptly with sublingual nitroglycerin.

▶ Clinical Findings

A. Symptoms and Signs

Workers exposed to excessive levels of nitrates typically experience headaches and have hypotension, tachycardia, and warm, flushed skin. With continued exposure, the symptoms and signs become less prominent. After 1–2 days without exposure to nitrates—generally on weekends—there may be signs of acute coronary ischemia ranging from mild angina at rest to manifestations of myocardial infarction (eg, nausea, diaphoresis, pallor, and palpitations associated with severe chest pain), or sudden death may occur.

B. Laboratory Findings and Cardiovascular Studies

During episodes of pain, the ECG may show evidence of acute ischemia: ST-segment elevation or depression with or without T-wave abnormalities. At other times, in the absence of pain, the ECG may be perfectly normal. Typical findings of myocardial infarction include development of a pathologic Q wave on ECG and elevation of serum troponin and other cardiac enzymes. Results of exercise stress testing and coronary angiography may be normal.

▶ Differential Diagnosis

Workers chronically exposed to nitrates also may have organic coronary artery disease, which must be identified.

▶ Prevention

Nitrates are extremely volatile and are absorbed readily through the lungs and skin. They can permeate the wrapping material of dynamite sticks, so workers who handle dynamite should be advised to wear cotton gloves. Natural rubber gloves should not be used because they tend to become permeated with nitrates and may enhance absorption.

With current automated processes in explosives manufacturing, direct handling of nitrates by employees is minimized. However, levels of nitrates in the workplace environment must be controlled by adequate ventilation and by air conditioning during periods of hot weather. The current OSHA permissible exposure limit (PEL) for nitroglycerin is 0.2 ppm parts of air (2 mg^3) as a ceiling limit. The OSHA PEL also bears a "skin" notation, which indicates that the cutaneous route of exposure (including mucous membranes and eyes) contributes to overall exposure, but even at lower levels (0.02 ppm), personal protective gear is recommended to avoid headache. Although there are no readily available biochemical measures to detect excessive nitrate exposure, findings of progressively decreasing blood pressure and increasing heart rate during the workday are suggestive of excessive exposure. Monitoring for these signs in employees also may help to prevent adverse effects of exposure to nitrates.

▶ Treatment

Treatment of myocardial ischemia caused by nitrate withdrawal includes cardiac nitrates (eg, nitroglycerin or isosorbide dinitrate) or calcium entry-blocking agents. Case reports indicate that ischemic symptoms may recur for weeks or months, indicating a persistent tendency to coronary spasm, so long-term cardiac nitrate or calcium blocker therapy may be needed. The worker should be removed from sources of organic nitrate exposure.

Course & Prognosis

In the absence of myocardial infarction or sudden death, anginal symptoms resolve fully after exposure to nitrate is stopped.

CARDIOVASCULAR ABNORMALITIES CAUSED BY HYDROCARBON SOLVENTS & CHLOROFLUOROCARBONS

Exposure to various solvents and propellants may result in cardiac arrhythmia, syncope with resulting accidents at work, or sudden death. Most serious cases of arrhythmia are associated with abuse of or industrial exposure to halogenated hydrocarbon solvents (eg, 1,1,1-trichloroethane and trichloroethylene) or exposure to chlorofluorocarbon (Freon) propellants. Nonhalogenated solvents and even ethanol present similar risks. Dilated cardiomyopathy, with or without histologic evidence of myocarditis, associated with severe cardiac failure has been reported in several people with occupational exposures to solvents, although causation is still unproven.

Exposure to solvents is widespread in industrial settings such as dry cleaning, degreasing, painting, and chemical manufacturing. Chlorofluorocarbons are used extensively as refrigerants and as propellants in a wide variety of products and processes. For example, a pathology resident developed various arrhythmias after exposure to chlorofluorocarbon aerosols used for freezing samples and cleaning slides in a surgical pathology laboratory.

Pathogenesis

Figure 20–3 illustrates two ways in which halogenated hydrocarbons and other solvents are thought to induce cardiac arrhythmia or sudden death. First, at low levels of exposure, these solvents "sensitize" the heart to actions of catecholamines. For example, experimental studies show that the amount of epinephrine required to produce ventricular tachycardia or fibrillation is reduced after the solvents are inhaled. Catecholamine release is potentiated by euphoria and excitement as a consequence of inhalation of the solvent, as well as by exercise. This, in combination with asphyxia and hypoxia, causes arrhythmia, which can result in death. Second, at higher levels of exposure, solvents may depress sinus node activity, thereby causing sinus bradycardia or arrest, or they may depress atrioventricular nodal conduction, thereby causing atrioventricular block. In some cases, they do both. Bradyarrhythmia then predisposes to escape ventricular arrhythmia or, in cases of more severe intoxication, to asystole. The arrhythmogenic action of solvents also may be enhanced by alcohol or caffeine.

Pathology

Most cardiovascular deaths following exposure to hydrocarbons are sudden deaths. Autopsies usually reveal no specific pathologic findings in sudden death cases but may reveal myocarditis in cases of dilated cardiomyopathy. The finding of a fatty liver suggests chronic exposure to high levels of halogenated solvents or to ethanol.

Clinical Findings

A. Symptoms and Signs

Symptoms of intoxication with hydrocarbon solvents or chlorofluorocarbons include dizziness, light-headedness, headaches, nausea, drowsiness, lethargy, palpitations, and syncope. Physical examination may reveal ataxia, nystagmus, and slurred speech. The heart rate and blood pressure

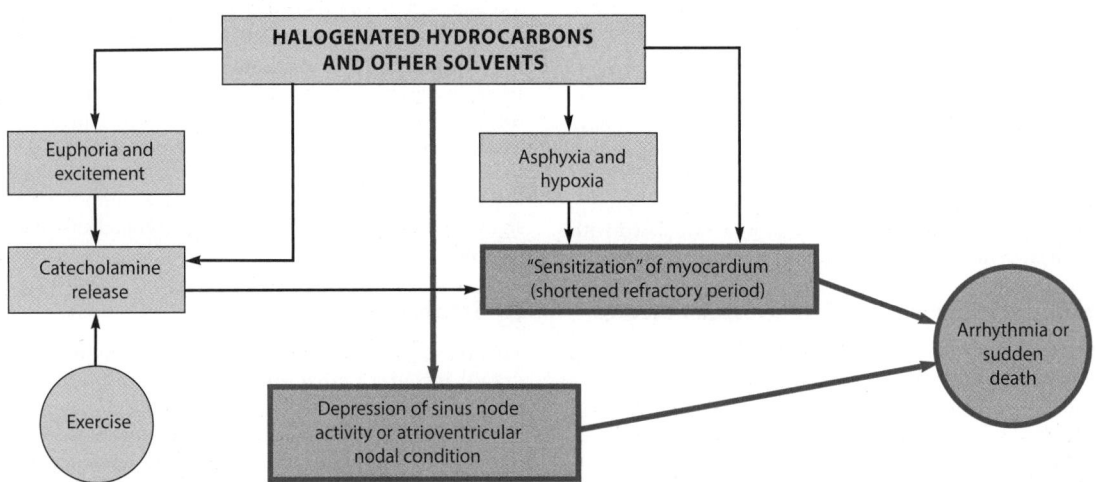

▲ **Figure 20–3.** Mechanisms of arrhythmia or sudden death following low-level exposure (light arrows) or high-level exposure (heavy arrows) to halogenated hydrocarbons and other solvents.

usually are normal, except at the time of arrhythmias, when a rapid or irregular heartbeat sometimes is accompanied by hypotension.

Convulsions, coma, or cardiac arrest may occur in severe cases of exposure to solvents. Workers who have heart disease or chronic lung disease with hypoxemia may be more susceptible to the arrhythmogenic actions of solvents.

B. Laboratory Findings

The concentrations of some hydrocarbons can be measured in expired air or in the blood.

C. Cardiovascular Studies

Arrhythmias induced by solvents or chlorofluorocarbons are expected to occur only at work, while the worker is exposed to these agents. The diagnosis is based on abnormalities observed during ambulatory electrocardiographic monitoring, which consist of one or more of the following: premature atrial or ventricular contractions, recurrent supraventricular tachycardia, and recurrent ventricular tachycardia. It is essential to monitor patients on both workdays and off days and to request a log of times of exposure to solvents or chlorofluorocarbons as well as a log of symptoms of palpitations or dizzy spells. A 12-lead ECG and an exercise stress test can help to determine the presence of coronary artery disease, which might increase sensitivity to hydrocarbon- or chlorofluorocarbon-induced arrhythmia.

▶ Differential Diagnosis

The diagnosis of solvent- or chlorofluorocarbon-induced arrhythmia is based on exclusion of other causes of arrhythmias at work (eg, the presence of a cardiac disease, metabolic disturbance, or drug abuse) and demonstration of a temporal relationship between episodes of arrhythmia and exposures to the toxic agent. The diagnosis is supported by industrial hygiene measurements documenting the level of exposure in the workplace and by objective and subjective evidence that the worker was intoxicated following exposure.

▶ Prevention

Preventive measures include proper handling of solvents and propellants, adequate ventilation in the workplace, and, in some cases, the use of protective respiratory equipment. Workers with heart disease—especially those with chronic arrhythmia—should be advised to avoid exposure to potentially arrhythmogenic chemicals.

▶ Treatment

If a worker collapses and resuscitation is required, use of epinephrine and other sympathomimetic drugs should be avoided, if possible, because they may precipitate further arrhythmia. β-Adrenergic blocking agents may be useful in managing solvent- or chlorofluorocarbon-induced arrhythmias. In cases of episodic arrhythmia, the worker should be removed from excessive exposure or advised to use protective respiratory equipment.

▶ Course & Prognosis

Arrhythmias are expected to resolve fully after exposure to hydrocarbons is stopped.

CARDIOVASCULAR ABNORMALITIES CAUSED BY ORGANOPHOSPHATE & CARBAMATE INSECTICIDES

Early cardiovascular manifestations of intoxication with organophosphate and carbamate insecticides include tachycardia and hypertension. Later, there may be bradycardia and hypotension. Delayed repolarization with QT-interval prolongation and episodes of ventricular tachycardia may be seen for up to 5–7 days after acute intoxication. The ECG also commonly shows nonspecific ST- and T-wave changes. A number of arrhythmias, including premature ventricular contractions, ventricular tachycardia and fibrillation, and heart block and asystole, have been observed.

Intensive cardiac and respiratory monitoring of patients for several days after exposure is recommended, with particular attention to the possible late development of arrhythmia or respiratory failure. High-degree heart block and polymorphous ventricular tachycardia with a prolonged QT interval are treated optimally with cardiac pacing. The use of antiarrhythmic drugs that depress conduction (eg, quinidine, procainamide, and disopyramide) and calcium channel blockers should be avoided.

CARDIOVASCULAR ABNORMALITIES CAUSED BY HEAVY METALS

Several metals are associated with disturbances in cardiovascular function, but their causative role is not fully established.

▶ Antimony

Therapeutic use of antimonial compounds for the treatment of parasitic infections produces electrocardiographic abnormalities—primarily T-wave changes and QT-interval prolongation—and has caused sudden death in some patients. Electrocardiographic changes also have been observed in workers exposed to antimony. Although these changes usually resolve after removal from exposure, a few studies report increased cardiovascular mortality rates in exposed workers. Studies in animals confirm that chronic exposure to antimony can produce myocardial disease.

▶ Arsenic

Subacute arsenic poisoning caused by ingestion of arsenic-contaminated beer is associated with cardiomyopathy and cardiac failure. Chronic arsenic poisoning has been reported to produce "blackfoot disease," which is characterized by claudication and gangrene, presumably secondary to spasms of the large blood vessels in the extremities. Arsenic exposure in drinking water is associated with an increased prevalence of hypertension. Acute arsenic poisoning can cause electrocardiographic abnormalities, and in one case it was reported to cause recurrent ventricular arrhythmia of the *torsade de pointes* type. A mortality study of copper smelters exposed to arsenic indicated that these workers have an increased risk of death as a result of ischemic heart disease.

▶ Arsine

Arsine gas causes red blood cell hemolysis. Massive hemolysis produces hyperkalemia, which can result in cardiac arrest. Electrocardiographic manifestations progress from high, peaked T waves to conduction disturbances and various degrees of heart block and then to asystole. Arsine also may directly affect the myocardium, causing a greater magnitude of cardiac failure than would be expected from the degree of anemia.

▶ Cadmium

Some earlier epidemiologic and experimental animal studies linked high-level cadmium exposure with hypertension, but recent epidemiologic studies do not support the association. Environmental exposure to cadmium, as assessed by blood or urine levels, is associated with an increased risk of peripheral arterial disease.

▶ Cobalt

In Quebec City, Canada, in 1965 and 1966, an epidemic of cardiomyopathy occurred in heavy drinkers of beer to which cobalt sulfate had been added as a foam stabilizer. The mortality rate in affected patients was 22%, and a major pathologic finding in those who died was myocardial necrosis with thrombi in the heart and major blood vessels. Other clinical features in affected patients included polycythemia, pericardial effusion, and thyroid hyperplasia. Cobalt is known to depress oxygen uptake by the mitochondria of the heart and to interfere with energy metabolism in a manner biochemically similar to the effects of thiamine deficiency. Because individuals receiving higher doses of cobalt for therapeutic reasons have not developed cardiomyopathy, it is possible that cobalt, excessive alcohol consumption, and nutritional deprivation acted synergistically to produce cardiomyopathy in this epidemic. Occupational exposure to cobalt has been associated with diastolic dysfunction on echocardiography. Several cases of cardiomyopathy in workers exposed to cobalt have been reported or patients who had hip implants that failed, releasing cobalt into tissue.

▶ Lead

Exposure to excessive levels of lead causes chronic renal diseases, and epidemiologic studies suggest that it also contributes to hypertension in the absence of renal disease. Some of the workplace studies of exposure to lead report an increased incidence of ischemic electrocardiographic changes and an increased risk of hypertensive or coronary artery disease and cerebrovascular disease in exposed workers. Nonspecific electrocardiographic changes and fatal myocarditis in the absence of hypertension have been observed in children with lead poisoning. Cardiomyopathy in moonshine drinkers is also attributed to lead exposure. Studies in animals indicate that lead may have direct toxic effects on the myocardium.

CARDIOVASCULAR ABNORMALITIES CAUSED BY PARTICULATE MATTER

Epidemiologic studies, by using time-series analysis, have demonstrated an association between the level of exposure to air pollution and increased mortality, including increased mortality from cardiovascular disease and stroke. Higher levels of air pollution are associated with more hospital admissions for cardiovascular disease. Several case-control studies of welders have reported increased risk of myocardial infarction and cardiovascular mortality. Welders inhale fumes containing gases and respirable particles (as well as metals such as zinc).

Inhalation of particulates has been shown to alter heart rate variability, with an increase in average heart rate, and to increase plasma viscosity. Gaseous pollutants include oxidizing gases that generate free radicals, which may result in generalized inflammatory responses, endothelial dysfunction, and enhanced blood coagulation. Hemodynamic stress, inflammation, and hypercoagulability are the suspected mechanisms for the link between air pollution and acute cardiovascular events.

REFERENCES

Burroughs Peña MS, Rollins A: Environmental exposures and cardiovascular disease: a challenge for health and development in low- and middle-income countries. Cardiol Clin 2017;35(1):71 [PMID: 27886791].

Genchi G, Sinicropi MS, Carocci A, Lauria G, Catalano A: Mercury exposure and heart diseases. Int J Environ Res Public Health 2017;14(1):74 [PMID: 28085104].

Kan H, Pan D, Castranova V: Engineered nanoparticle exposure and cardiovascular effects: the role of a neuronal-regulated pathway. Inhal Toxicol 2018;30(9-10):335 [PMID: 30604639].

Nigra AE, Ruiz-Hernandez A, Redon J, Navas-Acien A, Tellez-Plaza M: Environmental metals and cardiovascular disease in adults: a systematic review beyond lead and cadmium. Curr Environ Health Rep 2016;3(4):416 [PMID: 27783356].

Packer M: Cobalt cardiomyopathy: a critical reappraisal in light of a recent resurgence. Circ Heart Fail 2016;9(12):e003604 [PMID: 27852654].

Rajagopalan S: Air pollution and cardiovascular disease: JACC state-of-the-art review. J Am Coll Cardiol 2018;72(17):2054-2070 [PMID: 30336830].

Solenkova NV, Newman JD, Berger JS, Thurston G, Hochman JS, Lamas GA: Metal pollutants and cardiovascular disease: mechanisms and consequences of exposure. Am Heart J 2014;168(6):812-822 [PMID: 25458643].

■ SELF-ASSESSMENT QUESTIONS

Select the one correct answer for each question.

Question 1: Chronic exposure to carbon disulfide
  a. appears to accelerate atherosclerosis and/or precipitate acute coronary ischemic events
  b. increases serum thyroxine levels
  c. decreases serum cholesterol levels, particularly those of the very-low-density lipoproteins
  d. is reliably monitored in biologic fluids

Question 2: Carbon monoxide exposure
  a. enhances maximal exercise capacity in healthy workers
  b. may aggravate angina pectoris but not intermittent claudication
  c. has no effect on chronic obstructive lung disease
  d. may aggravate or induce cardiac arrhythmias

Question 3: Nitrates
  a. directly constrict blood vessels, including those of the coronary circulation
  b. deactivate the rennin-angiotensin system
  c. typically cause immediate chest pain
  d. appear to cause a 2.5- to 4-fold increase in the risk of cardiovascular death in workers handling explosives

Question 4: Organophosphate and carbamate insecticides
  a. can produce diverse cardiovascular disturbances, including tachycardia and hypertension, bradycardia and hypotension, heart block, and ventricular tachycardia
  b. stimulate acetylcholinesterase, which causes accumulation of acetylcholine at cholinergic synapses and myoneural junctions
  c. typically result in ataxia, nystagmus, and slurred speech
  d. invariably result in arrhythmias with chronic exposure

Question 5: Arsine gas
  a. causes red blood cell hemolysis
  b. leads to hypokalemia resulting in cardiac arrest
  c. electrocardiographic manifestations are diagnostic
  d. only indirectly affects the myocardium

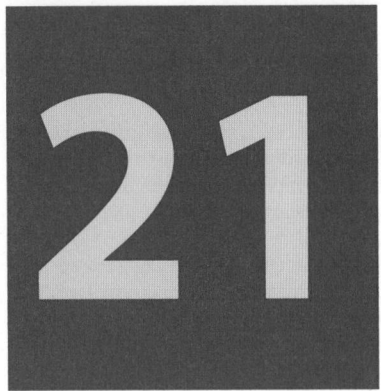

Liver Toxicology

Robert J. Harrison, MD, MPH

Sandeep Guntur, MD, MPH

The liver is the target organ of many occupational and environmental chemicals and plays a central role in their detoxification and elimination. Bacterial and viral infections and certain chemical and physical agents encountered in the workplace also affect the liver. Tables 21–1, 21–4, and 21–5 present the main causes of occupational liver disease.

DETECTION OF OCCUPATIONAL LIVER DISEASE

With the exception of a few chemicals that cause specific lesions (Table 21–1), hepatic injury as a consequence of industrial exposure does not differ clinically or morphologically from drug-induced damage (including damage caused by ethanol). Thus, it may be difficult to differentiate occupational from nonoccupational causes on the basis of screening tests.

Occupational liver disease may be of secondary importance to damage that occurs to other organs or may occur only at high doses after accidental exposure or ingestion. While acute toxic liver injury does occur, concern is focused increasingly on chronic liver disease resulting from prolonged low-level toxic exposure. In this respect, cancer is of central concern. Because chemical studies frequently are done on animals first, the occupational health practitioner must be able to evaluate—sometimes without the assistance of adequate human studies—the results of positive carcinogenesis studies in light of actual workplace exposures.

In individual cases, the clinician usually is first alerted to the presence of hepatic disease by routine enzyme tests and then must make a determination about whether the cause is occupational or nonoccupational. The occupational history and result of personal or workroom air sampling are crucial to formulation of a presumptive diagnosis. It is occasionally necessary to remove the affected worker from exposure to the suspected workplace toxic substance to establish the workplace relationship.

LIMITATIONS OF DETECTION

The detection of preclinical disease is made difficult by the lack of sufficiently sensitive and specific tests. It is common practice to measure liver enzymes periodically in workers exposed to a known or suspected hepatotoxin. This surveillance technique is complicated, however, by the problems of false-positive results (ie, elevated enzyme levels as a result of nonoccupational causes) and false-negative results (ie, normal values in the presence of biochemical dysfunction). In addition, little is known about the effects of multiple hepatotoxic exposures common to many occupations (eg, painters, printers, and laboratory technicians). (For a detailed discussion of these limitations, see "Medical Surveillance for Occupational Liver Disease.")

EPIDEMIOLOGIC EVIDENCE OF LIVER DISEASE

Epidemiologic studies have been performed on many groups of workers exposed to hepatotoxic agents. However, relatively few workplace hepatotoxic substances have been studied in humans. Epidemiologic studies, where available, generally provide the best evidence of toxicity; however, they may be limited by inadequate study design and other confounding factors, such as body mass index, alcohol ingestion, and medication use.

Serum Aminotransferase

Cross-sectional studies that include biochemical liver tests have been conducted among many groups of workers exposed to hepatotoxic agents. Serum aminotransferase elevations have been found in workers exposed to polychlorinated and polybrominated biphenyls (PCBs, PBBs) and polychlorinated naphthalenes. Hepatocellular liver enzyme abnormalities have been found among microelectronics equipment maintenance technicians, pharmaceutical industry workers exposed to mixed solvents, dry-cleaning operators, and petrochemical workers exposed to mixed

Table 21–1. Chemical agents associated with occupational liver disease.

Compound	Type of Injury	Occupation or Use
Arsenic	Cirrhosis, hepatocellular carcinoma, angiosarcoma	Pesticides
Beryllium	Granulomatous disease	Ceramics workers
Carbon tetrachloride	Acute hepatocellular injury, cirrhosis	Chemical manufacturing
1,2-dichloropropane	Biliary intraepithelial neoplasia and intraductal papillary neoplasm	Printing
1,4-dichlorobenzene	Acute hepatocellular injury	Insect repellant manufacture
1,1,2,2-tetrachloroethane (TTCE)	Acute hepatocellular injury	Glues
Dimethylacetamide	Acute hepatocellular injury	Spandex production
Dimethylformamide	Acute hepatocellular injury	Solvent, chemical manufacturing
Dimethylnitrosamine	Hepatocellular carcinoma	Rocket manufacturing
Dioxin	Porphyria cutanea tarda	Pesticides
Halothane	Acute hepatocellular injury	Anesthesiology
Hydrazine	Steatosis	Rocket manufacturing
Methylene dianiline (MDA)	Cholestasis	MDA production workers. Polyurethane foam insulation
2-nitropropane	Acute hepatocellular injury	Painters
Phosphorus	Acute hepatocellular injury	Munitions workers
Polychlorinated biphenyls	Subacute liver injury	Production, electrical utility
Tetrachloroethane	Acute or subacute hepatocellular injury	Aircraft manufacturing
Trichloroethylene	Acute hepatocellular injury	Cleaning solvent sniffing
Trinitrotoluene	Acute or subacute hepatocellular injury	Munitions workers
1,1,2,2-tetrachloroethane	Acute hepatocellular injury	
Vinyl chloride	Angiosarcoma	Rubber workers

aliphatic and aromatic hydrocarbons. Increased levels of liver enzymes have been found among chemical plant operators exposed to carbon tetrachloride. Hepatocellular damage with increased liver enzymes has been seen among coke oven workers exposed to coke oven emissions, with a greater risk among those with the cytochrome P450 MspI polymorphism. In a Chinese cohort, long-term exposure to coke oven emissions increased the risk of liver dysfunction, which was more prominent among those with higher body mass infection (BMI) and hepatitis virus infection. Solvent-exposed painters and paint makers have lifetime and peak solvent dose-related increases in serum transaminase and alkaline phosphatase activity, with a significant interaction with concurrent alcohol and hepatotoxic medication use. Increased levels of liver enzymes or bilirubin have been reported after occupational exposure to methylene chloride, polychlorinated naphthalenes, ethylene dichloride, hydrazine, antineoplastic drugs, dimethylacetamide (DMAc), and 2,3,7,8-tetrachlorodibenzo-p-dioxin (dioxin). Taxi drivers have recently been shown to have slightly elevated serum aminotransferases, possibly due to air pollution, as well as an increased risk for obesity and alcohol use.

Microsomal Enzyme Induction

By using the noninvasive antipyrine clearance test, induction of the microsomal enzyme system has been demonstrated in workers exposed to various pesticides (chlordecone, phenoxy acids, dichlorodiphenyltrichloroethane [DDT], lindane), halothane, PCBs, and various solvents. Functional abnormalities of liver metabolism, measured by antipyrine clearance or other noninvasive tests of liver function, are not accompanied by other clinical or laboratory signs of toxicity and so may provide a sensitive index of biological change.

Mortality Studies

Cohort mortality studies show an increased mortality rate from liver cirrhosis among newspaper pressmen, spray painters, chlorinated naphthalene workers, and oil refinery workers and from liver cancer among vinyl chloride, rubber, dye, and shoe factory workers. Case-control studies show a statistically significant association between primary liver cancer and exposure to chlorinated solvents, particularly among laundry workers, dry cleaners, gasoline service station attendants, printing industry workers, asphalt workers, automobile workers, and bartenders.

CHEMICAL AGENTS THAT CAUSE LIVER TOXICITY

Pathogenesis & Epidemiology

Occupational hepatotoxicity caused by chemicals is most frequently part of systemic toxicity involving other organ systems of primary clinical importance (eg, central nervous system depression, following exposure to hydrocarbon solvents). Occasionally, liver toxicity is responsible for the major clinical findings (eg, carbon tetrachloride intoxication associated with renal and central nervous system damage); rarely is liver disease the sole manifestation of toxicity.

The study of hepatotoxic potential in animals is an important first step for newly introduced chemicals. Differences among species, circumstances of exposure, and the difficulty in performing human studies may limit detection of experimental observations in the workplace. For example, while ingestion of arsenicals causes severe acute hepatic damage in both experimental animals and humans, there are reports of liver disease in humans in vintners exposed to arsenical pesticides.

There is no comprehensive repository of data on animal and human hepatotoxic agents. Identification of chemicals that may produce liver damage in humans has come about through a combination of experimental animal data, clinical observation, and epidemiologic studies. Some agents, such as trinitrotoluene (TNT), dimethylnitrosamine (DMA), tetrachloroethane, PCBs, and vinyl chloride, led to serious industrial hepatotoxicity before their effects on experimental animals were fully investigated. In the case of chlordecone (Kepone), human hepatotoxicity was found several years after experimental animal studies demonstrated clear evidence of liver damage following exposure.

Routes of Exposure

Inhalation, ingestion, and percutaneous absorption are the routes by which toxic chemicals can gain entry to the body. Inhalation is probably the most important route for hepatotoxic material, particularly for the volatile solvents. Several chemicals are lipophilic and may be absorbed through the skin in sufficient quantities to contribute to hepatotoxicity (eg, TNT, 4,4-diaminodiphenylmethane, tetrachloroethylene, PCBs, and dimethylformamide [DMF]). In cases of liver damage by industrial agents that are not airborne, it is often difficult to distinguish between contamination of ingested material, absorption from mucous membranes, and absorption through the skin. Oral intake of hepatotoxic agents is usually of importance only in the rare case of accidental ingestion, although mouth breathing and gum and tobacco chewing can increase the amount of gaseous substances absorbed during the workday.

Mechanisms of Toxicity

As Table 21–2 illustrates, chemical agents that cause hepatic injury may be classified into two major categories.

A. Intrinsically Toxic Agents

Agents intrinsically toxic to the liver—directly or indirectly—cause a high incidence of dose-dependent hepatic injury in exposed persons and similar lesions in experimental animals. Furthermore, the interval between exposure (under specified conditions) and onset of disease is consistent and usually short.

Table 21–2. Mechanisms of toxicity of chemicals causing hepatic injury.

Category of Agent	Incidence	Experimental Reproducibility	Dose Dependent	Example
Intrinsic toxin				
Direct	High	Yes	Yes	Carbon tetrachloride
Indirect				
Cytotoxic	High	Yes	Yes	Dimethylnitrosamine
Cholestatic	High	Yes	Yes	Methylene dianiline
Host idiosyncrasy				
Hypersensitivity	Low	No	No	Phenytoin
Metabolic abnormality	Low	No	No	Isoniazid

1. Direct hepatotoxins—Direct hepatotoxins or their metabolic products injure the hepatocyte and its organelles by a direct physicochemical effect, such as peroxidation of membrane lipids, denaturation of proteins, or other chemical changes that lead to destruction or distortion of cell membranes.

Carbon tetrachloride is the prototype and the best-studied example of the direct hepatotoxins, producing centrilobular necrosis and steatosis in humans and experimental animals. This agent appears to exert its hepatotoxic effects by the binding of reactive metabolites to a number of critical cellular molecules that interfere with vital cell function or cause lipid peroxidation of cell membranes. The toxicity of carbon tetrachloride is mediated by metabolism to the toxic trichloromethyl radical catalyzed by cytochrome P450 2EI. Damage to cellular membranes results in leakage of intracellular enzymes and electrolytes, leading to calcium shifts and lipid peroxidation.

Chloroform likewise may cause direct hepatic necrosis. A large number of haloalkanes (eg, trichloroethylene, carbon tetrabromide, tetrachloroethane, 1,1,1-trichloroethane, 1,1,2-trichloroethane, and hydrochlorofluorocarbons) produce hepatic injury ranging from steatosis to trivial or nondemonstrable liver damage. Their hepatotoxic potential is inversely proportional to chain length and bond energy and directly proportional to the number of halogen atoms in the molecule and to the atomic number of the halogen.

Most aromatic hydrocarbons are relatively low in hepatotoxic potential, with some evidence for acute hepatic injury caused by benzene, toluene, xylene, and styrene.

2. Indirect hepatotoxins—Indirect hepatotoxins are antimetabolites and related compounds that produce hepatic injury by interference with metabolic pathways. This may result in cytotoxic damage (degeneration or necrosis of hepatocytes) by interfering with pathways necessary for the structural integrity of the hepatocyte (morphologically seen as steatosis or necrosis) or may cause cholestasis (arrested bile flow) by interfering with the bile secretory process.

The cytotoxic indirect hepatotoxins include compounds of experimental interest (eg, ethionine and galactosamine), drugs (eg, tetracycline, asparaginase, methotrexate, and mercaptopurine), and botanicals (eg, aflatoxin, cycasin, mushroom alkaloids, and tannic acid). Ethanol belongs to this category by virtue of a number of selective biochemical lesions that lead to steatosis. Only one industrial chemical, 4,4-diaminodiphenylmethane (commonly known as *methylenedianiline* [MDA]), has been categorized as a cholestatic indirect hepatotoxin. Used as a plastic hardener—most commonly for epoxy resins—this agent has caused a number of epidemics (see "Acute Cholestatic Jaundice").

B. Agents Causing Liver Injury by Virtue of Host Idiosyncrasy

Chemically induced hepatic injury may be a result of some special vulnerability of the individual and not the intrinsic toxicity of the agent. In such cases, liver damage occurs sporadically and unpredictably, has low experimental reproducibility, and is not dose dependent. The injury may be a result of allergy (hypersensitivity) or of production of hepatotoxic metabolites. A well-established example is halothane, which causes acute hepatitis in a small percentage of individuals with a hypersensitivity immune response. The mechanism for halothane-induced hepatitis is thought to be a hypersensitivity reaction to liver neoantigens produced by the halothane metabolite 2-chloro-1,1,1-trifluoroethane. There appears to be a role for inherited susceptibility in halothane hepatitis.

▶ Hepatic Metabolism of Xenobiotics

The liver is especially vulnerable to chemical injury by virtue of its role in the metabolism of foreign compounds, or xenobiotics. The metabolism of xenobiotics is thus of central clinical interest. These chemicals, taken up by the body but not incorporated into the normal metabolic economy of the cell, are metabolized chiefly by the liver. Xenobiotic lipid-soluble compounds are well absorbed through membrane barriers and poorly excreted by the kidney as a result of protein binding and tubular reabsorption. Increasing polarity of nonpolar molecules by hepatic metabolism increases water solubility and urinary excretion. In this way, hepatic metabolism prevents the accumulation of drugs and other toxic chemicals in the body.

The strategic role of the liver as the primary defense against xenobiotics depends largely on cellular enzyme systems (mixed-function oxidases [MFOs]). The enzyme systems responsible for the metabolism of xenobiotics are attached to the membrane layers of the smooth endoplasmic reticulum. Although enzymes that catalyze the metabolism of nonpolar xenobiotics are present in the intestines, lungs, kidneys, and skin, the vast majority of metabolic conversions occur in the liver. Most xenobiotics that are toxic by the oral route are also hepatotoxic parenterally or by inhalation.

▶ Xenobiotic Agents Activated by the MFO System

Many hepatotoxic agents and hepatocarcinogens must be activated first by the MFO system to a toxic or carcinogenic metabolite. Examples include carbon tetrachloride, vinyl chloride, PCBs, bromobenzene, azo dyes, DMA, and allyl compounds. Electrophilic intermediates react with enzymes and regulatory or structural proteins and lead to cell death.

Many drugs, insecticides, organic solvents, carcinogens, and other environmental contaminants are known experimentally to stimulate some type of microsomal activity that is associated with the metabolism of xenobiotics. The administration of ethanol concomitantly with carbon tetrachloride enhances the toxicity of the latter, presumably via induction of the MFO system. Clinically, this may explain the well-documented synergistic effect between ethanol abuse and carbon tetrachloride toxicity in humans. Ethanol pretreatment in experimental human studies enhances the metabolic clearance of *m*-xylene and antipyrine by microsomal enzyme induction, and studies show that workers with prior alcohol consumption may be more likely to develop acute hepatotoxicity after occupational exposure to isopropyl alcohol, xylene, and toluene.

Other mechanisms may be at work as well because a single dose of alcohol given to animals several hours prior to administration of carbon tetrachloride potentiates toxicity. Experiments show that many other factors may affect the metabolism of xenobiotics: diet, age, sex, cigarette smoking, endocrine status, genetic factors, diurnal variations, underlying liver disease, and stress. There is considerable inter- and intraindividual variation in xenobiotic metabolism, and the relative importance of these factors in the occupational setting is not currently known. There is increasing evidence that tissue repair increases in a dose-dependent manner up to a threshold dose, but that this threshold can be lowered when one or more components of the mixture inhibit cell division and tissue repair. Enhanced microsomal enzyme function has been demonstrated in industrial workers exposed to hepatotoxins at levels below those shown to result in hepatic necrosis. Increasing attention has been directed to the use of noninvasive measurements of MFOs in the preclinical detection of liver disease (see next).

DISEASE PATTERNS & MORPHOLOGY OF HEPATIC INJURY

As Table 21–3 shows, occupational exposure to xenobiotics can lead to acute, subacute, or chronic liver disease. The clinical syndromes can be associated with several types of morphologic changes, as seen by light microscopy. Hepatic injury may be clinically overt or may be discovered only as a functional or histologic abnormality. Clinical evaluation of individuals with chronic liver disease caused by subtle repeated injury owing to workplace exposures has been of growing concern.

ACUTE HEPATIC INJURY

Acute liver disease was a cause of serious occupational liver disease in the first part of the twentieth century and may be still encountered. Acute hepatic injury has been reported as a result of exposure to agents listed in Table 21–4.

▶ Clinical Findings

Occupational exposure to xenobiotics may lead to degeneration or necrosis of hepatocytes (cytotoxic injury) or to arrested bile flow (cholestatic injury). The latency period is relatively short (24–48 hours), and clinical symptoms are often of extrahepatic origin. Anorexia, nausea, vomiting, jaundice, and hepatomegaly are often present. Severely exposed individuals who have sustained massive necrosis may have coffee-ground emesis, abdominal pain, reduction in liver size on examination, rapid development of ascites, edema, and hemorrhagic diathesis. This is often followed within 24–28 hours by somnolence and coma.

Morphologically, hepatic necrosis may be zonal, massive, or diffuse. Centrizonal necrosis is the characteristic lesion produced by the agents listed in Table 21–4, as well as by the toxins of *Amanita phalloides* and acetaminophen. Periportal or peripheral necrosis is produced by elemental phosphorus.

Table 21–3. Morphologic patterns of liver injury.

Type of Injury	Examples of Causes
Acute	
Cytotoxic	
Necrosis	
Zonal	Carbon tetrachloride, chloroform
Massive	Trinitrotoluene
Steatosis	Carbon tetrachloride, chloroform, phosphorus, dimethyl formamide, hydrazine
Cholestatic	Methylene dianiline, rapeseed oil
Subacute	Trinitrotoluene
Chronic	
Cirrhosis	Trinitrotoluene, polychlorinated biphenyls, tetrachloroethane
Sclerosis	Arsenic, vinyl chloride
Porphyria	Dioxin
Neoplasia	Arsenic, vinyl chloride
Steatosis	Dimethylformamide, carbon tetrachloride
Granuloma	Beryllium, copper

Table 21–4. Agents causing acute hepatic injury (partial list).

Anesthetic gases (halothane, methoxyflurane)
Bromobenzene
Carbon tetrabromide
Carbon tetrachloride
Chlorinated naphthalenes
Chloroform
Dichlorhydrin
Dimethylacetamide
Dimethylformamide
Elemental phosphorus
2-Nitropropane
Tetrachloroethane
Trichloroethane
Trichloroethylene
Trinitrotoluene
1,1,2,2-Tetrachloroethane

TNT, PCBs, and chloronaphthalenes can produce massive rather than zonal necrosis.

Various degrees of fatty change or steatosis also may be seen morphologically in association with toxicity owing to vinyl chloride, carbon tetrachloride, chloroform, tetrachloroethane, DMF, trichloroethane, styrene, hydrazine, and elemental phosphorus.

CARBON TETRACHLORIDE–INDUCED ACUTE HEPATIC INJURY

Carbon tetrachloride presents the classic example of an acute hepatotoxin. It was first recognized as such in the 1920s, when it was in common use as a liquid solvent, dry-cleaning agent, and fire extinguisher. Since then, hundreds of poisonings and fatalities have been reported, mostly from inhalation in confined spaces.

▶ Clinical Findings

Clinically, immediate nervous system symptoms of dizziness, headache, visual disturbances, and confusion are observed as a result of the anesthetic properties of carbon tetrachloride. This is followed by nausea, vomiting, abdominal pain, and diarrhea during the first 24 hours. Evidence of hepatic disease usually follows after 2–4 days but may appear within 24 hours. The liver and spleen become palpable, and jaundice develops, accompanied by elevated serum transaminase concentrations and prolonged prothrombin time. Renal failure may ensue a few days after the hepatic damage becomes manifest and in fact has been the cause of death in most fatal cases. Sequelae of hepatic failure such as hypoglycemia, encephalopathy, and hemorrhage may be complications. Some instances of carbon tetrachloride toxicity have occurred with accompanying ethanol intake, which may be a potentiating factor in hepatotoxicity.

Treatment with *N*-acetyl-L-cysteine (NAC) is effective in cases of massive carbon tetrachloride ingestion. Animal studies suggest that NAC may decrease the covalent binding of carbon tetrachloride–reactive metabolites, decrease the amount of carbon tetrachloride reaching the liver, or partially block lipid peroxidation.

ACUTE HEPATIC INJURY INDUCED BY OTHER XENOBIOTICS

Tetrachloroethylene causes acute hepatotoxicity when used as a dry-cleaning agent and causes acute centrilobular necrosis following recreational "solvent sniffing" of cleaning fluids. This may have been a result of contamination with dichloroacetylene rather than a consequence of tetrachloroethylene itself. In another case report, a 39-year-old man had acute liver failure due to tetrachloroethylene exposure. Histologic examination of the liver revealed massive hepatic necrosis, prominently, in zone 3 of the hepatic lobules. After supportive treatment including plasmapheresis, the individual improved clinically, but liver biopsy performed after

6 months showed architectural distortion with postnecrotic cirrhosis.

Both trichloroethylene and trichloroethane have been reported to cause acute, reversible hepatitis with fatty infiltration in several workers. A liver biopsy specimen from one trichloroethane-exposed printer showed focal bridging fibrosis and nodule formation with evidence of marked portal tract fibrosis, a pattern suggestive of macronodular or early cirrhosis.

A total of 18 Chinese factory workers were diagnosed with acute liver disease due to exposure to 1,1,2,2-tetrachloroethane (TTCE) in glue; one 18-year-old worker died due to liver failure after 3 months. The pattern of morphologic injury in these cases was similar to carbon tetrachloride, with histologic findings showing varying degrees of necrosis, fatty degeneration, and fibrosis in portal areas without cirrhosis. Patients with more severe jaundice had more severe pathologic changes, including piecemeal and bridge necrosis, and cholestasis.

Carbon tetrabromide caused a syndrome in chemists that is similar to acute carbon tetrachloride hepatotoxicity. DMAc caused acute, reversible hepatitis in one worker with severe inhalational and dermal exposure. Intentional nonoccupational exposure to the herbicide 2,4-dichlorophenoxyacetic acid (2,4-D) was reported to result in acute hepatitis with pronounced cholestasis, portal inflammation, and periportal edema. 2-Nitropropane, a nitroparaffin used as a solvent in epoxy-resin paints and coatings, has caused several cases of acute fulminant hepatitis following exposure in confined spaces. Exposure to mixed organic solvents (toluene, xylene, epoxy resin) has been reported to cause acute recurrent liver failure.

Hydrochlorofluorocarbons, increasingly used in industry as substitutes for ozone-depleting chlorofluorocarbons, have been reported to cause hepatocellular necrosis in workers after repeated exposure. The formation of trifluoroacetyl-adducted proteins may result in direct toxicity. The aromatic nitro amino compound 5-nitro-*o*-toluidine was reported recently to cause acute, reversible hepatitis among 15 hospitalized workers.

The solvent DMF has been reported to acutely cause increased levels of liver enzymes among workers involved in synthetic textile production and synthetic leather workers. In the study of synthetic leather workers, accidental skin contact with DMF led to significant DMF uptake. Liver biopsy specimens in acutely DMF-exposed workers showed focal hepatocellular necrosis with microvesicular steatosis. Liver biopsy specimens from workers with longer exposures showed macrovesicular steatosis without persisting acute injury or fibrosis. Abnormal liver function and chronic liver disease were associated with the glutathione *S*-transferase (GSTT-1) polymorphism. Progression to cirrhosis was not demonstrated up to 22 months following exposure. In a study of four synthetics production workers with DMF liver disease, the severity of the liver injury was related to the exposure levels. After removal of exposure, all patients recovered without specific treatment. In the past 10 years, increasing numbers of serious liver disease—including several deaths—have been reported among Chinese workers exposed to DMF.

Workers with concomitant alcohol use and infection with hepatitis B virus (HBV) had a greater risk of liver disease.

DMAc has been shown to cause acute hepatocellular injury among spandex production workers, with 90% decline of elevated alanine aminotransferase (ALT) within 31 days after cessation of exposure.

Fulminant hepatic failure has been reported in a recreational solvent abuser exposed to a mixture of isopropyl alcohol, methyl amyl alcohol, and butylated hydroxytoluene and in a worker following exposure to dichlorohydrin during tank cleaning.

TOXICANT-ASSOCIATED STEATOHEPATITIS

Toxicant-associated fatty liver disease (TAFLD) has been recently used to describe a form of liver injury pathologically similar to alcoholic liver disease (ALD) and nonalcoholic fatty liver disease (NAFLD). TAFLD occurs in nondrinking, nonobese subjects with occupational exposures to some industrial chemicals. Toxicant-associated steatohepatitis (TASH) is a more severe form of TAFLD characterized by hepatic steatosis, inflammatory infiltrate and fibrosis. In contrast to alcoholic steatohepatitis (ASH) and nonalcoholic steatohepatitis (NASH), which are typically associated with elevated serum aspartate aminotransferase (AST) and ALT, respectively, TASH may frequently be associated with normal liver enzymes. Since the current screening methodologies may not be sensitive for detection, TASH is likely to be more prevalent than is currently recognized.

TASH has been described among vinyl chloride production workers where the prevalence of steatohepatitis was 80% and of these, fibrosis was seen in 55%. Mean serum transaminases in these workers were normal, but total cytokeratin 18 (CK18) as a marker of cell death was elevated. The workers with TASH had insulin resistance with reduced adiponectin levels, as well markedly elevated serum tumor necrosis factor alpha and interleukin-1 beta, beta 6, and beta 8. Serum antioxidant activity was reduced. Necrotic, rather than apoptotic, hepatocellular death was noted in these VC workers with TASH.

ACUTE CHOLESTATIC JAUNDICE

Acute cholestatic jaundice is a rare manifestation of occupational toxicity. MDA was responsible for an epidemic of cholestatic jaundice observed in Epping, England (*Epping jaundice*), in 1965. This compound, used as a hardener for epoxy resin, had spilled from a plastic container onto the floor of a van that was carrying both flour and the chemical. Acute cholestatic injury was found subsequently in 84 persons who had eaten bread made from the contaminated flour. Onset was abrupt—with abdominal pain—in 60% of cases and was insidious in one-third. Histologic evidence of bile stasis with only slight parenchymal injury was seen in most cases, and all victims recovered without evidence of

persistent hepatic injury. An analysis 38 years later found no deaths from liver cancer or nonmalignant liver disease. Similar cases have been reported subsequently for industrial exposure during the manufacture and application of epoxy resins, and in a construction worker exposed to MDA during polyurethane foam production. Cholestatic liver injury has been reported after accidental ingestion of denatured rapeseed oil and after ingestion of moldy grain and nuts contaminated with aflatoxin.

SUBACUTE HEPATIC NECROSIS

This form of hepatic injury is characterized by a smoldering illness with delayed onset of jaundice. It usually follows repeated exposure to relatively small doses of a hepatotoxin. The onset of anorexia, nausea, and vomiting accompanied by hepatomegaly and jaundice may occur after several weeks to months of exposure and may lead variably to recovery or to fulminant hepatic failure. A few patients are reported to have developed macronodular cirrhosis, although clinical data are limited.

The histologic features of subacute hepatic necrosis consist of various degrees of necrosis, fibrosis, and regeneration. In cases where the clinical course is relatively brief (2–3 weeks), necrotic features predominate. In patients with a prolonged course of several months or more, postnecrotic scarring with subacute hepatic necrosis is seen. In the past, TNT caused many cases of both acute and subacute hepatic necrosis. Fortunately, subacute hepatic necrosis caused by occupational exposure is rare today.

CHRONIC HEPATIC INJURY

Several forms of chronic liver damage can result from continuing or repeated injury caused by prolonged exposure: cirrhosis and fibrosis, hepatoportal sclerosis, hepatic porphyria, and neoplasia.

CIRRHOSIS & FIBROSIS

The histologic pattern of progressive necrosis accompanied by regenerating nodules, fibrosis, and architectural distortion of the liver (*toxic cirrhosis*) is well described as part of the syndrome of subacute hepatic necrosis caused by TNT, tetrachloroethane, and the PCBs and chloronaphthalenes. Additionally, some survivors of TNT-induced injury were found to have macronodular cirrhosis.

Cirrhosis may occur after prolonged, repeated low-level exposure to carbon tetrachloride in dry-cleaning plants and to inorganic arsenical insecticides among vintners and from drinking arsenic-contaminated well water. Micronodular cirrhosis was described in a worker with repeated exposure to a degreasing solvent containing a mixture of trichloroethylene and 1,1,1-trichloroethane, and chronic active hepatitis was reported in a worker exposed to 1,1,1-trichloroethane.

Thirteen painters with no history of drug or alcohol ingestion exposed over 6–39 years to a variety of organic solvents had persistent biopsy-verified histologic changes of steatosis, focal necrosis, and enlarged portal tracts with fibrosis. Three nurses were reported to have irreversible liver injury after years of handling cytostatic drugs, with liver biopsies showing piecemeal necrosis in one and steatosis with fibrosis in the other two. The anesthetic agent halothane has been reported to cause cirrhosis and chronic active hepatitis after acute exposure.

A few studies of occupational cohorts exposed to acute hepatotoxins (eg, carbon tetrachloride and chlorinated naphthalenes) have demonstrated increased cirrhosis mortality, suggesting persistent subclinical injury after high exposures. Increased mortality as a consequence of cirrhosis has been observed among pressman, shipyard workers, metal fabrication employees, marine inspectors, and anesthesiologists. In some of these studies, limited data were available on the role of confounding factors such as ethanol consumption or viral hepatitis.

HEPATOPORTAL SCLEROSIS & HEPATIC PORPHYRIA

Portal and periportal fibrosis leading to portal hypertension (*noncirrhotic portal hypertension*) can be caused by exposure to inorganic arsenicals, thorium, and vinyl chloride. A few cases of porphyria cutanea tarda as a consequence of occupational exposure to the herbicide 2,4,5-trichlorophenoxyacetic acid, probably caused by contamination by dioxin, have been recorded. Turkish peasants developed liver disease and hepatic porphyria after ingesting wheat contaminated with the fungicide hexachlorobenzene.

GRANULOMATOUS DISEASE

Beryllium and copper exposure can result in granulomatous liver disease, with hepatic granulomas located near or within the portal tracts. Clinical liver disease usually is not significant, but granulomas occasionally result in hepatomegaly, necrosis, or fibrosis.

STEATOSIS

Steatosis is characterized morphologically by microvesicular or macrovesicular intracellular lipid formation. Steatosis from chemicals is a well-established phenomenon and may occur as a result of acute occupational exposure to elemental phosphorus, TNT, arsenical pesticides, DMF, toluene, aliphatic and aromatic organic solvents (white spirit, xylene, toluene, and styrene), chlordecone, and certain chlorinated hydrocarbons (eg, carbon tetrachloride, methyl chloroform, 1,1,1-trichloroethane, and tetrachloroethane). Nonoccupational causes include diabetes, hypertriglyceridemia, obesity, and smoking. Intracellular hepatic lipid formation results from xenobiotic effects on fat metabolism. Minimal to moderate elevation in transaminase levels is seen after acute occupational exposure, with resolution in several weeks after removal. Steatosis also may occur after chronic exposure to carbon tetrachloride or DMF. Progression from steatosis to

fibrosis or cirrhosis has not been documented. A large cohort study concluded that HBV infection was associated with lower risk of developing NAFLD indicating a possible effect of HBV infection on the pathogenesis of NAFLD development. A recent National Health and Nutrition Examination Survey (NHANES)–based cross-sectional study did not find an association between shiftwork and increased risk of NAFLD. A cross-sectional study among petrol station attendants in southern China concluded that exposure to methyl tertiary butyl ether (MTBE) was not a significant risk factor for the prevalence of NAFLD. A study in Taiwan examined the prevalence and factors related to NAFLD among occupational populations. Office and administrative support professions had a relative higher prevalence of NAFLD than laborers, peasants, and monks. Irregular lifestyle, eating habits, work stress, and physical inactivity were the likely cause for high prevalence of NAFLD.

NEOPLASIA

Hepatocellular Carcinoma

Hepatocellular carcinoma (HCC), which accounts for the majority of liver tumors, ranks fifth among types of human cancer. Liver cancer is the second leading worldwide cause of cancer-associated mortalities. Well-established risk factors for liver cancer include the hepatitis B and C viruses, aflatoxins, alcohol consumption, oral contraceptives, NASH, obesity, type 2 diabetes, cirrhosis, hemochromatosis, Wilson disease, and hemophilia. While many occupationally encountered chemical agents are known to cause HCC in experimental animals, only a relatively few studies have been performed in humans. Vinyl chloride, a halogenated aliphatic compound used since the 1940s in the production of polyvinyl chloride, was known to be an animal hepatotoxin in the early 1960s. Acro-osteolysis was reported in humans in 1966. In 1974, three cases of angiosarcoma, a rare liver tumor, were found in employees who had been exposed to vinyl chloride for up to 20 years. Subsequent reports and surveillance activities through the end of 2013 have recorded more than 200 cases of vinyl chloride–associated hepatic angiosarcoma. Epidemiologic studies confirm a strong relationship between cumulative vinyl chloride exposure and occurrence of liver and biliary cancer and hepatic angiosarcoma. Pathologically, hepatic damage in association with vinyl chloride exposure appears to progress sequentially from focal hepatocyte hyperplasia to sinusoidal dilatation to peliosis hepatis and sarcomatous transformation of the lining of the cells of sinusoids and portal capillaries. Studies indicate that vinyl chloride acts as a genotoxic carcinogen, with transformation of vinyl chloride into chloroethylene oxide (CEO) by cytochrome P450 isozyme 2E1. CEO can alkylate nucleic acid bases, with adducts leading to base-pair substitutions. Some evidence suggests that the *K-ras-2* mutation pattern or other genetic polymorphisms may increase the risk of developing hepatic angiosarcoma and HCC. Underlying HBV infection and alcohol intake appear to increase the risk of developing HCC owing to VCM exposure. In the past, liver disease usually was unrecognized until the late stages of histologic damage and with the victim only a few months from death. Recently, persistent serum transaminase elevations have been observed among workers previously exposed to vinyl chloride, with liver biopsies showing nonspecific fatty changes. Medical surveillance of vinyl chloride–exposed workers by using liver ultrasonography shows that workers exposed to 200 ppm for at least 1 year have a fourfold increased risk of developing periportal liver fibrosis. Most recently, two cases of angiosarcoma were reported in a hairdresser and barber exposed to hair sprays with VC as a propellant. A recent study of 1658 workers involved in VCM production and polymerization found that risk of death from liver cirrhosis and HCC increased with VCM exposure.

Hepatic angiosarcoma also has developed in vintners with long exposure to inorganic arsenic, in patients with psoriasis treated with inorganic potassium arsenite (Fowler solution) in the 1940s and 1950s, and in patients injected with a colloidal suspension of thorium dioxide (Thorotrast), used for carotid angiography and liver-spleen scans from 1930 to 1955. The increased risk of liver cancer has been demonstrated in animal studies and among occupational cohorts exposed to trichloroethylene, DMF, perchloroethylene, dioxins, PCBs, and PBBs, o-toluidine, 4,4′-methylene bis (2-chlorobenzenamine) (MOCA), organochlorine pesticides, and cadmium.

Case-control studies show elevated odds ratios for the development of liver cancer among workers in a variety of occupations such as chemical, clerical, automobile repair, dry cleaning and food service workers; transport equipment operators, and workers exposed to welding fumes. While some of these studies were not able to evaluate the significance of confounding factors such as alcohol and hepatitis B and C virus infection, taken as a whole, these studies indicate prolonged exposure to organic solvents represents a risk factor for liver cancer. The risk of liver cancer in a Nordic occupational cohort was slightly elevated in groups with high exposure to perchloroethylene (compared to occupationally unexposed subjects), with the risk increasing with increasing continuous exposure to the chemical. Among Finnish workers exposed to organic solvents, an elevated liver cancer incidence was observed in male printers, varnishers, and lacquerers; among men, the risk was increased in the highest exposure category of aromatic hydrocarbons, aliphatic/alicyclic hydrocarbons, chlorinated hydrocarbons and "other solvents." Among women, the risk was increased for the group "other solvents" that includes mainly alcohols, ketones, esters, and glycol ethers. A recent Taiwanese study found a significant dose-response relationship between the consumption of Chinese herbs containing aristolochic acid and HCC in patients with HBV infection, suggesting that aristolochic acid which may be associated with HBV plays an important role in the pathogenesis of HCC. There is mixed evidence suggesting that workers with higher serum levels of DDT were associated with increased HCC risk. A case-control study from China concluded that workers with airway exposure to Aspergillus flavus–contaminated dust had an elevated risk of hepatocellular cancer compared to those without exposure, requiring an urgent need for an intervention programs aimed at reducing exposure to inhalational aflatoxin B1 (AFB1).

Cholangiosarcoma

An outbreak of intrahepatic cholangiocarcinoma (ICC) was reported in 2013 among 17 workers exposed to chlorinated organic solvents used to remove ink residues (including 1,2-dichloropropane and dichloromethane in an offset color proof-printing department at a printing company in Japan. When compared to nonoccupational cases of ICC, the cases of occupational ICC were significantly younger, had higher levels of serum γ-glutamyl transpeptidase activity and regional dilatation of the bile ducts without tumor-induced obstruction. Pathologic examination of the occupational ICC cases showed precancerous or early cancerous lesions, such as biliary intraepithelial neoplasia and intraductal papillary neoplasm of the bile duct.

INFECTIOUS AGENTS CAUSING LIVER TOXICITY

Infectious hepatotoxic agents (Table 21–5) are of importance in the pathogenesis of both acute and chronic liver disease. In the past few decades, health care workers (HCWs) has substantial burden of hepatitis B and C infection. More recent estimates from the European Union suggest that HCWs may have a prevalence of hepatitis B and C comparable to that of general population. This is probably due to vaccination and adherence to universal precautions as an effective means to prevent occupational exposure.

Occupational exposure to infectious hepatotoxic agents also may occur among sewer workers; emergency health care personnel; animal-care, slaughterhouse, and farm workers; and laboratory workers.

Table 21–5. Infectious agents associated with occupational liver disease.

Hepatitis A virus	Nursery and kindergarten staff, sewer workers
Hepatitis B and C viruses	Health care workers with blood and body fluid contact
Hepatitis E virus	Swine containment workers
Cytomegalovirus	Pediatric health care workers
Coxiella burnetii	Animal care workers, farm workers, slaughterhouse workers
Leptospira icterohaemorrhagiae	Sewer workers, farm workers

HEPATITIS A

▶ Exposure

The cause of hepatitis A is the hepatitis A virus (HAV), a 27-nm RNA agent that is a member of the picornavirus family. Outbreaks of hepatitis A infection have been reported among personnel working with nonhuman primates, waste pickers, wastewater treatment plant workers, home health workers, food handlers, and in neonatal intensive care units. Serologic surveys suggest a higher prevalence of HAV antibodies among HCWs working in emergency rooms, surgery, laundry rooms, and children's psychiatry and among day-care workers and dentists. There are several case reports of HAV infection among waste water treatment plant workers, and some serologic studies have confirmed an increased risk in this population. Although day-care centers can be the source of outbreaks of occupationally acquired hepatitis A infection within some communities, disease within day-care centers more commonly reflects extended transmission within the community. There are no reports of hepatitis A outbreaks in correctional settings. While contaminated food and water are common epidemic sources, hepatitis A is transmitted primarily by person-to-person contact, generally through fecal contamination. Transmission of HAV is facilitated by poor personal hygiene and intimate household or sexual contact. Transmission by blood transfusion has occurred but is rare. Transmission in saliva has not been demonstrated. The recent outbreaks of hepatitis A in 2017 in California, Kentucky, Michigan, and Utah among persons who reported drug use or homelessness signaled a shift in hepatitis A epidemiology from point-source outbreaks associated with contaminated food to large community outbreaks with person-to-person transmission. On October 24, 2018, ACIP voted unanimously to add "homelessness" as an indication for ACIP-recommended HAV vaccination to halt ongoing outbreaks and prevent future outbreaks.

▶ Clinical Findings & Diagnosis

The incubation period for hepatitis A is 15–50 days (average: 28–30 days). The illness caused by HAV characteristically has an abrupt onset, with fever, malaise, anorexia, nausea, abdominal discomfort, and jaundice. High concentrations of HAV (10 particles/g) are found in stools of infected persons. Fecal virus excretion reaches its highest concentration during the incubation period and early in the prodromal phase; it diminishes rapidly once jaundice appears. Greatest infectivity is seen in the 2-week period immediately before the onset of jaundice or elevation of liver enzymes.

A chronic carrier state with HAV in blood or feces has not been demonstrated. The fatality rate among reported cases is approximately 0.3%. The diagnosis of acute hepatitis A is confirmed by the presence of immunoglobulin (Ig) M class anti-HAV in serum collected during the acute or early convalescent phase of the disease. IgG antibodies appear in the convalescent phase and remain positive for life, apparently conferring enduring protection against disease.

▶ Treatment

Treatment for hepatitis A is symptomatic, with rest, analgesics, and fluid replacement where necessary. Fulminant hepatic failure occasionally follows acute HAV infection. Orthotopic liver transplantation is well established as the appropriate treatment for severe cases.

▶ Prevention

HAV infections can be prevented by the following hygienic practices:

a) Handwashing (after using the bathroom, changing diapers, and before preparing or eating foods).

b) Avoiding tap water and raw foods in areas with poor sanitation.

c) Heating foods appropriately (the virus can be inactivated by heating to >185°F [>85°C] for 1 minute). Cooked foods can transmit HAV if the temperature during food preparation is inadequate to kill the virus or if food is contaminated after cooking.

d) Chlorine, iodine, and disinfecting solutions (household bleach 1:100 dilution) are effective for inactivation of HAV.

Numerous studies show that a single intramuscular dose of 0.02 mL/kg of immune globulin (immune serum globulin, gamma globulin) given before exposure or during the incubation period of hepatitis A is protective against clinical illness. The prophylactic value is greatest (80–90%) when immune globulin is given early in the incubation period and declines thereafter. In July 2017, the dose of GamaSTAN (immune globulin product available in the United States) for preexposure and postexposure prophylaxis was increased. Preexposure prophylaxis in persons who plan to travel in areas with high or intermediate hepatitis A endemicity depends on the duration of the travel (up to 1 month: 0.1 mL/kg; up to 2 months: 0.2 mL/kg; and 2 months or longer: repeat dose of 0.2 mL/kg every 2 months), and for postexposure prophylaxis, it is 0.1 mL/kg. This was a result of decreasing prevalence of previous HAV infection among plasma donors leading to declining anti-HAV antibody levels in donor plasma. Since hepatitis A cannot be diagnosed reliably on clinical presentation alone, serologic confirmation of hepatitis A in the index case is recommended before treatment of contacts. Once the diagnosis of acute infection is made, close contacts should be given HAV vaccine and/or immune globulin promptly within 2 weeks of exposure to prevent development of secondary cases. Such close contacts may include staff of day-care facilities, food handlers (in establishments with a food handler diagnosed with hepatitis A institutions for custodial care—or hospital staff if an unsuspected patient has been fecally incontinent.

Routine immune globulin administration is not recommended under the usual office or factory conditions for persons exposed to a fellow worker with hepatitis A or for teachers with schoolroom contact. Food handlers should receive immune globulin when a common-source exposure is recognized and restaurant patrons when the infected person is involved directly in handling uncooked foods without gloves. This is especially the case when the patrons can be identified within 2 weeks of exposure and the food handler's hygienic practices are known to be deficient. Serologic screening of contacts for anti-HAV antibodies to the HAV before giving immune globulin is not recommended because screening is more costly than immune globulin and would delay administration. Pregnancy or lactation is not a contraindication to immune globulin administration.

The inactivated hepatitis A vaccine is currently recommended for persons traveling to or working in countries with intermediate or high HAV endemicity, men who have sex with men (MSM), illicit drug users (injections and noninjection), laboratory workers with exposure to live virus, animal handlers with exposure to HAV-infected nonhuman primates, individuals with chronic liver disease, individuals with clotting factor disorders, individuals with close personal contact with an international adoptee from a country of high or intermediate endemicity during the first 60 days following arrival in the United States, and individuals with direct contact to others who have hepatitis A and homeless individuals. Prevaccination testing should be considered depending on the expected prevalence of immunity, cost of the vaccine compared with the cost of testing and age of the person being immunized. Immunogenicity studies show that virtually 100% of children, adolescents, and adults develop protective levels of antibody to HAV (anti-HAV) after completing a two-dose vaccine series (each given as an intramuscular injection of 1 mL of 1440 enzyme-linked immunosorbent assay [ELISA] units). (Protective antibodies remain for as long as 4 years, with kinetic models suggesting that protective levels of anti-HAV persist for at least 20 years.) In immunocompetent children and adults, the persistence of protective antibodies is greater than 85% more than 15–20 years and greater than 95% more than 20 years after vaccination, respectively. There is no need for HAV booster vaccination after completion of the primary two-dose vaccination series. For at-risk individuals who are allergic to hepatitis A vaccine or who are younger than 12 months, passive immunization via immune globulin may be given. Routine hepatitis A vaccination is not recommended for child-care workers, hospital workers, teachers, sewage treatment employees, correctional workers, or staff in institutions for the developmentally disabled. When outbreaks are recognized in these settings, use of HAV vaccine and/or immune globulin promptly within 2 weeks of exposure for persons in close contact with infected patients or students is recommended. Routine hepatitis A vaccination among restaurant employees is not recommended given the incidence of infection and present cost of the vaccine, even during epidemics.

An employee with symptoms and confirmed HAV infection should be restricted from work until symptoms subside or for 1 week after the onset of jaundice.

HEPATITIS B

▶ Exposure & Epidemiology

Hepatitis B infection is caused by the HBV, a major cause of acute and chronic hepatitis, cirrhosis, and primary HCC worldwide. HCWs with primary blood and body fluid contact are the primary group at risk. This includes workers with significant contact with blood, blood products, or body secretions: surgeons, oral surgeons, dental hygienists, pathologists, anesthesiologists, phlebotomists, medical technologists, respiratory therapists, emergency room personnel, and medical and surgical house staff. Medical waste handlers have also been found to have an increased risk of HBV infection. Also, persons not directly involved in patient care (eg, housekeeping, laundry, security, maintenance, and volunteers) but with potential exposure to infectious agents that can be transmitted between patients and HCWs is another important group that should be recognized as at risk group. In serologic studies in the United States in the 1970s, the annual rate of clinically manifest hepatitis B infection in hospital workers was approximately 0.1%, or about 10 times that of control populations. Hospital staff with frequent blood contact had a prevalence rate of hepatitis B surface antigen (HBsAg) of 1–2% and a prevalence rate of anti-HBV antibody (anti-HBs) of 15–30% compared with healthy controls, who had rates of 0.3% and 3–5%, respectively. Since the advent of standard precautions to prevent exposure to blood and other potentially infectious body fluids, along with preexposure vaccination against HBV, there has been a sharp decline in the incidence of HBV infection among HCWs. However, in many countries worldwide only a small percentage of HCWs have received the HBV vaccine.

The risk of infection with HBV depends on the titer of virions in the infectious fluid and correlates with the presence or absence of hepatitis e antigen in the source patient. The risk of infection following percutaneous injury with both HBsAg- and hepatitis B e-antigen (HBeAg)-positive blood is 22–31%; the risk of developing serologic evidence of HBV infection is 37–62%. Percutaneous injuries are the most efficient mode of HBV transmission, although in many nosocomial outbreaks HCWs cannot recall this history. Some HBV infections may result from infectious indirect blood or body fluid exposures onto nonintact skin (scratches, abrasions, or burns) or on mucosal surfaces. HBV is highly infectious, can be transmitted in the absence of visible blood, and remains infectious by surviving in dried blood at room temperature on environmental surfaces for at least 7 days. HBsAg-positive persons with elevated HBV DNA or those with HBeAg, a protein from the HBV that circulates in the blood and is a marker of infectivity, are most infectious. Persons with occult HBV infection (ie, those who test negative for HBsAg but have detectable HBV DNA) also may transmit infection.

Blood contains the highest titer of HBV, but HBsAg may be found in amniotic fluid breast milk, bile, cerebrospinal fluid, , ,pleural fluid, peritoneal fluid, pericardial fluid saliva, semen, synovial fluid, tears, and vaginal secretions. Urine, feces, vomitus, nasopharyngeal washings, sputum, and sweat are not efficient vehicles of transmission unless they contain blood because they contain low quantities of infectious HBV. HBsAg found in breast milk is also unlikely to lead to transmission, and hence HBV infection is not a contraindication to breastfeeding. Employment in a hospital without blood exposure carries no greater risk than that for the general population.

Most hospital workers experience accidental blood contact by needlestick injuries, usually during disposal of needles, administration of parenteral injections or infusion therapy, drawing blood, and handling linens and trash containing uncapped needles. To minimize the risk of bloodborne pathogen transmission, all HCWs should adhere to standard precautions, including the appropriate use of handwashing, protective barriers, and care in the use and disposal of needles and other sharp instruments. In the United States, the Needlestick Safety and Prevention Act of 2001 directed the Occupational Safety and Health Administration (OSHA) to revise the Occupational Exposure to Bloodborne Pathogens Standard and established detailed requirements for employers regarding the identification and use of effective and safer medical devices. This has resulted in a significant decline in percutaneous injuries among HCWs.

▶ Forms of Illness & Transmission

Three forms of hepatitis B are encountered in clinical practice: acute hepatitis B, inapparent sporadic episodes of unknown origin, and the chronic carrier state—detected by screening for HBsAg—in apparently healthy persons. Transmission occurs via percutaneous or permucosal routes when exposure to blood or potentially infectious body fluids occurs; HBV is not transmitted via the fecal-oral route or by contamination of food or water.

Among adults, HBV is transmitted primarily by percutaneous exposure to blood (eg, by injection-drug use) and sexual contact. HBV is transmitted efficiently by sexual contact both among heterosexuals and among MSM. Risk factors for sexual transmission among heterosexuals include having unprotected sex with an infected partner, having unprotected sex with more than one partner, and a history of another sexually transmitted infection (STI). Risk factors associated with sexual transmission among MSM include having multiple sex partners, history of another STI, and anal intercourse. Transmission can occur from interpersonal contact (eg, sharing a toothbrush or razor, contact with exudates from dermatologic lesions, or contact with HBsAg-contaminated surfaces) and in settings such as schools, child care centers, and facilities for developmentally disabled persons. Transmission of HBV from transfusion of blood or blood products is rare because of donor screening and viral inactivation procedures. Other possible sources of infection include contaminated medical or dental instruments, unsafe injections, needlestick injuries, organ transplantation, and dialysis.

▶ Course of Illness

The onset of acute hepatitis B is generally insidious, with anorexia, malaise, nausea, vomiting, abdominal pain fever, dark urine, changes in stool color, hepatomegaly, splenomegaly, and jaundice. Skin rash, arthralgia, and arthritis also can occur. The average incubation period is 60 days (range: 40–90 days) from exposure to onset of abnormal serum ALT levels and 90 days (range: 60–150 days) from exposure to onset of jaundice. Fulminant HBV infection is uncommon (<1%) but often results in death or liver failure necessitating liver transplantation. HBsAg can be detected in serum 30–60 days after exposure to HBV and persists for variable periods. Antibody to hepatitis B surface antigen (anti-HBs) develops after a resolved infection and indicates long-term immunity. The antibody to the core antigen (anti-HBc) develops in all HBV infections and persists indefinitely. The fatality rate among persons with reported cases of acute HBV infection is less than 1.5%, with the highest rates in adults 55 years or older. Because a substantial number of infections are asymptomatic and therefore are not reported, the overall fatality rate among all persons with HBV infection is likely lower.

The chronic carrier state is defined as the presence of HBsAg-positive serum on at least two occasions at least 6 months apart and is characterized by high levels of HBsAg and anti-HBc and various levels of serum transaminases, reflecting liver disease activity. Chronic infection occurs among 80%–90% of persons infected during infancy, 30% of persons infected before age 6 years, and less than 1–12% of persons infected as an older child or adult. Approximately 95% of primary infections in immunocompetent adults are self-limited, with elimination of the virus from blood and generally immunity to reinfection. Chronic infection develops more frequently in immunosuppressed persons (eg, hemodialysis patients and persons with human immunodeficiency virus [HIV] infection) and persons with diabetes. The natural course of HBsAg-positive chronic active hepatitis is progressive, frequently evolving to cirrhosis, HCC, and death owing to hepatic failure or bleeding esophageal varices.

(Depending on the country, the estimated relative risk for developing HCC after chronic HBV infection ranges from 6- to 100-fold.) Persons with chronic HBV infection are at 12–300 times higher risk of HCC than noncarriers. An estimated 1000–1500 persons die each year in the United States of hepatitis B–related liver cancer. HCC usually develops after 20–30 years of persistent HBV infection accompanied by hepatocellular necrosis, inflammation, and regenerative hyperplasia. Chronic hepatitis and liver cirrhosis are important endogenous factors in the development of HCC.

▶ Treatment

Treatment of acute HBV is dependent on the clinical setting and is mainly supportive. Tenofovir or entecavir are used to treat patients with a severe or a protracted course (eg, those who develop a coagulopathy [international normalized ratio (INR) >1.5], those with persistent symptoms or marked jaundice [bilirubin >10 mg/dL] for more than 4 weeks after presentation). Treatment can be stopped after confirmation that the patient has cleared HBsAg (two consecutive tests 4 weeks apart). Lamivudine or telbivudine can also be used, as the duration of treatment is generally short. However, since severe exacerbations of chronic HBV in previously undiagnosed patients can be difficult to differentiate from acute HBV, tenofovir or entecavir are preferred. Adefovir is not typically used because of its weak antiviral activity, and interferon should be avoided because of the risk of bacterial infections and a further increase in hepatic necroinflammation in patients with severe hepatitis or acute liver failure. The likelihood of liver failure from acute HBV is less than 1%, and in immunocompetent adults, the likelihood of progression to chronic HBV infection is less than 5%.

Therapeutic agents such as the pegylated interferon-alpha (IFNα, or PEG-IFNα) or nucleos(t)ide analogs (such as lamivudine, adefovir, entecavir telbivudine, and tenofovir) that have been approved for treatment of chronic hepatitis B can result in sustained suppression of HBV replication, loss of HBeAg and HBsAg and remission of liver disease in selected individuals. Periodic screening with α-fetoprotein or imaging studies can enhance early detection of HCC. Chronically infected persons with HCC who have undergone such screening have been reported to experience long-term survival after resection or ablation of small HCCs. Patients with chronic HBV should receive counseling on ways to prevent worsening liver disease (eg, avoid alcohol use, hepatitis A vaccination) and to reduce transmission to others. Persons with acute or chronic HBV infections should prevent their blood and other potentially infective body fluids from contacting other persons. They should not donate blood or share toothbrushes or razors with household members.

▶ Prevention

Postexposure prophylaxis should be based on the hepatitis vaccination status of the exposed person and whether the source of blood and the HBsAg status of the source are known or unknown. Multiple doses of hepatitis B immune globulin provides approximately 75% protection from HBV infection. Guidelines for hepatitis B prophylaxis following percutaneous exposure are given in Chapter 20.

Routine vaccination of infants, young children, and adolescents is expected to eliminate transmission of HBV eventually among adults in the United States. For individuals who have not been vaccinated previously and who are at risk for blood-borne pathogen exposure, vaccination should be done with the HBV vaccine, administered as a three-dose series via the intramuscular route in the deltoid muscle. For those workers who may be at risk for both hepatitis A and B infection, administration of the combination hepatitis A-B vaccine may be cost-effective. Protective immunity is conferred in more than 95% of vaccine recipients. The availability of recombinant hepatitis B vaccines has eliminated

previous, albeit unwarranted, concerns regarding the risk of blood-borne infections transmitted by plasma-derived vaccines. Nearly 90% of vaccine recipients have protective levels of anti-HBs 5 years after vaccination. Loss of detectable anti-HB levels after immunization does not imply loss of protection because studies show that exposure to HBV leads to an amnestic rise in anti-HB levels after natural infection. Therefore, routine booster doses of hepatitis B vaccine are not recommended.

Measurement of prevaccination anti-HB levels generally is not recommended but may be performed depending on the cost of screening and the prevalence of antibody in the group to be vaccinated. Screening is usually cost-effective, and should be considered for groups with a high risk of HBV infection (prevalence of HBV markers ≥20%), such as MSM, injection-drug users, and incarcerated persons. Screening is usually not cost-effective for groups with a low expected prevalence of HBV serologic markers, such as health professionals in their training years. Approximately 5% of immunocompetent adults fail to respond to the hepatitis B vaccine, with vaccine nonresponsiveness increasing with age greater than 40 years, obesity, and smoking. Postvaccination anti-HB testing (1–2 months after the third dose) is useful in establishing immune status for postexposure treatment or for administering booster doses to vaccine nonresponders. Nonresponders to the primary series have a 30–50% chance of responding to a second three-dose series. Revaccinated persons should be retested at completion of the second vaccine series. Nonresponders to vaccination who are HBsAg-negative should be counseled regarding the need to obtain hepatitis B immune globulin prophylaxis for known or probable parenteral exposure to HBsAg-positive blood. Screening by ultrasonography and serum α-fetoprotein measurement are indicated for patients at high risk for developing HCC.

The employee with HBV infection and liver disease should be advised to avoid exposure to other potentially hepatotoxic agents such as ethanol or workplace solvents.

HEPATITIS C

▶ Exposure & Epidemiology

Hepatitis C virus (HCV) is a single-stranded RNA virus of the family Flaviviridae. There are seven known genotypes, of which genotypes 1–6 are most commonly studied. The virus has a striking ability to persist in the host after infection, with chronic hepatitis occurring in approximately 70% of infected individuals. About 40% of infected persons progress to cirrhosis, leading to hepatic failure, HCC, and death from hepatic-related causes within 30 years. Viral persistence appears to be related to rapid mutation under immune pressure, with coexistence within the host as related but immunologically distinct strains. The high rate of mutation appears to be the primary mechanism underlying the absence of effective neutralization and the development of persistent infection. Globally, an estimated 71 million people have chronic HCV infection. Nearly 2.4 million Americans—1%

of the adult population—were living with HCV from 2013 through 2016. In 2017 in the United States, 38 states submitted 143,286 cases of chronic hepatitis C cases to the US Centers for Disease Control and Prevention, with 17,253 deaths nationwide.

HCV is spread primarily through parenteral exposures from blood transfusions or intravenous drug abuse. Up to 40% of cases in the United States have no identified exposure source. There is minimal evidence for sexual transmission or mother-to-infant transmission of HCV.

In contrast to HBV, the epidemiologic data for HCV suggest that environmental contamination with blood containing HCV is not a significant risk for transmission in the health care setting, with the possible exception of the hemodialysis setting, where HCV transmission related to environmental contamination and poor infection-control practices has been implicated. The risk of infection following occupational percutaneous exposure averages 1.8% (range: 0–7%) and is increased following deep injury or injury from a hollow-bore needle. In one longitudinal analysis at a large academic medical center between 2002 and 2015, the incidence of HCV infection was 0.1%.

Transmission rarely occurs from mucous membrane exposures (including conjunctivae) to blood, and no transmission in HCWs has been documented from intact or non-intact skin exposures to blood. The risk of transmission from tissues or other body fluids is not well characterized but is expected to be low.

▶ Clinical Findings & Diagnosis

Acute hepatitis C is usually a benign illness, with up to 80% of cases being anicteric and asymptomatic. The mean incubation period following transfusion-associated hepatitis C is 6–8 weeks. Mild elevations of transaminase levels occur in the acute phase; fulminant hepatic failure is rare. Persistent infection leads to liver cell destruction, possibly via direct cytopathic or immune-mediated mechanisms, with fluctuating levels of serum transaminases. Serum transaminase levels are a relatively poor indicator of the severity of disease as measured histologically.

Chronic active hepatitis or cirrhosis occurs in 3–20% of individuals with acute infection. Progression to cirrhosis appears to correlate with age at exposure, duration of infection, and degree of liver damage on biopsy. HCV is a major agent in the etiology of HCC throughout the world, with almost all cases occurring in the setting of cirrhosis. Alcohol appears to be an important cofactor in the development of complications from chronic HCV infection.

Diagnosis of HCV infection usually is based on detection of a reactive HCV antibody and the presence of HCV RNA. Several different antibody tests are available, including laboratory-based immunoassays, rapid point-of-care tests, and home-based tests, and all can be used as the initial assay for antibody testing for HCV. Nucleic acid tests (NATs) for detection of HCV RNA have been traditionally divided into two categories: qualitative and quantitative

assays. Quantitative HCV RNA tests should have a detection level of 25 IU/mL or lower to confirm the diagnosis of HCV infection. If the available quantitative test does not have that degree of sensitivity, then a qualitative test should be used for diagnosis. Anti-HCV antibodies become detectable an average of 12 weeks following exposure but may take as long as 6 months. First-generation anti-HCV assays used the c100-3 antigen and were highly effective in identifying HCV-positive blood donors. The anti–c100-3 assay failed to detect HCV-infected patients for several weeks after exposure, and some HCV-infected patients never developed anti-HCV antibody. Second-generation assays added two epitopes (c22-3 and c33c) to both the ELISA and the confirmatory recombinant immunoblot assay (RIBA-2). Antibodies to these epitopes develop much earlier after infection than do antibodies to c100-3. The second-generation assay is highly sensitive but relatively nonspecific for the detection of HCV. Nonspecificity is associated with aged sera, hypergammaglobulinemia, rheumatoid factor–positive sera, and sera from persons recently vaccinated for influenza. Because of the nonspecificity, ELISA reactivity should be confirmed with a supplemental RIBA-2. Its sensitivity is similar but higher than screening second generation immunoassays and is no longer available in the United States but may be available in other parts of the world.

The latest, third-generation EIAs (EIA-3) generally detect antibodies to recombinant antigens from the core, NS3, NS4, and NS5 proteins. These tests have very high sensitivity and high specificity.

The most sensitive method to detect HCV is measurement of HCV RNA by the polymerase chain reaction (PCR). HCV RNA is detectable by PCR in almost all patients within 1–2 weeks of exposure. In approximately 80% of individuals, HCV RNA persists with fluctuating serum transaminase levels. HCV RNA detection and quantification are essential tools in the diagnosis and management of individuals with chronic HCV infection.

Liver biopsy specimens from patients with chronic HCV infection may show portal inflammation, focal piecemeal necrosis, bile ductular proliferation, and characteristic lymphoid follicles within the portal tracts. Chronic HCV infection is associated with polyarteritis nodosa, membranous glomerulonephritis, and idiopathic Sjögren syndrome.

▶ Treatment

Studies assessing the effectiveness of immune globulin following HCV exposure are inconclusive, and immune globulin is not recommended for postexposure prophylaxis for HCV. No clinical trials have been performed to determine the efficacy of antiviral agents (interferon with or without ribavirin) after HCV exposure. No evidence currently supports the use of immediate postexposure prophylaxis with immune globulin, immune modulators, or antiviral agents. Existing data suggest that established HCV infection is needed before antiviral treatment can be effective. Some studies suggest that a short course of interferon early in the course of acute hepatitis C may be more effective in resolving infection than if antiviral treatment is initiated after chronic hepatitis C has been established. Direct-acting antivirals (DAAs) are licensed and target three viral proteins: the NS3-4A protease needed for processing the viral polyprotein, the NS5A phosphoprotein that regulates RNA replication and virus assembly, and the viral RNA-dependent RNA polymerase (NS5B) that catalyzes genome replication. Combination therapies cure more than 95% of treated patients. DAAs are highly effective, interferon-free (and in many cases, ribavirin-free) regimens appropriate for the majority of HCV-infected individuals. Regimen selection varies by genotype and other patient factors. Among patients with chronic HCV infection, antivirals have been effective against all genotypes (genotypes 1-6). Therapeutic trials have shown that combinations of interferons and ribavirin are more effective than monotherapy. Data on which to base recommendations regarding the use of antivirals in acute infection are insufficient because 15–25% of patients with acute HCV infection resolve their infection spontaneously, and antiviral treatment early in the course of chronic HCV infection may be as effective as acute treatment. Following percutaneous or mucosal occupational exposure to HCV, baseline (within 48 hours) and follow-up HCV antibody measurements should be performed to assess the risk of seroconversion (6 weeks, 3 months, and 6 months). Adding HCV RNA testing at baseline and within 3 weeks after the occupational exposure during follow-up of HCV antibody measurements is advantageous in early detection of HCV infection. During this follow-up period, the HCW should refrain from donating blood, plasma, organs, tissue, or semen. The exposed person does not need to modify sexual practices or refrain from becoming pregnant, and women may continue breast-feeding.

▶ Prevention

No vaccine is currently available for HCV. Prospects for vaccine development are challenging because of the transient efficacy of neutralizing antibodies, the high frequency of mutation in critical envelope protein regions, the high rate of persistent infection, and the possibility of reinfection with both homologous and heterologous strains.

HEPATITIS E

▶ Exposure & Epidemiology

Hepatitis E is an infectious inflammatory disease of the liver caused by the hepatitis E virus (HEV). HEV is a single-stranded, RNA-positive virus belonging to the family Hepeviridae. The most recently proposed classification system divides this family into two genera: Orthohepevirus and Pischihepevirus. Orthohepevirus B is found in birds, Orthohepevirus C infects rodents and carnivores, and Orthohepevirus D is found in bats. Orthohepevirus A is a relatively broader genus comprising seven genotypes of which five (HEV-1, -2, -3, -4, and -7) infect humans, two (HEV-3 and -4) infect pigs, one (HEV-3) infects rabbits, one (HEV-3)

infects deer, one (HEV-4) infects yak, four (HEV-3, -4, -5, and -6) infect wild boars, and one (HEV-7) infects camels. HEV has two discrete epidemiologic patterns: waterborne epidemics in developing countries only, caused by HEV genotypes 1 and 2, and sporadic zoonotic outbreaks in developing and developed countries caused by genotypes 3 and 4. Pigs, rabbits (second largest animal reservoir next to swine), wild deer, and wild boars serve as reservoirs for HEV. Direct contact with infected pigs, rabbits, and deer and consumption of contaminated deer and pig meat and meat products pose risks for HEV infection.

After the discovery of swine HEV in 1997, the risk of zoonotic transmission is a concern for public health. Acute hepatitis E occurs sporadically in the United States, Japan, and most European countries, but transmission pathways are unknown. Studies have demonstrated that HEV is mainly transmitted to humans through improperly cooked meat from deer and pigs.

HEV-3 foodborne chronic hepatitis infection in immunocompromised individuals (such as organ transplant recipients) is an important clinical problem linked with consumption of contaminated pork or deer. Chronic hepatitis E has almost exclusively been reported by genotype 3, with a case study of persistent hepatitis E in a child with HEV genotype 4. A recent zoonotic locally acquired acute hepatitis E caused by HEV-3 and -4 mix infection in Japan has corroborated these findings.

In addition to contaminated meat and milk, HEV-3 has also been found in bivalve mollusks in Japan, Thailand, and the United Kingdom, where human consumption of contaminated shellfish has been implicated as the cause of sporadic cases of acute hepatitis. Novel HEV-4–like gene fragment sequences have been identified in Chinese shellfish with sequence similarity to human and swine HEV strains. As a result, it is important to investigate shellfish as a source of human HEV infection as they are filter-feeders and thus may concentrate HEV, especially in more contaminated coastal areas. Camelids can also transmit HEV to people.

Animal body fluids may also be involved in zoonotic transmission of HEV. A recent report documented that HEV RNA was detected in the urine of experimentally infected pigs, and person-to-person blood transfusion-mediated hepatitis has been documented. HEV may be transmitted to people from infected bites or other forms of direct contact with animals, but these and other possible routes of zoonotic transmission have not been investigated. No reported cases of zoonotic fecal-oral transmission have yet been reported.

A rising rate of anti-HEV seroprevalence in swine workers has been reported in the United States and the Netherlands, Sweden, France and Moldova, Portugal, Norway, and among pork butchers. A higher seroprevalence rate has been documented among forestry workers in France and Germany, suggesting that stools from infected wild forest animals may be a source of transmission to humans. These findings suggest that factors other than direct contact with swine may be more important for zoonotic transmission of HEV to humans.

▶ Clinical Findings & Diagnosis

Transmission of HEV occurs predominantly by the fecal oral route although parenteral and perinatal routes have been implicated. Hepatitis E usually causes a self-limiting hepatitis in young adults with sporadic cases and occasional outbreaks involving hundreds or thousands of cases. Clinically the illness is indistinguishable from hepatitis A. The overall death rate among young adults and pregnant women is 0.5–3% and 20–25%, respectively. Death occurs in the third trimester from fulminant hepatic failure and obstetric complications such as eclampsia, with very high associated fetal loss.

Hepatitis E infection can be diagnosed by serologic testing and detecting viral RNA. Truncated capsid proteins of all four genotypes are available as ELISA coating antigens to detect anti-HEV IgG and IgM antibodies. Because there is strong antibody cross-reactivity toward diverse HEV genotypes, there is consensus that HEV has a single serotype. Several other detection reagents, such as viral RNA and anti-HEV IgG and IgM antibodies, have been used for HEV diagnosis, but these vary in sensitivity. Of the diagnostic assays which are commercially available, none has been formally approved in the United States by the Food and Drug Administration (FDA).

▶ Treatment

Ribavirin is currently the treatment for HEV infections in immunocompromised patients.

▶ Prevention

The most advantageous approach for interruption of HEV transmission from animals to humans is development of an effective animal HEV vaccine. Over the past two decades, various experimental HEV vaccines have been developed, but only one human vaccine has been clinically evaluated and approved in China. This subunit vaccine is based on a truncated capsid protein from human HEV genotype 1 that is expressed in *Escherichia coli* and confers full protection after three doses. Another vaccine, based on common key neutralizing epitopes located on N-truncated capsid proteins derived from rat, avian, and swine HEV strains, was only partially cross-protective in pigs challenged with a mammalian HEV-3. On the other hand, rabbits immunized with the Chinese human vaccine (HEV 239) and challenged with swine and rabbit HEVs experienced complete protection from homologous and heterologous HEV infection. Until an animal vaccine is developed which provides complete protection, human HEV 239 may be a strategy for interruption of the zoonotic transmission cycle.

OTHER INFECTIOUS AGENTS

Seroprevalence studies are inconsistent in demonstrating an increased risk of cytomegalovirus infection among potentially high-risk HCWs (pediatric and immunosuppressed adult units), kindergarten teachers, and child-care workers.

Cytomegalovirus may cause hepatitis, but the more serious consequence of infection for the pregnant worker may be a neonate with a congenital malformation. Nevertheless, hospital employers may consider that prudent policy is to reassign seronegative employees who wish to become pregnant to jobs where there is no contact with infected patients or their biological fluids.

Coxiella burnetii, the agent of Q fever, may cause acute infection among personnel exposed to infected sheep and goats. Persons at risk include animal-care technicians, laboratory research personnel, abattoir workers, and farmers. Acute hepatitis occurs in up to 50% of cases and usually is self-limited. The clinical picture of leptospirosis among farm and sewer workers because of exposure to *Leptospira icterohaemorrhagiae* also may be dominated by hepatic injury. Other causes of infectious hepatitis include yellow fever among forest workers (arbovirus) and schistosomiasis among agricultural workers (*Schistosoma mansoni*, *S japonicum*).

MEDICAL SURVEILLANCE FOR OCCUPATIONAL LIVER DISEASE

The choice of a surveillance test or tests to detect chemical liver disease in a working population exposed to potential hepatotoxins is determined by its specificity, sensitivity, and positive predictive value (see "Diagnostic Tests for Liver Dysfunction"). In an occupational setting, a screening test with high sensitivity (to correctly identify all those with disease) and specificity (to correctly identify all those without disease) is needed. Indocyanine green clearance and serum alkaline phosphatase have been suggested as the initial tests of choice for the surveillance of vinyl chloride workers (to reduce the number of false-positive results), followed by a test of high sensitivity such as serum γ-glutamyl transpeptidase (to reduce the number of false-negative results).

For most hepatotoxins, it is currently justified to base the choice of tests on practical criteria such as noninvasiveness, simplicity of test performance, availability, and adequacy of test analysis and cost. Although serum transaminases have a relatively high sensitivity for detection of liver disease, their low specificity limits the practical utility of periodic measurement in a worker population exposed to potential hepatotoxins. Nevertheless, serum transaminases remain the test of choice for routine surveillance of such populations.

Clearance tests have been used successfully in research settings but are not recommended for daily clinical or surveillance practice until further prospective studies in well-defined groups are completed. It is not known whether changes in microsomal enzyme activity in workers exposed to hepatotoxins may result in long-term liver damage.

So-called preemployment baseline measurement of serum transaminases may be helpful in establishing causality for purposes of workers' compensation where a claim is made alleging industrial liver disease. Routine medical surveillance involving measurement of serum transaminase levels should be conducted only when exposure assessment suggests a potential for hepatic injury. When the prevalence of liver disease in the population is low, the poor predictive value of an abnormal serum transaminase level after routine screening may lead to many costly diagnostic evaluations for nonoccupational liver disease.

Gray-scale ultrasonography of the liver has been used in surveillance of vinyl chloride–exposed workers but has not been applied routinely in other workplace settings for surveillance of hepatic disease. Hepatic parenchymal imaging by ultrasonography has been suggested as a sensitive marker for preclinical effects among solvent-exposed dry cleaners. The use of this technique as a routine tool for medical surveillance for hepatotoxin exposure remains to be determined.

Individuals with chronic elevations of serum transaminase levels may continue to work if exposure to potential hepatotoxins is minimized through appropriate workplace controls and exposure assessment.

DIAGNOSTIC TESTS FOR LIVER DYSFUNCTION

The ideal test for detection of liver dysfunction would be sensitive enough to detect minimal liver disease, specific enough to point to a particular derangement of liver function, and capable of reflecting the severity of the underlying pathophysiologic problem. Unfortunately, no such laboratory test is available, and "liver function tests" are used instead (Table 21–6).

Broadly speaking, these tests encompass tests of biochemical evidence of cell death and hepatic synthesis, as well as

Table 21–6. Tests for evaluation of liver disease.

Biochemical tests
Serum enzyme activity
Serum alkaline phosphatase
Serum lactate dehydrogenase
Serum bilirubin
Urine bilirubin
Tests of synthetic liver function
Serum albumin
Prothrombin time
α-Fetoprotein
Serum ferritin
Clearance tests
Exogenous clearance tests
Sulfobromophthalein
Indocyanine green
Antipyrine test
Aminopyrine breath test
Caffeine breath test
Endogenous clearance tests
Serum bile acid
Urinary D-glucaric acid
Proinflammatory cytokines
Cytokeratin 18 (CK18)

actual physiologic liver dysfunction. In addition, radiologic and morphologic evaluations are used often to delineate the nature of liver disease and, as such, may be viewed as tests of liver function. Biochemical tests and tests of synthetic function are indicated commonly for routine use; clearance tests are not widely available and are not indicated for routine use.

Epidemiologic studies in which measurement of serum enzyme levels is used to determine the hepatotoxicity of solvents have not included long-term outcomes such as chronic liver disease. Bile acids and other tests of metabolic function generally are more sensitive indicators of hepatic effect from organic solvents at levels of exposure below those expected to cause elevation of serum enzyme levels. It is not known if these more sensitive measures of hepatic function can predict subsequent disease in workers exposed to hepatotoxins.

Biochemical Tests for Liver Disease

A. Serum Enzyme Activity

The tests used most commonly to detect liver disease are AST and ALT determinations. Transaminase release is a consequence of release of enzyme protein from liver cells as a result of cell injury. Elevations of serum aminotransferase levels may occur with minor cell injury, making such determinations useful in the early detection and monitoring of liver disease of drug or chemical origin. However, transaminase levels may be elevated in viral, alcoholic, or ischemic hepatitis, as well as in extrahepatic obstruction, limiting the specificity of these tests. In addition, elevations of transaminase levels are found in obese individuals, and false-positive results have been reported in patients receiving erythromycin and aminosalicylic acid and during diabetic ketoacidosis. Conversely, significant liver damage may be present in individuals with normal levels of transaminases. There is some evidence that a serum AST:ALT ratio of greater than 1 may indicate occupational liver disease. The height of transaminase elevation in liver disease does not correlate with the extent of liver cell necrosis on biopsy and therefore has little prognostic value.

B. Alkaline Phosphatase

Serum alkaline phosphatase activity may originate from liver, bone, intestine, or placenta. Measurement of serum 5-nucleotidase may be used to determine the tissue origin of an elevated alkaline phosphatase; if elevated, it generally implies that the source of alkaline phosphatase is hepatobiliary, not bony. Toxic liver injury that results in disturbances in the transport function of the hepatocyte or of the biliary tree may cause elevation of serum alkaline phosphatase activity. Increased serum alkaline phosphatase levels also may be noted in the third trimester of pregnancy, as well as normally in persons older than 50 years and in patients with osteoblastic bone disorders and both intrahepatic and extrahepatic cholestatic disease.

Assay of alkaline phosphatase enzymatic activity in serum in anicteric individuals is particularly useful in detecting and monitoring suspected drug- or chemical-induced cholestasis; it is not helpful in screening individuals for toxic liver injury except when there is primary involvement of the biliary network.

C. Serum Bilirubin

Hyperbilirubinemia may be classified as conjugated or unconjugated. Conjugated hyperbilirubinemia indicates dysfunction of the liver parenchyma or bile ducts and may be found in Dubin-Johnson syndrome and Rotor syndrome and in viral hepatitis, drug- or toxin-induced hepatitis, shock liver, and metastatic disease of the liver. Unconjugated hyperbilirubinemia may be seen in Gilbert disease, uncomplicated hemolytic disorders, and congestive heart failure.

Serum bilirubin is of some value in detecting toxic cholestatic liver injury but is frequently normal in the presence of more common cytotoxic damage. It is probably most useful in the presence of severe acute liver damage; although patients with fulminant hepatitis may be anicteric, the level of serum bilirubin is of prognostic importance in chemical and alcoholic hepatitis, primary biliary cirrhosis, and halothane hepatitis.

D. Urine Bilirubin

Bilirubin in the urine is direct bilirubin because indirect bilirubin is tightly bound to albumin and not filtered by the normal kidney. A positive urine bilirubin test can confirm clinically suspected hyperbilirubinemia of hepatobiliary origin or may predate the appearance of overt icterus and thus serve as a useful screening test. Quantitative analysis of urine bilirubin is of no diagnostic significance.

E. Other Biochemical Tests

1. Serum γ-glutamyl transferase (SGGT)—SGGT is considered a more sensitive indicator than aminotransferases of drug-, virus-, chemical-, and alcohol-induced hepatocellular damage. Because of its lack of specificity, however, one must interpret abnormalities in conjunction with other tests.

2. Liver-specific enzymes—Liver enzymes, such as ornithine carbamyl dehydrogenase, phosphofructose aldolase, sorbitol dehydrogenase, and alcohol dehydrogenase, are less useful clinically than the aminotransferases, glutamyl transferases, or alkaline phosphatases.

3. Serum lactate dehydrogenase (LDH)—Serum LDH may originate from myocardium, liver, skeletal muscle, brain or kidney tissue, and red blood cells. Isoenzyme fractionation may determine the hepatic origin (LDH 5) but generally is too nonspecific for purposes of evaluating toxic chemical liver injury.

Tests of Synthetic Liver Function

Measurement of serum albumin concentrations may be a useful index of cellular dysfunction in liver disease. It is of little value in differential diagnosis.

Because all the clotting factors are synthesized by the liver, acute liver injury can result in prolongation of the prothrombin time, which depends on the activities of factors II, V, VII, and X. Measurement of prothrombin time is useful chiefly in fulminant hepatic failure, where a markedly elevated prothrombin time has prognostic significance, or in advanced chronic liver disease. It is a relatively insensitive indicator of liver damage and of little value in the differential diagnosis.

High serum concentrations of α-fetoprotein are present in 70% of patients with primary HCC in the United States, and serial determinations may aid in monitoring the response to therapy or in detecting early recurrence. α-Fetoprotein has no utility for surveillance in the occupational setting.

Serum ferritin levels accurately reflect hepatic and total-body iron stores. Serum ferritin is useful in screening for idiopathic genetic hemochromatosis as a cause of liver disease but has no utility for surveillance in the occupational setting.

Clearance Tests

Tests that measure the clearance of substances by the liver provide the most sensitive, specific, and reliable means of detecting the early phase of liver disease. Clearance tests may be used to determine the specificity of increased enzyme activity, to detect liver disease not reflected in abnormalities of serum enzymes, and to determine when recovery has occurred in reversible liver disease. This is especially the case when decreases in the functional state of the liver occur in patients with liver disease without active necrosis, including fatty liver, and in active cirrhosis in the absence of clinical abnormalities or abnormal enzymes.

In the occupational setting, measures of hepatic functional capacity have been used epidemiologically to demonstrate liver dysfunction in the absence of clinical or serologic abnormalities. The clinical utility of clearance tests in screening for chemical liver injury—or in confirming occupational etiology of disease in workers with known liver dysfunction—has not been demonstrated.

A. Exogenous Clearance Tests

Exogenous clearance tests are given to detect liver function by the administration of various test substances to the individual.

1. Bromsulfalein (BSP)—Practical use of hepatic clearance as a diagnostic measure began with BSP. Its use has been discontinued because of side effects of phlebitis, severe local skin reactions, and occasionally fatal anaphylactic reactions.

2. Indocyanine green—Hepatic uptake of indocyanine green, a tricarbocyanine anionic dye, is an active process depending on sinusoidal perfusion, membrane transport, and secretory capacity. The dye is not metabolized or conjugated by the liver and is excreted directly into the bile. After a single intravenous injection of indocyanine green, clearance is calculated from serial dye levels at 3, 5, 7, 9, 12, and 14 minutes or by ear densitometry. Unlike BSP, indocyanine green causes negligible toxicity or allergic reactions.

Studies of workers exposed to vinyl chloride show that indocyanine green clearance after a dose of 0.5 mg/kg is the most sensitive test for subclinical liver injury and has a specificity exceeded only by serum alkaline phosphatase. There is also a dose-response relationship between cumulative exposure to vinyl chloride and indocyanine green clearance. This has not been demonstrated in other groups of workers exposed to occupational hepatotoxins, and indocyanine green for detection of subclinical liver disease cannot be recommended for routine use.

3. Antipyrine test—This is the most widely used in vivo index of hepatic microsomal enzyme activity. Antipyrine is completely and rapidly absorbed from the gastrointestinal tract, distributed in total-body water, and almost completely metabolized by the liver via three major oxidative pathways. The rate of elimination is virtually independent of hepatic blood flow, with first-order kinetics of elimination and a half-life of approximately 10 hours in normal subjects. At 24–48 hours after an orally administered dose of 1 g, antipyrine clearance can be calculated by serial plasma or salivary measurements. Clearance can be calculated from a single salivary sample collected at least 18 hours after dosing, permitting a simpler, more convenient method of study. Repeat tests cannot be done less than 3 days apart, and to avoid the induction of antipyrine metabolism in the individual, an interval of 1 week is recommended.

The antipyrine test has undergone the most extensive study of all clearance tests in the detection of subclinical liver disease in occupational settings. It has been used to detect mean differences in hepatic enzyme activity between workers exposed to solvent mixtures and unexposed controls. Asymptomatic chlordecone-exposed workers had increased antipyrine clearance and biopsy-proved liver disease that normalized after exposure was terminated.

4. Aminopyrine breath test—The aminopyrine breath test has the advantage of being simple, noninvasive, safe, and relatively cheap. Clinical studies have documented the use of aminopyrine breath tests in patients with chronic advanced liver disease, but the sensitivity and specificity of the test for detection of subclinical chemical liver injury in asymptomatic populations have not been assessed.

After oral administration of about 2 µCi of [^{14}C]aminopyrine, the labeled methyl group is oxidized by the microsomal enzyme system and ultimately excreted as $^{14}CO_2$. Breath samples are collected 2 hours after administration, and the specific activity of $^{14}CO_2$ is measured in a liquid scintillation counter. The test requires physical rest from dose to breath sampling. For example, this test has been employed as a sensitive measure of increased microsomal enzyme activity among coke oven workers.

5. Caffeine breath test—Inhaled ^{14}C-labeled caffeine, labeled at one or all three methyl groups, followed by exhaled breath $^{14}CO_2$ measurement, was introduced recently as a noninvasive means of studying hepatic microsomal enzyme

function. It has not undergone evaluation in asymptomatic worker populations.

B. Endogenous Clearance Tests

1. Serum bile acids—Serum bile acid measurement has been used to detect subclinical liver dysfunction following halogenated hydrocarbon exposure and also may be useful in further medical workup for the individual with persistent enzyme abnormalities. Bile acids are synthesized by the liver and undergo enterohepatic circulation. Serum levels of bile acids are normally low in a fasting state (<6 µmol/L) and reflect only hepatic excretory function and not synthesis rate or volume distribution. Fasting bile acid levels are increased in relation to the degree of liver disease and impairment in excretion.

Depending on the population screened, the positive predictive value of an abnormal (>8.4 µmol/L) serum bile acid test ranges from 10% (general population) to 94% (hospitalized population with biopsy-proved hepatobiliary disease). In a large workplace study of vinyl chloride–exposed workers, measurement of serum bile acids had a sensitivity of 78%, a specificity of 93%, and a positive predictive value of 10%.

Serum bile acids have been suggested as a more sensitive indicator of hepatic dysfunction than biochemical tests for liver toxicity. Many animal studies have shown increased serum bile acids after exposure to aliphatic hydrocarbon solvents and the nonchlorinated aromatic hydrocarbon solvent toluene. A dose-dependent increase in the concentration of serum bile acids has been observed in workers exposed to hexachlorobutadiene and trichloroethylene, and among workers exposed to solvents in a paint factory. Other standard tests of liver function were normal in these workers, and bile acids had significant positive correlation with duration of exposure to organic solvents and lifetime hydrocarbon exposure score. The risk of increased bile acids in this study was influenced by gender, hepatitis B infection, alcohol consumption, and BMI. The significance of these findings and their clinical correlation with disease outcome has yet to be determined.

2. Urinary D-glucaric acid (UDGA)—UDGA has been used as an indirect measure of liver induction. D-Glucaric acid, a product of carbohydrate metabolism, is produced via the glucuronic acid pathway after initial xenobiotic metabolism. The mechanism for UDGA induction has not been elucidated, but UDGA excretion is correlated with microsomal enzyme content. Operating room personnel exposed to isoflurane and nitrous oxide have increased UDGA excretion.

Proinflammatory Cytokines

The use of Cytokeratin 18 (CK18) has recently been explored as a tool to assess occupational liver disease. CK18 is a cytoskeletal protein found in hepatocytes and other epithelial cells. Dying cells release CK18 into the extracellular compartment where they can be measured in serum. Both the whole

CK18 protein (CK18 M65) and the caspase 3-cleaved fragment (CK18 M30) may be measured. CK18 M65 measures total cell death, while CK18 M30 specifically measures caspase-3 dependent (apoptotic) cell death. While NASH and ASH are characterized by hepatocellular apoptosis, nonapoptotic death occurs in many forms of chemical hepatotoxicity. CK18 M65 has been studied as an emerging biomarker for TASH in the setting of normal liver enzymes ALT, AST, and CK18 M30. In one study, 30% of polymer workers exposed to acrylonitrile, 1,3-butadiene and styrene (ABS) had elevated CK18 M65 and had normal liver enzymes (AST/ALT). The observed CK18 elevations were generally not explained by obesity or ethanol, suggesting that this biomarker may be useful to detect cases of TASH.

CLINICAL MANAGEMENT OF OCCUPATIONAL LIVER DISEASE

▶ Occupational & Medical History

A careful occupational history of exposure to known human hepatotoxins should be obtained in every case of suspected occupational liver disease. Past medical history of liver disease should be noted. The review of symptoms should include those of acute central nervous system toxicity, such as headache, dizziness, and light-headedness, because the presence of these symptoms may indicate excessive solvent exposure.

Nonoccupational causes of liver disease should be evaluated carefully. Steroid use, glue sniffing, or other recreational solvent use should be determined. Travel to areas with endemic parasitic or viral diseases may be a significant risk for infectious hepatitis. A history of hobbies involving exposure to hepatotoxins should be taken. Previous blood transfusions, percutaneous exposures (eg, tattoos, needlesticks, ear piercing, or acupuncture), and intravenous drug use may be risk factors for viral hepatitis. A relationship between obesity and elevated liver enzyme levels has been well documented. Numerous medications may be hepatotoxic.

Use of protective work practices (such as respiratory protection, gloves, and work clothes) should be described because this may indicate the extent of pulmonary and skin absorption. Material data safety sheets should be obtained on the relevant products used. Airborne contaminant monitoring data (see Chapter 36) should be requested and reviewed for excessive exposure. Inquiry should be made of the employer about other employees with possible liver disease.

▶ Physical Examination

Acute liver disease owing to occupational exposure may present with right upper quadrant tenderness, hepatosplenomegaly, or jaundice. Mild hepatotoxicity may cause few physical findings. Examination of the respiratory tract or skin should be performed depending on the route of exposure. Chronic liver disease may result in stigmata such as spider angiomata, palmar erythema, testicular atrophy, ascites, and gynecomastia.

▶ Differential Diagnosis

Other causes of liver disease should be ruled out, particularly infectious and alcohol- and drug-induced hepatitis. The most common causes of elevated serum transaminase are ingestion of ethanol and obesity. If a history of excessive ethanol ingestion is elicited, the serum transaminase measurement should be repeated after 3–4 weeks of abstinence. If serum transaminase levels are normal on follow-up, ethanol should be suspected as the probable cause. Persistent serum transaminase elevation may represent chronic alcoholic hepatitis or continued occupational exposure.

The onset of liver transaminase elevations after exposure to a known or suspected hepatotoxin is suggestive of occupational liver disease, particularly if normal liver tests before exposure can be documented. Even if preexposure tests are normal, liver disease may develop coincidentally without relation to workplace exposure.

▶ Management of Acute Liver Disease

The most common clinical problem is that the individual with elevated serum transaminase levels on routine screening who may have occupational exposure to a known hepatotoxin. Nonoccupational causes of liver disease should be ruled out carefully and the workplace inspected for the presence of hepatotoxic exposures. If an occupational cause is suspected, the individual should be removed immediately from exposure for 3–4 weeks. The serum transaminase measurement then should be repeated; with few exceptions, serum transaminase concentrations will normalize following removal from exposure. A persistently elevated serum transaminase concentration suggests a nonoccupational cause of liver disease or, rarely, chronic occupational liver disease.

Although there is little evidence that individuals with nonoccupational liver disease are more susceptible to further liver damage as a consequence of occupational exposure, it is prudent to monitor these workers carefully for evidence of worsening liver damage. Appropriate engineering controls and personal protective equipment should be made available to reduce potential hepatotoxic exposures. If there is evidence of worsening liver disease or if exposure cannot be reduced satisfactorily, the individual should be reassigned. In one study of workers exposed to hydrocarbon solvents at a petrochemical plant, most workers with biopsy-proven NASH improved after removal from the work environment. Aside from removing the individual from exposure to the offending agent, there is no specific treatment for acute occupational liver disease.

▶ Management of Chronic Liver Disease

Persistent abnormalities in liver function tests after removal from exposure have been reported rarely, and a thorough search for other causes always should be conducted. Occasionally, chronic liver disease may follow acute chemical hepatitis or years of low-dose exposure.

Hepatic ultrasonography may show hepatic steatosis or periportal fibrosis. A recent study found that liver ultrasonography is a useful tool for the medical surveillance of vinyl chloride monomer workers, particularly among those exposed to VCM above 200 ppm for at least 1 year. Liver biopsy usually is not helpful in differentiating occupational from nonoccupational liver disease and is rarely indicated.

Treatment of HCC caused by occupational exposure does not differ from that of disease that is a result of other causes.

REFERENCES

Arafa A, Eshak ES: Medical waste handling and hepatitis B virus infection: a meta-analysis. Am J Infect Control 2020;48(3):316-319 [PMID: 31521422].

Auta A, Adewuyi EO, Kureh GT, Onoviran N, Adeloye D: Hepatitis B vaccination coverage among health-care workers in Africa: a systematic review and meta-analysis. Vaccine 2018;36(32 Pt B):4851-4860 [PMID: 29970299].

De Schryver A, De Schrijver K, François G, et al: Hepatitis E virus infection: an emerging occupational risk? Occup Med (Lond) 2015;65(8):667-672 [PMID: 26452392].

De Schryver A, Lambaerts T, Lammertyn N, François G, Bulterys S, Godderis L: European survey of hepatitis B vaccination policies for healthcare workers: an updated overview. Vaccine 2020;38(11):2466-2472 [PMID: 32057571].

Fedeli U, Girardi P, Gardiman G, et al: Mortality from liver angiosarcoma, hepatocellular carcinoma, and cirrhosis among vinyl chloride workers. Am J Ind Med 2019;62(1):14-20 [PMID: 30474170].

Hamano G, Kubo S, Takemura S, et al: Comparison of clinicopathological characteristics between patients with occupational and non-occupational intrahepatic cholangiocarcinoma. J Hepatobiliary Pancreat Sci 2016;23(7):389-396 [PMID: 27062258].

Henderson DK, Dembry L, Fishman NO, et al: SHEA guideline for management of healthcare workers who are infected with hepatitis B virus, hepatitis C virus, and/or human immunodeficiency virus. Infect Control Hosp Epidemiol 2010;31(3):203-232 [PMID: 20088696].

Ito D, Tanaka T, Akamatsu N, et al: Recurrent acute liver failure because of acute hepatitis induced by organic solvents: a case report. Medicine (Baltimore) 2016;95(1):e2445 [PMID: 26735550].

Joshi-Barve S, Kirpich I, Cave MC, Marsano LS, McClain CJ: Alcoholic, nonalcoholic, and toxicant-associated steatohepatitis: mechanistic similarities and differences. Cell Mol Gastroenterol Hepatol 2015;1(4):356-367 [PMID: 28210688].

Kubo S, Takemura S, Tanaka S, et al: Occupational cholangiocarcinoma caused by exposure to 1,2-dichloropropane and/or dichloromethane. Ann Gastroenterol Surg 2017;2(2):99-105 [PMID: 29863124].

Kuhar DT, Henderson DK, Struble KA, et al: Updated US Public Health Service guidelines for the management of occupational exposures to human immunodeficiency virus and recommendations for postexposure prophylaxis [published correction appears in Infect Control Hosp Epidemiol 2013;34(11):1238 Dosage error in article text]. Infect Control Hosp Epidemiol 2013;34(9):875-892 [PMID: 23917901].

Ledda C, Loreto C, Zammit C, et al: Non-infective occupational risk factors for hepatocellular carcinoma: a review (Review). Mol Med Rep 2017;15(2):511-533 [PMID: 28000892].

Lei Y, Xiao S, Chen S, Zhang H, Li H, Lu Y: N,N-dimethylformamide-induced acute hepatic failure: a case report and literature review. Exp Ther Med 2017;14(6):5659-5663 [PMID: 29285107].

Malaguarnera G, Cataudella E, Giordano M, Nunnari G, Chisari G, Malaguarnera M: Toxic hepatitis in occupational exposure to solvents. World J Gastroenterol 2012;18(22):2756-2766 [PMID: 22719183].

Maltezou HC, Botelho-Nevers E, Brantsæter AB, et al: Vaccination of healthcare personnel in Europe: update to current policies. Vaccine 2019;37(52):7576-7584 [PMID: 31623916].

Mundt KA, Dell LD, Crawford L, Gallagher AE: Quantitative estimated exposure to vinyl chloride and risk of angiosarcoma of the liver and hepatocellular cancer in the US industry-wide vinyl chloride cohort: mortality update through 2013. Occup Environ Med 2017;74(10):709-716 [PMID: 28490663].

Naggie S, Holland DP, Sulkowski MS, Thomas DL: Hepatitis C virus postexposure prophylaxis in the healthcare worker: why direct-acting antivirals don't change a thing. Clin Infect Dis 2017;64(1):92-99 [PMID: 27682067].

Nelson NP, Link-Gelles R, Hofmeister MG, et al: Update: recommendations of the Advisory Committee on Immunization Practices for use of hepatitis A vaccine for postexposure prophylaxis and for preexposure prophylaxis for international travel. MMWR Morb Mortal Wkly Rep 2018;67:1216-1220 [PMID: 30383742].

Qi C, Gu Y, Sun Q, et al: Low-dose N,N-dimethylformamide exposure and liver injuries in a cohort of Chinese leather industry workers. J Occup Environ Med 2017;59(5):434-439 [PMID: 28368964].

Schillie S, Vellozzi C, Reingold A, et al: Prevention of hepatitis B virus infection in the United States: recommendations of the Advisory Committee on Immunization Practices. MMWR Recomm Rep 2018;67(1):1-31 [PMID: 29939980].

Stanaway JD, Flaxman AD, Naghavi M, et al: The global burden of viral hepatitis from 1990 to 2013: findings from the Global Burden of Disease Study 2013. Lancet 2016;388(10049):1081-1088 [PMID: 27394647].

Syed SF, Zhao Q, Umer M, et al: Past, present and future of hepatitis E virus infection: zoonotic perspectives. Microb Pathog 2018;119:103-108 [PMID: 29621564].

Tavoschi L, Mason L, Petriti U, Bunge E, Veldhuijzen I, Duffell E: Hepatitis B and C among healthcare workers and patient groups at increased risk of iatrogenic transmission in the European Union/European Economic Area. J Hosp Infect 2019;102(4):359-368 [PMID: 30885816].

Wahlang B, Beier JI, Clair HB, et al: Toxicant-associated steatohepatitis. Toxicol Pathol 2013;41(2):343-360 [PMID: 23262638].

■ SELF-ASSESSMENT QUESTIONS

Select the one correct answer for each question.

Question 1: Direct hepatotoxins
  a. injure the hepatocyte and its organelles by a direct physicochemical effect
  b. may produce centrilobular necrosis but not steatosis
  c. such as chloroform cause indirect hepatic necrosis
  d. including benzene, toluene, xylene, and styrene cause massive acute hepatic injury

Question 2: Indirect hepatotoxins
  a. produce hepatic injury by interference with metabolic pathways
  b. increase bile flow
  c. include drugs such as antihistamines and aspirin
  d. do not include botanicals

Question 3: Mixed-function oxidases (MFOs)
  a. make the liver the primary defense against infections
  b. are cellular enzyme systems
  c. are attached to the membrane layers of the smooth endoplasmic reticulum
  d. do not defend against inhaled xenobiotics

Question 4: Carbon tetrachloride
  a. is an atypical or unusual form of hepatotoxin
  b. causes immediate anesthesia
  c. hepatic disease usually follows exposure by 2–4 hours
  d. causes renal failure after the hepatic damage becomes manifest

Question 5: Toxicant-associated steatohepatitis (TASH)
  a. describes hepatic steatosis, inflammation, and liver failure
  b. has occurred among vinyl chloride production workers
  c. reduces total CK18 as a marker of cell death
  d. causes insulin resistance with elevated adiponectin levels

Question 6: Hepatitis A
  a. is transmitted primarily by person-to-person contact, generally through fecal contamination
  b. outbreaks have been reported among day-care workers
  c. affects correctional settings and dentists
  d. primarily affects waste water treatment plant workers

Question 7: Hepatitis B
  a. affects only those HCWs with significant contact with blood
  b. is not transmitted via the fecal-oral route or by contamination of food or water
  c. causes a skin rash, but is unrelated to arthritis
  d. incubation period ranges from 45 to 60 hours

Question 8: Hepatitis C virus (HCV)
  a. has a marginal ability to persist in the host after infection
  b. infects nearly 1 million people annually in the United States
  c. is spread primarily through parenteral exposures from blood transfusions or intravenous drug abuse
  d. shows minimal evidence for sexual transmission

Question 9: Clearance tests
  a. provide the least sensitive and reliable means of detecting the early phase of liver disease
  b. fail to determine when recovery has occurred in reversible liver disease
  c. may demonstrate liver dysfunction in the absence of clinical or serologic abnormalities
  d. confirm occupational etiology of disease in workers with known liver dysfunction

Question 10: Cytokeratin 18 (CK18)
  a. has recently been explored as a tool to assess occupational liver disease
  b. is a cytoskeletal protein found in hepatocytes and renal cells
  c. is absorbed by dying cells
  d. detects cases of toxicant-associated liver cancer

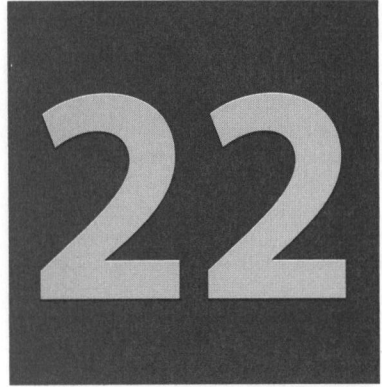

Renal Toxicology

German T. Hernandez, MD

Rudolph A. Rodriguez, MD

In the United States, 726,331 patients were treated for end-stage renal disease (ESRD) in 2016 at an annual cost near $50 billion in Medicare expenditures. Both the number of patients and the associated costs continue to grow annually. The etiology of the kidney injury in a significant percentage of these patients is never fully elucidated, and the diagnosis of renal disease of occupational origin is rarely considered. The true incidence of chronic kidney disease (CKD) secondary to occupational and environmental exposures in the United States is unknown. However, these exposures represent potentially preventable causes of CKD. Even if occupational and environmental exposures account for only a small percentage of the causes of ESRD in the United States, the significant morbidity, mortality, and costs associated with renal replacement therapy potentially could be prevented.

The kidney is especially vulnerable to occupational and environmental exposures. The kidneys receive approximately 20% of cardiac output and a fraction is filtered; this amount represents the glomerular filtration rate (GFR). The GFR is normally 125 mL/min or 180 L/d. Along the nephron, this filtrate is largely reabsorbed and then concentrated and acidified. Thus, occupational and environmental toxins can be highly concentrated in the kidney, and as the pH of the filtrate changes, some toxins can exist in certain ionic forms. These factors help to explain the pathophysiologic mechanisms involved in certain toxins. For example, lead and cadmium cause much of their renal ultrastructural damage in the proximal tubule, where two-thirds of the filtered load is reabsorbed.

Following relatively high-dose exposure to certain organic solvents, metals, or pesticides, acute kidney injury may develop within hours to days. The common renal lesion is acute tubular necrosis, and the clinical presentation is dominated by the extrarenal manifestations of these exposures with renal recovery as the rule if the other organ systems recover. CKD or ESRD also may develop after certain exposures. The common renal lesion in these cases is chronic interstitial nephritis, and lead nephropathy is a prime example. However, a rare presentation is a glomerular lesion seen after selected exposures such as to organic solvents or silicosis; in general, glomerular lesions after occupational or environmental exposures are very uncommon.

The renal evaluation of patients thought to have renal disease associated with an environmental or occupational exposure should be guided by the history, physical examination, and clinical presentation of the renal disease. The time course will help differentiate between acute and chronic kidney disease. In acute kidney injury, the urine sediment typically is diagnostic of acute tubular necrosis with evidence of tubular damage. Most CKDs associated with exposure to agents such as lead or cadmium present with chronic interstitial nephritis characterized by tubular proteinuria (usually < 2 g/24 h) and a urine sediment usually lacking any cellular elements. A nephritic urine sediment is suggestive of a proliferative renal lesion and has been associated with only a few exposures, such as to organic solvents. The nephrotic syndrome, characterized by more than 3.5 g protein per 24 hours, edema, and hypercholesterolemia, is also associated with exposure to some heavy metals, including mercury.

Monitoring workers for the possible renal effects of occupational exposures can be difficult because of the lack of sensitive and specific tests of renal injury. Serial measurement of traditional tests such as creatinine or blood urea nitrogen (BUN) is inadequate because these tests do not become abnormal until significant renal damage has occurred. Tests for use in adult studies correlate with the site of possible damage. Some of these tests detect possible glomerular injury (eg, urine albumin), proximal tubule damage (eg, retinol-binding protein, N-acetyl-β-D-glucosaminidase, and alanine amino peptidase), and distal tubule injury (eg, osmolality). Most of these tests were designed to detect early renal tubular damage. Unfortunately, their use is limited by many factors; for instance, some are unstable at certain urine pHs, others return to normal levels within a few days of the exposure despite renal damage, and others exhibit large interindividual variations. Most important, unlike microalbuminuria, which can predict future nephropathy in type 1 diabetes, the predictive value of these newer tests has not been validated.

More long-term studies are needed before these newer renal tests can be used routinely to monitor renal injury in the workplace.

The 2012 Kidney Disease Improving Global Outcomes (KDIGO) CKD Guidelines include a classification scheme and risk stratification framework for the evaluation and management of CKD. These guidelines suggest classifying patients with CKD based on cause, one of five estimated GFR categories, and one of three categories of albuminuria. Lower GFR and higher levels of albuminuria are associated with an increased risk of CKD progression and the development of complications.

ACUTE KIDNEY INJURY

Many occupational and environmental toxins can cause acute kidney injury, usually after high-dose exposure. Although the extrarenal manifestations of the toxic exposure generally dominate the clinical presentation and course, the characteristics and time course of the acute kidney injury are very similar in all exposures. In most cases, acute tubular necrosis is the kidney lesion that develops. Hours to days after the exposure, the acute tubular necrosis is manifested by decreased urine output, usually in the oliguric range of less than 500 mL/d. The urinalysis typically is diagnostic of acute tubular necrosis, with renal tubular cells, muddy brown granular casts, and little or no protein. Red blood cells, white blood cells, or casts of either cell type are not typically seen with acute tubular necrosis and their presence instead suggests a glomerulonephritis. Increases in BUN and creatinine and electrolyte abnormalities develop as expected in acute kidney injury, and patients may require dialysis until the renal function recovers. After 1–2 weeks, recovery from acute tubular necrosis usually is heralded by the onset of a diuresis.

Hemodialysis and/or hemoperfusion have almost no role in accelerating the clearance of occupational and environmental toxins. For these techniques to be effective, toxins must have a low apparent volume of distribution and molecular weight, a low affinity for plasma proteins, and low tissue-binding properties. For example, charcoal hemoperfusion can result in almost complete removal of circulating paraquat, but because of high tissue binding, only small amounts of total body paraquat are removed. Consequently, hemoperfusion does not affect the prognosis in paraquat poisoning. These extracorporeal techniques are effective only after a few intoxications, which include certain alcohols, salicylate, lithium, and theophylline.

ACUTE KIDNEY INJURY CAUSED BY HEAVY METALS

Significant exposure to any of the divalent metals—chromium, cadmium, mercury, and vanadium—can produce acute tubular necrosis. Of these metals, the only one encountered in industrial settings in high enough concentrations to produce acute tubular necrosis is cadmium. Exposure to cadmium in toxic amounts is usually through inhalation, and the classic history of exposure is that of workers welding cadmium-plated metals. Welders exposed to cadmium fumes present with coughing and progressive pulmonary distress leading to adult respiratory distress syndrome. Kidney injury occurs rapidly in the form of acute tubular necrosis. Severe exposure can produce bilateral cortical necrosis.

ACUTE KIDNEY INJURY CAUSED BY ORGANIC SOLVENTS

In the occupational setting, the lungs are the most common route of absorption of hydrocarbons. Inhaled hydrocarbons then quickly pass into the pulmonary circulation. Transcutaneous absorption is also an important route of absorption for solvents. Organic solvents are lipophilic and therefore are distributed in highest concentration in the fat, liver, bone marrow, blood, brain, and kidneys.

1. Halogenated Hydrocarbons

▶ Carbon Tetrachloride

Carbon tetrachloride (CCl_4) is used as an industrial solvent and as the basis for manufacture of fluorinated hydrocarbons. It was once used as a household cleaning agent and until the 1950s as a component of fire extinguisher fluid under the brand name Pyrene.

After acute exposure, patients typically present with confusion, somnolence, nausea, and vomiting. Mucous membrane irritant effects, such as burning eyes, may occur, although some workers may be symptom-free for several days following exposure and then present with complaints of vomiting, abdominal pain, constipation, diarrhea, and in some cases fever. Physical findings may be compatible with the acute abdomen at this stage of illness, and many patients have been improperly subjected to laparotomy.

After 7–10 days of illness, there may be a decline in urine output even to the point of anuria. Patients with carbon tetrachloride intoxication usually show signs of prerenal azotemia, as demonstrated by a low urinary sodium excretion, and if ischemic acute tubular necrosis does not supervene, the prerenal azotemia may improve after volume repletion. If the hepatotoxicity is severe, patients also may develop hepatorenal syndrome.

▶ Other Aliphatic Halogenated Hydrocarbons

Other aliphatic halogenated hydrocarbons are nephrotoxic, some to a greater and some to a lesser degree than carbon tetrachloride. Ethylene dichloride ($C_2H_4Cl_2$) is used as a solvent for oils, fats, waxes, turpentine, rubber, and some resins; as an insecticide and fumigant; and in fire extinguishers and household cleaning fluids. It is slightly less potent than carbon tetrachloride as a kidney toxin but causes greater central nervous system toxicity. Ingestion or heavy inhalation may produce acute tubular necrosis like that encountered with mercury poisoning.

Chloroform (CCl_3H) is more nephrotoxic than carbon tetrachloride and produces proximal tubule cell damage in animal models. Trichloroethylene (C_2HCl_3) has several industrial indications including use as an anesthetic agent. Acute kidney injury has followed inhalation of this agent and has occurred in persons using it as a solvent for cleaning. Although it is partially unsaturated, it has toxic effects comparable with those of carbon tetrachloride and chloroform.

Tetrachloroethane (1,1,2,2-tetrachloroethane, $C_2H_2Cl_4$) is an excellent solvent for cellulose acetate and is the most toxic of the halogenated hydrocarbons. Vinylidene chloride (1,1-dichloroethylene, $C_2H_2Cl_2$) is a monomer used in the manufacture of plastics and is not used as a solvent. Its toxicology is like that of carbon tetrachloride.

Ethylene chlorohydrin (2-chloroethyl alcohol, C_2H_4ClOH) is used as a solvent and as a chemical intermediate. It is more toxic than any of the other aliphatic halogenated hydrocarbons. Unlike the others, it penetrates the skin readily and is absorbed through rubber gloves. Its mechanism of toxicity is not well understood.

2. Nonhalogenated Hydrocarbons as a Cause of Acute Kidney Injury

▶ Dioxane

Dioxane is a cyclic diether; it is colorless, has only a faint odor, and is freely soluble in water. The vapor pressure of dioxane is quite low, so respiratory overexposure is rare. Although dioxane is less toxic than the halogenated hydrocarbons, toxicity can be insidious, and large amounts can be inhaled without warning. Injury may become apparent hours after exposure.

Clinically, patients present with anorexia, nausea, and vomiting. Jaundice is uncommon. In fatal cases, clinical presentation may resemble an acute abdominal emergency. Urine output decreases on about the third day of illness.

▶ Toluene

There are several reports of acute kidney injury occurring with toluene inhalation (glue sniffing); most case reports describe reversible acute tubular necrosis, with a few reports documenting acute interstitial nephritis. However, metabolic acidosis associated with toluene abuse has been well documented. The two mechanisms involved are overproduction of hippuric acid and reduction of excretion of net acid (primarily NH_4^+) in some abusers. Sodium and potassium depletion also occur in these patients contributing to a presentation with muscle weakness.

▶ Phenol

Phenol (carbolic acid) causes local burns and may be absorbed both through the lungs and skin. Although phenol causes severe local burns, systemic symptoms also may occur. These include headache, vertigo, salivation, nausea

and vomiting, and diarrhea. In severe intoxication, urinary albumin excretion may be increased. Red cells and casts are found in the urine. The potentially disastrous consequences of transdermal absorption should not be underestimated.

Patients may present with hypothermia, which is followed by convulsions. The urine may be dark, and oliguria may develop. Phenol is metabolized to hydroquinone, which, when excreted in the urine, may be oxidized to colored substances, causing the urine to change to green or brown (carboluria). Prolonged exposure has been reported to result in proteinuria.

▶ Pentachlorophenol

Pentachlorophenol (PCP) is banned in most countries; however, it is restricted from public use and available in a few countries. It is used as a preservative for timber and as an insecticide, herbicide, and defoliant. It is readily absorbed through the skin. In addition to causing acute kidney injury, PCP causes a hypermetabolic state, with hyperpyrexia and vascular collapse. Workers exposed to PCP in clearly subtoxic doses may present with reversible decreased proximal tubular function as manifested by reduced tubular resorption of phosphorus.

ACUTE KIDNEY INJURY CAUSED BY ARSINE

▶ Exposure

Arsine (AsH_3) is a heavy gas and is the most nephrotoxic form of arsenic. It is produced by the action of acids on arsenicals, usually during coal or metal-processing operations. Exposure to arsine may be insidious because even as simple an operation as spraying water on metal dross may liberate arsine. Arsine is also used in the semiconductor industry. It may be shipped over long distances with a potential for public health disasters as arsine is an extremely toxic gas.

▶ Clinical Findings

Arsine is primarily hemotoxic and is a potent hemolytic agent after acute or chronic exposure. The first signs of poisoning are malaise, abdominal cramps, nausea, and vomiting. This may take place immediately or after a delay of up to 24 hours. Renal failure results from acute tubular necrosis secondary to hemoglobinuria.

▶ Treatment & Prognosis

Acute tubular necrosis may be delayed by treatment with hydration with isotonic saline. Recovery from acute tubular necrosis induced by arsine may not be complete, and there is evidence that residual interstitial nephritis may result.

ARISTOLOCHIC ACID NEPHROPATHY & ANALGESIC NEPHROPATHY

When evaluating patients suspected of having CKD associated with environmental or occupational exposures, it is important to exclude herbal and analgesic nephropathy.

Both present with chronic interstitial nephritis, as do most occupationally related CKDs. Aristolochic acid nephropathy (previously known as Chinese herb nephropathy) was first described in 1991; physicians in Belgium noted an increasing number of young women presenting with ESRD following exposure to Chinese herbs at a weight-reduction clinic. The kidney tissue pathology includes extensive hypocellular interstitial fibrosis and tubular atrophy, and the renal disease is associated with urothelial carcinoma of the upper urinary tract. Aristolochic acid was the common denominator found in the weight-reduction formulas in Belgium. Cases of aristolochic acid nephropathy have been reported worldwide. Aristolochic acid exposure in rat models produce similar renal lesions as in humans, and aristolochic acid DNA adducts have been demonstrated in the kidney tissue of patients with aristolochic acid nephropathy. There is no treatment for aristolochic acid nephropathy except for CKD management and renal replacement therapy. Of note, patients considered for a kidney transplant may require bilateral nephroureterectomy due to the high incidence of urothelial carcinoma.

In general, herbal remedies are safe, but adulteration of these herbal remedies has been reported. The common contaminants that may cause renal disease include botanicals (eg, aristolochic acid), synthetic drugs (eg, nonsteroidal anti-inflammatory drugs [NSAIDs], and diazepam), and heavy metals (eg, lead and cadmium). Renal dysfunction because of NSAIDs and selective cyclooxygenase-2 inhibitors may present in three different forms. The most common form is hemodynamic kidney injury after the loss of prostaglandin-mediated afferent arteriolar vasodilatation. This then leads to afferent arteriolar vasoconstriction in patients with preexisting volume depletion or low effective circulating volume. NSAID's also can cause acute kidney injury secondary to acute interstitial nephritis, which usually is accompanied by nephrotic-range proteinuria. Both forms of kidney injury are reversible after discontinuation of the offending drug, but interstitial nephritis is usually more severe and may require dialysis support. The third form of renal dysfunction is papillary necrosis, which is not reversible, and occurs after many years of high doses of NSAIDs. Papillary necrosis occurs more commonly after chronic phenacetin use. Phenacetin is no longer available in the United States.

In addition to NSAIDs and aristolochic acid, herbal remedies may contain heavy metals, such as lead, cadmium, or mercury; the renal disease associated with these metals is discussed in the following sections.

BALKAN-ENDEMIC NEPHROPATHY

Balkan-endemic nephropathy (BEN) is a prototype for renal disease associated with environmental exposures. BEN highlights the difficulties involved in identifying specific toxins that may cause renal disease. In the late 1950s, BEN was first described as an interstitial nephropathy associated with urinary tract tumors. It is endemic to rural areas along the Sava, Danube, and Morava rivers in Serbia, Croatia,

Bosnia-Herzegovina, Bulgaria, and Romania. It strikes predominantly farm workers in the fifth to sixth decades. Most victims have resided for at least 20 years in villages where the disease is endemic, and children are not affected.

Patients present with abnormalities of tubular function, including renal tubular acidosis, glycosuria, and hyperuricosuria with hypouricemia. Proteinuria is usually less than 1 g/d, which is consistent with the absence of glomerular disease. Not all patients with CKD will progress to ESRD. Renal pathology includes interstitial fibrosis and periglomerular fibrosis; there is no inflammatory component, and glomeruli are normal. Papillary transitional-cell cancer is seen in 30–40% of patients with BEN. Anemia seems to be disproportionate to the degree of renal failure in these patients.

Aristolochic acid has been found in flour obtained from wheat contaminated with the seeds of *Aristolochia clematis* in areas of endemicity. In addition, aristolochic acid DNA adducts have been found in the kidney tissue of patients from endemic regions. Aristolochic acid exposure is now thought to be the cause of BEN. The term, aristolochic acid nephropathy, is used to describe the interstitial nephropathy caused by ingestion of plants containing aristolochic acid or of food with environmental contamination by aristolochic acid.

CKD OF UNKNOWN CAUSE IN AGRICULTURAL COMMUNITIES

Mesoamerican Nephropathy

There is an epidemic of CKD across Central America that disproportionately affects men in agricultural communities working in coastal lowland areas with high ambient temperatures. In addition to the absence of traditional risk factors such as hypertension and diabetes, the clinical manifestations include minimal proteinuria, hypokalemia, hyperuricemia, and small echogenic kidneys on ultrasound imaging. Agricultural workers in low altitudes seem to be particularly at risk for this form of CKD. The etiology is unknown, but most patients report recurrent dehydration due to strenuous work conditions in extreme heat and humidity. The etiology is likely multifactorial, but volume depletion with repeated episodes of heat-related acute kidney injury is an important contributor in the pathway to developing Mesoamerican nephropathy. Other etiologies are being investigated like toxins (agrochemicals, heavy metals, aristolochic acid, and medications), infections, and genetic causes, but the limited available data does not support any of these additional etiologies. Dialysis and transplantation is not an option for many in Central America and therefore many of these men die an early death due to CKD. Efforts are underway by many groups to identify the etiology of the CKD in this region. In the meantime, efforts to prevent Mesoamerican nephropathy focus on optimal hydration, limit work in high temperatures, avoid nonsteroidal anti-inflammatory drugs, and minimize exposure to nephrotoxic chemicals.

Table 22–1. Demographic and clinical characteristics of chronic kidney disease of unknown cause.*

Variable	Mesoamerican Nephropathy	Sri Lankan Nephropathy	Uddanam Nephropathy
Region	Pacific Coast, rural areas from Mexico to Panama	North Central Province	Central Indian states of Andhra Pradesh, Odisha, Chhattisgarh, Maharashtra
Demographic features	Age range, 20–50 y Male:female ratio, > 3:1	Age range, 40–50 y Male:female ratio, 1.3:1	Age range, 30–60 y More common in men
Affected population	Sugarcane workers, cotton workers, corn farmers, construction workers, port workers, miners, fishing industry workers, shrimp farm workers, brick workers	Rice farmers	Cashew, rice, and coconut farmers
Hypothesized Causes			
Heat exposure	Low-altitude areas with hot tropical climate, physical exertion, recurrent dehydration	Low-altitude areas with hot tropical climate	Coast and inland up to 60–70 m above sea level with hot tropical climate
Other	Toxic causes: pesticides, heavy metals, NSAIDs, tobacco use Infections: leptospirosis, hantavirus infection Gene-environment interactions	Cadmium, pesticides (glyphosate), hard water, high fluoride content in drinking water, arsenic, glyphosate chelation with metals, low water intake, malaria	Silica in groundwater, excessive use of painkillers, low water intake
Clinical Findings			
Acute phase	Fever, elevated serum creatinine level, muscle and joint pain, leukocytosis, leukocyturia, hematuria	Fever, fatigue, dysuria, joint pain, elevated serum creatinine level	Not described so far
Chronic phase	Insidious presentation (elevated serum creatinine level), low-grade or no proteinuria, hypokalemia, hyponatremia, hypomagnesemia, frequent hyperuricemia, reduced kidney size on ultrasound	Insidious presentation (elevated serum creatinine level), low-grade or no proteinuria, hypokalemia, hyponatremia, hypomagnesemia, frequent hyperuricemia, reduced kidney size on ultrasound	Insidious presentation (elevated serum creatinine level), low-grade or no hypertension, low-grade or no proteinuria, microscopic hematuria (rare), reduced kidney size on ultrasound

*NSAIDs denotes nonsteroidal anti-inflammatory drugs.
Source: Used, with permission, from Johnson RJ, Wesseling C, Newman LS: Chronic kidney disease of unknown cause in agricultural communities. N Engl J Med 2019;380(19):1843-1852.

Sri Lankan and Uddanam Nephropathy

CKD of unknown origin has also been observed in Sri Lanka and Uddanam, India among rice paddy, coconut, cashew nut, and rice farmers in rural areas. These workers present with clinical disease similar to those in Mesoamerica, with elevations of serum creatinine, minimal proteinuria, and chronic interstitial nephritis with variable glomerulosclerosis.

Table 22–1 compares the reported characteristics of the disease in Central America, Sri Lanka, and India.

▼ CHRONIC KIDNEY DISEASE

CKD CAUSED BY LEAD

Although organic lead, which was widely used as an additive to gasoline in the past, is not nephrotoxic, its combustion products are. At one time, lead was released into the environment at a rate of approximately 60 million kg/y as inorganic lead through the combustion of gasoline. Its environmental fate is unknown. Lead can be absorbed from the gastrointestinal tract or the lungs. Gastrointestinal absorption is approximately 10% in adults and 50% in children. Within 1 hour of absorption by the gut, lead is concentrated in bone (90%) and kidneys. The biologic half-life ranges from 7 years to several decades.

Although Lanceraux described the link between lead exposure and small contracted kidneys in 1863, the modern awareness of lead nephropathy originated with the Australian experience. Acute lead poisoning in childhood was very common in Queensland between 1870 and 1920, when lead paint was still being used. Twenty years later, a follow-up study of children hospitalized for acute lead poisoning found that more than 30% of these children had chronic nephritis, hypertension, or proteinuria. Gouty arthritis was noted in approximately 50% of patients. Epidemiologic data in the

United States also confirm the link between overt lead exposure and CKD, hypertension, and gout.

Experimental models of lead nephropathy found that administration of continuous high-dose lead to rats over a 1-year period resulted in a significant reduction in GFR, and the renal pathology revealed the characteristic proximal tubule intranuclear inclusions that are prominent early in human lead nephropathy. After 6 months of lead exposure, focal tubular atrophy and interstitial fibrosis appeared, and after 12 months, enlarged, dilated tubules were noted. Chelation of lead with dimercaptosuccinic acid (DMSA) resulted in an increase in GFR in rats, but the tubulointerstitial disease did not reverse. Continuous low-level lead exposure in rats did not produce significant changes in renal function and produced only mild alterations in renal morphology after 12 months.

Many studies have noted an approximate incidence of gout of 50% among subjects with lead nephropathy. The possible mechanisms of saturnine gout include decreased renal clearance of uric acid, crystallization at low urate concentrations, and lead-induced formation of guanine crystals. Human studies have found that patients with gout and CKD disease have significantly higher urinary lead excretion after chelation than do either subjects with gout and normal renal function or subjects with CKD and no gout. These findings implicate lead as the cause of both the gout and the CKD in these patients.

Acute lead intoxication is associated with hypertension, but the relationship between chronic lead exposure and hypertension remains controversial in the setting of mounting evidence. Despite the continued decline in lead exposure in the US population, a significant association between relatively low blood lead levels and hypertension remains among Mexican Americans and African-Americans in the United States. Many large population studies have found a direct correlation between blood lead levels and zinc protoporphyrin and blood pressure. The possible mechanisms linking lead and hypertension include increased intracellular calcium, inhibition of the Na^+, K^+-adenosine triphosphatase (ATPase) system, direct vasoconstriction, and alterations in the rennin-angiotensin-aldosterone axis.

Human studies also have investigated the role of lead in the association of hypertension and CKD. Early studies in patients with overt lead exposure, hypertension, and CKD have implicated lead as a cause of both the renal insufficiency and hypertension. However, these studies included patients with high-level lead exposure, including those with moonshine consumption. There is growing evidence that low-level lead exposure is associated with CKD among certain populations.

A recent population-based cohort study from Sweden has reported an association between low-level environmental lead exposure and decreased kidney function and incident CKD. Also, a Swedish case-control study of subjects with low-level exposure to lead found an association between increasing blood lead levels and the risk of ESRD.

Small studies from Taiwan recently have reported low-level environmental lead exposure as an independent risk factor for renal disease progression among patients with diabetic and nondiabetic CKD. Furthermore, intravenous chelation therapy with calcium ethylenediaminetetraacetic acid (calcium EDTA) seems to ameliorate the decline in renal function when compared with placebo in the same Taiwanese patients with diabetic and nondiabetic CKD.

▶ Presentation

The classic presentation for lead nephropathy is CKD accompanied by a history of hypertension and gout. However, the diagnosis of lead nephropathy also should be considered in patients with CKD and low-grade proteinuria, even without gout or significant hypertension. The urinalysis usually reveals 1+ to 2+ proteinuria but is otherwise normal, without cells or cellular casts. Twenty-four hour urine collection usually has non-nephrotic-range proteinuria in the range of 1–2 g, and renal ultrasonography typically shows small, contracted kidneys. Renal biopsy reveals nonspecific tubular atrophy, interstitial fibrosis, and minimal inflammatory infiltrates, and the arteriolar changes are indistinguishable from nephrosclerosis and appear even in patients with lead exposure and no history of hypertension. Electron microscopy shows mitochondrial swelling and increased numbers of lysosomal dense bodies within proximal tubule cells; intranuclear inclusion bodies usually are present in the early stages of lead exposure but often are absent after chronic exposure or after lead chelation.

▶ Diagnosis

The diagnosis is considered after documenting significant lead exposure. Whole blood lead levels are not useful unless elevated because low whole blood lead levels do not exclude chronic lead exposure. The calcium EDTA lead mobilization test correlates well with bone lead levels. One gram of calcium EDTA is given intravenously or 2 g of calcium EDTA with lidocaine are given intramuscularly in two divided doses 8–12 hours apart, and urine is then collected for 72 hours in patients with CKD or for 24 hours in patients with normal renal function. Early studies in patients with overt lead exposure demonstrated that a total excretion greater than 600 mcg lead chelate over 3 days was indicative of significant lead exposure. Studies of patients in Taiwan with low-level lead exposure raise the possibility that a total lead chelate excretion as low as 20–599 mcg may be significant. Tibial K x-ray fluorescence measurements also correlate well with bone lead levels and, if available, should replace the calcium EDTA mobilization test.

▶ Treatment

Overt lead nephropathy is one of the few preventable renal diseases. Whether renal function improves with treatment is controversial, but in some patients treatment has resulted in a modest improvement in GFR or, at the minimum, a slowing of the progression of the renal insufficiency even with low-level exposure. In addition, lead chelation treatment has led to increased urate excretion, which might have an impact on the management of gout in these patients. For patients with overt lead nephropathy, treatment consists of continued calcium EDTA injections thrice weekly, with the goal of normalizing the urinary lead chelate.

Among patients with CKD and low-level lead exposure (urine lead chelate excretion between 20 and 599 mcg), treatment is continued with weekly intravenous infusions of 1 g calcium EDTA until the urine lead chelate decreases to below 20 mcg. However, the safety and efficacy of calcium EDTA in patients with moderate to severe renal insufficiency have not been well studied, and calcium EDTA should be used with caution in these patients.

CKD CAUSED BY CADMIUM

Cadmium, which is found primarily as cadmium sulfide in ores of zinc, lead, and copper, accumulates with age, having a biologic half-life in humans in excess of 10 years. In the United States, the use of cadmium doubled every decade in the twentieth century because of its common use in the manufacture of nickel-cadmium batteries, pigments, glass, metal alloys, and electrical equipment.

Between 40% and 80% of accumulated cadmium is stored in the liver and kidneys, with one-third in the kidneys alone. Cadmium is also a contaminant of tobacco smoke, and in the absence of occupational exposure, accumulation is substantially greater in smokers than in nonsmokers. Nonindustrial exposure is primarily via food; only approximately 25% of ingested cadmium is absorbed. "Normal" daily dietary intake varies between 15 and 75 mg/d in different parts of the world, although only a small fraction of this amount (0.5–2.5 mg/d) is absorbed. The cadmium body burden of a 45-year-old nonsmoker in the United States is approximately 9 mg, whereas in Japan the total is approximately 21 mg. Although clinical disease has been recognized among the general population in Japan, this has not been the case in the United States, where cadmium generally has been regarded as an exclusively industrial hazard. This may represent a failure to assign the correct cause to conditions commonly regarded as the result of aging.

After exposure to cadmium, the blood concentration rises sharply but falls in a matter of hours as cadmium is taken up by the liver. In red blood cells and soft tissues, cadmium is bound to metallothionein, which is a low-molecular-weight polypeptide. This cadmium-metallothionein complex is filtered at the glomerulus, undergoes endocytosis in the proximal tubule, and is later degraded in the lysosomes. The adverse effects of cadmium on the proximal tubule are probably mediated by unbound cadmium, which can interfere with zinc-dependent enzymes.

The principal target organs for cadmium toxicity after chronic low-dose exposure are the kidneys and lungs. Once a critical concentration of 200 mcg/g of renal cortex is achieved, the renal effects, such as Fanconi syndrome, become evident. Hypercalciuria with normocalcemia, hyperphosphaturia, and distal renal tubular acidosis all contribute to the osteomalacia, pseudofractures, and nephrolithiasis seen in certain patients. Many of the symptoms usually originate from the increased calcium excretion that accompanies the renal tubular dysfunction. Ureteral colic from calculi is seen in up to 40% of patients subjected to industrial exposure. Itai-Itai ("ouch-ouch") disease is a painful bone disease associated with pseudofractures in Japan, and it is attributed to local cadmium contamination of food staples by polluted river water. The possible causes of osteomalacia include a direct effect of cadmium on bone, diminished renal tubular reabsorption of calcium and phosphate, and increased parathyroid hormone and the subsequent decreased hydroxylation of vitamin D.

The role of cadmium in the induction of chronic interstitial nephritis and CKD is controversial. A study of 1021 workers with low-level cadmium toxicity found that early kidney damage evidenced by tubular proteinuria was evident at levels thought to be safe by World Health Organization health-based limits. Although some studies demonstrate subtle declines in GFR or an increase in odds ratios of ESRD in cross-sectional studies, only a few studies demonstrate an increase incidence of severe CKD. A Swedish cohort study in a cadmium-polluted region found that the risk of developing ESRD over 18 years increased with higher levels of cadmium exposure.

Renal cadmium toxicity should be suspected in patients with low-molecular-weight proteinuria, urinary calculi, multiple tubular abnormalities, and a urine cadmium concentration greater than 10 mcg/g of urine creatinine. There is no definitive treatment as no chelating agent is effective in removing cadmium from the body. Supportive treatment with removal from the source of exposure and treatment of osteomalacia, if present, should be initiated.

CKD CAUSED BY MERCURY

▶ Exposure

Elemental, inorganic, and organic forms of mercury all can be renal toxic. Occupational mercury poisoning usually results from inhalation of metal fumes or vapor, although toxicity has been reported after exposure to oxides of mercury, mercurous or mercuric chloride, phenylmercuric acetate, mercuric oxide, and mercury-containing pesticides. Divalent mercury is quite nephrotoxic when ingested; it accumulates in the proximal tubule. Although acute tubular necrosis will result after administration of mercuric chloride ($HgCl_2$), such exposures are extremely rare as occupational hazards.

The two forms of renal disease resulting from mercury toxicity are acute tubular necrosis and nephrotic syndrome. In humans, acute tubular necrosis develops after ingestion of 0.5 g $HgCl_2$, and in rats, $HgCl_2$ is used routinely to produce an experimental model of acute tubular necrosis. There also have been sporadic case reports of nephrotic syndrome after mercury exposure. These may be idiosyncratic reactions, and accordingly, occupational studies have not been able to find an association between mercury exposure and proteinuria. Membranous nephropathy, minimal-change disease, and anti–glomerular basement membrane antibody deposition has been reported following mercury exposure.

Mercuric chloride can induce membranous nephropathy in certain rat strains. Before the development of the basement membrane immune deposits seen in membranous nephropathy, an autoimmune glomerulonephritis with linear immunoglobulin G (IgG) deposits along the glomerular capillary wall is first seen, but no pulmonary hemorrhage develops as seen in the Goodpasture syndrome. A T-cell-dependent polyclonal B-cell activation is responsible for the IgG deposits. As in humans, removal from mercury exposure, which can be in vapor or injections, results in reversal of the proteinuria in the rat models.

▶ Diagnosis

The clinical presentation in patients with acute tubular necrosis is usually dominated by the extrarenal manifestations of mercury toxicity. When the history of mercury exposure is available, the diagnosis of acute tubular necrosis from mercury toxicity is not difficult. On the other hand, it is more difficult to attribute glomerular disease such as membranous nephropathy to mercury exposure. Although elevated blood and urine mercury concentrations are consistent with significant exposure, these concentrations do not correlate with renal disease. Spontaneous resolution of the proteinuria following removal from the source of mercury exposure is consistent with mercury-mediated glomerular disease.

▶ Treatment

The mainstay of treatment is removal from the source of mercury exposure. For symptomatic patients who have urine or whole blood mercury concentrations of ≥ 100 mcg/L, treatment with chelation with the parenteral agent British anti-Lewisite (dimercaprol BAL) or with oral DMSA (succimer) should be considered. BAL is given as an initial dose of up to 5 mg/kg/dose every 4 hours for 48 hours, then 2.5 mg/kg/dose every 6 hours for 48 hours, then 2.5 mg/kg/dose every 12 hours for 7 days. DMSA is given at a dose of 10 mg/kg by mouth three times daily for 5 days, then twice daily for 14 days. In severe cases of mercury toxicity with anuric acute kidney injury, the use of hemodialysis with the prefilter infusion of DMSA has been reported to increase the removal of inorganic mercury.

CKD CAUSED BY BERYLLIUM

▶ Exposure

Beryllium is encountered in the manufacture of electronic tubes, ceramics, and fluorescent light bulbs, as well as in metal foundries. Because its absorption through the gut is very poor, beryllium's principal route of entry into the body is by inhalation.

▶ Clinical Findings

The main manifestation of berylliosis is as a systemic granulomatous disease involving primarily the lungs, as well as

the bone and bone marrow, the liver, the lymph nodes, and many other organs. Kidney damage occurs not as an isolated finding but only in conjunction with other forms of toxicity. In the kidneys, berylliosis can produce granulomas and interstitial fibrosis. Beryllium disease is associated with hypercalciuria and urinary tract stones.

CKD CAUSED BY URANIUM

Uranium can cause acute kidney injury in experimental models, and the pathologic changes are consistent with acute tubular necrosis. During the Manhattan Project, kidney disease occurred in subjects working on the atomic bomb. Whether uranium can cause CKD remains controversial. Although previous studies of Gulf War veterans exposed to depleted uranium and workers in a uranium-refining plant did reveal an increase in urinary β_2-microglobulin excretion, the studies did not document decreased renal function, and the urinary β_2-microglobulin levels were still in the normal range. In a study utilizing National Health and Nutrition Examination Survey (NHANES) 2001–2010 data, a high proportion of the U.S. population had exposure to environmental uranium documented with urine measurements, and there was an association between detectable urine uranium concentrations and microalbumin but not with decreased renal function.

CKD CAUSED BY SILICOSIS

Silicosis is a form of pneumoconiosis associated with pulmonary exposure to silica. Heavy exposure can result in a generalized systemic disease resembling collagen-vascular disease, such as systemic lupus erythematosus. Inhalation of silica may trigger an autoimmune response in sensitive individuals; in fact, the occurrence of positive antinuclear antibody and antineutrophil cytoplasmic autoantibodies is increased in patients with silicosis.

The association of silica and glomerulonephritis is suggested by animal studies, case-control studies, and multiple case reports. Animals experimentally exposed to silica developed acute interstitial nephritis with deposition of silica in the kidney. This fact led to speculation that silica may contribute to analgesic nephropathy as a result of the widespread use of silicates in analgesic preparations. The reported cases of silica-associated glomerular disease include glomerular proliferation with occasional crescents, subendothelial and membranous deposits, and tubular degeneration. A systematic review and meta-analysis of occupational exposure to silica and CKD found elevated standardized mortality ratios for kidney disease but without a dose-response relationship.

CKD CAUSED BY ORGANIC SOLVENTS

Solvent exposure may occur in many industries where there is use of paints, degreasers, and fuels, including the petrochemical and aerospace industries. There have been several interesting case reports over the last 40 years of anti–glomerular basement membrane antibody–mediated glomerulonephritis occurring after solvent exposure. However, it remains unclear whether the solvent exposure is truly causal in these cases. Membranous nephropathy also has been reported after long exposure to mixed organic solvents. Twenty-five case-control studies have investigated hydrocarbon exposure and renal disease, and although most of these studies have major limitations, 20 found an increased odds ratio between solvent exposure and a variety of renal diseases. Animal studies show that solvents can cause acute renal damage at high doses, and only mild chronic renal changes have been produced with chronic low-dose exposure. There are no animal models for immunologic renal disease caused by solvents.

Solvent exposure at high doses may lead to acute kidney injury, and multiple case reports suggest that solvent exposure is associated with glomerular disease. IgA nephropathy has been reported in a number of case reports of workers exposed to organic solvents, and studies support an association between organic solvent exposure and the progression of preexisting IgA to chronic renal failure or to ESRD.

CKD CAUSED BY CARBON DISULFIDE

▶ Exposure History & Clinical Findings

Carbon disulfide is used in the manufacture of viscose rayon. Accelerated atherosclerosis is an accepted consequence of long-term exposure to carbon disulfide, and the accelerated atherosclerosis may affect the renal circulation leading to renal dysfunction, hypertension, proteinuria, and renal insufficiency. A recent study reported the renal pathology of 10 workers with greater than 10 years of exposure to carbon disulfide. Most of the workers had proteinuria and half had CKD. The kidney biopsies findings were nonspecific, but all 10 workers had diffused mesangial cell proliferation and mesangial hyperplasia.

REFERENCES

Barnett LMA: Nephrotoxicity and renal pathophysiology: a contemporary perspective. Toxicol Sci 2018;164(2):379 [PMID: 29939355].

Harari F et al: Blood lead levels and decreased kidney function in a population-based cohort. Am J Kidney Dis 2018;72(3):381 [PMID: 29699886].

Jadot I: An integrated view of aristolochic acid nephropathy: update of the literature. Int J Mol Sci 2017;18(2):297 [PMID: 28146082].

Jelaković B: Balkan endemic nephropathy and the causative role of aristolochic acid. Semin Nephrol 2019;39(3):284 [PMID: 31054628].

Johnson RJ, Wesseling C, Newman LS: Chronic kidney disease of unknown cause in agricultural communities. N Engl J Med 2019;380(19):1843 [PMID: 31412197].

Min B, Kim G, Kang T, Yoon C, Cho SI, Paek D: IgA nephropathy in a laboratory worker that progressed to end-stage renal disease: a case report. Ann Occup Environ Med 2016;28:35 [PMID: 27504189].

Möhner M: Occupational exposure to respirable crystalline silica and chronic nonmalignant renal disease: systematic review and meta-analysis. Int Arch Occup Environ Health 2017;90(7):555 [PMID: 28409224].

Moody EC, Coca SG, Sanders AP: Toxic metals and chronic kidney disease: a systematic review of recent literature. Curr Environ Health Rep 2018;5(4):453 [PMID: 30338443].

Okaneku J: Urine uranium concentrations and renal function in residents of the United States—2001 to 2010. Clin Toxicol (Phila) 2015;53(10):931 [PMID: 26468995].

Orr SE: Chronic kidney disease and exposure to nephrotoxic metals. Int J Mol Sci 2017;2:18(5) [PMID: 28498320].

Ou S: Renal pathology in patients with occupational exposure to carbon disulphide: a case series. Nephrology (Carlton) 2017;22(10):755 [PMID: 27414474].

Satarug S: Chronic exposure to cadmium is associated with a marked reduction in glomerular filtration rate. Clin Kidney J 2019;12(4):468 [PMID 31384436].

■ SELF-ASSESSMENT QUESTIONS

Select the one correct answer for each question.

Question 1: The kidney
   a. is especially vulnerable to occupational and
      environmental exposures
   b. receives about half the cardiac output
   c. reabsorbs and dilutes filtrate
   d. prevents development of toxins in ionic forms

Question 2: Acute kidney injury
   a. occurs only after high-dose exposure
   b. always develops as acute tubular necrosis
   c. leads to a decrease in BUN and creatinine
   d. may require dialysis until the renal function recovers

Question 3: Chronic kidney disease (CKD)
   a. is rarely in the form of chronic interstitial nephritis
   b. does not include lead nephropathy
   c. does not follow exposures to organic solvents
   d. is characterized by tubular proteinuria

Question 4: Balkan-endemic nephropathy (BEN)
   a. is a form of aristolochic acid nephropathy
   b. is an interstitial nephropathy associated with urinary
      tract infections
   c. strikes farm workers at all ages
   d. affects children living on farms

Question 5: Lead nephropathy
   a. is an acute kidney disease accompanied by a history
      of hypertension and gout
   b. should not be considered in patients who do not
      have gout or hypertension
   c. ultrasonography typically shows small, contracted
      kidneys
   d. reveals no tubular atrophy on renal biopsy

Question 6: Overt lead nephropathy
   a. is one of the few preventable renal diseases
   b. treatment has no impact on the management of gout

   c. treatment consists of continued EDTA injections
      once weekly
   d. treatment is continued until urine lead chelate is
      below 20 mcg

Question 7: Cadmium
   a. primarily affects the kidneys and liver
   b. renal effects include the Fanconi syndrome
   c. symptoms usually result from the increased calcium
      excretion that accompanies the glomerular injury
   d. causes ureteral colic from calculi in most patients
      subjected to industrial exposure

Question 8: Silicosis
   a. can result in a generalized systemic disease resem-
      bling collagen-vascular disease
   b. is the most common cause of systemic lupus
      erythematosus
   c. decreases the occurrence of positive antinuclear
      antibody
   d. has no effect on the occurrence of antineutrophil
      cytoplasmic autoantibodies

Question 9: The epidemic of chronic kidney disease in Central America
   a. primarily affects automobile factory workers
   b. is caused by heavy metals
   c. disproportionately affects agricultural workers at
      lower, warm weather altitudes
   d. is a form of aristolochic acid nephropathy

Question 10: Toluene inhalation (glue sniffing)
   a. is a cause of nephrotic syndrome
   b. may lead to the development of respiratory acidosis
   c. is a cause of renal tubular acidosis
   d. is associated with Fanconi syndrome

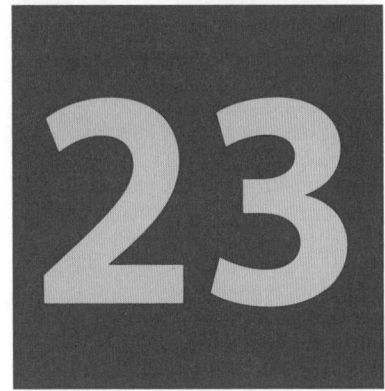

Neurotoxicology

Samuel M. Goldman, MD, MPH

Diseases of the nervous system are known for their diverse clinical manifestations. When the central nervous system (CNS) is affected, symptoms may include headache, cognitive and psychiatric disturbances, visual changes, seizures, ataxia, tremors, rigidity, weakness, and sensory manifestations. In peripheral nervous system diseases, pain, weakness, paresthesias, and numbness are common, and in some instances there may be additional autonomic disturbances.

The pattern of neurologic symptoms depends on the nature of the insult. For instance, excessive exposure to many industrial or environmental chemicals causes a generalized disorder of peripheral nerves, that is, peripheral neuropathy. This presents usually as a diffuse and symmetric clinical syndrome. In contrast, some occupations may predispose workers to physical injuries to peripheral nerves. Common examples are carpal tunnel syndrome from median nerve entrapment and lumbar radiculopathy from compression of the spinal roots. Single nerves or spinal roots are affected in these instances, leading to a localized pattern of neurologic symptoms and signs.

GENERAL PRINCIPLES

Neurologic evaluation of patients largely depends on history and physical examination, supplemented by traditional diagnostic tests such as computed tomography (CT) and magnetic resonance imaging (MRI) of the brain or spine, electroencephalography (EEG), nerve conduction study, electromyography (EMG), lumbar puncture, neuropsychologic testing, and specialized sensory testing (eg, audiology, color vision discrimination, olfactory perception). Toxicologic tests of blood or urine may provide evidence of recent exposures for some toxicants, whereas tests of hair or nail can sometimes clarify distant or chronic exposures. However, the increasingly common use of blood or urine testing to screen for low levels of metals and other toxicants without a clear toxicologic basis is of questionable value due to the lack of meaningful reference ranges and often unvalidated testing methods.

With few exceptions, the pathophysiology of most neurotoxic injuries is not well understood. Animal models of toxin exposure provide at best a rough guide to human disease. Moreover, it is nearly impossible to study the effects of toxins under controlled conditions in humans. Much of our current knowledge is gained from clinical observations of intense exposures during accidents or chronic heavy occupational exposures. Extrapolation of these classic observations to other situations is problematic. For instance, for many compounds, there is considerable uncertainty concerning the exposure level and duration necessary to cause neurologic injury. It has been especially difficult to ascertain the sequelae of chronic low-level exposure, a situation particularly likely to be encountered by today's physicians.

Despite our incomplete understanding in many of these diseases, several generalizations have been useful in the clinical approach to these disorders.

1. A dose-toxicity relationship exists in the majority of neurotoxic exposures. In general, neurologic symptoms appear only after an exposure reaches a time-dependent threshold level. Although dose-toxicity relationships may be multiphasic on a population level (eg, due to variation in genes encoding metabolic enzymes), individual susceptibility to most neurotoxicants varies over a limited range and idiosyncratic reactions seldom occur.

2. Exposure to toxins typically leads to a nonfocal or symmetric neurologic syndrome. Significant asymmetry such as weakness or sensory loss of one limb or one side of the body with sparing of the contralateral side should suggest an alternate cause.

3. There is usually a strong temporal relationship between exposure and the onset of symptoms, though to some extent this may reflect our inability to ascertain subtle deficits or syndromes with very long latencies. Immediate symptoms after acute exposure are often a consequence of the physiologic effects of the chemical (eg, the cholinergic effects of organophosphates [OPs]).

These symptoms subside quickly with elimination of the chemical from the body. Delayed or persistent neurologic deficits that occur after toxic exposures (eg, delayed neuropathy after OP poisoning) generally are a result of pathologic changes in the nervous system. Recovery is still possible, but it tends to be slow and incomplete.

4. The nervous system has a limited capability to regenerate, but some recovery is often possible after removal of the insulting agent. By contrast, worsening neurologic deficits more than a few months after cessation of exposure to a toxin generally argues against a direct causative role of the toxin.

5. Multiple neurologic syndromes are possible from a single toxin. Different neuron populations and different areas of the nervous system may react differently to a toxicant, depending on the intensity and duration of exposure, as well as physiologic variables such as the subject's age and genetic susceptibility. In particular, the clinical features of acute high-intensity exposures may manifest very differently from those of subacute or chronic lower-intensity exposures. A well-known example is lead toxicity, which may lead to an acute confusional state, chronic mental slowing, or a peripheral neuropathy.

6. Few toxicants present with a pathognomonic neurologic syndrome. Symptoms and signs may be mimicked by many psychiatric, metabolic, inflammatory, neoplastic, and degenerative diseases of the nervous system. It is therefore important to exclude other neurologic diseases with appropriate clinical examination and laboratory investigations.

A noteworthy caveat is the phenomenon of *coasting*—the continuing deterioration sometimes seen for up to a few weeks after discontinuation of toxic exposure. Coasting has been well documented in toxic neuropathies caused by pyridoxine (vitamin B_6) abuse, *n*-hexane toxicity, and vincristine chemotherapy. The delay reflects the time necessary for the pathophysiologic processes to evolve to neuronal injury and death.

Another qualification is illustrated by a hypothesis used to explain the pathogenesis of chronic degenerative diseases of aging such as Parkinson disease and Alzheimer dementia. It has been postulated that an environmental or toxic exposure may reduce the functional reserve of the brain. The patient, however, remains asymptomatic until aging or other biologic events further deplete the neuronal pool over many more years. Symptoms appear only when neuronal attrition reaches a threshold level. The hypothesis predicts a long latent period between toxic exposure and symptom manifestation, making these associations extremely difficult to characterize. Attrition may also explain the occasional observation of continuing deterioration for many years after cessation of a toxic exposure (eg, worsening many years after mercury poisoning in the Minamata Bay epidemic). Alternatively, extremely long latencies may reflect the slow evolution of a degenerative process such as through a prion-like seeding of misaggregated proteins initiated by a temporally remote toxic insult.

APPROACH TO PATIENTS

A confident diagnosis of a neurotoxic disorder can be made only after the documentation of all the following: (1) a sufficiently intense or prolonged exposure to the toxin, (2) an appropriate neurologic syndrome based on knowledge about the putative toxin, (3) evolution of symptoms and signs over a compatible temporal course, and (4) exclusion of other neurologic disorders that may account for a similar syndrome.

Exposure History

A detailed history of the nature, duration, and intensity of the exposure is essential in every evaluation. What are the potential toxins? What is the mode of exposure? How long and how intense are the exposures? Are there other confounding factors such as alcoholism, psychosocial issues, and possibility of secondary gains? Are coworkers similarly affected? Chronic exposures are especially difficult to assess. Not only is it essential to assess the average intensity and total duration of exposure, but intermittent peak exposures also are important to quantify.

Neurologic History

The toxicology history should be followed by a detailed characterization of the neurologic complaints. Patients frequently use descriptors such as *weakness, dizziness, forgetfulness, pain,* and *numbness* to refer to vastly different personal experience. Dizziness may mean vertigo from vestibular dysfunction, gait imbalance from sensory loss, or simply a nonspecific sense of ill feeling. Fatigue or asthenia may be referred to as weakness. Fatigue implies reduced endurance or a disinclination for physical activity rather than true weakness. Fatigue may be seen in association with depression, various systemic illnesses, and a wide range of neurologic diseases. The clinician must clearly understand the patient's symptoms and not simply accept their semantic characterization. It is especially useful to inquire about the functional consequences of the neurologic deficits. Questioning about activities of daily living is particularly useful both to better understand the nature of the complaints and to provide a reasonably objective measure of severity. A spouse or partner may provide insights into cognitive and sleep-related problems.

Documentation of the temporal course of the disease is very important. Symptoms may appear acutely (minutes or days), subacutely (weeks or months), or chronically (years). Fluctuating symptoms may suggest recurrent exposures or unrelated superimposed factors. Recovery after discontinuation of exposure helps to implicate the exposure. By contrast, a continuing progression of deficits beyond the "coasting" period may argue against an etiologic role of the exposure.

Central Nervous System

Symptoms and deficits depend on which groups of brain or spinal cord neurons are affected primarily (Table 23–1).

Table 23–1. Neurologic symptoms and signs.

Syndrome	Neuroanatomy	Symptoms and Signs	Examples
Acute encephalopathy	Diffuse; cerebral hemispheres	Varying combination of headache, irritability, disorientation, convulsions, amnesia, psychosis, lethargy, stupor, seizure, coma	Acute exposure to many toxins at sufficient doses
Chronic encephalopathy	Diffuse; cerebral hemispheres	Cognitive and psychiatric disturbances	Chronic exposure to many toxins
Ataxia	Cerebellum	Gait and balance disturbance	Ethanol, toluene, other solvents, methylmercury
Motor (voluntary) dysfunction	Spinal cord motor neurons; skeletal muscle fibers	Muscle atrophy, weakness; spasticity, tetanus	Botulinum toxin, tetrodotoxin, corticosteroids, lead Tetanus toxoid, hexachlorophene, organophosphates
Parkinsonism	Basal ganglia and other extrapyramidal motor pathways	Tremor, rigidity, bradykinesia, gait instability	carbon monoxide, hydrocarbon solvents, carbon disulfide, manganese, methyl-phenyl-tetrahydropyridine (MPTP)
Dysautonomia	Brainstem nuclei; nicotinic and muscarinic cholinergic ganglionic fibers	Tachycardia, bradycardia, diaphoresis, salivation, lacrimation, gastrointestinal, bladder	Organophosphates, carbamates, amphetamine, acrylamide, arsenic, inorganic mercury
Myeloneuropathy (myelopathy and polyneuropathy)	Spinal cord and peripheral nerves	Paresthesias, sensory loss, hyperreflexia, Babinski sign, gait ataxia	Nitrous oxide, organophosphates, n-hexane
Polyneuropathy	Peripheral sensory, motor and autonomic nerve fibers	Paresthesias, numbness, weakness, loss of deep tendon reflexes, more rarely, autonomic failure	Many toxins at sufficient doses (see Table 23–2)

Diffuse dysfunction of cortical or subcortical structures can result from a broad range of toxicants, manifesting along a continuum of altered mental status generally termed encephalopathy. Acutely, this may range from irritability to disorientation to delirium, coma or death. Acute ethanol poisoning provides a common example, and other acute intoxications, for example due to organic solvents, may erroneously be attributed to ethanol poisoning. Chronically, the primary symptoms may be cognitive and psychiatric. Some toxins cause relatively selective injury to the vestibular system or the cerebellum, resulting in disequilibrium, vertigo, and gait or limb ataxia. Basal ganglia involvement may lead to an extrapyramidal syndrome of bradykinesia, tremors, and rigidity that resembles Parkinson disease.

Evaluation of cognitive complaints should include at least a Mini–Mental State Examination (MMSE) or Montreal Cognitive Assessment (MoCA). Referral for neuropsychologic testing may be needed to better understand the pattern and severity of deficits in memory, attention, sensory, and psychomotor function. These tests are increasingly computerized and easier to administer, but good patient cooperation and an experienced interpreter are necessary to obtain meaningful results.

Patients with gait unsteadiness, dizziness, or vertigo should be examined for cranial nerve or cerebellar deficits. The evaluation should include testing of gait, tandem walk, and Romberg sign. The examiner also should note extraocular movements and the presence or absence of nystagmus, hearing deficits, limb ataxia, and sensory deficits. Tremors, if present, should be characterized with the outstretched hands (postural tremor), with the hands at rest, and with the hands performing pointing maneuvers (kinetic and/or intention tremors; eg, the finger-to-nose test). Tendon reflexes should be evaluated and muscle tone should be tested for rigidity. Rapid tapping of the fingers, hands, or feet is a useful test of the motor system. Along with formal strength testing, they should be part of the routine neurologic examination.

Laboratory tests, such as brain or spine imaging studies (eg, MRI or CT), lumbar puncture, electroencephalogram (EEG), and evoked potentials, are often needed to evaluate the anatomic integrity and physiology function of the CNS and to exclude neurologic diseases that may mimic a neurotoxic disorder. In some instances of neurotoxicity, various patterns of MRI signal abnormalities may be seen in the brain, although the appearance is rarely pathognomonic (see specific toxins). However, in many clinical settings and especially in the mildly affected patients, these studies may not show any abnormality.

Peripheral Nervous System

Peripheral nervous system disorders lead to sensory disturbances and weakness, often accompanied by impairment of the deep tendon reflexes on physical examination (see Table 23–1). Of the various components of the peripheral nervous system, the peripheral nerve is by far the most vulnerable to exogenous toxins. Because toxins reach the nerves systemically and affect all nerves simultaneously, the resulting syndrome is typically a symmetric peripheral neuropathy. This is also called a *polyneuropathy,* in contrast to the mononeuropathy that is more frequently the result of local mechanical injury. With few exceptions such as the myopathy caused by alcoholism and medical use of statins, toxic myopathy is uncommon.

The hallmark of most polyneuropathies is the distal distribution of the clinical symptoms and signs. The most common syndrome is subacute onset of tingling or numbness experienced in a symmetric stocking-and-glove distribution. Neuropathic pain is sometimes present and is described variously as burning, deep aching, or lancinating. Pain may be evoked by normally innocuous stimuli such as touching or stroking of the skin, a phenomenon known as *hyperpathia* or *allodynia.* Involvement of the motor nerve fibers manifests as muscle atrophy and weakness. These deficits may appear first in the distal-most muscles (ie, the intrinsic foot and hand muscles). More severe cases may involve muscles of the lower legs and forearms, leading to bilateral foot drop or wrist drop.

Physical examination of patients with peripheral nervous system disorders should include testing of muscle strength, sensation, and tendon reflexes of all four extremities. Are the sensory and motor deficits relatively symmetric? Are the feet more affected than the hands? Because the longest axons are the most vulnerable, neurologic deficits frequently are more severe in the feet than in the hands. Most polyneuropathies are accompanied by diminished or absent stretch reflexes of the Achilles tendons and demonstrable sensory impairment in the toes. Testing of these functions therefore should be included in any screening examination of the peripheral nervous system.

The clinical pattern of sensory and motor nerve involvement is useful in the differential diagnosis of peripheral neuropathy (Table 23–2). The most nonspecific syndrome is a distal symmetric sensorimotor polyneuropathy. This is indistinguishable from the neuropathies caused by common systemic diseases such as uremia, diabetes mellitus, and vitamin B$_{12}$ deficiency. Some toxins, such as lead, cause a neuropathy with prominent weakness. The differential diagnosis of such a neuropathy is relatively narrow and encompasses a few hereditary and immunologic neuropathies.

There are hundreds of causes of peripheral neuropathies. Nontoxic causes of neuropathy, such as those caused by systemic diseases, should be investigated and excluded.

Table 23–2. Toxic polyneuropathies.

Mostly sensory or sensorimotor polyneuropathy (little or no weakness)
  Acrylamide
  Carbon disulfide
  Ethylene oxide
  Metals: arsenic, lead, mercury, thallium
  Methyl bromide
  Polychlorinated biphenyls (PCBs)
  Thallium
Predominantly motor polyneuropathy or sensorimotor polyneuropathy with significant weakness
  Hexacarbons: *n*-hexane, methyl *n*-butyl ketone
  Metals: lead, arsenic, mercury
  Organophosphates
"Purely" sensory neuropathy (disabling sensory loss with no weakness)
  cis-Platinum
  Pyridoxine abuse
Cranial neuropathy
  Thallium
  Trichloroethylene (trigeminal neuropathy)
Prominent autonomic dysfunction
  Acrylamide
  n-Hexane (glue-sniffer)
  Thallium
  Vacor (PNU)
Possible association with neuropathies (mostly anecdotal)
  Benzene
  Carbon monoxide
  Dioxin
  Methyl methacrylate
  Pyrethrins

Approximately one-half of all polyneuropathies remain undiagnosed despite thorough investigation. Thus, the absence of an alternate etiology does not necessarily implicate a toxin. Aside from the presence of sufficient exposure and a compatible syndrome, the diagnosis depends on the documentation of progressive sensory or motor deficits during exposure and recovery of function months or years after cessation of exposure.

Nerve conduction studies and EMG are the primary tools in the laboratory evaluation of neuromuscular disorders. These two tests are often performed together, and the term *EMG* is often used loosely to refer to both tests. Nerve conduction and EMG studies, occasionally supplemented by nerve biopsy, are important in the pathophysiologic characterization of peripheral neuropathies. A fundamental categorization subdivides neuropathies into those with primary degeneration of nerve axons (axonal neuropathy) and those with significant myelin breakdown (demyelinative neuropathy). Diagnostic management of polyneuropathies is best left to experienced specialists.

There are several drawbacks to nerve conduction and EMG studies. These tests are at times painful and uncomfortable at best, with occasional patients tolerating them poorly. Another drawback is the need to use specialized and expensive equipment. Although simplified electronic devices have been advocated, especially in the setting of occupational health screening (eg, screening for carpal tunnel syndrome), there is an unavoidable compromise in accuracy. Furthermore, proper interpretation and performance of these tests require specialized training, and the expertise of providers may vary. Misleading conclusions from improper performance and interpretation are not uncommon.

Ultrasonography is gaining acceptance in the imaging of peripheral nerves, especially for visualization of the nerve at sites of entrapment, such as the carpal tunnel and the ulnar groove. Ultrasonography typically reveals enlargement and change in the echogenicity of compressed nerve. Resolution of these abnormalities may follow successful decompression, providing a way to follow patients in the course of treatment.

MRI and CT are important adjunctive tools to evaluate neuropathies. They are employed most frequently to assess cervical and lumbar radiculopathies, conditions that mimic neuropathy. The main limitation is their relative lack of specificity in diagnosing symptomatic disease. Asymptomatic but radiologically significant spondylitic disease is seen frequently in the normal population. Varying degree of MRI or CT abnormalities are encountered in more than 50% of asymptomatic subjects older than 50 years of age and in approximately 20% of those younger than 50 years of age. Thus, imaging studies should never replace a careful clinical evaluation.

NEUROLOGIC DISORDERS CAUSED BY SPECIFIC TOXINS

The reader is referred to the corresponding chapters on specific toxins for more detailed discussion on general toxicology and health effects. The following discussions are restricted to neurologic complications.

METALS

Arsenic

Arsenic compounds are used as wood preservatives, as gallium arsenide in the semiconductor industry, and as defoliants and desiccants in agriculture, in smelting and in glass manufacturing. Contamination of well water may result from leaching of arsenic by-products in smelting or heavy agricultural use of arsenicals. The valence states of arsenicals include elemental (0), arsenite (+3), and arsenate (+5), with organic or inorganic arsenites and arsenates being most toxic. The primary routes of absorption are gastrointestinal and respiratory. Arsenic freely crosses the blood-brain barrier. Trivalent arsenic binds to sulfhydryl groups in a variety of proteins, interferes with cellular respiration, and leads to increased lipid peroxidation and reduced glutathione levels.

Acute intoxication by arsenical compounds leads to nausea, vomiting, abdominal pain, and diarrhea. Dermatologic lesions, such as hyperkeratosis, skin pigmentation, skin exfoliation, and Mees lines, occur in many patients 1–6 weeks after onset of disease. Peripheral neuropathy is the most common neurologic manifestation of toxicity and may occur after either acute or chronic exposure. After a single massive dose, an acute symmetrical sensorimotor polyneuropathy develops within 1–3 weeks. This neuropathy mimics Guillain-Barré syndrome in many ways and respiratory failure may occur rarely. Symmetric paresthesias and pain, often initially noted in the soles of the feet, may occur in isolation or may be accompanied by distal weakness. With progression of neuropathy, sensory and motor deficits spread proximally. Shoulder and pelvic girdle weakness, as well as gait ataxia, are common in severe cases. Chronic exposure leads to a more insidious sensorimotor polyneuropathy, although there is no agreement for a threshold limit.

Intense exposure to arsenic may lead to mental confusion, psychosis, anxiety, seizure, or coma. Chronic low-level exposure to arsenic, often from environmental or occupational sources, has been associated with more subtle impairment of memory and concentration. In exposed children, there are also reports of lower verbal performance and hearing impairment.

EMG and nerve-conduction studies provide evidence of a nonspecific axonal neuropathy. Arsenic is detectable in blood and urine during ongoing exposure and may persist in urine for several weeks after a single massive exposure. With a low-level exposure, blood arsenic level returns to normal in about 12 hours, and urine arsenic clears within 48–72 hours after exposure. Arsenic remains detectable in hair and nails for months after exposure. Thus, hair or nail analysis can be useful. However, external arsenic contamination may give false-positive results. Pubic hair is preferable to scalp hair for its lesser susceptibility to contamination.

Lead

Neurotoxicity from lead has been recognized since at least the second century BCE. Lead exposure is a concern in a range of occupations and industries including auto repair, battery manufacturing, welding (on painted surfaces), construction workers, glass manufacturers, artists, miners, smelters, ceramics, painters, plumbers, shipbuilders and police officers (lead bullets), among others. Lead is present in paint, ceramic glazes, batteries, pipes, solder, ammunition, and cables. Nonindustrial sources include pottery, bullet fragments, and traditional folk remedies.

Lead neurotoxicity is not fully understood, but many of its effects may be due to its ability to compete for calcium-dependent processes, since they are similar-sized divalent cations. By substituting for calcium, lead can disrupt a huge range of enzymatic processes, impair intracellular and extracellular signaling of both neurons and glia, and damage mitochondria and other organelles.

Acute high-level exposure typically comes from accidental ingestion, inhalation, or industrial exposure. It results in a syndrome of abdominal colic and intermittent vomiting, accompanied by neurologic symptoms such as headache, tremor, apathy, and lethargy. Massive intoxication can lead to convulsions, cerebral edema, stupor, or coma and eventually to transtentorial herniation. Lead encephalopathy typically appears in adults at blood levels of 50–70 mcg/dL or higher. Children are more vulnerable than adults are to acute toxicity probably because of the immaturity of the blood-brain barrier. Behavioral disturbances and neuropsychologic impairment may be present at blood levels as low as 10 mcg/dL, although the exact threshold is debatable. Chronic low-level exposure to lead is responsible for impaired intellectual development in children, with observable decrements at levels as low as 1 mcg/dL, and no apparent threshold. Studies link early life exposure to decreased global IQ, as well as a wide range of behavioral disturbances, such as attention-deficit hyperactivity disorder, poor self-confidence, impulsive behavior, and shortened attention span.

Emerging data suggest that adults with higher lead levels may have a faster rate of cognitive decline, with a greater risk of Alzheimer disease and other dementias, particularly in persons who carry the APOE e4 genotype. Lead is sequestered in bone, and thus can provide a high chronic body burden as measured by x-ray fluorescence, despite having normal blood lead levels. The lead stored in bone potentially can be mobilized throughout life, particularly with bony fractures or osteoporosis. It remains to be seen whether the accelerated decline in cognition results from continuing exposure to lead or from accelerated aging or attrition of neuronal reserves. In animal studies, lead increases the expression of amyloid precursor protein, the primary constituent of beta-amyloid plaques of Alzheimer disease, perhaps through an epigenetic mechanism. High bone lead has also been associated with increased risk of Parkinson disease and amyotrophic lateral sclerosis (ALS, Lou Gehrig disease).

Peripheral neuropathy is a well-recognized complication of chronic lead poisoning in adults. Asymptomatic nerve-conduction-study abnormalities are detectable at lead levels greater than 40 mcg/dL. The best-known clinical syndrome is a predominantly motor neuropathy with little, if any, sensory symptoms. The classic description emphasizes bilateral wrist drop and foot drop. Toxicity also may manifest as a generalized proximal and distal weakness and loss of the tendon reflexes. Some patients have preserved reflexes, and their syndrome thus mimics a motor neuron disease such as ALS. In addition to the classic syndrome of motor neuropathy, some patients may present with distal limb paresthesias and no weakness. This is especially likely in patients with long-term low-level lead exposure.

In patients with acute lead-induced encephalopathy, brain CT or MRI may show focal areas of edema, most commonly in bilateral thalami and basal ganglia. Imaging studies, and sometimes autopsy, may detect intracranial calcification in patients with chronic lead toxicity. The radiologic findings are not specific to lead, and the differential diagnosis may include other causes of calcification, inflammation, and demyelination.

Manganese

Manganese is widely used in the manufacture of steel, alloys, and welding. Manganese is also found in alkaline batteries and various fungicides. Unlike the toxicants discussed above, manganese is an essential human nutrient, and thus has well-developed homeostatic processes. However, because these processes primarily regulate gastrointestinal sources, toxicity can still occur through respiratory routes. Poisoning occurs most commonly in the mining, smelting, milling, and battery-manufacturing industries, although there are occasional reports of environmental contamination. Manganese poisonings have also been reported among persons who intravenously administer the stimulant methcathinone (ephedrone), which is synthesized using potassium permanganate. Of recent interest is the potential risk of organic manganese in the form of methylcyclopentadienyl manganese tricarbonyl (MMT), an additive used in gasoline in some countries.

The classic syndrome of manganese poisoning, or manganism, was first described by Couper in 1837 in manganese ore grinders. It presents as an extrapyramidal disorder that resembles Parkinson disease, with tremor, rigidity, masked facies, and bradykinesias that develop slowly and may continue to progress after cessation of exposure. Unlike typical Parkinson disease, however, manganese-induced parkinsonism is usually symmetrical and includes atypical features such as facial grimacing, early foot dystonia and gait disturbance (so called "cock-walk"), and pronounced psychiatric features. Compared with Parkinson disease, the extrapyramidal symptoms of manganism are minimally responsive to dopaminergic therapy. Whether lower level chronic manganese exposures may result in subclinical neuropsychologic impairments is a hotly debated topic.

Manganese preferentially accumulates in the globus pallidus and selectively damages neurons in globus pallidus and the striatum. Because presynaptic projections from the substantia nigra are spared, dopamine transporter density on SPECT imaging is typically normal. On brain MRI, manganese accumulation can be visualized as increased signal on T_1-weighted images in the globus pallidus, a distinctive finding not seen in Parkinson disease and other forms of parkinsonism. These hyperintensities typically persist for 6 months after exposure cessation. In contrast, manganese levels in blood and urine reflect exposures incurred within the preceding few days. A variable syndrome of parkinsonism, cognitive impairment, and gait ataxia has been seen in patients with chronic liver failure. These patients also may have an abnormal T_1 signal in the globus pallidus and a mildly elevated blood manganese level. The liver is responsible for clearance of dietary manganese, and the neurologic abnormalities of these patients are also likely due to manganese toxicity. Because manganese and iron compete for transporter uptake into the CNS, iron deficiency may increase the risk of toxicity from manganese exposures.

Mercury

Mercury poisoning results from exposure to methyl mercury or other alkyl-mercury compounds, elemental mercury

(mercury vapor), and inorganic mercuric salts. Organic mercury is a particularly potent neurotoxin. Mercury is used in batteries, fungicides, electronics, chemical production, and other industries. Mercury in sludges and waterways is methylated by microbes into methyl mercury that is readily absorbed by humans.

Exposure to organic mercury occurs predominantly through ingestion of contaminated foods, though dermal exposures can rarely occur and are extremely hazardous. Exposure to inorganic and elemental mercury occurs most avidly through vapor inhalation, though gastrointestinal and dermal absorption may occur, the latter through use of contaminated cosmetic products. Elemental mercury freely crosses the BBB, though most is oxidized to Hg^{++} in red blood cells, whereas inorganic mercury may gain access to the CNS slowly through axonal retrograde transport. Ingested organic mercury is almost entirely absorbed from the gastrointestinal tract, where it binds to hemoglobin and distributes widely. It avidly crosses the BBB both through passive diffusion and bound to cysteine residues via the neutral amino acid transporter. Mechanisms of mercury toxicity are not well understood, but the affinity of mercury for enzyme sulfhydryl groups can disrupt cellular metabolism and enhance oxidative stress.

Several large endemics resulted from methyl mercury contamination in Minamata Bay (Japan) in the 1950s and 1960s, in Iraq in the 1970s, and in the Amazon River basin in the 1990s. Exposure occurred primarily through ingestion of contaminated fish. There is uncertainty concerning the neurologic effect of low-level mercury exposures such as that from dental amalgam and dietary fish consumption. Overall, there is no definitive evidence to associate low-level exposure with significant neurologic disease, although the developing nervous system is exquisitely sensitive to low levels of organic mercury.

Like many other toxins, mercury poisoning causes a diffuse encephalopathy. At moderate levels, particularly for organic mercury, this may primarily manifest as memory loss and impaired concentration. At higher levels, the encephalopathy is characterized by euphoria, irritability, anxiety, and emotional lability. More severe exposure leads to confusion and an altered level of consciousness. Cerebellar ataxia is common, and patients may develop a fine postural tremor that begins in the extremities and then involves the face and tongue. Hearing loss, visual field constriction, paresthesias, hyperreflexia, and Babinski sign may be present. CNS changes in both the cortex and cerebellum may be evident on MRI. Limb paresthesias and limb ataxia may result from early effects on dorsal root ganglia. All the preceding symptoms may be encountered in intoxication from organic mercury, metallic mercury, mercury vapor, or inorganic salts. A subacute predominantly motor neuropathy has been reported after metallic mercury or mercury vapor exposure. If acute, the syndrome resembles Guillain-Barré syndrome, whereas a more subacute syndrome may mimic ALS. Nerve-conduction study and nerve biopsy suggest a primary axonal loss.

SOLVENTS

Organic Solvents

Organic solvents include many hundreds of chemicals that share the property of readily dissolving other substances. They include alkanes, alkenes, esters, ethers, alcohols, ketones, and aromatic compounds among others. They may be halogenated, contain amine groups or other substitutions. Millions of workers are exposed daily to these compounds, often as complex mixtures. Some specific chemicals are discussed below, but in general, most organic solvents can produce similar acute neurotoxicity. Clinically important exposure to organic solvents occurs primarily as a result of industrial contact or volitional abuse. Most organic solvents possess acute narcotizing properties. Brief exposure at high concentrations causes a reversible encephalopathy. Coma, respiratory depression, and death occur after extremely high exposures. Chronic exposure to moderate or high levels of solvent can cause a dementing syndrome, with personality changes, memory disturbances, and other nonspecific neuropsychiatric symptoms. A sensorimotor polyneuropathy also may be present either as the only manifestation or in combination with CNS dysfunction. The better-known syndromes are either discussed under specific headings or are tabulated in Table 23–3.

Despite general agreement on the effects of moderate to high doses of organic solvents, the effect of chronic low-level exposure is less certain. The sequelae of this low-level exposure have been variously termed *painters' syndrome, chronic solvent encephalopathy,* and *psycho-organic solvent syndrome.* The neurologic symptoms are diverse and nonspecific and include headache, dizziness, asthenia, mood and personality changes, inattentiveness, forgetfulness, and depression. Many studies reported a higher-than-expected incidence of cognitive and psychiatric impairment, electrophysiologic abnormalities, and cerebral atrophy in chronically exposed subjects. Other studies have not identified significant differences between exposed subjects and controls. Several studies have found increased risk of neurodegenerative disorders in solvent-exposed workers, but associations with specific compounds have only rarely been studied.

Carbon Disulfide

Carbon disulfide is employed as a solvent in perfume production and varnishes, in soil fumigants and insecticides, and in industrial manufacturing. Neurotoxicity from carbon disulfide used in viscose rayon production has been recognized for over 100 years, yet large numbers of workers continue to be extensively exposed. A liquid at room temperature, carbon disulfide boils at 46°C. It is freely absorbed through all routes, though respiratory and dermal routes are most important.

Relatively brief inhalation exposure to a toxic level (≥ 300 ppm) of carbon disulfide causes dizziness and headache, followed by delirium, mania, or mental dulling. Concentrations

Table 23–3. Neurologic manifestations of other toxins.

Toxins	Acute Exposure	Chronic Exposure
Cyanides	Headache, vertigo, nausea, seizures, coma	Headaches, vertigo, tremor, weakness, optic neuropathy, myelopathy
Ethylene oxide	Encephalopathy	Sensorimotor polyneuropathy
1-methyl-4-phenyl-1,2,3,6-tetra-hydropyridine (MPTP)	Parkinsonism indistin-guishable from Parkin-son disease	Unknown
Organotin	Encephalopathy, visual disturbances	Encephalopathy, visual disturbances, hear-ing loss, vertigo
Selenium	Encephalopathy, periph-eral neuropathy	Fatigue, parasthesias
Tetrachloroethane	Narcosis, encephalopathy	Sensorimotor polyneu-ropathy, tremor
Thallium	Subacute polyneuropathy after massive expo-sure, encephalopathy	Sensorimotor polyneuropathy
Toluene	Euphoria or narcosis, encephalopathy	Cerebellar ataxia, tremor, encephalopathy
Vinyl chloride	Ataxia	Trigeminal neuropathy

above 400 ppm have a narcotizing effect and may lead to convulsion, coma, and respiratory failure.

Chronic exposure has been associated with both CNS abnormalities and peripheral neuropathy. The peripheral neuropathy presents with paresthesias and pain in the distal legs, loss of Achilles reflexes, and evidence of involvement of sensory and motor axons on nerve-conduction study. A nonspecific syndrome of fatigue, headache, and sleep disturbances is attributable to chronic low-level exposure to carbon disulfide. On MRI of the brain, some exposed patients have scattered abnormal foci in the subcortical white matter. The radiologic picture resembles that seen in patients with small-vessel disease and multiple subcortical strokes, although pathologic confirmation is not available. More extensive exposure, such as can occur in rayon production, may cause profound psychiatric disturbances including emotional lability and mania-like symptoms. Parkinsonism may also result from protracted high-level exposures to carbon disulfide, sometimes associated with white matter lesions in the basal ganglia. Partial slow recovery may occur, but persistent deficits are common.

Hexacarbons (n-Hexane & 2-Hexanone)

n-Hexane and 2-hexanone (also known as methyl n-butyl ketone) represent a group of widely used volatile organic compounds employed in homes and industries as solvents and adhesives. n-Hexane is commonly used as a cleaning agent in printing and furniture manufacturing, and in glues used in shoemaking and roofing. It was previously a common ingredient in brake-cleaning solutions used by mechanics, and has been found at very high levels in the discharge from oil and gas extraction sites. 2-hexanone was previously used in paint and paint thinner, to dissolve oils, and as a chemical intermediary. It is banned in most countries, but may still be present in older products. Occupational exposures may still occur in paper-making and oil and gas industries.

Chronic neurologic toxicity of these compounds is thought to result from the toxic intermediary g-diketone metabolite, 2,5-hexanedione, which is thought to cause axonal atrophy by reacting with lysine residues of neuronal proteins.

Toxic exposure results from inhalation, especially in poorly ventilated spaces, or excessive skin contact. Other solvents used in paints and adhesives, methyl ethyl ketone or acetone, may potentiate the neurotoxicity.

Like other organic solvents, the hexacarbons can induce an acute encephalopathy characterized by euphoria, hallucination, and confusion. The acute euphoric effect of hexacarbons leads to their abuse as a recreational drug. The most well-known syndrome is a distal symmetric sensorimotor polyneuropathy, the so-called glue-sniffer's neuropathy. Early symptoms are paresthesias and sensory loss. Weakness follows and involves distal muscles initially. Proximal musculatures are affected in more severe cases. Patients complain of easy tripping because of ankle weakness. Optic neuropathy and facial numbness may be present. Autonomic symptoms are uncommon and are present only in very severe cases. Nonspecific CNS symptoms, such as insomnia and irritability, may be present. On examination, sensory loss and weakness are readily demonstrable. Achilles stretch reflexes are lost early in the disease. Recovery begins after a few months of abstinence and may be incomplete. In some instances, spasticity and hyperreflexia appear paradoxically during the recovery stage. In these cases, there is probably degeneration of central axons, and the CNS signs are masked initially by the severe neuropathy.

A less dramatic polyneuropathy was recognized in the 1960s in workers in the shoe and adhesive industries, well before the recognition of glue-sniffer's neuropathy. The exposure to n-hexane was less intense and more chronic than that of glue sniffers. The clinical features are essentially similar, although the syndrome evolves more slowly and results in less severe deficits. Color vision deficits may also occur.

n-Hexane neuropathy has a distinctive neuropathology. Multiple foci of neurofilament accumulations form inside the nerve axons. Demyelination is common, but it is probably secondary to the axonal pathology. Because of this demyelination, nerve-conduction studies show slowing of motor nerve-conduction velocities. Cerebrospinal fluid (CSF) protein content is typically normal, in contrast to most other demyelinating neuropathies, which are associated with elevated CSF protein.

Methanol

Methanol is commonly used as a chemical intermediate, fuel, deicer, and solvent. The neurotoxicity of methanol is caused largely by formaldehyde and formate, the end products of its metabolism by alcohol dehydrogenase and aldehyde dehydrogenase. Formate inhibits mitochondrial cytochrome oxidase (complex IV), reducing ATP production and causing a metabolic acidosis. Most cases of poisoning result from accidental ingestion. Occupational exposures may also occur through inhalation or dermal routes. Neurologic symptoms usually appear after a latent period of 12–24 hours after intoxication. Patients suffer from headache, nausea, vomiting, and abdominal pain. Tachypnea, if present, indicates significant metabolic acidosis. Formate is directly toxic to the optic nerves, and visual symptoms appear within hours to days and range from blurring to complete blindness. These are accompanied by an encephalopathy, from mild disorientation to convulsion, stupor, or coma. In severely affected individuals, bilateral upper motor neuron signs such as hyperreflexia, weakness, and Babinski sign are present. Acute parkinsonian features have been occasionally reported after large intoxications. Brain CT or MRI may reveal infarction or hemorrhage localized in bilateral putamina, often accompanied by similar involvement of subcortical white matter. After recovery, neurologic sequelae may include ocular and extrapyramidal deficits.

Treatment of acute poisoning depends on control of the metabolic acidosis with sodium bicarbonate, competitive inhibition of the conversion of methanol to formaldehyde (by administration of fomepizole or ethanol), and swift removal of methanol by gastric lavage or hemodialysis.

Trichloroethylene & Tetrachloroethylene

Trichloroethylene (TCE) is used primarily as an industrial solvent and for metals degreasing. Until approximately 1980, it was also used for dry-cleaning, spot removal, coffee decaffeination, and as a surgical anesthetic. It is the most frequently reported organic contaminant in groundwater, found in up to one-third of US drinking water supplies. The structurally similar compound tetrachloroethylene, also known as perchloroethylene (PERC), has similar uses and has been the leading dry-cleaning solvent since the 1960s. Both compounds are rapidly and completely absorbed through inhalation or ingestion. Dermal absorption can occur but is thought to be a less significant route. Acute exposure to high levels of TCE causes a rapidly reversible CNS depression that may manifest as euphoria or narcosis. Trigeminal neuropathy has been rarely reported, more often with chronic exposures. PERC may produce deficits in visuospatial function and reaction time. Chronic low-level exposures are associated with modest reductions in reaction time and visual memory.

Possible latent effects may be of more concern. TCE was implicated in a cluster of Parkinson disease in a small manufacturing plant where workers had been exposed to open vapor degreasing vats for many years, as well as in several earlier case reports. A subsequent study in twin pairs discordant for Parkinson disease found a sixfold increased risk in the twin who had worked with TCE and a tenfold risk for PERC. Remarkably, TCE can produce a compelling rodent model of Parkinson disease, recapitulating the primary pathologic features of the disease. The proposed proximate toxic species for *both* TCE and PERC, which forms after CYP2E1-mediated oxidation, is 1-trichloromethyl-1,2,3,4-tetrahydro-β-carboline (TaClo), an extremely potent inhibitor of mitochondrial Complex 1, dopaminergic toxin, and structural analogue of the parkinsonism-producing compound MPTP. This hypothesis is strengthened by a recent study that detected endogenously formed TaClo in brains of mice fed TCE for 8 months.

PESTICIDES

Organophosphates

OPs are a very large class of compounds used commonly as insecticides and herbicides and, to a lesser extent, as petroleum additives, antioxidants, and flame retardants. At least 80 OP pesticides are currently in use, including malathion, parathion, chlorpyrifos, and diazinon. Well-known examples of particularly toxic OPs include the warfare agents Sarin and Soman. All are highly lipid soluble and are absorbed through skin contact or through mucous membranes via inhalation and ingestion. Exposures occur most frequently among pesticide applicators and farmworkers, and in attempted suicides. All the OPs share a common property of inhibiting the enzyme acetylcholinesterase (AChE). The more toxic OPs bind AChE more avidly, some essentially irreversibly through a process called *aging* (loss of an R group from the OP molecule). Once irreversibly bound, recovery from these more toxic OPs requires the de novo synthesis of AChE, which may take a week or more.

The acute neurologic effects of OPs are those of muscarinic and nicotinic overactivity. Symptoms usually are apparent within hours of exposure. These include abdominal cramps, diarrhea, increased salivation, sweating, miosis, blurred vision, and muscle fasciculations. Convulsions, coma, muscle paralysis, and respiratory arrest occur with severe intoxication. Unless there are complications from secondary anoxia or other insults to the brain, these symptoms improve either with atropine treatment or metabolism and excretion of the OP. Concurrent administration of AChE reactivators such as pralidoxime (2-PAM) may hasten recovery of AChE activity. Recovery from most OPs usually is complete within a few days, even though the AChE activity level may be restored only partially.

In some patients, an intermediate syndrome may occur within 12–96 hours of exposure. This is a result of excessive cholinergic stimulation of nicotinic receptors in skeletal muscles. This leads to blockade of neuromuscular junction transmission. Weakness of proximal muscles, neck flexors, cranial muscles, and even respiratory muscles may be evident. Sensory function is spared. Electrodiagnostic testing is useful in diagnosis, with the most characteristic finding being the presence of repetitive muscle action potentials after a single electrical stimulus applied to motor nerves. Another finding is a decremental motor response to repetitive nerve stimulation.

In some other patients, a delayed syndrome of peripheral neuropathy occurs 1–4 weeks after acute exposure, known as organophosphate-induced delayed polyneuropathy (OPIDP). There is little or no correlation between its onset and the severity of acute or intermediate symptoms. Paresthesias and cramping pain in the legs are often the first symptoms of OPIDP. Weakness begins distally and progresses to involve proximal muscles. Weakness dominates the clinical picture and at times may be very severe. Spasticity and other upper motor neuron signs suggesting concomitant spinal cord involvement are present in some patients. Recovery is slow and incomplete and depends on the degree of motor axons loss. The delayed neuropathy is likely due to inhibition of another enzyme, called neuropathy target esterase (NTE). Previously, it was thought that only compounds that lead to aging of the OP-NTE complex are capable of causing OPIDP, but more recent data suggest this may not be required for the delayed neuropathy to occur. Hens are particularly susceptible to OPIDP and are used to test commercially available OP pesticides for this propensity. All the neurotoxic compounds are phosphates, phosphoramidites, or phosphonates. Important examples are tricresyl phosphates (TCPs, eg, triorthocresyl phosphate), mipafox, leptophos, trichlorphon, trichlornate, dichlorvos, and methamidophos. Of these, triorthocresyl phosphate probably has caused the largest number of neuropathies. The so-called jake paralysis that likely affected tens of thousands was a result of drinking extracts of contaminated Jamaica ginger during the prohibition era. Other well-known outbreaks include contamination of cooking oil in Morocco and gingili oil in Sri Lanka.

By the time neuropathy appears, nerve-conduction studies show an axonal polyneuropathy affecting motor greater than sensory axons. These findings are not pathognomonic for OPs but are useful to distinguish this neuropathy from other causes of acute weakness such as Guillain-Barré syndrome and neuromuscular junction disorders.

Persistent subtle neuropsychologic impairment after an episode of acute poisoning may be more prevalent than previously thought. Also, chronic low-level exposure to OPs is linked to an encephalopathy with forgetfulness and other cognitive dysfunctions as chief complaints, although the clinical significance or severity of this effect is being debated. Several epidemiologic studies have suggested a link between OP and subsequent development of Alzheimer disease, ALS, and Parkinson disease.

The TCPs are inhibitors of NTE and are contained in jet engine oil that can contaminate aircraft cabin air as a result of mechanical problems (so-called "bleed air contamination"). Several case reports have shown residual neurologic impairment among flight attendants after bleed air contamination, and studies have demonstrated detectable levels of TCPs on aircraft cabin surfaces. Cabin crew can present with symptoms of headache, cognitive impairment, and paraesthesia; referral for neuropsychologic evaluation and nerve conduction studies/EMG should be considered.

Carbamates

Carbamate insecticides and fungicides comprise a structurally diverse class of pesticides that share similar toxic properties with the OPs. Insecticidal compounds include aldicarb, carbaryl, and methomyl; fungicidal compounds include benomyl, metam-sodium and maneb. Acute neurotoxicity from fungicidal carbamates has only rarely been reported and may reflect the toxicity of their associated metal ion (eg, maneb contains manganese) or their breakdown product (eg, metam-sodium degrades to methyl isocyanate). Like OPs, most insecticidal carbamates bind and inhibit the activity of AChE and thus their acute toxicity similarly manifests as a cholinergic syndrome. Because carbamates bind reversibly to AChE, the acute toxicity is usually self-limited as the enzyme regenerates, resolving within hours. Atropine and diazepam can be helpful, but the use of anti-aging agents such as pralidoxime is contraindicated in carbamate poisoning. Though neurotoxicity associated with chronic exposures has rarely been reported, several studies found higher risk of Parkinson disease associated with prior exposure to several carbamate pesticides, and animal models suggest they may be toxic to dopaminergic neurons.

Pyrethroids

Pyrethroid insecticides were initially extracted from the chrysanthemum flower, but now are predominantly synthetic. They are widely used for mosquito control and scabies treatment and in agriculture for a wide variety of crop pests. Their insecticidal activity derives from interaction with CNS voltage-gated Na+ channels. Absorption varies widely between compounds. Acute poisoning causes dizziness, headache, fatigue, and muscle fasciculations. This can progress to seizures and coma in severe cases. Complete recovery generally occurs over 2–3 weeks. Neurotoxicity associated with chronic use has not been well studied. There is limited epidemiologic evidence of association with neurodegenerative outcomes that require further study.

Paraquat

Paraquat is bipyridyl herbicide used extensively in the United States and much of the developing world, but banned in the European Union. It is structurally very similar to the parkinsonism-producing neurotoxin MPTP. A potent redox agent, it generates reactive oxygen species that damage cellular and organelle membranes. Acutely it causes pulmonary edema and fibrosis. Contrary to some early reports, paraquat does gain access to the CNS, probably via the neutral amino acid carrier, where it can activate microglia, damage mitochondria, and cause dopaminergic toxicity. Acute poisonings in humans have not been shown to cause consistent neurologic pathology. In animal models, however, paraquat produces a faithful animal model of Parkinson disease. Human epidemiologic evidence linking paraquat to an increased risk of Parkinson disease is increasingly consistent, and risk may be particularly high in the 20% of the population that lacks the Phase II metabolic enzyme glutathione-S-transferase T1.

Rotenone

Rotenone is a botanical insecticide and piscicide (kills fish) extracted from plants in the legume family. It has been used by indigenous peoples probably for centuries to hunt fish. It was previously used in a wide variety of garden and household products, but currently is used predominantly to kill invasive fish species in lakes and rivers. Rotenone acts by inhibiting mitochondrial Complex 1, thereby causing energetic collapse. Exposure is primarily respiratory; gastric absorption is thought to be limited. Acute toxicity is rarely reported. In rodents, rotenone produces an accurate model of Parkinson disease. The human epidemiology, though limited, finds a several-fold increased risk in rotenone applicators.

PERSISTENT ORGANIC POLLUTANTS

Polychlorinated biphenyls (PCBs)

PCBs comprise a family of congeners with two joined benzene rings substituted with chlorine molecules in varying number and position. They were used extensively in electrical transformers as coolants and for fire prevention, as well as in many other products and manufacturing applications from the 1930s until the late 1970s when their production in most developed nations was banned. Worldwide manufacture ended in 1993, but large quantities are still in use in existing applications, particularly in electrical capacitors. Because of their resistance to degradation, PCBs are ubiquitously detectable in air, water, and soil. They are highly lipid soluble and minimally metabolized, and they bioconcentrate up the food chain. Highly exposed individuals manifest distal extremity sensory loss and slowed nerve conduction velocity consistent with a peripheral neuropathy. Developmental toxicity is a concern, with some reports of developmental delay and hyperactivity. Human epidemiology and animal studies suggest dopaminergic toxicity with chronic exposures, particularly in women. Though data are sparse, several studies report associations with Parkinson disease and ALS.

Polybrominated diphenyl ethers (PBDEs)

PBDEs have been used in a broad range of products and industries for several decades, but were most ubiquitously used as flame retardants in polyurethane foams in furniture and mattresses during the 1980s–2000s particularly in the United States. PBDEs are environmentally very persistent and bioaccumulate in fatty tissues. Levels in household dust can be quite high, and infants may ingest relatively large quantities. PBDEs have estrogenic properties and are classified as potent endocrine disrupting chemicals, along with some of the PCBs, chemicals such as bisphenol A and many organochlorine compounds. Exposure to these compounds during gestation may have lifelong effects. Human epidemiology has found dose-related associations with behavioral abnormalities including poorer attention, reduced fine motor cognition, and cognitive deficits. In addition to endocrine disruption, PBDEs may be directly toxic to the nervous system through mechanisms involving oxidative damage and alterations of calcium signaling.

Per- and polyfuoroalkyl substances (PFAS)

PFAS are highly persistent fluorinated compounds used since the 1950s in a broad range of industries and products. Among others, these include carpeting, upholstery, fabrics, food wrappers, nonstick cookware, computer circuits, and fire-fighting foams. Although many PFAS have been banned for use in the United States, they are still prevalent in household dust and oral exposures in young children may be as high as several mg/day. Exposures may also be particularly high in proximity to industrial sites that manufactured fire-fighting foams. Like PCBs, PFAS are environmentally stable, lipid soluble, and bioconcentrate up the food chain. PFAS induce neurodevelopmental toxicity in animal studies, including reductions in spontaneous motor activity and reduced novelty seeking. Human epidemiology is sparse and inconsistent, but PFAS may be associated with childhood behavioral problems. In animals, brain PFAS levels correlate with decreased ACh and increased GABA receptor density.

Organochlorines

Organochlorines comprise a very broad class of insecticides and herbicides extensively used in agriculture and to kill human pests since the 1940s. Many compounds, such as DDT (dichlorodiphenyltrichloroethane), dieldrin, and heptachlor were largely phased out during the 1970s because of their extreme environmental persistence and ecotoxicity, and thus these compounds are discussed here rather than in the section on pesticides. Because of their persistence in the food chain and in adipose tissue, most humans on the planet still have measurable levels of these compounds in serum. Most organochlorines are highly lipid soluble, and thus are freely absorbed and passively cross the BBB, where they act as CNS stimulants. DDT acts by disrupting voltage-dependent Na^+ channels, causing axonal excitation. Other organochlorine mechanisms include interactions with GABA receptor function and calcium ATPases. DDT is relatively nontoxic to humans acutely, with large exposures causing facial and extremity paresthesias and tremor, confusion and malaise, with recovery over several days. Chronic exposures cause weakness, tremors, and psychiatric symptoms such as anxiety and irritability. Cyclodienes and many other organochlorines are more neurotoxic than DDT and may acutely cause seizures that can persist for weeks. DDT and many other organochlorines are endocrine disruptors and thus are thought to have developmental toxicity. Brain organochlorine levels have been found to be higher in postmortem analyses of persons with Parkinson disease, and several have been associated with risk of ALS.

MISCELLANEOUS COMPOUNDS

Acrylamide

Acrylamide (2-propenamide) and polyacrylamides are used as water-soluble thickeners and clarifying agents in a wide range of industrial processes, including production of plastics, permanent press fabrics, paper and dyes, and in wastewater treatment. The population most at risk of developing neurologic toxicity consists of workers who handle monomeric acrylamide in the production of polyacrylamides and those exposed to monomeric acrylamide used in grouting. Intoxication occurs by inhalation or skin absorption. Features of poisoning include local skin irritation, weight loss, lassitude, and neurologic symptoms of central and peripheral nervous system involvement.

Acute exposure typically causes a confusional state, manifesting as disorientation, memory loss, and gait ataxia. These symptoms are largely reversible, although irreversible dysfunction does occur after very intense exposure. Chronic lower-dose exposure sometimes leads to dizziness, increased irritability, emotional changes, and sleep disturbances. The primary site of action of acrylamide, however, is the peripheral nerve. A neuropathy may develop as a delayed manifestation a few weeks after acute exposure or insidiously after chronic exposure. Both sensory and motor nerves are affected, leading to sensory loss, weakness, ataxia, and loss of tendon reflexes. The loss of reflexes especially may be generalized, unlike other toxic neuropathies, in which only distal reflexes are lost. Autonomic involvement, such as hyperhidrosis and urinary retention, is common.

Unlike other type 2 alkenes, acrylamide is less reactive and less likely to form protein adducts in the peripheral tissues, and is thus more bioavailable to the nervous system. It causes presynaptic toxicity by binding to cysteine thiolate sites of specific nerve terminal proteins. This leads to abnormal accumulation of neurofilaments in axons. In this respect, its action is similar to that of organic solvents, notably the hexacarbons. Unlike hexacarbons, secondary demyelination does not occur. Nerve-conduction studies typically show a neuropathy accompanied by little or no slowing of nerve-conduction velocities, that is, a neuropathy predominantly with features of axonal degeneration.

Carbon Monoxide

Carbon monoxide is produced during incomplete combustion of hydrocarbons. It binds to hemoglobin 200-fold more avidly than does oxygen to form carboxyhemoglobin and causes neuronal hypoxia. Inhaling low concentrations (0.01–0.02%) of carbon monoxide, which produces COHb levels of 15–20% causes headache and mild confusion. A higher concentration of 0.1–0.2% (COHb levels of 30–40%) may result in somnolence or stupor, and inhalation of 1% for more than 30 minutes can be fatal. Early on, symptoms include headache, dizziness, and disorientation. More prolonged or severe hypoxia is accompanied by a varying combination of tremor, chorea, spasticity, dystonia, rigidity, and bradykinesia. Recovery from the hypoxia may be incomplete. Residual dementia, spasticity, cortical blindness, and parkinsonian features are relatively common. Early treatment with hyperbaric oxygen therapy may hasten recovery and reduce the likelihood of long-term sequelae.

Occasional patients recover completely after acute exposure only to worsen again 1–6 weeks later with acute disorientation, apathy, or psychosis. Neurologic examination often reveals an encephalopathy with prominent signs of frontal lobe and extrapyramidal dysfunction. Physical findings include bradykinesia, retropulsion, frontal release signs, spasticity, and limb rigidity. Risk factors for developing this delayed encephalopathy are a significant period of unconsciousness and an advanced age. CT or MRI most commonly shows abnormalities in bilateral subcortical white matter. Some patients also have involvement of the basal ganglia, especially the globus pallidus and the thalamus. Rarely, hemorrhagic infarction of the white matter or basal ganglia may be seen. Partial recovery is possible but may take one or more years. Some residual memory deficits and parkinsonism are common.

The effect of long-term exposure to low levels of carbon monoxide is unclear. A number of nonspecific symptoms—anorexia, headache, personality changes, and memory disturbances—are attributed to carbon monoxide, but a causal relationship has not been proven.

Methyl Bromide and Methyl Iodide

Organic bromides are thought to be more toxic than inorganic ones. Methyl bromide is used as a fumigant in greenhouses and fields for control of nematodes, fungi, and weeds. It has also been used as a refrigerant, solvent, and in fire extinguishers. Exposure is usually through inhalation. Acutely, methyl bromide (MeBr) can cause headache and dizziness followed by encephalopathic symptoms that usually present after a several hour latency period. These include dysarthria, ataxia, delirium, tremor, visual symptoms, and seizures. With chronic exposures, symptoms include a sensorimotor polyneuropathy along with cerebellar, pyramidal tract, and neuropsychiatric dysfunction. Toxicity may be due to disruption of cell membranes. Methyl iodide (MeI) has been used in various pharmaceutical and pesticide synthesis processes and for etching of electronic circuits. Reports of poisonings are uncommon. MeI is known to be a narcotic, and case reports have mentioned parkinsonism, cerebellar, and latent neuropsychologic sequelae similar to MeBr.

Nitrous Oxide

Prolonged heavy exposure to nitrous oxide, usually in the setting of substance abuse, causes a myeloneuropathy indistinguishable from vitamin B_{12} (cobalamin) deficiency. Toxicity likely results from inhibition of methionine synthesis from homocysteine, which is required as a methyl donor in many biosynthetic processes. How methionine deficiency interferes with B_{12} metabolism is unclear. Patients present with paresthesias in the hands and feet. Gait ataxia, sensory loss, Romberg sign, and leg weakness may be present. Tendon reflexes may be diminished or lost (peripheral neuropathy) or may be pathologically brisk (spinal cord involvement; ie, myelopathy). Serum vitamin B_{12} may be reduced, while the Schilling test is usually normal, and serum homocysteine may be elevated. Symptoms typically improve after cessation of exposure. Methionine and B_{12} supplementation may hasten recovery. Of interest is the observation that a brief exposure to nitrous oxide, for example during anesthesia, is sufficient to precipitate symptoms in patients with asymptomatic B_{12} deficiency.

Styrene

Styrene is used to make styrene polyesters and resins, fiberglass, and as a chemical intermediate. These compounds are used widely in manufacturing of automobiles, boats, bathtubs, insulation products, tires, and carpeting. Exposure to styrene is most likely to occur during the polymerization process and particularly among boat-builders. The primary route of absorption is respiratory, though its lipid solubility can also lead to rapid dermal absorption. Large acute exposures can cause headache, drowsiness, vertigo, weakness, and depression. Workers chronically exposed to levels over 50 ppm had reduced sensory nerve conduction velocity in a dose-dependent manner, slowed reaction times, and possibly slight deficits in color vision, all of which are thought to be reversible. Ototoxicity due to oxidative damage to cochlear hair cells has also been reported.

REFERENCES

Bowler RM, Lezak MD: Neuropsychologic evaluation and exposure to neurotoxicants. Handb Clin Neurol 2015;131:23-45.

Caudle WM: Occupational metal exposure and parkinsonism. Adv Neurobiol 2017;18:143-158.

Dickerson AS, Hansen J, Specht AJ, Gredal O, Weisskopf MG: Population-based study of amyotrophic lateral sclerosis and occupational lead exposure in Denmark. Occup Environ Med 2019;76(4):208 [PMID: 30705111].

Hageman G, Pal TM, Nihom J, Mackenzie Ross SJ, Berg MVD: Aerotoxic syndrome, discussion of possible diagnostic criteria. Clin Toxicol (Phila) 2019:1 [PMID: 31389264].

Karam C, Dyck PJ: Toxic neuropathies. Semin Neurol 2015;35(4):448 [PMID: 26502767].

Katona I, Weis J: Diseases of the peripheral nerves. Handb Clin Neurol 2017;145:453 [PMID: 28987189].

Lotti M, Aminoff MJ: Evaluating suspected work-related neurologic disorders (clinical diagnosis). Handb Clin Neurol 2015;131:9 [PMID: 26563780].

Naughton SX, Terry AV Jr: Neurotoxicity in acute and repeated organophosphate exposure. Toxicology 2018;408:101 [PMID: 30144465].

Park RM, Berg SL: Manganese and neurobehavioral impairment. A preliminary risk assessment. Neurotoxicology 2018;64:159 [PMID: 28803851].

Sharma A, Kumar S: Arsenic exposure with reference to neurological impairment: an overview. Rev Environ Health 2019;34(4):403. [PMID: 31603861].

■ SELF-ASSESSMENT QUESTIONS

Select the one correct answer for each question.

Question 1: Encephalopathy
   a. raises the level of consciousness
   b. symptoms may be cognitive but not psychiatric
   c. may be the result of toxins
   d. is never confused with parkinsonism

Question 2: Cognitive complaints
   a. should include at least a mini–mental state examination
   b. require referral to neuropsychologic testing
   c. mask the pattern and severity of the cognitive deficits
   d. are reliable symptoms of lead poisoning

Question 3: Peripheral nervous system disorders
   a. lead to sensory disturbances but no weakness
   b. are often accompanied by impairment of the deep tendon reflexes
   c. demonstrate heightened CNS vulnerability to toxins
   d. occur because toxins directly affect single nerves

Question 4: Polyneuropathy
   a. is a syndrome with asymmetric peripheral neuropathy
   b. frequently results from local mechanical injury
   c. is typically characterized by the distal distribution of the symptoms and signs
   d. has no neuropathic pain

Question 5: Peripheral neuropathy
a. has only a few known causes
b. is seldom caused by systemic diseases
c. often does not have an identified cause despite extensive testing
d. is almost always painful

Question 6: A focal neuropathy
a. produces localized motor and sensory disturbances
b. leads to generalized weakness
c. causes symmetrical atrophy of limb muscles
d. is usually caused by systemic exposures to toxins

Question 7: Acrylamide
a. exposure typically leads to irreversible dysfunction
b. acts primarily on the central nervous system
c. may produce a delayed neuropathy
d. rarely causes an autonomic involvement

Question 8: Arsenic
a. leads to peripheral neuropathy at only high-dose exposure
b. may produce an acute polyneuropathy within 1–3 hours

c. neuropathy precedes Guillain-Barré syndrome
d. chronic exposure leads to a more insidious sensorimotor polyneuropathy

Question 9: Mercury
a. poisoning causes a diffuse encephalopathy
b. exposure may present with euphoria, irritability, anxiety, and emotional lability
c. exposure may cause tremor but not cerebellar ataxia
d. causes Guillain-Barré syndrome

Question 10: Organophosphates
a. diminish muscarinic and nicotinic activity
b. with severe intoxication cause convulsions, coma, muscle paralysis, and respiratory arrest
c. intoxication typically lasts less than 12 hours
d. acetylcholinesterase activity must be restored before recovery occurs

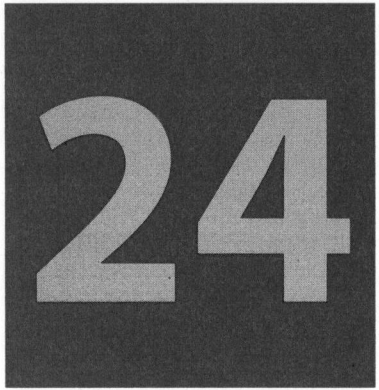

Occupational Hematology

Sammy Almashat, MD

Robert Harrison, MD

Exposure to hematotoxins may affect blood cell survival (denaturation of hemoglobin and hemolysis), porphyrin synthesis and metabolism (including some porphyrias), blood cell formation (aplasia), risk for hematopoietic neoplasms, or coagulation (through development of thrombocytopenia).

▼ DISORDERS ASSOCIATED WITH SHORTENED RED BLOOD CELL SURVIVAL

METHEMOGLOBINEMIA & HEMOLYSIS PRODUCED BY OXIDANT CHEMICALS

Methemoglobin is formed by the oxidation of ferrous (Fe^{2+}) hemoglobin to ferric (Fe^{3+}) hemoglobin. It was first recognized in the 1800s, when coal tars were converted into individual chemicals that served as precursors for many products ranging from explosives to synthetic dyes and perfumes. Overexposure to these chemicals—which included anilines, nitrobenzenes, and quinones—was common, and little was known about their potential toxicity. Workers in these plants came to be known as "blue workers" because they suffered from "blue lip" as a result of the chronic cyanosis from toxin-induced methemoglobinemia that developed in many of them. Gradually it was recognized that oxidation of hemoglobin was toxic to red blood cells and could be followed by an acute and life-threatening hemolysis known as *Heinz body anemia*. Heinz bodies are red blood cell inclusions that represent precipitated hemoglobin and are seen classically in individuals with a deficiency of glucose-6-phosphate dehydrogenase (G6PD) after exposure to an oxidant stress. Normal individuals exposed to large amounts of oxidant chemicals will develop methemoglobinemia and, occasionally, Heinz body hemolytic anemia.

▶ Pathophysiology of Methemoglobinemia & Oxidant Hemolysis

Hemoglobin is unique in its ability to combine reversibly with oxygen without oxidizing its iron moiety. The small amount of oxidized hemoglobin or methemoglobin produced is readily reduced by an efficient enzyme system linked to energy provided by glucose metabolism via the Embden-Meyerhof pathway (Figure 24–1).

Methemoglobin is dangerous because of its inability to bind oxygen and because it increases the oxygen affinity of the remaining heme groups in hemoglobin tetramer, thereby decreasing oxygen delivery to the tissues. Oxidation results in denaturation of hemoglobin with the formation of precipitated hemoglobin (Heinz bodies) within the red cell. The presence of Heinz bodies alters the surface membrane of the red cell, causing increased rigidity and leakage. Macrophages in the reticuloendothelial system of the spleen and liver (the extravascular compartment) sense the altered red cell surface and remove Heinz bodies via partial phagocytosis (extravascular hemolysis). Because the red cell surface is unable to reseal and form a spherocyte (as in autoimmune hemolysis), the red cell remains intact as a cell with a piece missing, the so-called bite, or blister, cell. Heinz bodies also may be formed from a second form of denatured hemoglobin, sulfhemoglobin. Unlike methemoglobin, sulfhemoglobin is irreversibly associated with the heme moiety.

The development of methemoglobinemia or oxidative hemolysis in an individual exposed to an oxidant stress depends on the route of exposure, the specific chemicals involved, the dose and duration of exposure, and most importantly, individual susceptibility. Inborn structural abnormalities (unstable hemoglobins)—or, much more commonly, disorders of normal reducing capabilities such as the X-linked deficiency of the oxidation-reduction enzyme G6PD—cause some individuals to be much more susceptible to oxidant stress than others. There are many varieties of both these abnormalities. Recognition of these high-risk individuals in the workplace is important to reduce their chance of particularly toxic exposures.

The normal individual has less than 1% circulating methemoglobin. Ninety-five percent of methemoglobin formed daily by the autoxidation of hemoglobin is reduced by $NADH_2$ (nicotinamide adenine dinucleotide [reduced

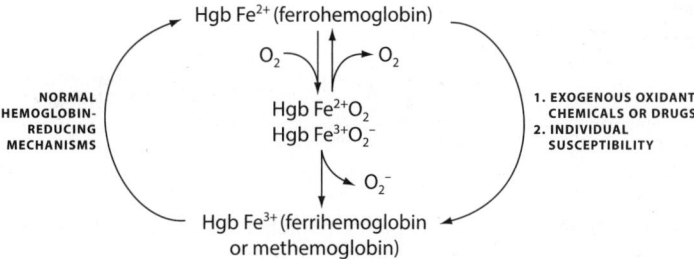

▲ **Figure 24–1.** Oxidation of hemoglobin by the Embden-Meyerhof pathway.

form]) generated by the dehydrogenation of phosphotriose by phosphotriose dehydrogenase. This reaction is catalyzed by NADH methemoglobin reductase (NADH cytochrome b5 reductase). A rare inborn deficiency of NADH methemoglobin reductase results in congenital cyanosis caused by methemoglobinemia (Figure 24–2).

An alternative methemoglobin reduction pathway exists that requires the presence of a redox cofactor such as methylene blue to achieve significant reducing capacity. In this reaction, nicotinamide adenine dinucleotide phosphate (NADPH) from the first two steps of the hexose monophosphate shunt converts methemoglobin to reduced hemoglobin. Because this pathway is normally responsible for so little reduction of methemoglobin, deficiency of the enzyme that catalyzes this reaction, NADPH methemoglobin reductase, does not result in methemoglobinemia or cyanosis. Because the formation of NADPH depends on G6PD, methylene blue, which is used to treat toxic and congenital methemoglobinemia, also can precipitate a hemolytic crisis in an individual with G6PD deficiency by competing for the NADPH necessary to maintain reduced glutathione, an essential protectant against erythrocyte oxidative stress. Additionally, methylene blue itself is an oxidant, but it is metabolized to the reducing agent leucomethylene blue. In normal individuals, the administration of a redox agent may increase the rate of reduction of hemoglobin dramatically so that it greatly exceeds that of the NADH-methemoglobin reductase reaction (Figure 24–3). This is the rationale for the effectiveness of methylene blue in toxic methemoglobinemia.

Two other pathways exist, but they reduce methemoglobin only to a small extent. Glutathione is responsible for conversion of less than 7–10% of ferrihemoglobin to ferrohemoglobin, and ascorbic acid in pharmacologic amounts also reduces oxidized hemoglobin. Because of the high redox potential of ascorbic acid, however, the rate of reduction is very slow, making it less effective in therapy. In physiologic concentrations, the contribution of ascorbic acid to methemoglobin reduction is insignificant.

Historically, most work-related episodes of methemoglobinemia primarily and less often hemolytic anemia were a result of exposure to aromatic nitro and amino compounds, including aniline. These compounds are used most extensively as intermediates in the synthesis of aniline dyes; they are also used as accelerators and antioxidants in the rubber industry and in the production of pesticides, plastics, paints, and varnishes. Table 24–1 lists chemicals that are associated with methemoglobinemia and/or oxidant hemolysis and their industrial uses. Many medicinal drugs are oxidants and can cause methemoglobinemia.

1. Aniline

The clinical presentation of methemoglobinemia is exemplified by aniline toxicity. Aniline, used in the manufacture of dyes and in the rubber industry, is the most common aromatic amine. It is fat-soluble and readily penetrates the intact skin, even through clothing. The vapor form also may gain entry to the body through the lungs. Ingestion is rare in the industrial setting but causes serious toxicity when it does occur. Aniline is converted by hepatic microsomes to phenylhydroxylamine, which behaves as a catalyst in mediating hemoglobin oxidation. Hepatic clearance

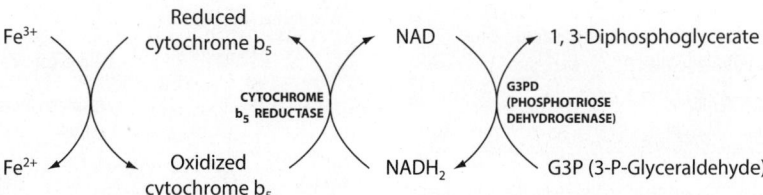

▲ **Figure 24–2.** Reduction of hemoglobin by NADH-methemoglobin reductase (NADH cytochrome b$_5$ reductase).

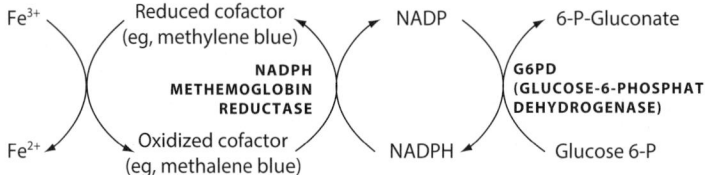

▲ **Figure 24–3.** Reduction of hemoglobin by NADPH-methemoglobin reductase can be accelerated by a redox agent such as methylene blue.

of phenylhydroxylamine is slow because its oxidized form, nitrosobenzene, is rapidly converted back to phenylhydroxylamine. Another clearance pathway gradually eliminates the amine from the body.

Clinical Presentation

Acute exposure usually is associated with spills or improper usage. Symptoms vary depending on the concentration of methemoglobin (Table 24–2). Most cases are mild and transient and present as asymptomatic blueness of the lips and nail beds. In more severe cases, the patient will appear deeply cyanotic. Freshly drawn blood appears dark maroon-brown and does not become red after exposure to air. Pulse oximetry may indicate normoxia or mild hypoxia not reflective of the

severity of methemoglobinemia. Arterial blood gases may show a normal oxygen tension (Po_2) but co-oximetry will reveal methemoglobinemia reliably. Often, because of differences in the measurement approach, there may be a "saturation gap," in which the oxygen saturation on arterial blood gases is substantially higher than that determined by pulse oximetry. Laboratory results may indicate hemolysis with an elevated reticulocyte count and variable degree of anemia. Examination of the peripheral blood smear shows evidence of reticulocytosis (polychromasia, possibly nucleated red cells) and may show bite or blistered red cells.

In chronic methemoglobinemia, polycythemia may be seen in response to chronic hypoxia. Hemolytic Heinz body anemia may or may not accompany methemoglobin formation or may follow resolution of cyanosis. Heinz bodies are detected easily by examining the peripheral blood smear stained with a supravital stain but will not be evident on a smear stained with Wright stain. Blood methemoglobin levels should be monitored closely.

▶ Prevention

The most important safeguard in preventing oxidative hemolysis is to minimize atmospheric and cutaneous exposure to potentially oxidizing chemicals such as coal tar products. The identification of susceptible individuals such as those with G6PD deficiency may help to avoid significant toxicity in high-risk job situations. Screening for G6PD deficiency must be done either before a hemolytic episode or 1–2 months after the hemolysis has resolved. Young red blood

Table 24–1. Chemicals associated with methemoglobinemia or oxidative hemolysis.

Chemical	Use
Aniline	Rubber, dyestuffs; production of MBI (methylene bisphenyl isocyanate)
Nitroaniline	Dyes
Toluidine	Dyes, organic chemicals
p-Chloroaniline	Dyes, pharmaceuticals, pesticides
o-Toluidine	Laboratory analytic reagent, production of trypan blue stain, chlorine test kits, test tapes, curing agent for urethane resins
Naphthalene	Fumigants used in clothing industry
Paradichlorobenzene	Fumigants used in clothing industry and in mothballs
Nitrates	Soil fertilizers
Trinitrotoluene	Explosives
Methyl nitrate	Oxidizing agent; intermediate in the production of phenylpropanolamine

Table 24–2. Symptoms of methemoglobinemia.

% Methemoglobinemia	Symptoms
10–30	Cyanosis, mild fatigue, tachycardia
30–50	Weakness, breathlessness, headache, exercise intolerance
50–70	Altered consciousness
> 70–80	Coma, death

cells, particularly reticulocytes, have normal G6PD levels in most G6PD-deficient individuals. During an acute hemolytic episode, older red blood cells are destroyed and replaced by young red blood cells. The result of a G6PD deficiency screen often will be normal in that acute setting. Biological monitoring in the workplace may be done by measuring methemoglobin levels and reticulocyte counts.

▶ Treatment

Treatment depends on rapid recognition of the problem. It is important to obtain as complete an exposure history as possible because it will guide treatment. The most important aspect of therapy is to ensure removal of the offending agent. Because of the fat-soluble nature of these compounds, it is essential that clothing be removed and the patient decontaminated thoroughly. For mild intoxication (< 20% blood methemoglobin), observation should be sufficient to watch for progression of symptoms. For moderate to severe intoxication (> 30% blood methemoglobin), 100% oxygen by mask is given to saturate the remaining hemoglobin, and the antidote, methylene blue, is administered. Care must be exercised in using methylene blue to avoid increasing methemoglobin from the oxidative potential of methylene blue itself or risk for hemolytic anemia, particularly in G6PD-deficient individuals (in whom it is ineffective).

For initial management of severe methemoglobinemia, methylene blue should be given intravenously as a 1% solution at a dose of 1–2 mg/kg over 5–10 minutes. The maximal effect should be seen within 1 hour. If no response is evident by this time, administration of methylene blue may be repeated at hourly intervals (in part, because of the short half-life of methylene blue in the body). Repeat doses, which may also be given orally, should be given for symptoms, not solely on the basis of the methemoglobin level. A patient who does not respond to methylene blue may have G6PD deficiency, and further administration could exacerbate hemolysis without reducing hypoxia.

Ascorbic acid may be given in conjunction with the oral dose of methylene blue at a dose of 300–400 mg orally, although its role for this purpose remains controversial. Its onset of action is slow, and its potential for urine acidification may potentiate renal toxicity in patients who are actively hemolyzing.

2. Chlorate Salts

Chlorate salts, used primarily in herbicides, cause an unusual form of methemoglobinemia and hemolysis that may be unresponsive to methylene blue. The denaturation of hemoglobin caused by chlorates is thought to be due to their direct oxidizing capacity and their ability to inhibit the hexose monophosphate shunt. Hemolytic anemia also has been seen in uremic patients undergoing hemodialysis when the water supply was found to contain chloramines, oxidant compounds made up of chlorine and ammonia now used in some public water supplies as a disinfectant. Treatment

for poisoning with chlorates is supportive although methylene blue has been reported as a successful antidote in a case report of a construction worker with methemoglobinemia resulting from inhalation of sodium chlorate fumes. Exchange transfusion has been advocated for severe toxicity.

HEMOLYSIS ASSOCIATED WITH EXPOSURE TO HEAVY METALS

After methemoglobinemia and oxidative hemolysis, transitional elements and heavy metals are the most important causes of work-related hemolytic anemia. These agents include arsenic, lead, mercury, copper, antimony, and others. The mechanism of hemolysis is unknown, but it is thought to be related to the affinity of these directly cytolytic metals to thiol groups such as are found on the surfaces of red blood cells and in the cysteine residues of hemoglobin. When the sulfhydryl-binding metals are exposed to red cells, the red cell membrane becomes permeable and takes on solute and water. This causes the red cell to swell and ultimately burst while in the vascular circuit (intravascular hemolysis).

1. Arsine

The most dramatic example of acute metal-induced hemolysis is that caused by arsine. Arsine is a volatile, colorless, nonirritating gas at room temperature. It is usually produced accidentally by the action of acid on a metal contaminated with arsenic. However, arsine gas is often used in the semiconductor industry to introduce small quantities of arsenic into the matrix of silicon wafers to impart semi-conductive properties into what will become computer chips.

Acute nonfatal arsine poisoning has been reported among workers cleaning a floor drain where residual arsenical herbicides containing arsenic trioxide reacted with hydrogen formed by the combination of sodium hydroxide and aluminum to form arsine, and in a worker engaged in recycling of gallium arsenide scrap. Chronic arsine poisoning has been described in workers at a zinc smelting plant and in workers engaged in the cyanide extraction of gold. These patients may be anemic, with chronic low-level hemolysis.

▶ Clinical Presentation

A. Symptoms and Signs

Many manifestations of acute arsine poisoning are caused by acute and massive intravascular hemolysis. Appearance of symptoms may be delayed for 2–24 hours after exposure. Symptoms include nausea and vomiting, abdominal cramping, headache, malaise, and dyspnea. Patients often are alarmed by the presence of tea-colored urine that is not associated with pain on urination, causing them to seek medical attention. Physical examination may reveal the peculiar garlicky odor of arsine, fever, tachycardia, tachypnea, and hypotension. Later in the course of hemolysis, the patient typically develops jaundice.

B. Laboratory Findings

The earliest laboratory finding is likely to be hemoglobin-uria. This occurs when the amount of free plasma hemoglobin exceeds normal haptoglobin binding and renal proximal tubular reabsorption. Accordingly, plasma haptoglobin levels fall, and free hemoglobin levels may be very high (> 2000 mg/dL have been reported; normal: < 1 mg/dL). The plasma may be brownish red from the presence of methemalbumin (oxidized hemoglobin bound to albumin). Although anemia may not be present on the first blood count, evaluation of the peripheral smear will reveal red cell fragmentation with marked poikilocytosis, basophilic stippling, and polychromasia. As the hematocrit falls, reticulocytosis develops. Total bilirubin is elevated, reflecting a rise primarily in the unconjugated or indirect form. When hemolysis is brisk, disseminated intravascular coagulation may occur, manifest as a low (or falling) fibrinogen level, a prolonged prothrombin time (caused by circulating fibrin split products), and the presence of schistocytes and thrombocytopenia. Renal function often is affected to various degrees, with an early rise in serum creatinine. This may be a result of both precipitated hemoglobin casts, causing renal tubular obstruction, and direct toxicity of arsine on the renal tubular and interstitial cells. Arsenic levels in blood and urine are useful as indicators of exposure rather than as guidelines for therapy.

▶ Treatment

Initial therapy should include vigorous hydration to ensure adequate renal perfusion. For severe hemolysis with plasma hemoglobin levels greater than 400–500 mg/dL, exchange transfusion has been advocated. Repeated exchange is indicated for increasing levels of hemoglobin.

Renal function may be preserved with hydration. However, should renal failure develop, acute hemodialysis may be required. All patients must be monitored closely until all evidence of hemolysis has resolved and renal function has stabilized. Some patients may be left with renal insufficiency or chronic renal failure requiring dialysis or transplantation. In chronic arsine poisoning, reduction of or ideally removal from exposure is the most important intervention.

2. Lead

Lead is more fully discussed in the section on porphyria. In addition to the suppression of erythropoiesis and heme synthesis described there, hemolytic anemia may occasionally be seen. The anemia of chronic lead toxicity, the primary hematologic effect of lead exposures, is enhanced by shortened red cell survival as well as by inhibition of hemoglobin synthesis.

It has been suggested that the pathogenesis of lead-induced hemolysis is related to its marked inhibition of pyrimidine-5 nucleotidase. The hereditary homozygous deficiency of this enzyme is marked by basophilic stippling of erythrocytes, chronic hemolysis, and intraerythrocytic accumulations of pyrimidine-containing nucleotides. These nucleotides perhaps compete with adenine nucleotides in binding to the active site of kinases in the glycolytic pathway, thereby altering red cell membrane stability. Because lead causes an acquired deficiency of this enzyme and the clinical findings are similar, severe toxicity has been likened to this hereditary disease.

3. Copper

Copper sulfate is used in the manufacture of wire, sheet metal, pipe, and other metal products, in agriculture as a fungicide, and as a preservative for wood, leather, and fabrics. Toxicity is typically a result of accidental ingestion and suicide attempts but also can occur via dermal absorption of copper sulfate solution through damaged (burned or cut), nonintact skin. Systemic toxicity can occur in the presence of only mildly elevated serum copper levels and results in intravascular hemolysis, methemoglobinemia, renal failure, and often death. Hemolysis also has been caused by hemodialysis with water contaminated by copper piping. In vitro data suggest that multiple mechanisms are involved, including inhibition of glycolysis, oxidation of NADPH, and inhibition of G6PD. No specific treatment exists other than supportive therapy, with transfusions and hemodialysis as indicated.

4. Cadmium

Cadmium exposure can occur in workers across many industries, including battery and solar cell manufacture, electroplating, silver soldering, demolition workers, work around cadmium-containing pigments and coatings, and, more recently, in e-waste workers in both the developed and developing worlds. Among its other long-established toxicity on several organ systems, most notably on its nephrotoxic effects, cadmium also has been implicated in causing acute anemia related, in part, to a hemolytic process. In studies in rats, cadmium altered the structure of red blood cells making them more prone to intra-splenic hemolysis. A case report described a worker in whom a very high cadmium blood concentration may have contributed, along with concomitant autoimmune hemolytic anemia, to a fatal hemolytic anemia and kidney failure. Although there is a mechanistic basis and at least one case report, occupational cadmium exposure has not yet been definitively implicated as a cause of hemolytic anemia in workers.

THE PORPHYRIAS

The porphyrias are a group of disorders characterized by abnormalities in the heme biosynthetic pathway (Figure 24–4) that result in the abnormal accumulation of heme precursors. Although these are genetic disorders (inherited or sporadic) of enzymatic activity, acquired porphyria has been described following exposure to various toxins. Heme biosynthesis occurs chiefly in the liver and bone marrow and to a certain extent in nervous tissue. The rate-limiting step in heme biosynthesis is the synthesis of δ-aminolevulinic acid from glycine and succinyl-coenzyme A (CoA) via δ-aminolevulinic acid synthetase. This step is under negative feedback control by heme. Clinically, symptomatic porphyria

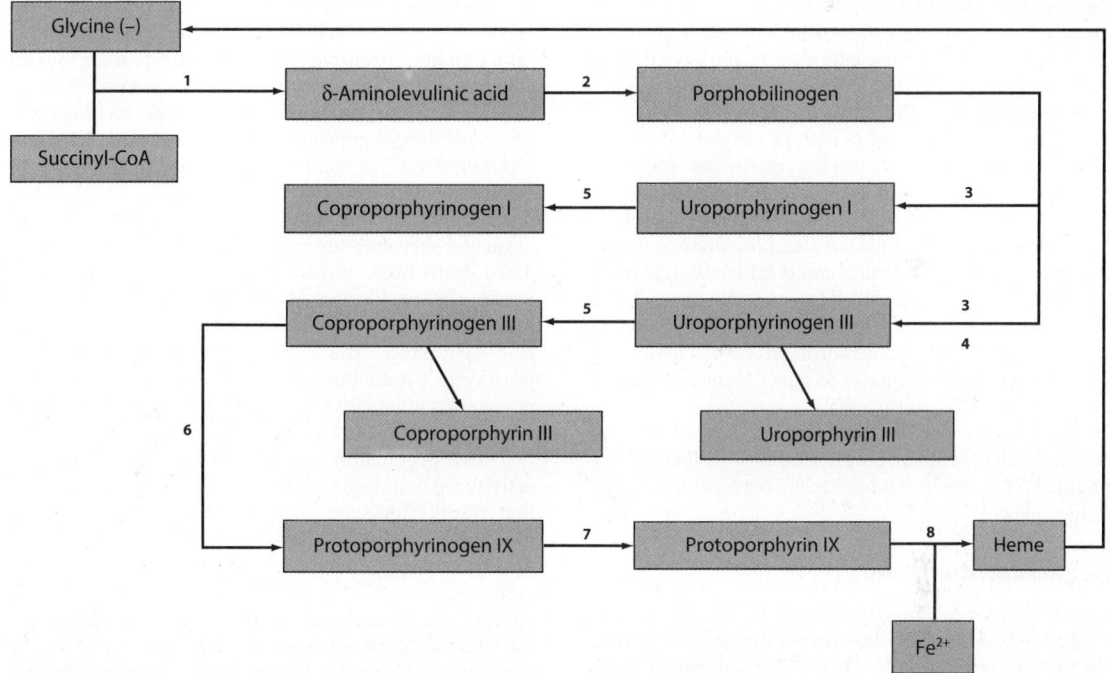

▲ **Figure 24–4.** The heme biosynthetic pathway. Heme is a feedback inhibitor of enzyme (1) δ-aminolevulinic acid synthetase. Other enzymes are (2) δ-aminolevulinic acid dehydrase, (3) uroporphyrinogen I synthase, (4) uroporphyrinogen III cosynthase, (5) uroporphyrinogen decarboxylase, (6) coproporphyrinogen oxidase, (7) protoporphyrinogen oxidase, and (8) ferrochelatase.

can occur either as a result of inadequate enzymatic function along any step in heme biosynthesis or as a result of inappropriate overstimulation of δ-aminolevulinic acid synthetase, usually in the setting of decreased heme concentration.

The clinical syndromes of porphyria are characterized by neurotoxicity or cutaneous photosensitivity (both may occur). Neurotoxicity—typically abdominal colic, constipation, autonomic dysfunction, sensorimotor neuropathy, and psychiatric problems—is considered the result of direct toxic effects of the urine-soluble heme precursors δ-aminolevulinic acid and porphobilinogen on nervous tissue. Neurotoxicity also may be the result of heme deficiency interrupting nervous tissue homeostasis. Cutaneous photosensitivity is manifested as repetitive vesiculation, scarring, and deformity, with hypertrichosis of sun-exposed areas of the skin. This is the result of the relatively urine-insoluble heme precursors uroporphyrin III, coproporphyrin III, and protoporphyrin IX fluorescing in the skin following absorption of 400-nm ultraviolet light. These fluorescing porphyrias also can cause discoloration of teeth and occasionally hemolysis of erythrocytes in which porphyrins accumulate.

A number of industrial and environmental toxins have induced toxic porphyrias similar to porphyria cutanea tarda in people heavily exposed to the agents (Table 24–3). These toxins, typically when absorbed in high doses, usually cause

liver injury and deranged hepatic heme synthesis. Although the exact metabolic effects of these agents are not entirely understood, unregulated stimulation of δ-aminolevulinic acid synthetase usually is demonstrable.

Table 24–3. Toxic substances associated with acquired porphyria in humans.

Toxin	Use
Hexachlorobenzene	Fungicide
2,4-Dichlorophenol	Herbicide
2,4,5-Trichlorophenol	Herbicide
2,3,7,8-Tetrachlorodibenzo-*p*-dioxin	Herbicide contaminant
o-Benzyl-*p*-chlorophenol	Cleanser and disinfectant
2-Benzyl-*p*-dichlorophenol	Commercial disinfectant
Vinyl chloride	Plastics
Lead	Paint compounds
Aluminum	Phosphorus binder

Because there is often no effective means of eliminating toxic environmental or industrial substances once they are incorporated into tissues, exposure to porphyrinogenic compounds must be avoided. Although no prospective data are available to support the use of phlebotomy for this purpose, this therapy may be of benefit in patients with toxic porphyria whose disease complex resembles porphyria cutanea tarda and in whom evidence of iron overload can be demonstrated. Patients with acute intermittent porphyria occasionally respond to high-dose carbohydrate infusions (400 g dextrose per day) or intravenous infusions of hematin (an iron-containing porphyrin). However, the use of hematin infusions in toxic porphyria may not be of benefit because, as in the case of hexachlorobenzene, the toxic agent may be interrupting the negative feedback signal by heme on δ-aminolevulinic acid synthetase.

For lead intoxication, prevention again is the best treatment. Unlike all other toxic porphyrias, specific therapy, recommended for severe lead intoxication, is available with lead chelating agents.

1. Hexachlorobenzene

In an outbreak of acquired porphyria in Turkey between 1955 and 1958, more than 3000 people developed a cutaneous porphyria syndrome that resembled congenital erythropoietic porphyria approximately 6 months following ingestion of wheat containing the fungicide hexachlorobenzene. The wheat was intended for planting and contained 10% hexachlorobenzene to control the fungus *Tilletia tritici.* Affected people demonstrated cutaneous photosensitivity with skin hyperpigmentation, hypertrichosis, bullae, weakness, and hepatomegaly, a condition termed *kara yara,* or "black sore." Porphyrinuria was nearly universal, with the urine being pigmented red or brown. The mortality rate was 10%. Breast-fed infants younger than 2 years of age had a 95% mortality rate when ingesting mother's milk contaminated with the fungicide. These infants developed weakness, convulsions, and cutaneous annular erythema, a condition termed *pembe yara,* or "pink sore." Excess porphyrins could not be detected in the urine of these infants. A similar result occurs in animal models of hexachlorobenzene-induced porphyria. Infant rats and mice die of neurologic toxicity from hexachlorobenzene without porphyrinuria, whereas adult rats and rabbits develop cutaneous photosensitivity and porphyrinuria following prolonged exposure to the chemical.

A follow-up study between 1977 and 1983 examined 204 patients who had previously suffered from hexachlorobenzene porphyria. The mean age of these individuals was 32 years, and the mean time from hexachlorobenzene exposure was 7 years. The mean duration of cutaneous porphyria symptoms was 2.4 years. At the time of study, 71% of people had hyperpigmentation and 47% had hypertrichosis. Residual scarring on sun-exposed areas of the skin was evident in 87%. Other features included perioral scarring, small hands, arthritis, short stature, weakness, paresthesias, and myotonia. Seventeen patients still had red urine and

demonstrated porphyrinuria (especially uroporphyrinuria). Hexachlorobenzene was measurable in 56 samples of human milk obtained from porphyric mothers at a mean value of 0.51 parts per million (ppm) (vs 0.07 ppm in controls).

The Turkish experience was the first associating exposure to an industrial chemical with acquired porphyria in humans. Not only were the symptomatic attack and mortality rates significant, but also the biochemical lesion persisted for decades in many survivors. The exact mechanism by which hexachlorobenzene induces porphyria remains to be elucidated. Most liver mitochondria of animals made porphyric by exposure to chlorinated benzenes, such as hexachlorobenzene, demonstrated increased activity of δ-aminolevulinic acid synthetase, the enzyme that controls the rate of porphyrin production. With the exception of mice made porphyric with diethyl-1,4-dihydro-2,4,6-trimethylpyridine-3,5-dicarboxylate, animal porphyric livers demonstrate an increased production of heme. Heme normally inhibits the activity of δ-aminolevulinic acid synthetase. This suggests that porphyrinogenic compounds are somehow interfering with the repressor signal of heme on δ-aminolevulinic acid synthetase. Other theories suggest that porphyrinogenic compounds induce δ-aminolevulinic acid synthetase by altering the intracellular oxidation state through action on the electron transport chain, thus stimulating succinyl-CoA production, depressing intracellular adenosine triphosphate levels, or both. In any event, the net result is overproduction of porphyrins mediated by unregulated δ-aminolevulinic acid synthetase activity.

The role of iron overload in the pathogenesis of hexachlorobenzene-induced porphyria has been examined. Most authorities believe that iron plays a permissive rather than a causative role in porphyrias. This is based on the fact that not all patients with porphyria cutanea tarda are iron overloaded, that porphyria cutanea tarda is rare in patients with hemochromatosis, and that phlebotomy does not correct the biochemical lesion in patients with porphyria cutanea tarda. In addition, rats made porphyric by hexachlorobenzene did not require iron overload for porphyria to develop, although the porphyria was worsened by iron overload. Thus, it remains unsettled whether iron overload is permissive or etiologic in patients exposed to porphyrinogenic toxins.

2. Herbicides

A number of herbicides clearly are associated with symptomatic porphyria. Workers exposed to 2,4-dichlorophenol and 2,4,5-trichlorophenol at a manufacturing plant exhibited chloracne hyperpigmentation, hirsutism, and skin fragility. They had increased excretion of urine porphyrins (uroporphyrin and coproporphyrin). Thus, these workers had developed an acquired porphyria cutanea tarda-like syndrome after variable exposure to these herbicides. A follow-up study of 73 workers at this same herbicide plant 6 years later found no people with the porphyric syndrome and only one with persistent uroporphyrinuria. The authors of the follow-up study hypothesized that the decrease in the syndrome was a result of improved personal safety habits of the workers and decreased exposure to the chemicals. An alternative explanation is that the true porphyrinogenic agent is perhaps 2,3,7,8-tetrachlorodibenzo-p-dioxin, a by-product of 2,4,5-trichlorophenol, and that this contaminant had been effectively eliminated from the chemical stores at the factory. The contaminant was strongly implicated in an outbreak of acquired porphyria cutanea tarda, chloracne, and polyneuropathy in 80 industrial workers producing herbicides in Czechoslovakia.

3. Disinfectants

The commercial disinfectants o-benzyl-p-chlorophenol and 2-benzyl-4,6-dichlorophenol were implicated as a cause of acquired porphyria cutanea tarda in one woman janitor exposed to these chemicals through inappropriate mixing of cleaning chemicals.

4. Aluminum

A porphyria cutanea tarda-like syndrome has been described in patients with chronic renal failure being maintained on regular hemodialysis. Plasma and urine uroporphyrins are increased in these patients, whereas plasma and urine coproporphyrins are often low. Because aluminum is known to inhibit some heme synthetic enzymes, and because many chronic renal failure patients on hemodialysis are aluminum overloaded, aluminum has been implicated, but without proof, as the cause of porphyria in these patients.

5. Vinyl Chloride

Vinyl chloride is a known hepatotoxin used in the production of plastics. A study of workers in a polyvinyl chloride production plant revealed significantly elevated urinary coproporphyrin levels. Exposure periods ranged from 2 to 21 years. The pathogenesis of coproporphyrinuria involves inhibition of coproporphyrinogen oxidase, inhibition of uroporphyrinogen decarboxylase (UD), and perhaps induction of δ-aminolevulinic acid synthetase. Workers with excess urinary coproporphyrin production also manifested thrombocytopenia, splenomegaly, esophageal varices, scleroderma-like skin changes, Raynaud syndrome, and acroosteolysis.

6. Lead

Lead intoxication (particularly with a blood lead level greater than 60 μg/dL) causes symptoms and signs remarkably similar to those associated with acute intermittent porphyria. The classic acute intermittent porphyria triad is abdominal pain, constipation, and vomiting—all representing the neurotoxic effects of excess δ-aminolevulinic acid and porphobilinogen. This triad is seen with equal frequency in lead intoxication. Other shared characteristics include neuromuscular pains, paresis or paralysis, paresthesias, diarrhea, and seizures. The major differences between the two diseases are (1) an increase in neuropsychiatric signs in acute intermittent porphyria compared with lead intoxication and (2) anemia, which is present in lead intoxication but virtually absent in porphyria. The anemia of lead poisoning is a characteristic microcytic anemia with basophilic stippling of erythrocytes and sideroblasts in the bone marrow.

The biochemical features of lead poisoning demonstrate why these two diseases are so similar clinically. Patients with lead intoxication have markedly elevated urinary δ-aminolevulinic acid levels, as in acute intermittent porphyria. Mild lead poisoning (pre-anemia stage) is associated with normal porphobilinogen excretion, but once anemia occurs, excess urinary porphobilinogen becomes demonstrable. Although mild elevations of urine coproporphyrins and uroporphyrin I are present, fecal uroporphyrin and coproporphyrin are normal in patients with lead poisoning. These alterations in porphyrins are present only in patients with inorganic lead intoxication, not in patients with organic lead intoxication. Excess accumulation of protoporphyrin IX also has been found in erythrocytes of lead-intoxicated patients. The effect of lead on heme synthesis disruption occurs at multiple steps in the synthetic pathway, with different individuals displaying different levels of sensitivity to lead exposure.

7. Polyhalogenated Aromatic Hydrocarbons, Including Dioxins

Polyhalogenated aromatic hydrocarbons (PHAHs) are another potential cause of porphyria in workers. Examples of PHAHs include polychlorinated biphenyls (PCBs), polychlorinated dibenzo-p-dioxins (PCDDs), polychlorinated dibenzofurans (PCDFs), dichlorodiphenyltrichlorethane (p,p′-DDT), and its metabolite 1,1-dichloro-2,2-bis(4-chlorophenyl) ethylene (p,p′-DDE).

PHAHs cause porphyria through the inhibition of hepatic UD, which is responsible for one of the enzymatic steps in the production of heme. Initially, a latent, asymptomatic coproporphyrinuria is induced, which can gradually progress into an overt symptomatic porphyria.

WORK-RELATED APLASTIC ANEMIA & MYELODYSPLASTIC SYNDROMES

1. Aplastic Anemia

Aplastic anemia, or medullary aplasia, is an acquired abnormality of the pluripotent hematopoietic stem cells (HSCs) resulting in pancytopenia (anemia, neutropenia, and thrombocytopenia). Many cases of aplastic anemia develop after the occurrence of dysplastic morphologic changes in hematologic cells with associated chromosomal abnormalities. The incidence of acute nonlymphocytic leukemia (ANLL) in patients with aplastic anemia who survive 2 years after diagnosis is approximately 5–10%; in patients with preceding dysplasia, the incidence may be higher. Chemicals that are capable of inducing bone marrow damage must also be assumed to be potential leukemogens.

The average incidence of fatal aplastic anemia per year in the United States is approximately 2 per million and rises with age to an annual age-specific mortality rate of about 10 per million in people older than age 65. Approximately 50% of cases of aplastic anemia in North America and western Europe are idiopathic; most of the remainder are termed *secondary aplastic anemias* and may be caused by drugs, chemicals, radiation, infection, and immunologic mechanisms. A small percentage of cases are caused by hereditary diseases. The largest category of secondary aplastic anemia is caused by therapeutic drugs, such as chloramphenicol, acetazolamide, phenylbutazone, phenytoin, and sulfonamides.

Three agents have been firmly established as a cause of aplastic anemia in occupational and environmental setting: benzene, ionizing radiation, and cytotoxic drugs such as antimetabolites and alkylating agents.

▶ Benzene

Benzene was first described as a cause of fatal aplastic anemia in 1897. Early unregulated exposure to benzene—used widely as a solvent in the production of many products, including fabrics and pesticides—led to many cases of acute and chronic toxicity. Workers historically at greatest risk of high concentration exposure are those involved in rubber manufacturing, shoemaking, petroleum and chemical production, and printing.

Before 1950, benzene was the single most common cause of toxic aplastic anemia. With chronic doses of greater than 100 ppm, isolated cytopenias and aplastic anemia were common. The cytopenias usually resolved after termination of exposure; even with persistent exposure, spontaneous remissions have been described. At exposures of 100 ppm or higher, some workers will develop fatal aplastic anemia. Great variation in susceptibility to exposure has been seen, with evidence of poisoning sometimes appearing only after weeks or years. Cases of cytopenia also have been seen several years after exposure has been terminated; these cases are less likely to resolve with time and may be part of a preleukemic syndrome. In severe chronic poisoning, decreased red cell survival with hemolysis has been reported.

The risk of aplastic anemia is often related to the amount and duration of exposure, although multiple scientific agencies and organizations have not identified a level below which benzene is considered without risk of hematologic disease. The diagnosis is made by examination of the bone marrow after an abnormal complete blood count is reported. The bone marrow will reveal hypocellularity with fatty replacement, although islands of hypercellularity may be seen. Although cytogenetic abnormalities are associated with benzene exposure, specific chromosome changes are not. The initial prognosis in benzene-related aplastic anemia is better than that for idiopathic aplastic anemia; up to 40% of patients may recover completely after removal from the source of exposure. If hypocellularity persists for more than several months, recovery is not likely to occur.

Treatment is supportive (ie, with transfusions and such growth factors as erythropoietin, granulocyte colony-stimulating factor, and granulocyte-macrophage colony-stimulating factor). Drugs such as androgens to stimulate hematopoiesis have not been used extensively in benzene-induced aplastic anemia but should be tried when no other treatment option exists (such as bone marrow transplantation or colony-stimulating factors). Allogeneic bone marrow transplantation is the only known cure for irreversible aplastic anemia but is hampered by donor availability, higher mortality risk with increasing patient age, and the toxicity of the transplant regimen.

▶ Ionizing Radiation

Ionizing radiation also has been associated with aplastic anemia in a dose-dependent manner. Internal exposure to absorbed alpha particles associated with aplastic anemia was demonstrated most strikingly in the radium watch dial workers who ingested radium by wetting their paintbrushes on their tongues. External exposure to radiation is much more common and may be in the form of whole-body exposure to a large dose, as in a nuclear accident or therapeutic radiation, or long-term exposure to small amounts, as may have occurred in the practice of radiology as a medical specialty prior to effective protection against radiation exposures.

Data from patients radiated for ankylosing spondylitis and from the survivors of the atomic bombings of Hiroshima and Nagasaki suggest that the risk of aplastic anemia is increased until 3–5 years after exposure, after which there is a marked decline in incidence. The most important late disturbance following irradiation of the bone marrow is leukemia. The ability to recover from a single dose of penetrating radiation depends on the fraction of surviving stem cells. Chromosomal aberrations are associated with exposure to ionizing radiation and rise in a linear manner as a function of the dose of radiation absorbed. The presence of these aberrations, including an increase in the number of sister chromatid exchanges, may signify excessive exposure but is not predictive of aplastic anemia or leukemia.

Strict regulation of exposure and monitoring with badges has virtually eliminated aplastic anemia caused by radiation except in cases of accidental overexposure. In this case, treatment again is primarily supportive. Recovery may be seen after a prolonged period of aplastic anemia lasting 3–6 weeks and may be predicted from the known total dose of radiation. If recovery does not occur, permanent injury to the stem cell population will result in chronic cellular hypoplasia or dysplasia or in leukemia. Treatment then may include bone marrow transplantation if a donor is available.

▶ Other Chemicals

Aplastic anemia has been reported following exposure to a variety of other chemicals listed in Table 24–4.

Two chemicals in particular deserve mention here. The aplastic anemia associated with trinitrotoluene may be accompanied by methemoglobinemia, oxidative hemolysis,

Table 24–4. Chemicals reported to cause aplastic anemia in an occupational setting.

Chemical	Use
Benzene	Intermediate in the synthesis of fabrics, pesticides, rubber; solvent for glues, varnishes, inks, paints; octane booster for gasoline
Trinitrotoluene (TNT)	Production of explosives
Hexachlorocyclohexane (lindane) Pentachlorophenol Chlorophenothane (DDT)	Pesticide
Arsenic	Manufacture of glass, paint, enamels, weed killers, tanning agents, pesticides
Ethylene glycol monomethyl or monobutyl ether	Production of paints, lacquers, dyes, inks, cleaning agents

liver damage, and dermatitis. The incidence of overexposure to arsenic has declined with its decreasing use and better controls over the recent decades. Fewer than 10 cases of overt arsenic poisoning are now reported annually in the United States. Complete spontaneous hematologic recovery usually is seen if the patient is promptly removed from the source of heavy exposure.

2. Myelodysplastic Syndromes

The myelodysplastic syndromes are a group of acquired genetic disorders of the blood-forming cells and characterized by ineffective hematopoiesis, clinically resulting in anemia, neutropenia, thrombocytopenia, or a combination of cytopenias. These syndromes are linked by the presence of bizarre hematopoietic morphology and the tendency to transform into acute leukemia. Specific syndromes associated with exposure to both occupational chemicals and cytotoxic drugs have a high incidence of progression to frank leukemia. Both benzene and ionizing radiation are known risk factors for myelodysplasia. Several case-control studies have suggested that other occupational risk factors, such as exposure to pesticides or solvents or employment in specific sectors such as farming, textile work, or the health professions, increase the risk of myelodysplasia. The median survival from these diseases is less than 12 months, and most patients eventually either develop leukemias or succumb to complications related to cytopenias. Exposure to benzene is specifically associated with a high incidence of deletions involving chromosomes 5 and 7.

Myelodysplastic syndromes are more common in men than in women, and 85% of patients are older than 40 years of age at the time of diagnosis. Laboratory features of myelodysplastic syndromes include cytopenias of various degrees

and often an increase in the red blood cell mean corpuscular volume. The marrow usually reveals dysplasia in all three cell lines (granulocyte/erythroid/megakaryocyte [platelet-forming]) and manifests abnormal marrow cellularity, usually hypercellular. There is an abnormal increase in the percentage of blast cells.

Several treatment options are available, although all have significant drawbacks. Allogeneic bone marrow transplantation (a transplant from a donor, usually a sibling or matched unrelated donor) is the only known cure but is limited primarily by patient age and carries a significant risk of treatment-related mortality. Transfusions and treatment of infections may be aided by the use of hematopoietic growth factors. The hypomethylating chemotherapy drug azacytidine is approved by the Food and Drug Administration for MDS, and two other agents, lenalidomide and decitabine, appear quite active, although none of these agents appears to be curative.

HEMATOPOIETIC CANCERS

1. Leukemia

▶ Occupations at Risk

- Workers exposed to ionizing radiation, including radiologists, nuclear industry workers, and military personnel
- Rubber workers, machinists, mechanics, printers, petroleum workers (refinery and upstream), gasoline delivery drivers, tankermen, and other workers exposed to benzene and solvents containing benzene

▶ General Considerations

The major forms of leukemia that have been linked to occupational exposures are ANLL; also known as acute myeloid leukemia, acute myelogenous leukemia, or acute myeloblastic leukemia [AML], chronic myelogenous leukemia (CML), and chronic lymphocytic leukemia (CLL). The acute leukemias are malignant diseases of the blood-forming organs characterized by a proliferation of immature blood cell progenitors in the bone marrow and other tissues. Together with replacement of the normal marrow with leukemic cells, there is a diminished production of normal erythrocytes, granulocytes, and platelets. The acute and chronic leukemias are classified morphologically by the World Health Organization according to the predominant cell line involved (lymphocytic and nonlymphocytic forms) and various clinical and pathological characteristics. The incidence rates for all types of leukemia vary widely by geographic areas and ethnic groups, but, in North America and Europe, they vary from about 8–12 cases per 100,000 person-years in men to about 5–8 cases per 100,000 person-years in women, with ANNL accounting for about 3–4 cases per 100,000 person-years in men and 1–2 cases per 100,000 person-years in women. The incidence of most leukemias increase with age with the highest rates above age 50.

Chronic leukemias are classified as lymphocytic and myelogenous. CML is a clonal myeloproliferative neoplasm derived from an abnormal multipotent HSC that has acquired the *BCR-ABL1* fusion gene, usually through t(9;22)(q34;q11), also known as the Philadelphia (Ph) chromosome. CML accounts for approximately 15–20% of leukemias in adults, with an annual incidence of 1–2 cases per 100,000, and with a slight male predominance. The average age at diagnosis of CML is around 64 years. CLL is one of the chronic lymphoproliferative disorders with accumulation of functionally incompetent lymphocytes, (monoclonal in origin). CLL is the same as the mature (peripheral) B-cell neoplasm small lymphocytic lymphoma (SLL), wherein CLL manifests primarily in the blood and SLL with primarily nodal involvement.

▶ Etiology

A differential etiology should be performed to determine whether occupational exposure likely caused or contributed to the development of leukemia. The risk for acute myeloid leukemia (AML) is increased following chemotherapy, with certain genetic or familial conditions, or with tobacco smoking. Risk factors for CML and CLL/SLL include genetics (family history) and infection (hepatitis C virus). There is also some evidence that obesity may increase the risk of ANNL and CML.

A. Radiation

Radiation remains the most conclusively identified leukemogenic factor in human beings. The earliest evidence began to accumulate soon after the discovery of x-rays, which were used mainly in the medical workplace; thus radiologists, radiation therapists, and radiation technicians were all at risk. Several studies showed an excess risk of leukemia among radiologists (approximately nine times that of other physicians) during the years 1930–1950, with a latency period of about 18 years. With the institution of dose limits, careful monitoring, and adequate shielding since that time, this excess risk has decreased significantly and should be eliminated.

The data from Hiroshima and Nagasaki atomic bomb survivors leave little doubt that the incidence of leukemia is increased following exposure to mixed gamma and neutron radiation and that the response is dose dependent. The risk of leukemia is increased in populations exposed to ionizing radiation at doses as low as 50–100 cGy. Between 100 and 500 cGy, there is a linear correlation between dose and leukemia incidence. The data suggest that the risk of leukemia is increased at a rate of 1–2 cases per million population per year per centigray. Maximal risk occurs approximately 4–7 years after exposure, and an increased risk has been seen in Japanese people as long as 14 years after exposure.

Whole-body exposure to radiation in single doses results in suppression of marrow growth, and a single whole-body dose of more than 400 cGy usually is fatal in humans. In sublethal exposure, cytopenias may occur, which gradually recover but indicate significant damage to the marrow precursor elements. Patients are then at risk to develop leukemia with a delay between exposure and disease of 8–18 years. Following radiation exposure, both acute and chronic myelogenous leukemia may occur. The specific rates per 100,000 for people within 1500 m (4921 ft) of the hypocenter are 8.1 for AML, 25.6 for CML, and 21.7 for acute lymphocytic leukemia.

Workers at risk secondary to exposure to ionizing radiation include military personnel in the vicinity of nuclear tests, uranium miners, and workers in nuclear power plants. Approximately 250,000 troops are estimated to have been present at multiple detonations of nuclear devices carried out by the United States from 1945 to 1976. In 1976, more than 3000 men exposed at the 1957 nuclear test explosion "Smoky" were studied, and a significant excess of leukemia was discovered. A review of death certificates of former workers at the Portsmouth Naval Shipyard in Portsmouth, New Hampshire (where nuclear submarines are repaired and refueled), revealed an observed-to-expected ratio of leukemia deaths of 5.62 among former nuclear workers.

B. Benzene

It is generally accepted in the scientific community that benzene or the various products that contain benzene is a cause of leukemia. Case reports of aplastic anemia and leukemia have been published for more than a century, and the petroleum industry recognized the toxicity of benzene on the blood system since the 1940s. There is extensive medical and scientific literature that shows that benzene causes cytogenetic damage and significantly increases the risk of AML in benzene-exposed workers. One of the most authoritative scientific bodies on the carcinogenic risk of chemicals—the World Health Organization International Agency for Research on Cancer (IARC)—has published over four decades *The Monographs on the Evaluation of Carcinogenic Risk to Humans*. IARC has concluded that benzene causes AML including acute myeloid leukemia in adults, and that there is limited evidence for CLL, non-Hodgkin lymphoma (NHL), and multiple myeloma (MM).

The Agency for Toxic Substances and Disease Registry (ATSDR)—an agency of the U.S. Federal Department of Health and Human Services had concluded: "Based on the results of the meta-analyses, the recent cohort studies and the finding that occupational benzene exposure is associated with reductions in both lymphoid and myeloid cell types, ATSDR concludes that there is sufficient evidence for causation for benzene and CLL, AML, and CML. Benzene is also recognized as a human carcinogen by all organizations that evaluate the carcinogenicity of chemicals and government agencies that classify chemicals as carcinogens, including the U.S. Environment Protection Agency (EPA) that classifies benzene as a human carcinogen, the U.S. National Institute for Occupational National Safety and Health (NIOSH) policy on occupational carcinogens, the U.S. National Toxicology Program (NTP), and the U.S. Occupational Safety and Health Administration (OSHA).

The level at which benzene exposure increases the risk of leukemia and other blood disorders has been demonstrated in the few ppm-year range, with significant increased risk also shown from frequent peak exposures in the same range. Cytogenetic abnormalities have been demonstrated at lower levels of benzene exposure as well. While some studies suggest that the increased risk of benzene exposure on AML and other blood disorders decline after more than 15 years latency, numerous other case reports and studies show that benzene exposure increases the risk of disease for several decades.

C. Other Agents

Chemicals other than benzene are known or suspected to cause leukemia. In 2012, IARC concluded that formaldehyde causes leukemia, supported particularly by studies demonstrating increased risk for professional workers, for example, embalmers and pathologists. The evidence is stronger for myeloid leukemias. Similarly, IARC concluded in 2012 that 1,3-butadiene, a monomer used in the production of synthetic rubber and polymers, causes hematolymphatic malignancies, with the evidence stronger for leukemia than for lymphoma. There is limited evidence according to IARC that ethylene oxide causes leukemia in humans. Exposure to ethylene oxide, used as a sterilant and in chemical processing, has been associated with an increased risk of lymphatic and hematopoietic cancers (specifically lymphoid tumors, ie, NHL, MM, and CLL). IARC also has classified the following agents as probably carcinogenic (Group 2A) with respect to leukemia: styrene, diazinon, and exposures resulting from petroleum refining work.

▶ Pathophysiology

A. Ionizing Radiation

The effects of radiation on human tissue depend on multiple factors, such as type of radiation, dose of radiation, length of exposure, body part exposed, and oxygen content of the exposed tissue. Damage secondary to radiation is greatest in rapidly dividing cells such as bone marrow stem cells, epithelial cells, and gamete-forming cells. The mechanism of radiation-induced injury at the cellular level involves direct and indirect damage to nucleic acids and proteins. DNA is a radiosensitive target, with even minor molecular damage resulting in profound effects on the cell and the organism. Radiation-induced molecular damage may be so severe that the cell no longer functions and cell death results. Cells exposed to radiation may survive with no effects (if only a small number of nonessential molecules are affected) or may survive with altered structure and function. If the alteration is within the DNA, clinical disease may not appear until after a latency period. Cancer induction appears to depend on an interaction of defective cellular repair and damage to the cell's regulator genes.

B. Benzene

There are likely multiple mechanisms by which benzene induces leukemia and other blood disorders. In experimental studies, including in human cells, benzene induces chromosomal aberrations and mutations. Workers exposed occupationally to benzene have exhibited chromosomal aberrations in peripheral lymphocytes. The leukemogenicity of benzene requires metabolism to other compounds in the liver and bone marrow, such as hydroquinone and 1,4-benzoquinone, which may be the active carcinogenic metabolites. Like certain chemotherapeutic drugs, known as topoisomerase-II inhibitors, benzene metabolites may act by inhibition of this enzyme that is responsible for the maintenance of proper chromosome structure. Hematotoxic effects from exposure to benzene, secondary immune system dysfunction, and epigenetic changes induced by benzene may also contribute to its leukemogenicity.

▶ Clinical Findings

The clinical findings, including symptoms, signs, and laboratory findings, in occupation- or environment-induced leukemias are not different from those observed in de novo leukemias. However, certain agents produce preceding toxic effects, which may be present prior to the development of leukemia.

1. *Radiation.* As noted earlier, 300–400 cGy of whole-body radiation is lethal in humans. Sublethal exposures will cause symptoms of nausea and vomiting, after which bone marrow suppression occurs. Thrombocytopenia, anemia, and neutropenia will develop, with their attendant symptoms. The development of leukemia occurs after a variable but relatively short latency period. When the disease progresses, symptoms are identical to acute leukemia.

2. *Benzene.* Benzene-induced hematotoxicity may lead to anemia, thrombocytopenia, and leukopenia, with attendant symptoms and clinical findings. Myelodysplasia may also precede the onset of AML, or AML may arise from benzene exposure without MDS. The presentation of leukemia due to benzene exposure is no different than that of de novo leukemia.

▶ Treatment & Prognosis

There have been recent major advances in the treatment of acute leukemias with the use of combination chemotherapy and bone marrow transplantation. The treatment of occupation-induced leukemia is essentially the same as that for spontaneous leukemias.

▶ Prevention

Avoidance of exposure to potential leukemogens, including ionizing radiation, benzene, and cigarette smoking, will reduce the occurrence of leukemia secondary to these agents.

A. Radiation

X-rays were discovered by Roentgen in 1895, and by 1902, the basic principles of radiation protection already had been elaborated: to minimize dose by reducing the time of exposure and by using shielding and distance. Since 1928, the International Council on Radiation Protection (ICRP) and the National Council on Radiation Protection have defined acceptable levels of radiation exposure for workers. The concept of dose equivalent or rem (Roentgen-equivalent man) is used because the same amounts of absorbed radiation energy can produce different levels of damage depending on the type of radiation present. Acceptable exposures for different organs vary, with a maximum permissible dose ranging from 5 rems of whole-body exposure to 30 rems of skin or bone exposure.

B. Benzene

In 1974, NIOSH published a recommended standard based on the evidence for hematotoxic effects: 10 ppm as an 8-hour time-weighted average (TWA), with a ceiling limit of 25 ppm. The current OSHA 8-hour time-weighted average workplace exposure limit is 1 ppm. Quantitative risk assessment analysis suggests that the risk of leukemia mortality from a working lifetime of exposure at this level would be about 1.7-fold compared to the background risk. NIOSH states that there is no known safe level of exposure to a carcinogen such as benzene, and advises reduction of worker exposure to chemical carcinogens as much as possible through elimination or substitution and engineering controls as the primary way to prevent occupational cancer. OSHA requires periodic medical surveillance annually, including a complete blood count, for workers exposed to benzene above the 8-hour TWA action level of 0.5 ppm.

2. Multiple Myeloma

MM is a chronic leukemia of differentiated B cells (termed *plasma cells*) that accounts for 15% of all hematologic cancers. It is always preceded by a chronic condition known as monoclonal gammopathy of unknown significance or MGUS, with MGUS carrying a 1% annual risk for transition to MM. It is characterized by anemia, painful lytic and osteopenic bone disease, monoclonal immunoglobulin production (in serum or urine or both), and hypogammaglobulinemia. Patients also may have hypercalcemia, renal failure, or neuropathy. Treatment involves a variety of agents, including thalidomide, chemotherapy (with such agents as melphalan, vincristine, vinblastine, doxorubicin, cyclophosphamide, and carmustine), and corticosteroids with the goal of alleviating bone pain, correcting complications of the disease, and prolonging life. Autologous bone marrow transplantation soon after diagnosis appears to improve both disease-free and overall survival. This less toxic form of therapy is available to a wider range of patients up to age 70 years.

The peak incidence of MM is between ages 55 and 65, and fewer than 2% of cases occur before the age of 40. MM is equally common in men and women but almost twice as common in blacks as in whites. The incidence of MM has been increasing over the last three decades in North American and European men, but this rise has not been noted in study populations in Minnesota and Sweden and simply may reflect an increase in our ability to diagnose the disease. The rise in incidence has aroused concern that myeloma might be associated with environmental or occupational factors.

The risks for MM include increasing age (MM risk increases with age, with most people diagnosed in their mid-60s), gender (men are more likely to develop MM than women), exposure to ionizing radiation, family history of MM, and tobacco smoking. There is also evidence that obesity increases the risk of MM.

Consideration of the studies and data using Sir Austin Bradford Hill's viewpoints as a framework for analysis shows that occupational exposure to benzene, including organic solvents containing benzene, is a cause of MM. Studies have also shown that benzene, petroleum products, paints, solvents, and other products that contain petroleum distillation fractions cause MM. Many epidemiologic studies also suggest that the risk of MM increases with various occupational exposures, such as petroleum products, organic solvents, heavy metals, asbestos, and pesticides. Workers at risk include agricultural workers, chemical workers, miners, smelters, stokers, and furniture workers.

Multiple studies have observed higher incidences of MM and its precursor, MGUS, in agricultural workers than in the general population, with pesticides among the suspected links. Carbaryl and captan are two in particular that have been identified in multiple studies as associated with increased MM risks in men.

IARC has concluded that benzene increases the risk of MM, based on increased risks for MM in workers exposed to benzene in several observational studies. A 2011 meta-analysis of occupational cohort studies found increased relative risks for MM in benzene-exposed workers, with higher risks in high-quality studies and in studies that also found significantly increased rates of acute myeloid leukemia (for which benzene is an established cause).

An important association between high-dose radiation exposure and MM has been observed in cohorts of controls and survivors of the atomic bombings of Hiroshima and Nagasaki for the period of 1950–1976. The relative risk for persons with an estimated air-dose exposure of 100 cGy or more was over four times higher than that of controls. This excess risk became apparent approximately 20 years after exposure.

3. Non-Hodgkin's Lymphoma

▶ Occupations at Risk

- Pesticide applicators mixing and spraying lindane or pentachlorophenol and any agricultural worker in frequent contact with these pesticides

- Workers involved in the manufacture of pentachlorophenol or in its application to wood or other products as a preservative

- Workers exposed to 1,3-butadiene in various industries, such as petroleum refining, manufacture of butadiene monomer, and plastics and rubber manufacture.
- Rubber workers, machinists, mechanics, printers, petroleum workers (refinery and upstream), gasoline delivery drivers, tankermen, and other workers exposed to benzene and solvents containing benzene

► General Considerations

NHLs are a variety of cancers involving the lymphocytes. NHL can arise from B lymphocytes (most common) or T lymphocytes. NHLs vary in terms of their aggressiveness, with follicular lymphomas the most common slow-growing, indolent NHLs and diffuse large B-cell lymphomas an example of a particularly aggressive form of NHL.

In the United States, an estimated 74,000 cases are diagnosed every year, with 20,000 annual deaths. Slightly more males than females are afflicted and, although a significant number of children and young adults are diagnosed every year, the risk is increased in the elderly. Whites have higher rates than minorities in the United States and the rates in developed countries, such as the United States and in Europe, are higher. Other nonoccupational risk factors include an NHL diagnosis in a first-degree relative, certain autoimmune diseases, immune-deficient states, infection with a number of viruses (human T-cell lymphotropic virus, Epstein-Barr virus, and human herpes virus 8), and tobacco smoking.

► Occupational Etiologies

A. Benzene

There are numerous occupations where significant exposure has occurred to solvents containing benzene. Consideration of the studies and data using Sir Austin Bradford Hill's viewpoints as a framework for analysis shows that occupational exposure to benzene, including organic solvents containing benzene, is a cause of NHL. The weight of the evidence supports a causal relationship between occupational exposure to benzene and benzene-containing organic solvents and the development of NHL. A summary review in 2010 highlights the WHO recognition that B-cell neoplasms are a group of related disorders, the mechanistic evidence for the genotoxicity of benzene, and the epidemiologic data. One meta-analysis supports an association between benzene exposure and NHL and two meta-analyses do not. An evolving and deeper understanding of the mechanisms of benzene-induced leukemia has emerged, and biomarkers of susceptibility to solvent- and benzene-induced NHL have also been studied in recent years.

B. Lindane

Lindane is the common name given to an isomer of hexachlorocyclohexane, a member of the class of pesticides known as halogenated aromatic hydrocarbons. In addition to its most prevalent, industrial use as an insecticide, it is also used in pharmaceutical creams and lotions that treat head lice and scabies.

In the United States, commercial production began in the 1940s and peaked in the 1950s. Lindane is now banned for industrial use in more than 50 countries, including the United States and the countries of the European Union, and its use is restricted in more than 30 others. However, its use persists in certain areas of the world, primarily as an insecticide for fruit and vegetable crops and for rodent control.

Workers can be exposed to lindane both during its formation and production, during its use for the treatment of wood structures and seed grain, and, most importantly, in the course of its use as a pesticide for livestock and crops. Occupational exposure occurs primarily through inhalation or dermal contact. Nonoccupational exposure has been reported in the general population through lindane residues in water supplies and on agricultural and livestock products contaminated with lindane.

C. Pentachlorophenol

Pentachlorophenol was first introduced in the 1930s as a wood preservative and this is still its most common use worldwide. The European Union banned pentachlorophenol's use for wood preservation and most other uses in 2009 and the United States and Canada have prohibited its use by consumers, so its main use remains as an industrial wood preservative in North America and other countries.

Because it is a solid at all but the highest temperatures, exposure to pentachlorophenol is mainly through dermal contact although absorption and inhalation exposure could theoretically occur if it is burned. Pentachlorophenol exposure by workers occurs during its manufacture; the spraying or mixing of pentachlorophenol as a pesticide; its application to wood as a preservative and during treatment of leather, pelts, or textiles; its presence in incinerated waste; and skin contact with materials already treated with pentachlorophenol. Because pentachlorophenol is a persistent organic pollutant, nonoccupational exposure occurs mainly through dietary ingestion, as the chemical bioaccumulates in the food chain.

D. 1,3-butadiene

1,3-butadiene is a compound used in the production of synthetic rubbers and polymers, which form components in the manufacture of a wide variety of industrial and consumer products, such as automobiles, appliance parts, construction materials, computers, telecommunication equipment, protective clothing, and various packaging and household articles. Occupational exposure to 1,3-butadiene can occur in many different manufacturing processes, such as petroleum refining, manufacture of butadiene monomer, and plastics and rubber manufacture.

The major evidence linking 1,3-butadiene to NHL comes from three cohort studies of workers at butadiene monomer production facilities, especially in workers employed during World War II when exposure levels were likely higher than in later years. The results from these studies are compelling as the workers, overall, had lower standardized mortality ratios for all-cause death than the general population, indicating that the workers were otherwise relatively healthy; and because in one study, hematolymphatic neoplasms, and in the two others, NHL specifically, were the only causes of death that were significantly elevated in the workers.

E. Glyphosate

The pesticide glyphosate has been deemed by IARC as probably the most heavily used herbicide in the world. It was first introduced for use in 1974 and is now found in more than 750 different products in the United States alone. It is primarily sprayed by large-scale agricultural establishments to control weed growth. Its use increased dramatically in recent years after the introduction of glyphosate-resistant crops in 1996 and the rise in non till farming practices that require more intensive weed control. Residential use of glyphosate for home gardens is also very widespread.

Occupations with potential exposure to glyphosate include pesticide handlers and agricultural workers coming into contact with glyphosate-treated crops. The main routes of exposure to glyphosate are inhalation and dermal exposure. Ingestion of foods with glyphosate residues is another potential, although less likely, route.

Glyphosate has been found to be significantly associated with an increased risk of NHL in several case-control studies, although a recent prospective cohort study found no association between glyphosate and any solid tumors or lymphoid malignancies overall, including NHL and its subtypes. Mechanistic studies have shown that glyphosate may induce DNA damage, oxidative stress, inflammation, and immunosuppression, as well as modulate cell proliferation and death and disrupt sex hormone pathways. A recent study has shown that glyphosate treatment, either at a chronic low dose or acute high doses, upregulates the expression of activation-induced cytidine deaminase (a B cell-specific genome mutator and a key pathogenic player in MM and NHL) in the bone marrow and spleen of mice. This mechanistic data strengthens the evidence that glyphosate increases the risk of B-cell lymphoid neoplasms.

▶ Pathology & Pathophysiology

Lindane is thought to exert its carcinogenic effects through systemic immunosuppressive effects and by inducing oxidative stress in lymphocytes. There is moderate, but uncertain, evidence that lindane is genotoxic, inducing chromosomal aberrations that may predispose to future cancers.

There is strong evidence that both pentachlorophenol and 1,3-butadiene act through genotoxic mechanisms. Pentachlorophenol also is thought to induce oxidative stress, alter cell proliferation and cell death mechanisms, and act through immunosuppressive and chronic inflammatory mechanisms.

There is strong evidence that glyphosate is mediated through genotoxic and oxidative stress mechanisms.

As discussed in section Leukemias, there are likely multiple mechanisms by which benzene induces leukemia and other blood disorders.

▶ Clinical Findings

A. Symptoms and Signs

Symptoms of NHL are varied and depend on site of origin and aggressiveness. Enlarged lymph nodes, chills, sweats, weight loss, and fatigue are common harbingers of disease. Lymphomas can originate in the chest, abdomen, brain, and skin, causing local symptoms. So-called "B symptoms" in certain types of lymphoma include relapsing-remitting fever, drenching night sweats, and unintentional weight loss. Physical examination can demonstrate enlarged lymph nodes under the skin, abdominal masses or hepatosplenomegaly, respiratory compromise, or focal neurologic symptoms.

B. Laboratory Findings

Blood tests can show anemia, leukopenia, thrombocytopenia, or pancytopenia. An elevated LDH also is often seen and measuring its levels can aid in both diagnosis and as a prognostic marker.

C. Imaging and Diagnosis

Definitive diagnosis of NHL is made through lymph node biopsy, usually consisting of surgical excision of a part of or the entire node. Needle aspiration is seldom done due to the risk of a lack of adequate tissue for definitive diagnosis.

▶ Medical Surveillance & Prevention

There are no validated screening tests for NHL. It is unknown whether certain workers with significant histories of exposure to lindane, pentachlorophenol, glyphosate, or benzene would benefit from medical surveillance, including periodic physical examinations and complete blood counts.

The most effective means of preventing occupational NHL is clearly to stop using carcinogens that could cause NHL in industrial processes. Otherwise, employers still using lindane, pentachlorophenol, and other potential NHL carcinogens should lower air concentrations to the lowest levels feasible, implement engineering controls, and require respiratory and skin protection.

▶ Treatment & Prognosis

NHL treatment varies by the specific subtype of lymphoma, but in most cases consists of chemotherapy, immunotherapy, radiation, or a combination of these modalities.

Roughly 40% of all NHL patients are diagnosed while still in Stage I or II disease, with 50% classified as Stage III-IV. Overall, 72% of US patients diagnosed with NHL survive 5 years after diagnosis, with five-year survival rates ranging from 62% for Stage IV disease to 83% for Stage I disease.

Table 24–5. Toxic agents associated with isolated thrombocytopenia.

Toxic Agent	Use	Mechanism
Toluene diisocyanate	Polymerizing agent	Immune
2,2-Dichlorovinyl dimethylphosphate	Insecticide	Megakaryocyte hypoplasia
Dieldrin		
Pyrethrin		
Hexachlorocyclohexane (lindane)		
Chlorophenothane (DDT)		
Turpentine	Organic solvent	Immune
Vinyl chloride	Plastics	Liver insufficiency with hypersplenism

TOXIC THROMBOCYTOPENIA

Unlike thrombocytopenia occurring as part of toxicant-induced aplastic anemia, isolated toxic thrombocytopenia occurs only rarely. A number of toxic exposures have been reported that resulted in isolated thrombocytopenia (Table 24–5). The pathophysiologic defect was enhanced peripheral platelet destruction, presumably on an immune basis (immune thrombocytopenic purpura). Benzene also causes thrombocytopenia in both isolated form and as part of a multi- or pancytopenia.

Some insecticides occasionally appear to cause a selective megakaryocyte aplasia in individuals with significant inhalation or ingestion exposure. Isolated thrombocytopenia has been reported after exposure to 2,2-dichlorovinyl dimethyl phosphate, dieldrin, pyrethrin, hexachlorocyclohexane (lindane), and chlorophenothane (DDT). These patients demonstrated absent or decreased bone marrow megakaryocytes. The likely pathophysiologic mechanism of thrombocytopenia appeared to be enhanced peripheral platelet consumption caused by hypersplenism.

Normal hemostasis depends both on the quantity of platelets present and on their ability to aggregate appropriately under physiologic stimulation. Qualitative disturbances in platelet function as a result of various occupational and environmental substances have been described. Some pesticides, such as p,p-DDE (2,2-bis-[p-chlorophenyl]-1,1-dichloroethylene) and Aroclor 1242 (a chlorinated biphenyl that is 42% chlorine), inhibit platelet aggregation in a dose-dependent manner by inhibiting platelet cyclooxygenase activity (an aspirin-like effect). Exposures to these substances could cause mucocutaneous bleeding in susceptible individuals. On the other hand, some environmental substances (eg, methyl mercury, cadmium, and triethyl lead) induce platelet aggregation and could result in hypercoagulation. These qualitative platelet disturbances have not yet been reported in humans subject to occupational exposure and remain theoretical risks.

REFERENCES

IARC: Benzene. Volume 120, 2018. http://publications.iarc.fr/.
Kuivenhoven M, Mason K: Arsenic (Arsine) Toxicity. StatPearls [Internet]. Treasure Island (FL): StatPearls Publishing. 2019, Apr 29.
Mitra P, Sharma S, Purohit P, Sharma P: Clinical and molecular aspects of lead toxicity: an update. Crit Rev Clin Lab Sci 2017;54(7-8):506-528 [PMID: 29214886].
Stölzel U, Doss MO, Schuppan D: Clinical guide and update on porphyrias. Gastroenterol 2019;157(2):365-381.e4 [PMID: 31085196].

■ SELF-ASSESSMENT QUESTIONS

Select the one correct answer for each question.

Question 1: Methemoglobin
 a. is like sulfhemoglobin since it is irreversibly associated with the heme moiety
 b. is dangerous because of its ability to bind oxygen
 c. decreases the oxygen affinity of heme groups in hemoglobin
 d. decreases oxygen delivery to the tissues

Question 2: Porphyrias
 a. are a group of disorders characterized by bluish discoloration of the skin
 b. result in the abnormal accumulation of hemoglobin in the skin
 c. are genetic disorders that affect only royal families
 d. can occur as a result of inappropriate overstimulation of δ aminolevulinic acid synthetase

Question 3: Acute intermittent porphyria causes
 a. symptoms and signs quite different than those associated with lead intoxication
 b. a classic triad of abdominal pain, constipation, and jaundice
 c. an increase in neuropsychiatric signs compared with lead intoxication
 d. a more pronounced anemia than occurs with lead intoxication

Question 4: Aplastic anemia
a. is distinct from medullary aplasia and secondary aplastic anemia
b. is largely an hereditary abnormality of the pluripotent hematopoietic stem cells
c. results in pancytopenia (anemia, neutropenia, and thrombocytopenia)
d. cases are largely caused by hereditary diseases

Question 5: Myelodysplastic syndromes
a. are a group of acquired nongenetic disorders of the blood-forming cells
b. are characterized by ineffective hematopoiesis
c. are characterized by a bizarre hematopoietic morphology confirming cancer
d. have in nearly all cases a progression to frank leukemia

Question 6: Multiple myeloma
a. is an acute leukemia of differentiated B cells (termed *plasma cells*)
b. accounts for 50% of all hematologic cancers
c. is characterized by anemia, painful lytic and osteopenic bone disease
d. has a long survival rate

Occupational Cancer

Sammy Almashat, MD, MPH

Robert Harrison, MD, MPH

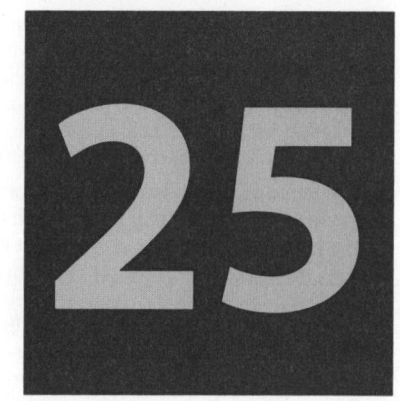

Millions of US workers are exposed to substances that are known to cause cancer in humans. The National Institute for Occupational Safety and Health (NIOSH) has estimated that 3–6% of cancers worldwide are caused by occupational exposures and that 46,000–92,000 US workers are afflicted with cancer due to past workplace exposures every year.

The identification of occupational carcinogens is important in part because most occupational cancers are completely preventable with appropriate exposure controls, personnel practices, and strict protective legislation. NIOSH has concluded that for carcinogens that are directly genotoxic, there is no threshold exposure level below which cancer risk disappears and, for others with indirect genotoxic or nongenotoxic mechanisms, while there may be a safe exposure threshold, such a threshold is typically very difficult to prove empirically.

DETERMINATION OF CARCINOGENICITY

Several governmental agencies and other organizations determine the carcinogenicity of chemical agents. The primary agencies are the International Agency for Research on Cancer (IARC), the National Toxicology Program (NTP) of the U.S. Public Health Service, the NIOSH, the American Conference of Governmental Industrial Hygienists (ACGIH), and, in California, the Office of Environmental Health Hazard Assessment (OEHHA) of the California Environmental Protection Agency (EPA), which determines those chemicals to be included on the list of chemicals known to the state to cause cancer pursuant to the Safe Drinking Water and Toxic Enforcement Act of 1986 ("Proposition 65").

The *IARC Monographs on the Evaluation of Carcinogenic Risks to Humans* are published by the World Health Organization's (WHO) IARC. Each monograph represents the consensus of an international working group of expert scientists. The monographs include a critical review of the pertinent peer-reviewed scientific literature as the basis for an evaluation of the weight of the evidence that an agent may be carcinogenic to humans. Published continuously since 1972, the scope of the monographs has expanded beyond chemicals to include complex mixtures, occupational exposures, lifestyle factors, physical and biological agents, and other potentially carcinogenic exposures. Through 2017, IARC had classified 47 occupational chemicals and other substances as "carcinogenic to humans" (group 1 classification) and at least an additional 19 as "probably carcinogenic to humans" (group 2A classification). Unfortunately, IARC has to-date evaluated less than 2% of chemicals manufactured or processed in the United States for carcinogenicity, meaning that virtually all chemicals to which workers are exposed on a daily basis are of unknown carcinogenic potential.

IARC classifies agents in five categories:

Group 1: Agents that are carcinogenic to humans

Group 2A: Agents that are probably carcinogenic to humans (agents for which there is limited evidence of carcinogenicity in humans and sufficient evidence of carcinogenicity in experimental animals)

Group 2B: Agents that are possibly carcinogenic to humans (agents for which there is limited evidence of carcinogenicity in humans and an absence of sufficient evidence of carcinogenicity in animals, or when there is inadequate evidence of carcinogenicity in humans, but there is sufficient evidence of carcinogenicity in experimental animals)

Group 3: Agents that are not classifiable as to carcinogenicity in humans (agents that do not fall in any other group)

Group 4: Agents that are probably not carcinogenic to humans (agents for which there is evidence suggesting lack of carcinogenicity in humans together with evidence suggesting lack of carcinogenicity in experimental animals)

The NTP of the U.S. Public Health Service categorizes chemicals of carcinogenic potential in two groups:

1. Chemicals known to be carcinogens (chemicals for which there is sufficient evidence of carcinogenicity from studies in humans, which indicates a causal relationship between the agent and human cancer)

2. Chemicals that are reasonably anticipated to be carcinogens. Chemicals are so categorized where:
(a) There is limited evidence of carcinogenicity from studies in humans, which indicates that causal interpretation is credible, but that alternative explanations, such as change, bias or confounding, could not adequately be excluded.

(b) There is sufficient evidence of carcinogenicity from studies in experimental animals, which indicates that there is an increased incidence of malignant tumors: (1) in multiple species or strains, or (2) in multiple experiments, or (3) to an unusual degree with regard to incidence, site or type of tumor, or age of onset. Additional evidence may be provided by data concerning dose-response effects, as well as information on mutagenicity or chemical structure.

For the US Occupational Safety and Health Administration (OSHA), a "potential occupational carcinogen means any substance, or combination or mixture of substances, which causes an increased incidence of benign and/or malignant neoplasms, or a substantial decrease in the latency period between exposure and onset of neoplasms in humans or in one or more experimental mammalian species as the result of any oral, respiratory, or dermal exposure, or any other exposure which results in the induction of tumors at a site other than the site of administration. This definition also includes any substance which is metabolized into one or more potential occupational carcinogens by mammals."

The Office of Environmental Health Hazard Assessment (OEHHA) of the California EPA identifies chemical agents that are known to the state to cause cancer and reproductive toxicity. Pursuant to the mandate of Proposition 65, the governor publishes a list of those chemicals so identified, which is commonly referred to as the "Proposition 65 list."

CARCINOGENESIS: CAUSES & FUNDAMENTAL PROPERTIES

The majority of cancers are multifactorial in etiology, the result of a combination of genetic and nongenetic factors. Genetic factors alone are estimated to cause only about 5% of cancers. Nongenetic factors, sometimes referred to as environmental factors, account for the majority of cancers. They include lifestyle factors such as tobacco use, alcohol consumption, poor diet, obesity, physical inactivity, and occupational and consumer exposures to myriad chemicals and product formulations, which collectively contribute to the occurrence of a substantial proportion of cancers.

Evidence suggests that cancers arise from a single abnormal cell. The initial stage in development of the abnormal cell appears to result from an alteration or mutation in the genetic material, deoxyribonucleic acid (DNA). This alteration may occur spontaneously or may be caused by exogenous factors, such as exposure to carcinogenic chemicals or radiation. Whether a tumor develops from this altered cell may depend on a variety of factors, such as the ability of the cell to repair the damage, the presence of other endogenous

or exogenous agents that foster or inhibit tumor development, and the integrity of the immune system.

Stages in Tumor Development

A variety of evidence indicates that cells undergo multiple heritable changes in the process of becoming a "cancer cell"; this process is termed *carcinogenesis*. Early animal studies investigating the etiology of cancer cell growth hypothesized that tumor development involved at least two distinct stages: initiation and promotion. A classic example of this process is the mouse skin tumor model. In this model, a small dose of a carcinogen, known as the *initiator* (in this case, typically a polycyclic aromatic hydrocarbon [PAH]) is applied to the skin. Although large doses of PAHs alone readily induced skin tumors, the smaller doses alone did not. However, application of a *promoter*, such as croton oil, following application of the initiator did result in tumor development. Clearly, there are limitations to the application of animal models of tumorigenesis to the etiology of common human tumors. However, these data have provided a framework to understand basic toxin-induced carcinogenesis (Figure 25–1).

Carcinogenesis is a multistep process including initiation, promotion, and progression. Initiation is thought to result from an irreversible change in the genetic material (DNA) of the cell arising from interaction with a carcinogen that is a necessary, but not sufficient, condition for tumor development. It is this somatic mutation that sets the stage for tumor development and is the basis for the somatic mutation theory of carcinogenesis.

Promotion consists of those processes subsequent to initiation that facilitate tumor development, presumably by stimulating proliferation of the altered cell. The mechanisms of promotion, sometimes referred to as *epigenetic mechanisms* (as opposed to the genotoxic or mutational effects of initiators), are incompletely understood. Promotion classically does not result from binding to and alteration of DNA but may result from production of or suppression of proteins that alter the way that DNA is transcribed. Promotion typically yields a benign tumor or group of preneoplastic cells that do not have the ability to invade stroma or metastasize; progression then creates those additional heritable changes necessary for the development of a malignant tumor.

Carcinogens are often divided into initiating agents, or genotoxic (DNA-reactive) "early stage" carcinogens, and promoting agents, or epigenetic "late stage" carcinogens. Table 25–1 lists the distinguishing features of initiating and promoting agents. Some agents (eg, cigarette smoke or asbestos) that seem to possess both initiating and promoting properties are termed *complete carcinogens*. However, it is also clear that damage from cigarette smoking may set the stage for a multiplicative relationship to carcinogenesis with exposure to carcinogens such as asbestos or nickel. Given the complexity of the multistage model and increasing experimental evidence that tends to blur the distinction between these categories, the value of categorizing specific agents probably is limited. In addition, owing to the time

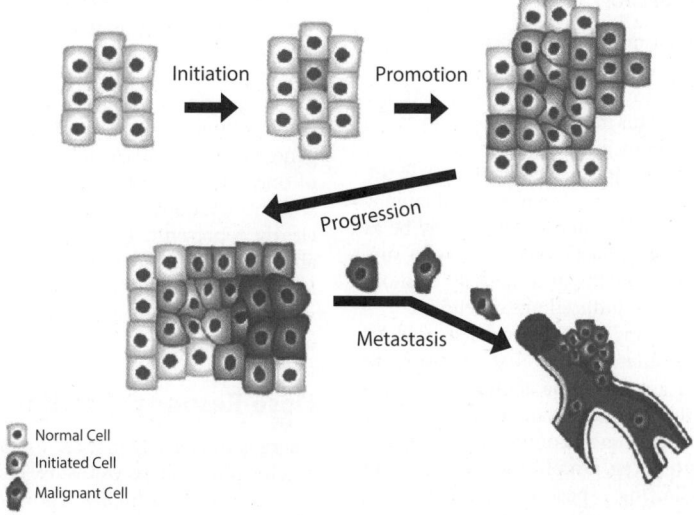

Normal Cell
Initiated Cell
Malignant Cell

▲ **Figure 25–1.** Carcinogenesis progression.

from exposure to an initiating agent to the subsequent development of visible cancer, identification of possible causal agents or contributing factors may be extremely difficult.

The mechanism by which carcinogen-induced alteration in DNA leads to initiation and ultimately to tumor development is related at least in part to mutations in protooncogenes and tumor-suppressor genes. Protooncogenes contain DNA sequences that, when altered by a mutational event into an oncogene, stimulate transformation and proliferation of an altered potentially neoplastic cell. In contrast, tumor-suppressor genes function as negative regulators of cell growth. A genetic change in one or more tumor-suppressor genes, which results in inactivation of a specific gene, may allow unregulated growth of the altered cell. The observation in experimental animals that tumors develop only after activation of one or more oncogenes and inactivation of one or more tumor-suppressor genes provides a mechanistic explanation for the multistep model of carcinogenesis.

For most toxic effects, the persistence or progression of damage requires the continued presence of the offending chemical agent. For cancer initiators, however, relatively short-term exposure in humans may, based on the results of animal studies, induce genetic damage in the cell sufficient to ultimately result in tumor development years after exposure has ceased.

Table 25–1. Distinctions between initiators and promoters of carcinogenesis.

Initiators	Promoters
Genotoxic	Not genotoxic; epigenetic mechanism
Carcinogenic alone	Not carcinogenic alone; active only after initiator exposure
Generally yield electrophilic compounds; highly reactive (often form free radicals)	Not electrophilic
Covalently bind to nucleophiles (eg, DNA), leading to irreversible alteration in genetic material	Generally do not bind to nor alter DNA; often act by induction of cellular proliferation; effects may be reversible
Generally active in short-term tests (mutagenic)	Not active in short-term tests
Existence of threshold dose cannot be verified	Threshold probably exists
Single exposure may be sufficient to induce subsequent cancer	Repeated exposures required

Induction-Latency Period

In both experimental animal models of cancer and human cancers with known causes, a significant interval of time is required from first exposure to the responsible agent to the development of malignancy. This interval is referred to as the *induction-latency* (or sometimes just *latency*) or *incubation period*. The requirement for multiple heritable changes in the cell may be at least partly responsible for prolonged latency intervals. Length of the induction-latency period may be as short as 2 years for radiation-induced leukemia (as in survivors of atomic bomb explosions) to as long as 40 or more years for some cases of asbestos-induced mesothelioma.

For solid tumors in humans thought to be caused by exposures, the minimum latency from first exposure to clinical evidence of cancer appears to be about 10–12 years or more. In contrast to the prolonged latency required for solid tumors, exposure-related cancers of the blood (eg, leukemia) and lymphatic system (eg, lymphoma) generally are seen within 3–7 years following exposure. Slower-growing hematologic cancers (eg, myelodysplasia or low-grade lymphomas) may be more delayed in appearance. The relatively long period of time may present a challenge for the clinician to uncover the relationship between a remote exposure and a newly found tumor.

THE QUESTION OF THRESHOLDS

Many toxic agents result in known adverse effects only when the exposure is above a certain threshold dose or duration. If this threshold dose is not exceeded, there are no demonstrable consequences to the health of the animal or human. With carcinogens, it is much more difficult to determine if such a threshold exists. Theoretically, if no threshold exists, there is no dose (other than zero) at which the incremental risk of cancer is zero.

Scientific evidence shows strong evidence for, and regulatory agencies generally accept, the nonthreshold model. Given that a single alteration (mutation) in DNA in one cell may set the stage for tumor development, it is theoretically possible that exposure of the cell to only one molecule of a carcinogen ultimately could lead to tumor formation. Although the probability of tumor formation tends to increase with increasing frequency and magnitude of exposure to the carcinogen, a single small exposure might be sufficient. For example, in the mouse skin tumor model described earlier, a single high-level exposure to a PAH has been shown to be capable of inducing a tumor. The NIOSH and other public health agencies typically evaluate risks with the assumption that there are no demonstrable thresholds for carcinogens. Many agencies, such as the United States Environmental Protection Agency (US EPA), set an allowable level of exposure at lifetime doses that theoretically would increase risk by an "acceptable" level, usually stated to be at 1 in 10,000 to 1 in 1,000,000. By contrast, worker safety and health regulators have taken a less safety-oriented approach when setting occupational thresholds for known carcinogens for workers.

The US OSHA has not typically set exposure limits for hazardous chemicals based on the compounds' carcinogenicity, instead focusing on noncarcinogenic acute and chronic effects. For all such chemicals, including carcinogens, OSHA has long deemed acceptable a risk of 1 in 1000 excess deaths when setting exposure limits for hazardous chemicals. As a general policy, OSHA has considered a lifetime excess risk of one death or serious illness per 1000 workers associated with occupational exposure over a 45 year working life as clearly representing a significant risk. However, as noted above, Benzene does not require OSHA to use such a rigid or formulaic criterion. Nevertheless, OSHA has taken a conservative approach and has used the 1:1000 example as a useful benchmark for determining significant risk.

Dose-Response Relationships

There is strong evidence for a dose-response effect for many carcinogens, where exposure to larger doses of a specific agent results in a higher risk of developing cancer than do smaller doses. While there has been some debate about the shape of the dose-response curve of carcinogen at relatively low doses of exposure, all major public health and scientific agencies support the view that there is linearity at low doses.

METHODS IN THE ASSESSMENT OF CARCINOGENICITY

Evidence to support the carcinogenicity of a chemical or physical agent for humans may be derived from three basic types of studies: human epidemiologic studies, experimental studies in animals, and mechanistic studies. In addition, structural similarity of a chemical to a known carcinogen may suggest that the agent could be a carcinogen.

Epidemiologic studies can provide unequivocal evidence of a carcinogenic hazard but often are not sufficiently sensitive to identify a carcinogenic hazard except when the risk is high or involves an unusual form of cancer. In addition, the latency period for cancer implies that many years of preventable human exposure would occur before informative epidemiologic studies are available. For these reasons, animal studies often provide the best means of assessing potential risks to humans. To answer questions about the similarity of response between animals and humans, studies of toxicokinetics and mechanisms have been employed. Toxicokinetic studies are done to allow cross-species comparisons of absorption, distribution, metabolism, and elimination but often are done in detail in only one species. Mechanistic studies are aimed at the goal of eventually elucidating the chemical species and cellular processes involved in cancer initiation and development.

In epidemiologic studies there are often limitations in the characterization of exposure, and the ability to identify and adjust for confounding exposures or genetic susceptibility. As a result, epidemiologic studies find associations between exposure and disease outcome but should not solely be used to conclude if these associations are causal. Statistically significant epidemiologic studies also require large populations of workers and other persons exposed to the toxicant at issue to reveal small but important effects of toxic chemicals. For many chemicals suspected to be causative of uncommon cancers, there are no sufficiently large populations of exposed workers to conduct epidemiologic studies that have sufficient statistical power to be scientifically valid.

Various toxic chemicals have been accepted within the medical community as causes of human disease, including cancer, even though there have been no epidemiologic studies conducted, which confirm or negate such causal associations due to the unavailability of sufficiently large populations to conduct scientifically valid epidemiologic studies, because other toxicologic evidence (eg, case reports, animal studies) exist, which sufficiently support such a causal association. Case reports and descriptive epidemiologic studies or case series may be used to elucidate causality, especially where the disease outcome in relatively rare. For example, mesothelioma (asbestos exposure) and angiosarcoma (vinyl chloride exposure) were initially described in case reports and series. In instances where exposure to a known carcinogen is demonstrated and there is a likely mechanism of disease, additional large-scale epidemiologic studies may not be needed to take to reduce/eliminate ongoing exposure and prevent further disease.

Moreover, epidemiologic studies require that cancer has already occurred, when it is more desirable to identify potential carcinogenic substances at an earlier stage before they have caused a large number of malignancies and thus become identifiable by epidemiologic studies. In this context, experimental animal studies and bioassays are very useful tools to identify human carcinogens and take public health action to prevent occupational and environmental exposures. IARC also considers mechanistic studies as an aide in interpreting the results of positive animal bioassays, and the US National Cancer Institute has found that epidemiology, animal, tissue culture, and molecular pathology should be seen as integrating evidences in the determination of human carcinogenicity.

Results from well-conducted animal bioassays can yield clear evidence to support the carcinogenicity of a compound in a particular animal species and have served as good predictors of human carcinogenicity. A large number of agents now known to be human carcinogens were first discovered to be carcinogenic in animals. Available evidence suggests that there is good correlation between animal and human results. As IARC stated in its preamble:

Although this association [between animal and human evidence] cannot establish that all agents that cause cancer in experimental animals also cause cancer in humans, it is biologically plausible that agents for which there is sufficient evidence of carcinogenicity in experimental animals (see Part B, Section 6b) also present a carcinogenic hazard to humans. Accordingly, in the absence of additional scientific information, these agents are considered to pose a carcinogenic hazard to humans.

In addition, IARC observes that "all known human carcinogens that have been studied adequately for carcinogenicity in experimental animals have produced positive results in one or more animal species."

IMPLICATIONS FOR REGULATORY ACTION & PREVENTIVE MEDICINE

When a sufficient body of evidence supporting carcinogenicity in humans exists, corrective action to protect public and worker health should proceed, even if there is some remaining uncertainty in the conclusions. Sufficient evidence of carcinogenicity in humans should prompt immediate protective interventions. Convincingly positive results from a well-conducted epidemiologic study or sufficient evidence of carcinogenicity in animals, as defined by IARC or NTP, should prompt attempts to reduce worker exposure as much as possible. The finding of limited evidence in animal bioassays or positive results in short-term tests should serve as a stimulus for further study of the suspect chemical. When the results in different studies are contradictory, results suggesting carcinogenicity generally outweigh the negative evidence. Given the limited sensitivity of epidemiologic methods, this principle for managing exposures should be considered when animal studies are clearly positive while epidemiologic studies do not appear to show increased risks (the precautionary principle).

Industry organizations, relying upon recommendations from occupational health and toxicology professionals, have the obligation, when warranted by the state of the evidence, to go further than the regulations require in using information regarding carcinogenicity to make decisions about chemical use and control. Unfortunately they rarely do so. On the contrary, industries may create uncertainty about scientific methods in order to delay any action that may affect their financial interests. For example, decisions to avoid the use of chemicals in IARC groups 1 and 2A (or those with evidence that would likely place them in these categories) or, alternatively, to tightly control exposures to these agents (to completely prevent exposure) would lead to reductions in the risk for occupational cancers. Pressure applied by chemical users on chemical manufacturers to study suspect chemicals and to develop safe alternatives to potential carcinogens is another effective approach to prevention of occupational and environmental cancer. Additionally, proper hazard communication should inform workers of potential carcinogens in their work area and provide them with the training and tools to prevent or minimize exposure.

Exposure to known or suspected carcinogens has probably declined in the United States and other economically developed countries as a result of both regulations that control exposure and changes in the chemicals produced and used and in the methods of production. Unfortunately, exposures to carcinogens in some developing countries are increasing in frequency and intensity. When measurements exist and are reported for workers in developing countries, exposure levels in given industries to carcinogens tend to be considerably higher than in developed countries. The transfer of hazardous industries to developing countries likely has further increased carcinogen exposure for workers in these countries. Recognizing the reduced ability of many developing countries to regulate these hazards effectively, it is incumbent on industrial concerns from developed nations to attempt to control these hazards for their workers (or contract workers) in developing countries.

IMPLICATIONS FOR CLINICAL PRACTICE

Medical Surveillance

The role of medical surveillance in workers currently or previously exposed to known or suspected carcinogens should follow well-established principles. Surveillance of populations at high risk of cancer is effective only if the screening test is sensitive and easy to perform, if it detects premalignant abnormalities or tumors at an early stage in their development, and if there is an effective intervention that reduces morbidity and mortality when applied to individuals at risk. For certain tumors not known to be associated with chemical exposures (eg, cervical cancer), screening techniques and effective therapy for early lesions have had a significant impact on the disease. There is some evidence that workers at high risk of bladder tumors, as a result of prior exposure to aromatic amines used in dyestuff manufacturing, can benefit from early detection by the use of urine cytology and cystoscopy as screening tools. The finding in the National Lung Screening Trial that screening of current and former high-risk cigarette smokers (≥ 30 pack year history) with low-dose computed tomographic (CT) scans reduced mortality from lung cancer by 20% raises the possibility that use of these tests might ultimately play a role in the screening of high-risk groups exposed to other carcinogens.

Despite these limitations, properly collected medical surveillance data combined with industrial hygiene data collection may prove useful in future epidemiologic studies and in the refinement of our knowledge regarding human dose-response relationships. If medical surveillance is to be performed, the protocol should be designed for each agent of concern based on the presumed target site from prior human and animal studies and the availability of screening tools. In practice, medical surveillance is required by OSHA standards for asbestos, arsenic, benzene, and a variety of other carcinogens, as listed in Table 25–2.

Determination of Cancer Causation

The practice of occupational medicine sometimes requires an assessment as to whether a cancer in an exposed worker is causally related to an exposure at work or to exposure. Such an assessment may occur informally in discussion with a concerned affected employee or more formally in the setting of a workers' compensation claim or toxic tort case.

The issue whether exposure to a particular chemical or class of chemicals can cause a particular disease is a scientific

Table 25–2. Carcinogens for which medical surveillance is required.

2-Acetylaminofluorene
Acrylonitrile
4-Aminodiphenyl
Arsenic (inorganic)
Asbestos
Benzene
Benzidine (and its salts)
Bis(chloromethyl) ether (BCME)
1,3-Butadiene
Cadmium
Coke oven emissions
1,2-Dibromo-3-chloropropane (DBCP)
3,3'-Dichlorobenzidine (and its salts)
4-Dimethylaminoazobenzene
Ethyleneimine
Ethylene dibromide (EDB)
Ethylene oxide
Formaldehyde[3]
Lead
4,4'-Methylelene-bis(2-chloroaniline) (MOCA)
Methylene chloride
Methyl chloromethyl ether (chloromethyl methyl ether [CMME])
Methylenedianiline (MDA)
α-Naphthylamine
β-Naphthylamine
4-Nitrobiphenyl
N-Nitrosodimethylamine
β-Propiolactone
Vinyl chloride

issue often referred to as "general causation," as opposed to "specific causation," which addresses the issue whether a particular chemical or class of chemicals caused a particular disease in a particular person.

The determination of general causation is a complex undertaking because such an endeavor requires extensive research in such fields of science as epidemiology, biostatistics, toxicology, pathology, molecular biology, carcinogenesis, cytogenetics, and other fields of medicine related to the particular disease of interest. The clinician or expert should consider published epidemiologic reports, as well as all relevant data, including human case reports, animal data, experimental studies, laboratory data, mechanistic data, and other types of data as well, including unpublished studies. It is important in this context to (1) identify all relevant studies, (2) read and critically evaluate all the relevant studies, (3) evaluate all the data based upon recognized scientific factors (the Bradford Hill viewpoints) and other factors relevant to the chemical and the disease; (4) exercise best professional judgment in reaching a conclusion on the issue of whether a particular chemical or class of chemicals can cause a particular disease; and (5) explain the factual basis and the reasoning supporting the conclusion.

Various authorities, beginning with Sir Austin Bradford Hill in 1965 and more recently IARC, have established viewpoints for evaluating causation from epidemiologic studies and assessing the degree of evidence supporting the designation of an agent as a carcinogen:

(a) *Consistency of the observed association.* A pattern of elevated risks observed across several independent studies would support or strengthen an inference of causality. Reproducibility of findings constitutes one of the strongest arguments for causality.

(b) *Strength of the observed association.* The finding of large, precise risks increases confidence that an association is not likely due to chance, bias, or confounding factors. A modest risk, however, does not preclude a causal association and may reflect a lower level of exposure, an agent of lower potency, or a common disease (eg, when there is a relatively high incidence rate of a disease in the general population, it is more difficult to reach a doubling of that incidence rate).

(c) *Specificity of the observed association.* As originally described, this refers to a single cause associated with a single effect. multiple causes. Thus, although the presence of specificity supports causality, its absence does not exclude it.

(d) *Temporal relationship of the observed association.* A causal interpretation is strengthened when exposure is known to precede development of the disease. Because some cancers have a latent period of 20 years or longer, it is important to ascertain whether the study included sufficient follow-up time after exposure.

(e) *Biological gradient (exposure-response relationship).* A clear exposure-response relationship (ie, increasing effects associated with increasing exposure) strongly suggests cause and effect, especially when such relationships are observed for both level and duration of exposure. Because an epidemiologic study may fail to detect an exposure-response relationship for several reasons (eg, a small range of observed exposure levels or exposure misclassification), the absence of an exposure-response relationship does not exclude a causal relationship.

(f) *Biological plausibility.* An inference of causality is strengthened by consistency with experimental data that show plausible biological mechanisms. A lack of mechanistic data, however, is not a reason to reject causality.

(g) *Coherence.* Other lines of evidence, for example experimental animal studies, toxicokinetic studies, short-term tests, and mechanistic studies, may strengthen an inference of causality. The absence of other lines of evidence, however, is not a reason to reject causality.

(h) *Experimental evidence (from human populations).* Experimental evidence is seldom available from human populations and exists only when conditions of human exposure are altered to create a "natural experiment" at different levels of exposure, or for medical treatments tested in randomized controlled trials with a sufficient follow-up period. Strong evidence for causality can be provided when a change in exposure brings about a change in disease frequency, for example, the decrease in lung cancer risk that follows cessation of smoking.

(i) *Analogy.* Evidence for causality can be strengthened by information on an agent's structural analogues.

Bradford Hill's viewpoints have been widely accepted in the scientific community. Scientific bodies that use most or all of these principles include the WHO, the IARC, the US EPA, the ACGIH, and the US Surgeon General.

Only one of Bradford Hill's factors, temporality, is essential to causality because exposure must precede the disease for exposure to be a factor in causing the disease.

In reaching an opinion regarding specific causation, the clinician or expert should follow standard methodology in the field of occupational medicine, which includes the abstraction and evaluation of medical records; evaluation of potential alternative causes for the claimed injury; analysis of diagnostic errors, including highlighting failures of differential diagnosis; evaluation of the extent of the exposure to the agent(s); and examination of temporal relationships, including latency.

Some of the same factors used in the assessment of the work-relatedness of any illness, largely derived from the medical and occupational history and medical, employment, and exposure records, are important in the assessment of a possible occupational cancer. It is critical to assess, to the extent possible, the nature of the agents involved and the intensity, setting, control, timing, and duration of the exposures, and other sources of exposure. Potential sources for this information include the individual, coworkers and managers, material safety data sheets or other sources of chemical use information, and if available, industrial hygiene data. Knowledge of the presence or absence of other symptoms or conditions that may be due to exposures may be helpful in establishing that substantial exposure had occurred. For some industries, there may be published exposure-assessment and dose-effect information. From these sources it may be possible to derive a qualitative or semiquantitative sense of the intensity, timing, and duration, as well as the potential health significance, of the exposures.

The medical history and medical records provide information about the cancer site and cell type and the presence of any other known risk factors for the cancer. Physical examination may be helpful, by demonstrating physical findings suggestive of other conditions associated with the exposure or other risk factors.

With the rare exception of certain tumors, such as mesotheliomas that almost universally stem from asbestos exposure, there is generally little about the appearance or behavior of a particular cancer that allows differentiation between work-related and spontaneous etiologies. The occurrence of some pathologic types of cancer may suggest a particular etiology.

Literature review can provide the descriptive epidemiology of the tumor type, including age, sex, and racial patterns of incidence, as well as information regarding known nonoccupational risk factors for the tumor type. Synthesis of this information first involves assessment of the quality of the epidemiologic and animal experimental evidence using the criteria discussed earlier.

All of the above information may be useful in developing a "differential assessment" of potential causative factors in an individual, akin to a differential diagnosis. In addition to an analysis of exposures, demographic features, latency period, and nonoccupational risk factors in the affected individual need to be factored into the assessment of causation.

In firefighters and police officers, there may be legislated presumptions in workers' compensation cases that cancers occurring during or after employment are considered to be work related. When such individuals, exposed to an agent known to be capable of causing cancer in humans, develop a cancer, it is presumed that the exposure caused the cancer unless there is evidence indicating that there is no "reasonable link" between the exposure and the cancer (thus the term, rebuttable presumption).

In workers' compensation and toxic tort cases, the standard of proof generally is reasonable medical probability (ie, that the exposure more likely than not caused the medical condition). Possible connections are not sufficient to establish causation.

Outside the medical/legal context, groups of employees may express concerns about whether they are at risk of developing cancer because of specific workplace exposures. Evaluation of these concerns initially involves similar assessments of the potential for general and specific causation related to the exposures. Risk communication efforts are then warranted to share meaningful information and provide perspective about possible risks. Application of the principles of risk communication, informed by scientific information and an understanding of the nature and magnitude of exposures, may help to interpret risk and to provide advice and reassurance, when appropriate.

Possible clusters of cancer in a working population pose somewhat different challenges to the occupational physician in terms of investigating causation and communicating risk. *Clusters* are defined as groups of like or similar illnesses, both pathologically and etiologically, aggregated in space and time within a group of individuals with the same occupation. A commonly encountered scenario involves the recognition by a group of workers that two or more individuals in their group have had cancer. The first challenge is to confirm that there is indeed a cluster, perhaps by interviewing members of the group or by reviewing medical records. Individuals may have distinctly different types of tumors that are typically etiologically unrelated (eg, breast cancer, Hodgkin lymphoma, and lung cancer). The individuals may not have shared the same space for very long, or one may have had cancer prior to joining the group. It is also important to assess exposure in the work area and to look for potential sources of exposure to carcinogens or other hazardous chemical or physical agents. If initial investigation does reveal that a true cluster might

exist, the next step is to confirm that the observed incidence exceeds what would have been expected in a population of comparable size and demographics (ie, that the apparent clustering did not occur by chance). This assessment requires appropriate statistical methods, typically using a Poisson distribution for low-frequency data, with comparison to cancer incidence data for a comparable population. There are several published investigations of "true" clusters where no plausible responsible environmental factor could be identified, even when the clusters did not appear to be due to chance. Thus, failure to determine an environmental cause after a thorough investigation should not be surprising. In the absence of known causes for observed clusters of cancer, careful and accurate presentation of the investigation results may help to ease concerns in the workforce.

▼ CLINICAL PRESENTATIONS

LUNG CANCER

ESSENTIALS OF DIAGNOSIS

- ▶ History of exposure to known lung carcinogens, such as asbestos, radon, chloromethyl ethers, PAHs, chromium, nickel, inorganic arsenic exposure, and many other agents.
- ▶ Cigarette smoking or exposure to cigarette smoke.
- ▶ Cough, hemoptysis, dyspnea, weight loss.
- ▶ Mass lesion, pulmonary infiltrate, hilar or mediastinal adenopathy on chest radiograph.
- ▶ Diagnosis usually made with one or more of the following: sputum cytology, bronchoscopy with brushings and biopsy, transthoracic needle biopsy; thoracotomy rarely required.

Occupations at Risk (Partial List)

- Asbestos-exposed workers, including miners, insulators, and shipyard workers
- Workers exposed to radon, for example, uranium miners
- Chemical production workers exposed to chloromethyl ethers
- Workers exposed to diesel exhaust/diesel particulate matter
- Workers exposed to PAHs, for example, aluminum reduction workers, coke oven workers, roofers, and rubber production workers
- Workers exposed to hexavalent chromium compounds, for example, in chromate production
- Workers exposed to nickel compounds, for example, in nickel mining and refining
- Workers exposed to inorganic arsenic compounds, for example, in arsenical pesticide production and use; and in copper, lead, and zinc smelting

▶ General Considerations

Lung cancer is the leading cause of cancer and cancer-related death worldwide, accounting for approximately 12% of new cancer diagnoses and 18% of cancer deaths. It is estimated that 236,000 Americans will be diagnosed with, and 132,000 will die from, lung cancer in 2021. There has been a decline in lung cancer seen most clearly in men; only recently has the decline become apparent among women in the United States. Unfortunately, in many parts of the world, especially in countries with developing economies, cigarette use continues to increase, and along with it, the incidence of lung cancers is also rising. While tobacco smoking remains the primary cause of lung cancer worldwide, more than 60% of new lung cancers occur in never smokers or former smokers, many of whom quit decades ago. Moreover, 1 in 5 women and 1 in 12 men diagnosed with lung cancer have never smoked.

▶ Etiology

Cigarette smoking is the most important and most preventable risk factor for cancer of the lung (and is a major risk factor for a number of other cancers). More than 80% of lung cancer deaths in the United States are attributable to cigarette smoking, although its relative importance may decline if recent trends toward reduced cigarette consumption continue. Secondhand smoke, also known as environmental tobacco smoke (ETS), also causes lung cancer, and occupations with a high smoking prevalence have an increased risk of cancer. This includes construction workers, mining workers, mechanics, drivers, restaurant cooks and servers, and others where smoking prevalence may be higher than 30%.

Exposures at work have been estimated to contribute to 10% of all lung cancer cases. There is a long list of occupational agents proven to be respiratory carcinogens. Those classified by IARC as group 1 carcinogens with sufficient human evidence that they cause lung cancer are arsenic compounds, asbestos, beryllium, bis(chloromethyl) ether, cadmium, chromium (hexavalent), coal tar pitch, nickel compounds, polyaromatic hydrocarbons (coke oven emissions and diesel exhaust), secondhand tobacco smoke, silica (crystalline), soot, and various forms of radiation, including from plutonium and radon-22, and x-radiation, and γ-radiation. Occupational agents suspected of causing lung cancer (including IARC group 2A agents, among others) include acid mists (strong inorganic), acrylonitrile, benzene, bitumens, alpha-chlorinated toluenes and benzoyl chloride (combined exposures), cobalt metal with tungsten carbide, creosotes, diazinon, fibrous silicon carbide, formaldehyde, hydrazine, insecticides (nonarsenical), mustard gas, 2,3,7,8-tetrachlorodibenzo-para-dioxin, talc (possible asbestos contamination in both mining and milling), and vinyl chloride.

Occupations that have been proven or suspected as causing lung cancer include those associated with the Acheson process, aluminum production, coal gasification, coke production, underground hematite mining, iron and steel founding, painting, rubber production, welding, certain types of glass manufacture, carbon electrode manufacture, printing processes, roofing, mastic asphalt work, and those involving close proximity to high-temperature frying. Workers at risk of radiation-related lung cancer include not only those involved in mining or processing uranium but also those exposed in underground mining operations of other ores where radon daughters may be emitted from rock formations.

The association of lung cancer with exposure to most of these agents appears to be independent of cigarette smoking. However, the effects of some known occupational carcinogens are greatly enhanced by smoking (eg, asbestos, radon).

More details on some of the major carcinogens described previously are as follows:

A. Asbestos

Asbestos is the substance generally considered to pose the greatest carcinogenic threat in the workplace. About 125 million people around the world are exposed to asbestos in their work environments, and many millions more workers have been exposed to asbestos in years past. NIOSH has estimated that current occupational exposures to asbestos will cause five deaths from lung cancer in every 1000 workers exposed for a working lifetime. About 20–40% of adult men report past occupations that may have entailed asbestos exposures. In the most highly affected age groups, mesothelioma may account for over 1% of all deaths. In addition to mesothelioma, 5–7% of all lung cancers are potentially attributable to occupational exposures to asbestos.

Asbestos refers to a group of fibrous silicates of several types. The minerals are divided into two classes: serpentine (chrysotile) and amphiboles (amosite, crocidolite, actinolite, anthophyllite, and tremolite). The three most common commercial forms are chrysotile, amosite, and crocidolite. Chrysotile represents 95% of all the asbestos ever used worldwide. All three commonly used forms of asbestos are known to increase the risk of lung cancer. Despite all that is known about the health effects of asbestos and the need for a global ban on production, (asbestos mine), production remains at over 1 million tons. Russia, China, and Kazakhstan are the three leading producers of asbestos.

Lung cancer is a major asbestos-related disease, accounting for 20% of all deaths in asbestos-exposed cohorts. A latency period of approximately 20 years has been noted before the majority of lung cancer cases are seen. Asbestos exposure increases the risk of lung cancer fivefold in nonsmokers. Several studies show evidence that cigarette smokers who were also exposed to asbestos have a much greater risk of developing cancer of the lung, indicating a synergistic effect between these carcinogens.

B. Radon

Radon exposure is known to increase the risk of lung cancer. This carcinogenic effect was discovered when increased mortality rates from lung cancer were identified in uranium miners. Large-scale mining of uranium began in the United States in 1948 because of the need for uranium to make nuclear weapons. By the 1960s, 20% of deaths in uranium miners in the United States were a result of lung disease. Excessive lung cancer in uranium miners is independent of cigarette smoking, although exposure to both is synergistic.

Ores containing uranium include all its decay products, which form a series of radionuclides, of which one is the inert gas radon. Radon diffuses out of the rock into the mine atmosphere, where it decays into radioisotopes of polonium, bismuth, and lead—termed *radon daughters*. These radionuclides are found in the air and then are inhaled as free ions or as attachments to dust particles. Epidemiologic studies of workers in US uranium mines demonstrate that the risk of lung cancer is proportionate to the cumulative radon daughter exposure. Increased risk of lung cancer also has been found in fluorspar miners, iron ore (hematite) miners, and hard-rock miners. Data from animal models support the carcinogenic effect of radon; respiratory tumors can be induced by inhaled radon daughter products.

Domestic radon exposure has been an issue of concern since 1984, when high radon levels were discovered in homes built on the Reading Prong geologic formation in Pennsylvania. The US EPA estimates that 21,000 people die from radon-induced lung cancer each year in the United States, with about 13% of annual US lung cancer deaths. The combined health effects of radon and tobacco exposure are synergistic. The US EPA recommends reducing radon in homes to less than 4 picocuries per liter (pCi/L) of air.

C. Chloromethyl Ethers

Exposure to multiple chemical substances can cause an increase in lung cancers in exposed workers. Among the most historically important of these are the chloromethyl ethers, which include chloromethylmethyl ether (CMME) and bischloromethyl ether (BCME). Chloromethyl ethers are produced in order to chloromethylate other organic chemicals in the manufacture of ion-exchange resins, bactericides, pesticides, dispersing agents, water repellents, solvents for industrial polymerization reactions, and flameproofing agents. The potential for chloromethyl ethers to cause cancer was first suspected in humans in 1962. In Philadelphia, cases of small-cell lung cancer occurred among approximately 45 men working in a single building of a large chemical plant. A large proportion of tumors occurred in young men and nonsmokers. Numerous other studies confirm these findings, with increased risk seen in workers with prolonged or intense exposure. Unlike other chemical carcinogens, which can cause a variety of cancers, the chloromethyl ethers are associated primarily with the induction of small-cell lung cancer. Inhalation studies in animals show that the chloromethyl ethers produce bronchial epithelial metaplasia and atypia, and both carcinogens are active alkylating agents. BCME is a more potent carcinogen than CMME.

D. Polycyclic Aromatic Hydrocarbons

PAHs, formed from the incomplete combustion of coal tar, pitch, oil, and coke, have long been recognized as carcinogens. In 1775, Sir Percival Pott reported an increased risk of scrotal cancer in chimney sweeps as a consequence of dermal exposure to soot. Creosotes, which are complex compounds made primarily from the distillation of coal tar, are another source of occupational PAHs. Epidemiologic evidence linking PAHs to lung cancer was provided in 1936, when a study of exposed workers in a coal carbonization plant in Japan revealed a marked increase in the rate of lung cancer.

Exposures to PAHs linked to an increased risk of lung cancer have been found in coke oven workers, roofers, printers, and truckers. Rubber plant workers and those employed in asphalt production, coal gasification, and aluminum reduction facilities are also at risk. The best-described occupational group is coke oven workers, where direct exposure to the coke oven emissions results in increased rates of lung cancer. A clear dose-response relationship has been described based on proximity of work to the ovens and the potential for exposure to PAHs.

E. Diesel-Engine Exhaust

Studies of miners, railroad workers, and truckers have demonstrated significant increases in the risk of lung cancer associated with exposures to diesel-engine exhaust. Further, this association has been observed in multiple case-control studies, including a large pooled analysis of 11 population-based case-control studies from Europe and Canada, which was adjusted for cigarette smoking. In 2012, IARC concluded, based on these studies, that there was sufficient evidence in humans for the carcinogenicity of diesel-engine exhaust. Similarly, IARC stated that animal bioassays demonstrated sufficient evidence of carcinogenicity. Diesel-engine exhaust contains a number of nitroarenes, which are nitro-substituted derivatives of PAHs (arenes). Many of these agents are animal carcinogens and are genotoxic.

F. Arsenic

Exposure to inorganic arsenic increases the risk of lung cancer; the first cases of arsenic-induced lung cancer were reported in 1930. Arsenic exposure in copper smelting, fur handling, sheep-dip compound manufacturing, and arsenical pesticide production and use has resulted in increased rates of lung cancer. Long latency periods of approximately 25 years are seen after exposure before the development of cancer. Arsenic is thought to act as a late-stage promoter of cancer and may interfere with DNA repair mechanisms. A dose-response relationship in exposed workers has been described. There is some evidence for a synergistic effect of smoking and arsenic exposure in increasing the risk of lung cancer.

G. Beryllium

Increased risks of lung cancer have been observed in studies of beryllium-processing workers. IARC concluded in 2012 that beryllium and beryllium compounds cause cancer of the lung in humans.

H. Cadmium

Increased risks of lung cancer have been reported in some studies of cadmium-processing workers, nickel-cadmium (Ni-Cd) battery workers, and workers in a cadmium recovery plant. Despite the possibility that coexposure to other lung carcinogens, such as cigarette smoke, arsenic, and nickel, could have contributed to excess risks, IARC concluded in 2012 that cadmium and cadmium compounds cause cancer of the lung in humans.

I. Chromium

Increased rates of lung cancer have been reported in industries, such as chromate production, chrome plating, and chrome-alloy production, which use chromium (VI) compounds, also known as hexavalent chromium compounds. Other lung carcinogens used in the electroplating industry, such as nickel and PAHs, may confound this relationship. IARC has concluded that chromium (VI) compounds cause cancer of the lung.

J. Nickel

Exposure to nickel in mining, refining, and subsulfide roasting facilities is associated with increased rates of lung and nasal cancer. While exposure to both soluble and insoluble nickel compounds has been associated with lung cancer risk, the evidence is strongest for water-soluble nickel compounds. IARC has concluded that there is sufficient evidence in humans for the carcinogenicity of mixtures that include nickel compounds and nickel metal.

K. Mustard gas

Studies of Japanese and German workers in factories that manufactured mustard gas during World War II show an excess of respiratory cancers. This is consistent with the finding that mustard gas can produce lung tumors in laboratory animals. There may be a higher rate of squamous cell cancer of the lung in humans.

L. Silica

In a number of occupational settings, workers exposed to crystalline silica had increased risks for lung cancer, including in quarries and granite works and in refractory brick and diatomaceous earth industries. Studies of individuals with documented silicosis have also demonstrated increased lung cancer risk. Based on this information, IARC concluded in 1997 that there is sufficient evidence in humans for the carcinogenicity of inhaled crystalline silica in the form of quartz or cristobalite from occupational sources.

▶ Pathology

The four major types of lung cancer are squamous cell (epidermoid) carcinoma, adenocarcinoma, large-cell carcinoma, and small-cell (oat-cell) carcinoma. All histologic types of lung cancer are linked to occupational exposures. Even in studies of workers exposed to CMME or BCME, who are much more likely to develop the relatively uncommon

small-cell histology, other types of lung cancer have been observed. Although early work suggested that the peripheral distribution of asbestos fibers was associated with a higher incidence of adenocarcinomas in this region, this has not been found in recent, more thorough studies. Lung cancers in asbestos-exposed persons occur equally throughout the lung, and all pathologic types are seen.

▶ Clinical Findings

A. Symptoms and Signs

- 75–90% are symptomatic at diagnosis.
- Presentation depends on
  - Type and location of tumor
  - Extent of spread
  - Presence of distant metastases and any paraneoplastic syndromes
- Anorexia, weight loss, and asthenia in 55–90%.
- New or changed cough in up to 60%.
- Hemoptysis in 5–30%.
- Pain, often from bony metastases, in 25–40%.
- Local spread may result in endobronchial obstruction and postobstructive pneumonia, effusions, or a change in voice due to recurrent laryngeal nerve involvement.
- Superior vena cava (SVC) syndrome.
- Horner syndrome.
- Liver metastases are associated with asthenia and weight loss.
- Possible presentation of brain metastases.

Symptoms and signs and laboratory and imaging procedure findings in occupational lung cancer generally do not differ from lung cancers of nonoccupational etiology. In some cases, an imaging or other finding may suggest a particular etiology; for example, the presence of pleural plaques, in conjunction with a lung tumor, would suggest heavy asbestos exposure as the cause.

▶ Prevention

Avoidance of exposure to lung carcinogens is the most important preventive measure, but complete avoidance is typically not possible, especially for those agents that occur naturally in the environment such as asbestos, arsenic, and silica. The most effective method of reducing the mortality rate for lung cancer is primary prevention. This includes identification of etiologic agents in the workplace, adherence to strict workplace standards, and worker education. Because tobacco use is known to increase the incidence of lung cancer in occupationally exposed groups, aggressive antismoking campaigns in the workplace are critically important.

Recent evidence shows that low-dose CT screening for lung cancer among high-risk workers (such as former nuclear weapons production and maintenance workers and construction workers*) leads to a favorable yield of early-stage lung cancers, and that occupation can be used in combination with age and smoking to identify populations that provide a similar screening yield and lung cancer stage distribution as was demonstrated in the National Lung Screening Trial study. These data are consistent with the guidelines from the National Comprehensive Cancer Network, which recommends lung cancer screening for people aged 50 or older with a ≥ 20 pack-year smoking history if they have an additional risk factor (such as history of exposure to radon or occupational lung carcinogens). A similar approach was recommended by an international group convened under the auspices of the Finnish Institute of Occupational Health in 2014. Low-dose CT screening for lung cancer should now be considered as an option for any older, tobacco smoking worker with a history of significant exposure to known occupational lung carcinogens.

There is lack of evidence supporting the use of chemoprevention for lung cancer in high-risk populations. A study of primary chemoprevention of lung cancer, using retinol and beta carotene, in current and former smokers and asbestos workers was discontinued after increases in risk were observed.

▶ Treatment & Prognosis

Therapy of occupationally induced lung cancers is no different from treatment for each of the specific cell types of lung cancer that may be seen in other settings. In general, even in patients with localized disease, long-term survival is the exception rather than the rule.

▶ Other Lung Carcinogens

The following substances are classified by IARC as those with "sufficient" (group 1) or "probable" (group 2A) evidence of overall carcinogenicity and that *may* increase the risk of lung cancer specifically:

- Acid mists
- Art glass
- Cobalt metal with tungsten carbide
- Diazinon

MESOTHELIOMA

ESSENTIALS OF DIAGNOSIS

- ▶ Asbestos exposure (20+ years earlier) may cause pleural or peritoneal mesotheliomas. Erionite is another etiologic agent implicated in both forms of mesothelioma.
- ▶ Unilateral, nonpleuritic chest pain, dyspnea, dry cough, weight loss.
- ▶ Pleural effusion or pleural thickening or both on chest radiographs.
- ▶ Malignant cells in pleural fluid or tissue biopsy.
- ▶ Diagnosis by open thoracotomy with multiple biopsies.

Occupations at Risk (partial list)

- Asbestos miners
- Construction workers
- Workers exposed to insulation materials in production, installation, and removal
- Shipyard workers
- Asbestos textile manufacturing
- Welders, plumbers, electricians
- Workers involved in the mining, production, and use of zeolites, such as erionite

▶ General Considerations

Mesothelioma is uncommon, accounting for only a small fraction of deaths caused by cancer, but it and other asbestos-related diseases have been of great interest to occupational health physicians and to public health professionals. This is because both community-based and industrial exposures to asbestos and asbestiform fibers increase risks for mesothelioma. Exposure to asbestos from the use of construction materials that contain asbestos is a serious and often neglected problem throughout the world.

In the United States in 2015, there were 3209 new cases of mesothelioma and 2404 mesothelioma deaths; incidence and mortality rates were higher for men (1.5 cases per 100,000 and 1.2 deaths per 100,000, respectively) than women (0.4 cases per 100,000 and 0.2 deaths per 100,000, respectively). From 2000 to 2015, mesothelioma incidence declined somewhat for men but held steady for women. The global mesothelioma burden is estimated to be in the range of 36,300–38,400 annual deaths.

▶ Etiology

Diffuse malignant mesotheliomas of the peritoneum and pleura are considered "sentinel tumors" or pathognomonic of exposure to asbestos. Asbestos is the dominant cause of human malignant mesothelioma and is responsible for at least 85–90% of pleural malignant mesothelioma among men. Malignant mesothelioma is caused by all types of asbestos (chrysotile, crocidolite, amosite, anthophyllite, tremolite, and actinolite). The latency period from asbestos exposure to the diagnosis of mesothelioma is often 30 years or more. Higher quantitative asbestos fiber content of dried lung has been found in some patients with mesothelioma. Further evidence of the etiologic role of asbestos has been shown in experimental animals in which intrapleural injection or administration by inhalation of asbestos fibers causes mesothelioma that is histologically identical to human tumors.

Epidemiologic data show that variable levels of exposure to asbestos can result in mesothelioma, despite the known dose-response relationship. While most cases occur in individuals with a history of heavy asbestos exposure, some cases occur in individuals with relatively trivial contact at work or in the home environment (eg, exposure of wives washing their husbands' contaminated work clothes). Malignant mesotheliomas have been documented among neighborhood residents of asbestos-using factories; community residents of asbestos mining areas, and household residents of asbestos workers.

In addition to asbestos, IARC has concluded that there is sufficient human and animal evidence that the asbestiform-like agent erionite causes mesothelioma. Erionite is what is known as a natural fibrous zeolite, found in volcanic ash. Although erionite is structurally similar to asbestos, it has different chemical and physical properties. Nonoccupational exposure to erionite has been documented in the Cappadocia region of Turkey where extremely high rates of pleural and peritoneal mesothelioma were linked to high erionite levels in the surrounding environment. Occupational exposure has decreased since the 1980s when the use of erionite for industrial applications made way for synthetic substitutes. However, workers involved in the mining, production, and use of other zeolites can be at risk for erionite exposure.

There is suggestive but not yet definitive evidence that certain forms of ionizing radiation also may cause malignant mesothelioma. Cigarette smoking does not increase the risk of malignant mesothelioma. Unlike lung cancer, there is no evidence for synergy between cigarette smoking and asbestos exposure in the development of this tumor.

▶ Pathogenesis

All types of asbestos are capable of causing mesothelioma. The mechanisms of induction are unknown. Cancer development is related to the physical properties (ie, fiber size and dimension). In work done in rats, long, thin fibers of a variety of types have proved carcinogenic, whereas short fibers and those with a relatively broad diameter have failed to produce mesothelioma. Inhaled fibers are expectorated or swallowed. Short fibers are cleared more readily than long fibers and are more likely to end up in the pleura. Fibers remain accumulated in the lower lung, adjacent to the pleura. The pathogenesis of peritoneal mesothelioma is thought to be similar to that of pleural tumors. Fibers of asbestos are transported in lymphatics to the abdomen, and asbestos is also transported across the mucosa of the gut after ingestion.

▶ Pathology

A major area of difficulty in the study of mesothelioma has been distinguishing its pathologic features. Many tumors metastasize and spread to the mesothelial lining of the chest and abdomen. This has led to misdiagnosis of mesothelioma when it was, in fact, a metastatic tumor, such as an adenocarcinoma, and the reverse is true as well. Confusion also exists because of the tumor's diverse microscopic appearance.

Two types of mesothelioma have been described: benign solitary and diffuse malignant. The benign solitary type remains localized, although it may become large and compress neighboring thoracic structures. This tumor has not been associated with asbestos exposure; it is a benign tumor arising from fibroblasts and other connective-tissue elements in the areolar submesothelial cell layers of the pleura and is not occupational

in origin. By contrast, diffuse malignant mesothelioma arises from either the pluripotential mesenchymal cell or the primitive submesothelial mesenchymal cell, which retains the ability to form epithelial or connective-tissue elements.

Malignant mesothelioma is a diffuse lesion that spreads widely in the pleural space and usually is associated with extensive pleural effusion and direct invasion of thoracic structures. On gross examination, numerous tumor nodules may be noted, and in advanced cases, the tumor has a hard, woody consistency. Microscopically, malignant mesotheliomas consist of three histologic types: an epithelial (or epithelioid) type that may resemble metastatic adenocarcinoma, a mesenchymal type, and a mixed type. Histochemical and immunohistochemical techniques that use Alcian blue stains and a panel of antibodies to specific cellular antigens, respectively, can be employed to help distinguish mesothelioma from metastatic adenocarcinoma. Studies with the electron microscope have defined certain characteristic features that are also helpful in differentiating the tumor from metastatic disease.

▶ Clinical Findings

A. Symptoms

Symptoms in diffuse pleural mesothelioma may be entirely absent or minimal at the time of onset of the disease. Disease progression results in the most common symptom of a persistent gnawing chest pain on the involved side, which may radiate to the shoulder and arm. In most patients, pain becomes the most incapacitating symptom. Dyspnea on exertion, dry cough (occasionally hemoptysis), and increasing weight loss are frequent accompanying symptoms. Some patients have low-grade fever, which can result in an incorrect diagnosis of chronic infection. The symptoms of peritoneal mesothelioma are nonspecific but may include increased abdominal girth, pain, and weight loss.

B. Signs

Physical findings vary with the stage of disease. Most patients present with pleural effusion. Local tumor growth may depress the diaphragm and displace the liver or spleen, giving the impression of hepatomegaly or splenomegaly. In advanced disease, there may be obvious enlargement of the affected hemithorax, with bulging of the intercostal spaces and displacement of the trachea and mediastinum to the unaffected side. After removal of pleural fluid, a pericardial or pleuroperi-cardial rub may be heard. Advanced signs also may include mediastinal lymph node enlargement, subcutaneous nodules in the chest wall, and clubbing. Encroachment on the mediastinal structures may lead to neuropathic signs such as vocal cord paralysis or Horner syndrome. Congestion and edema may develop in the upper trunk or lower limbs secondary to compression of the superior or inferior vena cava.

C. Laboratory Findings

Laboratory findings are nonspecific but may include anemia and thrombocytosis.

D. Imaging

Radiographic studies of the chest most commonly show unilateral pleural effusion. After thoracentesis, the pleura may show thickening or nodularity, seen usually at the bases. CT scanning, which is the most sensitive test for evaluating the pleural surface, may show thickened tumor along the chest wall, and late in the disease, tomograms or an overpenetrated film will show compressed lung surrounded on all sides by a tumor 2–3 cm thick. Extrapleural extension can result in soft-tissue masses or radiologic evidence of rib destruction. Signs of asbestosis such as interstitial pulmonary fibrosis, pleural plaques, and calcification are valuable findings when present.

E. Special Examination

1. Sputum Cytology—Microscopic examination of sputum rarely shows malignant cells unless the tumor has invaded lung parenchyma. Asbestos bodies may be seen.

2. Thoracentesis—The considerable force necessary to enter the pleural space with a thoracentesis needle may be a clue to the presence of pleural mesothelioma. Pleural fluid is serosanguineous or hemorrhagic in 30–50% of cases but is commonly straw-colored. Cytologic examination of pleural fluid is not typically helpful diagnostically. Mesothelial hyperplasia is not uncommon in benign pleural effusions and easily can be mistaken for malignant cells.

3. Pleural Biopsy—Because of the limitations of pleural fluid cytologic examination, biopsy confirmation is required. A CT-guided pleural biopsy may permit diagnosis in some cases. Thoracoscopy (pleuroscopy) with biopsy of pleural masses can be an effective technique and is less invasive than an open biopsy. Pleurodesis (obliteration of the pleural space) with insufflation of talc to reduce recurrence of pleural effusions can be performed as part of this procedure. An open thoracotomy with multiple biopsies from different pleural areas is sometimes required for diagnosis.

▶ Differential Diagnosis

The major disorders that must be differentiated from mesothelioma are inflammatory pleurisy, primary lung cancer, and metastatic adenocarcinoma or sarcoma. Inflammatory pleurisy is suggested by the associated clinical picture and by typical findings in the analysis of sputum and pleural fluid. In primary lung cancer, the more prominent symptom of cough, the less common presence of severe chest pain, the presence of parenchymal tumors, and the absence of pleural abnormalities after thoracentesis help to differentiate between these two types of cancer. Primary tumors of the pancreas, gastrointestinal tract, or ovary should be excluded because these tumors can metastasize to the pleural or peritoneal space and mimic mesothelioma.

▶ Prevention

Avoidance of exposure to asbestos is the most effective means to prevent mesothelioma. The exposures to asbestos that lead to mesothelioma may be less intense and of shorter duration than the exposures that lead to asbestosis or lung cancer. Recommendations for levels of asbestos in the air of occupational settings were first established in the 1940s, but it was not until 1970 that federal regulations began as a result of the passage of the Occupational Safety and Health Act (OSHAct) and the Clean Air Act. The current OSHA standard is 0.1 fibers/cc of air on an 8-hour time-weighted average (TWA) basis, although adherence to this standard may not be fully protective against the development of mesotheliomas.

▶ Treatment

A. Surgical Measures

Surgery has been used with some success as the primary method of treatment in pleural mesotheliomas, both for tumor debulking and for palliation of symptoms. Even with tumors with extensive infiltration of adjoining viscera, partial surgical resection has led to an apparent increase in longevity, although it is not curative. Subtotal pleurectomy with decortication is the accepted procedure. More radical surgeries such as pleuropneumonectomy (extrapleural pneumonectomy) may be appropriate for selected patients. Postoperative adjuvant chemotherapy and radiation therapy sometimes are used, but there are no studies to support their use. Surgical resection of all visible disease is believed to be the treatment of choice. Surgical excision has no role in the management of peritoneal mesothelioma unless the tumor is localized.

B. External Radiotherapy

Radiation therapy clearly has been shown to be of benefit in controlling pain and pleural effusion in mesothelioma. Although antitumor efficacy has been noted using high-dose radiation, this modality is relatively ineffective in altering the dismal survival statistics for this disease.

C. Chemotherapy

There has been no systematic study of the role of cytotoxic drugs in mesothelioma. While there are well-documented reports of definite antitumor effects in some patients, chemotherapy is not curative. Pemetrexed (a folate antimetabolite), cisplatin, gemcitabine (a nucleoside analog), methotrexate, and other drugs, sometimes in combination, have been used. The U.S. Food and Drug Administration has approved combination treatment with pemetrexed and cisplatin for malignant pleural mesothelioma that is not surgically resectable.

▶ Course & Prognosis

The median survival for malignant pleural mesothelioma is less than 1 year, and the prognosis has not improved over the past four decades. Several factors correlate with improved survival in mesothelioma. Patients whose tumors are in the pleura survive twice as long as those with peritoneal tumors;

survival is longer for patients with epithelial types than for those with mixed or fibrosarcomatous types; and survival is longer for patients younger than 65 years, those who respond well to chemotherapy, and those able to undergo surgical resection.

CANCER OF THE NASAL CAVITY & SINUSES

ESSENTIALS OF DIAGNOSIS

▶ Presenting symptoms are unilateral nasal obstruction, nonhealing ulcer, and occasional bleeding.

▶ More frequent in men than in women (2:1).

▶ Usually squamous cell histology.

Occupations at Risk (partial list)

- Wood and other dusts
  - Boot and shoe manufacturing
  - Furniture workers
  - Carpenters and joiners
  - Textile manufacturing
- Nickel
  - Nickel refinery workers
- Chromium
  - Chromate pigment manufacturing
  - Metal plating workers
  - Isopropyl alcohol production workers
- Formaldehyde
  - Numerous manufacturing processes, including furniture and textile finishing, garment industry
  - Embalming

Cancers of the nasal cavity and sinuses are rare and account for fewer than 10 cases per million in the United States per year. This disease is uncommon in younger than 40–50 years of age, and rates increase with age. Evidence suggests a fairly steady incidence over the years. Over 50% of all sinonasal tumors are squamous cell, while about 10% are adenocarcinomas. Both these histologies are linked to occupational exposures. Other histologic types include other carcinoma, sarcoma, and melanoma.

▶ Etiology

Many different occupational exposures are linked to cancer of the nasal cavity and paranasal sinuses. These include wood and leather dust, nickel, radium, and isopropyl alcohol production (by the strong acid process), for which IARC has concluded that there is sufficient evidence in humans. Agents or industries, for which IARC has concluded that

there is limited evidence in humans (and sufficient evidence in animal studies) for causation of these tumors, include hexavalent chromium compounds, formaldehyde, carpentry and joinery, and textile manufacturing (possibly due to textile dusts, dyes, and/or formaldehyde). Employment in several other industries, including furniture and shoe manufacturing, with corresponding exposures to wood and leather dusts, respectively, also has been associated with these cancers. Cigarette smoking also increases the risk of nose and paranasal sinus cancer.

A. Wood and Other Organic Dusts

Many studies have shown an increased incidence of carcinoma of the sinonasal area in persons exposed to wood dust. Adenocarcinoma of the ethmoids and middle turbinates is the most frequent cell type encountered in these workers. The exact substance in wood dust responsible for carcinogenesis has not been identified.

An excess of both adenocarcinomas and squamous cell carcinomas of the nasal sinuses also has been observed among workers in the boot and shoe industry, exposed to leather dust. As in the case of woodworkers, the specific etiologic agent in leather dust is unknown. Dusts involved in the textile industry and flour dusts in bakeries and flour mills also have been associated with the development of sinonasal cancers.

B. Nickel

Both nasal cancer and lung cancer are linked to occupational nickel exposure. Most studies have been done on nickel refinery workers exposed to complex particulates (insoluble nickel sulfide dust, nickel oxides, and soluble nickel sulfate, nitrate, or chloride) and gaseous nickel carbonyl. Nickel and nickel carbonyl are carcinogenic under experimental conditions, yet epidemiologic evidence points away from the nickel carbonyl process and incriminates exposure to dust from the preliminary processes. The mean latency period between exposure and diagnosis of cancer in refinery workers is 20–30 years.

C. Other Occupational Exposures

Tumors of the nasal epithelium and mastoid air cells have been noted in women exposed to radium used for painting dials of watches and in radon chemists. Chromium is known to cause ulceration and perforation of the nasal septum, and there is an excess risk of sinonasal cancer in workers involved in manufacturing chromate pigments. Mustard gas, cutting oils (mineral oils), and formaldehyde are also linked to excess cancers of the nasal cavity and paranasal sinuses.

▶ Clinical Findings

The earliest symptoms of nasal cavity neoplasms are a low-grade chronic infection associated with discharge, obstruction, and minor intermittent bleeding. The patient often complains of "sinus trouble" and may have been treated inappropriately with antibiotics for prolonged periods before the true diagnosis was known. Subsequent symptoms depend on the pattern of local growth. Maxillary sinus tumors develop silently when they are confined to the sinus, producing symptoms only with extension outside the walls. With extension into the oral cavity, pain may be referred to the upper teeth. Nasal obstruction and bleeding are common complaints, along with "sinus pain" or "fullness" of the involved antrum.

▶ Diagnosis & Treatment

In all cases, the patient should receive careful inspection and palpation of the facial structures, with attention to the eye and especially the extraocular movements. The nasal and orbital cavities should be examined closely. Helpful radiologic studies include facial bone or sinus radiograph series and CT scan of the involved areas. Biopsies are required for diagnosis.

Therapy is the same for occupational cancers as with other nasal and sinus cancers, including surgical therapy and radiation therapy, with chemotherapy reserved for advanced disease. The prognosis is better for nasal cavity cancers because they tend to be diagnosed at an early stage.

CANCER OF THE LARYNX

ESSENTIALS OF DIAGNOSIS

- ▶ Hoarseness is an early presenting symptom.
- ▶ Much more frequent in men than in women (4.5:1), usually middle aged or older.
- ▶ Usually squamous cell histology.

Occupations at Risk

- Asbestos-exposed workers, including miners, insulators, and shipyard workers
- Workers exposed to strong inorganic acid mists
- Workers in the rubber production industry

Cancer of the larynx is more common than sinonasal cancer, representing about 2% of the total cancer risk in the United States. In the United States, there is evidence that the incidence of cancer of the larynx is decreasing.

▶ Etiology

Laryngeal cancer is primarily a disease of older individuals with incidence rates rising sharply after age 50. At the time of diagnosis, approximately 60% are localized, 30% show regional spread, and 10% have distant metastases. Laryngeal tumors in the United States are classified into three groups

according to anatomic site of origin, with about 30–40% supraglottic, 60% glottic, and 1% subglottic cancers. Nearly all are squamous cell carcinomas.

IARC has concluded that there is sufficient evidence in humans that occupational exposure to asbestos increases the risk of laryngeal cancer. Asbestos exposure in a variety of occupations, including miners, asbestos product manufacturers, and insulators, is associated with high rates of laryngeal cancers. Similarly, IARC has concluded that there is sufficient evidence in humans that strong inorganic acid mists cause laryngeal cancer. Occupational agents or industries for which IARC has concluded that there is limited evidence in humans are mustard gas (sulfur mustard) and rubber production. Cigarette smoking and alcohol use are the major nonoccupational risk factors.

▶ Clinical Findings

Symptoms of laryngeal carcinoma vary depending on the site of involvement. Any patient who complains of persistent hoarseness, difficulty in swallowing, pain on swallowing, a "lump in the throat," or a change in voice quality should be examined promptly by indirect laryngoscopy. Limitation of motion or rigidity should be noted, and direct laryngoscopy with biopsy of suspicious lesions is necessary. Lateral soft-tissue radiographs of the neck and CT scanning are also useful, especially to delineate extent of disease.

▶ Treatment

Therapy is no different for work-related laryngeal cancers than for other laryngeal cancers.

BLADDER CANCER

ESSENTIALS OF DIAGNOSIS

- ▶ Presenting complaints of hematuria and vesical irritability.
- ▶ Diagnosis by urine cytologic examination and cystoscopy.

Occupations at Risk (partial list)

- Workers exposed to inorganic arsenic compounds, for example, in arsenical pesticide production and use; and in copper, lead, and zinc smelting
- Work with aromatic amines, such as 2-naphthylamine (also known as β-naphthylamine), 4-aminobiphenyl, benzidine, and *ortho*-toluidine
- Dye/pigment manufacturing and use
- Workers in rubber manufacturing industries
- Painters
- Workers in rubber production
- Workers exposed to diesel exhaust

▶ General Considerations

Bladder cancer accounts for approximately 5% of all malignant tumors in the United States. In the United States, more than 80,000 cases are diagnosed each year. The male-to-female ratio is about 4:1. The highest incidence of bladder cancer occurs in industrialized countries with lower incidence in less developed countries. Cigarette smoking is the most important known preventable cause of bladder cancer, with half of all cases attributed to this risk factor. Smokers have at least three times the risk of bladder cancer compared with nonsmokers. The increased frequency in men may reflect slightly higher smoking rates but, because of increasing parity in smoking rates between men and women recently, the persistently higher rates of bladder cancer in men currently are now mainly due to more men working in hazardous occupations than do women. Nonsmokers exposed to secondhand smoke in the workplace also may be at risk. In a 2018 meta-analysis of 14 observational studies, secondhand smoke exposure was associated with a 22% increased risk of bladder cancer among nonsmokers. As with most cancers, the incidence of bladder cancer increases with age, with most cases occurring in individuals 65 years and older.

▶ Occupational Etiology

Aromatic amines are the major occupational cause of bladder cancer, mostly through inhalation, but also in some cases through dermal absorption. The chemicals were first used on a mass scale in the dye industry, beginning in the 19th century in Germany. It was not long before the first reports were published, in 1895, of occupational bladder cancer in a series of workers at a German dye plant. Further reports of workers with bladder cancer emerged in the United States in the 1930s and 1940s after the country began mass-producing the chemicals in World War I. Currently, IARC has classified four aromatic amines, 2-naphthylamine, benzidine, orthotoluidine, and 4-aminobiphenyl, as causative of bladder cancer. Eventually, companies relocated much of their dye production to the developing world, where the extent of aromatic-amine-induced occupational bladder cancer has not yet been determined. Exposure may still occur in industrialized countries, including in laboratories where certain aromatic amines are used in cancer research, fumes in foundries or heated cooking oils, or in the production of pesticides, rubber materials, and pharmaceuticals.

IARC also has classified the following occupational agents and occupations as causing bladder cancer in humans: ionizing radiation (x- and γ-radiation), and work in painting, aluminum, auramine, magenta, and rubber production. Occupational exposures with evidence for causing bladder cancer in humans include 4-chloro-ortho-toluidine, 2-mercaptobenzothiazole, coal-tar pitch, soot, tetrachloroethylene, diesel engine exhaust, and work in dry cleaning, hairdressing (perhaps due to hair dyes), printing, and textile manufacturing.

▶ Pathogenesis

Most occupation-related urinary tract tumors are thought to be caused by contact of the bladder epithelium with carcinogens in the urine. Because of the concentrating ability of the kidney, the bladder is exposed to higher concentrations of these materials than other body tissues. Recent data indicate that hereditary polymorphisms of the arylamine N-acetyltransferase gene may play a role in the etiology of bladder cancer by modulating the effect of as well as the interaction between carcinogens, including cigarette smoke and aromatic amines. The risk of cancer appears to be the highest in slow acetylators, suggesting that individual mechanisms of detoxification play an important role in the risk of toxin- induced bladder cancer.

▶ Pathology

The vast majority of bladder cancers arise from the urothelial cells lining the inside of the bladder and are known as transitional cell carcinomas. Much less common subtypes are squamous cell carcinomas, small cell carcinomas, adenocarcinomas, and sarcomas. Tumors may be papillary or flat, in situ or invasive, and are graded according to degree of cellular differentiation, with poorly differentiated cancers carrying worse prognoses.

Multiple genetic changes have been associated with bladder cancer, such as expression of the *RAS* and *FGFR* proto-oncogenes and the tumor-suppressor gene *p53*, some of which are correlated with an increased risk of disease progression.

▶ Clinical Findings

The most common presenting symptom of bladder cancer is hematuria, which occurs in 80–90% of patients and usually is painless and gross. More than 20% of patients have vesical irritability, with increased frequency, dysuria, and urgency. Urine cytology has low sensitivity for low-grade and early-stage cancers. Definitive diagnosis relies on cystoscopy and transurethral biopsy of the suspicious areas.

Bladder cancer generally spreads by local extension through invasion of the muscular wall, through lymphatics, or by hematogenous dissemination. Clinical sites of metastatic disease include the pelvic lymph nodes, lungs, bones, and liver (in decreasing order of occurrence). Once the diagnosis has been confirmed by biopsy, a chest radiograph, radionuclide bone scan, and liver and renal function studies should be done. CT scans are extremely useful in staging. Current staging depends on depth of involvement, nodal involvement, and the presence or absence of distant metastases.

▶ Prevention

Prevention of exposure to known carcinogens is the most effective means of preventing occupational bladder cancer.

The use of urinalysis for microscopic hematuria and urinary cytologic examinations followed by cystoscopy when indicated can be used for medical monitoring. Screening of high-risk occupational groups may detect bladder cancer at an earlier stage, but there have been no consistent studies demonstrating favorable impact on relevant outcomes or survival.

► Treatment

Initial treatment for nonmetastatic disease is surgical. Carcinoma in situ and superficial lesions are treated with transurethral resection of the malignant areas, occasionally followed by intravesical immunotherapy or chemotherapy. More advanced disease requires more aggressive approaches, including partial or radical cystectomy, systemic chemotherapy and/or radiation.

Prognosis is generally better than for other cancers when the cancer is diagnosed early, with 5-year survival rates of 97% for in situ lesions and 70% for localized cancers. These rates decline to 36% and 5% for cancers with regional spread and distant metastases, respectively.

LIVER CANCER: HEPATIC ANGIOSARCOMA & HEPATOCELLULAR CARCINOMA

ESSENTIALS OF DIAGNOSIS

▶ For hepatic angiosarcoma, major causative occupational exposures are vinyl chloride and arsenic compounds, with occupations at risk including polyvinyl chloride (PVC) manufacture and vintners, respectively. Vinyl chloride and arsenic compounds also likely cause hepatocellular carcinoma (HCC).

▶ Right upper quadrant abdominal pain, weight loss.

▶ Hepatomegaly on physical examination.

▶ Diagnosis by hepatic arteriogram and open liver biopsy.

Liver Carcinogens, With Occupations at Risk

- Vinyl chloride
  - Workers involved in manufacture of PVC
- Arsenic
  - Vintners
  - Arsenical pesticide production and use
  - Copper, lead, zinc smelting
  - Sheep-dip manufacturers (contamination of drinking water)

► General Considerations

Liver cancer involves any of the cell types in the liver, with HCC by far the most common type. HCC has the seventh highest age-adjusted rate of cancer and fourth highest rate of cancer death worldwide and has several nonoccupational causes, including chronic hepatitis B and C infection, chronic excessive alcohol use, and other illnesses that lead to hepatic inflammation and cirrhosis.

Angiosarcoma of the liver is a rare tumor caused by exposure to vinyl chloride and arsenic. Thorotrast (thorium dioxide) exposure was a major nonoccupational risk factor when this agent was used as a radiographic contrast agent from about 1930 to 1955. This cancer occurs most commonly in middle-aged men, with a male-to-female ratio of 4:1. The mean age at presentation is 53 years. Characteristic features of the disease include a long period of asymptomatic laboratory abnormalities, difficulty in diagnosis, and poor response to treatment.

► Occupational Etiologies

Vinyl chloride is the raw material with which the common plastic PVC is made. In 1974, a cluster of cases of angiosarcoma of the liver in men was reported by an alert physician in Louisville, Kentucky. The men were all workers at a local industrial plant that polymerized vinyl chloride. By 1981, 10 cases of hepatic angiosarcoma were identified among 1855 employees older than 35 years, with no other cases of angiosarcoma identified in the Louisville area. In one review of 20 patients with angiosarcoma of the liver after vinyl chloride exposure, the mean time from first exposure to development of tumor was 19 years, with a range of 11–37 years. In addition to the Louisville experience, cancer in other patients from plants elsewhere producing vinyl chloride has been noted. Similar hepatic lesions in experimental animals exposed to high concentrations of vinyl chloride also have been observed.

Workers in the vinyl chloride industry also have been found to be at increased risk of HCC in several large cohort studies. Vinyl chloride workers with concomitant hepatitis B infection or higher alcohol use may be at especially high risk. Dose-response and duration-response relationships were observed.

Although the evidence is not as striking, both hepatic angiosarcoma and HCC are also associated with arsenic compounds, including arsenical pesticides, arsenic-contaminated wine, and Fowler solution used medicinally. These associations have been mostly seen in Taiwanese communities exposed to groundwater with extremely high levels of arsenic.

While IARC has concluded that aflatoxins, which are produced mainly by the fungus species *Aspergillus flavus* and *A parasiticus*, cause HCC, the extent to which carcinogenic exposure occurs in workers is unclear. Occupational exposure occurs during the processing and handling of contaminated grains, especially animal feed and several studies have detected aflatoxins through airborne sampling of agricultural grain storage facilities. The main route of exposure, and that which has been studied as an etiologic pathway for aflatoxin-induced HCC, is ingestion of aflatoxin-contaminated agricultural products.

DDT and trichloroethylene (TCE) are other occupational agents classified by IARC as probable causes of liver cancer based on human and animal evidence. The major source of occupational exposure to TCE is metal degreasing operations, while DDT's use is now limited to its use as an insecticide in developing countries that deploy it for malaria prevention.

▶ Pathology & Pathophysiology

The two distinctive hepatic lesions seen after exposure to vinyl chloride are hepatic fibrosis and angiosarcoma. The hepatic fibrosis is characterized by three features: a nonspecific portal fibrosis, capsular and subcapsular fibrosis in a nodular form (the most characteristic lesion), and focal intralobular accumulation of connective tissue fibers. The neoplasm is hemorrhagic and cystic and replaces most of the normal tissue. The carcinogenicity of the vinyl chloride monomer is related to the metabolic formation of reactive metabolites.

Hepatic angiosarcomas caused by Thorotrast and inorganic arsenicals show many of the histologic features observed in the evolution of the hepatic angiosarcoma in the vinyl chloride workers.

▶ Clinical Findings

A. Symptoms and Signs

The symptoms of hepatic angiosarcoma and HCC are nonspecific, and some patients may be asymptomatic. Abdominal pain is the most common symptom, usually in the right upper quadrant. Fatigue, weakness, and weight loss are seen in 25–50% of patients. Physical examination may reveal hepatomegaly with ascites, jaundice, and splenomegaly.

B. Laboratory Findings

Patients may have some abnormality of liver function testing, including elevation of serum alkaline phosphatase and α-fetoprotein, although laboratory studies may be uniformly normal, especially in early-stage cancers.

C. Imaging and Diagnosis

Routine abdominal radiographs and gastrointestinal contrast studies usually are normal. Radionuclide liver scans are abnormal in most patients, but the findings can range from distinct filling defects to nonspecific nonhomogeneous uptake (which can be confused with cirrhosis and splenomegaly). Hepatic arteriograms are the most helpful diagnostic tool, usually demonstrating normal-sized hepatic arteries that may be displaced by tumor, peripheral tumor stain, puddling during the middle of the arterial phase, and a central area of hypovascularity. Hepatic ultrasonography also may

demonstrate a hepatic mass. Definitive diagnosis of angiosarcoma is best made by thoracoscopic liver biopsy. Because of the difficulty in making the diagnosis and rapid clinical deterioration, more than 50% of hepatic angiosarcomas are diagnosed only after death.

D. Screening Tests

▶ Medical Surveillance & Prevention

As part of the US OSHA standard for vinyl chloride, exposed employees should receive periodic testing, including history and physical examination and liver function tests. Further testing such as imaging tests (ultrasound, liver scan), angiography, and biopsy should be performed as indicated for significant abnormalities. Preventive measures for hepatic angiosarcoma and HCC include stringent limitations on employee exposure to vinyl chloride and arsenic compounds.

▶ Treatment & Prognosis

For hepatic angiosarcoma, partial hepatectomy with intent to cure is possible in only a very limited number of patients because of extensive fibrosis in the uninvolved liver. No forms of treatment, including radiation, chemotherapy, or liver transplantation have been shown to improve survival. Overall survival usually is measured in months, with the median survival approximately 6 months and only a small percentage of patients surviving 2 years. The major cause of death is irreversible, rapidly progressive hepatic failure.

HCC has a somewhat better prognosis but one that is still poor, with 5-year survival rates of 31% for localized cancers to 2% for cancers with distant metastases. A small percentage of HCCs are surgically resectable, but most are treated with one or more of chemotherapy, radiation, chemoembolization, immunotherapy, or liver transplantation.

BILE-DUCT CANCER

ESSENTIALS OF DIAGNOSIS

▶ Causative occupational exposures are 1,2-dichloropropane (1,2-DCP; also known as propylene dichloride) and dichloromethane (also known as methylene chloride), with major occupations at risk being workers in printing plants or printing presses; paint and furniture stripping; and bathtub refinishing. At-risk workers are those in plastic and chemical manufacturing plants and agricultural workers, including pesticide applicators in developing countries.

▶ Often asymptomatic in early stages; symptoms in advanced stages include jaundice, pruritus, dark urine, light-colored stools, right upper quadrant abdominal pain.

▶ Diagnosis by imaging and endoscopic, laparoscopic, or open abdominal biopsy.

General Considerations

Bile-duct cancers, also known as cholangiocarcinomas, are rare cancers involving any portion of the intrahepatic (10%) or extrahepatic (90%) bile ducts. Just 8000 cases are diagnosed every year in the United States, though the incidence in Southeast Asia is considerably higher due to the endemic "liver flukes" *Opisthorchis viverrini* and *Clonorchis sinensis* parasites that can increase the risk of cholangiocarcinomas. Other major nonoccupational risk factors are primary sclerosing cholangitis, chronic ulcerative colitis, and choledochal cysts.

Occupational Etiology

Occupational risks for cholangiocarcinoma were first detected in Japanese printing-plant workers, where a cluster of cholangiocarcinoma cases led to the identification of 1,2-dichloropropoane (1,2-DCP; also known as propylene dichloride) and dichloromethane (also known as methylene chloride) as likely causes. According to IARC, one or both of 1,2-DCP and dichloromethane are used in a variety of industrial and commercial uses, such as chemical intermediates in the production of other organic chemicals such as propylene, carbon tetrachloride, and tetrachloroethylene; as textile stain removers, including use in bathtubs; oil and paraffin extractants; scouring compounds; metal cleaners; solvents; paint- and stain-removers; and as a grain and soil fumigant. Occupational exposure to both 1,2-DCP and dichloromethane occurs mainly through inhalation, and to a lesser extent through dermal contact. IARC has classified 1,2-DCP as group 1 (carcinogenic to humans) and dichloromethane as group 2A (probably carcinogenic to humans) chemicals.

In the Osaka, Japan, printing plant in which a cholangiocarcinoma cluster was first detected, 1,2-DCP and dichloromethane were used as cleaners in offset-printing processes. The workers in whom cholangiocarcinoma was diagnosed were responsible for removing ink from rollers using volatile solvents containing 1,2-DCP and/or dichloromethane hundreds of times a day in a poorly-ventilated room. Workers wore gloves but no respiratory protection. The average airborne concentration of 1,2-DCP was estimated at 100–670 ppm while that of dichloromethane ranged from 80 to 540 ppm.

Of 73 workers who had worked in this room for at least one year from 1991 to 2006, 11 were diagnosed with cholangiocarcinoma. All were men diagnosed at age 45 or younger. All 11 patients had been exposed to 1,2-DCP for 7–17 years and were diagnosed 7–20 years after first exposure. In addition, all but one of the patients were also exposed to dichloromethane for 1–13 years. With the exception of a silent gallstone found in one patient, none had any risk factors for cholangiocarcinoma.

A follow-up cohort study of 111 current and former workers in the same printing plant found an additional 6 cases of cholangiocarcinoma, all in men 45 years or younger. Of the total 17 cases of cholangiocarcinoma at the plant, all

were exposed to 1,2-DCP, 11 to dichloromethane, and 8 to a third chemical, 1,1,1-trichloroethane. Notably, 10 of the 17 patients had intrahepatic-type cholangiocarcinoma.

While all of the workers at the Osaka plant had been exposed to 1,2-DCP, another Japanese study identified three workers at another printing plant diagnosed with cholangiocarcinoma that had previously been exposed to dichloromethane but not 1,2-DCP.

These epidemiologic studies led to the conclusion that both 1,2-DCP and dichloromethane were the most likely etiologic agents in the occupational cholangiocarcinoma cases. Other chemicals present in the affected workplaces had been ruled out as suspects due to shorter/lower exposure levels and use in various other industries without inducing known occupational cancers. As of 2018, 42 cases of occupational cholangiocarcinoma had been confirmed in Japan.

Pathology & Pathophysiology

The pathway for the carcinogenicity of 1,2-DCP is as yet unclear. Dichloromethane is metabolized through the hepatic cytochrome P450 system into highly reactive metabolites, including formaldehyde, carbon dioxide, and S-(chloromethyl) glutathione, which are thought to be genotoxic and carcinogenic. The distinctive bile duct lesions seen after exposure to 1,2-DCP and dichloromethane are signs of chronic bile duct injury along with DNA damage, precancerous/preinvasive lesions such as biliary intraepithelial neoplasia (BilIN) and intraductal papillary neoplasm of the bile duct (IPNB) at various sites within the bile ducts. Of note, patients with occupational cholangiocarcinoma have been reported to exhibit regional biliary ductal dilatation without visible tumor-induced obstruction more often than have patients with nonoccupational cholangiocarcinoma.

Clinical Findings

A. Symptoms and Signs

Symptoms and signs of cholangiocarcinoma often depend on the location of the tumor but typically present at an advanced stage. Extrahepatic tumors can cause symptoms of bile obstruction, such as jaundice, pruritus, light-colored/greasy stools, and dark urine. Intrahepatic disease typically presents even later in the disease course, after the cancer has advanced enough to cause systemic symptoms such as weight loss and fatigue. Physical examination can demonstrate the above signs in addition to right upper quadrant tenderness and possibly a palpably enlarged gallbladder (Courvoisier sign).

B. Laboratory Findings

Patients can have abnormal liver function testing indicating cholestasis with elevated levels of alkaline phosphatase and total and conjugated bilirubin. Tests for the nonspecific gastrointestinal malignancy markers α-fetoprotein, carcinoembryonic antigen, and CA19-9 might also be positive.

C. Imaging and Diagnosis

Transabdominal ultrasound is the modality of first choice when cholangiocarcinoma is suspected and can detect dilated, obstructed bile ducts proximal to the tumor in addition to potential liver metastases. For further imaging, magnetic resonance imaging (MRI), CT, magnetic resonance cholangiography (MRCP), and/or endoscopic retrograde cholangiopancreatography (ERCP) can be used to visualize the biliary tree. Biliary ductal dilatation without an obvious tumor obstruction may be seen in occupational cholangiocarcinoma. For a definitive diagnosis, ERCP or percutaneous abdominal fine needle aspiration can be used to obtain a biopsy of suspected tumor tissue.

D. Screening Tests

▶ Medical Surveillance & Prevention

US OSHA's federal regulation on 1,2-DCP consists of an 8-hour TWA exposure limit of 75 ppm (350 mg/m³), while several European countries (10 ppm or 47 mg/m³) and Japan (1 ppm or 4.6 mg/m³) have much lower limits. The Japanese government has initiated a medical surveillance program for current and former workers exposed to high levels of 1,2-DCP.

For dichloromethane, US OSHA has an 8-hour TWA exposure limit of 25 ppm, which is lower than the PELs of any other developed country (35–100 ppm). OSHA's short-term exposure limit (STEL) of 125 ppm also is lower than most countries, with the exception of Sweden and Denmark (75 ppm). In addition, the OSHA dichloromethane standard is more extensive than exists for most other toxic chemicals, requiring exposure monitoring, regulated areas, personal protective equipment, medical surveillance, among other measures.

The most effective means of preventing both 1,2-DCP and dichloromethane-related health effects is to ban the use of the chemicals, as has been done for 1,2-DCP for agricultural fumigation in the United States and for dichloromethane for consumer (but not occupational) uses in the United States and Europe. Otherwise, employers still using 1,2-DCP or dichloromethane should lower air concentrations to levels that do not pose a risk to employees, require respiratory and skin protection, and have periodic medical surveillance of exposed employees, among other measures.

▶ Treatment & Prognosis

Because cholangiocarcinoma is typically detected at an advanced stage, treatment is often provided to stem the progression of the disease rather than an intent to cure. For nonmetastatic disease, surgical resection of the bile duct, sometimes with removal of surrounding lymph nodes and portions of the liver, pancreas, and/or stomach, is typically performed, followed by chemotherapy and radiation. For advanced disease, palliative surgery and chemotherapy or radiation can be given to improve quality of life.

Five-year survival rates after diagnosis range from 1% to 24% depending on the location and stage of the disease at the time of diagnosis.

KIDNEY CANCER

ESSENTIALS OF DIAGNOSIS

▶ Exposure to TCE is the major occupational risk factor.

▶ Presenting complaints of hematuria and vesical irritability.

▶ Diagnosis by urine cytologic examination and kidney biopsy.

▶ General Considerations

Kidney cancers are cancers involving any portion of the kidneys. An estimated 74,000 cases are diagnosed every year in the United States, with 15,000 annual deaths. Renal cell carcinoma accounts for 90% of all kidney cancers, with transitional cell carcinomas of the renal pelvis and ureter much less common subtypes. Major nonoccupational risk factors include smoking, obesity, and certain inherited syndromes.

▶ Occupational Etiologies

The major occupational causes of kidney cancer is TCE, also known as 1,1,2-trichloroethene and ethylene trichloride. TCE is a chemical first mass produced for commercial use in the 1920s as a metal degreaser and was briefly used as a dry-cleaning agent but, due to its harsh effects on clothes, was largely (but not entirely) replaced by tetrachloroethylene in the 1950s. The major source of occupational exposure to TCE is in metal degreasing operations, which are of two types: cold degreasing, which involves the dipping of greasy metal parts into TCE solutions and vapor degreasing, a process that heats and evaporates TCE with its vapor condensing on and cleaning metal parts. Cold degreasing results in higher occupational TCE exposures than vapor degreasing. It also is used as a remover of spots and stains on textiles, including on upholstery and to a minor extent in dry-cleaning. In these capacities, TCE is used in a variety of industries, including metal and machine production (including electrical machinery, appliances, and transport equipment), construction, wholesale and retail sectors, restaurants and hotels, and personal and household services, including dry-cleaning shops.

Occupational exposure to TCE occurs mainly through inhalation of vapors and skin absorption of TCE vapors and liquids. IARC has classified TCE as carcinogenic to humans (group 1) specifically with regards to kidney cancer, while the US NTP also has concluded that TCE causes kidney cancer. The IARC and the NTP conclusions were based on robust and consistent epidemiologic evidence demonstrating an increased risk of kidney cancer in workers exposed to TCE, primarily in workers in a variety of industries, such as aerospace and metal-parts manufacture, using TCE in metal degreasing. Cohort studies, case-control studies, and multiple meta-analyses have confirmed the association. The types of kidney cancer found to be caused by TCE have been renal cell carcinoma and, in some studies, all kidney cancers combined as a single outcome.

Other Potential Occupational Carcinogens

IARC has concluded that arsenic, cadmium, printing processes, and welding fumes also are probably carcinogenic (group 2A) to the human kidney, based on sufficient animal evidence and limited evidence from human studies. Exposure to tetrachloroethylene (perchloroethylene), a chlorinated solvent widely used in dry cleaning, has also been associated with an increased risk of kidney cancer in a US population–based case-control study.

Pathology & Pathophysiology

The mechanism of TCE's carcinogenicity is not completely understood but is thought to be due to both mutagenic and cytotoxic effects on the kidney. Once absorbed, TCE is metabolized via glutathione- (GSH-) mediated pathways that result in genotoxic and nephrotoxic metabolites that are both generated in and delivered to the kidneys. Chronic renal tubular damage may be a precursor to TCE-induced renal carcinogenicity.

Clinical Findings

A. Symptoms and Signs

Symptoms of kidney cancer include hematuria, unilateral low back or flank pain, fatigue, and unexplained weight loss. Physical examination can demonstrate costovertebral angle tenderness, a palpable low back, flank, or abdominal mass, or, in cases of significant renal insufficiency, peripheral edema.

B. Laboratory Findings

Blood tests can show acute or chronic renal insufficiency and anemia. Urinalysis can demonstrate hematuria and proteinuria and urine cytology may be positive for dysplastic cells.

C. Imaging and Diagnosis

For renal cell carcinoma, CT is the imaging method of choice for initial visualization and diagnosis. MRI, ultrasound, PET or PET/CT, intravenous pyelogram, or angiography also can be used to supplement the CT images or to look for regional lymph node or vascular involvement. Unlike with most other cancers, imaging is often sufficient for diagnosis with no need for a diagnostic biopsy. The same imaging modalities are used, with the addition of ureteroscopy/cystoscopy and, if feasible, biopsy.

Medical Surveillance & Prevention

The US OSHA standard for TCE consists of an 8-hour TWA exposure limit of 100 ppm and a STEL of 200 ppm, both of which are less protective than virtually every other developed country (8-hour TWA exposure limits mostly ranging from 10–50 ppm and STEL mostly at 20–100 ppm).

The US Preventive Services Task Force does not provide recommendations regarding routine screening for kidney cancer for the general public. However, workers with significant histories of exposure to TCE may benefit from medical surveillance, including periodic physical examinations, urinalysis, and blood work monitoring hemoglobin and kidney function.

The most effective means of preventing TCE-related health effects is to use a safer substitute. Employers still using TCE should lower air concentrations to levels that do not pose a risk to employees, require respiratory and skin protection, and have periodic medical surveillance of exposed employees.

Treatment & Prognosis

For renal cell carcinomas detected before spread to lymph nodes or metastasis, radical nephrectomy is the treatment of choice and often curative. Cancers that spread to lymph nodes are still treated with radical nephrectomy though not as successfully, while stage IV cancers with distant metastases are almost always incurable, with palliative care the focus. For all patients, common nonsurgical options include external beam radiation therapy, arterial embolization, and anti-angiogenic and immunotherapies. For localized transitional cell carcinomas of the renal pelvis or ureter, nephroureterectomy including resection of the bladder cuff is indicated, while treatment for disease with regional or distant metastatic spread is often limited to radiation or chemotherapy.

Because renal cell carcinoma is usually diagnosed early in the disease process, 5-year survival rates are relatively high, at 75%, but this decreases dramatically to just 12% with the presence of distant metastases. Five-year survival rates for transitional cell carcinomas of the renal pelvis or ureter are 80–100% if localized but just 5–30% with any infiltration of the pelvic wall or regional or distal spread.

OVARIAN CANCER

ESSENTIALS OF DIAGNOSIS

- ▶ Exposure to asbestos is the major occupational risk factor.
- ▶ Often asymptomatic in early stages. Presenting complaints in later stages include nonspecific symptoms such as pelvic or abdominal pain, abdominal bloating, vaginal bleeding, dysuria, or early satiety.
- ▶ Diagnosis by imaging (ultrasound, CT, and/or MRI), CA-125 blood levels, and biopsy.

General Considerations

Ovarian cancers are those involving any of the cell types in the ovary. Worldwide, it is the eighth most commonly diagnosed cancer in women, with 295,000 new cases and 185,000 deaths every year. Epithelial cancers account for up to 90% of all malignant tumors, with stromal and germ cell tumors much less common subtypes. Major nonoccupational risk factors include genetic predisposition, especially the presence of BRCA1 and BRCA2 mutations, increased number of lifetime ovulations, and increased body mass index.

Occupational Etiologies

The major occupational cause of ovarian cancer is asbestos, which has been used commercially for more than 100 years for a wide variety of uses. Asbestos refers to a group of fibrous silicates of several types. The minerals are divided into two classes: serpentine (chrysotile) and amphiboles (amosite, crocidolite, actinolite, anthophyllite, and tremolite). The three most common commercial forms are chrysotile, amosite, and crocidolite. Chrysotile represents 95% of all the asbestos used worldwide. All three commonly used forms of asbestos are known to cause an increased risk of cancer.

Workers are exposed to asbestos primarily through inhalation and, to a lesser extent ingestion, in a number of industries, including the mining and milling of asbestos, the manufacture or use of products containing asbestos, the construction and automotive industries, and in the asbestos-abatement industry. It is estimated that 125 million workers around the world are exposed to asbestos in the course of their jobs.

IARC has classified asbestos as carcinogenic to humans (group 1) specifically with regards to ovarian cancer (among other cancers) and that a causal relationship is "clearly established." This conclusion was based on evidence from at least five strongly positive cohort studies in women with high occupational exposures to asbestos and was further supported by at least two epidemiologic studies demonstrating a positive, though not statistically significant association between environmental, nonoccupational exposure to asbestos and ovarian cancer. A 2011 meta-analysis of 18 cohort studies of occupational exposure to asbestos among women confirmed the association. In most of the studies, crocidolite and chrysotile asbestos were the specific fiber types implicated, with crocidolite asbestos conferring the highest risk of ovarian cancer. However, several studies in which the type of asbestos fiber was not known still demonstrated an increased aggregate risk of ovarian cancer.

In addition to asbestos, ionizing radiation also has been linked to the development of ovarian cancer, based primarily on the Life Span Study of Japanese atomic bomb survivors.

Pathology & Pathophysiology

The mechanism of asbestos' carcinogenicity in ovaries is not completely understood. Once inhaled or ingested, asbestos is cleared into the pleural or peritoneal cavities and can accumulate and persist for years in many different body tissues, including the ovaries. A histopathologic study found "significant asbestos fiber burdens" in the ovaries of most women whose husbands had documented exposure to asbestos whereas such findings were about half as frequent in women with no known asbestos exposure history.

Clinical Findings

A. Symptoms and Signs

Symptoms of ovarian cancer often do not manifest until the cancer has metastasized and are usually nonspecific. They can include pelvic or abdominal pain, abdominal bloating, vaginal bleeding, dysuria, nausea and early satiety, fatigue, and unexplained weight loss. Physical examination can demonstrate a palpable adnexal mass on pelvic examination, abdominal distension, or in cases of advanced disease, ascites, pleural effusion, or bowel obstruction.

B. Laboratory Findings

An elevated CA-125 is seen in most women with epithelial ovarian cancer, but less often in early-stage cancers. In addition, this biomarker is nonspecific and can be elevated due to a variety of cancerous and noncancerous conditions. Serial tracking of CA-125 levels may be useful to monitor the progress of treatment.

C. Imaging and Diagnosis

Transvaginal ultrasound is the imaging method of choice for initial visualization and diagnosis of ovarian cancer. Subsequent CT or MRI is recommended for better visualization of suspicious masses and to look for regional lymph node or peritoneal spread. Fine needle aspiration or percutaneous biopsy of suspicious ovarian masses is not routinely recommended due to the potential to spread ("seed") any still-localized cancer to the peritoneal cavity. Definitive diagnosis is made through laparoscopic or open surgical techniques. In advanced disease in the setting of ascites, aspiration and cytologic analysis of peritoneal fluid can be performed.

Medical Surveillance & Prevention

The US Preventive Services Task Force recommends against routine screening of asymptomatic women for ovarian cancer, without a high-risk genetic cancer syndrome.

The most effective means of preventing asbestos-related health effects is to remove asbestos from all workplaces and to protect asbestos-abatement workers responsible for removing asbestos to the fullest extent possible. The US EPA attempted to ban most uses of asbestos in the United States in 1989, but this was overturned by a judicial ruling 2 years later. To this day, the production, import, and use of asbestos remain legal in most countries around the world. In the absence of a total ban, employers with workers potentially exposed to asbestos must at a minimum abide by regulatory authorities' requirements for occupational asbestos exposures, which in the United States includes an 8-hour TWA of 0.1 fibers per cubic meter of air, engineering controls, respiratory protection, exposure and medical monitoring, and hazard communication, among other measures.

▶ Treatment & Prognosis

Surgery and chemotherapy are indicated for almost all patients with ovarian cancer. For early-stage cancers, surgery usually consists of a hysterectomy, bilateral salpingo-oophorectomy, and omentectomy, along with biopsies and followed by chemotherapy. For more advanced cancers, this protocol is accompanied by removal of as much cancerous tissue as possible.

Because most ovarian cancers are diagnosed after the tumor has metastasized, the overall 5-year survival rate is low, at 48%. This increases to 92% for the minority of patients with localized disease at diagnosis and is just 29% for patients with distant metastases.

SKIN CANCER (NONMELANOMATOUS)

ESSENTIALS OF DIAGNOSIS

▶ Major risk is ultraviolet (UV) radiation.

▶ Skin findings: crusting, ulceration, easy bleeding, changing pigmented lesion.

▶ Fair complexion increases risk.

Skin Carcinogens, With Occupations at Risk

- Solar (UV) radiation
  - Outdoor workers
- PAHs, including those from creosotes
  - Workers exposed to coal-tar, coal-tar pitch and soot, such as roofers
  - Workers exposed to untreated or mildly treated mineral oils, for example, metal workers
- Workers exposed to shale oil and those in the petroleum refining industry
- Arsenic
  - Arsenical pesticide production and use
  - Copper, lead, zinc smelting
  - Sheep-dip manufacturers (contamination of drinking water)
- Ionizing radiation
  - Uranium miners
  - Health workers

▶ General Considerations

Neoplastic diseases of the skin are commonly divided into melanoma and nonmelanomatous skin cancer (NMSC), which consists mainly of basal cell and squamous cell carcinoma. NMSC is currently the most common form of cancer in the white population of the United States, accounting for one-third of all diagnosed cases of cancer. Although the dominant risk factor for NMSC (UV light) has been established, epidemiologic study of skin cancer has been limited. NMSC has an excellent prognosis, with 96–99% cure rates, making death certificate reviews useless.

There is an incorrect perception that skin cancer other than melanoma is a trivial disease. In addition, patients are rarely hospitalized, with the result that they are commonly not included in cancer registries. Because of failure to register or record skin cancers, much of the data on incidence are from surveys conducted many years ago. It is projected that more than 80,000 Americans will develop NMSC each year. Basal cell cancer is more than three times as common as squamous cell cancer.

Globally, NMSC is the most common form of cancer, more common than all other cancers combined. Most of these cancers are due to solar (UV) radiation and occur at high rates in people who work or play in the sunlight or use tanning booths and tanning lights.

▶ Etiology

The primary causes of skin cancer in industry include UV radiation, PAHs, arsenic, and ionizing radiation. The information presented below refers primarily to NMSC. An increased risk of melanoma is associated with UV light exposure.

A. UV Radiation

The major risk factor for skin cancer in lightly pigmented persons is radiation from the sun. The experiment of nature in which different intensities of UV radiation occur at different global latitudes has provided the opportunity for many epidemiologic studies to show an increased incidence of NMSC in whites at latitudes closer to the equator. The earliest realization that excess sun exposure leads to skin cancer was made on the basis of occupation in 1890, when Unna described changes of the skin of sailors, including skin cancer that resulted from prolonged exposure to the weather.

There are approximately 4.8 million outdoor workers in the United States, with certain occupations at greater risk, such as those in agriculture and professional sports. In experimental animals, the most carcinogenic wavelength is in the range of 290–300 nm (sunlight does not include wavelengths < 290 nm). The actual carcinogenic spectrum for humans is unknown. It is also notable that in experimental animals, a variety of foreign substances, including phototoxic chemicals (eg, coal tar, methoxsalen), chemical carcinogens (eg, benzo[a]pyrene), and nonspecific irritants (eg, xylene), under suitable conditions augment UV carcinogenesis.

B. Polycyclic Aromatic Hydrocarbons

Although chemical carcinogenesis of the skin does not seem to be nearly as frequent a cause of NMSC as UV radiation, it was described more than a century earlier. Percival Pott described the increased incidence of scrotal cancer in chimney sweeps in 1775, but it was not until the 1940s that a PAH, benzo[a]pyrene, was shown to be a constituent of soot. These hydrocarbons have the ability to induce skin cancers in laboratory animals, and mixtures of them are found in coal tar, pitch, asphalt, soot, creosotes, anthracenes, paraffin waxes, and lubricating and cutting oils. Exposures to untreated or mildly treated mineral oil containing PAHs have been linked to skin and scrotal cancers among mule spinners, wax pressmen, metal workers exposed to poorly refined cutting oils, and machine operators using lubricating oils. Latent periods between exposure to PAHs and skin cancer vary from about 20 (coal tar) to 50 years or more (mineral oil).

C. Arsenic

Arsenic causes cancer in experimental animals and is a well-recognized human carcinogen. Skin tumors associated with arsenic occur following ingestion, injection, or inhalation, as well as from skin contact. Medicinal inorganic arsenicals and arsenic in drinking water are the sources most commonly implicated. Detailed studies in Taiwan established that use of well water with high arsenic concentrations resulted in skin cancer, with a dose-response relationship. An estimated 1.5 million workers in the United States are exposed to inorganic arsenic in such diverse trades as copper and lead smelting, the metallurgical industry, and the production and use of pesticides; however, skin tumors attributed to occupational arsenic exposure are very uncommon. It is thought that some of the cases cited in the literature of agricultural workers with arsenic-induced skin cancers may be the result of other carcinogenic influences, such as sunlight and tars. The simultaneous presence of arsenical hyperkeratoses or hyperpigmentation, which occurs at lower exposure levels, strongly implicates arsenic as the etiologic agent in an individual with NMSC. In addition, cancers tend to be multiple and occur in younger patients than those attributable to UV light.

D. Ionizing Radiation

Roentgen radiation-induced skin carcinoma was first reported in 1902, shortly after the discovery of x-rays, in those who worked the machines. There was an excess in skin cancer deaths among radiologists in the period 1920–1939, and an excess risk also has been found for uranium miners. Patients receiving radiation for acne, tinea capitis, and facial hair in the past had an increased risk of invasive skin cancers. The latent period for radiation-induced skin cancers varies inversely with the dose, with the overall range from 7 weeks to 56 years (average 25–30 years), and the skin cancers often occur in areas with chronic radiation dermatitis. Although epidemiologic studies do not give reliable data on dose-response relationships, the risk from exposures under 1000 cGy appears to be small, and skin cancer may be induced by dose equivalents of 3000 cGy. There are now strict controls on industrial and occupational exposure to ionizing radiation, and currently, it appears that ionizing radiation is not responsible for much cutaneous carcinogenesis.

E. Shale Oil and Petroleum Refining

Workers in the shale oil and petroleum refining industries (both IARC group 2A carcinogens) also are at risk for skin cancer. In the early twentieth century, increased rates of skin cancer, mainly in the scrotum, were found in British workers in the shale oil industry and in cotton-textile workers who used shale oil as a lubricant. Petroleum refining workers are exposed to a wide range of potentially carcinogenic substances, including PAHs and mineral oils, and have been found to have higher rates of skin cancer, mainly squamous cell carcinoma but also, in a few cases, melanoma, leading to IARC's classification of petroleum refining as a probable skin carcinogen.

▶ Pathophysiology

Early studies elucidated the two-stage theory of carcinogenesis. They found that a single application of a potent carcinogen such as benzo[a]pyrene applied in a quantity insufficient to cause tumors allowed tumor development after subsequent application of croton oil, which by itself produced no tumors at all. The authors theorized that the production of a tumor was initiated by the carcinogen but that its subsequent development could be promoted nonspecifically. It appears that initiation is permanent and irreversible, but promotion, up to a point, is reversible.

UV light fits into this theory of chemical carcinogenesis in that it appears to be both an initiator and a promoter for carcinoma of the skin. Two major effects of UV radiation on the skin that seem likely to be responsible for the carcinogenic effects are photochemical alteration of the DNA and alterations in immunity. Certain immunologic defects, both in skin and in lymphocytes, can be induced by UV radiation. Exposure to UV light depletes the dermis of Langerhans cells and renders it unable to be sensitized to potent allergens. Alterations at the level of DNA are also thought to be responsible for ionizing radiation-induced skin cancers.

▶ Pathology

The histologic types of skin lesions associated with sun exposure include solar keratoses, basal cell epitheliomas, squamous cell carcinomas, keratoacanthomas, as well as malignant melanomas. Solar keratoses contain morphologically cancerous cells, but they are considered premalignant because invasion is limited to the most superficial part of the dermis. Approximately 13% of all solar keratoses develop into squamous cell carcinomas, but these are rarely aggressive.

The estimated incidence of metastases from all sun-induced squamous cell carcinomas is 0.5% or less. Almost all squamous cell carcinomas in whites occur in highly sun-exposed areas, but 40% of basal cell epitheliomas occur on shaded areas of the head and neck.

Regardless of the source of exposure, certain features are common in all cases of arsenic-induced skin cancers. Punctate keratoses of the palms and soles and hyperpigmentation are seen frequently. The skin tumors are of several types. Squamous cell carcinomas arise either from normal skin or from keratoses. Basal cell epitheliomas, including multiple superficial squamous cell and basal cell epitheliomas, as well as areas of intraepidermal (in situ) squamous cell carcinoma (Bowen disease), have been described. Multiple tumors, most of which are found on unexposed areas, are the rule. Cancer of the scrotum, which is seen following topical exposure to PAHs, is rare.

Early radiation workers with heavy exposure from uncalibrated machines developed predominantly squamous cell carcinomas, found mainly on the hands and feet and occasionally on the face. More recently, basal cell cancers have been described following repeated occupational exposures. Radiation-related tumors usually arise in areas of chronic radiation dermatitis, and whether they can occur on clinically normal skin is a matter of dispute.

▶ Clinical Findings

Basal cell epithelioma frequently presents as a nodular or nodular-ulcerative lesion on the skin of the head and neck and only 10% of the time on the skin of the trunk. It is much less common on the upper extremities and very uncommon on the lower extremities. The lesion generally is smooth, shiny, and translucent, with telangiectatic vessels just beneath the surface. It is usually not painful or tender, even with ulceration, except when crusting or bleeding is seen with minor trauma. Basal cell carcinomas rarely metastasize, but they can invade widely and deeply, extending through the subcutaneous tissue to involve neurovascular structures and occasionally erode into bone.

Squamous cell carcinoma presents first in a premalignant stage characterized by actinic keratosis, a rough, reddened plaque on sun-exposed skin. There is then an in situ stage, which appears as a well-demarcated, slightly raised erythematous plaque with more substance and scaling than actinic keratosis. Squamous cell cancers arising in sun-exposed areas of the body tend to be on the most highly irradiated areas, such as the tip of the nose, the forehead, the tips of the helices of the ears, the lower lip, or the backs of the hands. Metastases are more common than from basal cell cancer, and squamous cell cancers on mucosal membranes metastasize more frequently than do those found on the skin surface.

▶ Prevention

The most important step in prevention of occupation-related skin cancers is avoidance of UV light. This is especially true for workers who are more susceptible to UV light, such as those with fair complexions or with certain hereditary diseases (eg, albinism and xeroderma pigmentosum).

Protective clothing, such as wide-brimmed hats and long sleeves, is the most effective barrier to UV radiation exposure in outdoor workers. Sunscreens that provide protection in the UVA and UVB spectrum should be used daily. The effectiveness of sunscreens in preventing NMSC and melanoma is unknown, though their effectiveness for avoidance of erythema has been proved. Periodic examinations are recommended to detect the presence of malignant and premalignant skin lesions among those at risk.

The incidence of scrotal cancer is now rare because of preventive measures. Good personal hygiene should include compulsory showering and changing of clothes when entering and leaving the plant, as well as washing of exposed skin after leaving contaminated areas. Isolated or closed-system operations, protective clothing, and employee education are also critical in avoidance of skin cancer induced by PAHs.

Currently, the maximum allowable dose equivalent of ionizing radiation for occupational exposure to the skin is 30 rems in any year, except that forearms and hands are allowed 75 rems in any year (because there is little red marrow in the forearms and hands). These recommendations are based mainly on avoidance of hematologic disease and may need to be revised in order to prevent skin cancer. Exposure can be limited further by the use of shielding devices such as lead gloves and aprons.

▶ Diagnosis & Treatment

Biopsy is necessary in all cases of suspected skin carcinoma. Treatment for occupationally induced skin cancers is not different from other skin cancers.

OTHER CANCERS

A number of agents are known to cause certain other cancers in humans. Work in the rubber production industry is causally associated with stomach cancer, as well as leukemia, lymphoma, and lung and urinary bladder cancers. Ionizing radiation, specifically x- and γ-radiation, is known to cause a number of cancers in humans—salivary gland, esophagus, stomach, colon, lung, bone, skin (basal cell), female breast, kidney, urinary bladder, brain and central nervous system, thyroid, and leukemia (excluding chronic lymphocytic leukemia). Occupational lead exposure has been shown, in an observational study of two large cohorts of workers in Finland and Great Britain, to be associated with increased risks of brain, lung, laryngeal, stomach cancers, and Hodgkin lymphoma. IARC has classified lead as "probably carcinogenic to humans." Many other cancers are reported to be associated with specific occupational or environmental exposures in humans, most with limited evidence based upon epidemiologic studies. Semiconductor workers demonstrate excess risks for non-Hodgkin lymphoma, leukemia, brain tumor, and breast cancer. There is evidence that exposure to asbestos increases the risk of cancers of the pharynx, stomach, and colorectum.

REFERENCES

3M: Regulation Update—Methylene Chloride. April 20, 1997: http://multimedia.3m.com/mws/media/276354O/regulations-update-20-methylene-chloride.pdf. Accessed March 20, 2019.

ACS. Bladder Cancer Risk Factors. https://www.cancer.org/cancer/bladder-cancer/causes-risks-prevention/risk-factors.html.

ACS: Kidney Cancer, Tests: https://www.cancer.org/cancer/kidney-cancer/detection-diagnosis-staging/how-diagnosed.html.

ACS. What Causes Bladder Cancer? https://www.cancer.org/cancer/bladder-cancer/causes-risks-prevention/what-causes.html.

American Cancer Society. Risk Factors for Kidney Cancer. https://www.cancer.org/cancer/kidney-cancer/causes-risks-prevention/risk-factors.html.

American Cancer Society. Survival rates for bile duct cancer. https://www.cancer.org/cancer/bile-duct-cancer/detection-diagnosis-staging/survival-by-stage.html.

American Cancer Society. Treatment of Liver Cancer by Stage. https://www.cancer.org/cancer/liver-cancer/treating/by-stage.html.

American Cancer Society. Liver Cancer Survival Rates. https://www.cancer.org/cancer/liver-cancer/detection-diagnosis-staging/survival-rates.html.

American Cancer Society. Kidney Cancer Survival Rates. https://www.cancer.org/cancer/kidney-cancer/detection-diagnosis-staging/survival-rates.html.

American Cancer Society. What Is Bladder Cancer? https://www.cancer.org/cancer/bladder-cancer/about/what-is-bladder-cancer.html.

American Cancer Society. Tests for Kidney Cancer. https://www.cancer.org/cancer/kidney-cancer/detection-diagnosis-staging/how-diagnosed.html.

American Cancer Society. Cancer Statistics Center. Lung and Bronchus. https://cancerstatisticscenter.cancer.org/?_ga=2.265743750.866082910.1550537740-1664590862.1550537740#!/cancer-site/Lung%20and%20bronchus. Accessed February 18, 2019.

American Cancer Society. Health Risks of Secondhand Smoke. https://www.cancer.org/cancer/cancer-causes/tobacco-and-cancer/secondhand-smoke.html. Accessed February 18, 2019.

American Cancer Society. Key Statistics for Bile Duct Cancers. https://www.cancer.org/cancer/cancer-causes/infectious-agents/infections-that-can-lead-to-cancer/parasites.html; and Parasites that Can Lead to Cancer. https://www.cancer.org/cancer/cancer-causes/infectious-agents/infections-that-can-lead-to-cancer/parasites.html.

Bray F, Ferlay J, Soerjomataram I, Siegel RL, Torre LA, Jemal A: Global cancer statistics 2018: GLOBOCAN estimates of incidence and mortality worldwide for 36 cancers in 185 countries. CA Cancer J Clin 2018;68(6):394-424 [PMID: 30207593].

Bray F et al: Global cancer statistics 2018: GLOBOCAN estimates of incidence and mortality worldwide for 36 cancers in 185 countries. CA Cancer J Clin 2018;68(6):394-424.

Camargo MC et al: Occupational exposure to asbestos and ovarian cancer: a meta-analysis. Environ Health Perspect 2011;119(9):1211-1217.

Canadian Cancer Society. Diagnosis of cancer of the renal pelvis or ureter. https://www.cancer.ca/en/cancer-information/cancer-type/renal-pelvis-and-ureter/diagnosis/?region=on.

Cancer.net. ASCO. Bladder Cancer: Stages and Grades. https://www.cancer.net/cancer-types/bladder-cancer/stages-and-grades.

Centers for Disease Control and Prevention. What Are the Risk Factors for Lung Cancer? https://www.cdc.gov/cancer/lung/basic_info/risk_factors.htm. Accessed February 18, 2019.

Centers for Disease Control and Prevention. Smoking is down, but almost 38 million American adults still smoke. January 18, 2018. https://www.cdc.gov/media/releases/2018/p0118-smoking-rates-declining.html. Accessed February 18, 2019.

EPA Actions to Protect the Public From Asbestos. https://www.epa.gov/asbestos/epa-actions-protect-public-exposure-asbestos. Accessed May 31, 2019.

Farioli A et al: Radiation-induced mesothelioma among long-term solid cancer survivors: a longitudinal analysis of SEER database. Cancer Med 2016;5(5):950-959 [PMID: 26860323].

Federal Register 2014 Oct 10;79(197):61422.

GESTIS International Limit Values. 1,2-Dichloropropane. https://limitvalue.ifa.dguv.de/WebForm_ueliste2.aspx. Accessed April 28, 2019.

GESTIS International Limit Values. Dichloromethane (CAS 75-09-2). http://limitvalue.ifa.dguv.de/WebForm_ueliste2.aspx. Accessed March 20, 2019.

Ghouri YA, Mian I, Rowe JH: Review of hepatocellular carcinoma: epidemiology, etiology, and carcinogenesis. J Carcinog 2017;16:1.

Heller DS, Gordon RE, Westhoff C, Gerber S. Asbestos exposure and ovarian fiber burden. Am J Ind Med 1996;29(5):435-439. https://onlinelibrary.wiley.com/doi/full/10.3322/caac.21492.

https://www.who.int/news-room/fact-sheets/detail/cancer.

IARC Monograph: Erionite. 2018. https://monographs.iarc.fr/wp-content/uploads/2018/06/mono100C-12.pdf.

IARC Monographs for: Orthotoluidine (https://monographs.iarc.fr/wp-content/uploads/2018/06/mono100F-11.pdf), 2-naphthylamine (https://monographs.iarc.fr/wp-content/uploads/2018/06/mono100F-10.pdf), benzidine 2010 (https://monographs.iarc.fr/wp-content/uploads/2018/06/mono99-10.pdf), and 4-aminobiphenyl (https://monographs.iarc.fr/wp-content/uploads/2018/06/mono100F-6.pdf).

IARC. Monograph: 2-naphthylamine. https://monographs.iarc.fr/wp-content/uploads/2018/06/mono100F-10.pdf.

IARC Monograph. Vinyl Chloride. PDF pp. 5-6.

IARC Monograph. Arsenic.

IARC Monograph. Aflatoxins. https://monographs.iarc.fr/wp-content/uploads/2018/06/mono100F-23.pdf.

IARC. Shale oil monograph. https://monographs.iarc.fr/wp-content/uploads/2018/06/mono100F-20.pdf.

IARC. Petroleum refining monograph. https://publications.iarc.fr/Book-And-Report-Series/Iarc-Monographs-On-The-Identification-Of-Carcinogenic-Hazards-To-Humans/Occupational-Exposures-In-Petroleum-Refining-Crude-Oil-And-Major-Petroleum-Fuels-1989.

IARC. Inorganic and organic lead compounds. Monograph 87. 2006. https://monographs.iarc.fr/iarc-monographs-on-the-evaluation-of-carcinogenic-risks-to-humans-34/.

IARC's 2012 Asbestos Monograph: https://monographs.iarc.fr/wp-content/uploads/2018/06/mono100C-11.pdf.

IARC's 2012 Asbestos Monograph, PDF p. 38: https://monographs.iarc.fr/wp-content/uploads/2018/06/mono100C-11.pdf.

IARC's 2014 Monograph on TCE: https://monographs.iarc.fr/wp-content/uploads/2018/06/mono106-001.pdf.

IARC's 2012 Asbestos Monograph: https://monographs.iarc.fr/wp-content/uploads/2018/06/mono100C-11.pdf.

IARC Monograph on Radiation. https://monographs.iarc.fr/wp-content/uploads/2018/06/mono100D.pdf.

IARC's 2012 Asbestos Monograph, PDF p. 38: https://monographs.iarc.fr/wp-content/uploads/2018/06/mono100C-11.pdf.

Johns Hopkins School of Medicine. Cholangiocarcinoma: Introduction. https://www.hopkinsmedicine.org/gastroenterology_hepatology/_pdfs/pancreas_biliary_tract/cholangiocarcinoma.pdf.

Kinoshita M et al: Occupational cholangiocarcinoma diagnosed 18 years after the end of exposure to 1,2-dichloropropane and dichloromethane at a printing company: a case report. Surg Case Rep 2019;5(1):65 [PMID: 31016414].

Kubo S et al: Case series of 17 patients with cholangiocarcinoma among young adult workers of a printing company in Japan. J Hepatobiliary Pancreat Sci 2014;21(7):479-488.

Kubo S et al: Occupational cholangiocarcinoma caused by exposure to 1,2-dichloropropane and/or dichloromethane. Ann Gastroenterol Surg 2017;2(2):99-105.

Kumagai S, Kurumatani N, Arimoto A, Ichihara G: Cholangiocarcinoma among offset colour proof-printing workers exposed to 1,2-dichloropropane and/or dichloromethane. Occup Environ Med 2013;70(7):508-510.

Loomis D, Guha N, Hall AL, Straif K: Identifying occupational carcinogens: an update from the IARC monographs. Occup Environ Med 2018;75(8):593-603 [PMID: 29769352].

Mahdavifar N, Ghoncheh M, Pakzad R, Momenimovahed Z, Salehiniya H. Epidemiology, incidence and mortality of bladder cancer and their relationship with the development index in the world. Asian Pac J Cancer Prev 2016;17(1):381-386 [PMID: 26838243].

Marant MC et al: Occupational exposures and cancer: a review of agents and relative risk estimates. Occup Environ Med 2018;75(8):604-614 [PMID: 29735747].

Mayo Clinic. Kidney Cancer. https://www.mayoclinic.org/diseases-conditions/kidney-cancer/symptoms-causes/syc-20352664.

Medscape. Bladder Cancer: Signs and Symptoms. https://emedicine.medscape.com/article/438262-overview.

Medscape. HCC. Workup. https://emedicine.medscape.com/article/197319-workup#c5.

Medscape: Ovarian Cancer. Revised October 2018. https://emedicine.medscape.com/article/255771-overview.

National Cancer Institute. Bile Duct Cancer (Cholangiocarcinoma) Treatment (PDQ®)–Health Professional Version. https://www.cancer.gov/types/liver/hp/bile-duct-treatment-pdq. Accessed April 28, 2019.

National Cancer Institute. Bile Duct Cancer. https://www.cancer.gov/types/liver/patient/about-bile-duct-cancer-pdq.

National Cancer Institute. Bile Duct Cancer (Cholangiocarcinoma) Treatment (PDQ®)–Patient Version. https://www.cancer.gov/types/liver/patient/bile-duct-treatment-pdq. Accessed April 28, 2019.

National Cancer Institute. Cancer Stat Facts: Kidney and Renal Pelvis Cancer. https://seer.cancer.gov/statfacts/html/kidrp.html.

National Cancer Institute. Ovarian Cancer: Treatment. https://www.cancer.gov/types/ovarian/hp/ovarian-epithelial-treatment-pdq#_676_toc.

National Cancer Institute. Cancer Fast Stats: Ovarian Cancer. https://seer.cancer.gov/statfacts/html/ovary.html.

National Cancer Institute. Renal Cell Cancer Treatment (PDQ®)–Health Professional Version. https://www.cancer.gov/types/kidney/hp/kidney-treatment-pdq#_31.

National Cancer Institute. Transitional Cell Cancer of the Renal Pelvis and Ureter Treatment (PDQ®)–Health Professional Version. https://www.cancer.gov/types/kidney/hp/transitional-cell-treatment-pdq#_49.

National Cancer Institute. Five year survival rates: renal pelvis and ureter cancer. https://training.seer.cancer.gov/kidney/intro/survival.html.

National Toxicology Program. Report on Carcinogens: TCE. 2015. https://ntp.niehs.nih.gov/ntp/roc/monographs/finaltce_508.pdf. PDF p. 24

National Toxicology Program. Report on Carcinogens: TCE. 2015. https://ntp.niehs.nih.gov/ntp/roc/monographs/finaltce_508.pdf. PDF p. 198.

NCI. Bladder and Other Urothelial Cancers Screening (PDQ®)–Health Professional Version. https://www.cancer.gov/types/bladder/hp/bladder-screening-pdq#_60.

NCI. Bladder Cancer Treatment. https://www.cancer.gov/types/bladder/patient/bladder-treatment-pdq#_134.

NCI. Cancer Stat Facts: Bladder Cancer. https://seer.cancer.gov/statfacts/html/urinb.html.

NCI. Cancer Stats: Bladder. https://seer.cancer.gov/statfacts/html/urinb.html.

NCI. Liver Cancer Prevention. https://www.cancer.gov/types/liver/patient/liver-prevention-pdq#section/_28.

NIH. Smoking and Bladder Cancer. 2011. https://www.nih.gov/news-events/nih-research-matters/smoking-bladder-cancer.

NIOSH (2016). Current intelligence bulletin 68: NIOSH chemical carcinogen policy. By Whittaker C, et al, on behalf of the NIOSH Carcinogen and RELs Policy Update Committee. Cincinnati, OH: U.S. Department of Health and Human Services, Centers for Disease Control and Prevention, National Institute for Occupational Safety and Health, DHHS (NIOSH) Publication No. 2017-100, p. 19.

NIOSH. Occupational Cancer. https://www.cdc.gov/niosh/topics/cancer/default.html. Accessed April 8, 2019.

NTP 2015 report. See Zhao2005 cohort study on Boeing aerospace workers and Charbotel2005 case control study on screw cutting plant workers. PDF pp. 307-320.

NTP 2015 report, PDF pp. 113-116.

NTP 2015 report, PDF p. 84.

NTP 2015 report, PDF p. 127.

OSHA. PELs. 1910.1000. Table Z-1. https://www.osha.gov/laws-regs/regulations/standardnumber/1910/1910.1000TABLEZ1. Accessed April 28, 2019.

OSHA. PELs. 1910.1000. Table Z-2. https://www.osha.gov/dsg/annotated-pels/tablez-2.html. Note absence of any reference within table to a more detailed standard, as there are for formaldehyde and methylene chloride.

OSHA Asbestos Regulation. 1910.1001. https://www.osha.gov/laws-regs/regulations/standardnumber/1910/1910.1001.

PAHO. History of Aromatic Amines and Occupational Bladder Cancer. http://www.bvsde.paho.org/bvsast/i/fulltext/training_problembased/case8_table7.htm.

Reid BM, Permuth JB, Sellers TA. Epidemiology of ovarian cancer: a review. Cancer Biol Med 2017;14(1):9-32. doi:10.20892/j.issn.2095-3941.2016.0084.

Rushton L: The global burden of occupational disease. Curr Environ Health Rep 2017 Sep;4(3):340-348 [PMID: 28733964].

Siacon A. EPA ban on popular toxic paint strippers: what to know. USA Today. March 16, 2019. https://www.usatoday.com/story/news/nation/2019/03/16/methylene-chloride-epa-bans-chemical-used-popular-paint-strippers/3190041002/. Accessed March 20, 2019.

Steenland K, et al. Cancer incidence among workers with blood lead measurements in two countries. Occup Environ Med 2019;76(9):603-610.

Thomas LB, Popper H. Pathology of angiosarcoma of the liver among vinyl chloride-polyvinyl chloride workers. Ann N Y Acad Sci 1975;246:268-277.

USPSTF Published Recommendations: Cancer. https://www.uspreventiveservicestaskforce.org/BrowseRec/Index. Accessed May 2, 2019.

USPSTF Published Recommendations: Ovarian Cancer. https://www.uspreventiveservicestaskforce.org/Page/Document/RecommendationStatementFinal/ovarian-cancer-screening1#Pod8. Accessed May 31, 2019.

Welch LS et al: Early detection of lung cancer in a population at high risk due to occupation and smoking. Occup Environ Med 2019;76(3):137-142 [PMID: 30415231].

WHO. Key Statistics on Cancer (updated September 2018).

Yamada K, Kumagai S, Endo G. Chemical exposure levels in printing workers with cholangiocarcinoma (second report). J Occup Health 2015;57(3):245-252.

Yan H, et al. Secondhand smoking increases bladder cancer risk in nonsmoking population: a meta-analysis. Cancer Manag Res 2018;10:3781-3791.

■ SELF-ASSESSMENT QUESTIONS

Select the one correct answer for each question.

Question 1: Latency period
a. is different than the induction-latency or incubation period
b. is unrelated to the general requirement for multiple heritable changes in the cell before a cancer develops
c. is the interval of time required from first exposure to the responsible agent to the development of malignancy
d. for most occupational cancers in humans is typically 2–8 years

Question 2: Epidemiologic studies
a. provide the strongest evidence for human carcinogenicity
b. evaluate effects on animals and human subjects
c. involve a small and discrete number of individuals
d. typically confirm carcinogenic effects

Question 3: Short-term tests
a. provide evidence of carcinogenicity or the ability to induce chromosomal damage by chemicals
b. assessed endpoints exclude gene mutation and induction of DNA damage and repair
c. rely solely on the fact that carcinogens covalently bind to DNA and thereby induce DNA damage
d. include the Ames test

Question 4: Tests for DNA repair
a. can demonstrate that DNA damage has occurred following exposure to a chemical
b. include cytogenetic tests that assess changes in the morphologic structure of chromosomes
c. consistently can be indicative of the effects of both genotoxic and nongenotoxic carcinogens
d. include chromosomal translocations and the formation of micronuclei

Question 5: DNA or protein adducts
a. are a potentially valuable tool in the measurement of levels of specific carcinogens covalently bound to DNA or proteins
b. are detectable only in white blood cells
c. do not quantify internal dose better than older available methods such as air monitoring or measuring blood or urine levels of an agent
d. help identify smokers in occupationally exposed groups

Question 6: Lung cancer
a. has a latency period of approximately 10 years
b. is readily detected by screening studies
c. is a major asbestos-related disease, accounting for 20% of all deaths in asbestos-exposed cohorts
d. is increased 10-fold in smoking asbestos-exposed workers

Question 7: Diesel-engine exhaust
a. has been demonstrated to increase the risk of lung cancer solely in studies of miners and railroad workers
b. is not considered a human carcinogen
c. in animal studies provides equivocal results
d. contains a number of nitroarenes, which are nitro-substituted derivatives of PAHs (arenes)

Question 8: Cancers of the nasal cavity and paranasal sinuses
- a. are common wherever smoking is prevalent
- b. are common in younger than 40–50 years
- c. are primarily adenocarcinomas
- d. are linked to many different occupational exposures

Question 9: All benzidine-derived dyes
- a. cause bladder cancer in the highest incidence in developing countries
- b. are ultimately metabolized to form nitroarenes, which are the active carcinogenic agent derived from the dyes
- c. cause bladder cancer with a mean latency period of about 10 years
- d. should be considered to be potential human carcinogens

Question 10: Arsenic
- a. is suspected to be a human carcinogen, although it has not been definitively confirmed through epidemiologic studies
- b. skin tumors associated with arsenic occur exclusively from skin contact
- c. induced skin cancers tend to be isolated and singular
- d. cancers occur in younger patients than those attributable to UV light

Question 11: Acute nonlymphocytic leukemia (ANLL)
- a. decreases with age with the highest rates in younger than 50
- b. and chronic myelogenous leukemia (CML) are linked to occupation
- c. is characterized by a diminished number of immature blood cell progenitors in the bone marrow
- d. due to benzene exposure is distinct from de novo leukemia

Genetic Toxicology

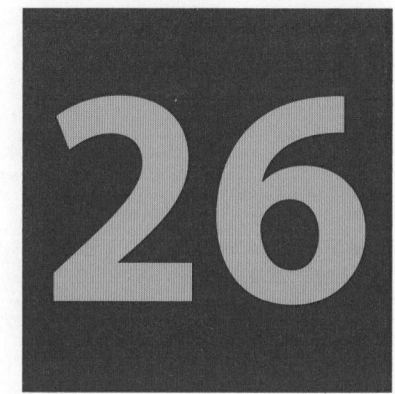

Ulrike Luderer, MD, PhD, MPH

WHAT IS GENETIC TOXICOLOGY?

Genetic toxicology is the study of the actions of chemical and physical agents on DNA. It encompasses genotoxicity, mutagenesis, and epigenetic alterations. Mutagenicity refers to induction of alterations in the DNA sequence that can be transmitted to daughter cells during cell division. Genotoxicity is a broader term that includes formation of DNA adducts, DNA strand breaks, sister chromatid exchanges, and unscheduled DNA synthesis. Epigenetic modifications are transmissible during cell division, but do not involve changes in the DNA sequence. Epigenetic alterations include changes in DNA methylation, histone modifications, and micro RNA expression. Potential health impacts of genotoxicity include cancer, genetic disorders, developmental toxicity, and epigenetically mediated transgenerational effects.

HISTORY

Early genetic toxicology studies focused on mutagenesis by environmental chemicals and radiation. Mutagenesis induced by x-rays was first discovered in the 1920s, and chemical mutagenesis by mustard gas was discovered in the 1940s, both in *Drosophila*. The first demonstration of mutagenesis in a mammal, by x-rays in mice, was published in 1951. Discovery of the structure of DNA in 1953 led to research into how chemicals and physical agents interact with DNA and development of *in vivo* and *in vitro* assays to identify mutagenic agents. The National Toxicology Program (NTP) was established in response to a Congressional recommendation to "launch a program of testing mutagenicity of all compounds produced in commercial quantities" in the National Institute of Environmental Health Sciences (NIEHS), one of the National Institutes of Health (NIH).

The field of (quantitative) structure-activity relationship (SAR and QSAR) modeling began in the early 1960s and grew as the database of molecular structures, reactivity, and toxicity, as well as computational methods grew in the subsequent decades. In the 1970s and 1980s, numerous relatively rapid *in vitro* and *in vivo* genotoxicity and mutagenicity tests were developed. Perhaps the most well-known of these is the so-called Ames test for mutagenicity utilizing the bacterium *Salmonella typhimurium*. In the 1980s and 1990s, much basic research focused on identifying molecular pathways involved in mediating toxicity. With the advent of transgenic mouse models, studies of global or tissue-specific and/or inducible deletion or overexpression of genes became possible *in vivo*. Epidemiologic research focused on the roles of specific genes in modulating toxicity, so-called gene-environment interactions. A large focus was on analyzing the impact of specific common genetic polymorphisms in xenobiotic metabolizing enzymes on susceptibility to diseases caused by occupational or environmental exposures.

Since the first draft sequence of the human genome in 2000 and the completion of the human genome sequence in 2003, there has been rapid development of so-called 'omics technologies that allow for global analyses of biological molecules within samples. Application of these technologies to toxicology holds promise for more efficient identification of genotoxic chemicals and deciphering of mechanisms of genotoxicity.

TYPES OF GENOTOXICITY AND CELLULAR DNA DAMAGE RESPONSES

Genotoxicity

Figure 26–1 shows the structure of DNA deoxyribonucleosides, which consist of a nitrogenous base (adenine, guanine, cytosine, or thymine) attached to a deoxyribose sugar. DNA can be modified by reactive chemicals, including metabolically activated xenobiotics, as well as by reactive oxygen and nitrogen species (ROS and RNS) generated as byproducts of oxidative phosphorylation and other cellular processes or during xenobiotic metabolism (Figure 26–2). Table 26–1 shows commonly modified sites in DNA.

Chemicals, the metabolism of which results in ROS generation, include polycyclic aromatic hydrocarbons (PAHs)

Purines

Pyrimidines

deoxyguanosine

deoxycytidine

deoxyadenosine

thymidine

▲ **Figure 26–1.** Chemical structure of deoxyribonucleo-sides. Nucleosides consist of nucleobases and a 5-carbon sugar, which in DNA is deoxyribose (dR). Nucleobases adenine and guanine are derived from purine, while nucleobases cytosine and thymine are derived from pyrimidine.

Table 26–1. Major nucleophilic sites in nucleic acids.

Nucleotide	Location
=N-guanine	N^3, N^7
Adenine	N^1, N^3, N^7
Cytosine	N^3
-NH-guanine	N^1
Thymidine	N^3
-NH$_2$-guanine	N^2
Adenine	N^6
Cytosine	N^4, C=O
Guanine	O^6
Cytosine	O^2
Thymidine	O^2, O^4
Any	P=O deoxyribose phosphate

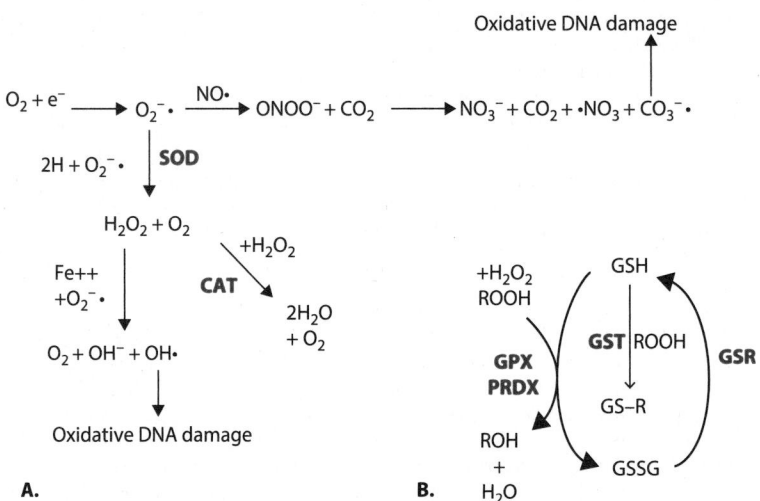

▲ **Figure 26–2.** ROS and RNS generation and detoxification. **A.** ROS are formed by the sequential addition of electrons to molecular oxygen, forming superoxide anion radical ($O_2^-\bullet$), H_2O_2, and hydroxyl radical. Peroxynitrite ($ONOO^-$) is formed when superoxide anion radical reacts with nitric oxide (NO). Carbonate anion radical ($CO_3^-\bullet$) is formed when peroxynitrite reacts with CO_2. Key antioxidant enzymes (in bold) and the reactions they catalyze are shown. CAT, catalase; SOD, superoxide dismutase. **B.** The tripeptide glutathione (GSH) acts as a cofactor for GPXs and GSTs to reduce peroxides. GSH can also scavenge free radicals through direct chemical reactions. GSR reduces the oxidized form of GSH (GSSG, Glutathione disulfide); GPX, glutathione peroxidase; GSR, Glutathione reductase; GST, Glutathione-S-transferase; PRDX, peroxiredoxin.

and menadione, which can be metabolized to redox cycling semiquinones and quinones cycling of quinones and semiquinones. Indirect ionization of water with resulting generation of ROS is responsible for about two-thirds of the DNA damage caused by ionizing radiation, while direct ionization of DNA is responsible for about a third of the DNA damage caused by ionizing radiation. Moreover, disruption of cellular processes involved in production and metabolism of ROS by ionizing radiation can result in persistently increased ROS generation lasting days to years.

Purine and pyrimidine deoxyribonucleosides in DNA can be oxidized by hydroxyl radicals (OH•), formed by the Fenton reaction in the presence of ferrous iron and hydrogen peroxide, by singlet oxygen ($^1O_2$), or by peroxynitrite-(ONOO-) derived carbonate anion radicals (see Figure 26–2A). The most common oxidized base in DNA is 8-oxo-7,8-dihydro-2′-deoxyguanosine (8-oxo-dG), due to guanine having the lowest oxidation potential of the four bases. In addition to single, oxidized bases, OH• and ionizing radiation can cause tandem base lesions between a pyrimidine radical and adjacent base, DNA inter-strand cross-links, DNA double-strand breaks, and complex oxidatively generated clustered DNA lesions.

Many genotoxic chemicals that directly bind covalently with DNA or are metabolized to reactive intermediates that bind to DNA are electrophilic and will therefore react with nucleophilic centers in DNA, such as N^7 and O^6 of guanine and phosphate groups (see Table 26–1). However, mutagenic activity in vitro and carcinogenicity in vivo do not correlate well with electrophilicity alone. Nucleophilic selectivity is also important, with monofunctional alkylating agents that exhibit low selectivity among nucleophiles being more tumorigenic than those exhibiting high selectivity for nucleophiles with high reactivity. This is because the sulfur containing sites on proteins, such as thiols in cysteine, have the highest nucleophilicity. So high selectivity monofunctional alkylating agents, such as methyl bromide or ethylene oxide, bind chiefly to proteins and not to DNA. Low-selectivity monofunctional alkylating agents, such as N-methyl-N-nitrosourea, N-ethyl-N-nitrosourea, temozolomide, N-methyl-N-nitro-N-nitrosoguanidine (MNNG), N-ethyl-N-nitro-N-nitrosoguanidine (ENNG) alkylate DNA bases, which can decrease the strength of the bond between the base to the deoxyribose, resulting in an apurinic or apyrimidinic site (AP site, also called abasic site). Polyfunctional alkylating agents such as nitrogen mustards (cyclophosphamide, ifosfamide, chlorambucil, melphalan), nitrosoureas (carmustine/BCNU, lomustine/CCNU), and alkyl sulfonates (busulfan) can generate inter- or intra-strand cross-links. Activation of N-nitrosamines, which are common contaminants in various foods and beverages, as well as in tobacco smoke and fuel combustion products, results in formation of alkylating agents.

Bulky DNA adducts include large DNA adducts of carcinogens such as electrophilic metabolites of PAHs, heterocyclic aromatic amines (HAAs), and aflatoxins. Platinum containing agents, such as cisplatin, carboplatin, and oxaliplatin, form bulky DNA adducts, but are often grouped with polyfunctional alkylating agents because they bind to and cross-link DNA. These adducts can hinder DNA polymerases, inducing errors in DNA replication, and they can block transcription. Both of these can trigger apoptosis.

Base or nucleoside analogs such as 2-aminopurine, an analog of adenine, or 5-azacytidine, an analog of cytidine can be incorporated into DNA. These base analogs mis-pair more frequently than the normal base.

DNA Damage Response

Sensing DNA Damage

It is estimated that the endogenous level of DNA damage is in the order of more than 50,000 lesions per cell, about 30,000 of which are abasic sites. To maintain the integrity of the genome in the face of constant DNA damage, organisms have evolved a network of DNA damage responses (Figure 26–3). Poly(ADP-ribose) polymerase 1 (PARP1) is highly activated within seconds by both single and double-strand DNA breaks and catalyzes the poly ADP-ribosylation of proteins near the damage site, consuming NAD+ in the process. This recruits subsequent DNA damage response sensors, and poly(ADP)ribosylation is then removed within minutes. Single-strand DNA damage is sensed by the 9-1-1 complex of RAD9 checkpoint clamp component, RAD1 checkpoint DNA exonuclease, and HUS1 checkpoint clamp component. Double-strand breaks are recognized by the MRN complex consisting of MRE11 homolog double-strand break repair nuclease, RAD50 double-strand break repair protein, and nibrin (NBN).

Once DNA damage is sensed, the key signal transducers are the phosphatidylinositidyl-3-kinase (PIK)-like proteins ataxia telangiectasia mutated (ATM) and ATM-Rad3-related (ATR), which are recruited by the MRN complex and 9-1-1 complex, respectively. ATM is the primary orchestrator of the response to double-strand DNA breaks via regulation of check-point pathways and DNA repair pathways, while ATR mainly responds to other types of DNA damage, such as single-strand breaks, DNA cross-links, and stalled DNA replication forks (due to DNA damage or other causes). ATM and ATR phosphorylate histone 2AX (H2AX; once phosphorylated, it is called γH2AX) near double-strand breaks or stalled replication forks, altering the chromatin conformation to make it more accessible for repair.

Activated ATM and ATR also phosphorylate and thereby increase levels of the p53 transcription factor and tumor suppressor protein, and they phosphorylate the E3 ubiquitin protein ligases MDM2 protooncogene and MDM4 regulator of p53, the key negative regulators of p53. Numerous posttranslational modifications of p53 allow for exquisite modulation of its functions. This enables p53 to promote cell cycle arrest, cellular senescence, apoptotic cell death or DNA repair, depending on the specific cellular context. Generally, more extensive DNA damage is more likely to result in prolonged activation of p53 and cell death, while less extensive

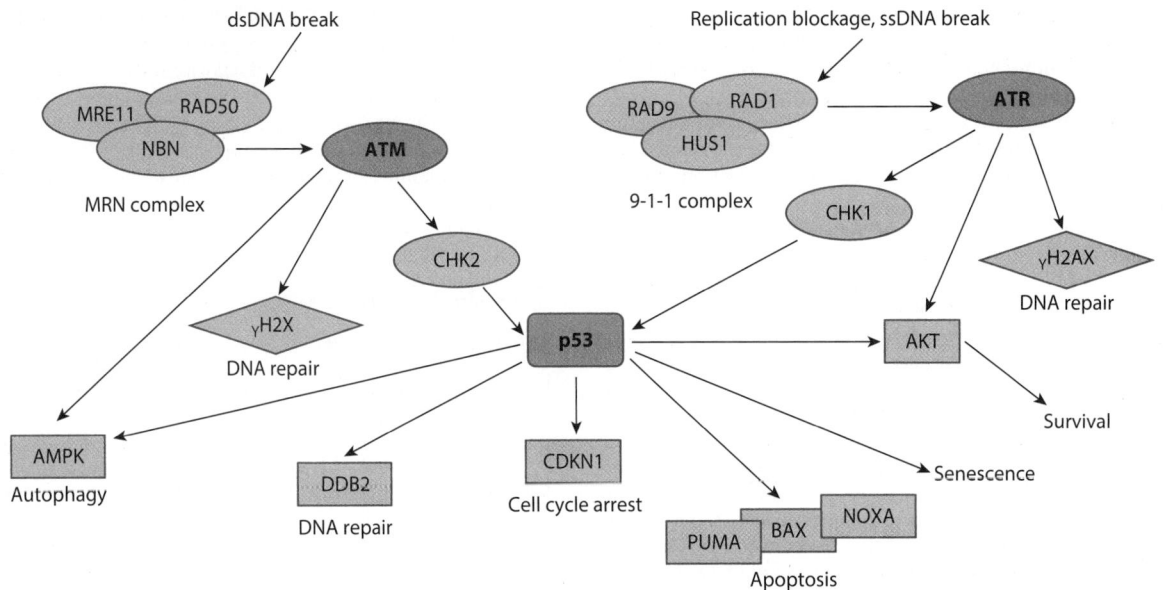

▲ **Figure 26–3.** Overview of DNA damage responses. The major sensors of DNA damage are the MRN complex for dsDNA breaks and the 9-1-1 complex for ssDNA breaks and replication blockage. Major transducers are ATM, ATR, CHK1, and CHK2. γH2AX is a mediator. Effectors are shown in rectangles. See text for additional details.

damage leads to short-term p53 activation and DNA repair. In the absence of DNA damage signaling, MDM2 and MDM4 ubiquitinate p53, which results in its subsequent proteasomal degradation. Depending on the posttranslational modification, p53 can induce cell cycle arrest via activation of CDKN1 (also known as p21) or can induce autophagy via activation of AMP-activated protein kinase (AMPK). ATM and ATR phosphorylation of the checkpoint kinases, CHK1 and CHK2, are additional routes through which DNA damage leads to cell cycle arrest. ATM also stimulates AMPK, a major regulator of autophagy, and ATR activates mitogen-activated protein kinase kinase kinase (MAPKKK), which via JNK (mitogen-activated protein kinase 8) signaling also activate autophagy. Cell cycle arrest and autophagy buy time and resources, respectively, to repair DNA damage, but if the damage is too severe, ultimately one of several cell death pathways may be activated or senescence, an irreversible cell cycle arrest, may be induced. PAR due to PARP activation can cause ATP depletion and loss of mitochondrial transmembrane potential leading to parthanatos, a nonapoptotic form of cell death. Activation of p53 can trigger apoptotic cell death or a regulated form of necrotic cell death called mitochondrial permeability transition pore (MPTP)-dependent regulated necrosis.

DNA Repair

Major DNA repair pathways include O⁶-methylguanine-DNA methyltransferase (MGMT), base excision repair (BER), nucleotide excision repair (NER), mismatch repair (MMR), nonhomologous end-joining (NHEJ), and homologous repair (HR). These pathways are briefly described in the following discussion. There are multiple other DNA repair pathways, such as alternative end-joining and single-strand annealing, which are error-prone and are engaged by products of defective NHEJ or HR or in situations when there is overwhelming DNA damage, resulting in complex DNA lesions such as chromosomal rearrangements.

MGMT accepts a methyl group from O⁶-methylguanine at Cys¹⁴⁵, resulting in inactivation and proteasomal degradation of MGMT.

The canonical MMR pathway repairs base-base mismatches and insertion-deletion loops. MMR starts with recognition of the mismatch by MutSα, a heterodimer of MSH2 (MutS protein homolog 2) and MSH6, or MutSβ, a heterodimer of MSH2 and MSH3. MutSα is mainly involved in repairing mismatched bases and short insertion-deletion loops, while MutSβ is mainly involved in repairing long insertion-deletion loops up to 16 nucleotides. PCNA (proliferating cell nuclear antigen) is thought to recruit MutS to mismatches. MutLα (MSH1 plus PMS2) or MutLβ (MSH1 plus PMS1) is recruited by MutS. MutS and MutL have ATPase activities. When they are complexed together, MutL acts as an endonuclease and completes the mismatch excision in the 3′ to 5′ direction, while it works together with exonuclease 1 to excise nucleotides in the 5′ to 3′ direction. The final steps of MMR are DNA resynthesis by DNA polymerase δ together with PCNA followed by DNA ligation by DNA ligase 1.

BER repairs N-methylated DNA bases, such as N^7-methylguanine, N^3-methylguanine, and N^3-methyladenine, as well as 8-oxo-dG. Efficiency of repair is generally faster for methyl (eg, MNU) versus ethyl adducts (eg, ENU). BER starts with recognition of the modified base, leading to recruitment of downstream BER proteins. First, the damaged base is excised by a DNA glycosylase, leaving an apurinic site. Oxoguanine glycosylases (OGGs) are the specific glycosylases that recognize and excise 8-oxo-dG. The phosphodiester bond of the apurinic site is next cleaved by AP endonuclease (APE1), leaving a DNA strand break with 5'-deoxyribose-5-phosphate and 3'OH. Repair of the strand break requires poly(ADP) ribosylation by PARP1 and PARP2 and insertion by DNA polymerases (Pol) of nucleotides (Polβ for single nucleotide BER and Polε or Polδ with PCNA for multinucleotide BER). DNA ligase III, together with X-ray cross complementing 1 (XRCC1) for single nucleotide repair or DNA ligase I for multinucleotide repair then ligates the strand ends. Since single-strand breaks are formed during BER, there is a risk of double-strand breaks occurring, if, for example, multiple lesions requiring BER occur in close proximity or if the cell enters S (synthesis) phase of the cell cycle before the single-strand break is repaired. If there is massive DNA damage, PARP activation consumes cellular nicotinamide adenine dinucleotide (NAD+) and thereby also depletes ATP, which can trigger a form of necrotic cell death.

NER repairs intra-strand cross-links and bulky DNA adducts. There are two kinds of NER, one repairs lesions in actively transcribing genes, and the other repairs lesions anywhere in the genome. These differ by the proteins that are involved in detecting lesions. The key actors in excising lesions and synthesizing and ligating DNA in both kinds of NER are ERCC1 (Excision repair 1, endonuclease noncatalytic subunit), ERCC2 and ERCC3 (Excision repair 2 and 3, TFIIH core complex helicase subunits), and ERCC4 (Excision repair 4, endonuclease catalytic subunit, also known as XPF).

NHEJ involves the direct joining (ligation) of DSB ends. Repair of DSBs by canonical NHEJ begins with binding of a Ku70-Ku80 heterodimer to the DNA break ends. Ku70-Ku80 then recruit DNA-dependent protein kinase catalytic subunit (DNA-PKcs) to form a long-range synapse connecting the two DNA ends. Then scaffolding factors XRCC4, XRCC4-like factor (XLF), paralogue of XRCC4 (PAXX), and DNA ligase IV bring the two DNA ends close together to form a short-range synapse, which permits DNA end processing by the nuclease Artemis, DNA polymerases, and other enzymes, and end ligation. NHEJ occurs throughout the cell cycle.

HR is an error-free process that repairs DSBs and blocked replication forks; most commonly utilizing recombination between sister chromatids. HR begins with end resection of up to 300 nucleotides of a strand that ends at a DSB, initiated by the MRN complex together with CtBP-interacting protein (CtIP); this also displaces Ku70-Ku80 from the DNA ends. Next long-range resection occurs in which exonuclease 1, endonuclease DNA2, and Bloom syndrome protein (BLM) work together to digest the 5' strand of the DNA end. These two processes result in a long 3' ssDNA tail. This 3' tail is coated with RPA (replication protein A) complexes, which protect it from interacting with other nearby ssDNA. For repair to continue, the RPA complexes must be replaced by RAD51, which requires mediation by BRCA2 DNA repair associated (BRCA2) in partnership with BRCA1, BRCA1-associated RING domain protein 1 (BARD1), and partner and localizer of BRCA2 (PALB2). PARP1 and PARP2 stabilize the so-called RAD51 filaments at damaged replication forks, facilitating DNA repair. The RAD51-ssDNA nucleoprotein complex invades duplex DNA molecules to seek out homologous sequences, mediated by BRCA1-BARD1. In somatic cells this mainly results in conservative, noncrossover synthesis-dependent strand annealing, while in meiotic cells formation of a so-called double Holliday junction intermediate, a branched DNA structure that can mediate exchange between two homologous DNA molecules, can result in crossing over. ATM and ATR activate key proteins required for HR, including BRCA1, BRCA2, and BLM. Unlike NHEJ, HR occurs only during S phase and G2 phase. This is due in part to regulation of DNA end resection by cell cycle dependent kinase (CDK) activity, which increases during S phase. CDK phosphorylates CtIP, allowing it to more efficiently activate the nuclease activity of the MRN complex to initiate end resection. In addition, as cells enter S phase, DNA helicase B, which suppresses DNA end resection, is inactivated, and expression of HR genes is increased. During G1 phase, PALB2 is degraded, which suppresses the assembly of the complex that allows RAD51 to replace RPA.

If DNA damage is not repaired and cell death is not induced, then mutagenesis can occur. Therefore, the balance between DNA damage and repair determines mutation rate.

MUTAGENESIS

As discussed earlier, DNA damage results from the reaction of a mutagen (or its metabolite) with DNA. A mutation occurs when the adduct results in erroneous replication of DNA so that the daughter cells do not contain the same base sequence as the parent cell contained prior to exposure.

DNA replication is carried out by the DNA replisome protein complex, which contains DNA polymerase(s), helicase (separates DNA strands), single-strand DNA binding protein (keeps strands from reannealing), primase (lays down RNA primer), ligase (joins DNA segments), and other proteins. DNA synthesis is coordinated between the so-called leading strand (forms from 5' to 3' end via addition of complementary nucleotides by polymerase) and lagging strand (forms 5' to 3' in short segments called Okazaki fragments primed by RNA primase). Humans have at least 19 DNA synthesis enzymes, including DNA polymerases belonging to the A, B, X, and Y DNA polymerase families. A-family members are high fidelity polymerases whose active sites only accommodate standard base pairs. Y-family polymerases, which are involved in translesion DNA synthesis, have active sites that are less specific, allowing them to bypass DNA damage, including bulky DNA adducts. During normal DNA replication with A-family polymerases, only the correct dNTP will bind to the DNA polymerase for base pairing; however, DNA adducts alter the conformation of the DNA, which can block or alter the incorporation of dNTPs. It must be noted that mammalian DNA replisomes are very complex with numerous protein-protein interactions within the replisome. Therefore, the replisome handles DNA damage differently from the isolated DNA polymerases on which much data has been based.

There are three major proposed mechanisms by which DNA damage results in mutations: decreased replication fidelity, replication blockage, and frameshifts.

Replication fidelity can be decreased if incorporation of the correct dNTP is reduced, if incorporation of incorrect dNTPs is increased, or if both occur. O^6-methylguanine and N^2-methylguanine are examples of DNA adducts that result in decreased incorporation of the correct dNTP, leading to a decrease in the ratio of correct to incorrect pairings. O^6-methylguanine inhibits incorporation of dCTP by several orders of magnitude, which allows relatively more dTTP to be incorporated, resulting in a G:C to A:T point mutation if not repaired. The oxidative DNA lesion 8-oxo-dG both decreases incorporation of dCTP opposite the 8-oxo-dG and increases misincorporation of dATP to an even greater extent, resulting in high rates of G:C to T:A transversion mutations. In contrast, N^7-methylguanine adducts are not cytotoxic or mutagenic because they do not block DNA replication and are read as guanine.

Replication blockage can occur if the DNA adduct allows binding of the dNTP to the active site of DNA polymerase, but not by standard Watson–Crick pairing (adenine pairs with thymine via two hydrogen bonds; guanine pairs with cytosine via three hydrogen bonds). It can also occur if the adduct causes the dNTP to be repulsed away from the active site or if the adduct is so bulky that it cannot fit into the active sites of DNA polymerases. Examples of the latter include PAH- and nitro PAH-DNA adducts, cyclobutene pyrimidine dimers formed by UV radiation, DNA-protein crosslinks, and DNA-DNA cross-links.

Frameshift mutations occur when nucleotides are deleted or added to the new strand during DNA replication. These can occur by multiple mechanisms. One mechanism is stabilized misalignment due to stacking interactions with the incoming dNTP, as can occur with large planar cyclic DNA adducts like N^2-ethenoguanine. Slippage of the DNA template strand during replication generates frameshift mutations in repetitive DNA sequences. Incorporation of an incorrect dNTP, followed by misalignment of the template strand is another mechanism by which frameshifts occur. Apurinic or apyrimidinic sites cannot pair with an incoming dNTP, causing the site to loop-out from the strand and allowing the dNTP to pair with the next template base, resulting in a frameshift.

Mutagenesis can also occur in the absence of exposure to chemical or physical mutagens when the normal ratios of the four dNTPs are altered or when the absolute concentrations of dNTPs are increased.

Table 26–2. Oncogenes and their functions.

Oncogene(s)	Gene Category and Function
HRAS, KRAS	Regulatory GTPases, regulate proliferation
SIS	Growth factor, encodes platelet derived growth factor (PDGF)
Src-family, BTK family	Cytoplasmic tyrosine kinases, mediate signals for cell growth, differentiation, migration, survival
EGFR, PDGFR, KDR (VEGFR), ERBB2 (HER2/neu)	Receptor tyrosine kinases, mediate signals for cell growth, differentiation, survival
MYC, FOS	Transcription factors, regulate genes involved in proliferation
MOS, RAF	Serine/threonine kinases, activate signaling cascades involved in differentiation, proliferation, survival

Oncogenes and Tumor Suppressors

A protooncogene is a normal cellular gene that will not transform cells without an alteration, such as a mutation, that activates it to an oncogene. Mutations of oncogenes are generally dominant; mutation of only one allele is sufficient to convert a protooncogene to an oncogene. Examples of oncogenes and the functions of the gene products of their protooncogene precursors are listed in Table 26–2, and include HRAS protooncogene, a GTPase. Protooncogenes regulate cellular growth, proliferation, differentiation, and survival. Mutation of HRAS results in loss of GTPase activity and thereby loss of termination of growth factor signaling via the HRAS-coupled receptor.

A tumor suppressor gene is one whose normal function is DNA damage repair, inhibition of growth or proliferation and/or induction of apoptotic death, while loss of function of the gene promotes tumor growth and survival. Tumor suppressor gene inactivation was previously thought to require that both alleles be mutated or epigenetically inactivated. However, more recent work has demonstrated that transcriptional regulation, proteasomal degradation, or aberrant subcellular location can also contribute to inactivation. In familial cancer syndromes, such as familial retinoblastoma, one allele is inactivated in the germ line, while inactivation of the second allele occurs in somatic cells. In nonfamilial cancer, both alleles are silenced in the somatic cells, giving rise to the cancer. Examples of tumor suppressor genes are listed in Table 26–3 and include RB1, the gene that is inactivated in retinoblastoma, and TP53. The tumor suppressor function of p53 is relatively independent of its response to DNA damage in that it requires the action of the alternative reading frame (ARF) protein, which increases p53 levels in

Table 26–3. Tumor suppressor genes and their functions.

Gene(s)	Gene Category and Function
TP53	Regulates cell cycle, apoptosis
RB1, p16 (INK4a)	Regulate cell cycle
CHK1, CHK2	Protein kinases, regulate G1 cell cycle
APC	Inhibits beta catenin signaling
TSC1	Interacts with tuberin
BRCA1, BRCA2	DNA repair
MSH2, MLH1	DNA mismatch repair
PTEN	Regulates PI3 kinase/AKT signaling
BCL2	Regulates apoptosis

APC, adenomatous polyposis coli; CHK, checkpoint kinase; PTEN, phosphatase and tensin homolog; RB1, retinoblastoma transcriptional corepressor 1; TSC, tuberous sclerosis.

response to hyperproliferative signals by blocking the E3 ubiquitin ligase activity of MDM2 and sequestering it in the nucleolus, away from p53. Mice lacking p53 spontaneously develop tumors, and mutations in the *TP53* gene or mutations in other genes that prevent activation of p53 are among the most common events in human cancers. Notably, many *TP53* mutations in cancer are gain of function mutations that contribute to genetic instability and metastasis. Thus, while wild type p53 is a tumor suppressor, these mutated forms of p53 are oncogenes.

EPIGENETICS

Epigenetic modifications are heritable changes in gene expression that do not involve changes in the DNA sequence. The epigenetic cellular components that control gene expression include methylation of DNA, various posttranslational histone modifications, and noncoding RNAs.

Methylation of DNA occurs predominantly at the 5 position of cytosine in so-called CpG islands, stretches of DNA about 1 kb long that are rich in CpG and GpC nucleotides. It is estimated that 50–60% of promoter regions of genes have multiple CpG islands. When these are methylated, this generally inhibits expression of the gene. DNA is methylated by DNA-methyltransferase (DNMT) enzymes. *De novo* methylation of DNA is carried out by DNMT3A and DNMT3B. DNA methylation is maintained during DNA replication by DNMT1. The parent DNA strand is used as a template for cytosine methylation of the daughter strand immediately after replication. The DNMTs use S-adenosylmethionine (SAM) as the methyl donor. Demethylation of DNA is a multistep process carried out by ten-eleven translocation (TET) enzymes, which demethylate 5-methylcytosine (5mC)

by converting it to 5-hydroxymethylcytosine (5hmC), then converting 5hmC to 5-formylcytosine, and converting 5-formylcytosine to 5-carboxycytosine. The latter can be converted to cytosine by terminal deoxynucleotidyl transferase.

DNA within cells that are not transcriptionally active is maintained in a compact, supercoiled state (heterochromatin) in which 145–147 pairs of DNA bases are wrapped around a histone protein complex that consists of four pairs of proteins, H3, H4, H2A, and H2B. Transcriptionally active DNA (euchromatin) is less coiled, allowing access to transcription proteins. Posttranslational histone modifications occur on the *N*-terminal histone tails and include methylation, acetylation, phosphorylation, sumoylation, and ubiquitylation. These modifications serve to relax chromatin and promote transcription or compact chromatin and inhibit gene expression. Acetylation is catalyzed by histone acetyl transferases (HATs), while deacetylation is catalyzed by histone deacetylases (HDACs). Several different protein lysine methyltransferases catalyze histone methylation, including the Polycomb repression complex, while histone demethylases catalyze demethylation. Methylation and acetylation predominantly occur on H3 and H4. Acetylation of H3 and H4 eliminates positive charges on histones, allowing the DNA to separate from them, promoting transcription. Methylation can either promote or inhibit transcription depending on which lysines (K) are methylated. H3K27 and H4K20 methylation are associated with inhibition of transcription, while H3K4 and H3K36 are associated with activation of transcription. Histone phosphorylation generally increases compaction of chromatin.

Small noncoding RNAs (sncRNAs) include micro-RNAs (miRNAs), small interfering RNAs (siRNAs), piwi-associated RNAs (piRNAs), and transfer RNA (tRNA) fragments. miRNAs and siRNAs are about 20 nucleotides long in mammals. Both miRNAs and siRNAs are generated in the nucleus and transported to the cytoplasm where both interact with the RNA-induced silencing complex (RISC). Once loaded onto RISC, miRNAs bind to complementary sequences in 3′ untranslated regions of mRNAs, preventing translation of the mRNAs. When siRNAs are loaded onto RISC, they also bind to complementary target mRNAs, but this results in cleavage of the target mRNA to prevent its translation. piRNAs are 23–29 nucleotides long sncRNAs that repress transposons both at the transcriptional and posttranscriptional level.

Role in Carcinogenesis

A mutation is not necessary for carcinogenesis if a DNA adduct results in the heritable alteration of the expression of one or more critical genes via epigenetic modifications, such as DNA methylation. A bulky adduct on guanine in a CpG island that is normally methylated can interfere with methylation during cell replication, potentially resulting in expression of a gene that is normally repressed. Ethionine, the antimetabolite of methionine, greatly inhibits the synthesis of SAM, which blocks maintenance methylation of DNA.

This is critical for liver carcinogenesis by ethionine. Similarly, mice fed a choline or methionine-deficient diet develop liver cancer due to decreased SAM synthesis and global hypomethylation of DNA, resulting in increased expression of oncogenes, as well as mutations in *Tp53*.

It is now well-established that epigenetic silencing of tumor suppressor genes and DNA damage repair genes by DNA methylation, chromatin modifications that repress transcription, and miRNAs are common in human cancers. Examples include epigenetic silencing via promoter methylation of *MGMT, XRCC1, ERCC1, BRCA1/2, CDKN2A/B, MLH1, MSH2,* and *RB1*; targeting of *TP53* by miR-155 and of *RB1* by miR-17; and inhibition of the expression of *CDKN1* by deacetylation of H3 and H4 or by *H3K4* methylation. In addition, in several cancers somatic mutations have been found in genes that are involved in regulating epigenetic modifications. For example, mutations in *TET2* or isocitrate dehydrogenase (*IDH1/2*) cause high levels of CpG island methylation in certain low-grade glioblastomas and acute myeloid leukemia. *TET2* requires 2-oxoglutarate as a cofactor to convert 5mC to 5hmC. Cells with the *IDH1/2* mutation make 2-hydroxyglutarate, which cannot serve as a cofactor for *TET2*, instead of 2-oxoglutarate. Genes that code for proteins involved in histone modifications are also frequently mutated in cancers. Examples include mutations of histone methyltransferases *MLL2* and *EZH2* in lymphomas and histone demethylase *UTX* in several different cancers.

Role in Transgenerational Effects

In the past decade there has been an explosion of studies demonstrating that parental exposures to stressors including various toxicants, over- or undernutrition, and psychologic stress can alter expression of genes in a heritable manner not mediated by mutations in the germline. These heritable changes in gene expression have been associated with increased risk of obesity, diabetes, cardiovascular disease, infertility, and other disorders in multiple generations. In order for effects to be deemed transgenerational, as opposed to merely multigenerational, they must be demonstrated in the third filial generation (F3) for *in utero* exposures via the pregnant mother and in the F2 generation for exposures to the father. This is because exposure of F1 embryos developing *in utero* exposes not just the embryo but also the germ cells in the gonads of the embryo, which will give rise to the F2 generation. Therefore, the F3 generation will be the first unexposed generation. Similarly, the sperm of an exposed male will give rise to the F1 generation, and the F2 generation will be the first unexposed generation. Such transgenerational effects are thought to be mediated by heritable epigenetic alterations in the germline, but the specific mechanisms by which these epigenetic modifications escape erasure during development remain largely unknown.

Epigenetic reprogramming occurs in primordial germ cells, the precursors to gametes, and during early embryogenesis. Reprogramming of primordial germ cells involves extensive demethylation of DNA, as well as removal of histone modifications and reactivation of the inactive X-chromosome. The methylation and histone modifications are reestablished during the last stages of gametogenesis. During early post-fertilization development both the maternal and paternal pronuclei undergo extensive demethylation of DNA. This is an active process in the male pronucleus (mediated by TET enzymes) and passive in the female pronucleus (due to lack of methylation of newly synthesized DNA strands during cell division). Histone modifications are also removed from the maternal pronucleus and paternal protamines are replaced with maternal histones in the male pronucleus. *De novo* DNA methylation and histone modifications occur after the embryo has implanted.

The focus of transgenerational inheritance has therefore been on regions which escape this nearly global epigenetic reprogramming. These include imprinted regions and metastable epialleles. The expression of clusters of imprinted genes are epigenetically regulated by imprinting control regions (ICRs) via methylation, sncRNAs, and histone modifications. Imprinted genes are either maternally imprinted (repressed via the maternal ICR and expressed from the paternally inherited allele) or paternally imprinted (repressed via the paternal ICR and expressed from the maternally inherited allele). Over 150 imprinted genes have been discovered, and many are critically important for prenatal and postnatal growth and metabolism. Parental imprints are removed and reset during the gametic and embryonic epigenetic reprogramming events. The metastable locus *Agouti viable yellow* (*Avy*) is an example of epivariation. In this mouse model, an endogenous retrovirus element of the intracisternal particle class is found within the *Agouti* locus and provides an alternative promoter that controls fur color. Methylation of this promoter is very stable within individuals and highly variable even among genetically identical individuals. Notably, methylation of this promoter can be altered by gestational exposures to diet rich in methyl donors or the environmental toxicant Bisphenol A, and these changes in methylation persist into adulthood. However, to date there is a relative lack of strong evidence that environmentally mediated alterations in DNA methylation are transmitted transgenerationally.

Most histones are replaced during spermatogenesis with protamines which allows for the nucleus of mature sperm to be highly compacted compared to somatic cells. About 1–4% and 4–15% of histones persist in mature mouse and human sperm, respectively. Moreover, several histone methylation marks, including H3K27me3, have been reported to escape epigenetic reprogramming in the sperm. These are candidates for transgenerational transmission of epigenetic information. One well-characterized example is the *tm1Alf* mutation which blocks expression of the *Kit* gene. This mutation causes white fur on the tail tips and feet in heterozygotes, due to decreased expression of the KIT tyrosine kinase receptor (homozygotes die shortly after birth). Interestingly, wild type offspring of heterozygous parents display the abnormal phenotype for several generations due to inheritance of miRNAs that target *Kit* RNA via the sperm. Exposure of males to ionizing radiation, high fat diet, and other stressors have been reported to alter sperm miRNA and/or tRNA fragment profiles.

CARCINOGENESIS

The multistage model of carcinogenesis begins with exposure to a carcinogen, resulting in an initiation event that alters the genome of a cell (mutation and/or epigenetic change), followed by growth and promotion to a differentiated neoplasm and ultimately progression to undifferentiated cancer.

GENETIC TOXICOLOGY TESTING

Standard *In Vivo* and *In Vitro* Tests

For most of the second half of the twentieth century genetic toxicity testing was focused primarily on identifying carcinogens, with a lesser emphasis on germline mutations. In recent decades, genomic alterations, including heritable alterations described earlier in the discussion of transgenerational effects, have been causally associated with other disease outcomes besides cancer. The "gold standard" genetic toxicology tests have been the 2-year rodent cancer bioassays in rats and/or mice, such as the Organization for Economic Cooperation and Development (OECD) Guideline 451, which requires daily administration of the test substance at three dose levels plus control to 50 animals of each sex per group. All animals are subjected to full detailed gross necropsy, with microscopic examination of all tissues in the control and high dose groups, as well as all tissues that have macroscopic abnormalities. These assays are extremely expensive and time-consuming, utilize large numbers of animals, and provide little to no mechanistic data. Therefore, many *in vitro* and short-term *in vivo* genetic toxicology tests have been developed which are used to screen chemicals in development and to prioritize chemicals for cancer bioassay testing. The most commonly used test batteries include the Ames bacterial mutagenesis test, *in vitro* cytogenetics assays, and an *in vivo* mammalian assay for chromosome damage.

The Ames test utilizes the bacterium *S typhimurium* to detect reverse mutations in histidine genes. The assay is performed with and without the rat liver microsome metabolizing system (S9) in order to identify mutagens that require metabolic activation, as well as those that do not. This test is estimated to be 60% predictive of rodent carcinogens. Commonly used *in vitro* cytogenetics assays measure chromosome aberrations in cultured human peripheral blood lymphocytes, Chinese Hamster Ovary cells, or mouse lymphoma cells. In addition to DNA damage, positive results in these assays can result from inhibition of DNA repair, cytotoxicity, apoptosis induction, poor culture conditions, and other causes. The most widely used *in vivo* mammalian assay for chromosome damage is the rodent bone marrow micronucleus formation assay. Notably, these and other screening tests perform relatively well at identifying genotoxic chemicals, but generally fail to identify non-genotoxic carcinogens.

Twenty-First Century Genetic Toxicology Testing

In 2007, the National Research Council published *Toxicity Testing in the 21st Century*, which called for a new approach to improve toxicity testing that would "provide broader coverage of chemicals and their mixtures, endpoints, and life-stage vulnerabilities," while also reducing testing time and cost, using fewer animals, and providing detailed mechanistic and dosimetry information. The report further called for accomplishing this through a comprehensive array of *in vitro* tests combined with computational models. Progress has been made towards this vision, and a brief discussion of the applications to genetic toxicity testing follows.

Computational Modeling

Tools to calculate physicochemical characteristics and (quantitative)structure-activity relationships, (Q)SAR, are often used to screen chemicals for potential reactivity and toxicity and prioritize them for further testing. However, most (Q)SAR models are applicable to small to moderately sized organic molecules, not to inorganic or organometallic molecules or chemical mixtures. In addition, the various commercially available and proprietary (Q)SAR programs rely on different training sets of chemicals, and each is only useful for chemicals with similar structural domains as those in the training set. Also, because they rely on data from similar chemicals, (Q)SAR models are less useful for highly novel molecules. That said, progress is being made on QSAR of peptides, manufactured nanoparticles, among others. Moreover, both chemical structure annotation errors and errors in annotation of experimental measurements are common in publications and therefore also in databases used for QSAR. Recognition of the prevalence of such errors has led to increased emphasis on curation of chemical data to be used in QSAR modeling. Examples of curated databases include the US Environmental Protection Agency's (EPA) toxicity reference database, ToxRefDB, and Distributed Structure-Searchable Toxicity (DSSTox) project.

High-Throughput Assay Panels

Over the past decade and a half, numerous governmental and private entities have established high-throughput screening initiatives and screened chemicals for toxicity using various *in vitro* high-throughput assay panels. The US EPA ToxCast research program is one of the largest of these efforts. ToxCast has screened over 3800 chemicals with hundreds of assay endpoints. ToxCast is part of the Tox21 consortium, which also includes the NTP at the NIEHS, the NIH National Center for Advanced Translational Sciences, and the Food and Drug Administration. Taken together the Tox21 program has screened about 10,000 chemicals in approximately 70 high-throughput assays. ToxCast predictive signatures have been identified for rat liver cancer, reproductive toxicity, and developmental toxicity using chemicals in the ToxCast chemical library for which *in vivo* studies performed according to regulatory guidelines have demonstrated these toxicities. For example, the liver cancer predictive signature suggests that perturbation of the peroxisome proliferator activated receptor gamma (PPARγ) pathway combined with at least one of PPARα activation, upregulation of the cytokine CCL2, androgen antagonism, or oxidative stress pathways is associated with likelihood of being a rat liver carcinogen.

Many of the ToxCast endpoints are relevant to cancer and genetic toxicity. Cancer related endpoints include cell proliferation, cell cycle arrest, mitochondrial mass and membrane potential, histone phosphorylation, nuclear size, protein content, nuclear p53 localization, c-Jun phosphorylation, and alterations in specific downstream protein levels in response to upstream effectors known to be involved in cancer. Two independent groups have mapped ToxCast assays to the Key Characteristics (KCs) of Carcinogens. Both groups mapped assays to 5 of the 10 KCs of carcinogens; four of these were common to both studies, while two KCs were only mapped by one group each. Both groups found that the KCs "alters DNA repair or causes genomic instability," "is immunosuppressive," or "causes immortalization" were not covered by the ToxCast assays. They also found that known carcinogens that require metabolic activation received very low scores when ranked according to the number of positive assay endpoints they produced. This highlights the known low metabolic capacity of ToxCast assays. Other technical limitations of the ToxCast assays, as well as other high-throughput assay approaches, are requirements that test substances have sufficient solubility in the chosen vehicle (dimethyl sulfoxide for ToxCast), do not bind strongly to plastic, and are not volatile.

Many data sharing resources have been created to make high-throughput toxicity data publicly available for analysis, with PubChem being the largest. As of 2014 more than 47 million compounds, 700,000 bioassays and 13 billion data points were archived on PubChem. Since then the amount of data available on this and other resources has continued to increase rapidly, as have efforts to develop data mining methods to extract, integrate, visualize, and analyze data from the various datasets.

'Omics: Genomics, Transcriptomics, Epigenomics, Proteomics, Metabolomics

The term 'omics is used to describe global analysis of biological molecules within a biological sample. Genomics refers to global analysis of DNA, transcriptomics to global analysis of RNA transcripts, proteomics to global analysis of proteins, metabolomics to the global analysis of small molecule metabolites. Epigenomics includes global analysis of the DNA methylome (methylomics), global analysis of histone modifications, global analysis of sncRNAs, and global analysis of chromatin accessibility. Toxicogenomics refers to the utilization of 'omics technologies to study adverse effects of chemicals on human health and the environment.

Early 'omics applications utilized microarray technology to quantify mRNAs or to identify single nucleotide polymorphisms in the DNA sequence. These microarrays consist of quartz chips spotted with DNA oligonucleotides complementary to known mRNAs or single nucleotide polymorphisms. Fragmented and fluorescently labeled mRNA or DNA samples hybridize to complementary oligonucleotides on the chip, and the intensity of fluorescence is measured using a detection system. Protein microarrays consist of a support surface onto which antibodies are spotted and probed with a sample lysate. Microarray technologies are now largely being replaced by high-throughput sequencing technologies for DNA and RNA and mass spectrometry for proteins and metabolites. High-throughput sequencing methods generally involve fragmenting the DNA, sampling fragments randomly, and utilizing parallel sequencing processes whereby thousands or millions of sequences are read concurrently. The reads from the fragments then have to be assembled based on overlapping regions. Analysis of RNA via sequencing generally requires a reverse transcription step to make complementary DNA (cDNA), which is then sequenced using the same sequencing methods as for genomic DNA. Whole genome DNA reference sequences have been assembled for several species by sequencing multiple individuals within a species and generating a representative sequence for each species. Sequences from RNA-sequencing are aligned to the appropriate reference genome to determine which genes were expressed in the samples and relative expression levels.

During the past decade, use of toxicogenomic data for dose-response and mode of action (MOA) determination in risk assessment has been developed. Until now most of these studies have utilized transcriptomic data integrated into standard *in vivo* and *in vitro* toxicologic tests. MOAs are sequences of key events leading from an exposure to a toxicant to an adverse health outcome. Several studies have compared dose-response data obtained from *in vivo* toxicology studies with dose-response curves obtained from toxicogenomics studies to derive points of departure (PODs) for quantitative risk assessment. No observed adverse effect levels (NOAELs) and lowest observe adverse effect levels (LOAELs) have traditionally been used by regulatory agencies as PODs for deriving recommended exposure limits. More recently benchmark dose (BMD) modeling is being used to derive PODs. BMDs are dose levels with confidence limits corresponding to specific response levels near the low end of the observable range of data. The lower confidence limit on the BMD is designated BMDL. BMD/BMDLs are derived from all the concentration response data and convey more information than NOAELs and LOAELs.

As an illustrative example, Moffat et al (2015) derived PODs and developed MOAs for benzo[a]pyrene from *in vivo* toxicology studies alone, from transcriptomic data only, or using a "genomics-informed" approach, which combined both methods. They derived BMD/BMDLs using dose-dependent changes in gene expression for all significantly affected genes from transcriptomic data from various tissues of orally dosed mice, then calculated the average BMD/BMDLs for significantly altered pathways identified using Ingenuity Pathway Analysis. They chose the BMD/BMDLs for pathways associated with DNA adducts and DNA damage, which is an early key event in the MOA prior to the irreversible event of mutagenesis. They found that the BMDLs for traditional and transcriptomic approaches were very similar, differing by at most one order of magnitude. Moreover, the transcriptomic approach, even when using only transcriptomic data from a cultured human cell line, identified many of the key events in the known genotoxic MOA by which BaP induces cancers in multiple tissues. An alternative approach to choosing the BMD/BMDL utilizes the BMD/BMDL for the most sensitive endpoint without consideration of MOA; this approach has been suggested to be the preferred approach for chemicals with nonselective mechanisms that perturb many pathways. When applied to the same data by Moffat et al, this approach resulted in very similar BMD/BMDLs as the MOA approach.

The National Toxicology Program (NTP 2018) undertook a similar comparison of genomic dose response with apical endpoint dose response for 13 compounds that had been tested in 2-year cancer or 28-day subchronic developmental toxicity guideline bioassays. They compared the half log interval around the BMD for the most sensitive apical endpoint to the BMDL-BMD-BMDU (95% confidence limit around the BMD) values for the most sensitive gene set-level biological effect or pathway from transcriptomic analyses of the same tissue in 5-day in vivo dosing studies. Gene sets were identified from two curated collections, Gene Ontology Biological Processes and MSigDB pathways. They found that the intervals overlapped for all but one study for which the BMDL-BMD-BMDU values were slightly more sensitive. The overall conclusion of these and other similar studies is that in vivo genomic dose-response studies yield similar POD concentrations and MOAs as do those derived from traditional in vivo bioassays.

Progress is also being made to combine high-throughput assays with toxicogenomics and QSAR in genetic toxicology. One example is the work of Li et al (2017), who have defined an in vitro transcriptomic biomarker, called TGx-DDI (toxicogenomic-DNA damage-inducing), which consists of a panel of 64 genes that discriminate between genotoxic and non-genotoxic agents. They combined this panel with a high-throughput, direct digital counting technology that allows for direct quantification of RNA transcripts in cell lysates without the need for RNA extraction. A validation study showed that the assay correctly identified 100% of direct DNA-reactive agents, more than half of indirect-acting DNA damage inducing agents, and more than 90% of non-DNA damage-inducing agents. Another example is the MOA QSAR approach, which uses chemical structure- and physicochemical property-based features and biological descriptors from high-throughput assays to identify "chemotypes." Chemotypes are sets of chemical classes that are highly enriched within a group of related MOAs, thus linking biological key events and chemical structures.

Challenges to completely replacing in vivo toxicology studies with high-throughput and toxicogenomic assays include that concentrations used in vitro are often not relevant to the in vivo situation; that absorption, distribution, metabolism, and excretion in vivo need to be understood to translate an in vitro concentration to a human dose; and that statistically significant transcriptomic changes in pathways may or may not be indicative of adverse effects in humans.

USES OF GENETIC TOXICOLOGY IN OCCUPATIONAL AND ENVIRONMENTAL MEDICINE

There are several intersections of genetic toxicology and clinical occupational medicine practice. Occupational medicine physicians may assist in designing safety programs for and conduct medical surveillance of workers who are potentially exposed to chemical, physical, or biological agents that are genotoxic. Genetic toxicology research has played and continues to play an important role in identifying genotoxic hazards, deciphering their modes and mechanisms of action, and understanding exposure-response relationships. This research is critical for risk assessment of occupational and environmental genotoxic hazards. Other research in the field has identified genetic variations, including polymorphisms and mutations, that increase susceptibility to occupational diseases. However, screening for such variants has not entered occupational medicine practices for reasons discussed in the following discussion, and occupational exposure limits generally are not designed to protect these sensitive subpopulations.

There is extensive scientific literature documenting genotoxicity in workers exposed to various genotoxic agents, including anticancer drugs (healthcare, manufacturing), ionizing radiation (healthcare, nuclear power industry), heavy metals (lead, mercury, manganese), formaldehyde, urinary bladder carcinogens, solvents (benzene, trichloroethylene), nanomaterials, and PAHs (road paving, coke oven plants, diesel exhaust). Commonly used assays in these studies include cytogenetic assays (micronuclei, sister chromatid exchanges, and chromosome aberrations), comet assay for DNA strand breaks, ^{32}P post-labeling assay for DNA or protein adducts, and mutation frequency in various gene loci. Analyses are generally performed on peripheral blood lymphocytes or buccal epithelial cells. Current guidelines, however, do not recommend biomonitoring for genotoxicity in routine medical surveillance of exposed workers due to inter-individual variability and difficulty in interpreting individual results, as well as concerns about reproducibility of some of the assays. On the other hand, both personal and environmental exposure monitoring are recommended and are routinely conducted for workers with ionizing radiation exposure. Environmental exposure monitoring is recommended for healthcare settings with hazardous drug exposures to evaluate the effectiveness of preventive measures designed to prevent exposure of workers.

One of the clearest linkages of a genetic variant with an occupational disease is the association of the

HLA-DPB1-Glu[69] polymorphism with susceptibility to beryllium sensitization and chronic beryllium disease. This polymorphism in the gene that codes for the HLA-DP β_1 chain of the Major Histocompatibility Complex is found in 75% of patients with chronic beryllium disease. Silver and Sharp (2006) used ethical and clinical criteria to evaluate employer-sponsored voluntary screening programs for this polymorphism. They estimated, based on disease prevalence and carrier frequency in one of the largest beryllium-using facilities in the United States, that the longitudinal positive predictive value of this genetic marker for development of disease is 12%. Considering this relatively low predictive value, the difficulty of protecting confidential information, and concerns about possible coercion to undergo testing, the authors concluded that even voluntary screening programs for this polymorphism were not indicated. The 2014 American Thoracic Society Statement on beryllium sensitivity and chronic beryllium disease diagnosis and management does not recommend screening of workers for this polymorphism.

Several international bodies, such as the European Group on Ethics in Science and New Technologies have concluded that it is not ethically acceptable to conduct genetic screening in the context of preemployment medical examinations. The US Congress passed the Genetic Information Nondiscrimination Act (GINA) in 2008. GINA prohibits employers from using genetic information for decisions regarding hiring, firing, promotions, or terms of employment. However, GINA does not prevent employers from collecting genetic information for medical surveillance and research purposes. Collection of genetic information for surveillance under GINA requires that written notice be provided to the employee, that the employee give written authorization for the collection of the data, and that the employee must be informed of the results. In addition, GINA specifies that only aggregate results can be provided to the employer.

The GINA requirement that only aggregate results are permitted to be provided to the employer may not be possible when the number of workers undergoing surveillance is small because individuals are likely to be readily identifiable. An example of such a situation was recently discussed as regards astronauts employed by the US National Aeronautics and Space Administration (NASA; Reed and Antonsen, 2018). NASA functions as employer, primary care provider, and research investigator in relation to the astronaut corps. The authors argued that GINA provides an exception for circumstances that make data aggregation impossible, such as small numbers of employees. NASA conducts occupational surveillance to understand the health hazards of space travel and to develop preventive measures to counter those adverse health effects. Space travel, especially outside of the Earth's protective magnetosphere, entails exposure to ionizing radiation, which is a known genotoxic agent. Therefore, in the future it may be important to use genotoxicity assays in medical surveillance of astronauts. The authors argue that data aggregation would render the surveillance data useless because in order to identify hazards and develop preventive measures, genetic information must be associated with an astronaut's individual exposures. The authors make a similar argument for collection of individualized genetic data for clinical purposes. In both of these cases, the authors emphasize that the data must be properly safeguarded and must not be considered when making space flight selection decisions.

REFERENCES

Chepelev, N. L., I. D. Moffat, S. Labib, J. Bourdon-Lacombe, B. Kuo, J. K. Buick, F. Lemieux, A. I. Malik, S. Halappanavar, A. Williams and C. L. Yauk (2015). "Integrating toxicogenomics into human health risk assessment: lessons learned from the benzo[a]pyrene case study." Critical Reviews in Toxicology 45(1): 44-52. [PMID: 25605027].

Dearfield, K. L., B. B. Gollapudi, J. C. Bemis, R. D. Benz, G. R. Douglas, R. K. Elespuru, G. E. Johnson, D. J. Kirkland, M. J. LeBaron, A. P. Li, F. Marchetti, L. H. Pottenger, E. Rorije, J. Y. Tanir, V. Thybaud, J. van Benthem, C. L. Yauk, E. Zeiger and M. Luijten (2017). "Next generation testing strategy for assessment of genomic damage: A conceptual framework and considerations." Environmental and Molecular Mutagenesis 58(5): 264-283. [PMID: 27650663].

Iyer, S., N. Pham, M. Marty, M. Sandy, G. Solomon and L. Zeise (2019). "An Integrated Approach Using Publicly Available Resources for Identifying and Characterizing Chemicals of Potential Toxicity Concern: Proof-of-Concept With Chemicals That Affect Cancer Pathways." Toxicological Sciences 169(1): 14-24. [PMID: 30649495].

Lee, M. P. (2019). "Understanding Cancer Through the Lens of Epigenetic Inheritance, Allele-Specific Gene Expression, and High-Throughput Technology." Frontiers in Oncology 9: 794. [PMID: 31497535].

Liu, B., Q. Xue, Y. Tang, J. Cao, F. P. Guengerich and H. Zhang (2016). "Mechanisms of mutagenesis: DNA replication in the presence of DNA damage." Mutation Research. Reviews in Mutation Research 768: 53-67. [PMID: 27234563].

Meek, D. W. (2015). "Regulation of the p53 response and its relationship to cancer." Biochemical Journal 469(3): 325-346. [PMID: 26205489].

Ronson, G. E., A. L. Piberger, M. R. Higgs, A. L. Olsen, G. S. Stewart, P. J. McHugh, E. Petermann and N. D. Lakin (2018). "PARP1 and PARP2 stabilise replication forks at base excision repair intermediates through Fbh1-dependent Rad51 regulation." Nature Communications 9(1): 746 [PMID: 29467415].

Scully, R., A. Panday, R. Elango and N. A. Willis (2019). "DNA double-strand break repair-pathway choice in somatic mammalian cells." Nature Reviews Molecular and Cell Biology. 20(11): 698-714. [PMID: 31263220].

Vannini, I., F. Fanini and M. Fabbri (2018). "Emerging roles of microRNAs in cancer." Current Opinion in Genetics and Development 48: 128-133. [PMID: 29429825].

Xavier, M. J., S. D. Roman, R. J. Aitken and B. Nixon (2019). "Transgenerational inheritance: how impacts to the epigenetic and genetic information of parents affect offspring health." Human Reproduction Update 25(5): 518-540. [PMID: 31374565].

■ SELF-ASSESSMENT QUESTIONS

Select the one correct answer for each question.

Question 1: Mutagenicity refers to the
   a. study of the actions of chemical and physical agents on DNA
   b. changes in DNA methylation, histone modifications, and micro RNA expression
   c. induction of alterations in the DNA sequence that can be transmitted to daughter cells during cell division
   d. Study of genotoxicity, mutagenesis, and epigenetic alterations

Question 2: DNA can be modified
   a. by reactive chemicals, including metabolically activated xenobiotics
   b. if mutagenesis does not occur

   c. if DNA damage is repaired
   d. to affect the mutation rate

Question 3: A proto-oncogene is
   a. one whose normal function is DNA damage repair
   b. a normal cellular gene that will not transform cells without an alteration, such as a mutation, that activates it to an oncogene
   c. an example of genetic instability and metastasis
   d. a heritable change in gene expression that does not involve changes in the DNA sequence

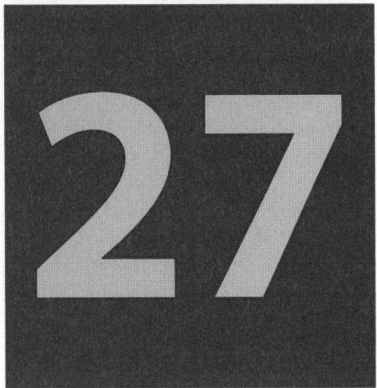

Female Reproductive Toxicology

Sarah Janssen, MD, PhD, MPH

Michael Shahbaz, MD, MPH

The occurrence of adverse reproductive outcomes is of fundamental concern to the individuals and families affected. This is especially true if the individuals perceive that they are living or working in areas with potential exposure to hazardous agents over which they have little or no control. Concern has been fueled by incidents such as the contamination of fish with methyl mercury in Minamata Bay, Japan, which was caused by a release from a manufacturing plant. Consumption of the contaminated fish by pregnant women resulted in an epidemic of mental retardation, cerebral palsy, and developmental delay in their offspring. Use of polychlorinated biphenyl (PCB)–contaminated cooking oil in Taiwan resulted in intrauterine growth retardation and hyperpigmentation of the skin in infants of exposed women. Effects on that cohort continue to be uncovered today, including on offspring pubertal development. In recent years, there have been concerns about the reproductive effects of occupational exposure to solvents, pesticides, and video-display terminals or electromagnetic fields (EMFs). A new area of research has sprung up to identify and study chemicals that may act to disrupt the endocrine system, affecting both wildlife and humans.

Only a few substances are known to have strong associations with adverse reproductive outcomes in humans, but relatively little research has been devoted to these outcomes until the last few decades. A larger number of agents are suspected to cause reproductive harm based on the animal literature and toxicologic assessment. In addition to the emotional stress on affected families, the societal burden of these adverse health outcomes includes high medical costs for compromised children and the increasing use of advanced technology to achieve conception and monitor pregnancy. Another reason to better understand reproductive outcomes is that they may act as sentinels for detecting occupational and environmental hazards because of the relatively short latency between exposure and clinical health event. If workers or community residents are protected from exposures that are harmful to the fetus, they usually will be protected from other health effects associated with these exposures as well. Measures that can be taken to prevent further exposure include substitution or containment of the suspect hazard. Thus, preventing exposure should be a primary goal in the health care provider's overall assessment of the patient's situation.

POPULATION AT RISK

Women comprise 47% of the workforce in the United States, with a majority employed in the following job categories: office and administrative support, education/library, health care provider or support, and personal care and service. Some of the leading occupations for women have potential exposures to known reproductive toxicants (eg, large numbers of women work in the nursing profession or health service occupations with potential exposure to chemotherapeutic agents, anesthetic gases, ionizing radiation, and biologic agents). In addition, there is an increasing number of women in occupations traditionally held by men where there is potential for exposure to reproductive hazards. When women are employed in jobs traditionally held by men, there can be difficulty in obtaining personal protective equipment that fits, accessing separate changing rooms and wash areas, and getting health and safety information that is gender-specific, where appropriate.

Women also may be exposed to reproductive hazards in the environment, which can be more difficult to detect than in the workplace. Often these environmental hazards may be local exposures, but some are of nationwide interest, such as the widespread use of pesticides that persist in the environment and food chain. In addition, exposure to fetuses or children may have lasting effects, so these represent a wider population at risk.

REPRODUCTIVE OUTCOMES & RATES

A number of adverse reproductive effects may result from exposure to chemical and physical agents either pre- or postconception. These effects range from infertility to birth

Table 27–1. Prevalence of selected adverse pregnancy outcomes in the United States.

Endpoint	Frequency per 100	Unit
Infertility	12–13	Couples
Recognized spontaneous abortion	10–20	Women or pregnancies
Birth weight < 2500 g	7–9	Livebirths
Preterm (≤ 37 wk)	11–13	Livebirths
Fetal death (or stillbirth)	0.7–1	Stillbirths and livebirths
Infant death (< 1 y)	0.7	Livebirths
Birth defects (through 1 y of life)	3	Livebirths
Chromosomal anomalies in livebirths	0.2	Livebirths

defects in the infant. Several of these outcomes are quite frequent and represent a serious public health concern (Table 27–1). Accurate data on the rates of these outcomes can be difficult to obtain because of the lack of national monitoring systems and methodologic differences between individual epidemiologic studies. Approximately 10% of couples in the United States are infertile, which is defined as an inability to conceive during 12 months of unprotected intercourse. Additional couples may experience periods of subfertility or delayed conception. After conception, a continuum of reproductive loss may occur from the time of implantation to delivery. Up to 50% of embryos may be lost after implantation (the earliest time at which conception can be detected), with approximately 15–20% of pregnancies ending in clinically detected spontaneous abortion (SAB) and approximately 1% ending in fetal death. Of all liveborn infants, 7–9% are of low birth weight (LBW), approximately 11% are born prematurely, and approximately 3% will have a congenital anomaly. Whereas rates of fetal and infant death have decreased over the past few decades, rates of LBW and preterm delivery have not, and in some areas they have shown slight increases. Some of the observed risk patterns for these outcomes include (1) older maternal age associated with increased rates of infertility, SAB, and some birth defects and (2) black race associated with nearly doubled rates of LBW, preterm delivery, and fetal death. Ethnic differences may reflect in part unequal access to regular or early prenatal medical care. Other reproductive endpoints that may be affected by exogenous exposures include menstrual function and age at menopause or menarche. Recent studies indicate trends to earlier onset of puberty in girls; about 12% of white girls and 28% of black girls in the United States enter puberty by age 8.

REPRODUCTIVE & DEVELOPMENTAL PHYSIOLOGY & SENSITIVE PERIODS

Germ Cell Development & Menstrual Cycle Function

The female reproductive cycle is a complex process regulated by the autonomic nervous and endocrine systems and mediated by the hypothalamic-pituitary-gonadal axis (Figure 27–1). Unlike males, the female germ cells (oogonia) develop and begin the first meiotic division in utero, with no new generation after birth. The oocytes remain arrested until follicular activation occurs 15–40 years later. Under gonadotropin hormone stimulation at the start of each menstrual cycle, a group of primary follicles begins to develop. Increased levels of the follicle-stimulating hormone (FSH) lead to the selection and growth of a dominant follicle, which produces estrogen to support proliferation of endometrial tissue. A midcycle release of the gonadotropins, FSH, and luteinizing hormone (LH) results in the release of the ovum, or ovulation. The remaining corpus luteum secretes increasing amounts of progesterone and other hormones to prepare for implantation, exerting a negative feedback on the gonadotropins. In the absence of fertilization, the corpus luteum degenerates. The subsequent decrease in ovarian steroids leads to sloughing of the endometrium, as well as to rising levels of FSH, and menstruation occurs after a 12- to 14-day luteal phase. Although this general pattern of menstrual function is known, there is much interwoman variation, and the exact mechanisms are not well understood. If a sperm successfully fertilizes an ovum, the ovum completes a second meiotic division and forms a zygote. This zygote undergoes several rapid cell divisions as it is transported down the fallopian tube to the uterus.

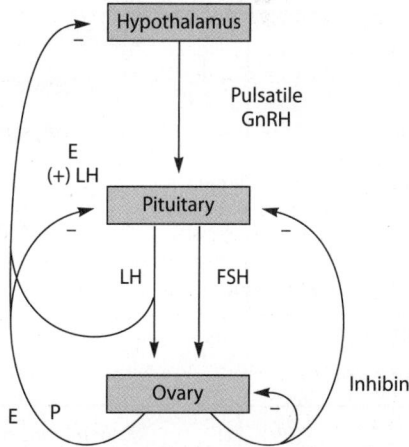

▲ **Figure 27–1.** Feedback regulation of the hypothalamic-pituitary-ovarian axis. E, estrogens; FSH, follicle-stimulating hormone; GnRH, gonadotropin-releasing hormone; LH, luteinizing hormone; P, progesterone.

Endocrine control of the reproductive process might be disrupted by chemicals that, in turn, could lead to menstrual disorders and infertility. This is especially true for those chemicals with steroid-like activity (eg, certain pesticides and dioxins; see later). Because the germ cells are present from birth and many exposures occur during a woman's life, there is great potential for genetic or cytotoxic harm to the oocytes. It is postulated that the cumulative effects of occupational, environmental, and other exposures may explain the increased incidence of chromosomal abnormalities and SAB that occurs as maternal age increases. But because the greatest potential for genetic damage is most likely to occur during replication and division of the genetic material, the actual sensitivity during the relatively long dormant period is unknown. Genetic damage could result in lack of fertilization or unsuccessful implantation, which can be seen clinically as infertility, or could lead to later fetal loss. Preconception mutagenesis also might result in a birth defect in an infant. Certain mutagenic chemicals are in use in industry, such as organic solvents, ethylene oxide, and metals (eg, arsenic and nickel). Oocyte destruction by chemicals such as polyaromatic hydrocarbons (PAHs) could lead to infertility or to early menopause.

Development of the Fetus

The dividing zygote reaches the uterus approximately 1 week after fertilization, and approximately 1 week later,

implantation is complete. The placental villi secrete human chorionic gonadotropin (hCG), which is necessary to maintain pregnancy, and the placenta also takes over the secretion of estrogen and progesterone. The next 6 weeks are called the *embryonic period* and are the most critical for development because all the major organ systems are formed in precise sequence (Figure 27–2). During the subsequent fetal period, growth and organ maturation continue until term. In particular, the central nervous, genitourinary, and immune systems continue to develop throughout pregnancy. The period of most rapid fetal growth is considered to occur during the last trimester. Full term is typically 38 weeks after conception, with a normal fetal weight of 6.6–7.9 lb (3000–3600 g) and a length of 19–20 in (360 mm).

Exposures during weeks 1 and 2 after conception may cause early pregnancy loss if they interfere with tubal transport, implantation, or endocrine control or if they are cytotoxic to the fetus itself. Such a loss may appear only as a late or heavy menstrual flow. With increasingly sensitive laboratory assays available, women trying to conceive or being studied for pregnancy outcome can have these very early losses detected by a short rise and subsequent fall in hCG. The embryo may be less sensitive to structural damage at this time because differentiation has not yet begun, and damage is potentially correctable by the rapidly dividing cells. Thus, congenital anomalies are unlikely to result from very early embryo exposures.

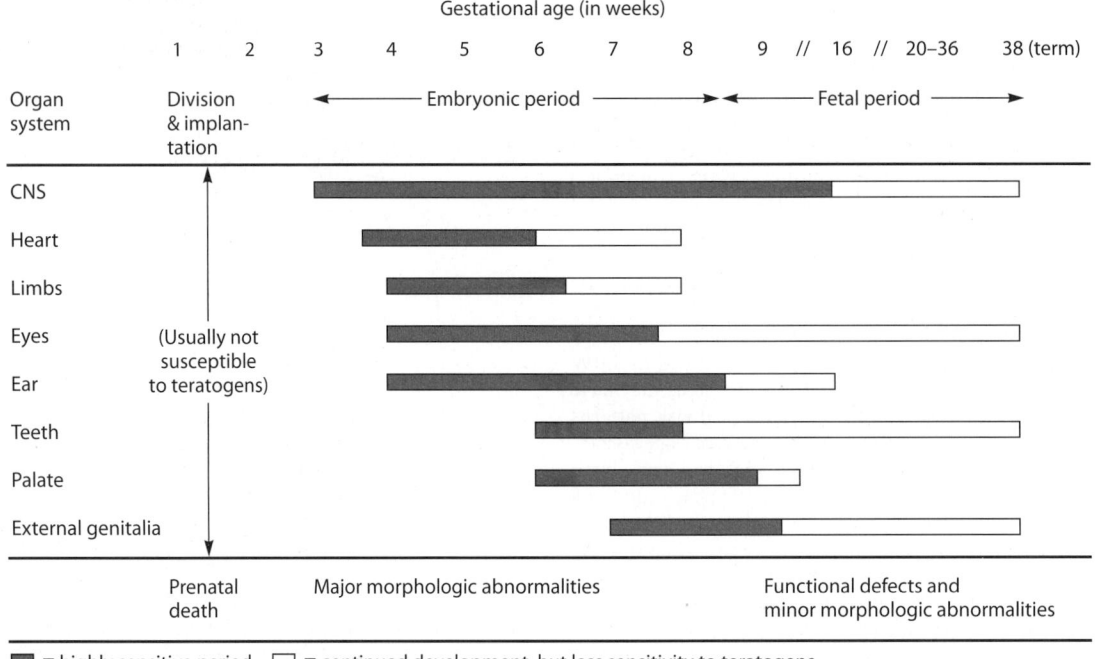

▲ **Figure 27–2.** Critical periods of fetal development by organ system.

The greatest susceptibility to teratogenic agents occurs during the embryonic period, or organogenesis, when major morphologic abnormalities may be induced. The timing of an effect can be very specific. Although different agents administered at the same time may cause the same anomaly, the same agent given at two different times may induce different anomalies. Known or suspected human teratogens include antineoplastic drugs, diethylstilbestrol (DES), lead, and ionizing radiation (Table 27–2). The embryonic period is when the highest rates of pregnancy loss occur, with approximately 60–75% of recognized losses in the first trimester. Approximately 35% of aborted conceptuses are karyotypically abnormal, and another 30% have morphologic abnormalities.

Exposure after the first trimester may induce minor morphologic abnormalities or growth deficits. Since the endocrine, central nervous, and other systems are still developing, their respective function might be affected by exposures during this time. Organic mercury, tobacco smoke, and lead are examples of substances that have adverse effects with exposure later in pregnancy. Potentially, carcinogens could cross the placenta and exert an effect at any stage of development.

Table 27–2. Human evidence for adverse female reproduction or developmental effects of selected agents.

Agent	Human Outcomes	Common Occupations at Risk
Anesthetic gases Nitrous oxide	Subfertility, SAB, BDs	Anesthesiologists, dental hygienists, veterinarians

Antineoplastic drugs
  Cyclophosphamide
  Paclitaxol
  Vismodegib
  Uracil Mustard
	SAB/BDs	Pharmacists, nurses

Arsenic	SAB, LBW	Electronic recyclers, copper smelter workers, miners
Bromopropane(s)	Infertility, menstrual disorders	Dry cleaners, foam cushion gluers
Cadmium	LBW	Silver solder operators, electroplating technicians, battery production workers
Carbon disulfide	SAB, menstrual disorders	Rubber, cellophane, and rayon fabric workers
Carbon monoxide	SAB, LBW	Welders, garage mechanics

Chlorination by-products
  Chloroform
  Dichlorobromomethane
  Dibromochloromethane
  Bromoforms
	SAB, LBW, menstrual disorders	Electronic testing technicians

Chromium	Preterm, LBW, SGA	Welders, spray painters, chrome plating bath operators
Dioxins	Menstrual disorders, SAB, BDs	Metallurgical workers
Electromagnetic fields (EMF)	SAB, childhood cancer	Machinists, electricians, welders
Ethylene glycol ethers Ethylene oxide	SAB	Medical equipment sterile processing technicians
Lead	Infertility, SAB, preterm, neurobehavioral, delayed puberty	Construction workers (renovations/demolitions), solder operators
Mercury (Inorganic)	Menstrual disorders, CNS malformation, cerebral palsy, neurobehavioral	Amalgam, barometer and battery makers, gold miners

(continued)

Table 27–2. Human evidence for adverse female reproduction or developmental effects of selected agents. (Continued)

Agent	Human Outcomes	Common Occupations at Risk
Mercury (Organic)	Menstrual disorders, infertility	

Pesticides/herbicides/fungicides/insecticides
  Atrazine
  Carbaryl
  Dichlorodiphenyltrichloroethane
  Simazine
  Thiophanate-methyl
	Fertility, fetal loss, menstrual
	  disorders, BDs
		Agricultural workers

Physical stress	Preterm, LBW, SAB	Inadequate staffing levels, long work hours, shift work, role ambiguity

Phthalates
  Dibutyl phthalate
	Preterm, structural anomaly,
	  premature thelarche
		Manicurists

Polyaromatic hydrocarbons (PAHs)	LBW, SGA	Asphalt, aluminum production, and coking plant workers
Polychlorinated biphenyls (PCBs)	LBW, hyperpigmentation, menstrual disorders	Repair and maintenance workers of PCB transformers
Radiation, ionizing	Infertility, menstrual disorders, SAB, BDs, childhood cancer	Radiology technicians, radiologists, miners, nuclear plant workers
Organic solvents	Menstrual disorders, fertility, SAB, BDs	Semiconductor and microelectronics workers, laboratory workers
Tobacco smoke (Direct)	Fertility, fetal loss, LBW, SIDS	Construction, transportation, repair and maintenance workers
Tobacco smoke (Secondhand)	Menstrual disorders, fertility, preterm, SAB, BDs	

BDs, birth defects; LBW, low birth weight; SAB, spontaneous abortion; SGA, small for gestational age.

Postnatal Development & Lactation

The young infant continues development after birth, with general body growth and central nervous system maturation the most obvious changes. In children, prenatal exposures may result in deficits in growth or behavior and mental function (eg, fetal alcohol syndrome). Prenatal maternal cigarette smoking is strongly related to sudden infant death syndrome and is thought to be related to growth. In addition, prenatal exposures may exert effects manifested during reproductive maturation of the offspring, with early pubertal development an increasing concern in industrialized countries. Prenatal exposures or conditions are also being investigated for long-term effects into adulthood.

Child development also may be affected by postnatal exposures. Environmental exposures may be present in the residence or community, and parental occupational exposures may be brought home on clothing or delivered through breastfeeding. Contamination of breast milk occurs primarily by passive diffusion. Thus low-molecular-weight lipophilic nonpolar substances can have higher concentrations in breast milk than in maternal serum. Substances with higher milk-to-plasma ratios (> 3) include the PCBs and dichlorodiphenyltrichloroethane (DDT) residues. Lactation is the main route of excretion for toxicants that bioaccumulate in maternal adipose tissue. Although acute toxicity in infants from contaminated breast milk has been reported (eg, PCBs), the effects of low-level chronic exposures have not been well studied. Therefore, most pediatricians would continue to recommend the benefits of breastfeeding, except for unusual exposure circumstances.

Maternal Physiologic Changes

A number of physiologic changes and medical complications can occur in the pregnant woman that might be affected by occupational or environmental exposures. These changes are also noteworthy to the physician for the way in which they may modify fetal exposures or require accommodation in the workplace. For example, increased tidal volume and respiratory rate of the pregnant woman may increase the absorbed dose of aerosolized chemicals. An increased metabolic rate also may lead to changes in metabolism of specific compounds, leading to a different effective dose. Pregnant women also can experience fatigue and nausea. The nausea may increase sensitivity to substances with strong odors or tastes. Thus, potential changes in exposure dose and common consumption patterns (eg, caffeinated or alcoholic beverages) could occur.

SCIENTIFIC LITERATURE

Toxicologic risk assessment is the means of characterizing health effects of hazards in the workplace or environment by combining evidence from scientific studies with likely exposure scenarios using mathematical modeling. When evaluating a patient, the clinician will identify potential exposures via a detailed environmental and occupational history. Existing databases should be consulted for information about reproductive hazards; however, many chemicals and physical hazards have not been studied adequately with respect to reproduction. Because the clinician may need to consult the original literature, this section provides an explanation of basic issues in conducting or interpreting experimental and epidemiologic studies.

As a consequence of the scarcity of human data dealing with reproductive effects, regulatory and oversight agencies often must rely on animal studies when identifying toxicants. Animal studies are applicable to humans with respect to whether there is any harm but are not necessarily predictive of specific human effects. Furthermore, animal studies generally use a range of doses extending well beyond typical human exposures that may involve different routes of exposure and examine endpoints not seen in humans (eg, fetal resorptions). In the evaluation of the animal literature and its relevance to humans, the following aspects need to be considered: species tested; route, timing, and dose of exposure; endpoints examined; systemic or maternal toxicity; litter effects; consistency among animal studies; concordance with reproductive biology; and biologic plausibility of the mechanism of action. From the higher-quality animal studies, the dose-response relationship is assessed to set standards for exposure levels. One goal is to try to ascertain the no-observed-adverse-effect level (NOAEL), which is the highest dose level at which no biologically adverse effects occur, or alternatively, the lowest-observed-adverse-effect level (LOAEL). Then it is customary to apply uncertainty factors (or safety factors) to this level when estimating the "safe" exposure level for humans.

Epidemiologic Studies

Well-conducted epidemiologic studies should provide the best means of evaluating whether a specific agent or group of agents adversely affects human reproduction and development but are less often used for setting standards. Human studies have many limitations, so certain criteria or a weight-of-evidence type of scheme is often used in evaluating whether a substance reasonably can be considered as having an adverse effect. Besides performing qualitative comparison of consistency of results, quality of studies, and biologic plausibility, this might involve conducting a meta-analysis where results from several studies are combined statistically.

A. Study Designs

The basic study designs used to examine the association of an exposure and possible outcomes include the cross-sectional, case-control, and cohort studies. The cross-sectional design is the simplest and has been used often in occupational and environmental reproductive studies. In these studies, there is potential selection bias because the population existing in the workplace at the time of study may not be representative of the workforce during the time of previous exposure. For example, women with live births may leave the workforce temporarily to care for their infants, whereas women experiencing SABs may continue to work and are at greater risk for subsequent SABs. On the other hand, women who experience adverse outcomes that they associate with a workplace exposure may change jobs. The case-control study is most appropriate for evaluating relatively rare diseases (eg, birth defects or childhood cancers). Because the outcome of interest is specified at the onset, the continuum of reproductive effects that may result from a given exposure cannot be evaluated. The cohort study is the preferred study design for most reproductive outcomes. A prospective cohort study allows specific measures of an exposure and potential confounders to be ascertained at the etiologically relevant time periods, before the health endpoint is ascertained.

The cohort and case-control studies are considered hypothesis-testing studies and usually are conducted after a possible association has been suggested. For example, an acute clinician may recognize a series of cases that seem to have a factor in common. This situation is most likely to occur with a rare disease or new syndrome and was instrumental in identifying such associations as thalidomide and severe limb defects and DES and vaginal clear-cell carcinoma. A reported cluster of adverse outcomes occurring in a group of persons is a common way for environmental and occupational problems to be brought to attention, but such clusters often remain unexplained on further investigation.

Valuable data could be obtained from surveillance systems, but there are few established systems in place for adverse reproductive outcomes other than birth defects and, very recently but on a limited basis, autism and other developmental disabilities. Reasons for this include the fact that not all outcomes attract medical attention or require hospitalization (eg, SABs and subfertility), so they are more difficult to ascertain routinely.

B. Exposure Assessment

Although the methods used to measure occupational or environmental exposure are beyond the scope of this chapter, a brief overview of issues specific to evaluating exposure with respect to reproductive outcomes is presented. It should be kept in mind that the exposures of three individuals may be involved (eg, each parent and the fetus/offspring).

To cause reproductive damage, an agent must be absorbed into the bloodstream, and to harm the fetus directly (eg, changes in maternal hormones could affect the fetus) it also must cross the placenta. This process is affected by individual metabolism and the molecular structure of the compound. Some chemicals react with the first tissues they encounter, such as the lungs or skin, and are not absorbed into the bloodstream unless they are ingested (eg, acids, chlorine, and asbestos). Once in the bloodstream, agents that are of low molecular weight, are lipophilic, and are in a non-ionized state are most likely to cross the placenta. Maternal metabolism may result in a metabolite that is more or less toxic to the fetus than the original substance. Unless chronic exposure results in a steady-state level in the body, the rapidity with which a substance is cleared also can affect its toxicity. Often these issues are beyond the scope of epidemiologic studies but should be considered within the overall body of evidence about the toxicity of a substance. When evaluating epidemiologic studies, an association with an exposure at the critical time is more relevant to establishing causality. In addition to timing, a dose-response relationship is examined if exposure data are sufficiently detailed. However, this relationship may not be evident with reproductive outcomes because different doses may result in different outcomes (eg, birth defect versus fetal death).

In epidemiologic studies, exposures can be ascertained from interviews, existing records, or biomarkers. If exposure history is obtained by retrospective interview, the possibility of biased recall among cases or misclassification because of a lack of records or diminished memory is of concern. Ascertainment of current exposure status for cohort studies limits possible recall bias, but women may not be aware of all their exposures, and asking one spouse about the other may not provide sufficiently accurate information.

Existing records often do not provide detailed information but rather serve to group women broadly. For example, residence on the birth certificate might be used to assign likelihood of an environmental exposure. However, residence at delivery may not reflect residence in the first trimester, nor does it account for individual behavioral differences, such as how much time is spent away from the area. Similarly, occupational registries may be used to group women by broad exposures, but specific worksite practices will be unknown. The most accurate occupational exposures are obtained by an industrial hygienist, but such studies are also more costly and often limited in sample size to allow for more detailed study.

Laboratory measurement of exposure provides a quantification of exposure that is less likely to be biased. Techniques for measuring environmental levels in air, water, and soil have been developed for many agents, including radon, EMFs, solvents, pesticides, metals, and particulate levels. Measurements on biologic samples provide an indication of internal dose, which would be more biologically relevant. For example, cotinine (a metabolite of nicotine) is used to assess tobacco smoke exposure. Biologic monitoring requires a prospective study unless stored samples are available. A number of difficulties can arise with such studies, for example, small sample size or selection bias because of the higher costs and greater participation required of subjects. Sampling at one point in time may not reflect the critical exposure period, particularly if the substance is metabolized rapidly.

C. Health Endpoints & Study Design Issues

Numerous endpoints have been examined in reproductive and developmental toxicity studies. Table 27–3 summarizes the definition and ascertainment of these outcomes as well as potential confounders. For a factor to be a confounder, it must be related to both the endpoint and the exposure in the study of interest. Lack of control for one of the variables in the list does not imply that the study is deficient if the investigators found that this factor did not act as a confounder in their study.

Many of the pregnancy outcomes in Table 27–3A are relatively frequent and lend themselves to a prospective study design. One design is to enroll women when they come in for a prenatal visit and then ascertain pregnancy outcomes by medical records, vital records, or both. However, the detection of SAB depends on the time at which the pregnancy is recognized. Women who have had prior losses and are worried about an exposure may seek medical attention sooner than other women, and thus more of their losses will be detected. A case-control design also can be used to study SAB, but when SABs are ascertained from medical or laboratory records, a certain percentage of early losses will be missed, which may be related to exposure status. Studies have been conducted that collect urine samples for the measurement of hCG and early pregnancy loss (or for ovulation detection). These studies are very labor intensive, and the types of participants may represent a selected population.

In contrast to fetal loss, specific congenital anomalies are not common, and thus a case-control study design is usually used. The primary concerns with these types of studies are ascertainment of relevant cases, selection of appropriate control subjects, and possible recall bias. Classification of defects is problematic because they may have varying etiologies, but any single defect is extremely rare. Many defects are not evident at birth; therefore, additional postnatal follow-up may be necessary for identification.

Because birth weight is recorded fairly accurately and is associated with subsequent mortality and morbidity, it has been the subject of much perinatal research using a variety of study designs. Mean birth weight can be examined, or it is often categorized as LBW (< 2500 g). However, this category includes infants who are born prematurely, as well as those who are growth retarded for their age. These two groups may be etiologically different and experience different risks of mortality. To distinguish these, investigators can examine LBW among only term infants or small for gestational age infants (SGA; usually defined as births below the tenth percentile on standard-weight-for-gestational-age curves).

Perinatal deaths include a variety of causes with a number of classification schemes developed to summarize them. For occupational or environmental factors, it is useful to distinguish between prepartum and peripartum stillbirths because a toxic effect is more likely to be related to death in utero. When infant deaths are examined, neonatal deaths are found to be more likely to be related to exposures or conditions of pregnancy, whereas postnatal deaths also reflect conditions of infancy.

Table 27–3. Developmental and reproductive outcomes, definitions, and source of ascertainment in epidemiologic studies.

Outcome	Definition	Source of Ascertainment	Possible Confounders
A. Developmental Outcomes			
Clinical spontaneous abortion	Fetal loss by 20 wk	Interview, MDs or MRs pregnancy test	Maternal age, prior SAB, smoking, alcohol, gestational age at pregnancy recognition
Early, or subclinical loss	Loss by 6–8 wk Short rise and fall in hCG level	Urinary assay (days 5–20 after ovulation)	Same as clinical (unknown)
Congenital anomalies	Varies—structural, physiologic, genetic, major and minor	Problematic—vital records incomplete; MRs, MDs, or registries	Few known—maternal age, prior hx, gender, race (defect specific)
Fetal growth	LBW: < 2500 g SGA: ≤ 10th percentile weight-for-age Preterm: < 37 wk	Vital records (accuracy of gest. age), MRs, interview	Maternal age, race, SES, parity, maternal weight and gain, prior hx, prenatal care, gestational age, gender, multiple birth, nutrition, smoking, stress
Fetal, neonatal, or infant death	FD: 21 wk-term ND: First month of life ID: First year	Vital records (underreport FDs), MRs, interview	Vary by timing and cause: maternal age, race, SES, parity, infant gender, multiple birth, birth weight, and gestational age
B. Reproductive Outcomes			
Infertility	No conception in 12 mo unprotected intercourse or specific dx (eg, tubal disease, ovulatory factor, cervical factor, endometriosis)	Interview or survey Vital records crude	Maternal age, STD hx, IUD or OC use hx, smoking, weight (?), stress (?)
Time to conception	Continuous = months of unprotected intercourse, or Categorize (3, 6, 12 mo)	Interview Diary	See above, frequency of intercourse
Age at puberty	Age at menarche, breast or pubic hair development	Interview, physical examination, MRs	Race, body size, birth weight, exercise, diet (unknown)
Menstrual cycle dysfunction	Cycle length (or categorize; < 24, > 34 days), bleed characteristics, pain, anovulation, long FP or short LP	Interview, BBT or cervical mucous test, hormone measurements in serum or urine	Maternal age, obesity, alcohol abuse, smoking, stress, exertion, some drugs or medical conditions (more work needed)
Age at menopause	Cessation of menstruation: mean about 50 y, but perimenopausal many years prior	Interview, MRs, hormone levels	Smoking, age at menarche, pregnancy hx

BBT, basal body temperature; dx, diagnosis; FD, fetal death; FP, follicular phase; hx, history; ID, infant death; IUD, intrauterine device; LBW, low birth weight; LP, luteal phase; MD, medical doctor, physician records; MR, medical (hospital) records; ND, neonatal death; OC, oral contraceptives; SAB, spontaneous abortion; SES, socioeconomic status; SGA, small for gestational age; STD, sexually transmitted disease.

The reproductive endpoints in Table 27–3B are less well studied epidemiologically than are pregnancy outcomes. This is partly because the population at risk is harder to determine, and such outcomes only recently have come under more public concern. Infertility and subfertility often are studied retrospectively because it is difficult to assemble a population of women trying to become pregnant. The definition of infertility is based on waiting time and may include some people in whom no physiologic change has occurred. If cases are limited to a medically diagnosed population, the study may be biased by a differential likelihood of seeking treatment after varying waiting times, potentially dependent on suspected exposures. Often control subjects are difficult to select for these studies. Because the label of infertility ignores the potential continuum of effects, time to pregnancy is a preferred measure. Retrospectively, women who are pregnant or have delivered recently can be questioned about past use of contraception. The choice of a reference date about when exposures are determined in controls is critical. If the time of conception is used, women who had been trying unsuccessfully before that time may have changed their exposures, and the true period at risk (when contraception is stopped) will not be included. Prospective studies may be conducted by having women keep diaries of when their menstrual periods occur, when they have intercourse, and when they use contraception to identify cycles truly "at risk" of pregnancy, as well as monitoring conception by hormone tests. Menstrual cycle function is the least well investigated but is best studied prospectively with the use of diaries to record signs and symptoms. Cycle length can be used as a crude measure of function, but normal lengths may mask such problems as insufficient luteal phase and progesterone production. Studying such defects requires accurate determination of day of ovulation and measurement of hormone patterns. These types of studies have become relatively easier to conduct in population-based groups by the recent development of cost-efficient serial-sample laboratory assays of urinary hormone metabolites. Such studies may be well suited to an occupational cohort in which a well-defined worker population is assembled and has the advantage of including more women, not just those who are pregnant. The ages at menarche and menopause define the length of natural reproductive capacity and are also related to other endpoints such as breast cancer. Age at menarche is relatively well recalled, even by adults, but other measures of puberty are determined most accurately by trained physical examiners, so prospective or cross-sectional studies would be necessary.

Selected Reproductive Hazards

As noted, few chemicals have been studied adequately in terms of their reproductive effects, and most exposure standards are not based on reproductive effects. Nevertheless, a number of potential reproductive or developmental hazards have been identified in humans. In fact, a number of agents have been added onto the Safe Drinking Water and Toxic Enforcement Act of 1986 (Proposition 65) as reproductive toxicants. Many of the toxic agents in Table 27–2 have been examined in occupational settings where exposures tend to be higher than those encountered in the environment and relatively easier to document. However, some of these hazards are encountered environmentally from long-term use and disposal by industry, natural occurrence, or acute releases. After brief discussion of the evidence for some of these, the following section presents three more detailed examples of accumulating epidemiologic data.

Some of the agents that have been shown conclusively to be reproductive toxicants in humans, other than medications, include anesthetic gases, diethylstilbestrol (DES), polychlorinated biphenyls (PCBs), vinyl chloride, ionizing radiation, mercury, solvents, and lead. Health care workers may be exposed to other hazards, including biologics and antineoplastic drugs, associated with increased risks of SAB.

Workers involved in the manufacture of these and other pharmaceuticals also may be put at risk. Pesticides are used commonly worldwide and represent different classes, such as insecticides, herbicides, and fungicides, some of which may be endocrine disruptors (see later). General exposure to pesticides most likely occurs via the diet or home use, but worker exposures tend to be the highest. In addition to diet, chemicals in air and water may lead to environmental exposures. Increasing evidence shows that air pollutants may be associated with adverse pregnancy outcomes on a population level, including LBW, preterm delivery, stillbirth, and infant death.

Reports of clusters of malformations in women working with video-display terminals (VDTs) in the early 1980s led to extensive public and scientific interest. A review of subsequent analytical studies from several countries did not generally support much association of adverse reproductive outcomes with VDT work; a meta-analysis found a pooled odds ratio of 1.0 for VDT use and SAB. However, a Finnish report released later showed an elevated risk (odds ratio [OR]: 3.4) among women who used VDTs with a high level of extremely low-frequency magnetic fields. The concern shifted to EMFs that are present in all workplaces and homes. The next generation of EMF studies examining electric appliance use, residential wire coding, and residential spot measurements yielded inconsistent results with respect to SAB and little evidence of increased risk for birth defects. Two studies with better exposure measures (eg, the subjects wore measuring devices for 24 hours) subsequently found increased risks of SAB (OR: 1.7–1.8) associated with various EMF metrics. These findings led the California EMF Program to conclude in their risk-evaluation document that EMFs were a possible risk for miscarriage and that further research to study the nature of changing or high magnetic fields was warranted.

Whether employment per se has a harmful effect on pregnancy outcome has been evaluated, with the general consensus that it does not. Physical exertion at work has been a cause of concern because of the extreme effects seen in professional athletes and dancers. The American College of Obstetricians and Gynecologists published guidelines on exertion levels during later stages of pregnancy indicating that moderate or light exertion levels should be safe throughout pregnancy. Heavy lifting, prolonged standing, or repetitive stooping and bending are recommended to be discontinued early during the second trimester. The most consistent adverse effect of physical exertion seems to be on preterm delivery and possibly LBW and SAB, with less consistent results seen for fecundability and menstrual disorders. Several studies show that shift work, or working irregular hours, is associated with a moderately increased risk of SAB, with similar results for LBW and decreased fecundability or longer time to pregnancy.

A. Endocrine-Disrupting Chemicals

In the last two decades, concern has risen about a variety of compounds that may affect the endocrine system by mimicking or antagonizing endogenous hormones. Hormones act as chemical messengers, directing a wide variety of biologic functions through gene expression, and are particularly important during fetal development. Alterations were first noticed in the 1980s among various wildlife populations and later confirmed experimentally. Disruption of the hormone system by chemical contaminants now has been seen in a wide range of species from birds to fish, mollusks, frogs, alligators, and polar bears. Effects in both males and females have been observed, with one unusual but predominant finding being the development of intersex reproductive systems, with both male and female aspects. Originally focused on chemicals that interfered with estrogen receptor pathways, research from a variety of disciplines during the last 5 years has revealed a number of other actions such as antiandrogens, progesterone blockers, or interference with thyroid hormone.

These so-called endocrine-disrupting chemicals (EDCs) or hormonally active agents (HAAs) vary structurally, from persistent pesticides such as DDT/dichlorodiphenyl dichloroethylene (DDE) to PCBs and plasticizers such as phthalates, perfluorinated compounds (PFCs), triclosan, parabens, and bisphenol-A. Because some of these compounds persist for years in the environment and have entered the food chain, low exposure may continue despite bans on the use of some of them in the United States. Immigrants from Southeast Asia or Latin America have higher body burdens of persistent pesticides such as DDT, as well as ongoing exposure to other pesticides in agricultural work. Thyroid hormone disruption and neurodevelopmental deficits have been found in animal studies. These compounds are used widely as flame retardants in plastics used in electrical appliances, computers, building materials, and furnishings. Exposure may occur in manufacturing and dismantling of these products as well as from their degradation in the environment. Another class of compounds with similar manufacturing uses owing to their chemical stability that are now being measured in the environment and wildlife are perfluorinated organic compounds (PFOCs).

A number of studies have focused on bisphenol-A (BPA), a synthetic chemical utilized in the manufacturing of everyday consumer products, such as water bottles, epoxy resins for the lacquer lining of food and beverage cans, and polycarbonate plastic bottles for babies. Exposure to BPA can occur through dermal absorption, inhalation, or ingestion; in fact, when BPA containing products are exposed to light or heat, this chemical leaches into food or beverages. BPA can impair female fertility as it impacts oocyte development and implantation. Triclosan is often added into personal care products such as toothpaste and soaps as an antibacterial agent, impacting thyroid and sex hormone homeostasis. Similarly, parabens are commonly used for their antimicrobial properties in personal care products and have estrogenic activity. PCBs and mercury have been associated with adverse neurodevelopmental effects in prenatally exposed children. Polybrominated biphenyl (PBB) and PCB exposure in utero also have been associated with earlier menarche, whereas lead exposure has been associated with delayed puberty. Thus, a variety of effects from these ubiquitous compounds may be revealed in humans as the research progresses, including other reproductive endpoints such as infertility and tumorigenesis.

Some unique aspects of EDCs are that effects may occur not only at high doses but also lower doses, making classic high-dose experiments potentially misleading. Furthermore, the developing fetus is exquisitely sensitive to both natural hormone signals and exogenous chemical signals. Besides guiding the fetus through critical developmental pathways, these early interactions also help to set its sensitivity to subsequent hormonal signals, leading to potential lifelong consequences. These compounds also may act by creating changes that are permanent to the lineage, leading to transgenerational effects.

B. Solvents

Solvents may well be one of the most pervasive chemical exposures of women because they include many compounds used in the workplace and the home. In the early 1980s, solvent exposure was considered a potential reproductive hazard when increased risks for adverse outcomes were identified among laboratory workers in Scandinavia. In some industries (eg, dry-cleaning and pharmaceutical industries), use of specific solvents, such as perchloroethylene, methylene chloride, toluene, xylene, and glycol ethers, has been associated with concurrent elevation in SAB risk. Several case-control studies show associations of solvent exposure and cardiac and other congenital anomalies.

A meta-analysis that combined raw data from five studies for each outcome found that the odds for major malformations increased 64% (eg, OR: 1.64) and for SAB increased 25% with solvent exposure. Confounding and dose-response patterns were not assessed. Suggestive study findings indicate a potential association between solvent use and fetal growth or preterm delivery. Studies have found that offspring of pregnant women occupationally exposed to organic solvents obtained lower scores on various behavioral assessments. These results would be consistent with effects of heavy maternal alcohol consumption. Because alcohol is a type of solvent, a "fetal solvent syndrome" has been proposed. Many of the epidemiologic studies suffer from crude exposure assessment, making definitive conclusions difficult, but animal data support the findings. Some studies have examined menstrual patterns, but few consistent results have emerged. At least one study reported reduced fecundability among women with daily or high solvent exposure. Exposures in the semiconductor industry, which employs a largely female workforce, have demonstrated an increased risk of SAB, reduced fecundability, and menstrual cycle length increased in exposed workers. The investigators found risk of exposure to photoresist and developer solvents (eg, glycol ethers and xylene) and fluoride compounds as the primary etiologic agents.

C. Tobacco Smoke Exposure

Active smoking has been causally associated with a number of developmental and reproductive endpoints; infants of women who smoke during pregnancy are estimated to have twice the risk of LBW or a decrement in mean birth weight of 150–200 g compared with infants of nonsmokers. Other adverse developmental outcomes associated with maternal tobacco smoking include preterm delivery, fetal and infant death, and behavioral deficits in offspring. Tobacco smoking is also associated with infertility, menstrual disorders, and earlier age at menopause. In the workplace or other environments, nonsmokers may be exposed to passive smoke, also called *environmental tobacco smoke* (ETS). Tobacco smoke contains thousands of compounds; those with potential reproductive toxicity include nicotine, carbon monoxide, PAHs, heavy metals, aromatic solvents, and others. Based on studies measuring biomarkers in the early to mid-1990s, from 40% to nearly 100% of nonsmokers may be exposed to some ETS, with working representing, on average, 35% of exposure time.

Reviewing the evidence for adverse effects of ETS exposure on reproduction, over 30 studies have examined mean birth weight, with the better studies indicating a weight decrement ranging from 25 to 100 g. In an earlier meta-analysis, the adequate studies conducted among nonsmoking mothers yielded a pooled weight decrement of 31 g (CL: −42, −20). Studies based on measurement of cotinine (a metabolite of nicotine) in nonsmokers yield even greater weight decrements, particularly as assays have gotten more sensitive so that a truly not (or very low) exposed comparison group can be identified. Of the studies that examined dose-response effects, several found evidence for such trends, further strengthening the argument for causality. At least 20 studies of LBW or SGA have been conducted; the higher-quality studies of LBW yielded a pooled OR of 1.4, or a 40% increase. Some evidence suggests that specific subsets of women may be more susceptible to effects, including older women and nonwhites.

Reviews by several agencies generally conclude there is a consistent slight effect of ETS exposure on reducing mean birth weight (or slightly increasing the risk of growth retardation). There is also good evidence that ETS exposure can lead to sudden infant death syndrome in offspring and may be associated with preterm delivery, SAB, and adverse effects on cognition and behavior. There is a lack of studies of effects of ETS exposure on adult reproductive function, although a few have consistently found earlier mean age at menopause. Therefore, women who are pregnant or attempting it should be counseled to avoid areas where exposure to ETS is likely. In the workplace, other exposures, such as particulates or chemicals, may interact to magnify the effects of ETS. Exposure in other places, such as in commuting or recreation, may become more important sources of exposure as workplace restrictions on smoking are increasingly imposed.

REPRODUCTIVE ASSESSMENT

The medical evaluation of the patient with potential exposure to a reproductive hazard follows the traditional components of history taking, physical examination, and laboratory assessment. In addition, special consideration is needed in the evaluation, communication, and management of reproductive risk for the patient.

Medical Evaluation

In the clinical setting, infertility is defined as an inability to conceive after 12 months of unprotected intercourse. Potential causes for infertility in the female include ovulatory dysfunction, tubal or pelvic factors, and uterine or cervical factors. It is estimated that the cause of infertility is a result of male factors in 40% of affected couples, a result of female factors in 40–50% of affected couples, and of no known etiology in 10–20% of the affected couples. Therefore, for the infertility workup, the male partner needs to be assessed concurrently. Adverse pregnancy outcomes include SAB, stillbirth, prematurity, congenital birth defects, LBW, and developmental disorders (see Tables 27–1 and 27–3). A full discussion of the diagnosis and treatment of various obstetric/gynecologic or pediatric conditions is beyond the scope of this chapter. However, the following is a general overview of the types of evaluation techniques that can be used to assess the female reproductive system.

▶ Interview

The patient interview should start with the following areas: demographic data, general medical history, and reproductive history (including age at puberty, menstrual function, past pelvic surgeries or gynecologic procedures, pregnancy and birth outcomes, sexually transmitted diseases, contraception, and familial illness). In addition, it should cover lifestyle habits (such as smoking and alcohol consumption, exercise, and stress), work history and current job tasks and exposures, and potential environmental exposures (eg, ETS; commuting; residential proximity to industry, waste sites, or heavy traffic; and possibly hobbies or home products use).

▶ Physical Examination

This examination should assess the physical integrity of the reproductive system and rule out any extraneous mass or structural abnormality.

▶ Laboratory

A hormonal profile can be obtained for the assessment of potential fetal loss (hCG and LH), ovarian function (progesterone and estrogen metabolites), and pituitary function (LH and FSH). A wide range of tests and assays is available and needs to be selected based on the medical conditions under consideration. During field biologic monitoring studies, urine samples are relatively easy to collect for hormonal assays. Exposure burden for some hazards may be measured in biologic tissues (eg, exhaled breath, blood, or urine), but few of these lead to diagnostic interpretation.

Risk Evaluation

The steps generally conducted in the toxicologic risk assessment may be adapted in simplified form for the clinical workup, including

1. Hazard identification of any hazardous agents the patient may be exposed to from a detailed occupational and environmental history during interview

2. Hazard evaluation to determine whether a given substance or physical agent may be a reproductive hazard by consulting databases and the literature

3. Exposure assessment, which is performed by estimating the level of exposure from patient work history, product labels, material safety data sheets, industrial hygiene data, environmental sampling, or biologic monitoring results, as well as potential routes of exposure and consistency of symptoms

4. Risk characterization with respect to effects on the reproductive system (This activity is based on information gathered in the first three steps and considers toxicity, timing, and extent of exposure, potency, severity of outcome, and degree of uncertainty in animal and human studies.)

Often, not all the needed information is available, and an educated guess is necessary. It is very helpful to have established contacts for additional consultation when a more difficult risk assessment is involved. Potential contacts include local or state health departments, university medical centers, poison control centers, NIOSH, Environmental Protection Agency (EPA), Agency for Toxic Substances and Disease Registry (ATSDR), Occupational Safety and Health Administration (OSHA), and the Association of Occupational and Environmental Clinics (AOEC). Access to online literature databases is very useful (eg, REPRORISK, REPROTOX, and TERIS; see references).

Risk Communication

Building on the information gathered during the risk-assessment process, risk communication is the logical follow-up by which the involved person or persons obtain the information needed to make informed and independent decisions about health and safety risks. In general, there is an underlying principle that needs to be acknowledged and dealt with sensitively: the threat or actual fact of adverse reproductive outcome has a profound impact on an individual's life. All questions must be answered truthfully and completely. A description of the limitations in knowledge may be needed. The timing of exposure and of the first contact with the involved person is very important. When possible, the risk communication is conducted prior to actual exposure in order to intervene at the primary prevention stage. The options available for the female worker should be presented in such a way that the medical impact and the economic consequences of decisions are understood and discussed. The clinician may need to communicate the risks to an employer as well in order to resolve the situation, but the medical confidentiality of the involved individual must be maintained.

Risk Management

A comprehensive workplace reproductive health policy should be developed and implemented for both female and male workers, and should be coordinated by a committee composed of representatives from management and labor and consultants in occupational medicine and industrial hygiene. Remediation should occur before conception (which is not always planned) to provide protection during organogenesis, as well as to prevent fertility problems. Furthermore, it may be important to extend protection postpartum during lactation. This may require a written request from the personal physician.

The following components should be included as part of a comprehensive reproductive health program: (1) Exposure reduction or elimination, replacement of hazards with safer agents, improved engineering controls, safer work practices, and personal protective equipment (the latter should not be the primary mode of protection). Exposure reduction or elimination is the most desirable option and should be attempted in all situations involving a reproductive hazard. (2) Temporary job transfer: remove individual from work environment in which reproductive hazard exists. Problems may occur when there is no nonexposed job location. Thus, this option should be considered when there is a high-risk situation and exposure reduction/elimination is not possible. (3) Disability leave: paid leave is subject to company policy, and temporary pregnancy disability leave must be treated the same as any other medical disability leave. The early embryo sensitivity period already has occurred during potential workplace exposure by the time a disability leave is granted. There is no guarantee that the medical disability will be approved, and benefits rarely are equivalent to the individual's current wage. This option should be considered when there is a high-risk situation in which the employer will not reduce exposure and a temporary transfer is not possible (see also Chapter 7). (4) Remove individual from work: This is the least desirable action. It is illegal for an employer to terminate the affected individual because of pregnancy. A woman may choose to quit work because of personal reasons, but it is important to help her evaluate all options and to understand the possible consequences. This option is to be considered only when all other options have been explored and the woman is comfortable with the possible consequences.

If an environmental exposure is of concern, options for individual amelioration are less but generally follow the principles just outlined (eg, substitution, safer practices, and removal). Since some exposures may act synergistically, reducing those possible for an individual in the workplace, the home, or the diet is desirable. Additionally, this points to the need to control other environmental exposures at the population level.

LEGAL ISSUES & WORKPLACE STANDARDS

In the lawsuit involving International Union, UAW versus Johnson Controls, Inc., the U.S. Supreme Court held that an employer violated Title VII's ban on sex discrimination by excluding from production jobs in a lead-battery factory all women who could not prove their sterility. The Court indicated that a policy directed only at fertile women is overt discrimination on the basis of sex regardless of the scientific evidence of heightened safety concerns for mothers or potential mothers. In addition, any policies or actions taken by the employer must not violate existing laws prohibiting discrimination on the basis of pregnancy, childbirth, or related medical conditions. Employers cannot require that an individual be sterilized as a condition of employment. If an employee disabled by pregnancy, childbirth, or a related medical condition transfers to a less hazardous job, an employer must allow her to return to her original job or to a similar one when the disability has resolved.

OSHA has the mandate to promulgate standards that protect workers from adverse health effects (including reproductive effects) resulting from workplace hazards. However, only a few agents have OSHA standards that are based partially on reproductive effects. Included among these agents are dibromochloropropane (DBCP), lead, ethylene oxide, glycol ethers, and ionizing radiation. There are OSHA standards requiring reporting of employee exposure to hazardous chemicals and training of employees using these chemicals. But it should be recognized that many chemical and physical agents found in the workplace are not covered by an OSHA standard and that those standards that do exist for the most part are not based on reproductive endpoints. This is why the simplified risk evaluation process should be implemented at any worksite that has potential reproductive hazards present.

REFERENCES

Costet N et al: Correction to: occupational exposure to organic solvents during pregnancy and childhood behavior: findings from the PELAGIE birth cohort (France, 2002-2013). Environ Health 2018;17(1):71 [PMID: 30053883].

Govarts E et al: Prenatal exposure to endocrine disrupting chemicals and risk of being born small for gestational age: pooled analysis of seven European birth cohorts. Environ Int 2018;115:267-278 [PMID: 29605679].

Hamra GB et al: Prenatal exposure to endocrine-disrupting chemicals in relation to autism spectrum disorder and intellectual disability. Epidemiology 2019;30(3):418-426 [PMID: 30789431].

Henrotin JB et al: Deprivation, occupational hazards and perinatal outcomes in pregnant workers. Occup Med (Lond) 2017;67(1):44-51 [PMID: 27821643].

Karwacka A, Zamkowska D, Radwan M, Jurewicz J: Exposure to modern, widespread environmental endocrine disrupting chemicals and their effect on the reproductive potential of women: an overview of current epidemiological evidence. Hum Fertil (Camb) 2019;22(1):2-25 [PMID: 28758506].

Lenters V et al: Early-life exposure to persistent organic pollutants (OCPs, PBDEs, PCBs, PFASs) and attention-deficit/hyperactivity disorder: a multi-pollutant analysis of a Norwegian birth cohort. Environ Int 2019;125:33-42 [PMID: 30703609].

Ma Y et al: Effects of environmental contaminants on fertility and reproductive health. J Environ Sci (China) 2019;77:210-217 [PMID: 30573085].

Matuszczak E, Komarowska MD, Debek W, Hermanowicz A: The impact of bisphenol A on fertility, reproductive system, and development: A review of the literature. Int J Endocrinol 2019;2019:4068717 [PMID: 31093279].

Padula AM et al: A review of maternal prenatal exposures to environmental chemicals and psychosocial stressors-implications for research on perinatal outcomes in the ECHO program. J Perinatol 2020;40(1):10-24 [PMID: 31616048].

Rim KT: Reproductive toxic chemicals at work and efforts to protect workers' health: a literature review. Saf Health Work 2017;8(2):143-150 [PMID: 28593069].

Rock KD, Patisaul HB: Environmental mechanisms of neurodevelopmental toxicity. Curr Environ Health Rep 2018;5(1):145-157 [PMID: 29536388].

Serra H, Beausoleil C, Habert R, Minier C, Picard-Hagen N, Michel C: Evidence for bisphenol B endocrine properties: scientific and regulatory perspectives. Environ Health Perspect 2019;127(10):106001 [PMID: 31617754].

Sifakis S, Androutsopoulos VP, Tsatsakis AM, Spandidos DA: Human exposure to endocrine disrupting chemicals: effects on the male and female reproductive systems. Environ Toxicol Pharmacol 2017;51:56-70 [PMID: 28292651].

Warembourg C et al: Prenatal exposure to glycol ethers and sex steroid hormones at birth. Environ Int 2018;113:66-73 [PMID: 29421409].

Zhang S et al: Association of perfluoroalkyl and polyfluoroalkyl substances with premature ovarian insufficiency in Chinese women. J Clin Endocrinol Metab 2018;103(7):2543-2551 [PMID: 29986037].

Zhu W et al: Triclosan and female reproductive health: a preconceptional cohort study. Epidemiology 2019;30 Suppl 1:S24-S31 [PMID: 31181003].

■ SELF-ASSESSMENT QUESTIONS

Select the one correct answer for each question.

Question 1: Chemical exposures
  a. during weeks 1 and 2 after conception may cause early pregnancy loss if they interfere with tubal transport, implantation, or endocrine control
  b. predictably appear as a late or heavy menstrual flow
  c. cause a short rise and subsequent plateau in hCG
  d. are likely to cause congenital anomalies from very early embryo exposures

Question 2: Chemical exposures
  a. later in pregnancy spare the endocrine, central nervous, and other systems
  b. that are of less concern later in pregnancy are organic mercury, tobacco smoke, and lead
  c. after the first trimester may induce minor morphologic abnormalities or growth deficits
  d. to carcinogens are of no concern because they do not cross the placenta

Question 3: Endocrine-disrupting chemicals (EDCs)
  a. do not vary structurally to persistent pesticides such as DDT and plasticizers such as phthalates and bisphenol-A
  b. are hormonally active agents (HAAs)

  c. may persist for years in the environment but do not enter the food chain
  d. are not implicated in thyroid hormone disruption

Question 4: Solvents
  a. include many compounds used in the workplace but seldom in the home
  b. are considered a potential reproductive hazard only among laboratory workers
  c. such as perchloroethylene, methylene chloride, toluene, xylene, and glycol ethers have been associated with concurrent elevation in SAB risk
  d. show associations with cardiac but no other congenital anomalies

Question 5: Tobacco smoking
  a. is always associated with a number of developmental and reproductive endpoints
  b. results in 10 times the risk of low birth weight compared with infants of nonsmokers
  c. does not induce preterm delivery, fetal and infant death, and behavioral deficits in offspring
  d. is associated with infertility, menstrual disorders, and menopause at earlier age

Male Reproductive Toxicology

Sarah Janssen, MD, PhD, MPH

In studying male reproductive toxicants, the ultimate aim is to protect the reproductive health of men and the health of their offspring, which is fundamentally important for the health of future generations. The occurrence of adverse reproductive outcomes is of great concern to the individuals and families involved. This is especially true if the individuals perceive that they are living or working in areas with potential exposure to hazardous agents. Adverse reproductive effects can be very stressful for affected families. Existing human information on this subject is very sparse and inadequate for the reproductive assessment of most suspect compounds and physical agents.

Another reason to better understand male reproductive functions is that they may act as sentinels for detecting occupational and environmental hazards. Reproductive effects have a relatively short latency between exposure and detectable health event (such as abnormal semen profile) as compared with the long latency for cancer. If workers or community residents are protected from exposures that are harmful to reproduction, they usually will be protected from other health effects associated with these exposures as well. While the extent to which workplace and environmental hazards affect reproductive function is unknown, these hazards are potentially preventable. Measures that can be taken to prevent further exposure include substitution or containment of the suspect hazard. Thus, preventing exposure should play a primary role in the health care provider's overall assessment of the patient's situation.

REPRODUCTIVE OUTCOMES & RATES

Definitions

A number of adverse reproductive effects may result from male exposure to chemical and physical agents. These effects range from infertility to birth defects in the infant. Infertility is present when a couple has not conceived after 1 year of unprotected sexual intercourse. Male sexual dysfunction may involve changes in libido (interest in sexual activity),

erectile dysfunction, or ejaculatory problems. Semen abnormalities can include azoospermia (complete absence of sperm), oligospermia (decreased sperm count), teratospermia (abnormally shaped sperm), and asthenospermia (sperm showing decreased motility). Abnormal birth outcomes include spontaneous abortion (SAB) (fetal loss prior to the twenty-eighth gestational week), stillbirth (fetal loss after the twenty-eighth week), death (infant: younger than 1 year of age; neonatal: younger than 28 days of age; or postneonatal: 28 days to 11 months of age), congenital defect (abnormal appearance or function at birth), prematurity (birth prior to the thirty-seventh week of gestation), low birth weight (LBW) (weight < 2500 g at birth), and very low birth weight (weight < 1500 g at birth).

Population Rates

Precise rates for these types of pregnancy loss are difficult to obtain because of a lack of national monitoring systems and methodologic differences in individual epidemiologic studies. Nevertheless, a range of prevalence rates can be estimated (Table 28–1). Approximately 10% of couples in the United States are infertile. Additional couples may experience periods of subfertility or delayed conception. After conception, a variety of reproductive losses may occur at any time from conception to full term. Up to 50% of embryos may be lost after implantation (the earliest time at which conception can be detected), with approximately 15% of pregnancies ending in a clinically detected SAB. Of all liveborn infants, 7.8% are of LBW, and approximately 3% will have a clinically detectable congenital anomaly. The causes for most of these outcomes are unexplained. However, there are a few known risk factors for women, such as older maternal age (associated with increased rates of SAB), certain infectious agents (eg, cytomegalovirus, hepatitis B virus, human immunodeficiency virus [HIV], rubella, toxoplasmosis, varicella-zoster virus, and human parvovirus), cancer treatment (eg, methotrexate), strenuous physical labor, and certain environmental agents (eg, lead and ionizing radiation).

Table 28–1. Prevalence of selected adverse reproductive events, United States.

Endpoints	Rate per 1000 Live Births	Average Annual Number of Cases	Reference Population
Birth Defects			
Spina bifida	.35	1460	U.S., 2004–2006
Anencephaly	.21	959	U.S., 2004–2006
Transposition of great arteries	.30	1252	U.S., 2004–2006
Down syndrome	1.45	6057	U.S., 2004–2006
Deaths			
Infant (< 1 y of age)	5.96	23,446	U.S., 2013
Neonatal (< 28 d)	4.04	15,893	U.S., 2013
Postneonatal (28 d to 11 mo)	1.92	7553	U.S., 2013
Birth Weight			
Low birth weight (< 2500 g)	50.26	316,597	U.S., 2013
Very low birth weight (< 1500 g)	219.56	56,585	U.S., 2013
Other outcomes			
Recognized spontaneous abortion	100–200	Pregnancies or women	Estimated U.S.
Infertility	100–150	Couples	Estimated U.S.
Abnormal sperm morphology	40.00	Men	Estimated U.S.
Azoospermia	10.00	Men	Estimated U.S.

REPRODUCTIVE PHYSIOLOGY

Although this section focuses on male-mediated exposure associated with reproductive and developmental abnormalities, it is important to note that maternal and fetal exposures also need to be assessed for a complete evaluation. It is recognized that more prolonged direct sources of exposure to the products of conception occur in the woman and that maternal exposure can continue postnatally during lactation. However, changes in fertility have been reported in both sexes, and genetic changes can be transmitted by either parent.

Male Reproductive System

Adequate hormonal regulation is necessary for proper functioning of the male reproductive system (Figure 28–1). For this to occur, coordinated hypothalamic, pituitary, and gonadal interactions are critical. These include (1) hypothalamic production of gonadotropin-releasing hormone (GnRH), (2) pituitary gland production of follicle-stimulating hormone (FSH) and luteinizing hormone (LH), and (3) testis production of spermatozoa (germ cells) from the germinal epithelium, testosterone from the Leydig cell, and inhibin B from the Sertoli cell. GnRH release stimulates the pituitary gland production of FSH and LH. FSH acts on the Sertoli cell within the seminiferous tubules to stimulate spermatogenesis and produce inhibin B (which inhibits pituitary gland hormones). The action of LH is to stimulate testosterone production in the Leydig cell. Conversely, testosterone has a negative-feedback effect on the pituitary and hypothalamic hormones, as well as the production of germ cells (sperm) and Sertoli cell activity. Testosterone is found bound to sex hormone–binding globule (SHBG) or albumin and may be converted to the more potent dihydrotestosterone or estradiol in the circulatory system.

In males, puberty is due to adequate testosterone levels and manifested by reproductive system maturity and development of secondary sexual characteristics (eg, increased muscle mass, beard growth, axillary and pubic hair, deepening of the voice, libido, and external genitalia growth).

In general, spermatogenesis involves two major sites within the testis. Starting from a germ cell, it takes 74 days for development through the stages of spermatogonium, spermatocyte, and spermatid into a mature spermatozoon (or sperm) in the seminiferous tubules of the testis. During the next 12 days, the sperm travels along the epididymis for eventual ejaculation. Thus approximately 3 months are required to complete the maturation and transport of the sperm.

Teratology

There are important issues in teratology to be considered when evaluating male reproductive function. Preconception exposure may act directly on the germ cell (sperm). This condition could lead to either no fertilization or an aberration of the zygote and an eventual SAB (possibly clinically undetected) or birth defect. The reproductive toxicant may affect the embryo even when exposure occurs prior to conception either to the mother or to the father. Thus one must consider infertility, SABs, and birth defects when assessing men exposed to suspect reproductive toxicants.

Another important aspect to consider is that spermatogenesis involves a continuously replicating cell population (in

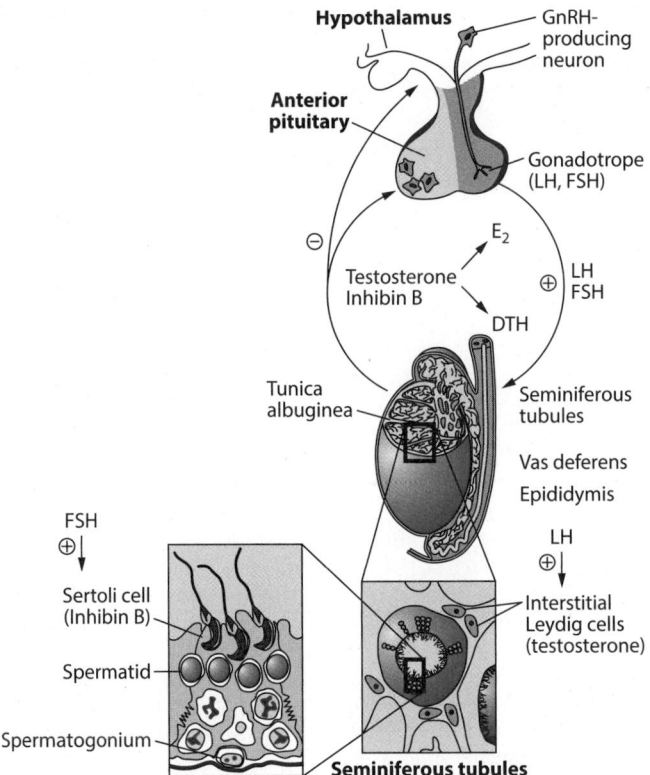

▲ **Figure 28–1.** Hypothalamic, pituitary, and testicular interactions involved in hormonal homeostasis necessary for adequate male reproductive function. DHT, dihydrotestosterone; E$_2$, estradiol; FSH, follicle-stimulating hormone; GnRH, gonadotropin-releasing hormone; LH, luteinizing hormone.

the billions), whereas oogenesis occurs prenatally with a finite population at birth (only approximately 400 oocytes ovulated during the reproductive years) that is depleted at around age 50 years. Therefore, chemical or physical agents whose toxicity depends on cell division will have greater effect on the male germ cell. A complete evaluation of a male exposed to a reproductive hazard should take into account the large variability in individual susceptibility to reproductive agents; the environmental, occupational, and lifestyle factors of both parents; and the possibility that a toxic effect may lead to a clinically nondetectable abnormality at the birth of the offspring.

Potential Mechanisms of Action

Most male reproductive hazards can be characterized by having one or more of the following potential mechanisms of action: central nervous system or endocrine abnormality (decreased libido and fertility as possible adverse reproductive effects), direct testicular toxicity (decreased fertility), spermatogenesis or germ cell damage in the form of morphologic change, decreased cell number, abnormal motility or chromosomal abnormality (decreased fertility, fetal

loss, congenital malformations, childhood developmental disabilities, and cancers), and toxicants in the semen leading to abnormal sperm motility or direct action on the uterus or fetus (all the prior possible effects or outcomes). Although the focus of this chapter is on direct male reproductive effects, the potential for take-home exposure from the workplace leading to family member exposure needs to be assessed concurrently in the evaluation of a worker.

SCIENTIFIC LITERATURE

Human risk assessment of reproductive or other hazards in the workplace or environment involves the following components: hazard identification, dose-response assessment, exposure assessment, and risk characterization. The clinician may be involved in one or more of these steps when evaluating the health risk for a patient or worker.

Informational Sources

When evaluating a patient with potential exposure to reproductive hazards, the clinician needs to identify biologic, chemical, and physical agents in the workplace or environment via the patient exposure history and any available informational material such as warning signs, product labels, material safety data sheets, and purchase orders. These documents may identify the agents to which a person is potentially exposed but usually provide very little information on reproductive hazards. The US Environmental Protection Agency (EPA) estimates that more than 80,000 chemicals are being used in industry, with only 4000 of these having been evaluated in animals (with a much smaller number studied in humans). Adding to this problem is the approximately 2000 new chemicals being introduced into the workplace each year. Many of these chemicals lack adequate premarket reproductive assessment. Some informational sources on animal and human studies are available for those hazards that have been evaluated, such as the Registry of Toxic Effects of Chemical Substances (RTECS), REPROTOX (reproductive hazard information database), Shepard's Catalog of Teratogenic Agents, and the Teratogen Information System (TERIS). All these sources review the human and animal literature for toxic effects of environmental chemicals and, for the latter three databases, drugs. Because of the scarcity of human data dealing with reproductive effects, it is important to know where this type of information can be obtained. In addition to the research databases listed, there are government-based efforts to evaluate the existing scientific literature with respect to reproductive hazards. In California, there is a state-mandated program that evaluates chemicals known to cause cancer or reproductive toxicity. As of June 2020, there were 78 pharmaceutical or environmental compounds determined to have male reproductive toxicity by this program (Table 28–2).

Epidemiologic Studies

Well-conducted epidemiologic studies should provide the best means of evaluating whether a specific agent or group of agents adversely affects *human* reproduction and development. Human studies cannot be controlled, as can animal experiments, so certain criteria or a weight-of-evidence type of scheme often is used in evaluating whether a substance reasonably can be considered as having an adverse effect.

A. Study Designs

The basic study designs used to examine the association of an exposure and possible outcomes include the cross-sectional, case-control, and cohort studies, which are discussed thoroughly in the Appendix. The cross-sectional design is the simplest and has been used often in occupational and environmental reproductive studies. If the mechanism of action is thought to be interference with spermatogenesis, this study design is useful because there is a relatively short 3-month lag period between exposure and abnormal health outcome. However, if direct germinal epithelium damage is being considered as the mechanism of action, there is potential selection bias because the population existing in the workplace at

the time of study may not be representative of the workforce during the time of prior exposure. For example, testicular biopsy among the workers exposed to chronic and high levels of dibromochloropropane (DBCP) demonstrated tissue scarring. This could result in permanent decreased sperm concentration, even after exposure has ended. The case-control study is most appropriate for evaluating relatively rare diseases in large populations (eg, birth defects or childhood cancers). Because the outcome of interest is specified at the onset, the continuum of reproductive effects that may result from a given exposure cannot be evaluated. The cohort study is the preferred study design for most reproductive outcomes. A prospective cohort study allows specific measures of an exposure and potential confounders to be ascertained at the etiologically relevant time periods. In addition, a cohort design allows repeated test measurements (eg, semen analysis) that tend to have relatively high individual variability.

The cohort and case-control studies are considered hypothesis-testing studies and usually are conducted after a possible association has been suggested by previous observations or a documented group exposure. For example, an acute clinician may recognize a series of cases that seem to have a factor in common. This situation is most likely to occur with a rare disease or new syndrome and was instrumental in identifying associations such as thalidomide and severe limb defects and diethylstilbestrol (DES) and vaginal clear-cell carcinoma. A reported cluster of adverse outcomes occurring in a group of people is a common way for environmental and occupational problems to be brought to attention, but such clusters often remain unexplained on further investigation.

Valuable data could be obtained from surveillance systems, but there are few established systems in place for adverse reproductive outcomes other than birth defects. Reasons for this include the fact that not all outcomes attract medical attention or require hospitalization (eg, semen abnormalities, SABs, and subfertility). As a result, these outcomes are more difficult to ascertain and are associated with a smaller financial impact for society.

B. Exposure Assessment

Although the methods used to measure occupational or environmental exposure are beyond the scope of this chapter, a brief overview with issues specific to evaluating male exposure associated with reproductive outcomes is presented. In addition, it should be kept in mind that the exposures of three individuals may be involved (ie, each parent and the embryo/fetus/offspring).

To affect fertility or spermatogenesis, an agent must reach the appropriate organs via the bloodstream (eg, chemical agent) or physical change (eg, radiation or excessive heat). Some chemicals react with the first tissues they encounter, such as the lungs or skin, and are not absorbed into the bloodstream unless they are ingested (eg, acids, chlorine, and asbestos). Unless a chronic exposure results in a steady-state level in the body, the rapidity with which a substance

Table 28–2. Chemicals known to cause male reproductive toxicity.[a]

Abiraterone acetate	Ethylene glycol monoethyl ether
Acrylamide	Ethylene glycol monoethyl ether acetate
Altretamine	Ethylene glycol monomethyl ether
Amiodarone hydrochloride	Ethylene glycol monomethyl ether acetate
Anabolic steroids	Ethylene oxide
Benomyl	Ganciclovir
Benzene	Ganciclovir sodium
Bromacil lithium salt	Gemfibrozil
1- and 2-Bromopropane	Goserelin acetate
1,3-Butadiene	Hexafluoroacetone
2,4-D Butyric acid	n-Hexane
Cadmium	2,5-Hexanedione
Carbaryl	Hydramethylnon
Carbon disulfide	Idarubicin hydrochloride
2-Chloropropionic acid	Lead and lead compounds
Chromium (hexavalent compounds)	Leuprolide acetate
Cidofovir	Methyl chloride
Colchicine	Methyl-n-butyl ketone
Hydrogen cyanide (HCN) and cyanide salts (CN salts)	Molinate
Cyclophosphamide (anhydrous or hydrated)	Myclobutanil
o,p'- and p,p'-DDT	Nickel (soluble compounds)
Di(2-ethylhexyl)phthalate (DEHP)	Nifedipine
Di-n-butyl phthalate (DBP)	Nitrobenzene
Di-n-hexyl phthalate (DnHP)	Nitrofurantoin
1,2-Dibromo-3-chloropropane (DBCP)	Oxydemeton methyl
Ethylene dibromide	Paclitaxel
Dichloroacetic acid	Quizalofop-ethyl
DDE (Dichlorodiphenyldichloroethylene)	Ribavirin
DDT (Dichlorodiphenyltrichloroethane)	Sodium fluoroacetate
N,N-Dimethylacetamide	Streptozocin (streptozotocin)
p-Dinitrobenzene	Sulfasalazine
m-Dinitrobenzene	Thiophanate methyl
o-Dinitrobenzene	Tobacco smoke (primary exposure)
2,6-Dinitrotoluene	Triadimefon
2,4-Dinitrotoluene	Trichloroethylene
Dinitrotoluene (technical grade)	Uracil mustard
Dinoseb	Vinyl cyclohexene dioxide (4-vinyl-1-cyclohexene diepoxide)
Doxorubicin hydrochloride (adriamycin)	4-Vinylcyclohexene
Epichlorohydrin	Vismodegib

[a]Source: California Environmental Protection Agency: Proposition 65 list of chemicals known to cause cancer or reproductive toxicity, https://oehha.ca.gov/proposition-65/proposition-65-list.

is cleared also can affect its toxicity. Often these issues are beyond the scope of epidemiologic studies but should be considered within the overall body of evidence about the toxicity of a substance.

In epidemiologic studies, exposures can be ascertained from interviews, existing records, or biomarkers. If exposure history is obtained by retrospective interview, there is the possibility of biased recall among cases or misclassification because of a lack of monitoring records or diminished memory. Recall may be affected by changes in exposures. Ascertainment of current exposure status for cohort studies limits

possible recall bias, but men may not be aware of all their exposures. In interview studies, asking one spouse about the other may not provide sufficiently accurate information. Also, obtaining residence at time of delivery many not reflect timing of importance for sperm development.

Existing records often do not provide detailed information but rather serve to group men broadly. For example, the residence listed on a birth certificate might be used to assign the likelihood of an environmental exposure. However, residence at delivery may not reflect residence of the father, nor does it account for individual differences, such as how much time is spent out of the area at work. Similarly, occupational registries may be used to group men by broad exposures, but specific work-site practices will be unknown. The most accurate occupational exposures would be obtained by an industrial hygienist, but such studies are also likely to cost more or be limited in sample size to allow for more detailed study.

Laboratory measurement of exposure may be done in a prospective study or on stored biologic samples and provides a quantification of exposure that is less likely to be biased. Techniques for measuring environmental levels have been developed for many agents, including radon, electromagnetic fields (EMFs), solvents, pesticides, metals, and dust levels. Measurements on biologic samples provide an indication of internal dose, which would be more biologically relevant. A number of difficulties can arise with these types of studies, including small sample size or selection bias owing to the higher costs and greater participation required of subjects. Sampling at one point in time may not reflect the critical exposure period, particularly if the substance is cleared rapidly.

As noted earlier, it is important to consider the timing of exposure in an epidemiologic study. An association with an exposure at the critical time is more relevant, and such information may be useful for excluding the possibility of a particular effect if the timing is wrong. In addition to timing, a dose-response relationship usually is examined.

In summary, exposure assessment in epidemiologic studies may involve problems with unknown exposure levels, unknown biologic indicators, poor sources of information on exposure, imprecise exposure timing, and multifactorial exposure sources.

C. Biologic Outcomes

There is variable quality in the detection and measurement of biologic endpoints for male reproductive toxicity studies. For specific male reproductive conditions and male-mediated reproductive outcomes, the range of conditions includes sexual dysfunction, endocrine changes, semen abnormalities, chromosomal anomalies, infertility, and abnormalities in the fetus and offspring. Case ascertainment methods can include the following: birth certificates, hospital records, surveillance programs (eg, birth defects registries), medical insurance forms, reproductive history questionnaires, and semen analyses. The latter two methods tend to be the most useful type of case ascertainment because of relatively more precise male information as opposed to the usually inadequate paternal information found in birth outcome records.

D. Statistical Issues

For selected reproductive endpoints, the necessary number of study participants for adequate statistical power is shown in Table 28–3. One advantage of conducting studies of semen analysis is that relatively fewer participants are needed, and there is a direct measurement of the abnormality being studied (eg, abnormal number, motility, and shape of sperm). It should be noted that the general population normal ranges for these semen endpoints are unreliable because of differences in laboratory proficiency and techniques. It is preferable to test for internal trend within a given worker group or community group or to obtain an appropriate control group. Although fewer participants are needed for semen studies, there may be a problem in selecting the most appropriate comparison group.

E. Confounding Factors

Potential confounders need to be considered in the evaluation of men exposed to occupational or environmental reproductive hazards. For a factor to be a confounder, it must be related to both the endpoint and the exposure in the study of interest. Lack of control for a known confounder in prior

Table 28–3. Sample sizes needed to detect a relative risk of 2.0 among exposed and unexposed groups for selected reproductive endpoints (95% confidence level and 80% power).

Outcome	Estimated Prevalence in Unexposed Group[a]	Unit	Sample Size Needed		
			Exposed Group	Nonexposed Group	Study Total
Fetal loss (recognized spontaneous abortions + stillbirths)	15.0%	Pregnancies	133	133	266
Infertility	12.5%	Couples	167	167	334
Low birth weight	7.8%	Live births with known birth weight	290	290	580
Major congenital malformation	3.0%	Live births + fetal deaths	814	814	1628
Sperm with abnormal morphology	40.0%	Men	27	27	54

[a]Prevalence rates derived from estimated general population values in Table 28–1; and Lawson C: Occupational reproductive research agenda for the 3rd millennium. Environ Health Perspect 2003;111:584 [PMID: 12732741].

studies does not imply that the study is deficient if the investigators found that this factor did not act as a confounder in their study or had reason to believe that the factor would not be associated with the exposure of interest. Potential confounding factors in male reproductive studies include personal characteristics (eg, paternal age), medical conditions (eg, recent infection, trauma to the gonads, impaired autoimmune status, high fever, mumps orchitis, diabetes, prostatitis, varicocele, and hydrocele), drug use (eg, marijuana, estrogen, chlorambucil, cyclophosphamide, and nitrofurantoin), and habits (eg, tobacco use, alcohol use, and frequent sauna or hot tub use). In addition, there is the possibility of a potential synergistic health effect from two or more coexisting exposure or risk factors. In conducting occupational studies, a potential confounder may be an environmental agent, such as exposure to solvents, metals, pesticides, excess heat, ionizing radiation, and neurotoxins in non-workplace settings. Conversely, one needs to assess workplace hazards when conducting community-based reproductive studies.

Selected Examples of Reproductive Hazards

Few chemicals have been studied adequately in terms of their reproductive effects. Most exposure standards are not based on reproductive effects. More evidence is available from animal than human studies, but direct extrapolation to the human cannot always be made. Although epidemiologic studies can be more difficult to interpret because of the methodologic issues described earlier, a number of potential reproductive or developmental hazards have been identified (Table 28–4).

The majority of toxic agents in Table 28–4 have been examined in occupational settings where exposures tend to be of higher concentrations than those encountered in the environment and relatively easier to document. In the literature, most occupational events involving high-level exposures and documented adverse reproductive effects have occurred in male workers (eg, dibromochloropropane and exogenous estrogens). In addition, known reproductive hazards have been encountered environmentally from long-term use and disposal by industry, as well as from acute releases.

A. Declining Semen Quality and Environmental Factors

Several studies have noted a historical decrease in sperm count, with one report providing data as far back as 50 years. Over time, the method for evaluating sperm count (unlike the other semen-quality parameters) has not changed and is thought to be less susceptible to chronologic changes in laboratory technique. However, most of these retrospective trend analyses have been conducted at fertility centers that include semen donors, vasectomy candidates, or infertility clinic patients and thus may not be representative of the general male population. Furthermore, geographic differences and lack of information for known risk factors usually are

associated with these older studies. Despite these limitations, various studies demonstrate decreased sperm concentrations in many European countries and in various US regions. The International Study of Semen Quality in Partners of Pregnant Women found significant differences in mean sperm count between men in Copenhagen, Paris, Edinburgh, and Turku, Finland. In the United States, a four-city prenatal clinic study (Los Angeles, Minneapolis, Columbia, Missouri, and New York City) is being conducted that uses identical clinical evaluation, data collection, and semen analysis techniques as the European study. Preliminary findings from the US study show a significantly lower sperm count among fertile men in Columbia, Missouri, in comparison with those in the other three cities. It is interesting to note that Columbia is in a more agricultural area than the other cities. Possible explanations given for the lower sperm count include estrogen exposure in utero, diet, lifestyle factors, and environmental pollution as a result of the increased worldwide use of chemicals (especially compounds with estrogen-like activity. Further follow-up of these multicenter studies will help to better explain this difference.

B. Dibromochloropropane

DBCP (1,2-dibromo-3-chloroporpane) is noteworthy for its role in the first documented outbreak of a male reproductive hazard in the workplace. DBCP is a nematocide that is associated with reproductive and developmental abnormalities in animals. These animal effects include oligospermia, asthenospermia, and testicular and seminiferous tubule atrophy. Workers exposed to DBCP in chemical production facilities have shown exposure-dependent testicular toxicity. The following associations have been noted in DBCP-exposed workers: azoospermia, oligospermia, increased plasma FSH levels, and histologic abnormalities of the testicular tissue (decrease or absence of germ cells in seminiferous tubules). Decreased fertility was experienced among workers with testicular changes, and the most extreme FSH elevations were found in workers who did not recover after a period of no exposure. Thus, this compound represents one of the few well-established male reproductive toxicants and provided the stimulus for subsequent increased activity in male-mediated reproductive research in the work setting.

C. Lead

Lead is one of the most studied occupational and environmental agents and has a broad range of effects on multiple organ systems. Male reproductive effects have been found with both organic and inorganic lead exposures. Organic lead compounds, unlike the inorganic form, can be absorbed dermally. Sexual dysfunction (eg, decreased libido, abnormal erectile function, and premature ejaculation) has been noted in case reports after ingestion of fuels containing organic lead. A case series of tetraethyl lead–intoxicated men revealed reversible semen abnormalities: oligospermia, azoospermia, asthenospermia, and teratospermia. Inorganic

Table 28–4. Established or highly suspect relationships between male reproductive abnormalities and selected environmental and occupational agents or processes, based on human studies.

Agent	Oligospermia	Teratospermia	Asthenospermia	Hormonal or Sexual Dysfunction	Other Effects
Alcohol	X (azoospermia)				Testicular atrophy
Boron	X				
Bromine vapor	X	X	X		
2-Bromopropane	X (azoospermia)				
Cadmium					Decreased fertility
Carbon disulfide	X	X	X	X	
Carbaryl (Sevin)		X			
Chlordecone	X	X	X		
Dibromochloropropane	X (azoospermia)			X	Testicular atrophy
2,4-Dichlorodiphenoxyacetic acid (2,4-D)	X (azoospermia)	X	X		
DDT (dichlorodiphenyl-trichloroethane)					Found in semen of infertile men
Estrogens	X				
Ethylene dibromide	X	X	X		
Ethylene glycol ethers (eg, 2-ethoxyethanol)	X	X			
Heat, excessive	X		X		
Lead	X	X	X	X	
Manganese				X	
Mercury, inorganic	X	X	X	X	
Perchloroethylene			X		
Radiation, ionizing	X	X	X	X	
Radiation, microwave	X	X	X		
Styrene	X				
Toluene diamine & dinitrotoluene	X				
Vinyl chloride				X	
Process					
Greenhouse work	X	X		X	
Nuclear power plant cleanup (Chernobyl)	X	X	X	X	
Oral contraceptive manufacturing				X	
Plastic production (styrene & acetone)		X			
Welding		X	X		

Compiled from multiple sources, including NIOSH, CDC: National Occupational Research Agenda: Fertility and Pregnancy Abnormalities.

lead case reports have noted decreased libido (including erectile problems) and abnormal ejaculations. Endocrine changes (decreased testosterone and increased LH levels) have been observed in clinic-based case series. In men not exposed to high levels of lead, detectable lead concentrations in sperm have been reported that are less than those found in whole blood but greater than those of serum.

Epidemiologic studies have used semen analyses to better quantify male reproductive outcomes. A cross-sectional survey of 150 male lead battery workers was conducted in Romania. Blood lead levels ranged from 23–75 mcg/dL, with a mean lead exposure duration of 3.5 years. Oligospermia, asthenospermia, and teratospermia were noted in a dose-response fashion. There were certain methodologic problems with this study: (1) Both masturbation and coitus interruptus were allowed in semen collection. The latter method is not normally accepted because of the potential of semen mixing with the body fluids of the partner. (2) No environmental exposure data were presented. (3) The dose-response curve was constructed allowing multiple results from the same subject. And (4) the controls included 50 plant technicians and office workers who were not assessed for comparability. This study provided the basis for the consideration of reproductive effects in establishing the Occupational Safety and Health Administration (OSHA) lead standard.

Lead exposure was evaluated among 18 battery workers and 18 cement workers in Italy. There was a statistically significant decrease in median sperm count and an increase in the prevalence of oligospermia among the battery workers. Participation rates were low, with 47% for the exposed and 22% for the comparison group. The exposed group had a mean blood lead level (BLL) of 61 mcg/dL and a mean zinc protoporphyrin (ZPP) level of 208 mcg/dL. In contrast, the nonexposed group had a mean BLL of 18 mcg/dL and a mean ZPP of 24 mcg/dL. Oligospermia was noted at a BLL as low as 40 mcg/dL.

In summary, semen abnormalities (ie, oligospermia, asthenospermia, and teratospermia) have been detected in the blood lead range of 40–139 mcg/dL. Also, hormonal disturbances have been documented for men at BLLs as low as 44 mcg/dL (testosterone) and 10 mcg/dL (FSH and/or LH).

D. Endocrine Disruptors

The term *endocrine disruptor* is used to refer to a variety of manufactured chemicals that may cause health abnormalities by interfering with the normal hormonal balance of humans or animals. The most commonly studied chemicals that may fit this category are polychlorinated biphenyls (PCBs), dioxins, and persistent pesticides. The four main disease categories attracting the most attention in endocrine disruptors research are reproductive, carcinogenic, neurologic, and immunologic health outcomes. Because of the complexity of the male reproductive system, each of these diseases may have an impact on this system.

There appears to be an increased incidence for endocrine-mediated cancers such as breast, testicular, and prostate tumors. Thus far no specific chemical has been identified as the cause for the increase in these tumors.

Current studies are concentrating on several suspect chemical groups that may act via an endocrine-mediated neurotoxicity: PCBs, dioxins, DDT, and other chlorinated pesticides and metals. It should be noted that for the male reproductive system to function normally, an intact neurologic system is necessary. Thus, the results of these studies may have an impact on related reproductive research.

The suggestion of possible immunosuppression comes from the fact that certain endocrine disruptors (eg, DES, PCBs, and dioxins) alter the types of lymphocytes present in the bloodstream. Laboratory animals and wildlife have demonstrated such changes in association with exposure to DES, PCBs, carbamate, organochlorine pesticides, and organic and heavy metals. As was noted earlier, infection and associated immunologic disturbances are considered a risk factor for male infertility.

There are well-documented reports of human reproductive effects (semen abnormalities) from exposure to endocrine disruptors. For example, kepone exposure at a US pesticide factory led to workers with oligospermia. DES use during pregnancy can increase the incidence of nonmalignant genital abnormalities in both male and female offspring. Also, wildlife and experimental animals with offspring showing feminization, demasculinization, and abnormalities in sexual behavior and development demonstrate endocrine-disrupting chemicals in their environment. Further studies are being conducted to better understand this situation.

Phthalates represent a newer type of chemical being considered as an endocrine disruptor. The CDC National Report on Human Exposure to Environmental Chemicals has shown that urinary phthalate metabolites are detectable in the general population at all ages and in different regions of the country. Phthalates are used in the production of hundreds of items, such as food packaging, plastic clothing, personal care products, detergents, adhesives, and vinyl flooring. More recent research looked at boys aged 2–36 months old and found that concentrations of four phthalate metabolites (prenatal urinary monoethyl, mono-*n*-butyl, monobenzyl, and monoisobutyl phthalates) were inversely related to anogenital distance. Also, the median concentrations for each of the metabolites associated with short anogenital distance and incomplete testicular descent are below the corresponding median levels seen among women in the National Exposure Survey. Animal studies support this potentially hazardous human health effect. These preliminary results may suggest that current widespread exposure to phthalates may cause human male reproductive damage at levels found in the general population.

Another endocrine disruptor with possible male reproductive effects is 2,2'4,4'5,5'-hexachlorobiphenyl (CB-153). This chemical is a persistent organochloride pollutant and has been associated with decreased sperm motility among fishermen having a diet high in fatty fish. Although the association in this study was not statistically significant, there is much interest in evaluating any possible reproductive effect from this persistent environmental contaminant, as well as other categories of endocrine disruptors.

REPRODUCTIVE ASSESSMENT

The medical evaluation of the patient with a potential exposure to a reproductive hazard follows the traditional components of history taking, physical examination, and laboratory assessment with an emphasis on both health and exposure parameters. In addition, special consideration is needed in the assessment, communication, and management of reproductive risk for the patient, as well as possible environmental evaluation and sampling at the work site or other location of potential exposure.

Medical Evaluation

In the clinical setting, infertility is defined as an inability to conceive after 12 months of unprotected intercourse. It is estimated that the cause of infertility is related to male factors in 40% of the affected couples, female factors in 40–50% of the affected couples, and no known etiology in 10–20% of the affected couples. For the infertility and adverse pregnancy outcome workup, the female partner needs to be assessed concurrently. A full discussion of the diagnosis and treatment of various urologic and other related medical conditions is beyond the scope of this chapter. However, the following is a general overview of the types of evaluation techniques that can be used to assess the male reproductive system.

A. Medical History

The patient interview should cover the following areas: demographic data (eg, both maternal and paternal age if birth outcome is being assessed), general medical history (eg, febrile illnesses, trauma, infections and structural abnormalities of the genitourinary system, and past surgeries), drug use (including medications, street drugs, alcohol, and tobacco), habits (eg, sauna and hot tub use), work history, and reproductive history (eg, past problems of infertility and pregnancies and birth outcomes for each sexual partner). It is important to ask about potential occupational and environmental exposure to any of the known or suspected reproductive hazards cited in Table 28–4. More complete details for an environmental and occupational history can be found in Chapter 2.

B. Physical Examination

This examination should focus on the physical integrity of the genital system to rule out any extraneous mass or abnormality and the presence of secondary sex traits (eg, hair growth pattern and possible gynecomastia). A physical abnormality may impede spermatogenesis, ejaculation, and erection (eg, varicocele, hydrocele, hypospadias, and cryptorchism). It is important to evaluate testicular size, prostate tenderness, and the presence of any structural anomalies. Testicular size

averages 4.6 cm in length (range 3.5–5.5 cm) and 12–25 mL in volume, with the seminiferous tubules accounting for 95% of the testicular volume. Hypovirilization and infertility can indicate Klinefelter syndrome (47,XYY, often associated with small testes and occurring in 0.2% of adult men) or viral orchitis.

C. Hormonal Profile

A number of hormonal tests are available, and selection needs to be based on the medical conditions under consideration. A preliminary hormonal profile that can be obtained for field surveys includes FSH, LH (pituitary function), and testosterone (testicular function). For field biologic monitoring surveys, blood samples are relatively easy to collect for hormonal assays, but care must be taken to obtain samples at standardized times to avoid diurnal variability problems. The FSH is increased in individuals with azoospermia, such as the DBCP episode. With a normal testosterone level and an increased FSH level, a decrease in spermatogenesis occurs, which is usually associated with severe germinal epithelium damage. If there is a sperm abnormality with normal LH and testosterone, then an obstruction to the reproductive system can be ruled out. If both LH and testosterone are low, then a hypothalamic or pituitary abnormality is likely. In the situation where low testosterone and high LH concentrations are seen, there is the possibility of a primary defect at the testicular level. When there is a high level of testosterone and a low level of LH, an autonomous or exogenous source of testosterone needs to be considered. Finally, having both LH and testosterone elevated would suggest an autonomous LH secretion or resistance to testosterone action. One additional hormone being studied for utility in screening situations is inhibin B, which is reduced when damage to the seminiferous tubules occurs.

D. Semen Analysis

Analysis of semen parameters can be conducted by both traditional and computer-aided semen analysis (CASA) methods. The basic parameters of interest are ejaculate volume, sperm count or concentration, motility, morphology, swim velocity (direct measurement obtainable via CASA), and the presence of any suspect toxicant. The subsequent normal ranges discussed are to be used as general guidelines for the interpretation of a semen profile. There is much variability in the quality of semen analysis by laboratory, and the CASA may not be available at all reproductive/infertility laboratories. Because the normal ranges for semen characteristics may vary by laboratory, it is important to review the ranges provided by the laboratory being used.

The sperm concentration refers to the number of sperm per milliliter of ejaculate, with a normal level of more than 20 million per milliliter. Normal ejaculate volumes are 1.5–5.5 mL. Sperm motility is the percentage of motile sperm, with a normal sample showing greater than 40% motile sperm. Morphology refers to the percentage of normal (oval) and abnormal sperm head, midpiece, and tail shapes. The 10 general categories of sperm morphology are oval/normal, microcephalic, macrocephalic, tapered head, double head, headless, no head or tail, amorphous head, immature forms, and abnormal tails. Normal morphology is greater than 50% normally shaped sperm if using the World Health Organization (WHO) classification system and greater than 14 if using the stricter Kruger classification.

When semen analyses are used for epidemiologic or screening purposes, certain aspects need to be addressed. There is a need to conduct concurrent motility and count measures because most cells are nonmotile or poorly motile. Thus, sperm count alone is not recommended. For count and motility, it is important to note the time since last ejaculation (48–72 hours maximum for accurate reading). Also, all semen analyses should be conducted at the same laboratory because of the high interlaboratory variability. Optimally, a semen sample should be analyzed within 1 hour of production so that the sperm remain viable for analysis. A standardized semen collection procedure needs to be established and followed by the individual being evaluated. Masturbation is recommended (preferably with no sexual partner, condom, or lubricant use), with the collection of semen in specially provided containers. It is extremely important that the entire volume of ejaculate be collected and that the specimen not be subjected to extreme temperatures in transport to the analysis site. Multiple samples from the same individual can show much variability; therefore, serial measurements are preferred. Most infertility evaluations involve three subsequent samples on separate days. Finally, there are three potential barriers to cooperation from individuals being recruited for participation in a study. (1) Highly motivated subjects are needed for the study, yet the individual is usually asymptomatic and may not understand the usefulness of an evaluation. (2) Religious and cultural taboos may be encountered. And (3) there may be a lack of available sperm because of a preexisting medical condition such as vasectomy.

E. Other Tests

Other male reproductive tests are available for further clinical evaluation but are not usually included in epidemiologic field studies. These tests include GnRH challenge, thyroid profile, testicular biopsy, postcoital test, and sperm-oocyte interaction. Some more recent evaluation methods involve sperm DNA, chromosome and maturity bioassays, and biologic markers for fertilization function (eg, sperm antigen). In azoospermia or severe oligospermia, a testicular biopsy can assess the seminiferous tubules and Leydig cell histology for fibrosis and lack of spermatogenesis. The postcoital test involves the interaction of sperm examined in mucus following intercourse. If the index sperm penetrates a donor mucus but not the sexual partner's mucus, the mucus of the sexual partner may be a problem. The patient's sperm is considered abnormal if no penetration of either mucus occurs. The sperm-oocyte interaction test uses the zona pellucida of a hamster oocyte to evaluate if the patient's sperm is able to fuse (the capacitation and acrosomal reaction needed for eventual conception). Antisperm antibodies on the sperm surface are a form of immunologic infertility and sometimes are a result of prior surgical reversal of a vasectomy. Furthermore, a wide range of medical tests and assays may be indicated for the underlying medical conditions thought to be present. Lastly, the assessment of body burden for certain exposures may be estimated via exhaled breath, blood, urine, semen, and other biologic tissue measurements.

To allow comparison among different studies, the WHO has published two manuals on a standardized approach for evaluating infertile men. One manual deals with the investigational process, diagnosis, and management of infertile males. Included are a patient data-collection form and a diagnostic decision flow diagram to facilitate the analysis of data between different clinicians. The laboratory manual describes procedures for examining human semen and provides lower limits for the normal range of various tests. These lower limits include 2.0 mL for semen volume, 20 million sperm per milliliter for concentration, and 40 million for number of sperm per ejaculate, 50% with progressive motility and 30% with normal morphology.

Occupational and Environmental Health Consultation

The health risk assessment process may prove to be difficult because of inadequate exposure or a lack of toxicologic or medical information. It is very helpful to have established professional contacts with expertise in occupational or environmental health consultation when a more difficult risk assessment is involved. Potential contacts may include local or state health departments, university medical centers or schools of public health, poison control centers, National Centers for Disease Control and Prevention (CDC, including the National Institute for Occupational Safety and Health and the National Center for Environmental Health), U.S. Environmental Protection Agency, Agency for Toxic Substances and Disease Registries, OSHA, and the Association of Occupational and Environmental Clinics. Access to online literature databases also can be very useful such as REPROTOX and TERIS (see "Informational Sources" above for more details).

Communication Regarding Reproductive Hazards

There is an underlying principle that needs to be acknowledged and sensitively dealt with: The threat or actual fact of reproductive dysfunction or adverse reproductive outcome has a profound impact on an individual's life and his or her family. All questions must be answered truthfully and completely. A description of the limitations in knowledge may be needed. The timing of exposure for the male and of the first contact with the involved female partner is very important. Whenever possible, the risk communication is conducted prior to actual exposure in order to intervene at the primary prevention stage. The options available for the male worker should be presented in such a way that the medical impact and the economic consequences of decisions are understood and discussed. The medical confidentiality of the involved individual should be maintained at all costs. If an occupational situation, it is imperative that the employer, involved employee(s), and medical consultant work together in resolving a particular exposure, as well as in developing a general policy on reproductive hazards in the workplace that involves both genders. Ideally, this policy should be developed within a health and safety committee composed of representatives from management and labor and consultants in occupational medicine and industrial hygiene.

Recommendations for Controlling Exposure

In the evaluation of the patient, a clinician can play an important consultative role in the control or elimination of exposure in the home, workplace, or other site of high risk. Working with the key health personnel or public health officials involved in this process, the following actions may be considered for men exposed to reproductive toxicants.

A. Exposure Reduction or Elimination

Replace hazards with safer ones; improved engineering controls, safer work practices, and personal protective equipment (this latter item should not be the primary mode of protection—emphasis should be placed on the other actions). Exposure reduction or elimination is the most desirable option and should be attempted in all situations where a reproductive hazard exists.

B. Temporary Job Transfer or Removal From Area of Exposure

Remove the individual from work environment, residence, or other site where the reproductive hazard exists. This option should be offered to men exposed to reproductive toxicants who are considering having children.

C. Permanent Removal of Individual from Work or Exposure Setting

This should be considered for male workers exposed to reproductive toxicants where reassignment is not possible. For female workers, it is illegal for an employer to terminate an affected woman because of pregnancy. An individual may choose to quit work for personal reasons, but it is important to help the individual to evaluate all the other options and to understand the possible consequences. In the residential setting, there have been permanent relocation of populations owing to environmental contamination. The permanent removal of an individual from a residence, work setting, or other exposure site is considered after all the other options have been explored.

LEGAL ISSUES & WORKPLACE STANDARDS

In the lawsuit International Union, UAW versus Johnson Controls, Inc., the U.S. Supreme Court held that an employer violated Title VII's ban on sex discrimination by excluding from production jobs in a lead-battery factory all women who could not prove their sterility. The Court indicated that a policy directed only at fertile women is overt discrimination on the basis of sex regardless of the scientific evidence of heightened safety concerns for mothers or potential mothers. In addition, any policies or actions taken by the employer must not violate existing laws prohibiting discrimination on the basis of pregnancy, childbirth, or related medical conditions. Employers cannot require that an individual be sterilized as a condition of employment. If an employee disabled by pregnancy, childbirth, or a related medical condition transfers to a less hazardous job, an employer must allow the employee to return to the employee's original job or a similar one when the disability has resolved. Thus, the workplace must be made safe, and reproductive hazard information must be provided to both men and women.

OSHA has the mandate to promulgate standards that protect workers from adverse health effects (including reproductive effects) resulting from workplace hazards. However, there are only four agents with OSHA standards that are based partially on reproductive effects: dibromochloropropane (DBCP), lead, ethylene oxide, and ionizing radiation. It should be recognized that many chemical and physical agents found in the workplace are not covered by an OSHA standard and that those standards that do exist for the most part are not based on reproductive endpoints. This is why the risk assessment process discussed earlier should be implemented at any work site that has potential reproductive hazards present.

REFERENCES

Caporossi L et al: Cross sectional study on exposure to BPA and phthalates and semen parameters in men attending a fertility center. Int J Environ Res Public Health 2020;17(2):489 [PMID: 31940982].

Choi KH, Kim H, Kim MH, Kwon HJ: Semiconductor work and adverse pregnancy outcomes associated with male workers: a retrospective cohort study. Ann Work Expo Health 2019; 63(8):870-880 [PMID: 31421636].

Kumar S, Sharma A: Cadmium toxicity: effects on human reproduction and fertility. Rev Environ Health 2019;34(4):327-338 [PMID: 31129655].

Mai CT, Kirby RS, Correa A, Rosenberg D, Petros M, Fagen MC: Public health practice of population-based birth defects surveillance programs in the United States. J Public Health Manag Pract 2016;22(3):E1-E8 [PMID: 25905668].

Matthews TJ, MacDorman MF, Thoma ME: Infant mortality statistics from the 2013 period linked birth/infant death data set. Natl Vital Stat Rep 2015;64(9):1-30 [PMID: 26270610].

Ren J et al: Low-level lead exposure is associated with aberrant sperm quality and reproductive hormone levels in Chinese male individuals: results from the MARHCS study low-level lead exposure is associated with aberrant sperm quality. Chemosphere 2020;244:125402 [PMID: 31809925].

Talibov M et al: Parental occupational exposure to low-frequency magnetic fields and risk of leukaemia in the offspring: findings from the Childhood Leukaemia International Consortium (CLIC). Occup Environ Med 2019;76(10):746-753 [PMID: 31358566].

Zamkowska D, Karwacka A, Jurewicz J, Radwan M: Environmental exposure to non-persistent endocrine disrupting chemicals and semen quality: an overview of the current epidemiological evidence. Int J Occup Med Environ Health 2018;31(4):377-414 [PMID: 30160090].

■ SELF-ASSESSMENT QUESTIONS

Select the one correct answer for each question.

Question 1: Semen abnormalities can include
  a. azoospermia (low sperm count)
  b. oligospermia (increased sperm count)
  c. teratospermia (abnormally motile sperm)
  d. asthenospermia (sperm showing decreased motility)

Question 2: Male reproductive toxicants
  a. include DBCP, ionizing radiation, mercury, and lead
  b. are of concern only in occupational settings
  c. mostly involve low-level exposures
  d. include DBCP and exogenous estrogens

Question 3: DBCP
  a. is a nematocide that is associated with reproductive and developmental abnormalities
  b. exposed workers exhibit azoospermia, oligospermia, and decreased plasma FSH levels
  c. causes decreased sperm fertility among all exposed workers
  d. exposure may result into a permanent azoospermia in some workers

Question 4: Inorganic lead
  a. is the only form of lead with male reproductive effects
  b. has been implicated in cases of increased libido
  c. presents in some males as endocrine changes (decreased testosterone and increased LH levels)
  d. is frequently detected in the sperm of workers with low-level exposure

Question 5: Phthalates
  a. should not be considered as an endocrine disruptor
  b. metabolites are detectable in the general population at all ages
  c. are associated with short anogenital distance together with incomplete testicular descent
  d. may cause human male reproductive damage at levels found in the general population

Metals

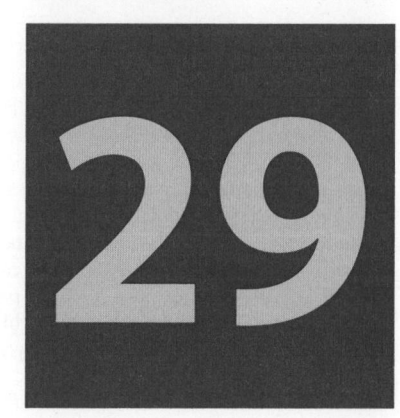

Richard Lewis, MD, MPH

Michael J. Kosnett, MD, MPH

The diverse physical properties of metals have resulted in their extensive use in industry. These naturally occurring materials have long been recognized for their ability to impart a variety of valuable characteristics to finished goods. Metals are used in the construction, automotive, aerospace, electronics, glass, and numerous other manufacturing industries. Metals are major sources of pigments and stabilizers for paints and plastics. Metals are also used as catalysts and intermediates in the chemical and pharmaceutical industries. Occupational and environmental exposure to metals may occur during the manufacture or fabrication of finished products, as well as later in the product life cycle during modification, physical disturbance, or disposal. For some metals, such as arsenic in drinking water, significant exposure may occur primarily as the consequence of geologic rather than anthropogenic activity.

Metals are used rarely in their pure form, usually being present in alloys. They also may be bound to organic materials, altering their physical characteristics and potential toxicity. Some compounds, such as hydrides and carbonyls, are highly toxic and may be formed accidentally when the parent metal reacts with acids. Metals may be altered by burning and smelting or after uptake by biologic systems. The chemical structure of the metal or organometallic compound alters absorption, distribution, and toxicity.

Metals exert biologic effects through numerous modes of action. These may include chemical interactions, such as binding to sulfhydryl groups, that alter the structure and function of many proteins and enzyme systems. Metals may react with cellular structures and macromolecules in ways that may induce oxidative stress, alter gene expression, disturb the function of essential cations, and trigger immune responses. Certain metals, such as zinc, copper, chromium, cobalt, molybdenum, and manganese, are essential for normal metabolism. Others, such as lead, mercury, arsenic, and cadmium, serve no recognized biologic purpose, raising public health concerns owing to their ubiquitous presence in living organisms.

General population exposure to most metals arises primarily from ingestion in food and water, with lesser degrees of exposure from inhalation of contaminated air. Hazardous levels of exposure from inhalation is more commonly encountered in occupational settings. Familiarity with the potential health effects of metals in different settings is helpful not only for the occupational health and safety professional but also for primary and specialty care medical providers.

Because metals may perturb biochemical and physiochemical functions in cells throughout the body, overexposure to metals should often be considered in the differential diagnosis of patients presenting with multisystemic signs or symptoms. Health care providers should also be aware that low levels of metal exposure not associated with overt manifestations or symptoms may nonetheless contribute to deleterious effects such as cancer, adverse reproductive and developmental outcomes, immune dysfunction, and latent neurodegeneration.

ARSENIC

ESSENTIALS OF DIAGNOSIS

▶ Acute effects

- Gastrointestinal distress (nausea, vomiting, diarrhea, abdominal pain).
- Hypotension, metabolic acidosis.
- Cardiopulmonary dysfunction (prolonged QT interval, arrhythmias, congestive cardiomyopathy, noncardiogenic pulmonary edema).
- Anemia and leukopenia.
- Sensorimotor peripheral neuropathy.

▶ Chronic effects

- Constitutional (fatigue, malaise).
- Anemia and leukopenia.
- Hyperkeratosis and hyperpigmentation.
- Sensorimotor peripheral neuropathy.
- Cardiovascular disease (coronary heart disease and stroke).
- Peripheral vascular disease.
- Cancer of the skin, lung, and bladder.

General Considerations

Arsenic is a naturally occurring metalloid that occurs in a variety of chemical forms and valence states. The elemental form, which seldom exists in nature and is of low solubility, is a rare cause of human toxicity. Inorganic arsenic is encountered in commerce predominantly as the trivalent (As+3) or pentavalent (As+5) oxides, sulfides, or salts. Trivalent forms generally have greater acute toxicity than the pentavalent species, but *in vivo* interconversion may occur, and compounds of both valences are capable of exerting a similar pattern of acute and chronic intoxication. Organoarsenicals, which occur naturally and in many synthetic forms, vary widely in their toxicological attributes, from the virtually nontoxic natural compound arsenobetaine widely encountered in seafood, to the highly toxic vesicant warfare agent lewisite (dichloro [2-chlorovinyl] arsine). Arsine, a hydride gas (AsH_3) is a potent hemolytic agent.

Use

Arsenic is used principally in the United States in the production of chromated copper arsenide (CCA) wood preservatives for industrial applications (eg, marine timbers and utility poles); its widespread former use as a preservative for residential lumber was voluntarily discontinued in 2003. Arsenic is used as a minor constituent of metal alloys, such as the hardening of lead in battery grids, bearings, and ammunition, and in the manufacture of certain types of glass. With the exception of monosodium methanearsonate (MSMA) as a herbicide, virtually all the domestic use of arsenic as a pesticide or herbicide has been discontinued. High-purity arsenic is used in the manufacture of gallium arsenide chips and circuit boards incorporated in products in the electronics, aerospace, and telecommunications sectors. Arsenic trioxide was introduced to the US Pharmacopoeia in 2000 as a drug for cancer chemotherapy. The use of phenylarsenic compounds as feed additives for poultry and swine was terminated in the United States in 2015. Inorganic arsenic is occasionally encountered in folk remedies and tonics, particularly some of Asian origin.

Occupational & Environmental Exposure

Occupational exposure to arsenic may occur in the smelting of lead, copper, gold, and other nonferrous metals. Readily volatilized arsenic trioxide is concentrated in flue dust and can be condensed and recovered in a cooling chamber. Furnace and flue maintenance operations carry risk of exposure. Arsenic also may be found in fly and bottom ash from coal combustion, and exposure is possible during coal boiler maintenance. In the microelectronics and glass industries, workers may be exposed to arsenic from source materials, finished products, or maintenance operations. Arsine gas is used in semiconductor manufacturing and also may be formed accidentally when compounds or products containing inorganic arsenic come in contact with hydrogen or reducing agents in aqueous solution.

General population exposure to inorganic arsenic occurs primarily through ingestion of foodstuffs that contain arsenic as a consequence of its natural crustal occurrence or anthropogenic contamination. The US Food and Drug Administration in 2016 proposed action levels for arsenic in apple juice and rice in an effort to reduce dietary arsenic exposure, particularly to young children (https://www.fda.gov/food/metals/arsenic-food-and-dietary-supplements). In various parts of the world, inorganic arsenic of geologic origin may be found in artesian well water at concentrations that exceed the US Environmental Protection Agency (EPA) maximum contaminant level of 10 mcg/L by one or more orders of magnitude. Arsenic may also leach into groundwater from certain landfills or surface impoundments containing coal combustion waste. Seafoods (fish, mollusks, and seaweeds) may often contain small amounts of inorganic arsenic, and relatively higher levels of naturally occurring nontoxic organoarsenicals such as arsenobetaine, or various arsenosugars and arsenolipids. The toxicologic risk posed by the latter two compounds and their metabolites, which include DMA (see later) is a topic of research interest.

Absorption, Metabolism, & Excretion

Soluble arsenic compounds are well absorbed after ingestion or inhalation. Percutaneous absorption is limited, but may be of clinical significance after extensive exposure to concentrated reagents. Inorganic arsenic undergoes *in vivo* biomethylation to monomethylarsonic acid (MMA) and dimethylarsinic acid (DMA), which are predominantly excreted, together with residual inorganic arsenic, in the urine. Approximately 10–30% appears in the urine as inorganic arsenic, 10–20% as MMA, and 60–70% as DMA. Genetic, dietary, and dose factors appear to influence the extent of biomethylation, and a relatively higher percentage of MMA in the urine may reflect increased susceptibility to arsenic-related disease. When chronic daily absorption of inorganic arsenic is less than 1000 mcg, approximately two-thirds of the absorbed dose is excreted in the urine within 2–3 days. Arsenic binds to sulfhydryl groups present in keratinized tissue, and small amounts are excreted by incorporation into the hair and nails. Arsenic compounds are believed to exert their hazardous effects through multiple modes of action, including inhibition of enzymes vital to cell metabolism, induction of oxidative stress, and alterations in gene expression and cell signal transduction. Arsine gas uniquely induces massive hemolysis by forming a reactive intermediate with oxyhemoglobin that alters transmembrane ion flux.

Clinical Findings

A. Symptoms and Signs

1. Acute exposure—Acute exposure to several hundred milligrams or more of a soluble inorganic arsenic salt may result in a constellation of multisystemic signs and symptoms that emerge over a period of hours to weeks. Early prominent signs include gastrointestinal distress, including nausea, vomiting, diarrhea, and abdominal pain. Diffuse capillary leak may result in hypotension, tachycardia, decreased urine output, and shock. Central nervous system findings are highly variable, and range from none to seizures and encephalopathy. If the patient survives the initial phase, a second phase within 1 day to 1 week may feature cardiac arrhythmias, congestive cardiomyopathy, and noncardiogenic pulmonary edema. A third phase that emerges 1–4 weeks post ingestion may include anemia and leukopenia, and sensorimotor peripheral neuropathy.

Arsine gas is nonirritating, and inhalation yields no immediate symptoms. A garlic-like odor is occasionally but not invariably noted. After a dose-dependent latent interval of 2–24 hours, massive hemolysis may ensue, accompanied by constitutional symptoms of headache, malaise, fever, chills, and gastrointestinal distress. Hemoglobinuria imparts a reddish color to the urine, and elevated plasma hemoglobin may result in a bronze discoloration of the skin. Oliguria and acute renal failure, which emerge within 1–3 days, are often major complications.

2. Subacute and chronic exposure—Subacute arsenic intoxication associated with absorption of weeks to months of more than 0.05 mg/kg/d may also result in multisystemic effects including fatigue, gastrointestinal symptoms, depressed hemoglobin, liver enzyme elevation, peripheral neuropathy, and prolonged QT interval, possibly associated with ventricular arrhythmias. Chronic arsenic ingestion of more than 0.01 mg/kg/d over a period of years may result in the emergence of a distinctive pattern of spotted hyperpigmentation and palmarplantar hyperkeratosis, a sensory predominant peripheral neuropathy, vascular disease, and noncirrhotic portal hypertension. Epidemiologic data suggest a link between chronic arsenic ingestion and diabetes mellitus, hypertension, increased cardiovascular disease incidence and mortality, nonmalignant respiratory disease, and adverse reproductive outcomes. Chronic arsenic inhalation may cause lung cancer, and chronic arsenic ingestion may cause cancer of the skin, lung, and bladder.

B. Laboratory Findings

Early in the phase of severe acute arsenic poisoning there may be laboratory evidence of metabolic acidosis and rhabdomyolysis. As intoxication progresses, there may be anemia and leukopenia, hepatic transaminase elevation, and QT segment prolongation and arrhythmias on the electrocardiogram.

Measurement of urine arsenic is helpful in confirming recent exposure. In the first 2–3 days following acute symptomatic arsenic intoxication, *total* urine arsenic concentration is typically much greater than 1000 mcg/L and depending on the severity of poisoning may not return to back ground values for several weeks. Ingestion of seafood, which may contain nontoxic organoarsenicals such as arsenobetaine and arsenosugars, may greatly elevate total urine arsenic concentration for up to 3 days. It may sometimes be useful to have urine arsenic reported as inorganic arsenic plus its primary human metabolites MMA and DMA—the sum of these three species is usually less than 20 mcg/L in the general population from background dietary and environmental exposure. Segmental analysis of arsenic in the hair and nails may sometimes offer forensic evidence of elevated arsenic exposure months after urine arsenic concentration has normalized, but values should be interpreted cautiously owing to the potential of external contamination. Blood arsenic, which has a highly variable relationship to exposure and is subject to rapid clearance, is rarely of value for clinical diagnosis or biological monitoring.

▶ Prevention

Because arsenic is a known human carcinogen, workplace exposure should be reduced as much as feasible by a program of engineering and administrative controls, and personal protective equipment. Biological monitoring of arsenic in urine may yield information on recent airborne or inhalation exposure to soluble arsenic compounds, but may have limited utility after inhalation of poorly soluble arsenic aerosols.

▶ Treatment

Management of acute arsenic intoxication should combine intensive supportive care of metabolic acidosis, hypotension, and other cardiovascular derangements with prompt administration of chelating agents. Intravenous unithiol (DMPS), the chelating agent of choice, may be of limited availability in the United States. Other useful agents include oral succimer (DMSA) and intramuscular dimercaprol (BAL). Gastric decontamination should be considered. Prolonged inpatient support and monitoring may be indicated for initially symptomatic patients due to delayed cardiopulmonary and neurologic complications. Management of chronic arsenic intoxication should focus on removal from sources of exposure and supportive care. Oral chelation with unithiol or succimer can be empirically considered in individuals with high urine arsenic concentrations, as may folate supplementation in deficient individuals.

Treatment of arsine gas poisoning should focus on vigorous intravenous hydration, possibly supplemented by osmotic diuresis with mannitol, to maintain urine output and reduce the acute risk of hemoglobinuric renal failure. Elevation of plasma or serum hemoglobin levels of 1.5 g/dL or higher, and/or signs of renal insufficiency should prompt exchange transfusion with whole blood. Hemodialysis may be indicated for renal failure, but is not a substitute for the exchange transfusion-mediated removal of the arsenic-hemoprotein complexes thought to contribute to ongoing hemolysis. Chelation is of uncertain value in the management of arsine intoxication.

BERYLLIUM

ESSENTIALS OF DIAGNOSIS

- ▶ Tracheobronchitis, pneumonitis (acute).
- ▶ Granulomatous pulmonary disease.
- ▶ Dermatitis (ulceration and granulomas).
- ▶ Eye, nose, and throat irritation.
- ▶ Lung cancer.

General Considerations

Beryllium is a lightweight gray metal with high tensile strength. It is extracted from beryl ore after grinding and heating using electrolytic reduction. Bertrandite ($4BeO \cdot 2SiO_2 \cdot H_2O$), although lower in beryllium content (0.1–3%), provides a source of acid-soluble beryllium that is more easily extracted. Beryllium occurs naturally in soils, associated with aluminum.

Use

The unique properties of beryllium are ideally suited for the production of hard, corrosion-resistant alloys for use in the aerospace industry. Beryllium alloys (primarily copper) are used in tools, bushings, bearings, and electronic components. Beryllium is used in nuclear reactors as a neutron moderator and a fuel source. Beryllium oxide combines high thermal conductivity with high electrical resistance for use in ceramics, microwave tubes, and semiconductors. Beryllium has been used in the manufacture of fluorescent and neon lamps in the past, leading to the first cases of chronic beryllium disease (CBD) recognized in the United States.

The risks for the development of beryllium sensitization and CBD remain an important occupational concern due to uncertainties regarding specific exposure and susceptibility factors. Mining of beryl ore appears to result in a relatively low risk of CBD. In contrast, the purification and use of refined beryllium compounds, particularly beryllium oxide, continues to result in a substantial risk of sensitization and disease in the aerospace, nuclear, electronics, and beryllium alloy industries. In 1999, the United States Department of Energy adopted an exposure limit of 0.2 mcg/m^3 as an 8-hour time weighted average, and this was adopted by OSHA in a standard promulgated in 2017. The short-term (15 minute) exposure limit is 2.0 mcg/m^3.

Beryllium compounds are poorly absorbed after inhalation, ingestion, or skin contact. Beryllium may be retained in the lung, resulting in a potential prolonged latency between exposure and the development of health effects. The development of sensitization and CBD appear to be related to solubility, particle size, and individual sensitivity. Gene–environment interaction studies reveal that certain genotypes, particularly HLA-DPBI, enhance susceptibility to beryllium sensitization and CBD. Pathologically, CBD primarily results in interstitial lung disease evidenced by the presence of fibrosis and noncaseating granulomas.

1. Acute or subacute exposure—Acute or subacute exposure to beryllium dusts, gas, or fumes has irritant effects on the eyes, mucous membranes, and respiratory tract, although these appear to require exposures substantially higher (likely > 100 mcg/m^3) than current short-term exposure limits. Death has occurred as a result of pulmonary edema and respiratory failure. Acute respiratory and systemic symptoms may be followed by the development of CBD.

2. Chronic exposure—Sensitization and CBD may develop months, years, or decades after exposure. Asymptomatic

Table 29–1. Beryllium regulations in the United States.

	DOE (1999)	OSHA (2018)
Exposure		
Permissible exposure limit	0.2 mcg/m³ as 8 h TWA	0.2 mcg/m³ as 8 h TWA
Short-term exposure limit	2.0 mcg/m³	2.0 mcg/m³
Medical Surveillance		
Application	Current Be exposure	Current/Be affected[a]
History and examination	Annual	Every 2 y
BeLPT	Annual	Every 2 y
Pulmonary function	Baseline/examiner discretion	Not required
Chest x-ray/B-reading	Every 5 y	Not required
Low-dose CT scan	Not required	Examiner discretion
Past Exposure	Be-associated[b]	
Exam/BeLPT	Every 3 y	Not specified
Chest x-ray/B-reading	Every 5 y	Not specified

[a]OSHA Beryllium-affected workers exhibit signs or symptoms of beryllium exposure (sensitization or CBD).
[b]DOE Beryllium-associated workers may have been exposed to airborne concentrations of beryllium at a DOE facility or exhibit signs or symptoms of beryllium exposure (sensitization or CBD).

sensitization is detected through the Beryllium Lymphocyte Transformation Test (BLPT). With the development of CBD there is exertional dyspnea accompanied by fatigue, weight loss, cough, and chest pain. On physical examination, there may be rales, hepatosplenomegaly, lymphadenopathy, and clubbing. Beryllium compounds are considered human carcinogens, leading to an excess risk of lung cancer. After skin contact, beryllium may cause an irritant or allergic dermatitis characterized by erythema, papules, and vesiculation. Beryllium skin testing is not recommended due to the risk of inducing sensitization.

Acute pneumonitis is manifested by arterial hypoxemia with diffuse pulmonary infiltrates. CBD is a respiratory irritant with pulmonary function studies showing either an obstructive or restrictive pattern. The first sign may be a drop in diffusing capacity. Radiographic findings include diffuse bilateral nodular or linear infiltrates, often with bilateral hilar adenopathy. Bronchoalveolar lavage may demonstrate lymphocyte alveolitis with an increase in T cells. Biopsy of affected tissues reveals noncaseating granulomas.

The BeLPT (beryllium lymphocyte proliferation) is a specialized testing process used to confirm sensitization. Mononuclear cells are placed in culture in the presence of beryllium sulfate, across a range of concentrations, with cell proliferation measured after day 4 or 5 and day 6 or 7. Results are presented as positive, negative, borderline, or uninterpretable. The current consensus is that two abnormals, one abnormal and one borderline, or three borderline results indicate sensitization.

While standard exposure control measures appear to be effective in the processing of beryl ores, prevention of beryllium sensitization and CBD in other industry sectors remains a challenge. Standard medical surveillance required by the DOE and OSHA includes periodic BeLPT and pulmonary function testing every 1 or 2 years, respectively. Chest x-rays (DOE) or low-dose spiral CT scans (OSHA) are also used in medical surveillance.

▶ Treatment

Persons with beryllium sensitization or CBD should be restricted from any potential beryllium exposure. CBD disease may respond to corticosteroids. Asymptomatic sensitized workers should undergo periodic medical monitoring with annual chest radiograph and pulmonary function studies to detect the onset of CBD.

▶ Prognosis

An estimated 40–60% of workers with beryllium sensitization will go on to develop CBD. Asymptomatic sensitized workers should undergo periodic medical monitoring with annual chest radiograph and pulmonary function studies to detect the onset of CBD.

CADMIUM

ESSENTIALS OF DIAGNOSIS

▶ Acute effects
  • Chemical pneumonitis.
  • Acute renal failure.
▶ Chronic effects
  • Proteinuria.
  • Osteomalacia.
  • Emphysema.
  • Anemia.
  • Anosmia.
  • Lung cancer.

▶ General Considerations

Cadmium is a soft, silver-white electropositive metal that provides unique properties to metal coating, glass, paints, and pigments. Pure cadmium sulfide (greenockite) is rare; however, cadmium is commonly present in zinc, lead, and copper ores. Cadmium is produced as a by-product of the smelting and refining of these ores and is recovered by electrolysis and distillation. Cadmium is a nonessential biologic contaminant.

▶ Use

Cadmium compounds are used extensively in electroplating. Cadmium imparts corrosion resistance to steel, iron, and a variety of other materials for use in automotive parts, aircraft, marine equipment, and industrial machinery. Cadmium alloys are used in high-speed bearings, solder, and jewelry. Cadmium sulfides and selenides are used as pigments in rubber, inks, plastics, paints, textiles, and ceramics, particularly where heat stability and alkali resistance are desirable. Nickel-cadmium batteries are used in motor vehicles and rechargeable household appliances. Cadmium is also used in photoelectric cells and in semiconductors.

▶ Occupational & Environmental Exposure

The refining of cadmium ores is associated with potential exposure to both dusts and fume. Workers may have exposure to cadmium in the smelting of zinc, lead, and copper. Cadmium is used in the manufacture of batteries, paints, and plastics. Workers may be exposed to cadmium mist from plating baths, as well as to fine dust when machining cadmium-plated parts. Welders may be exposed to harmful fumes when working with cadmium-containing silver solders.

Nonoccupational exposure occurs primarily through dietary intake. Liver and meat by-products, shellfish, and vegetables are potential sources of cadmium. The tobacco plant accumulates environmental cadmium, and cigarette smoke is an important source of chronic cadmium exposure. Air and water contamination may be significant in areas surrounding zinc smelters. Irrigation of rice paddies with contaminated water in Japan led to an epidemic of osteoporosis in postmenopausal women (Itai-Itai disease) in the 1940s.

▶ Absorption, Metabolism, & Excretion

Cadmium is absorbed primarily through inhalation or ingestion. After inhalation, 10–40% may be absorbed, depending on particle size and chemical composition. Gastrointestinal absorption is usually 5% but may be increased in the presence of iron, protein, calcium, or zinc deficiencies. Absorbed cadmium is bound to plasma proteins. Cadmium accumulates in the liver and kidneys, where binding to metallothionein protects against cellular damage. Liver stores are released slowly and taken up by the kidney. There is a gradual increase in the body burden of cadmium, peaking at age 60 years.

Excretion is primarily renal, with a biologic half-life of 8–30 years. Transient peaks in urinary excretion also may occur after short-term, high-dose exposure. Renal excretion of cadmium increases after chronic exposure because of impaired proximal tubular reabsorption, a manifestation of cadmium-induced nephrotoxicity.

▶ Clinical Findings

A. Symptoms and Signs

1. Acute exposure—Acute inhalation of cadmium oxide fume has resulted in industrial fatalities. After a delay of several hours, victims complained of sore throat, headache, myalgias, nausea, and a metallic taste. Fever, cough, dyspnea, and chest tightness progress to a fulminant chemical pneumonitis and death from respiratory failure. Hepatic and renal injury also may occur following acute exposure. Ingestion of cadmium compounds results in nausea, vomiting, headache, abdominal pain, liver injury, and acute renal failure.

2. Chronic exposure—The most frequent manifestation of chronic exposure to cadmium is proteinuria. Initially, there is increased excretion of low-molecular-weight proteins, such as β_1- and β_2-microglobulins. With continued exposure, this can progress to Fanconi syndrome, with aminoaciduria, glycosuria, hypercalciuria, and phosphaturia. Cadmium-induced renal failure may be difficult to distinguish from diabetic nephropathy. Renal tubular dysfunction can result in nephrolithiasis and osteomalacia. Bone pain and pathologic fractures may occur owing to renal calcium and phosphorus loss and impaired synthesis of vitamin D. Chronic inhalation of cadmium dusts and fumes also may result in pulmonary fibrosis and emphysema. Other effects that have been reported include anosmia and anemia. Cadmium is potentially neurotoxic and also may cause testicular injury. Cadmium is a human carcinogen and is associated with an excess risk of lung cancer and prostate cancer. There are associations between cadmium exposure and tumors at other locations including kidney, breast, and prostate.

B. Laboratory Findings

1. Acute inhalation—Evaluation of acute inhalations should include an arterial blood gas evaluation, a chest radiograph, spirometry, and assessment of renal and hepatic function. Hypoxemia, diffuse pulmonary infiltrates, and a reduction in lung function and diffusing capacity indicate acute cadmium oxide exposure and impending respiratory failure. In subacute cases, bronchopneumonia may develop. Normal blood and urine cadmium levels are 1 mcg/L and 1 mcg/g of creatinine, respectively. After acute cadmium fume inhalation, these may rise as high as 3 and 0.36 mg/L.

2. Chronic exposure—Workers exposed to cadmium should participate in periodic biologic monitoring and medical examinations. The biologic monitoring should include urine and blood cadmium levels, as well as measurement of urinary β_2-microglobulin levels. Tables 29–2 and 29–3 summarize the requirements of the programs for cadmium-exposed workers in the United States.

β_1- and β_2-microglobulin levels are a sensitive indicator of cadmium nephrotoxicity, although exercise, febrile illness, nephrotoxic medications, and other kidney disorders also may affect these tests. A loss of sense of smell, mild anemia, and airway obstruction also may be observed in workers with chronic exposure.

▶ Prevention

Process enclosure, local exhaust ventilation, and personal protective measures will minimize exposure to cadmium fume and dust. Workplace and personal hygiene are critical in preventing chronic exposure. Smoking must be prohibited in work areas that use cadmium. Welding on cadmium-treated metal or brazing with cadmium solders should be performed only in areas that are properly ventilated. Air-supplied respirators must be used in enclosed spaces.

Biologic monitoring should focus on the minimizing cadmium exposure to prevent proteinuria. Urine cadmium levels should be kept below 3 mcg/g of creatinine to prevent chronic renal damage. Because of the long biological half-life of cadmium, the biological monitoring of workers who have had significant past exposure is difficult.

Table 29–2. Biologic monitoring program for cadmium.

Actions	Biologic Monitoring Result
Annual biologic monitoring Medical examination every 2 y	Urine cadmium < 3 mcg/g creatinine β_2-Microglobulin < 300 mcg/g creatinine Cadmium in blood < 5 mcg/L whole blood
Semiannual biologic monitoring Medical examination annually Exposure assessment Exposure control	Urine cadmium 3–7 mcg/g creatinine β_2-Microglobulin 300–750 mcg/g creatinine Cadmium in blood 5–10 mcg/L whole blood
Mandatory removal Medical examination Exposure assessment	Urine cadmium > 7 mcg/g creatinine β_2-Microglobulin > 750 mcg/g creatinine Cadmium in blood > 10 mcg/L whole blood

Table 29–3. Medical examination for cadmium workers.

Medical and occupational history
Focusing on cadmium exposure; smoking; renal, cardiovascular, musculoskeletal, and respiratory conditions; reproductive concerns; use of nephrotoxic medications, recent physical exercise, recent febrile illnesses

Physical examination
Blood pressure, respiratory system, genitourinary system, prostate examination (men older than 40 y), respirator medical clearance

Diagnostic testing
Pulmonary function testing
Chest radiograph
Complete blood count
Blood urea nitrogen, creatinine
Urinalysis, urinary protein measurements

Treatment

After acute inhalation of cadmium oxide fumes workers should be evaluated for evidence of acute lung injury. In severe poisoning, chelation with calcium disodium edetate ($CaNa_2$ EDTA) may enhance cadmium excretion. Renal function should be monitored closely. Dimercaprol should not be used. Individuals with evidence of chronic cadmium toxicity should be removed from further exposure.

CHROMIUM

ESSENTIALS OF DIAGNOSIS

- Sinusitis, nasal septum perforation.
- Allergic and irritant dermatitis, skin ulcers.
- Respiratory irritation, bronchitis, asthma.
- Lung cancer.

General Considerations

Chromium is a hard, brittle gray metal that is widely distributed as chromite ($FeOCr_2O_3$) or ferrochromium. Chromium metal is produced through reduction of chromic oxide with aluminum. Chromates are produced by high temperature roasting of chromite in an oxidizing atmosphere. Chromium toxicity is based on the valence state. Hexavalent chromium [Cr(VI)] is the most toxic form and is carcinogenic. In contrast, trivalent chromium [Cr(III)] is an essential element for normal glucose metabolism in man.

Use

Chrome plating is used on automotive parts, household appliances, tools, and machinery, where the coating imparts corrosion resistance and a shiny, decorative finish. Chromium-iron alloys, alone or combined with nickel or manganese, produce a variety of durable, high-strength stainless steels. Chromium compounds confer heat resistance in refractory materials. Chromate pigments are added to paints, dyes, textiles, rubber, plastics, and inks. Medically, chrome-based orthopedic devices are used for joint replacement and radioisotopic ^{56}Cr is used in nuclear medicine to label erythrocytes.

Occupational & Environmental Exposure

Mining and crushing operations result in exposure primarily to chromic oxide. The greatest occupational hazards historically have been in chromate production, where exposure to Cr(VI) resulted in a high incidence of lung cancer. Exposure to chromium fumes occurs in the production and welding of stainless steel. Electroplaters are exposed to chromic acid mist. Erosion of the nasal septum occurred in chrome plating without proper ventilation. Workers may be exposed to chromates through their use in the paint, textile, leather, glass, and rubber industries and in lithography, printing, and photography. Certain cements have a high chromium content. Chromium is found in low concentrations in water, urban air, and a variety of foods. Chromium in jewelry is a common cause of skin allergies.

Absorption, Metabolism, & Excretion

Chromium compounds may be absorbed after ingestion, inhalation, or skin contact. The soluble Cr(VI) forms are absorbed much more readily than the insoluble trivalent forms. Cr(VI) readily enters cells, where it is converted to Cr(III). Intracellular Cr(III) binds to proteins and nucleic acids. Ingested Cr(III) is absorbed less readily and crosses into cells much more slowly. Chromium generally does not accumulate in tissues, although inhaled insoluble forms may remain in the lung. Excretion is primarily renal.

Clinical Findings

A. Symptoms and Signs

Acute exposure to high concentrations of chromic acid or chromates will cause immediate irritation of the skin, eye, nose, throat, and respiratory tract. Chronic exposure may cause ulceration, bleeding, and erosion of the nasal septum. Cough, chest pain, and dyspnea may indicate exposure to irritant levels of soluble chromium compounds or the development of chromium-induced asthma.

Dermatologic manifestations are common in chromium workers. Penetration of the skin will cause painless erosive ulceration (chrome holes) with delayed healing. These occur commonly on the fingers, knuckles, and forearms. Chromates are skin allergens causing erythematous or vesicular lesions at points of contact. Generalized eczematous dermatitis, particularly of the hands, should suggest sensitization.

Ingestion of chromium compounds has caused nausea, vomiting, abdominal pain, and prostration. Death is a result of uremia.

Cr(VI) is a known human carcinogen. Workers involved in chromate production, chrome plating, and chrome alloy work all have been found to have an increased incidence of lung cancer.

B. Laboratory Findings

With massive exposure, there will be evidence of renal and hepatic damage. Proteinuria and hematuria precede anuria and uremia. A reduction in airflow may be seen after acute irritant exposure or in workers with chromium-induced asthma. Skin allergy can be confirmed by patch testing. Persistent cough, hemoptysis, or a mass lesion on chest radiograph in a chromium worker should prompt a thorough evaluation for possible lung cancer.

Prevention

Reduction of exposure to Cr(VI) will reduce the respiratory and nasal complications. Surveillance for nasal irritation or septal perforation will identify high-risk jobs to direct exposure-control efforts. Avoidance of skin contact—particularly contact with damaged or inflamed skin—will reduce the risk of developing chrome ulcers or skin sensitization. Prompt evaluation for skin sensitization will prevent the development of severe or chronic dermatitis.

Exposure to Cr(VI) should be reduced to the lowest feasible levels to reduce the risk of lung cancer. Chromium workers also should be encouraged to stop smoking. Biologic monitoring of urine chromium levels may be useful as an assessment of recent exposure. Exposure to 0.05 mg/m^3 of Cr(VI) in air will result in levels of 30–50 mcg/g of creatinine at the end of the workweek.

▶ Treatment

After acute inhalation injury supplemental oxygen and bronchodilators may be required. Careful attention to fluid and electrolyte balance is indicated in the setting of acute renal injury. Chromium-induced nasal and skin ulcerations should be treated with a 10% ointment of CaNa$_2$ EDTA and an impervious dressing with frequent application to prevent formation of persistent ulcers. Persons who develop chromium respiratory or skin allergy should be removed from further exposure if they cannot be protected adequately.

LEAD (INORGANIC)

ESSENTIALS OF DIAGNOSIS

▶ Acute effects
- Central nervous system (fatigue, headache, encephalopathy).
- Gastrointestinal (constipation, abdominal pain).
- Hematologic (hemolytic; hypochromic, normocytic, or microcytic anemia).

▶ Chronic effects
- Constitutional (fatigue, malaise, insomnia, anorexia, weight loss, decreased libido, arthralgias, myalgias).
- Cardiovascular (hypertension; increased cardiovascular morbidity and mortality).
- Hematologic (normochromic or microcytic anemia).
- Central nervous system (impaired concentration and cognition, headache, diminished visual-motor coordination, tremor, encephalopathy).
- Peripheral motor neuropathy.
- Renal (chronic interstitial fibrosis; hyperuricemia and gout).
- Reproductive and developmental (impaired growth and neurocognitive development; adverse reproductive outcomes, altered sperm formation and function).

▶ General Considerations

Lead is a soft, malleable, blue-gray metal characterized by high density and corrosion resistance. The ores of commercial interest include the sulfide (galena), the carbonate (cerussite), and the sulfate (anglesite). Lead is concentrated through flotation and smelted in a three-step process: blending, sintering, and furnace reduction. Raw lead is further refined to remove copper, arsenic, antimony, zinc, tin, bismuth, and other contaminants.

Lead serves no useful biologic function in humans. Lead exerts its toxic effects by interfering with the action of essential cations (eg, calcium, zinc, iron) and macromolecules (enzymes, receptors, membranes, transcription factors) in cells throughout the body. This may result in alterations in mitochondrial and cellular membranes, neurotransmitter synthesis and function, cellular redox status (oxidative stress), nucleotide metabolism, and endocrine signaling. Because these myriad biochemical actions impact cells throughout the body, subclinical or overt impacts in multiple organ systems are a hallmark of lead toxicity.

▶ Use

Lead is among the most extensively recycled of any commodity metal. Secondary smelting accounts for approximately 80% of US domestic lead consumption, approximately 90% of which is used in the production of lead acid batteries. Although lead acid batteries are used primarily in the automotive industry, their use in uninterrupted power supplies for computers and telecommunications is increasing worldwide, especially in the developing world. Additional uses of lead include ammunition; pigments, glass, and ceramics; alloys in steel, brass, bronze, and solder; and sheet lead for construction, industrial tanks and vessels, and radiation shielding (Table 29–4). Global production and consumption of lead has been increasing over the past decade concurrent with a growing demand for storage batteries.

▶ Occupational & Environmental Exposure

According to data collected by the National Institute for Occupational Safety and Health (NIOSH) approximately 95% of all elevated blood lead levels among adults in the United States are work-related. Industry subsectors with the highest numbers of lead-exposed workers have included battery manufacturing, secondary smelting and refining of nonferrous metals, and painting and paper hanging. Although most lead exposure occurs in manufacturing sectors, construction work disproportionately contributes cases with very high blood lead levels (≥ 40 mcg/dL). Construction workers may sporadically encounter high lead exposure during demolition, sandblasting, sanding, or mechanical or torch cutting of structures or components fabricated with lead or covered with lead paint or coatings. Inhalation of lead dust or fume has been the predominant pathway of occupational lead exposure, but incidental ingestion of dust may be significant in some cases. Prominent nonoccupational exposures to lead by adults include shooting firearms;

Table 29–4. Lead sources in occupations and industries.

Ammunition/explosives production
Artisanal gold mining
Automotive repair shops
Battery manufacturing and recycling
Brass, bronze, copper, or lead foundries
Bridge, tunnel, and elevated highway/subway construction
Cable/wire stripping, splicing or production
Ceramic manufacturing
Firing range work
Glass recycling, stained glass, and glass manufacturing
Home renovation/restoration
Lead abatement
Lead production or smelting
Machining or grinding lead alloys
Manufacturing and installation of plumbing components
Manufacturing of industrial machinery and equipment
Metal scrap yards and other recycling operations
Motor vehicle parts and accessories (including radiator repair)
Occupations using firearms
Pipe dope (lubricants)
Plastics manufacturing
Pottery or ceramic manufacturing
Production and use of chemical preparations
Radiation shielding
Rubber manufacturing
Sandblasting, sanding, scraping, burning, or disturbing lead paint
Use of lead-based paints
Welding or torch-cutting painted metal

Table 29–5. Hobbies, activities, and other sources that may result in lead exposure.

Beauty products such as kohl eye makeup, certain hair dyes
Bronze casting
Cookware or tableware fabricated from imported bronze, brass, or pewter
Casting ammunition, fishing weights, or lead figurines
Collecting, painting, or playing games with lead figurines
Copper enameling
Electronics with lead solder
Folk remedies or traditional medicines
Furniture refinishing
Glassblowing with leaded glass
Hunting and target shooting
Imported children's jewelry
Jewelry making with lead solder
Liquor distillation (moonshine)
Pottery and ceramic production with lead glazes and paints
Print making and other fine arts
Remodeling/renovating homes built before 1978
Retention of lead bullets or shrapnel
Stained glass craftwork and painting on stained glass

remodeling, renovating, or painting; retained bullets (gunshot wounds); and lead casting (Table 29–5).

In the United States, children are predominantly exposed to lead by ingestion of deteriorated residential lead-based paint applied many years in the past and lead contaminated house dust and soil. Children may also be exposed to lead dust carried home on the contaminated clothing of adults with occupational exposure and lead in consumer products. The latter may include certain imported home remedies and cosmetics, imported candies or foods, toys, imported or handmade lead-glazed pottery or tableware, and inexpensive children's jewelry. Corrosion of lead in older plumbing may increase the lead content of tap water. Historical automotive emissions from leaded gasoline continues to contaminate certain soils, particularly near major roadways, and there is ongoing exposure to airborne or settled lead emitted from active or inactive point sources such as smelters, metal working, or mining sites. Air lead emissions have declined drastically (> 99%) in the United States over the past four decades, and the largest overall source of emission nationwide is piston engine aircraft operating on leaded aviation gasoline.

▶ Absorption, Metabolism, & Excretion

Inhalation and ingestion are the primary routes of lead absorption. Airborne particle size influences overall transfer of inhaled lead to the blood, because as particles become larger they have an tendency to deposit in the upper airway and be translocated to the gut, rather than to deposit in the lower airway and undergo direct respiratory absorption. Toxicokinetic modeling of empiric data suggests that in workplace settings, approximately 35–40% of inhaled lead is ultimately absorbed to the bloodstream. The extent to which ingested lead is absorbed to the blood is influenced in part by particle solubility (soluble particles undergo greater absorption), the mass of lead ingested, and the extent of coingestion with liquids or solid food (food in the gut decreases absorption). An estimated 15% of ingested soluble lead is absorbed in adults, compared to approximately 40–50% in young children. Iron-deficiency and low calcium diets may increase gastrointestinal absorption.

In the blood, approximately 99% of lead is bound to erythrocytes and 1% is present in the plasma. Lead is initially distributed to soft tissues such as the bone marrow, brain, kidney, liver, muscle, and gonads; subsequently to the subperiosteal surface of bone; and ultimately to bone matrix. Lead also crosses the placenta and poses a potential risk to the fetus. The clearance of lead from the body follows a multicompartment model composed predominantly of the blood and soft tissues with a half-life of 1–2 months and bone with a half-life of years to decades. Approximately 70% of lead excretion is via the urine, with lesser amounts eliminated through the bile, skin, hair, nails, sweat, and breast milk. The fraction not undergoing prompt excretion, approximately half of the absorbed lead, may be incorporated into the skeleton, the site of greater than 90% of the body lead burden in most adults. In patients with a high burden of lead in bone, slow redistribution to the blood may elevate blood lead concentrations for years after exposure ceases. Skeletal lead mobilization may be accelerated during conditions associated with increased bone turnover, such as hyperthyroidism, immobilization osteoporosis, and pregnancy and lactation.

▶ Clinical Findings

A. Symptoms and Signs

1. Acute exposure—Acute symptomatic lead intoxication is now a rare occurrence and usually requires several days or weeks of intense exposure. In occupational settings, this may be associated with exposure to lead oxide fume or high concentrations of lead in dust. Children may present with acute lead intoxication following ingestion of lead present in paint chips, toys, ornaments or other small objects. Both adults and children may sustain acute massive exposure from contaminated food, beverage, or folk medicines. The signs and symptoms are usually neurologic—ranging from headache to ataxia to diminished sensorium or consciousness and convulsions (encephalopathy)—and/or gastrointestinal—nausea, constipation, and crampy abdominal pain (lead colic). In children with encephalopathy, there may be antecedent or concurrent evidence of decreased visual acuity or abnormalities of the third or sixth cranial nerves.

The diagnosis of acute lead intoxication may be challenging, and depending on the presenting signs and symptoms it has sometimes been misdiagnosed as appendicitis, peptic ulcer, biliary colic, pancreatitis, pelvic inflammatory disease, or meningitis. Subacute presentations featuring anorexia, malaise, myalgias, arthralgias, headache, and intermittent abdominal cramps have been mistaken for a flu-like viral illness. Lead poisoning should be a prominent consideration in the differential diagnosis of patients presenting with abdominal pain, headache, and anemia, and to a lesser extent, in those with motor neuropathy, gout, and renal insufficiency. Lead encephalopathy should be considered in adults or children presenting with delirium or convulsions (particularly with coexistent anemia).

2. Chronic exposure—Chronic symptomatic lead intoxication is characterized by the insidious onset of dose-dependent multisystemic signs and symptoms. Constitutional findings may include fatigue, malaise, arthralgias, myalgias, anorexia, insomnia, loss of libido, irritability, and depressed mood. Neurologic symptoms may begin with decrements in concentration and headache and possibly progress after high exposure to frank encephalopathy. Tremor may occur. Gastrointestinal disturbances may include constipation and crampy abdominal pain. Months to years of high-dose lead exposure (eg, blood lead concentrations > 80 mcg/dL) may be associated with a predominantly motor peripheral neuropathy, and nephropathy, the latter characterized by interstitial fibrosis and nephrosclerosis. Chronic renal effects also include hyperuricemia and gout. Adverse reproductive effects associated with high lead exposure include spontaneous abortion or stillbirth in females and diminished or aberrant sperm production in males. An impact of low-level exposure on reproductive outcomes such as preterm delivery, low birth weight, and spontaneous abortion has been inconsistently observed in epidemiologic studies. Chronic lead poisoning should be considered in any child with neurobehavioral or neurocognitive deficits or developmental delay.

The subclinical effects of chronic lead exposure are of considerable public health concern. Low-level lead exposure has deleterious effects on the neurocognitive development of the fetus and young child, and no blood lead threshold for this impact has been identified. In adults, chronic lead exposure associated with blood lead concentrations in the range of 10–25 mcg/dL is an established risk factor for elevated blood pressure, and exposure of this magnitude has been linked to increased cardiovascular mortality in large epidemiologic studies. Animal and epidemiologic studies suggest that early and mid-life lead exposure may be associated with an increased risk of neurodegenerative processes later in life.

B. Laboratory Findings

Whole blood lead concentration is the most common and useful laboratory test to confirm exposure. Lead in blood is a reasonable reflection of the lead content of most soft tissues. However, because blood lead is influenced by recent exogenous exposure as well as by redistribution of skeletal lead stores, knowledge of the temporal pattern of exposure is invaluable when evaluating blood lead measurement in workplace biomonitoring. The geometric mean blood lead concentration for the general United States population in 2015–2019 was 0.820 mcg/dL (95th percentile 2.75 mcg/dL). Noninvasive K x-ray fluorescence measurement of lead in bone, a biomarker of long-term cumulative lead exposure, is used predominantly as a research tool. Measurement of lead in urine following a dose of a chelating agent (chelation challenge testing) correlates satisfactorily in most cases with blood lead test results, and is seldom indicated in clinical practice.

An elevation in erythrocyte protoporphyrin (often measured as zinc protoporphyrin or ZPP) reflects lead-induced inhibition of heme synthesis. Because there is a time lag of several weeks associated with lead-induced elevation in ZPP, the finding of a blood lead of more than or equal to 30 mcg/dL with no concurrent increase in ZPP suggests that the lead exposure was of recent onset.

Acute high-dose lead exposure may induce a hemolytic anemia, (or anemia with basophilic stippling if exposure has been subacute). Hepatic aminotransferases may be elevated. Chronic lead intoxication may result in a hypochromic anemia that is either normocytic or microcytic. Elevated BUN and serum creatinine may reflect transient azotemia associated with acute or subacute high-dose lead exposure, or the irreversible renal insufficiency of chronic lead nephropathy. Radiographically, abdominal x-rays may show opacities consistent with recent lead ingestion, and a head CT scan revealing cerebral edema may aid in the diagnosis of lead encephalopathy.

Prevention

Prevention of occupational overexposure to lead can be accomplished through a careful program of product substitution, engineering controls, personal protective equipment, and work practices such as assiduous handwashing and post-shift showering. Current OSHA lead standards that require medical removal from elevated workplace lead exposure when blood lead levels exceed 50 or 60 mcg/dL were enacted several decades ago and offer insufficient protection. An expert panel in 2007 recommended that removal be initiated for a single blood lead level greater than 30 mcg/dL, or when two successive blood lead levels measured over a 4-week interval are more than or equal to 20 mcg/dL. The longer-term goal should be for workers to maintain blood lead levels less than 10 mcg/dL (Table 29–6).

In 2010, the US Centers for Disease Control and Prevention issued guidelines for the identification and management of lead exposure in pregnant and lactating women that recommended prompt action to reduce lead exposure in women with prenatal blood lead levels more than or equal to 5 mcg/dL, and medical removal from workplace exposure of any woman with a prenatal blood lead level of more than or equal to 10 mcg/dL.

If workplace blood lead concentrations are maintained below 20 mcg/dL, it may be sufficient to implement a streamlined medical surveillance regimen in which laboratory testing is limited to blood lead measurements every 6 months if blood lead levels remain less than 10 mcg/dL, and every 3 months if blood lead levels are 10–19 mcg/dL. Additional recommended program elements include annual measurement of blood pressure, an annual questionnaire regarding medical conditions (such as renal insufficiency) that might increase the risk of lead-related adverse health effects, and periodic worker education regarding the nature of lead hazards and controls.

In 2012, CDC recommended parental education, environmental investigation, and additional medical monitoring for all children with blood lead concentrations more than or equal to 5 mcg/dL. In 2015, CDC designated an adult blood lead of more than or equal to 5 mcg/dL as elevated for purposes of medical surveillance. EPA regulations effective since 2010 require contractors performing renovation, repair, and painting projects that disturb lead-based paint in pre-1978 residences and child-occupied facilities to undergo certification and to adhere to specific work practices to prevent lead contamination.

Treatment

The essential first step in the management of lead intoxication is identification and elimination of the sources of overexposure. Chelating agents, such as parenteral calcium disodium EDTA (calcium versenate) or oral dimercaptosuccinic acid (DMSA, succimer), decrease lead concentration in the blood and certain tissues and greatly accelerate urinary lead excretion. However, there are no randomized placebo-controlled trials of chelation that indicate it improves the therapeutic outcome of patients. In general, chelation in adults should be reserved for those with markedly elevated blood lead concentrations (eg, > 80–100 mcg/dL), or possibly symptomatic individuals with blood lead concentration

Table 29–6. Medical surveillance recommendations for lead-exposed workers.

Category of Exposure	Recommendation
All lead-exposed workers[a]	Baseline or preplacement medical history and physical examination; baseline BLL, serum creatinine. Annual BP measurement, health questionnaire
BLL < 10 mcg/dL	BLL every month for first 3 mo of placement, or upon change in task to higher exposure, then BLL every 6 mo. If BLL increases ≥ 5 mcg/dL, evaluate exposure and protective measures. Increase monitoring if indicated. For BLL 5–9, reduce exposure for women who are or may become pregnant
BLL 10–19 mcg/dL	As above for BLL < 10 mcg/dL, plus: BLL every 3 mo. Evaluate exposure, engineering controls, and work practices. Consider removal from exposure to avoid long-term risks if exposure control over an extended period does not decrease BLL < 10, or if medical condition present that increases risk with continued exposure. Revert to BLL every 6 mo after 3 BLLs < 10 mcg/dL. Remove pregnant women from exposure
BLL ≥ 20 mcg/dL	Remove from exposure if repeat BLL measured in 4 wk remains ≥ 20 mcg/dL, or if first BLL ≥ 30 mcg/dL. Monthly BLL testing. Consider return to lead work after 2 BLLs < 15 mcg/dL a month apart, then monitor as above

BLL, blood lead level.
[a]Lead-exposed means handling or disturbing materials with a significant lead content in a manner that could reasonably be expected to cause potentially harmful exposure through inhalation or ingestion.

more than 50 mcg/dL. The CDC recommends chelation of children with blood lead concentrations more than or equal to 45 mcg/dL. Chelation of asymptomatic children or adults with low blood lead concentrations is not recommended. Chelation, as well as the supportive care and decontamination required for symptomatic patients, should be conducted under the guidance of an experienced specialist in occupational medicine or medical toxicology. Adjunctive measures include treatment of coexisting iron deficiency anemia, and provision of adequate dietary calcium.

MANGANESE

ESSENTIALS OF DIAGNOSIS

▸ Manganese-induced parkinsonism.

▸ Behavioral changes, psychosis.

▸ Respiratory symptoms and disease.

▸ General Considerations

Manganese is a brittle gray metal that is abundant in soils and sediments. The most important source of manganese for commercial use is manganese dioxide, occurring as pyrolusite. Manganese is an essential trace element in humans with an average daily requirement of 2–5 mg for adults.

▸ Use

Ferromanganese, an iron alloy containing more than 80% manganese metal, is used in steel production. Manganese serves as a depolarizer in dry-cell batteries and an oxidizing agent for chemical syntheses. Manganese is used in the manufacture of matches, paints, and pesticides (Maneb). The manganese carbonyls, particularly methylcyclopentadienyl manganese tricarbonyl (MMT), have been used as antiknock agents in fuel and as sources of manganese in the electronics industry.

▸ Occupational & Environmental Exposure

Exposure to manganese dioxide occurs in the mining, smelting, and refining of manganese ores. Manganese exposure also occurs near crushing operations and reduction furnaces engaged in the production of alloys and steel. These operations historically had the highest levels of exposure and the greatest risk for manganese toxicity.

Exposures may occur in battery production, chemicals plants, and the electronics industry. Workers engaged in the manufacture of fuels containing MMT may have respiratory or skin contact with this highly toxic liquid. Combustion of manganese-containing fuels results in environmental release of manganese oxides. Welding rods and steel alloys are important sources of occupational manganese exposure.

▸ Absorption, Metabolism, & Excretion

Manganese may be absorbed after inhalation of smaller particles (< 10 μm) or ingestion of larger particles or aggregates of fume. Iron deficiency increases manganese absorption, as well as deposition in the basal ganglia.

Manganese is excreted primarily in the bile. The biologic half-life of manganese is approximately 30 hours. Blood, urine, and hair levels are elevated in exposed workers, but individual results do not correlate with symptoms or toxicity. Variations in manganese or iron homeostasis may account for variable individual susceptibility to toxicity.

▸ Clinical Findings

A. Symptoms and Signs

1. Acute exposure—Dermal and respiratory exposure to MMT results in slight burning of the skin followed by headache, a metallic taste, nausea, diarrhea, dyspnea, and chest pain. Acute overexposure to MMT can cause chemical pneumonitis and hepatic and renal toxicity.

2. Chronic exposure—Industrial exposure to manganese can result in accumulation of manganese in the basal ganglia causing Mn-induced parkinsonism. Psychiatric abnormalities, such as emotional disturbances, memory loss, compulsive behavior, delusions, and disorientation may be the initial presenting symptoms. Episodes of excitability, garrulousness, and sexual arousal have been termed manganese psychosis. With continued exposure, there is development of dystonia, slowed speech, masked facies, bradykinesia, gait dysfunction, and micrographia. Tremor is less pronounced in manganese-induced parkinsonism. Salivation, sweating, and vasomotor disturbances also may occur. There are phenotypic distinctions between Mn-induced parkinsonism and idiopathic Parkinson disease.

B. Laboratory Findings

Laboratory findings usually are normal. Minor decreases in leukocyte and red blood cell counts may be seen. Liver enzyme elevations also have been reported. T1-weighted images on magnetic resonance imaging (MRI) demonstrate high signal changes in the globus pallidus indicating manganese accumulation. Measurement of elevated urine or blood manganese levels confirms exposure. These measurements can discriminate exposed from nonexposed groups but do not correlate well with individual exposure or the degree of toxicity.

▸ Prevention

Manganese exposure should be reduced by the use of closed systems, local exhaust ventilation, and respiratory protection. Dermal and respiratory exposure to MMT should be prevented through the use of proper personal protective equipment. Medical surveillance should focus on the nervous system and the respiratory system. Careful neurologic examinations and pulmonary function testing should be performed routinely on all exposed workers. Workers with exposure to MMT also should have periodic assessment of respiratory, liver, and kidney function.

► Treatment

Workers suspected of having manganese-induced parkinsonism should be removed from exposure. Unlike idiopathic Parkinson disease, manganese-induced symptoms are resistant to treatment with levodopa.

After skin contact with MMT, the affected areas should be cleansed immediately to reduce skin absorption. Workers who develop respiratory symptoms after inhalation of MMT should be admitted to the hospital for observation. Liver and kidney function should be monitored.

MERCURY

ESSENTIALS OF DIAGNOSIS

► Elemental mercury
- Acute respiratory distress.
- Tremor.
- Neuropsychiatric disturbances and erethism (shyness, emotional lability).
- Gingivostomatitis.

► Inorganic mercury salts
- Hemorrhagic gastroenteritis.
- Oliguric renal failure.
- Proteinuria.

► Organic mercury (alkyl mercury compounds)
- Paresthesias (peri-oral and distal extremities).
- Constriction of visual fields.
- Ataxia and gait disturbance.
- Dysarthria and hearing loss.
- Cognitive dysfunction.
- Adverse neurodevelopmental effects.

► General Considerations

Elemental mercury is a heavy silvery-white metal that is a liquid at room temperature. The high vapor pressure of mercury results in continuous release into the atmosphere, a major factor contributing to occupational exposure and environmental contamination. Mercury is recovered primarily from cinnabar ore (HgS). The release of mercury into the atmosphere from both natural sources, such as volcanoes and wild fires, and from industrial emissions, particularly coal-burning power plants has led to global distribution of this element. Rainwater captures oxidized mercury and

returns the element to bodies of water, where it is taken up and biomethylated by marine organisms. From there it enters the food chain, resulting in accumulation in animals and humans. Mercury is not an essential element in humans, and reducing environmental exposure continues to be an international concern.

► Use

Elemental mercury is used in control instruments, tubes, rectifiers, thermometers, barometers, batteries, and electrical devices. Mercury in brine cells catalyzes the electrolytic production of chlorine. Historical use of alkyl mercury compounds (methyl mercury and ethyl mercury) as grain fumigants caused serious human poisoning. Use in the felt industry in the nineteenth century led to extensive poisoning ("mad as a hatter"). The use of mercury in artisanal gold mining continues to be a significant source of occupational exposure and environmental contamination in some developing countries. Despite declining utilization, mercury dental amalgams remain an important source of low-level exposure. Almost all use of the organomercury preservative thimerosal in the preparation of vaccines has been discontinued. Mercurous mercury salts have been used in skin lightening creams leading to exposure and toxicity.

The international Minamata Convention on Mercury, signed by 128 countries since 2013, will result in a worldwide phase-out by 2020 of mercury in numerous products including batteries, switches and relays, fluorescent lamps, pesticides, biocides and antiseptics, measuring instruments (eg, thermometers, sphygmomanometers), and manufacturing processes such as chloralkali production (by 2025).

► Occupational & Environmental Exposure

Workers involved in the extraction and recovery of mercury are at high risk for exposure to mercury vapor. Maintenance work on furnaces and flues is another source of exposure. Chloralkali workers can have significant exposure from contamination if workplace hygiene is not maintained.

Mercury is being phased out of medical equipment, although health care workers still may be exposed from damaged or broken equipment or past workplace contamination. Dentists and dental technicians may have short-term peak exposures during certain dental procedures.

Two historic epidemics of overt methylmercury poisoning occurred owing to environmental contamination of food sources. Release of mercury wastes from a chemical plant into Minamata Bay in Japan from 1932 to 1968 led to accumulation of methyl mercury in seafood. *Minamata disease* resulted in neurologic impairment and birth defects in thousands of the affected area residents. Distribution of grain treated with methylmercury fungicides similarly poisoned over 50,000 persons in Iraq in the early 1970s. The largest contemporary source of mercury exposure to the general population consists of dietary methylmercury in fish and shellfish. High-end consumption of seafood with elevated levels of methylmercury, particularly by women of reproductive age and young children, has been associated with subclinical developmental neurotoxicity. FDA and EPA have advised pregnant women, women who might become pregnant, nursing mothers, and young children to avoid consumption of fish with elevated mercury levels (eg, swordfish), to limit consumption of albacore tuna and selected other fish with moderate amounts of mercury to four ounces a week and to otherwise consume 8–12 ounces of a variety of low mercury fish per week (see http://www.fda.gov/Food/FoodborneIllnessContaminants/Metals/ucm393070.htm).

▶ Absorption, Metabolism, & Excretion

Elemental mercury is efficiently absorbed after the inhalation but not ingestion. Soluble mercurial salts and aryl mercury compounds undergo gastrointestinal absorption; absorption by inhalation is rare but possible. Alkyl mercury compounds are absorbed readily through all routes, including skin contact.

Inorganic and aryl mercury compounds are distributed to many tissues, although the brain and kidney are the primary target organs. There they bind to sulfhydryl groups and interfere with numerous cellular enzyme systems and membranes. Metallothionein, a family of proteins rich in cysteine containing sulfhydryl groups, binds numerous metals including mercury and may exert a protective effect in the kidney. Alkyl mercury in the bloodstream is taken up rapidly by red blood cells and also accumulates in brain tissue.

Both organic and elemental mercury compounds readily cross the placenta and are secreted in breast milk. Peak exposures to both organic and inorganic mercury compounds are more hazardous because of the intense effects on the central nervous system. Mercury compounds are principally eliminated in the urine (major route for inorganic and elemental) and feces (major route for organic mercury). Elimination follows a biphasic pattern, initially rapid, then slow. The urinary elimination half-time is approximately 40 days for inorganic mercury. The half-time of methylmercury in blood is variable but averages 50 days. Sectional analysis of mercury in hair has been used as a biomarker of methylmercury exposure in epidemiologic studies.

▶ Clinical Findings

A. Symptoms and Signs

The spectrum of clinical effects associated with mercury compounds depends strongly on their chemical form, which in turn influences their uptake and distribution to target organs.

1. Inorganic mercury—Inhalation of high concentrations of elemental mercury vapor, particularly when heated, may result in a life-threatening pneumonitis and noncardiogenic pulmonary edema. Acute gingivostomatitis may also occur. Less intense inhalation exposure, particularly in a subchronic or chronic pattern, may result in the classic triad of tremor, neuropsychiatric disturbance, and gingivostomatitis. Neuropsychiatric manifestations, including fatigue, insomnia, anorexia, and memory loss are common. There may be an insidious change in mood to shyness, withdrawal, and depression along with explosive anger or blushing, a behavioral pattern referred to as erethism. Mercurial tremor typically begins as a fine intention tremor of the fingers, but may progress to involve the face and choreiform movements of the limbs. Subclinical changes in peripheral nerve function may occur but overt sensorimotor peripheral neuropathy is rare. Low-level exposure to elemental mercury vapor may be associated with subclinical neurologic deficits.

In contrast to the neurologic manifestations associated with elemental mercury inhalation, ingestion of mercury salts, particularly mercuric chloride, may result in the abrupt development of a corrosive gastroenteritis, accompanied by abdominal pain and bloody diarrhea, and in severe cases by shock, intestinal necrosis, and death. Oliguric renal failure from acute tubular necrosis may appear after an interval of several hours to days. Chronic exposure to inorganic salts may result in neurologic and renal effects, the latter sometimes manifested by proteinuria.

Acrodynia is a rare idiosyncratic reaction that may appear after chronic inorganic mercury exposure. Occurring predominantly in exposed children, the presentation features hypertension, pain in the extremities that is often accompanied by pinkish discoloration and desquamation, profuse sweating, anorexia, insomnia, irritability and/or apathy, and a miliary rash.

2. Organic mercury—Exposure to alkyl mercury compounds results in the delayed (weeks to months) insidious onset of progressive nervous system damage that may be fatal. The earliest symptoms are of numbness and tingling of the extremities and perioral region. Loss of motor coordination follows, with gait ataxia, tremor, and deficits in fine motor control. Constriction of the visual fields, dysarthria, and central hearing loss occur, and behavioral changes and intellectual impairment may be prominent. Developmental neurotoxicity in infants exposed in utero in the Minamata Bay epidemic resembled cerebral palsy. Developmental deficits may occur in the absence of overt maternal toxicity. Severe poisoning with thimerosal, or its mercurial metabolite ethylmercury, has been associated with nephrotoxicity as well as neurotoxicity.

B. Laboratory Findings

After acute high-dose inhalation, there may be hypoxemia and diffuse infiltrates on chest x-ray. Acute tubular necrosis from ingestion of inorganic mercury salts may be accompanied in early stages by hematuria and proteinuria, and subsequently by increasing serum BUN and creatinine as oliguric renal failure ensues.

Most individuals without occupational exposure will have a urine mercury concentration less than 1.5 mcg/L and a blood mercury concentration less than 5 mcg/L. Overt neurologic effects have been observed in individuals with chronic urine mercury levels of 100–200 mcg/L, although lower values may be noted in pediatric cases of acrodynia. After methylmercury exposure, symptoms have been observed at whole blood mercury concentrations in excess of 200 mcg/L; however, subclinical neurodevelopmental deficits may occur at lower concentrations. Measurement of whole blood and urine mercury concentration is useful in assessing exposure to mercury. Blood mercury is the key biomarker of methylmercury exposure (which undergoes minimal renal excretion). Shortly after initial overexposure to elemental and inorganic mercury blood values may increase more rapidly than urinary levels.

Prevention

Awareness of the constant hazard of mercury vapor exposure along with proper handling of materials and meticulous attention to workplace hygiene will reduce potential exposures. Use of proper ventilation and respiratory protection is required in all operations that use mercury compounds. Special attention should focus on maintenance workers. Care in the handling and disposal of mercury compounds will prevent inadvertent contamination of the workplace. Because of its high vapor pressure, even minute spills of metallic mercury (eg, 1 mL) may result in a chronic inhalation hazard in a residence, school, or commercial building. Agency for Toxic Substances and Disease Registry (ATSDR) offers guidance on the management of mercury spills in residences, commercial buildings, and vehicles (https://www.atsdr.cdc.gov/emergency_response/action_levels_for_elemental_mercury_spills_2012.pdf). EPA provides instructions for the cleanup of small spills, for example, the amount in a mercury thermometer (https://www.epa.gov/mercury/what-do-if-mercury-thermometer-breaks), as well as somewhat larger spills, for example, up to two tablespoons (https://www.epa.gov/mercury/what-do-if-you-spill-more-mercury-amount-thermometer). Elemental mercury spills resulting in release of more than 1 lb (2 tablespoons) to the environment require mandatory notification of the EPA National Response Center, and in most cases will require remediation by a specialized hazardous response contractor.

In 2013, the American Conference of Governmental Industrial Hygienists (ACGIH) revised its biological exposure index for elemental mercury to a preshift urine value of 20 mcg/g creatinine to minimize the risk of neurologic and renal toxicity.

Treatment

After acute exposure to elemental mercury droplets, contaminated clothing and footwear should be removed, enclosed in airtight bags, and professionally discarded. Skin should be thoroughly irrigated. Individuals potentially exposed to high airborne levels should be observed for several hours for the delayed presentation of pneumonitis or pulmonary edema. After acute ingestion of mercuric salts, anticipate severe gastroenteritis and delayed renal failure and treat supportively with vigorous IV fluid replacement. Prompt chelation with intravenous unithiol (DMPS) or intramuscular dimercaprol (BAL) may mitigate nephrotoxicity after mercuric salt ingestion. Oral succimer (DMSA) may also be considered, although its oral bioavailability in the setting of severe gastroenteritis and shock is uncertain. Unithiol or succimer may accelerate the renal elimination of mercury following elemental mercury exposure, but the impact on clinical outcome is uncertain. In methylmercury intoxication, sparse data suggest that oral succimer and N-acetylcysteine (NAC) may be effective in decreasing mercury levels in the tissues, including the brain. Dimercaprol (BAL) may redistribute mercury to the brain and should be avoided after intoxication with elemental mercury or methylmercury since the brain is a key target organ.

OTHER METALS

1. Antimony

General Considerations

Antimony is a soft metal that is found as oxides and sulfides in a variety of ores. Antimony metal is used in semiconductors and antimony oxide in nanoparticles. Antimony alloys are used in battery grids, type castings, bearings, and cable sheaths. Antimony compounds have application in munitions, glass and pottery, fire retardants, paints and lacquers, rubber compounds, chemical catalysts, and solder. Pentavalent antimonials are used medicinally in the treatment of leishmaniasis, schistosomiasis, and filariasis.

Occupational & Environmental Exposure

Mining and smelting operations have resulted in significant worker exposure to antimony dusts and fumes. Health effects attributed to exposure to antimony during refining include respiratory tract irritation and pneumoconiosis. Antimony trioxide and antimony trichloride used in the microelectronics industry are strong irritants.

Stibine gas (SbH_3), a hemolytic toxin similar to arsine, may be formed when antimony alloys are processed with certain reducing acids. Stibine is also used as a grain fumigant. Parenteral administration of antimonial compounds for medicinal purposes is associated with electrocardiographic changes, alterations in liver function, and hemolysis. Soluble forms of antimony are readily absorbed after inhalation. Antimony is excreted largely in the urine. Urinary antimony levels have been correlated with possible sleep disturbances.

Clinical Findings

Acute exposure to antimony dusts and fumes causes intense irritation of the eyes, throat, and respiratory tract. Stibine gas toxicity leads to jaundice and anuria as a consequence of massive hemolysis. Chronic skin exposure to antimony compounds may cause pustular dermatitis. Antimony is suspected of being a human carcinogen.

Hemoglobinuria and red blood cell casts are a sign of stibine-induced hemolysis. Electrocardiographic changes after therapeutic use or industrial exposure include T-wave changes and rhythm disturbances.

Acute inhalation of antimony trichloride can cause pulmonary edema. Rounded opacities in the middle lung fields on chest radiograph or CT scan are consistent with antimony pneumoconiosis. The presence of antimony in urine is diagnostic of past exposure but not with severity of exposure or health effects.

► Prevention

Chelation with dimercaprol or penicillamine is indicated when significant cardiovascular, pulmonary, or hepatic impairment occurs after acute exposure. Stibine-induced hemolysis requires exchange transfusion.

Personal protective devices should be worn where there is potential exposure to antimony dusts or fumes. Biologic monitoring of urinary antimony levels confirms exposure.

2. Nickel

► General Considerations

Nickel is a hard, silver-white, malleable, magnetic metal that has wide industrial application. Nickel is refined by electrolysis or the Mond process, in which treatment with carbon monoxide leads to the formation of nickel carbonyl [$Ni(CO)_4$]. Nickel occurs naturally in a variety of vegetables and grains.

The major use of nickel is in the production of stainless steel. Nickel alloys provide durability for use in food and dairy processing equipment. Coins, tableware and utensils, springs, magnets, batteries (nickel–cadmium), and spark plugs use nickel alloys. Nickel salts are used in electroplating to impart lustrous, polishable, corrosion-resistant surfaces to parts and equipment. Nickel compounds are also used as catalysts and pigments.

► Occupational & Environmental Exposure

Exposure to nickel compounds may occur during mining, milling, and refining operations. In the Mond process, workers also may be exposed to highly toxic nickel carbonyl gas. In electroplating shops, workers may have respiratory and skin exposure to soluble nickel salts. Workers using nickel as a catalyst may be exposed to nickel powders.

Nickel is poorly absorbed from the gastrointestinal tract. Soluble nickel compounds and nickel carbonyl are readily absorbed after inhalation. Absorbed nickel does not accumulate in tissues and is excreted in the urine with a half-life of approximately 1 week. Insoluble nickel compounds may accumulate in the respiratory tract—a factor that may contribute to carcinogenicity.

► Clinical Findings

The most common manifestations of exposure to soluble nickel compounds are dermatologic. Nickel is a common cause of allergic contact dermatitis. Exposure to high levels of soluble nickel aerosols also may cause rhinitis, sinusitis, and anosmia. Cough and wheezing should suggest the possibility of nickel-induced asthma. Exposure to nickel carbonyl causes headache, fatigue, and nausea followed by delayed interstitial pneumonitis, delirium, seizures, and coma. Nickel is considered a human respiratory tract carcinogen. Nickel skin allergy is confirmed by patch test.

► Treatment & Prevention

Nickel dermatitis is treated with topical steroids and avoidance of contact exposure. Acute nickel carbonyl poisoning is treated with sodium diethyldithiocarbamate (ditiocarb sodium) or disulfiram.

Skin and respiratory protection should be used where there is potential exposure to nickel dusts, fumes, or soluble nickel aerosols and liquids. Medical surveillance should concentrate on the skin and respiratory system, with prompt removal of those who develop dermal or respiratory allergy. A biologic threshold level of 10 mcg/L in plasma is recommended for workers exposed to nickel compounds. A maximum level of 10 mcg/L in the urine is recommended for workers exposed to nickel carbonyl.

3. Selenium & Tellurium

► General Considerations

Selenium and tellurium are distributed widely in mineral ores, particularly in sulfur and copper deposits. Selenium is an essential trace element in humans, preventing oxidative damage in erythrocytes. Tellurium is not an essential trace element for humans.

Selenium is used in the manufacture of glass and plastics to impart a red tint or to neutralize green discoloration. The photoconducting properties of selenium are useful in rectifiers and solar cells. Selenium is used in paint pigments, animal feeds, and veterinary medicines. It is used medicinally in dandruff shampoos and topical antifungal lotions and is promoted as a dietary supplement. Tellurium is used in the vulcanization of rubber to increase durability. Like selenium, tellurium is finding increasing use in electronics, primarily in the manufacture of photocells and semiconductors.

► Occupational & Environmental Exposure

Workers engaged in the refining of copper and silver may be exposed to airborne selenium and tellurium fumes and dust. Selenium and tellurium are encountered in the electronics, glass, ceramics, plastics, and rubber industries. Formulators may be exposed to selenium in the production of pharmaceuticals and animal feed. Agricultural use of sodium selenite as a pesticide and selenium contamination of phosphate fertilizers has led to soil and groundwater contamination.

Selenium and tellurium compounds may be absorbed through the lungs, gastrointestinal tract, or damaged skin. Selenium is metabolized to organic forms in the liver.

Dimethyl selenium and dimethyl telluride are excreted through the lungs and impart a garlic odor to the breath. Tellurium accumulates in liver and bone, and excretion may be prolonged after exposure.

▶ Clinical Findings

Acute inhalation of selenium or tellurium fumes, oxide dusts, halide vapors, hydrogen selenide, or telluride may cause severe respiratory irritation, resulting in cough, chest pain, and dyspnea. Neurologic, hepatic, and renal damage may occur. Selenium oxide may cause severe skin burns. Both can cause a garlicky odor of the breath, and tellurium exposure often causes a blue-black discoloration of the skin.

Chronic exposure to selenium and tellurium compounds may result in nonspecific complaints of fatigue and lassitude. There is often a strong garlic odor to the breath and sweat. Chronic airborne selenium exposure may cause conjunctivitis, termed *rose eye*. Dermatologic manifestations include irritant or allergic dermatitis, painful paronychia, and loss of hair and nails. Reddish skin and hair discoloration also may be present.

Laboratory evaluation usually is nondiagnostic. Liver enzyme elevations and anemia may be seen. Measurement of selenium in the urine will confirm overexposure, normal concentrations being less than 150 mcg/L.

▶ Treatment & Prevention

Prompt evacuation and resuscitation should be undertaken in cases of acute inhalation. Burns of the skin should be irrigated with a solution of 10% aqueous sodium thiosulfate followed by use of a 10% sodium thiosulfate cream. Administration of ascorbic acid may lessen the offensive garlic odor of exposed individuals. Chelation is contraindicated and may cause renal damage.

Respiratory and skin protection should be used where exposure to high levels of airborne selenium and tellurium compounds cannot be controlled through other means. Medical surveillance should focus on gastrointestinal and dermatologic complaints. Urine selenium should remain below 100 mcg/L in individuals exposed to air levels of 0.1 mg/m^3. Urinary tellurium levels should be kept below 0.05 mg/L. Pregnant women should not work directly with tellurium compounds.

4. Thallium

▶ General Considerations

Thallium is found in iron, copper, sulfide, and selenide ores. Thallium is prepared as water-soluble (sulfate, acetate) and water-insoluble (halide) salts. Thallium sulfate was used as a medicinal agent in the treatment of syphilis, gonorrhea, gout, and tuberculosis in the nineteenth century and as a depilatory in the 1920s. Thallium salts were once added to pastes and grains as rodenticides leading to numerous accidental, homicidal, and suicidal poisonings. Currently, thallium

is finding increasing uses in the manufacture of electronic components, optical lenses, imitation jewelry, dyes, and pigments. [^{201}Tl]Cl is used in myocardial imaging.

▶ Occupational & Environmental Exposure

Workers may encounter thallium in the thallium salt production, electronics, and optical industries. Smelting operations can expose maintenance workers and result in air and water contamination.

▶ Clinical Findings

Thallium is absorbed readily through the gastrointestinal tract, skin, and respiratory system. Thallium binds avidly enzyme systems interferes with cellular respiration and protein synthesis. With acute exposure or ingestion gastrointestinal symptoms predominate early, followed by cardiac and neurologic manifestations, particularly painful dysesthesias. An ascending paralysis may follow. Alopecia occurs at the end of the first week. In chronic intoxication, alopecia and dry skin may be the only complaint. Fatigue, asthenia, insomnia, and behavioral dysfunction may be presenting symptoms. Nerve-conduction studies are consistent with axonal degeneration and the diagnosis is confirmed by demonstrating elevated thallium levels in the urine. Normal levels range from 0 to 10 mcg/L and levels in workers should be maintained below 50 mcg/L. In acute cases, treatment with Prussian blue will bind secreted thallium in the gut. Potassium chloride will exchange with thallium in cells and increase renal excretion. Chelating agents have not been shown to be effective in chronic intoxication. Recovery generally is complete, although permanent blindness and hair loss have been reported.

▶ Prevention

Proper skin and respiratory protection are essential. Eating and smoking should not be permitted in areas where thallium compounds are handled. Thallium is a cumulative toxin, and biologic monitoring of urine levels should be considered where there is chronic exposure to thallium compounds. The banning of thallium-containing pesticides has reduced the frequency of thallium poisoning in the United States, but these compounds still may be encountered and are still available in other countries.

5. Vanadium

▶ General Considerations

Vanadium is a soft gray metal that is derived commercially from vanadium sulfide ores. Vanadium is found in fossil fuels, contributing to environmental contamination. Vanadium imparts strength and elasticity to steel and durability for high-speed tool bits. Vanadium is also used as a catalyst for plastics, a mordant in dyeing, and a colorant in ceramics and glass.

Occupational & Environmental Exposure

Exposure to vanadium pentoxide dusts and fumes may occur during milling and roasting. An inhalation hazard exists in cleaning fuel dusts from oil and coal. Fossil-fuel-burning power stations may emit vanadium compounds, resulting in environmental contamination and air pollution. Vanadium compounds are absorbed after inhalation or ingestion. Excretion is primarily renal, with little bioaccumulation.

Clinical Findings

Acute exposure to high levels of vanadium pentoxide dusts or fume results in eye irritation, epistaxis, cough, and bronchitis. Pneumonia may follow acute exposures. Sensitivity to vanadium may result in occupational asthma or allergic dermatitis. An unusual presentation of chronic exposure is a green discoloration of the tongue. Patch testing may be used to confirm dermal sensitization to vanadium compounds.

Treatment & Prevention

Persons who develop respiratory or dermatologic allergy should be permanently removed from exposure. Proper respiratory protection is critical when handling vanadium compounds and during the cleaning of oil and coal furnace flues. Medical surveillance focuses on respiratory and dermatologic complaints, looking for respiratory or skin sensitization. Biologic monitoring of vanadium in urine (end of shift/end of workweek) may be useful in controlling exposure.

WELDING

Welding is a joining process with wide application in manufacturing and the building trades. Through the application of heat or pressure, welding joins metals with a lightweight bond, with strength and resistance approaching that of the parent metal. Welding is a labor-intensive activity. Even though automated welding methods are finding increasing applications, manual arc welding remains the principal industrial welding process.

Health Hazards of Welding

Welders work with a wide variety of materials under varied conditions and are exposed to many health hazards, including air contaminants (metal fumes, particulates, gases); physical agents such as radiation (infrared, ultraviolet), noise, and electricity; and ergonomic stress. Tables 29–7 and 29–8 list the common air contaminants of different welding processes. Shielded metal arc (SMA) welding of mild steel, or "stick welding," is the most common use of welding. The main exposure is to iron oxide, and pulmonary deposition of this nonfibrogenic particulate has resulted in the development of a benign pneumoconiosis. Exposure to manganese and fluoride fumes may be considerable when certain welding rods are used.

The corrosion-resistant properties of stainless steel are a result of a high concentration of chromium (18–30%). Nickel

Table 29–7. Air contaminants of selected welding processes.

Process	Base Metal	Contaminants
Shielded metal arc (stick welding)	Mild steel	Dust, iron oxide, manganese
Shielded metal arc (stick welding)	Stainless steel	Chromium, nickel, manganese, fluorides
Gas metal arc (MIG)	Stainless steel	Chromium, nickel, manganese, nitrogen oxides, ozone
Tungsten inert gas (TIG)	Aluminum	Ozone, aluminum oxide
Gas, brazing, cutting	Variable	Nitrogen oxides, cadmium oxide, metal fume

and manganese also may be present in different stainless steel alloys. Exposure to chromium (including CrVI), nickel, and manganese may be considerable, particularly with gas metal arc processes. The stainless steel surface reflects ultraviolet radiation, with formation of oxides of nitrogen and ozone. Low-hydrogen welding of stainless steel generates high concentrations of fluoride fumes.

Most aluminum welding uses the tungsten inert gas method. As with stainless steel, the gas-shielded process results in formation of ozone as a consequence of the action of ultraviolet radiation on the nascent oxygen in the atmosphere. Total dust and aluminum oxide generation are also considerable.

Table 29–8. Potential hazards of welding processes.

Air contaminants	
Metals	
Iron oxide	Benign pneumoconiosis
Manganese	Neurotoxicity, pneumonia
Cadmium oxide	Acute lung injury
Zinc oxide	Metal fume fever
Chromium	Lung cancer, allergy
Nickel	Lung cancer, allergy
Fluoride	Skin or respiratory irritation
Gases	
Ozone	Respiratory irritation, asthma
Nitrogen oxides	Acute lung injury
Carbon monoxide	Systemic poisoning
Physical hazards	
Radiation	
Ultraviolet	Photokeratitis, skin erythema
Infrared	Burns, cataracts(?)
Electricity	Electric shock, electrocution
Noise	Hearing loss
Ergonomic stress	Muscle strain

Brazing and gas welding both generate metal fume. An acetylene torch is used to generate an intense flame. Exposure to cadmium oxide from cadmium-containing silver solder has caused acute lung injury and death after brazing in enclosed spaces. Similar consequences have occurred from generation of the oxides of nitrogen during gas welding. In all cases, improper ventilation was the critical factor in creating the hazard.

Radiation and heat result in the most common injuries to welders: photokeratitis (welder's flash) and thermal burns. These are often related to improper use of protective goggles, gloves, and screens. Flying sparks or debris may cause burns or eye injury as well. Noise exposure may exceed 80 dB in welding processes, particularly cutting or gouging operations; in plasma welding (where intense heat is generated), levels may approach 120 dB. Environmental conditions also will influence noise generation. Electrical shock is a constant hazard and requires careful grounding and shielding of cables and equipment. Most manual processes place isometric stress on the welder, particularly involving the shoulders and the upper extremities.

Coatings or contaminants may present additional hazards (Table 29–9), particularly when their presence and potential hazard are unknown or unsuspected. The formation of toxic gases, fumes, or vapors usually is due to the heating of a coated or treated metal, although phosgene exposure is related to the action of ultraviolet radiation or heat on chlorinated hydrocarbon vapors (similar to the formation of ozone from oxygen and oxides of nitrogen from nitrogen).

Soldering is not associated with significant exposure to metal fumes because the temperatures are low. Potential contamination of the workplace with lead dust requires careful attention to hygiene. Some fluxes, such as rosin, are skin sensitizers and may cause allergic dermatitis or asthma.

▶ Clinical Findings

A. Acute Exposure

1. Photokeratitis—Photokeratitis is the result of exposure of the cornea to ultraviolet B radiation (UVB) in the range of 280–315 nm. The duration of exposure necessary to induce this effect varies with the distance from the arc and the light intensity. Following exposure of the unprotected eye to the welding arc for several seconds, the worker develops pain, burning, or a feeling of "sand or grit" in the eye. Physical examination shows conjunctival injection, and slit-lamp examination may reveal punctate depressions over the cornea. The condition is self-limited, resolving in several hours. Careful examination for foreign bodies or evidence of thermal ocular injury is mandatory.

2. Metal fume fever—Metal fume fever is a benign, self-limited condition characterized by the delayed onset (8–12 hours) of fever, chills, cough, myalgias, and a metallic taste. A history of welding on galvanized metal suggests the diagnosis.

3. Upper respiratory irritation—Upper respiratory tract irritation may result from exposure to a variety of welding contaminants, including dusts, ozone, aluminum oxide, nitrogen oxides, cadmium oxide, and fluorides. Asthma also may be triggered as a result of nonspecific irritation or allergy (chromium, nickel).

4. Acute lung injury—While unusual, exposure to oxides of nitrogen and cadmium oxide may cause acute lung injury and delayed pulmonary edema. A history of gas welding or brazing in enclosed or poorly ventilated spaces or sheet metal work should raise this concern and serve as an indication for careful medical evaluation and observation.

5. Work-related asthma—Exposure to sensitizing agents or irritants in welding fumes can result in work-related asthma.

B. Chronic Exposure

1. Siderosis—Siderosis results from accumulation of nonfibrogenic iron oxide particles in the lung. While the radiographic appearance may be dramatic, with evidence of diffuse reticulonodular densities, reports of deficits of pulmonary function are inconsistent, suggesting a mild or minimal effect. In welders who also have been exposed to crystalline silica or asbestos, radiographic differentiation of hemosiderosis from pulmonary fibrosis is difficult. Pleural thickening or calcification has not been related to welding in the absence of asbestos exposure.

2. Other chronic effects—Welders report an excess of respiratory symptoms and have increased work absences from respiratory diseases. Welding fumes can result in a decrease in lung function and increased risk of COPD, and diffuse interstitial fibrotic disease has been reported. Welding has been associated with an increased risk of pneumonia, and a recent study shows an increased risk of invasive pneumococcal disease. The International Agency for Research on **Cancer** (IARC) has concluded that exposure to **welding** fumes causes **lung cancer** in humans, especially due to exposure to the carcinogens hexavalent chromium (Cr[VI]), and nickel.

▶ Prevention

Most acute injuries or poisonings related to welding processes are preventable. Strict adherence to appropriate safety

Table 29–9. Coatings and contaminants encountered in welding.

Galvanized metal	Zinc oxide
Paints	Lead, cadmium, isocyanates, aldehydes, epoxies
Biocides	Organic mercury, organic tin
Chlorinated solvents	Phosgene
Rustproofing	Phosphorus, phosphine
Alloys, sheet metal	Cadmium, nickel, manganese, beryllium
Solders	Rosin, colophony

procedures will prevent burns, eye injuries, and electric shock. Awareness of the potential hazards, with attention to the provision of adequate ventilation, is the best safeguard against accidental overexposure to air contaminants. In enclosed spaces, air-supplied respirators are essential, particularly with processes that result in generation of nitrogen oxides. Pneumococcal vaccination should be considered for welders in light of the increased risk of invasive pneumococcal disease.

▶ Treatment

The primary treatment for metal fume fever is supportive with oral hydration and the use of antipyretics and anti-inflammatory medications (eg, nonsteroidal anti-inflammatory drugs and aspirin). Welders suspected of having acute overexposure to nitrogen oxides, phosgene, or cadmium oxide should be observed for possible development of pulmonary edema. Treatment of pulmonary edema and respiratory insufficiency related to these agents is supportive. Individuals with work-related asthma caused by welding should be removed from the source of exposure. Engineering controls (ventilation) and/or respiratory protection may not be feasible to protect against work-related asthma, and the individual may need to be reassigned to another job (if possible).

REFERENCES

Baker BA et al: Arsenic exposure, assessment, toxicity, diagnosis and management. Guidance for occupational and environmental physicians. J Occup Env Med. 2018;19:e634 [PMID: 30358658].

Balmes JR et al: An official American Thoracic Society statement: diagnosis and management of beryllium sensitivity and chronic beryllium disease. Am J Respir Crit Care Med 2014;190(10):e34 [PMID: 25398119].

Centers for Disease Control and Prevention (CDC): Guidelines for the Identification and Management of Lead Exposure in Pregnant and Lactating Women. CDC, 2010. http://www.cdc.gov/nceh/lead/publications/LeadandPregnancy2010.pdf.

Centers for Disease Control and Prevention (CDC): Low Level Lead Exposure Harms Children, 2012. http://www.cdc.gov/nceh/lead/ACCLPP/Final_Document_030712.pdf.

Cherrie JW, Levy L: Managing occupational exposure to welding fume: new evidence suggests a more precautionary approach is needed. Ann Work Expo Health 2020;64(1):1 [PMID: 31686108].

Environmental Protection Agency. Integrated Science Assessment for Lead. EPA: Research Triangle Park, NC. 2013. http://epa.gov/ncea/isa/lead.htm.

Gibb HJ: Extended followup of a cohort of chromium production workers. Am J Ind Med 2015;905 [PMID: 26041683].

Honaryar MK et al: Welding fumes and lung cancer: a meta-analysis of case-control and cohort studies. Occup Environ Med 2019; 76(6):422 [PMID: 30948521].

Kosnett MJ et al: Recommendations for medical management of adult lead exposure. Environ Health Perspect 2007;115:463 [PMID: 17431500].

Kwakye G: Manganese-induced Parkinsonism and Parkinson's disease: shared and distinguishable features. Int J Environ Res Public Health 2015;12(7):7519 [PMID: 26154659].

Lin G: Clinical characteristics and treatment of thallium poisoning in patients with delayed admission in China. Medicine (Baltimore). 2019;98(29):e16471 [PMID: 31335706].

■ SELF-ASSESSMENT QUESTIONS

Select the one correct answer for each question.

Question 1: Chronic arsenic ingestion
a. may result in chronic renal failure
b. causes severe CNS disturbances and mental illness
c. causes arthralgias and myalgias
d. may cause cancer of the skin, lung, and bladder

Question 2: Chronic berylliosis
a. seldom presents with exertional dyspnea
b. may develop following a single acute exposure
c. does not cause chest pain
d. is associated with parkinsonism

Question 3: The beryllium lymphocyte proliferation test (BeLPT)
a. confirms sensitization
b. leaves no room for error or misinterpretation
c. requires only one borderline test to confirm sensitization
d. requires two borderline tests to confirm sensitization

Question 4: Chronic exposure to cadmium
a. may lead to diabetes mellitus
b. may result in diabetic nephropathy
c. can result in nephrolithiasis and osteomalacia
d. is associated with an excess risk of testicular cancer

Question 5: Exposures to chromic acid or chromates
a. always lead to immediate symptoms
b. do not result in cough, chest pain, and dyspnea
c. may result in chromium-induced asthma
d. are associated with an increased incidence of bone cancer

Question 6: Acute high-dose lead exposure
  a. may induce a hemolytic anemia
  b. depresses hepatic aminotransferases
  c. causes persistent azotemia
  d. may cause bronchospasm

Question 7: Chronic lead intoxication
  a. presents with classic symptoms that lead to rapid diagnosis
  b. affects the peripheral nervous system only in children
  c. primarily results from workplace exposure in adults
  d. may result in gastrointestinal bleeding

Question 8: Workers should be removed from workplace lead exposure
  a. for a single blood lead level greater than 20 mcg/dL
  b. when two successive blood lead levels measured over a 4-week interval are equal to or greater than 10 mcg/dL
  c. when the ZPP exceeds 25 mcg/dL
  d. with a prenatal blood lead level of equal to or greater than 10 mcg/dL

Question 9: Industrial exposure to manganese
  a. results in chronic nervous system stimulation without damage
  b. may cause fatigue, headache, apathy, but no observable behavioral changes
  c. may lead to a clinical syndrome that is similar to idiopathic parkinsonism
  d. causes a tremor that is more pronounced than parkinsonism

Question 10: Mercury
  a. is an essential element in humans
  b. exposure in the environment is of no consequence
  c. is a powdery gray metal at room temperature
  d. emissions have led to global distribution of this element

Question 11: Nickel
  a. is nontoxic
  b. is a common cause of allergic contact dermatitis
  c. may cause septal perforation
  d. may cause brain cancer

Chemicals

Robert J. Harrison, MD, MPH

ACIDS & ALKALIS

Acids and alkalis are of great importance as industrial chemicals. When ranked by volume of production, the inorganic acids and alkalis (including chlorine and ammonia) are 5 of the 10 major chemicals produced yearly in the United States.

1. Acids

ESSENTIALS OF DIAGNOSIS

▶ Acute effects
  • Irritative dermatitis, skin burn.
  • Respiratory irritation, pulmonary edema.
▶ Chronic effects
  • Hydrofluoric acid: osteosclerosis.
  • Nitric acid (oxides of nitrogen): bronchiolitis fibrosa obliterans.
  • Chromic acid: nasal ulceration, perforation, skin ulceration.
  • Sulfuric acid: laryngeal cancer.

▶ General Considerations

An inorganic acid is a compound of hydrogen and one or more other elements (with the exception of carbon) that dissociates to produce hydrogen ions when dissolved in water or other solvents. The resulting solution has the ability to neutralize bases and turn litmus paper red. Inorganic acids of greatest industrial use are chromic, hydrochloric, hydrofluoric, nitric, phosphoric, and sulfuric acids. Inorganic acids share certain fire, explosive, and health hazards.

Organic acids and their derivatives include a broad range of substances used in nearly every type of chemical manufacture. All have primary irritant effects depending on the degree of acid dissociation and water solubility.

▶ Use, Production, & Occupational Exposure

A. Inorganic Acids

1. Sulfuric acid—Sulfuric acid is the leading chemical in production volume. It is less costly than any other acid, can be handled easily, reacts with many organic compounds to produce useful products, and forms a slightly soluble salt with calcium oxide or calcium hydroxide. The majority of sulfuric acid is used in the manufacture of phosphate and other fertilizers, petroleum refining, production of ammonium sulfate, iron and steel pickling, manufacture of explosives and other nitrates, synthetic fiber manufacture, and as a chemical intermediate. Workers with potential exposure to sulfuric acid include electroplaters, jewelers, metal cleaners, picklers, and storage-battery makers. Occupational exposure can occur both by skin contact and by inhalation of sulfuric acid mist.

2. Phosphoric acid—Phosphoric acid is used predominantly in the manufacture of fertilizers and agricultural feeds, in water treatment, and as a component of detergents and cleansers. Other uses include the acid treatment (pickling) of sheet metal, chemical polishing of metals, as a tart flavoring agent for carbonated beverages, as a refractory bonding agent, and for boiler cleaning, textile dying, lithographic engraving, and rubber latex coagulation. Occupational exposure occurs primarily to the liquid acid by skin contact.

3. Chromic acid—Chromic acid is produced by roasting chromite ore with soda ash and treatment with sulfuric acid to form chromic acid anhydride, chromic acid (chromium trioxide), and dichromic acid. Chromic acid is used in chromium plating, process engraving, cement manufacturing, anodizing, metal cleaning, tanning, and the manufacture of ceramic glazes, colored glass, inks, and paints. Without local exhaust ventilation, occupational exposure to chromic acid mist during metal-plating operations can range up to several milligrams per cubic meter.

4. Nitric acid—Nitric acid is produced from the oxidation of ammonia in the presence of a catalyst to yield nitric oxide, which is then further oxidized and absorbed in water to form an aqueous solution of nitric acid. Nitric acid is used to produce ammonium and potassium nitrate, explosives, adipic acid, isocyanates, fertilizers, nitroparaffins, and nitrobenzenes. Occupational exposure can occur by topical contact with the liquid acid, as well as by inhalation of nitrogen oxides evolved when nitric acid reacts with reducing agents (eg, metals or organic matter) or during the combustion of nitrogen-containing materials (eg, welding, glass blowing, underground blasting, and decomposition of agricultural silage). Reports of occupational exposure to nitric acid are limited to measurements of nitrogen oxides that evolved by these reactions.

5. Hydrochloric acid—Hydrochloric acid is an aqueous solution of hydrogen chloride and is used in steel pickling, chemical manufacturing, oil- and gas-well acidizing, and food processing. Hydrochloric acid gas also may evolve from thermal degradation of polyvinyl chloride, a hazard to firefighters.

6. Hydrofluoric acid—Hydrofluoric acid (hydrogen fluoride) is a colorless liquid manufactured by reaction of sulfuric acid with calcium fluoride in heated kilns. It evolves as a gas and then is condensed as liquid anhydrous hydrogen fluoride. Hydrofluoric acid is used as an intermediate in the production of fluorocarbons, aluminum fluoride, and cryolite; as a gasoline alkylation catalyst; and as an intermediate in the production of uranium hexafluoride. It is used in metal cleaning, glass etching, polishing applications, and semiconductor manufacturing. Occupational exposure can occur both by direct skin contact and by inhalation of fumes.

7. Organic acids—Among the saturated monocarboxylic acids, formic acid is used mainly in the textile industry as a dye-exhausting agent, in the leather industry as a deliming agent and neutralizer, as a coagulant for rubber latex, and as a component of nickel plating baths. Propionic acid is used in organic synthesis, as a mold inhibitor, and as a food additive. The unsaturated monocarboxylic acid, acrylic acid, is used widely in the manufacture of resins, plasticizers, and drugs. The aliphatic dicarboxylic acids like maleic, fumaric, and adipic acids find use in the manufacture of synthetic resins, dyes, surface coatings, inks, and plasticizers. The halogenated acetic acids are highly reactive chemical intermediates used in glycine, drug, dye, and herbicide manufacture. Glycolic acid and lactic acid are used widely in the leather, textile, adhesive, and plastics industries, and lactic acid is also used as a food acidulant.

▶ Metabolism & Mechanism of Action

Both inorganic and organic acids, by virtue of their water solubility and acid dissociation, will cause direct destruction of body tissue, including mucous membranes and skin. The extent of direct skin damage depends on the concentration of acid and length of exposure, whereas the damage to the respiratory tract by inhalation of acid mists will depend on particle size. Hydrofluoric acid, one of the most corrosive of

the inorganic acids, readily penetrates the skin and travels to deep tissue layers, causing liquefaction necrosis of soft tissues and decalcification and corrosion of bones. The intense pain that may accompany hydrogen fluoride burns is attributed to the calcium-precipitating property of the fluoride ion, which produces immobilization of tissue calcium and an excess of potassium that stimulates nerve endings. The fluoride ion also may bind body calcium, causing life-threatening systemic hypocalcemia after acute skin exposure or osteosclerotic bone changes after chronic exposure to hydrogen fluoride mist.

▶ Clinical Findings

A. Symptoms and Signs

1. Acute exposure—All acids act as primary irritants of the skin and mucous membranes.

A. Skin—All acids on contact with the skin cause dehydration and heat release to produce first-, second-, or third-degree burns with pain. Sensitization is rare. Hydrofluoric acid solutions of less than 50% may cause burns that may not become apparent for 1–24 hours; stronger solutions cause immediate pain and rapid tissue destruction, appearing reddened, pasty-white, blistered, macerated, or charred.

B. Respiratory effects—Inhalation of vapors or mists causes immediate rhinorrhea, throat burning, cough, burning eyes, and conjunctival irritation. High concentrations may cause shortness of breath, chest tightness, pulmonary edema, and death from respiratory failure. Inhalation of acid vapors or mists generally causes immediate symptoms because of high water solubility in mucous membranes, but respiratory effects may be delayed for several hours. Noncardiogenic pulmonary edema has been reported following acute inhalation exposure to sulfuric acid fumes, with almost complete recovery except for slightly decreased diffusion capacity on pulmonary function testing. For nitric acid exposure with oxides of nitrogen, overexposure tends to produce delayed symptoms 1–24 hours after inhalation, beginning with dyspnea followed by pulmonary edema and cyanosis. Rapidly progressive pulmonary edema of delayed onset may follow the inhalation of fumes from accidental nitric acid exposure. In these cases, postmortem electron microscopy of lung tissue suggests increased permeability as a result of microvascular injury.

Chlorine species are highly reactive, resulting in a variety of dose-related lung effects ranging from respiratory mucous membrane irritation to pulmonary edema. Obstructive or restrictive pulmonary defects can result immediately following exposure, with complete resolution over a few days to weeks in most individuals. A few patients have long-term, persistent obstructive or restrictive pulmonary deficits or increased nonspecific airway reactivity after high-level exposure to chlorine gas.

Exposure to lower levels of acid vapors or mists over months may increase the risk of developing irritant-associated asthma. Aluminum potroom workers with exposure to fluorides have an increased risk of respiratory symptoms, with a greater prevalence of airway responsiveness as measured by nonspecific airway challenge. Occupational asthma also has been reported following exposure to chloramines in indoor swimming pool air.

C. SYSTEMIC EFFECTS—Several deaths have been reported as a result of persistent hypocalcemia and hypomagnesemia following exposure to concentrated hydrofluoric acid, with the exposures involving as little as 2.5% of total body surface area. Systemic toxicity involving gastrointestinal hemorrhage, acute renal failure, and hepatic injury has been reported following chromic acid ingestion.

2. Chronic exposure—

A. SKIN—Chromate compounds can be allergens and can cause pulmonary as well as skin sensitization, but chromic acid results only in direct irritant dermatitis. Ulceration of the skin and ulceration and perforation of the nasal septum have been reported following chronic exposure to chromic acid.

B. DENTAL EROSION—Exposure to inorganic and organic acid fumes is reported to cause tooth surface loss. An increase in periodontal pockets but not oral mucous membrane lesions was found among acid-exposed workers.

C. RESPIRATORY EFFECTS—Bronchiolitis obliterans, a chronic interstitial lung disease, has been described after acute pneumonitis from nitric acid and oxides of nitrogen. No significant change in lung function has been found among workers exposed to phosphoric acid while refining phosphorus. Acids and a variety of other irritants have been recognized to cause vocal cord dysfunction, with chronic symptoms of hoarseness and loss of voice.

D. SYSTEMIC EFFECTS—Osteosclerosis has been found in workers exposed to hydrofluoric acid and fluoride-containing compounds. Farmers with formic acid exposure have increased renal ammoniagenesis and urinary calcium excretion, possibly as a result of interaction with the oxidative metabolism of renal tubular cells.

E. CANCER—Studies of workers exposed to sulfuric acid mists show an excess risk of laryngeal and nasopharyngeal cancer. The International Agency for Research on Cancer (IARC) concludes that there is sufficient evidence that occupational exposure to strong inorganic acid mists containing sulfuric acid is carcinogenic (group 1). Battery manufacturers and steel workers exposed to mineral acid mists have an increased risk of upper aerodigestive tract cancer. For chromic acid, IARC concludes that there is sufficient evidence of carcinogenicity in humans and animals (group 1). Airborne hexavalent chromium exposure results in an increased risk of lung cancer among chromium platers. The National Institute for Occupational Safety and Health (NIOSH) recommends that chromic acid be regulated as a carcinogen. An increase in the number of sister-chromatid exchanges has been found in lymphocytes of workers exposed to acid aerosols at a phosphate fertilizer factory. IARC finds that hydrochloric acid is not classifiable in terms of carcinogenicity to humans (group 3). The cancer risk was not increased among cohorts of chemical manufacturing workers exposed to hydrogen chloride and nitric acid.

B. Laboratory Findings

In cases where inhalation exposure may cause more extensive mucosal irritation, the chest radiograph may show interstitial or alveolar edema, and hypoxemia may be evident by arterial blood gas analysis. Nonspecific abnormalities in liver and kidney function have been reported following massive inhalation exposures to sulfuric acid and hydrofluoric acid. Urine fluoride levels can be used as biologic indices of exposure in hydrofluoric acid intoxication, with a normal mean value of 0.5 mg/L in urine (recommended occupational postshift urinary biologic standard of 7 mg/L).

▶ Differential Diagnosis

There are many respiratory irritants, including gases such as ammonia, phosgene, halogens (chlorine, bromine), sulfur dioxide, and ozone; solvents such as glycol ethers; and dusts such as fibrous glass. The symptoms and clinical course of lung disorders caused by these substances and by the acids discussed in this chapter do not differ; thus, the history is essential. Likewise, hundreds of industrial chemicals may cause direct irritant dermatitis.

▶ Prevention

A. Work Practices

When possible, highly corrosive acids should be replaced by acids that present fewer hazards, and if use of corrosives is essential, only the minimum concentration should be used. Proper storage practices should include fire-resistant buildings with acid-resistant floors, retaining sills, and adequate drainage; containers should be adequately protected against impact, kept off the floor, and labeled clearly. Wherever possible, handling should be done through sealed systems or the substances transported in safety-bottle carriers. Decanting should be done with special siphons or pumps. The potential for violent or dangerous reactions (eg, when water is poured into nitric acid) can be avoided by appropriate training.

Where processes produce acid mists (as in electroplating), local exhaust ventilation should be installed. Workers potentially exposed to splashes or spills must wear acid-resistant hand, arm, eye, and face protection, and respiratory protection should be available for emergency use. Emergency showers and eyewash stations should be strategically located.

B. Medical Surveillance

Preplacement and periodic examinations should include medical history of skin and respiratory disease and examination of the skin, teeth, and lungs. For potential hydrofluoric acid exposure near or above the permissible exposure limit, periodic postshift urinary fluoride in excess of 7 mg/L (adjusted for urine specific gravity of 1.024) may indicate excessive exposure. Elemental analysis of hair for fluoride has been correlated with fluoride levels in serum and urine.

Treatment

Immediate on-site first aid treatment of acid burns to the eye or skin includes copious flushing with running water with removal of all contaminated clothing. First- or second-degree burns involving a small area generally can be treated at the on-site medical facility with debridement and application of suitable burn dressings. All other acid burns should be treated at a hospital emergency facility.

For hydrofluoric acid burns, the definitive treatment is aimed at deactivation of the fluoride ion in tissue with calcium, magnesium, or quaternary ammonium solution. If the hydrogen fluoride concentration is 20% or more, if the patient has been exposed to a long delay of a lower concentration, or if a large tissue area has been affected by a lower concentration, then calcium gluconate solution should be used. Calcium gluconate solution is prepared by mixing 10% calcium gluconate with an equal amount of saline to form a 5% solution and is infiltrated with a small needle in multiple injections (0.5 mL/cm^2 of tissue) into and 5 mm beyond the affected area. Dramatic pain relief should occur. Vesicles and bullae should be debrided carefully, with removal of necrotic tissue; if periungual or ungual tissues are involved, the nail should be split to the base. A burn dressing then is applied along with calcium gluconate 2.5% gel or magnesium sulfate paste. Hydrofluoric acid burns of the hand have been treated successfully with repeated application of an occlusive glove over topical calcium carbonate gel. Repeated intra-arterial infusion over 4 hours with 10 mL of 10% calcium chloride diluted with 40 mL of normal saline also has been recommended for the treatment of hydrofluoric acid extremity burns. Careful monitoring of serum magnesium and calcium levels is required. If the hydrogen fluoride concentration is 20% or less and only a small surface area is involved, the burn can be flushed with water and then treated with 10% magnesium sulfate solution under a soft dressing. The eye burned with hydrogen fluoride should be irrigated copiously and then evaluated by an ophthalmologist. Calcium gluconate 1% in normal saline can be used as an irrigant.

Systemic effects from absorption should be anticipated from skin burns from hydrogen fluoride of greater than 50% concentration or from extensive burns at any concentration. Hypocalcemia can be life-threatening and should be monitored by repeated measurement of serum calcium and electrocardiography for QT-interval prolongation. Calcium gluconate 10% intravenously with adequate hydration should be used for calcium depletion.

For inhalation of acid vapors or mists, the victim should be removed immediately from the source of exposure and treated on-site with 100% oxygen. If there are symptoms of shortness of breath, chest tightness, or persistent cough, the patient should be evaluated at the hospital. Patients who are

minimally symptomatic with normal peak expiratory flow rate and oxygen saturation values can be discharged from the emergency department after several hours of observation and instructed to return if dyspnea occurs. Upper body or facial burns are a clue that inhalation may have occurred with possible serious lower airway damage. Evaluation should include a chest radiograph and arterial blood gas analysis for oxygen. Hypoxemia should be treated with 100% oxygen by mask or by intubation in the event of severe hypoxemia, acidosis, or respiratory distress. Fluid balance should be monitored carefully and intracardiac pressure measured directly, if necessary. Bronchospasm may be treated with inhaled bronchodilators or intravenous aminophylline and steroids if necessary. The benefits of steroids in the management of noncardiogenic pulmonary edema caused by acid inhalation are unknown, but the drugs may be used empirically to speed recovery and prevent the subsequent development of interstitial lung disease. Nebulized calcium gluconate 5% solution has been used successfully for treatment of inhalational exposure to hydrofluoric acid.

2. Alkalis

ESSENTIALS OF DIAGNOSIS

- Acute effects
  - Skin and eye burns.
  - Respiratory irritation.
- Chronic effects
  - Corneal opacities of the eye (untreated).
  - Obstructive lung disease.

General Considerations

Alkalis are caustic substances that dissolve in water to form a solution with a pH higher than 7. These include ammonia, ammonium hydroxide, calcium hydroxide, calcium oxide, potassium hydroxide, potassium carbonate, sodium hydroxide, sodium carbonate, and trisodium phosphate. The alkalis, whether in solid form or concentrated liquid form, are more destructive to tissue than most acids. They tend to liquefy tissues and allow for deeper penetration, depending on concentration, duration of contact, and area of the body involved.

Use, Production, & Occupational Exposure

In the United States, all sodium hydroxide (caustic soda) is produced by the electrolysis of sodium or potassium chloride in mercury cells. In this process, pure saturated brine is decomposed by electric current to liberate chlorine gas at the anode and sodium metal at the cathode. The latter reacts with water to form sodium hydroxide. Most caustic soda is produced as a 50% aqueous solution. Sodium hydroxide is used in pulp and paper production, water treatment, and manufacture of a wide variety of organic and inorganic chemicals, soaps and detergents, textiles, and alumina.

Sodium carbonate (soda ash) is produced by the ammonium chloride process, by the reaction of sodium chloride and sulfuric acid, or by leaching out of rock deposits. Sodium carbonate is used in glass manufacturing, as a component of cleaning-product formulations, in pulp and paper processing and water treatment, and as a chemical intermediate.

Potassium carbonate (potash) is produced by carbonating potassium hydroxide solutions obtained by electrolysis. Potassium carbonate is used in the manufacture of soap, glass, pottery, and shampoo; in tanning and finishing leather; in photographic chemicals, fire-extinguishing compounds, and rubber antioxidant preparations; and as an alkalizer and drainpipe cleaner.

Potassium hydroxide (caustic potash) is produced by electrolysis of potassium chloride solution and is used as a chemical intermediate in the manufacture of potassium carbonate, potassium phosphate, soaps, tetrapotassium pyrophosphate, liquid fertilizers, dyestuffs, and herbicides.

Calcium oxide (quicklime) is made by calcining limestone. Calcium oxide is used in metallurgy as a flux in steel production, for ammonia recovery in the Solvay process for sodium carbonate, in construction applications and water purification and softening, in beet and sugar cane refining, in kraft paper pulp production, and in sewage treatment.

▶ Metabolism & Mechanism of Action

Occupational exposure to the alkalis is primarily by direct contact with the eyes, skin, and mucous membranes. Inhalation of caustic mists generally is limited by the irritant properties of the compound. Contact of the eyes with alkalis causes disintegration and sloughing of corneal epithelium, corneal opacification, marked edema, and ulceration. Alkaline compounds will combine with skin tissue to form albuminates and with natural fats to form soaps. They gelatinize tissue and result in deep and painful destruction. Accidental or intentional ingestion of alkalis may cause severe esophageal necrosis with subsequent stenosis.

▶ Clinical Findings

A. Symptoms and Signs

1. Acute exposure—In contrast to acids, skin contact with the alkalis may not elicit immediate pain but may start to cause immediate damage with erythema and tissue necrosis within minutes to hours. Splashes of alkali to the eyes, if not treated within minutes, may result in corneal necrosis, edema, and opacification.

Irreversible obstructive lung injury has developed after acute inhalation of sodium hydroxide in a poorly ventilated space. Workers have suffered severe skin and inhalational injuries following exposure to "black liquor" used in the pulp and paper industry. Fatal injury has occurred after a relatively brief inhalation and dermal contact with a hot concentrated caustic solution. Acute tracheobronchitis and respiratory failure as a result of high-dose ammonia inhalation may result in permanent, severe, and fixed airways obstruction. Bronchiolitis obliterans caused by occupational exposure to incinerator fly ash has been reported.

2. Chronic exposure—Chronic exposure to caustic dusts does not increase the mortality rate significantly. Long-term sodium hydroxide inhalation has been reported to cause severe obstructive airway disease with significant air trapping. Chronic exposure to ammonia of over 7.5 ppm is associated with pulmonary function decrements among swine production facility workers. An increased prevalence of coughing, wheezing, and ocular and nasal irritation was reported among community residents exposed to alkali dust. Corneal opacities have resulted from untreated corneal alkali burns. An increased risk of nasopharyngeal carcinoma has been observed among Chinese textile workers exposed to acid and caustics.

B. Laboratory Findings

No specific laboratory tests are of value in the diagnosis and management of problems resulting from alkali exposure.

▶ Differential Diagnosis

Many other industrial chemicals, including acids, may cause eye and skin burns.

▶ Prevention

A. Work Practices

Insofar as possible, solutions of caustics should be handled in closed systems that will prevent contact with or inhalation of the chemical. All persons with potential exposure to caustics should wear proper protective clothing and equipment, such as a full-face shield, safety goggles, apron or suit, rubber gloves, and boots. Emergency showers and eyewashes must be located where eye or skin contact may occur.

B. Medical Surveillance

Medical examination of the eyes, skin, and respiratory tract is recommended for all workers with caustic exposure.

▶ Treatment

Sodium and potassium hydroxide may cause more extended and deeper damage as a result of rapid penetration through ocular tissues. Alkali burns of the eye and skin should be treated within minutes by copious irrigation with tap water and removal of all contaminated clothing. Irrigation with a weak acid such as 5% acetic acid also has been suggested. First aid treatment with prompt and continuous eye irrigation is essential to prevent permanent corneal damage and visual loss. Topical use of a synthetic metalloproteinase inhibitor has been shown to reverse or stop the progression of corneal ulceration following an experimental alkali burn.

A relatively new hypertonic, polyvalent, amphoteric chelating compound (Diphoterine) also appears to be of benefit for emergent eye and skin decontamination. A physician or health practitioner should be consulted for eye burns and careful examination of the eye performed. If eye damage is suspected, follow-up with an ophthalmologist is recommended. Intensive topical steroids, antibiotics, and amniotic membrane transplantation may be required.

ACRYLAMIDE & ACRYLONITRILE

1. Acrylamide

ESSENTIALS OF DIAGNOSIS

► Acute effects
  • Dermatitis.
► Chronic effects
  • Peripheral neuropathy.

► General Considerations

Pure acrylamide is a white crystalline solid at room temperature and is highly soluble in water. It is a vinyl monomer with high reactivity with thiols and with hydroxy and amino groups. Commercial acrylamide is shipped in 50% aqueous form in stainless steel drums, tank trucks, and cars. Acrylamide manufacture is from the catalytic hydration of acrylonitrile.

► Use

The major use of acrylamide monomer is in the production of polymers, which are useful as flocculators. Polyacrylamides are used for waste and water treatment flocculants, in products for sewage dewatering, and in a variety of products for the water treatment industry. Other uses include strengtheners for papermaking and retention aids, drilling-mud additives, textile treatment, and surface coatings. One of the more important uses is as a grouting agent, particularly in mining and tunnel construction.

► Occupational & Environmental Exposure

Monomer manufacturing workers are potentially exposed to acrylamide, as are papermaking workers, soil-stabilization workers, textile workers, tunnel workers, and well drillers. Biomedical laboratory workers can be exposed to acrylamide used to make polyacrylamide gels. Intoxication has been reported in the manufacture of acrylamide monomer, in the handling of a 10% aqueous solution in a mine, in the production of flocculators, in the use of a resin mixture containing residual monomer, in the production of polymers while manufacturing paper coating materials, and during the use of acrylamide in grouting materials. One nonoccupational incident occurred in Japan, where a family ingested well water containing 400 ppm acrylamide.

Acrylamide may be formed at elevated temperatures in cooking, particularly of carbohydrate-rich foods such as potatoes (eg, crisps, chips, and fries). Residual levels of acrylamide also can be found in cosmetic products.

► Metabolism & Mechanism of Action

Acrylamide is absorbed easily in animals following all routes of administration. The peripheral nerve terminal is a primary site of acrylamide action, with possible inhibition of membrane-fusion processes impairing neurotransmitter release. Quantitative data on absorption or excretion in humans are not available. Following intravenous administration in rats, acrylamide is distributed throughout total body water within minutes and then excreted largely in the urine with a half-life of less than 2 hours. Protein-bound acrylamide or acrylamide metabolites have a half-life in blood and possibly in the central nervous system of about 10 days. The primary metabolite of acrylamide is N-acetyl-S-(3-amino-3-oxypropyl) cysteine, and it is excreted predominantly in the urine.

► Clinical Findings

A. Symptoms and Signs

Acrylamide polymer may cause dermatitis. The monomer can produce numbness and tingling of hands and weakness of the hands and legs. Acrylamide is neurotoxic in many experimental animals, causing distal axonopathy and central neuronal degeneration.

More than 60 cases of acrylamide-associated neurotoxicity have been reported in humans. Subclinical peripheral neuropathy has been found in tunnel workers exposed to acrylamide during grouting work. Similar to the neuropathy associated with the hexacarbons n-hexane and methyl-n-butyl ketone, acrylamide neuropathy is considered a typical example of a dying-back disorder, where degeneration begins at the distal ends of the longest and largest fibers and spreads proximally. In most cases, toxicity results from skin contact and dermal absorption, although acrylamide may be absorbed by inhalation as well. The cellular and molecular site of acrylamide neurotoxicity may involve alterations in fast anterograde transport or sulfhydryl groups on presynaptic proteins. The neurologic features of acrylamide intoxication vary depending on the speed of intoxication. In the Japanese family that ingested contaminated well water, encephalopathy with confusion, disorientation, memory disturbances, hallucinations, ataxia, and peripheral neuropathy developed in approximately 1 month. Reported time to onset of symptoms in occupational cases has varied from 4 weeks to approximately 24 months. Clinically, acrylamide peripheral neuropathy affects both motor and sensory nerve fibers predominantly in the distal limbs. Difficulty in walking and clumsiness of the hands are usually the first symptoms, followed by numbness of the feet and fingers. Distal weakness is found on examination, with loss of tendon reflexes and vibration sensation. Evidence of excessive sweating affecting predominantly the extremities has been reported commonly, along with redness and exfoliation of the skin. In acute cases, central nervous system involvement may result in truncal ataxia, lethargy, and dysarthria. Major histologic findings are swelling of axons and/or a decrease in large-diameter axons. The axonopathy is reversible slowly over time, but complete recovery depends on the severity of intoxication.

Acrylamide has been found to increase the tumor yield in mice and is genotoxic in animal studies. Acrylamide reacts with hemoglobin to form DNA adducts and heritable translocations in animal studies. Human studies have shown increased DNA adducts and chromosomal aberrations among workers exposed to acrylamide. High acrylamide intake is associated with increased risks of ovarian and endometrial cancers in a relatively linear manner, especially among never smokers. Occupational exposure to acrylamide has been associated with excess mortality from pancreatic cancer. There is some evidence to suggest that acrylamide results in adverse developmental or reproductive effects in animal studies.

The State of California has listed acrylamide as a carcinogen since 1990. The IARC has concluded that there is sufficient evidence in experimental animals for acrylamide to be classified as a carcinogen (group 2A).

B. Laboratory Findings

Electrophysiologic studies of workers with signs and symptoms of neurotoxicity have shown only a slight effect on maximal conduction velocity of either motor or sensory fibers. Sensory nerve action potentials usually are reduced and are the most sensitive electrophysiologic test.

Sural nerve biopsies performed on two patients during recovery from acrylamide neuropathy showed axonal degeneration affecting mainly large-diameter fibers. Recent studies have suggested the use of urinary *S*-carboxyethyl cysteine and mercapturic acid metabolites of acrylamide for biomonitoring use in the workplace and general populations, respectively.

▶ Differential Diagnosis

The combination of truncal ataxia with peripheral neuropathy—predominantly motor—accompanied by excessive sweating and redness and peeling of the skin makes the diagnosis of acrylamide-associated neurotoxicity likely. Other occupational toxic agents associated with peripheral neuropathy must be considered, along with the presence of other underlying metabolic diseases, drug use, and endocrine disorders.

▶ Prevention

A. Work Practices

Mechanized bag loading of polymerization reactors, closed-line transfer of liquid acrylamide, and other closed-system processes are important to minimize exposure. Where necessary, personal protective equipment designed to prevent dermal and inhalation exposure to acrylamide should be available. General population consumption of acrylamide in foods can be reduced by changes in food-manufacturing raw materials and preparation methods.

B. Medical Surveillance

Preplacement and periodic examinations should exclude symptomatic peripheral neuropathies. Hemoglobin adducts have been used to monitor occupational exposure to both acrylamide and acrylonitrile. A neurotoxicity index involving electrophysiologic measures was correlated with urinary 24-hour mercapturic acid levels, hemoglobin adducts of acrylamide, employment duration, and vibration sensitivity. Vibration threshold may be a sensitive indicator of early neurotoxicity caused by acrylamide exposure.

▶ Treatment

Skin contaminated with acrylamide should be washed immediately with soap and water, and contaminated clothing should be removed. There is no known treatment for acrylamide intoxication. Removal from exposure is the only effective measure that can be taken. Full recovery has been observed in most cases after 2 weeks to 2 years, although in severe cases some residual neurologic abnormalities have been noted.

2. Acrylonitrile

ESSENTIALS OF DIAGNOSIS

▶ Acute effects
- Respiratory irritation, nausea, dizziness, and irritability, followed by convulsions, coma, and death.

▶ Chronic effects
- Nausea, dizziness, headache, apprehension, fatigue.

▶ General Considerations

Acrylonitrile is a volatile colorless liquid with a characteristic odor resembling that of peach seeds, discernible at 20 ppm or less. It is a highly reactive compound. Pure acrylonitrile polymerizes readily in light, and storage requires the addition of polymerization inhibitors. Its vapors are explosive and flammable and may release hydrogen cyanide on burning.

▶ Use

Acrylonitrile was not an important product until World War II, when it was used in the production of oil-resistant rubbers. Nearly all world production of acrylonitrile is now based on a process where propylene, ammonia, and air react in the vapor phase in the presence of a catalyst. Hydrogen cyanide and acrylonitrile are the chief by-products formed; the latter undergoes a series of distillations to produce acrylonitrile.

Much of acrylonitrile monomer is used for the manufacture of acrylic fibers for the apparel, carpeting, and home furnishings industries. Acrylonitrile-containing plastics, particularly the resins acrylonitrile-butadiene-styrene (ABS) and styrene-acrylonitrile (SAN), are used in pipe and pipe fittings, automotive parts, appliances, and building components. Nitrile elastomers are used for their oil- and hydrocarbon-resistant properties in the petrochemical and automobile industries. Acrylonitrile is also used to make acrylamide.

▶ Occupational & Environmental Exposure

Potential exposure to acrylonitrile may occur in monomer-, fiber-, resin-, and rubber-producing plants. Potential exposure to acrylonitrile in acrylic fiber production is greatest when the solvent is removed from newly formed fibers and during decontamination of acrylonitrile processing equipment, loading, surveillance of the processing unit, and product sampling. Acrylonitrile exposure may also occur from fine particles emitted during 3-D printing that use ABS filaments.

▶ Metabolism & Mechanism of Action

Acrylonitrile is absorbed readily in animals following ingestion or inhalation. There is a biphasic half-life of 3.5 hours and 50–77 hours, with elimination predominantly in the urine. Acrylonitrile is metabolized to cyanide, and its metabolites are eliminated in the urine. In humans, absorption can occur through both inhalation and skin contact. The acute toxicity of acrylonitrile in humans is thought to be due to the action of cyanide, and thiocyanate is detected in blood and urine of workers. Acrylonitrile is an electrophilic compound and binds covalently to nucleophilic sites in macromolecules. Hemoglobin adducts have been used for exposure assessment in experimental animal studies and for follow-up of acute exposure to acrylonotrile in accidentally exposed workers. It has been postulated that the mutagenic effect of acrylonitrile is caused by glycidonitrile, a reactive intermediate able to alkylate macromolecules.

▶ Clinical Findings

A. Symptoms and Signs

A few deaths have been reported from acrylonitrile exposure, with respiratory distress, lethargy, convulsions, and coma at 7500 mg/m³. Acrylonitrile was implicated in four cases of toxic epidermal necrosis that developed 11–21 days after the victims returned to houses fumigated with a 2:1 mixture of carbon tetrachloride and acrylonitrile. One patient had measurable blood cyanide levels at autopsy. Symptoms of acute poisoning are described as irritability, respiratory irritation, limb weakness, respiratory distress, dizziness, nausea,

cyanosis, collapse, convulsions, and cardiac arrest; these resemble cyanide poisoning.

Chronic human toxicity has been reported in rubber workers exposed to 16–100 ppm of acrylonitrile for periods of 20–45 minutes, with complaints of nasal irritation, headache, nausea, apprehension, and fatigue. A case of asthma has been reported following exposure to fine particles emitted during 3-D printing that use ABS filaments. Acrylonitrile is carcinogenic in rats after 2 years of feeding and inhalation, inducing brain tumors and stomach papillomas. An excess risk of colon and lung cancers occurred among acrylonitrile polymerization workers from a textile fibers plant. Epidemiologic studies suggest that acrylonitrile is associated with an increased lung cancer risk as well as possible increased risk for death due to bladder cancer and pneumonitis. The IARC has concluded that there is sufficient evidence in experimental animals for acrylonitrile to be classified as a carcinogen (group 2A).

B. Laboratory Findings

The use of biomarkers such as chromosomal aberrations and hemoglobin adducts has shown some promise as a tool to understand susceptibility for health effects and to monitor acutely exposed workers. Elevated serum cyanide or urine thiocyanate levels may be found in cases of acute intoxication.

▶ Differential Diagnosis

Acute poisoning with acrylonitrile may mimic cyanide intoxication.

▶ Prevention

A. Work Practices

Controls have proved effective in reducing employee exposure to acrylonitrile. NIOSH has recommended that acrylonitrile be handled in the workplace as a potential human carcinogen and has published detailed recommendations for adequate work practices.

B. Medical Surveillance

Preplacement and annual medical examinations should include special attention to the skin, respiratory tract, and gastrointestinal tract, as well as to the nonspecific symptoms of headache, nausea, dizziness, and weakness that may be associated with chronic exposure. Treatment kits for acute cyanide intoxication should be immediately available to trained medical personnel at each area where there is a potential for release of or contact with acrylonitrile.

Biologic monitoring may be useful to reflect exposure to acrylonitrile. The relationship between the degree of exposure to acrylonitrile and the urinary excretion of thiocyanate and acrylonitrile was determined in Japanese workers from acrylic fiber factories. A mean postshift urine thiocyanate concentration of 11.4 mg/L (specific gravity 1.024) was found to correlate with an 8-hour average acrylonitrile exposure of

4.2 ppm. Normal urinary thiocyanate levels in nonsmokers do not exceed 2.5 mg/g of creatinine. Mean urinary acrylonitrile levels of 30 mcg/L in Dutch plastics workers were found to correlate with a mean 8-hour time-weighted average (TWA) exposure level of 0.13 ppm and were used to monitor adequate work practices.

▶ Treatment

Treatment of acute intoxication with acrylonitrile is similar to that of cyanide poisoning. A combination of *N*-acetylcysteine with sodium thiosulfate has been suggested as an appropriate measure for acrylonitrile intoxication.

AROMATIC AMINES

ESSENTIALS OF DIAGNOSIS

▶ Acute effects
  • Dermatitis.
  • Asthma.
  • Cholestatic jaundice.
  • Methemoglobinemia.
▶ Chronic effects
  • Bladder cancer.

▶ General Considerations

The aromatic amines are a class of chemicals derived from aromatic hydrocarbons, such as benzene, toluene, naphthalene, anthracene, and diphenyl, by the replacement of at least one hydrogen atom by an amino group. Some examples are shown below.

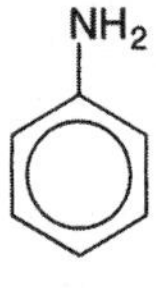

Aniline 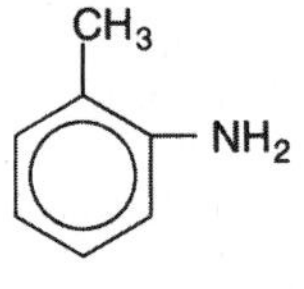   o-Toluidine

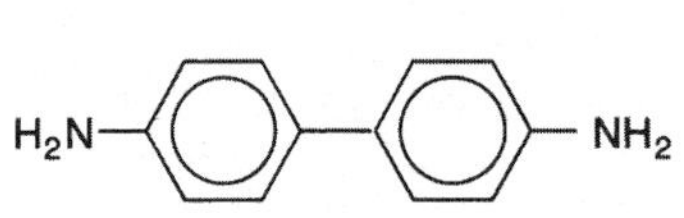

Benzidine

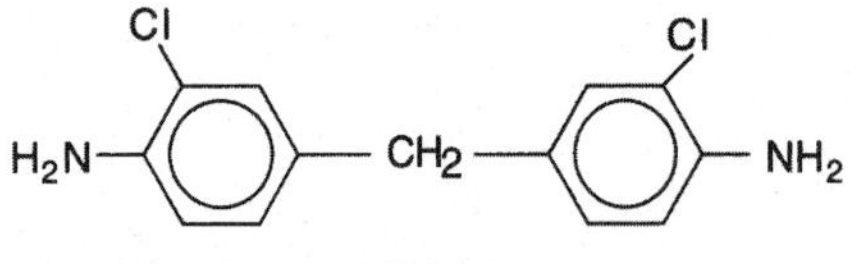

MBOCA

▶ Use

Aromatic amines are used mainly in the synthesis of other chemicals. The principal commercial use of benzidine was as a chemical intermediate in dye manufacture, especially for azo dyes in the leather, textile, and paper industries. Benzidine once was used in clinical laboratories for the detection of blood, but this has been discontinued because of safety concerns. Benzidine is no longer produced for commercial sale in the United States. Any benzidine production must be captive consumption and maintained in closed systems.

Aniline is used as a chemical intermediate in the production of methylene diisocyanate, rubber products, dyes, pesticides, pigments, and hydroquinones. *p,p′*-Methylene dianiline is used as a chemical intermediate in the production of polyurethanes, dyes, and polyamide and polyimide resins and fibers and as a laboratory analytic reagent. *o*-Toluidine is used as a component of printing textiles, in the preparation of ion-exchange resin, as an antioxidant in rubber manufacture, and in the synthesis of dyestuffs. 1,4-Phenylenediamine may be found in some hair dyes. 4,4-Methylenebis(2-chloroaniline) (MBOCA) has been used as a curing agent in urethane and epoxy resins. It is no longer manufactured commercially in the United States.

Because of the demonstrated carcinogenicity of *b*-naphthylamine, its manufacture and use have been banned in many countries. Production of *b*-naphthylamine ceased in the United States in 1972.

▶ Metabolism & Mechanism of Action

The aromatic amines are nearly all lipid-soluble and are absorbed through the skin. Metabolism is largely via the formation of hydroxylamine intermediates. These metabolites are transported to the bladder as *N*-glucuronide conjugates and hydrolyzed by the acid pH of urine to form reactive electrophiles that bind to bladder transitional epithelial DNA. The polymorphic enzyme *N*-acetyltransferase-2 is involved in the metabolism of the aromatic amines; slow acetylator status is a genetic risk factor for bladder cancer. Increased susceptibility for bladder cancer also may be related to glutathione *S*-transferase M1 gene deficiency. Urine pH (influenced by diet) may have a strong effect on the presence of free urinary aromatic compounds and on urothelial cell DNA adduct levels.

▶ Clinical Findings

A. Symptoms and Signs

1. Acute exposure—

A. DERMATITIS—Because of their alkaline nature, certain amines constitute a direct risk of dermatitis. Many aromatic amines can cause allergic dermatitis, notably *p*-aminophenol and *p*-phenylenediamine. The latter was known as *fur dermatitis* and caused asthma among fur dyers and currently may cause contact dermatitis among hairdressers.

B. Respiratory effects—Asthma caused by *p*-phenylenediamine has been reported.

C. Hemorrhagic cystitis—Hemorrhagic cystitis can result from exposure to *o*- and *p*-toluidine and 5-chloro-*o*-toluidine. The hematuria is self-limited, and no increase in bladder tumors has been noted.

D. Hepatic injury—Cholestatic jaundice has resulted from industrial exposure to diaminodiphenyl methane, which also caused toxic jaundice as a consequence of contaminated baking flour (*Epping jaundice*). The hepatitis is reversible after cessation of exposure. Acute liver dysfunction has been reported among workers exposed to 5-nitro-*o*-toluidine.

E. Methemoglobinemia—Acute poisoning by aniline and its derivatives results in the formation of methemoglobin. A significant elevation of methemoglobin levels has been demonstrated in adult volunteers after ingestion of 25 mg aniline. The mean lethal dose is estimated to be between 15 and 30 g, although death has followed ingestion of as little as 1 g aniline. It has been postulated that a toxic metabolite, phenylhydroxylamine, is responsible for the methemoglobin. Peak levels of methemoglobin are observed within 1–2 hours of ingestion. Cyanosis becomes apparent at levels of methemoglobin of 10–15%, and headache, weakness, dyspnea, dizziness, and malaise occur at levels of 25–30%. Concentrations of methemoglobin greater than 60–70% may cause coma and death.

2. Chronic exposure—An excess of bladder tumors was recognized in 1895 among German workers who used aromatic amines in the production of synthetic dyes. British dyestuffs workers had a high risk for the development of bladder cancer. In the United States, bladder cancer has occurred in workers exposed to β-naphthylamine or benzidine in the manufacture of dyes and in chemical workers exposed to *o*-toludine.

Workers involved in the production of auramine and magenta from aniline and those working with 4-aminobiphenyl have an increased risk of bladder tumors. Workers exposed to 4-chloro-*o*-toluidine have a 73-fold excess of bladder cancer. Animal studies show an increased risk of bladder tumors after exposure to benzidine, *o*-toluidine, *o*-dianisidine-based dyes, MBOCA, and other aromatic amines. European studies of individual susceptibility to the development of aromatic amine–associated bladder cancer suggest some modulation by genetic polymorphisms.

The IARC considers benzidine carcinogenic to humans (group 1A) and MBOCA probably carcinogenic to humans (group 2A). The IARC has concluded that there is sufficient evidence in experimental animals for the carcinogenicity of *o*-toluidine and *p,p′*-methylene dianiline (group 2B) and finds limited evidence for the carcinogenicity of aniline in animals (group 3).

Results from cohort and case-control studies strongly support the association between occupational aromatic amine exposure (ie, benzidine, naphthylamines, MBOCA, and *o*-toluidine) and bladder cancer. An outbreak of 10 cases of bladder cancer was reported among approximately 40 workers at a Japanese plant that produces organic dyes and pigment intermediates. These cases were exposed primarily to *o*-toluidine, paratoluidine, ortho-anisidine, aniline, 2,4-xylidine, and orthochloroaniline. Meta-analysis also show evidence of association between occupational benzidine and beta-naphthylamine exposure and lung cancer.

B. Laboratory Findings

Methemoglobin levels can help in the detection of excess absorption of the single-ring aromatic compounds. Normal individuals have methemoglobin concentrations of 1–2%. A biologic threshold limit value (TLV) of 5% has been proposed.

Determination of the metabolites *p*-aminophenol and *p*-nitrophenol can be useful to monitor exposure to aniline and nitrobenzene. After 6 hours of exposure to 1 ppm nitrobenzene, the urinary concentration of *p*-aminophenol should not exceed 50 mg/L, and the recommended biologic threshold value is 10 mg/L. Levels of free MBOCA in the urine can be used to monitor exposure to this compound. Levels of free MBOCA in urine should be minimized to the limit of detection and used as an index of the adequacy of existing work practices and engineering controls. For workers exposed to the known or suspected carcinogenic aromatic amines, periodic screening of urine for red blood cells and evidence of dysplastic epithelium may detect early bladder cancer.

▶ Differential Diagnosis

Aliphatic nitrates (eg, ethylene glycol dinitrate), aliphatic nitrites, inorganic nitrites, and chlorates also may cause methemoglobinemia. Occupation-associated bladder cancer may account for 10–15% of all cases of bladder cancer. Exposure to arsenic in drinking water also causes an increased risk of bladder cancer. Cigarette smoking, with inhalation of carcinogenic arylamines (eg, 2-aminonaphthalene), is also a significant risk factor.

▶ Prevention

A. Work Practices

Every effort should be made to eliminate use of the carcinogenic aromatic amines by substitution of safer alternatives. Appropriate engineering controls for manufacturers of polyurethane products who use MBOCA—particularly the use of automated systems and local exhaust ventilation—can reduce the potential for exposures successfully. Because most cases of aniline exposure occur through skin and clothing contamination, emphasis should be placed on providing appropriate gloves and protective clothing. Hygiene surveys that can demonstrate surface contamination and biological monitoring can be useful tools to determine exposure to MBOCA.

For the benzidine-based dyes, worker exposure should be reduced to the lowest feasible levels through appropriate engineering controls, including the use of closed-process and liquid metering systems, walk-in hoods, and specific local exhaust ventilation. Dust levels can be minimized by the use of dyes in pellet, paste, or liquid form. Restricted access to areas with potential exposure and provision of suitable protective clothing and respirators should be instituted.

B. Medical Surveillance

Preemployment and periodic measurement of postshift urinary p-aminophenol is useful for biologic monitoring of aniline exposure. Similarly, periodic postshift urine samples for free MBOCA can be an important adjunct to industrial hygiene measures of exposure.

The American Conference of Governmental Industrial Hygienists (ACGIH) recommended biologic exposure limit (BEL) for o-toluidine, MBOCA, and aniline is methemoglobin in blood in excess of 1.5% during or at the end of the work shift. Biologic monitoring by high-pressure liquid chromatographic (HPLC) methods for analysis of urinary o-toluidine, aniline, and MBOCA may be useful. Measurement of methylene dianiline (MDA) using the sensitive gas chromatography–mass spectrometry (GC-MS) assay in urine correlates with hemoglobin adducts of MDA in polyurethane production workers and may serve as a sensitive index of exposure (particularly for dermal exposure) at levels below air-monitoring-detection limits. Hemoglobin adducts also have been used for biologic monitoring of workers exposed to 3-chloro-4-fluoroaniline.

High-risk populations with past or current exposure to carcinogenic aromatic amines should be screened on a periodic basis with exfoliative bladder cytology. Positive findings are followed up with direct urologic examination. Biomolecular screening using voided urine samples for DNA ploidy, bladder tumor–associated antigen p300, and a cytoskeletal protein has been used in one cohort of workers exposed to benzidine.

▶ Treatment

The definitive treatment of methemoglobinemia caused by aniline poisoning is administration of the reducing agent methylene blue. However, an excessive amount of methylene blue may itself provoke the formation of methemoglobin. Additionally, the ability of methylene blue to reduce methemoglobin can be impaired by hereditary glucose-6-phosphate dehydrogenase (G6PD) deficiency and can precipitate frank hemolysis. The recommended dose of methylene blue for the initial management of methemoglobinemia is 1–2 mg/kg of body weight intravenously, equivalent to 0.1–0.2 mL of a 1% solution. Maximal response to methylene blue usually occurs within 30–60 minutes. Repeated doses should be spaced about 1 hour apart and based on methemoglobin levels; most patients, unless they are anemic, can tolerate a level of 30% or less. Methylene blue administration should be discontinued if either a negligible response or an increase in methemoglobin levels results after two consecutive doses or if the total dose exceeds 7 mg/kg. It is advisable

to continue to monitor methemoglobin levels even after an initial response to methylene blue because there is a potential for continued production of methemoglobin by aniline.

Treatment of bladder cancer associated with aromatic amine exposure is identical to that of nonoccupationally associated bladder tumors. Early detection through screening programs may improve prognosis.

CARBON DISULFIDE

ESSENTIALS OF DIAGNOSIS

▸ Acute effects
  • Irritability, manic delirium, hallucinations, paranoia.
  • Respiratory irritation.
▸ Chronic effects
  • Coronary artery disease.
  • Neurobehavioral abnormalities.
  • Retinal microaneurysms.
  • Peripheral neuropathy with ascending symmetric paresthesias and weakness.

▶ General Considerations

Carbon disulfide is a colorless volatile solvent with a strong, sweetish aroma. The average odor threshold of 1 ppm is below the permissible exposure limit; therefore, carbon disulfide is a material with good warning properties. It evaporates at room temperature and its vapor is 2.6 times heavier than air; it may form explosive mixtures in a range of 1–50% by volume in air.

▶ Use

Carbon disulfide is used in the manufacture of rayon, cellophane, carbon tetrachloride, and rubber chemicals and as a grain fumigant.

▶ Occupational & Environmental Exposure

In the production of viscose rayon, carbon disulfide is added to alkali cellulose to yield sodium cellulose xanthate. The latter is dissolved in caustic soda to yield viscose syrup, which can be spun to form textile yarn, tire yarn, or staple fiber or cast to form cellophane. Exposure to high concentrations of carbon disulfide can occur during the opening of sealed spinning machines and during cutting and drying.

▶ Metabolism & Mechanism of Action

Inhalation is the major route of absorption in occupational exposure, and 40–50% of carbon disulfide in inhaled air is retained in the body. Excretion of carbon disulfide by the lung accounts for 10–30% of absorbed dose, and less than 1% is excreted unchanged by the kidney. The remainder is excreted in the form of various metabolites in the urine.

Carbon disulfide is metabolized by formation of dithio-carbamates and reduced glutathione conjugates, as well as by oxidative transformation. Thiourea, mercapturic acids, and the glutathione conjugate 2-thiothiazolidine-4-carboxylic acid (TTCA) can be detected in urine of exposed workers. Formation of dithiocarbamate may account in part for the nervous system toxicity of carbon disulfide, whereas oxidation yields carbonyl sulfide, a hepatotoxic metabolite. Carbon disulfide reacts with protein amino functions to form adducts of dithio-carbamate, which then undergo oxidation or decomposition to an electrophile, which reacts with protein nucleophiles to result in protein cross-linking. Cross-linked neurofilaments then may accumulate within axonal swellings.

▶ Clinical Findings

A. Symptoms and Signs

1. Acute exposure—Acute carbon disulfide intoxication was described in the 1920s among workers in the viscose rayon industry, involving exposure to concentrations of hundreds or thousands of parts per million. Signs and symptoms included extreme irritability, uncontrolled anger, rapid mood changes (including manic delirium and hallucinations), paranoid ideas, and suicidal tendencies.

Exposure to 4800 ppm of carbon disulfide for 30 minutes may cause rapid coma and death. High concentrations of vapor may cause irritation of the eyes, nose, and throat; liquid carbon disulfide may cause second- or third-degree burns.

2. Chronic exposure—Chronic effects of lower-level exposure to carbon disulfide include the following:

A. EYE—Viscose rayon workers have been reported to have a high incidence of eye irritation. A high incidence of retinal microaneurysms and delayed fundal peripapillary filling by fluorescein angiography has been reported in workers exposed to carbon disulfide. Color vision has been reported to be disturbed in Chinese workers below the current TLV.

B. EAR—Carbon disulfide exposure enhances noise-induced high-frequency hearing loss. Vestibular symptoms of vertigo and nystagmus also may occur.

C. HEART—Epidemiologic studies indicate that workers exposed to carbon disulfide are at increased risk for cardiovascular disease mortality. There is a correlation between blood pressure, elevated triglyceride, and decreased lipoprotein levels and exposure to carbon disulfide. The pathophysiologic mechanism is unclear but may include an effect on oxidative stress in plasma or alteration of arterial elastic properties. Carbon disulfide may cause increased heart rate variability with persistent effects after exposure has ended. A greater risk of ischemic electrocardiographic changes has been seen in a longitudinal study of viscose rayon workers.

D. NERVOUS SYSTEM—Studies show persistent neurobehavioral changes in psychomotor speed, motor coordination, and personality in workers exposed to low concentrations (5–30 ppm) of carbon disulfide. There is a reduction in peripheral nerve conduction on exposure to less than 10 ppm, although clinical symptoms of polyneuropathy are not present. Distal latency, motor nerve-conduction velocity, and sensory amplitude were found to be sensitive indicators of polyneuropathy in viscose rayon workers exposed to carbon disulfide. Lower levels of exposure have been correlated with decreased slow-fiber-conduction velocity with prolongation of the refractory period of the peroneal nerve. Impaired motor and sensory nerve conduction has been demonstrated in prospective studies of workers exposed to carbon disulfide near the TLV. Cerebellar atrophy with extrapyramidal symptoms with atypical parkinsonism and cerebellar signs has been reported. Small-vessel disease with cerebral lesions in the basal ganglia, subcortical white matter, and brainstem has been reported. Peripheral nerve signs and symptoms may persist for as long as 3 years after exposure has ceased.

E. REPRODUCTIVE EFFECTS—Carbon disulfide exposure was associated with a significant effect on libido and potency but not on fertility or semen quality. Women exposed to concentrations of less than 10 ppm may have an increased rate of menstrual abnormalities, spontaneous abortions, and premature births. No other effects on general endocrine function have been observed.

B. Laboratory Findings

Nonspecific elevations of liver enzymes and creatinine have been reported in acute intoxication. With chronic exposure, peripheral nerve-conduction velocity can be decreased, and neurobehavioral testing may show abnormalities in psychomotor skills and measures of personality function.

Urinary metabolites that catalyze the reaction of iodine with sodium azide can be used to detect exposure above 16 ppm (iodine-azide reaction). The concentration of end-of-shift urinary TTCA is related to exposure and can detect uptake as low as 10 ppm over the whole working shift. The ACGIH BEI is 5 mg TTCA per gram of creatinine in urine at the end of a shift. Heavy physical work and greater skin contact are correlated with higher TTCA levels. Biopsy of the sural nerve in cases of suspected peripheral nerve damage may be indicated and may show degeneration of both axon and myelin with a predominant loss of large myelinated fibers.

▶ Differential Diagnosis

Cardiac disease from carbon disulfide intoxication must be differentiated from atherosclerotic heart disease from other causes. Peripheral polyneuropathy should be distinguished from that caused by alcohol, drugs, diabetes, and other toxic agents. Neuropsychiatric symptoms may be a result of depression, posttraumatic stress syndrome, or other toxic exposures such as organic solvents.

▶ Prevention

A. Work Practices

Control of exposure must rely largely on engineering controls, with enclosure of processes and machines and proper use of ventilation systems. Operator rotation and respiratory protection during peak exposures should be implemented. Potential sources of ignition are prohibited in areas where carbon disulfide is stored or handled, and the substance must not be allowed to accumulate to concentrations higher than 0.1%. Impervious clothing, gloves, and face shields should be worn to prevent skin contact.

B. Medical Surveillance

Initial medical examination should include the central and peripheral nervous systems, eyes, and cardiovascular system. Visual acuity and color vision should be measured and a baseline electrocardiogram obtained. Periodic medical surveillance to detect early signs or symptoms of toxicity should include questions regarding cardiac, nervous system, and reproductive function, with evaluation of blood pressure, peripheral nerve function, and mental status. Neurobehavioral testing, exercise electrocardiography, and nerve-conduction velocity testing may be indicated. Reduced color discrimination may be a sensitive marker for carbon disulfide neurotoxicity. Measurement of finger tremor frequencies may provide an early indication of chronic carbon disulfide intoxication. Magnetic resonance imaging (MRI) may show periventricular hyperintensity and lacunar infarct, which may be of diagnostic use in selected patients with neurobehavioral effects from carbon disulfide exposure.

Measurement of TTCA in urine collected at the end of the work shift following the first workday is the test of choice for biologic monitoring. Skin disease and increased absorption of carbon disulfide may be important in exposure assessment. Five milligrams per gram of creatinine corresponds to an 8-hour exposure (TWA) to the current TLV. The widely used iodine-azide test is insensitive at carbon disulfide levels of less than 16.7 ppm. The presence of preexisting neurologic, psychiatric, or cardiac disease should be considered relative contraindications for individual exposure.

Treatment

Skin and eye contact with carbon disulfide should be treated immediately by washing with large amounts of water, and all contaminated clothing should be removed. No specific treatment is available for chronic carbon disulfide toxicity.

CHLOROMETHYL ETHERS

ESSENTIALS OF DIAGNOSIS

► Acute effects
  • Respiratory irritation.
  • Skin rash.
► Chronic effects
  • Lung cancer.

General Considerations

The haloethers bis(chloromethyl) ether (BCME) and chloromethylmethyl ether (CMME) are highly volatile, colorless liquids at room temperature, miscible with many organic solvents. The haloethers are alkylating agents that are highly reactive *in vivo*. Technical-grade CMME contains 1–8% BCME as an impurity.

Use

BCME is formed when formaldehyde reacts with chloride ions in an acidic medium. It has been used in the past primarily for chloromethylations (eg, in the preparation of ion-exchange resins), where a polystyrene resin is chloromethylated and then treated with an amine.

Occupational & Environmental Exposure

Occupational exposure to the chloromethyl ethers occurs in anion-exchange resin production. Beginning in the 1940s, workers have been exposed to BCME in ion-exchange resin manufacture, where exposure levels ranged from 10 to 100 ppb. Small quantities are produced in the United States and only in closed systems to make other chemicals.

BCME also may be a potential hazard in the textile industry, where formaldehyde-containing reactants and resins are used in fabric finishing and as adhesives in laminating and flocking fabrics. Thermosetting emulsion polymers containing methylacrylamide as binders may liberate formaldehyde on drying and curing and then form BCME in the presence of available chloride. A NIOSH study of textile finishing plants found from 0.4 to 8 ppb BCME in the workroom air. This led to the use of low-formaldehyde resins and chloride-free catalysts.

Clinical Findings

A. Symptoms and Signs

1. Acute exposure—The chloromethyl ethers are potent skin and respiratory irritants. There are no reported cases of acute overexposure to either BCME or CMME.

2. Chronic exposure—Both BCME and CMME are carcinogenic and mutagenic in animal and cellular test systems. When rats are exposed to 0.1 ppm BCME by inhalation for 6 hours a day, 5 days a week, a high incidence of esthesioneuroblastomas and squamous cell carcinoma of the respiratory tract is observed. Both BCME and CMME produce skin papillomas and squamous tumors on direct application or subcutaneous injection. In humans, an excess of lung cancer has been suspected. An industry-wide survey of plants using chloromethyl ethers has documented a strikingly increased risk of lung cancer in exposed workers. More than 60 cases of BCME-associated lung cancer have been identified, with oat cell the principal histologic type. The historical average time-weighted exposure in these cases is estimated to be between 10 and 100 ppm, and the latency period between exposure and lung cancer ranges from 5 to 25 years. An increasing incidence is observed with intensity and length of exposure.

In addition, the risk of lung cancer is increased in smokers versus nonsmokers. The mortality rate from respiratory tract cancer is significantly (almost three times) higher among chloromethyl ether–exposed workers, with a latency of 10–19 years. The risk of cancer among exposed workers declines after 20 years from first exposure. NIOSH recommends that BCME be regulated as a potential human carcinogen. The IARC considers BCME carcinogenic to humans (group 1A).

B. Laboratory Findings

The lung carcinoma associated with BCME and CMME presents in similar fashion to nonoccupationally associated carcinoma. Chest radiography may show a mass that should lead to appropriate diagnostic testing. Alternatively, sputum cytology may be abnormal in the presence of a normal chest radiograph and thus may be useful as a screening technique in individual cases. Sputum cytology may be of limited value in the follow-up of workers exposed to known carcinogens who remain at risk for many years following exposure.

▶ Differential Diagnosis

Known occupational lung carcinogens include asbestos, arsenic, chromium, and uranium; consequently, a careful occupational history should be obtained from an individual who presents with lung carcinoma.

▶ Prevention

A. Work Practices

Enclosed chemical processes are essential to reduce exposure below 1 ppb, and continuous monitoring has been used successfully to warn of excessive exposures to BCME and CMME. Since the number of potentially exposed workers has markedly declined since the 1970s, medical follow-up of past exposed workers has assumed a greater role.

B. Medical Surveillance

Preplacement and annual lung examination should be included in medical surveillance of exposed workers. Periodic sputum cytology may be of limited value in detecting early lung cancer.

▶ Treatment

The treatment of lung carcinoma associated with BCME/CMME exposure does not differ from that of nonoccupational cases.

DIBROMOCHLOROPROPANE

ESSENTIALS OF DIAGNOSIS

▶ Acute effects
  • Oligospermia, azoospermia.

▶ General Considerations

Dibromochloropropane (DBCP) is a brominated organochlorine nematocide that was used extensively since the 1950s on citrus fruits, grapes, peaches, pineapples, soybeans, and tomatoes. Millions of pounds were produced in the United States. In 1977, employees at a California pesticide formulation plant were found to be infertile, and further investigation documented azoospermia and oligospermia among workers exposed to DBCP. In the United States, its use has been restricted since 1980 to a soil fumigant against plant-parasitic nematodes in pineapples. However, two American companies continued to export DBCP to less developed countries for use on bananas. This practice has largely stopped in recent years, but DBCP is one of many pesticides still in use in developing countries that lack regulation and enforcement. DBCP may remain persistent in soil and continues to be detected as a groundwater contaminant in areas of high past use.

In DBCP-exposed men with both azoospermia and elevation of follicle-stimulating hormone (FSH) levels, follow-up evaluation generally has shown permanent destruction of germinal epithelium. A 17-year follow-up of DBCP-exposed workers found sperm count recovery at 36–45 months in three of nine azoospermic and three of six oligozoospermic men, with no improvement thereafter. A significant increase in plasma levels of FSH and luteinizing hormone was found in the most severely affected workers, with incomplete recovery of sperm count and motility.

In vitro, in vivo, and human genotoxicity studies indicate that DBCP can act as a mutagen and clastogen. No correlation has been found between DBCP contamination in drinking water and mortality rates from leukemia or gastric cancer. Birth outcomes (low birth weight and birth defects) did not differ among DBCP-exposed workers or community residents exposed to DBCP-contaminated drinking water.

NIOSH recommends that DBCP be regulated as a potential human carcinogen. The IARC finds that there is sufficient evidence of carcinogenicity in animals (group 2B).

DIMETHYLAMINOPROPIONITRILE

Dimethylaminopropionitrile was a component of catalysts used in manufacture of flexible polyurethane foams. In 1978, NIOSH reported urinary dysfunction and neurologic symptoms among workers at facilities that used dimethylaminopropionitrile. Workers at polyurethane-manufacturing plants developed neurogenic bladder dysfunction after the introduction of a catalyst containing dimethylaminopropionitrile. Workers had urinary retention, hesitancy, and dribbling. Examination showed a pattern of decreased sensation confined to the lower sacral dermatomes, abnormal retention of contrast material on intravenous pyelogram, or abnormal cystometrograms. Nerve-conduction velocity studies were normal. Symptoms of persistent sexual dysfunction were found 2 years after the original epidemic, and one worker had residual sensorimotor neuropathy. Following these findings, production of catalysts containing dimethylaminopropionitrile was discontinued voluntarily.

Dimethylaminopropionitrile appears to be a unique example of a neurotoxin that produces localized autonomic dysfunction without peripheral nervous system damage. Urotoxic effects may be related to metabolism via a cytochrome P450–dependent mixed-function oxidase system, with formation of reactive intermediate metabolites that interfere with axoplasmic transport. The discovery of this toxicity by an alert clinician underscores the role of the community practitioner in the discovery of new occupational diseases.

ETHYLENE OXIDE

ESSENTIALS OF DIAGNOSIS

▶ Acute effects
- Respiratory tract irritation.
- Skin rash.
- Headache, drowsiness, weakness.

▶ Chronic effects
- Increased sister chromatid exchanges in lymphocytes.
- Possible increased risk of cancer.

▶ General Considerations

Ethylene oxide is a colorless flammable gas with a characteristic ether-like odor. At elevated pressures, it may be a volatile liquid. It is completely miscible with water and many organic solvents. The threshold of detection in humans is about 700 ppm but is quite variable, and smell cannot be relied on to warn of overexposure. To reduce the explosive hazard of ethylene oxide used as a fumigant or sterilant, it is often mixed with carbon dioxide or halocarbons (15% ethylene oxide and 85% dichlorofluoromethane).

▶ Use

Ethylene oxide is used in the manufacture of ethylene glycol (used for antifreeze and as an intermediate for polyester fibers, films, and bottles), nonionic surface-active agents (used for home laundry detergents and dishwashing formulations), glycol ethers (used for surface coatings), and ethanolamines (for soaps, detergents, and textile chemicals). It is used as a pesticide fumigant and as a sterilant in hospitals, medical products manufacture, libraries, museums, beekeeping, spice and seasoning fumigation, animal and plant quarantine, transportation vehicle fumigation, and dairy packaging.

▶ Occupational & Environmental Exposure

Most ethylene oxide is used as a chemical intermediate in plants where closed and automated processes generally maintain exposure levels below 1 ppm. The greatest potential for worker exposure occurs during loading or unloading of transport tanks, product sampling, and equipment maintenance and repair.

Ethylene oxide is the most common method of sterilization of medical devices in the United States with use in approximately 50% of devices that require sterilization. Field surveys of hospital gas sterilizers generally have found that 8-hour TWA exposures to ethylene oxide are below 1 ppm. However, occupational exposure may be several hundred parts per million for brief periods during the opening of the sterilizer door, in the transfer of freshly sterilized items to the aeration cabinet or central supply area, during tank changes, and at the gas-discharge point. Ethylene oxide may also be released into the air and increase the risk to surrounding communities. As a result, closures of ethylene oxide sterilization facilities in the United States has led to consideration of alternatives including hydrogen peroxide, peracetic acid, radiation, and nitrogen dioxide.

▶ Metabolism & Mechanism of Action

Ethylene oxide is absorbed through the skin and respiratory tract. It is an alkylating agent that binds to DNA and may cause cellular mutation.

▶ Clinical Findings

A. Symptoms and Signs

1. Acute exposure—Ethylene oxide is irritating to the eyes, respiratory tract, and skin, and at high concentrations it can cause respiratory depression. Symptoms of upper respiratory tract irritation occur at between 200 and 400 ppm, and above 1000 ppm ethylene oxide may cause headache, nausea, dyspnea, vomiting, drowsiness, weakness, and incoordination. Direct contact of the skin or eyes with liquid ethylene oxide can result in severe irritation, burns, or contact dermatitis.

2. Chronic exposure—

A. Reproductive effects—Ethylene oxide is toxic to reproductive function in both male and female experimental animals. Retrospective studies of reproductive function show a higher rate of spontaneous abortions and preterm birth in women exposed to ethylene oxide.

B. Carcinogenic effects—Ethylene oxide is genotoxic in a variety of animal test systems. Chronic inhalation bioassays in rats have shown that ethylene oxide results in a dose-related increase in mononuclear cell leukemia, peritoneal mesothelioma, and cerebral glioma. Intragastric administration of ethylene oxide in rats produces a dose-dependent increase of squamous cell carcinomas of the forestomach. Studies show a dose-related increase in chromosomal aberrations, sister chromatid exchange in lymphocytes and micronuclei in bone marrow cells of exposed workers; and a dose-related increase in the level of hemoglobin adducts. The GSTT1-null genotype is associated with increased formation of hemoglobin adducts in relation to ethylene oxide exposure, suggesting that individuals with homozygous deletion of the *GSTT1* gene may be more susceptible to the genotoxic effects of ethylene oxide.

Retrospective cohort mortality studies have suggested an excess of lymphatic and hematopoietic, and breast cancers in ethylene oxide–exposed workers. The IARC considers ethylene oxide to be carcinogenic to humans (group 1). NIOSH recommends that ethylene oxide be treated as a potential human carcinogen.

C. Neurologic toxicity—Impairment of sensory and motor function has been observed in animals exposed to 357 ppm ethylene oxide over 48–85 days, and four cases of peripheral neuropathy were described among workers exposed to a leaking sterilizing chamber for 2–8 weeks. Central neurotoxicity has been reported following chronic ethylene oxide exposure, including neuropsychologic abnormalities, lower P300 amplitude, and peripheral neuropathy.

D. Other—Occupational asthma also has been reported following acute exposure.

B. Laboratory Findings

No specific finding is characteristic of ethylene oxide exposure. Lymphocytosis has been noted after acute exposure. Where inhalation results in respiratory symptoms, the chest radiograph may show interstitial or frank alveolar edema. Where suspect, a complete blood count may be helpful in the diagnosis of leukemia. Cytogenetic analysis (ie, sister chromatid exchange) of peripheral lymphocytes cannot be used in individual cases to quantitate exposure or estimate cancer risk.

▶ Differential Diagnosis

The mixture of chlorofluorocarbons found in sterilant cylinders also may produce upper respiratory symptoms on inhalation exposure. Many other genotoxicants, including cigarette smoke and other alkylating agents, can cause an increase in sister chromatid exchanges and chromosomal aberrations.

▶ Prevention

A. Work Practices

Proper engineering controls are essential for reducing short-term exposures to hospital sterilizer staff during procedures where ethylene oxide levels have been found to be greatest. A NIOSH survey found that engineering controls are extremely effective in hospitals in reducing ethylene oxide exposure during sterilization. These controls include effective sterilization chamber ethylene oxide purging, local exhaust ventilation at the sterilizer door, adequate ventilation of floor drains, efficient handling of product carts from sterilizer to aerator, and installation of ethylene oxide tanks in ventilated cabinets. Self-contained breathing apparatus or airline respirators are the only respirators acceptable for ethylene oxide and must be worn when concentrations of ethylene oxide are

unknown, such as when entering walk-in chambers or for emergency response. With the implementation of effective engineering controls, work shift exposures to ethylene oxide may decrease, but intermittent peak excursions and accidental exposures still may occur.

B. Medical Surveillance

Preplacement and periodic examinations should include attention to the pulmonary, hematologic, neurologic, and reproductive systems. Consistent changes in hematologic parameters have not been demonstrated among workers monitored for ethylene oxide exposure. The mean absolute numbers of eosinophils and red blood cells and percentage of hematocrit were significantly elevated among a group of workers with higher cumulative doses of ethylene oxide. Other studies have not demonstrated the utility of the complete blood count as a screening test for medical surveillance of ethylene oxide–exposed hospital workers. Biologic monitoring studies of ethylene oxide–exposed workers show an increase in chromosomal aberrations, sister chromatid exchanges, micronuclei, and hemoglobin adducts. Personnel trained in emergency response for use of self-contained breathing apparatus should be evaluated for cardiorespiratory fitness with pulmonary function or exercise testing.

▶ Treatment

Removal from the work environment after inhalation of the gas should be immediate. If respiratory symptoms are evident, oxygen should be administered and the victim brought to the emergency room. Any contaminated clothing should be removed immediately and, where appropriate, the skin thoroughly washed with soap and water. A chest radiograph should be obtained if warranted by respiratory symptoms, and the patient should be observed for several hours for the onset of pulmonary edema. No other specific treatment is indicated.

FORMALDEHYDE

ESSENTIALS OF DIAGNOSIS

▶ Acute effects
  • Eye irritation causing lacrimation, redness, and pain.
  • Cough, chest tightness, shortness of breath.
  • Skin irritation, contact dermatitis.
▶ Chronic effects
  • Bronchitis, exacerbation of asthma.

▶ General Considerations

Formaldehyde is a colorless flammable gas with a pungent, irritating odor. Known to physicians as a tissue preservative and disinfectant, formaldehyde is a basic feedstock of the modern chemical industry. It also may be encountered as formalin (37–50% formaldehyde), methyl aldehyde, methanal (methanol-formaldehyde mixture), methylene glycol, paraform, or paraformaldehyde (a linear copolymer of formaldehyde).

▶ Use

The largest use of formaldehyde is the manufacture of urea-formaldehyde and polyacetal and phenolic resins and as an intermediate in the manufacture of ethylenediaminetetraacetic acid, methylene dianiline, hexamethylenetetramine, and nitriloacetic acid. Other important uses include wood industry products, molding compounds, foundry resins, adhesives for insulation, slow-release fertilizers, manufacture of permanent-press finishes of cellulose fabrics, and formaldehyde-based textile finishes. Formaldehyde is used in relatively small quantities for preservation and disinfection. It is a by-product of the incomplete combustion of hydrocarbons and is found in small amounts in automobile exhaust and cigarette smoke.

▶ Occupational & Environmental Exposure

Occupational exposure to formaldehyde above 1 ppm occurs in the production of formaldehyde resin and plastics and in the manufacture of apparel, plywood particle board and wood furniture, paper, and paperboard; workers at risk include urea-formaldehyde foam insulation dealers and installers, mushroom farmers, embalmers, and laboratory workers. NIOSH industrial hygiene surveys have found formaldehyde levels of up to 8 ppm in hospital autopsy rooms and up to 2.7 ppm in gross anatomy laboratories. Wildland firefighters may be exposed to formaldehyde as a result of vegetation combustion. Hairdressers may be chronically exposed to high concentrations of formaldehyde in the workplace due to the use of this chemical in hair smoothing agents.

Residential exposure to formaldehyde to several parts per million occurs from urea-formaldehyde foam insulation (UFFI) and particle board in mobile homes. Levels of formaldehyde are highest in new residences and decline with a half-life of 4–5 years for mobile homes and of less than 1 year for UFFI homes. Mean levels for mobile homes are about 0.5 ppm and for UFFI homes about 0.1 ppm. Diurnal and seasonal variations in exposure levels may occur.

▶ Metabolism & Mechanism of Action

Formaldehyde is formed intracellularly as N_5,N_{20}-methylenetetrahydrofolic acid, an important metabolic intermediate. Exogenous formaldehyde can be absorbed by inhalation, ingestion, or dermal absorption. More than 95% of an inhaled dose is absorbed and metabolized rapidly to formic acid by formaldehyde dehydrogenase. Formaldehyde disappears from plasma with a half-life of 1–1.5 minutes, so an increase cannot be detected immediately following inhalation exposure to high concentrations. Most formaldehyde is converted to CO_2 via formate, and a small fraction is excreted in the urine as formate and other metabolites. Formaldehyde interacts with macromolecules such as DNA, RNA, and protein. This probably accounts for its carcinogenic effect.

▶ Clinical Findings

A. Symptoms and Signs

1. Acute exposure—Formaldehyde vapor exposure causes direct irritation of the skin and respiratory tract. Both direct irritation (eczematous reaction) and allergic contact dermatitis (type IV delayed hypersensitivity) occur. After a few days of exposure to formaldehyde solutions or formaldehyde-containing resins, the individual may develop a sudden urticarial eczematous reaction of the skin of the eyelids, face, neck, and flexor surfaces of the arms. Allergic contact dermatitis may occur from exposure to phenol-formaldehyde resins, water-based paints, or photographic products. There appears to be no relationship between cutaneous disease from formaldehyde and personal or family history of atopy. Direct irritation of the eyes, nose, and throat occurs among most people exposed to 0.1–3 ppm of formaldehyde vapor.

The odor threshold is 0.05–1 ppm; some individuals may note irritation of the upper respiratory tract at or just above the odor threshold. Shortness of breath, cough, and chest tightness occur at 10–20 ppm. Exposure to 50–100 ppm and above can cause pulmonary edema, pneumonitis, or death. Irritant symptoms caused by formaldehyde exposure do not elicit a consistent immunologic response with elevated levels of immunoglobulin (Ig) E or IgG antibody to formaldehyde–human serum albumin.

Several studies show respiratory irritation from exposure to formaldehyde and wood dust. Embalmers report more frequent symptoms of respiratory irritation with exposures during embalming exceeding permissible limits. Formaldehyde exposures in gross anatomy dissection may exceed exposure limits, causing significantly increased upper respiratory symptoms and decrements in airflow during exposure. Respiratory irritant effects are significantly associated with formaldehyde exposure in mobile homes. Residents of homes insulated with urea-formaldehyde foam had a higher prevalence of respiratory symptoms than did residents of control homes but had no demonstrated changes in various hematologic or immunologic parameters.

2. Chronic exposure—

A. Cancer—Squamous cell carcinomas of the nasal epithelium were induced in rats and mice exposed for prolonged periods (up to 2 years). Biochemical and physiologic studies in rats have shown that inhaled formaldehyde can depress respiration, inhibit mucociliary clearance, stimulate cell proliferation, and cross-link DNA and protein in the nasal mucosa.

Generally consistent results have been found in studies of nasopharyngeal and hypopharyngeal cancer and exposure to formaldehyde, with several studies showing an increased risk of sinonasal cancer (particularly adenocarcinoma) with exposure to formaldehyde. Three cases of malignant melanoma of the nasal mucosa have been reported in persons occupationally exposed to formaldehyde. An increased risk of pancreatic cancer has been observed among embalmers exposed to formaldehyde. The IARC has found sufficient evidence to conclude that formaldehyde is carcinogenic in humans (nasopharyngeal cancer), and in 2009 added leukemia to the list of neoplasms caused by formaldehyde. The latter finding is supported by significant increases in the frequencies of monosomy, trisomy, tetrasomy, and sister chromatid exchanges in formaldehyde exposed workers. The National Toxicology Program of the National Institute of Environmental Health Sciences considers formaldehyde to be a known human carcinogen and NIOSH recommends that formaldehyde be regulated as a potential human carcinogen.

B. Respiratory—Occupational asthma has been reported as a result of exposure to formaldehyde resin dust, with studies reporting workers with asthma and positive specific bronchial challenge to formaldehyde. However, exposure-chamber studies have not demonstrated increased airway responsiveness among asthmatics following formaldehyde challenge. Tests of formaldehyde-specific IgE antibodies and cutaneous reactivity also generally have been negative, and formaldehyde sensitization does not correlate with symptoms. A study of students exposed to formaldehyde showed short-term decrements in peak expiratory flow rates. Workers exposed to formaldehyde have significantly greater cross-shift reduction in forced expiratory volume in 1 second (FEV_1) and significantly lower respiratory symptoms than do unexposed controls. There is increasing evidence that indoor exposure to formaldehyde increases the risk of asthma in both children and adults.

C. Other effects—Chronic formaldehyde exposure has been linked in case reports to a variety of neuropsychologic problems, but cohort studies have not been performed to confirm these findings. Spontaneous abortions in cosmetologists and laboratory workers have been associated with the use of formaldehyde-based disinfectants and formalin, respectively. Wood workers exposed to formaldehyde had significantly delayed conception. However, a meta-analysis does not confirm these findings. A large population case-control study suggests that formaldehyde exposure, or employment in formaldehyde-exposed occupations, is related to the risk of ALS.

B. Laboratory Findings

1. Liver and kidney—Routine tests of hepatic and renal function generally are unremarkable. Measurement of formic acid in the urine generally is not helpful because of the short half-life of formaldehyde.

2. Skin—If contact dermatitis is suspected, patch testing should be performed with appropriate concentrations of formaldehyde.

3. Respiratory system—Cough, shortness of breath, or wheezing may be associated with decreased FEV_1 by pulmonary function testing. Peak-flow recordings while at work may show a decrease in maximal airflow during or after exposure to formaldehyde. After exposure to over 20–30 ppm of formaldehyde, chest radiographs may show interstitial or alveolar edema with a resulting reduction in arterial oxygen content on blood gas analysis.

▶ Differential Diagnosis

Numerous workplace gases and vapors may produce symptoms of upper respiratory tract irritation. Symptoms of eye and throat irritation among office workers may be a result of inadequate ventilation, cigarette smoke, or glues and solvents emitted from newly installed synthetic materials. Asthmatics may be particularly sensitive to the effects of formaldehyde exposure to indoor environments.

▶ Prevention

A. Work Practices

Ventilation engineering controls are effective at significantly reducing exposure to formaldehyde in anatomy laboratories and during embalming procedures. Safety goggles or a full-length plastic face mask should be worn where splashing is possible. At air concentrations above the permissible exposure limit, a full-facepiece respirator with organic vapor cartridge is required. Protective neoprene clothing and boots and gloves impervious to formaldehyde should be worn to prevent skin contact.

B. Medical Surveillance

A preplacement history of asthma or allergy should be obtained, along with a baseline FEV_1 and forced vital capacity (FVC). Biologic monitoring using urinary formate concentration is not useful with the possible exception of populations where ambient formaldehyde concentrations are greater than 1 ppm.

Low-level exposure to formaldehyde during embalming is associated with cytogenetic changes in epithelial cells of the mouth and in blood lymphocytes. These cytogenetic effects may be useful markers in biologic monitoring of formaldehyde-exposed workers. Various pathologic changes have been observed in the nasal mucosa of formaldehyde-exposed workers, including ciliary loss, goblet cell hyperplasia, squamous metaplasia, and mild dysplasia.

▶ Treatment

In case of eye and skin contact, immediately flush the contaminated area with water for 15 minutes and remove any contaminated clothing. Immediate removal to fresh air is required for inhalation exposure, with administration of oxygen for shortness of breath or hypoxemia. For formaldehyde exposure exceeding 20–30 ppm, emergency department observation with periodic evaluation of respiratory status is necessary for 6–8 hours.

NITRATES: NITROGLYCERIN & ETHYLENE GLYCOL DINITRATE

ESSENTIALS OF DIAGNOSIS

▶ Acute effects
- Headache.
- Angina.
- Fall in blood pressure.

▶ Chronic effects
- Sudden death.
- Increased incidence of ischemic heart disease.

▶ General Considerations

Nitroglycerin (glyceryl trinitrate, trinitro propanetriol) and ethylene glycol dinitrate (dinitroethanediol) are liquid nitric acid esters of monohydric and polyhydric aliphatic alcohols. Those of the tetrahydric alcohols (erythritol tetranitrate, pentaerythritol tetranitrate) and the hexahydric alcohol (mannitol hexanitrate) are solids. They are less stable than aromatic nitro compounds.

Nitroglycerin is readily soluble in many organic solvents and acts as a solvent for many explosive ingredients, including ethylene glycol dinitrate. It is an oily liquid at room temperature with a slightly sweet odor. The sensitivity of nitroglycerin decreases with decreasing temperature, so ethylene glycol dinitrate may be added to nitroglycerin-bearing dynamites to depress the freezing point. Explosions of nitroglycerin may occur when the liquid is heated or when frozen nitroglycerin is thawed. Ethylene glycol dinitrate is an oily colorless liquid that is more stable and less likely than nitroglycerin to explode when it burns.

▶ Use, Production, & Occupational Exposure

Alfred Nobel first used a mixture of nitroglycerin with diatomaceous earth and later a more stable mixture of nitroglycerin, sodium nitrate, and wood pulp to form dynamite. The major application of nitroglycerin is in explosives and blasting gels, as in low-freezing dynamite in mixture with ethylene glycol dinitrate. Other explosive uses are in cordite in mixture with nitrocellulose and petroleum and in blasting gelatin with 7% nitrocellulose. Nitroglycerin also has medical therapeutic applications for the treatment of angina.

Nitroglycerin may be manufactured by a process in which glycerin is added to a mixture of nitric and sulfuric acids. Dynamite is formed by adding "dope," or mixtures of sodium nitrate, sulfur, antacids, and nitrocellulose. Ethylene glycol dinitrate is made by nitration of ethylene glycol with mixed acid.

Occupational exposures to nitroglycerin and ethylene glycol dinitrate can occur during their manufacture and during the manufacture and handling of explosives, munitions, and pharmaceuticals. Skin absorption for both nitroglycerin and ethylene glycol dinitrate has not been quantified but is generally greater than respiratory absorption. Air sampling in dynamite plants where both nitroglycerin and ethylene glycol dinitrate are manufactured and used to produce explosives has shown that short-term higher exposures (in the range of 2 mg/m^3 of ethylene glycol dinitrate) occur among mixers, cartridge fillers, and cleanup or maintenance workers.

▶ Metabolism & Mechanism of Action

Both nitroglycerin and ethylene glycol dinitrate pass readily through the skin. Although there is an excellent correlation between blood nitrate ester levels and airborne exposures, skin absorption is more significant. Both nitroglycerin and ethylene glycol dinitrate are hydrolyzed to inorganic nitrates. The biologic half-life of both nitroglycerin and ethylene glycol dinitrate is about 30 minutes. Both act directly on arteriolar and venous smooth muscle, causing vasodilation within minutes with a consequent drop in blood pressure and an increase in regional myocardial blood flow. The headache associated with nitrate esters is secondary to cerebral vessel distension.

The tolerance that develops after 2–4 days of continuous exposure appears to be the result of an increased sympathetic compensatory mechanism. The pathogenesis of sudden death caused by nitroglycerin and ethylene glycol dinitrate is postulated to be a rebound vasoconstriction resulting in acute hypertension or myocardial ischemia. NIOSH recommends that workplace exposure to nitroglycerin and ethylene glycol dinitrate be controlled so that workers are not exposed at concentrations that will cause vasodilation, as indicated by the development of throbbing headaches or decreases in blood pressure. At this exposure level, workers should be protected against work-related angina pectoris, other signs or symptoms of ischemia or cardiac damage, and sudden death.

▶ Clinical Findings

A. Symptoms and Signs

1. Acute exposure—Symptoms of acute illness include loss of consciousness, severe headache, difficulty breathing, weak pulse, and pallor. Tolerance to these effects develops in dynamite production workers after 1 week of exposure, but symptoms recur on return to work after an absence of 2 days or more. The headache associated with nitroglycerin (*powder headache*) frequently begins in the forehead and moves to the occipital region, where it can remain for hours or days. Associated symptoms include depression, restlessness, and sleeplessness. Alcohol ingestion may worsen the headache.

An acute drop in mean blood pressure of 10 mm Hg systolic and 6 mm Hg diastolic occurs on return to work after

2–3 days off. Mean blood pressure measurements increase over the week as compensatory mechanisms develop.

Blood pressure reduction has been noted after exposure to 0.5 mg/m^3 for 25 minutes, and some workers develop headaches after inhalation exposure of more than 0.1 mg/m^3. Both irritant and allergic contact dermatitis as a consequence of nitroglycerin exposure have been reported.

2. Chronic exposure—Angina pectoris and sudden death have been described among dynamite workers handling nitroglycerin and ethylene glycol dinitrate. In affected workers, the angina usually occurs on the weekend or early in the work shift following periods away from work. The angina is relieved by reexposure to nitroglycerin or ethylene glycol dinitrate in contaminated clothes or by taking nitroglycerin sublingually. Sudden deaths without premonitory angina also have been recorded in dynamite workers. There is an excess risk of cardiac disease among nitroglycerin and ethylene glycol dinitrate workers.

Other reported chronic effects include symptoms of Raynaud phenomenon and peripheral neuropathy. At high concentrations, the aliphatic nitrates may give rise to methemoglobinemia. A retrospective cohort mortality study of munitions workers exposed to nitroglycerin and dinitrotoluene showed an increase in ischemic heart disease mortality for those younger than age 35 years.

B. Laboratory Findings

Coronary angiography has shown normal coronary arteries in workers with angina, and atheromatous coronary vessels generally have not been found on autopsy of workers who died suddenly. The incidence of ectopy is not increased in dynamite workers, and electrocardiograms may be normal. Abnormalities in digital plethysmography show changes in the digital wave pulse with inhalation exposures of $0.12–0.41$ mg/m^3.

▶ Differential Diagnosis

An increased incidence of cardiovascular disease has been found in carbon disulfide–exposed workers. Sudden cardiac death may occur after exposure to carbon monoxide or to hydrocarbon solvents.

▶ Prevention

A. Work Practices

Avoidance of headaches, blood pressure reduction, angina, or sudden death is achieved by reduction of exposure through proper work practices. Control of exposure is best accomplished by closed systems, local ventilation, and the use of proper seals, joints, and access ports. The danger of detonation can be minimized by the use of nonsparking equipment, prevention of smoking and open flames, and other safety measures. Natural and synthetic rubber gloves accelerate absorption of nitrate esters, so only cotton or cotton-lined gloves should be worn. Dermal contact with nitrates should

be minimized because this may be an important route of absorption.

B. Medical Surveillance

Preplacement and periodic examination should stress a history of cardiovascular disease and physical examination of cardiac abnormalities. Urinary glycerol dinitrates may have potential as a biologic monitoring tool. A small experimental study in humans has shown that urinary N-methylnicotinamide may have potential as a biomarker for nitrate exposure, but further studies are necessary to determine its importance in the occupational setting. Methemoglobin is not sensitive for routine monitoring of exposure.

▶ Treatment

Treatment of cardiac symptoms caused by nitrate ester exposure does not differ from that of symptoms of coronary insufficiency caused by underlying coronary artery disease. Sublingual nitroglycerin should be used immediately for anginal symptoms. New-onset angina or a change in anginal patterns should be evaluated by noninvasive cardiac imaging or angiography if indicated.

NITROSAMINES

ESSENTIALS OF DIAGNOSIS

▶ Acute effects
  • Liver damage.
▶ Chronic effects
  • Probable human carcinogen (selected).

▶ General Considerations

N-Nitrosamines have the general structure shown below:

where R′ and R can be alkyl or aryl or aryl, for example, N-nitrosodimethylamine (NDMA), N-nitrosodiethylamine (NDEA), N-nitrosodiethanolamine (NDELA), and N-nitrosodiphenylamine (NDPhA). Derivatives of cyclic amines also occur, for example, N-nitrosomorpholine (NMOR) and N-nitrosopyrrolidine (NPyR). N-Nitrosamines are volatile solids or oils and are yellow because of their absorption of visible light by the NNO group.

Reactions of nitrosamines involve mainly the nitroso group and the CH bonds adjacent to the amine nitrogen.

Enzymatic reactions leading to the formation of carcinogenic metabolites are thought to occur at the alpha carbon.

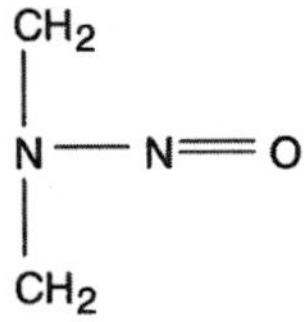

NDMA 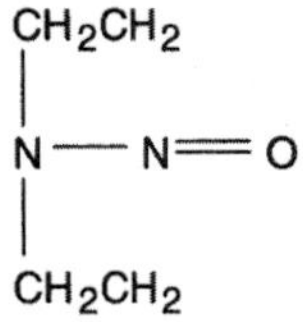   NDEA 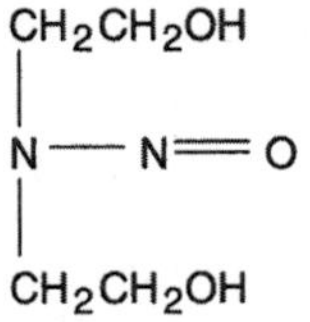   NDELA

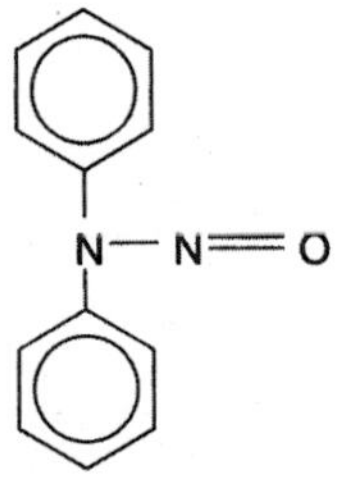

NDPhA 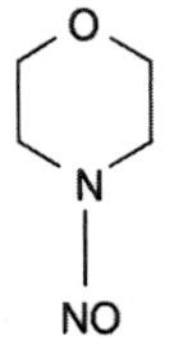   NMOR 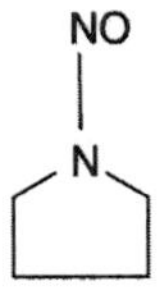   NPyR

Use, Production, & Exposure

Nitrosamines are formed by the reaction of a secondary or tertiary amine with nitrite ion in an acidic medium, according to the general equation shown below:

$$NH + NO_2 \xrightarrow{H^+} N - N = O$$

Appreciation of the carcinogenicity of the nitrosamines has led to their characterization in many occupational and environmental circumstances. Humans may be exposed to nitrosamines in several ways: formation in the environment and subsequent absorption from food, water, air, or industrial and consumer products; formation in the body from precursors ingested separately in food, water, or air; from the consumption or smoking of tobacco; and from naturally occurring compounds. There is no commercial production in the United States of nitrosamines. Prior to 1976, NDMA was used in the production of dimethylhydrazine, a rocket propellant. NDMA now is used primarily as a research chemical. Other uses of NDMA include the control of nematodes, inhibition of nitrification in soil, as a plasticizer for rubber and acrylonitrile polymers, in the preparation of thiocarbonyl fluoride polymers, as a solvent in the plastics and fiber industry, and as an antioxidant. NDELA is a known contaminant of cosmetics, lotions, shampoos, certain pesticides, antifreeze, and tobacco. NDEA is used primarily as a research chemical, a gasoline and lubricant additive, an antioxidant, a stabilizer in plastics, a fiber industry solvent, a copolymer softener, and a starting material for synthesis of

1,1-diethylhydrazine. The major uses of NDPhA have been in the rubber industry as an antiscorching agent or vulcanization retarder. NDPhA reacts with other amines in the rubber to form N-nitrosamines.

The largest nonoccupational exposure to preformed nitrosamines is derived from tobacco products and tobacco smoke, which may contain NDMA, NDEA, NPyR, and others. Nitrosamine content is greater in sidestream smoke and from cigars. Low levels of nitrosamines occur in several types of food, including cheese, processed meats, beer, and cooked bacon. Many cosmetics, soaps, and shampoos are contaminated with NDELA as a result of the nitrosation of triethanolamine by bactericides.

Nitrate can be reduced to nitrite *in vitro* and in human saliva *in vivo*. The reaction of ingested nitrites with amines will yield *in vivo* nitrosamines in the acidic medium of the stomach. Main contributors to gastric nitrite load are vegetables, cured meats, baked goods, cereals, fruits, and fruit juices.

Occupational Exposure

NDMA has been detected in the workroom air of a rubber sealing factory, fish meal producer, manufacturer of surface-active agents, rubber footwear plant, and chrome and leather tanneries. N-nitroso-piperidine and N-nitroso-phenylamine exposure has been documented among road paving asphalt workers. There are many thousands of workers employed by cutting-fluid manufacturing firms, and an undetermined number of machine shop workers have the potential to be exposed to nitrosamines in cutting oils. Direct contact with cutting fluids and the presence of airborne mists provide the opportunity for ingestion or skin absorption.

The greatest exposure to the population as a whole occurs from cigarette smoking and the ingestion of nitrite-preserved meats. Third hand smoke (THS) has been shown to contain mutagenic and carcinogenic substances, including nitrosamines. Certain classes of pesticides have been found to contain identifiable N-nitroso contaminants formed during synthesis or as a result of interaction with nitrate fertilizers applied simultaneously to crops. The Environmental Protection Agency (EPA) requires testing for nitrosamines of suspect formulation. NDMA has been found in drinking water, probably associated with the chloramine drinking water disinfection process when nitrogen species are added for chloramination.

Metabolism & Mechanism of Action

The nitrosamines are metabolized rapidly after skin or gastrointestinal absorption with a biologic half-life for NDMA of several hours. NDMA is enzymatically demethylated to form monomethylnitrosamine, which then yields an unstable diazohydroxide. The carcinogenic action of the nitrosamines is attributed to this electrophilic species, which can react covalently with DNA.

▶ Clinical Findings

A. Symptoms and Signs

1. Acute exposure—Two cases of industrial poisoning caused by NDMA were reported in 1937 in chemists producing an anticorrosion agent. They developed headaches, backache, abdominal cramps, nausea, anorexia, weakness, drowsiness, and dizziness; both workers developed ascites and jaundice, and one died with diffuse hepatic necrosis. Five family members who ingested lemonade accidentally contaminated with NDMA developed nausea, vomiting, and abdominal pain within a few hours, and two died 4 and 5 days later with generalized bleeding. Postmortem examination showed hepatic necrosis.

2. Chronic exposure—Approximately 85% of more than 200 nitrosamines tested in animals are carcinogenic, inducing tumors of the respiratory tract, esophagus, kidney, stomach, liver, and brain. N-Nitrosodimethylamine, NDMA, NDEA, NDPhA, NDELA, NPyR, and NMOR are carcinogenic in many animal species and are transplacental carcinogens. Animal evidence shows that N-nitrosamines and similar xenobiotic compounds are pancreatic carcinogens, although an Australian case control study did not find an increased risk of pancreatic cancer in humans.

Analyses of lung tissue have found higher levels of 7-methyl-dGMP (a metabolic product of N-nitrosamines) in association with specific genotypes. Genetic polymorphisms may be predictive of carcinogen adduct levels and therefore may predict the risk of cancer following carcinogen exposure. Exposure to nitrosamines among rubber workers is associated with a significantly increased mortality from cancers of the esophagus, oral cavity, and pharynx. Studies of workers exposed to metalworking fluids indicate an association between metalworking fluid and stomach, pancreatic, laryngeal, liver, and rectal cancer. Although it remains to be determined which specific constituents of metalworking fluids are responsible for the increased risk of various cancers, N-nitrosamines are one of the suspect chemicals. The IARC considers that NDEA and NDMA are probably carcinogenic to humans (group 2A) and that NDELA, NMOR, and NPyR are possibly carcinogenic to humans (group 2B). NIOSH recommends that NDMA be regulated as a potential human carcinogen.

Nitrates may be found in drinking water and have been associated in epidemiologic studies with a greater risk of gastric cancer. Case-control studies of gastric cancer and occupational exposures have suggested a slight increase in risk associated with exposure to nitrosamine. Maternal dietary exposure to N-nitroso compounds (NOC) or to their precursors during pregnancy has been associated with risk of childhood brain tumors.

Liver cirrhosis has been reported following chronic exposure to NDMA.

B. Laboratory Findings

In the few fatalities reported, elevated liver enzymes consistent with hepatic necrosis were noted.

▶ Prevention

A. Work Practices

Nitrosamines should be handled in well-ventilated fume hoods. To minimize the potential for formation of nitrosamines, nitrate-containing materials should not be added to metalworking fluids containing ethanolamines. Reduction of nitrosamine exposure in the rubber industry includes the avoidance of compounds that give rise to nitrosamines. Adequate engineering controls should be instituted for working with raw polymers, elastomers, and rubber parts containing dialkylamine compounds that may emit nitrosamine when heated.

B. Medical Surveillance

Increased single-strand DNA breaks in peripheral mononuclear cells have been found in metalworkers exposed to NDELA in cutting fluids. Screening for mutagenicity of cutting fluids containing nitrite and NDELA has been suggested as a means to assess risk of hazardous exposure. Use of biologic samples for exposure to NDELA has been employed to monitor exposure of workers to metalworking fluids. No specific medical surveillance for nitrosamines is recommended.

▶ Treatment

There is no treatment for nitrosamine exposure.

PENTACHLOROPHENOL

ESSENTIALS OF DIAGNOSIS

▶ Acute effects
- Skin and respiratory tract irritation.
- Systemic collapse.

▶ Chronic effects
- Skin rash (chloracne secondary to chlorodibenzodioxin).

▶ General Considerations

Pentachlorophenol (PCP) is a crystalline solid with low water solubility and a characteristic pungent phenolic odor. Its commercial production proceeds by the direct chlorination of phenol in the presence of chlorine and a catalyst or by the alkaline hydrolysis of hexachlorobenzene; both processes result in 4–12% tetrachlorophenol and less than 0.1% trichlorophenol in the final product. In addition, the required elevated temperatures to produce PCP result in the formation of condensation products, including the toxic dimers dibenzo-p-dioxin and dibenzofuran. Analyses of commercial PCP have reported ranges of chlorinated dioxins and furans from 0.03 to 2510 ppm. Tetrachlorodibenzodioxin has been found in a commercial sample of PCP, but not the most toxic

2,3,7,8-isomer. High serum dioxin levels have been reported among chlorophenol workers after occupational exposures. Thus, evaluation of the health effects of PCP must be considered separately from those of its impurities.

Use

PCP is used as a wood preservative, herbicide, defoliant, fungicide, and chemical intermediate in the production of pentachlorophenate. A 0.1% solution in mineral spirits, fuel oil, or kerosene is commonly applied as a wood preservative. PCP is used in pressure treatment of lumber at a 5% concentration. About 80% of PCP is used by the wood-preserving industry to treat products such as railway ties, poles, pilings, and fence posts. Treated wood products have a useful product life five times that of untreated wood, resulting in significant economic savings and conservation of timber resources. PCP is usually applied to wood products as a 5% solution in mineral spirits, fuel oil, or kerosene. In the United States, commercial and industrial use of PCP as a preservative is concentrated in the South, Southeast, and Northwest. The remaining 20% is used in production of sodium PCP, in plywood and fiberboard waterproofing, in termite control, and as an herbicide for use in rights of way and industrial sites. PCP is registered by the EPA as a termiticide, fungicide, herbicide, algicide, and disinfectant and as an ingredient in antifouling paint. It can be applied as a microbial deterrent in the preservation of wood pulp, leather, seeds, rope, glue, starch, and cooling-tower water. It may not be used for domestic purposes because it is a restricted-use pesticide by the EPA.

Because of the risk of teratogenicity and fetotoxicity, the EPA, since 1984, has required that PCP products in concentrations of 5% or less be used only by certified applicators and has restricted the use of PCP on products that may come in contact with bare skin, food, water, or animals.

Occupational & Environmental Exposure

Occupational exposure to PCP occurs primarily in the gas, electric service, and wood preservative industries. Newer automated processes and closed systems at larger facilities are generally reducing exposure. Acute exposure may occur with the opening of pressure-vessel doors or in tank cleaning, solution preparation, and the handling of wood after treatment. Hand application of PCP also may pose a risk of overexposure. Dermal exposure is the principal route, either through direct contact with PCP or through contact with treated wood.

Nonoccupational exposure to PCP can occur after the wood has been treated and shipped, where handling may result in dermal exposure. Six months after treatment, PCP will be present on the wood surface at a concentration of about 0.5 mg/ft^2. Elevated levels of PCP have been found in the blood and urine of residents of log homes where the logs have been dipped in PCP prior to construction; air samples showed an indoor air concentration of up to 0.38 mcg/m^3 5 years after construction.

▶ Metabolism & Mechanism of Action

Absorption of PCP in the occupational setting is largely through inhalation and skin absorption. The latter is increased when PCP is dissolved in organic solvents. Metabolic studies in rodents and human liver homogenates indicate that PCP undergoes oxidative dechlorination to form tetrachlorohydroquinone, which results in lipid peroxidation and cell death. PCP is excreted mainly in urine as free PCP and as a conjugate with glucuronic acid. Pharmacokinetics are characterized in a single-dose oral administration study by first-order absorption, enterohepatic circulation, and first-order elimination, with 74% of the oral dose of PCP excreted unchanged within 8 days. The half-life for elimination was approximately 30 hours. However, in chronically exposed workers during 2- to 4-week vacations, the terminal half-life of elimination ranges from 30 to 60 days.

Acute intoxication with PCP is caused by interference with cellular electron transport and the uncoupling of oxidative phosphorylation in mitochondria and endoplasmic reticulum. Interaction with energy-rich phosphate compounds results in hydrolysis and free-energy release, leading to a hypermetabolic state with peripheral tissue hyperthermia.

▶ Clinical Findings

A. Symptoms and Signs

1. Acute exposure—

A. Skin—Commercial PCP can cause skin irritation after single exposures to more than a 10% concentration of the material or after prolonged or repeated contact with a 1% solution. Skin sensitization has not been demonstrated. Chloracne may occur after exposure to PCP contaminated with dioxins and dibenzofurans, particularly associated with direct skin contact.

B. Eye, nose, and throat—Irritation can occur at levels above 0.3 mg/m^3.

C. Systemic intoxication—Systemic intoxication caused by PCP became evident in the 1950s after two workers died following cutaneous exposure in a wood-dipping operation. Since that time, fatalities from PCP have occurred among chemical production workers, herbicide sprayers, and wood manufacturers. A unique poisoning tragedy occurred in 20 babies wearing diapers inappropriately laundered in 23% sodium pentachlorophenate; two babies died.

Acute intoxication is characterized by the rapid onset of profuse diaphoresis, hyperpyrexia, tachycardia, tachypnea, weakness, nausea, vomiting, abdominal pain, intense thirst, and pain in the extremities. An intense form of muscle contraction is observed before death. Postmortem examination of one acutely intoxicated worker showed cerebral edema with fatty degeneration of the viscera. The minimum lethal dose of PCP in humans is estimated to be 29 mg/kg.

2. Chronic exposure—Long-term exposure to PCP is associated with conjunctivitis, sinusitis, and bronchitis. Chloracne

may occur among PCP-exposed workers and may persist for years after exposure has ceased. Occupational exposure to PCP does not cause adverse effects on the peripheral nervous system, and consistent immunologic effects have not been demonstrated following prolonged exposure to PCP.

Paternal exposure to chlorophenate wood preservatives is associated with congenital anomalies in offspring of sawmill workers. Bone marrow aplasia has been reported after exposure to PCP. Cytogenetic studies of PCP-exposed workers have not demonstrated increased sister chromatid exchanges or chromosomal breakage.

An increased risk for non-Hodgkin lymphoma has been observed following exposure to PCP and phenoxyacetic acids. The IARC finds *sufficient evidence* in humans (group 1) for the carcinogenicity of PCP (non-Hodgkin lymphoma). The US EPA concludes that the use of PCP poses a risk of oncogenicity because of the contaminants hexachlorodibenzodioxin and hexachlorobenzene. PCP and its contaminants cause teratogenic and fetotoxic effects in test animals, but little is known concerning adverse reproductive outcomes in humans.

B. Laboratory Findings

Acute intoxication with PCP can result in elevation of blood urea and creatinine, with metabolic acidosis and increased anion gap. Increased serum lactic acid dehydrogenase activity and reduced creatinine clearance have been measured in chronically PCP-exposed workers.

Blood levels of PCP in fatal cases have ranged from 40 to 170 mg/L. Urine levels have ranged from 29 to 500 mg/L in fatal cases and from 3 to 20 mg/L in nonfatal cases of intoxication. In PCP-exposed workers, mean urine PCP levels were 0.95–1.31 mg/L. In nonoccupationally exposed individuals in the United States, urine values of PCP average 6.3 mcg/L, with a range from 1 to 193 mcg/L and an average of 15 mcg/L in hemodialysis patients.

▶ Differential Diagnosis

Acute intoxication can be confused with hyperthermia from other causes, including heat stroke or sepsis. Symptoms of respiratory irritation may be due to the solvent carrier or other occupational irritants. Chloracne is associated with polychlorinated biphenyls, polychlorinated dibenzodioxins, or polychlorinated dibenzofurans.

▶ Prevention

A. Work Practices

Appropriate respiratory protection must be worn where exposure to PCP may exceed permissible limits, particularly in higher-risk operations such as formulating plants and pressure-vessel and tank maintenance. Gloves of nitrile and polyvinyl chloride provide the best protection against both aqueous sodium pentachlorophenate and PCP in diesel oil. Clothing contaminated with PCP must be removed, left at the workplace, and laundered before reuse. Washing and showering facilities should be available to prevent contamination of food, drink, and family. Coating PCP-treated logs of home interiors with a sealant will reduce PCP exposure to the residents.

B. Medical Surveillance

Preemployment urine analysis for PCP should be performed and repeated at intervals. Samples should be collected prior to the last shift of the work week and PCP measured by methods that incorporate hydrolysis. The recommended ACGIH BEI is 2 mg of total PCP per milligram of creatinine in urine or 5 mg of free PCP per milligram of creatinine in plasma before the last shift of work. Discontinuation of PCP exposure will not result in persistent excretion of total PCPs in urine.

Routine medical surveillance should include attention to skin rash and mucous membrane irritation. Hot weather appears to be a predisposing factor for PCP intoxication, so exposure to PCP should be minimized during those times. Significant skin absorption of PCPs may occur and can be documented by urinary PCP monitoring.

▶ Treatment

Solutions of PCP spilled on the skin are treated with prompt and thorough washing with soap and water. Eyes contaminated with PCP should be flushed for 15 minutes with water. All contaminated shoes and clothing should be removed immediately.

In the event of acute PCP intoxication, adequate intravenous hydration and efforts to maintain normal body temperature are essential to prevent cardiovascular collapse. Rapid onset of muscular spasms may prevent intubation and resuscitation, so careful monitoring of respiratory status is critical. Metabolic acidosis should be treated with sodium bicarbonate. Atropine sulfate is contraindicated.

POLYCHLORINATED BIPHENYLS

ESSENTIALS OF DIAGNOSIS

- ▶ Acute effects
  - Skin rash (chloracne).
  - Eye irritation.
  - Nausea, vomiting.
- ▶ Chronic effects
  - Weakness, weight loss, anorexia.
  - Skin rash (chloracne).
  - Numbness and tingling of extremities.
  - Elevated serum triglycerides.
  - Elevated liver enzymes.

General Considerations

Polychlorinated biphenyls (PCBs) are a large family of chlorinated aromatic hydrocarbons prepared by the chlorination of biphenyl. Commercial products are a mixture of PCBs with variable chlorine content and are named according to the percentage of chlorine. In addition, all PCBs are contaminated with small but highly toxic concentrations of polychlorinated dibenzofurans.

Use

Between 1930 and 1975, approximately 1.4 billion pounds of PCBs were produced in the United States. The fire-resistant nature of PCBs, combined with their outstanding thermal stability, made them excellent choices as hydraulic and heat-transfer fluids. They also were used to improve the waterproofing characteristics of surface coatings and were used in the manufacture of carbonless copy paper, printing inks, plasticizers, special adhesives, lubricating additives, and vacuum-pump fluids. In the United States, commercial PCBs were marketed under the name Aroclor. In 1977, Congress banned the manufacture, processing, distribution, and use of PCBs.

Occupational & Environmental Exposure

Leakage of PCBs from capacitors and transformers while in storage, shipment, or maintenance results in transient exposure risks for utility repair crews, railroad maintenance workers, building engineers, and custodians. Improper storage of used PCB electrical equipment may result in environmental contamination and community exposure. Electrical fires occurring in transformers containing PCBs may release polychlorinated dibenzofurans and polychlorinated dibenzodioxins formed through incomplete combustion of PCBs and chlorinated benzenes. Incidents of widespread building contamination caused by PCB transformer fires have occurred in many cities. The EPA maintains a database of PCB transformers that were in use or in storage for reuse that may pose a significant risk to the general public if leakage or fire should occur.

Metabolism & Mechanism of Action

Chlorinated biphenyl compounds are readily absorbed through the respiratory tract, gastrointestinal tract, and skin. Distribution is primarily into fat. Biphenyls are metabolized in the liver as the primary site of biotransformation. PCB mixtures cause induction of the hepatic microsomal monooxygenase systems. Induction is related to chlorination, and PCB mixtures containing higher percentages of chlorine are more potent than mixtures with lower levels of chlorination. More highly chlorinated isomers are also more resistant to metabolism and therefore are more persistent. Hydroxy metabolites can be detected in bile, feces, and breast milk, but urinary excretion is quite low. This leads to bioaccumulation in fat at low exposure levels and the persistence of PCBs in fatty tissue years after exposure. The formation of electrophilic arene oxide metabolites may cause DNA damage and the initiation of tumor growth.

Clinical Findings

A. Symptoms and Signs

1. Acute—Acute exposure to PCBs results in mucous membrane irritation and nausea and vomiting. Transient skin irritation may result from direct handling of PCBs containing mixtures of solvents.

In the mass food poisoning incident, which was a result of rice oil contamination, in western Japan in 1968 (*yusho*, or *rice oil disease*), ingestion of PCBs resulted in chloracne. Chloracne probably results from interference with vitamin A metabolism in the skin, with disturbances of the epithelial tissues of the pilosebaceous duct. Typical chloracne presents with cystic or comedonal lesions over the face, ear lobes, retroauricular region, axillae, trunk, and external genitalia and may occur at any age. Yusho patients also showed dark pigmentation of the gingivae, oral mucosa, and nails, with conjunctival swelling. It is not clear whether all or some of these findings were a result of trace contamination of the PCBs with dibenzofurans; the latter compound may have increased during cooking.

2. Chronic—In addition to the acute symptoms of upper respiratory tract irritation, chronic workplace exposure to PCBs also has resulted in chloracne. The relationship between dose of exposure and the appearance of chloracne is inconsistent, although chloracne persists for years after exposure has ceased.

PCBs have an efficient transplacental transfer, and adverse reproductive effects of PCBs have been reported in many animal species; these include failure of implantation, increased number of spontaneous abortions, and low birth weight of litters. In *yu-cheng* (*oil disease*), mothers were exposed to PCBs and their heat-degradation products from the ingestion of contaminated rice oil in 1979. Children of these mothers were born growth retarded, with dysmorphic physical findings, delayed cognitive development, and increased activity levels. Rare cases of chloracne and, more commonly, nail abnormalities have been found in *yu-cheng* children. Higher prenatal exposure to PCBs predicts poorer cognitive abilities, impaired development, and endocrine abnormalities in the offspring of women with exposure to PCBs in the environment or from eating PCB-contaminated fish; these effects appear long-lasting in follow-up studies. In a large pooled study of children in seven European birth cohorts, there was no association between pre- or postnatal exposure to persistent organic pollutants (including PCBs) and the risk of attention-deficit/hyperactivity disorder before the age of 10 years. Another study found no association between any specific endocrine disruptor biomarkers (including PCBs) in maternal prenatal serum and the odds of autism spectrum disorder or intellectual disability.

Cytogenetic analysis of peripheral blood lymphocytes has shown increased chromosome aberrations and sister chromatid exchanges among PCB-exposed workers. PCBs fed to test animals produce hepatocellular carcinomas. Cohort studies and case reports of workers exposed to PCBs show an increased risk of malignant melanoma and brain, liver, biliary, stomach, thyroid, hematopoietic, and colorectal cancer. Case control studies show that PCBs significantly increase the risk of non-Hodgkin lymphoma.

PCBs are known as environmental endocrine-disrupting chemicals, with a variety of end-organ hormonal effects. For example, low doses of PCBs potentially can interfere with thyroid hormone receptor–mediated transactivation and alter prenatal steroid hormones. Some PCBs exert dioxin-like activity mediated through receptors that can interfere with sexual hormone–mediated processes. To determine whether these exert an important clinical effect, several studies of environmental PCB exposure and breast cancer incidence have been performed over the past several years. A significant association between PCB levels and breast cancer risk has been demonstrated in some but not all studies.

In a community-based prospective study around a chemical factory that produced PCBs and other organochlorines, a dose-response relationship was observed between PCB serum levels and the onset of hypertension and dementia.

B. Laboratory Findings

Mild elevations of serum triglyceride concentrations have been found in *yusho* patients and occupationally exposed individuals. PCB-exposed workers have been reported to have significant correlations between the serum PCB level and the g-glutamyl transpeptidase level.

If exposure to PCB is suspected, serum or fat levels of PCBs may be measured to document absorption. In a steady state, serum is as good a reflection of body burden as is fat. Results must be interpreted in light of established normal values for geographic area and laboratory technique. PCBs can be measured in human tissue by a variety of analytic methods and have been variously reported as total PCB content related to a commercial mixture, as quantification of chromatographic peaks, or by characterization of specific congeners. Analysis of coplanar mono-*ortho*-substituted and di-*ortho*-substituted PCB levels in human blood may be useful following acute or chronic exposure. These more toxic congeners contribute significantly to dioxin toxic equivalents in blood from US adults. Normative PCB values among US adults have been published by the Centers for Disease Control and Prevention (CDC).

▶ Differential Diagnosis

Occupational exposure to PCBs may be accompanied by exposure to chlorinated dibenzodioxin and dibenzofuran contaminants and may be responsible for chronic toxicity. Concurrent exposure to solvents is important because these substances may cause chronic fatigue and elevated liver enzymes. Mild chloracne should not be confused with other papular rashes. A biopsy may be necessary to establish the diagnosis.

▶ Prevention

A. Work Practices

Work practices to avoid exposure to PCBs include the use of special PCB-resistant gloves and protective clothing. Adequate ventilation should be maintained during spill cleanup or maintenance of vessels containing PCBs; if this is not possible, approved respirators should be provided. Provision should be made for proper decontamination or disposal of contaminated clothing or equipment. Locations where PCBs are stored should be clearly posted as required by law. Environmental sampling may be necessary to ensure adequate worker protection or safety for public reentry to contaminated areas. Reentry or cleanup levels have been established for dioxins and PCBs to protect workers who reoccupy buildings following a PCB fire.

B. Medical Surveillance

Workers intermittently exposed to PCBs should have a baseline skin examination and liver function tests. Follow-up examination can be limited to symptomatic individuals and those exposed as a consequence of accidental contamination. Routine serum measurements are not recommended.

▶ Treatment

Acute exposure should be treated by immediate decontamination of the skin with soap and water to prevent skin absorption. No specific measures are available for respiratory tract or skin absorption. No treatment is available for chronic PCB toxicity. Chloracne is treated with topical therapy for symptomatic relief.

POLYCYCLIC AROMATIC HYDROCARBONS

ESSENTIALS OF DIAGNOSIS

▶ Acute effects
- Dermatitis, conjunctivitis (coal tar pitch volatiles).

▶ Chronic effects
- Excess cancer rates in selected occupations.

▶ General Considerations

Polycyclic aromatic hydrocarbons (PAHs) are organic compounds consisting of three or more aromatic rings that contain only carbon and hydrogen and share a pair of carbon atoms. They are formed by pyrolysis or incomplete combustion of such organic matter as coke, coal tar and pitch, asphalt, and oil. The composition of the products of pyrolysis depends on the fuel, the temperature, and the time in the hot area. PAHs are emitted as vapors from the zone of burning and condense immediately on soot particles or form very small particles themselves. Such processes always lead to a mixture of hundreds of PAHs. Compounds with three or four aromatic rings predominate. Carcinogenic PAHs are found among those with five or six rings. The simplest fused ring is naphthalene. Some important PAHs in the occupational environment are shown below:

Naphthalene   Anthracene

Benzo(a)pyrene

▶ Use, Production, & Exposure

Pure PAHs have no direct use except for naphthalene and anthracene. Anthracene is used in the manufacture of dyes, synthetic fibers, plastics, and monocrystals; as a component of smoke screens; in scintillation counter crystals; and in semiconductor research. Benzo(a)pyrene (BaP) is used as a research chemical and is not produced commercially in the United States. Bitumens are contained in road-paving, roofing, and asphalt products. The majority of carbon black is used as a pigment for rubber tires, with the remainder used in a variety of products such as paint, plastics, printing inks, pigment in eye cosmetics, carbon paper, and typewriter ribbons.

Creosote is used extensively as a wood preservative, usually by high-pressure impregnation of lumber, and as a constituent of fuel oil, lubricant for die molds, and pitch for roofing. Creosote contains over 300 different compounds, the major components of which are PAHs, phenols, cresols, xylenols, and pyridines.

Coal tar pitch is used as a raw material for plastics, solvents, dyes, and drugs. Crude or refined coal tar products are used for waterproofing, paints, pipe coatings, roads, roofing, and insulation; as a sealant, binder, and filler in surface coatings; and as a modifier in epoxy resin coatings.

Naphthalene is used as a chemical intermediate in the production of phthalic anhydride, carbamate insecticides, naphthol, sulfonic acids, and surfactants and as a moth repellent and tanning agent. PAHs as contaminants can be found in air, water, food, and cigarette smoke, as well as in the industrial environment.

▶ Occupational Exposure

A. Coal Tars & Products

Exposures to PAHs may occur among carbon black production workers, wildland firefighters, petroleum tanker deck crews, meat smokehouse workers, and printing press room operators. The most important source of PAHs in the air of the workplace is coal tar. Tars and pitches are black or brown liquid or semisolid products derived from coal, petroleum, wood, shale oil, or other organic materials. Coal tars are by-products of the carbonization of coal to produce coke or natural gas. The coke-oven plant is the principal source of coal tar. Coal tar pitch and creosote are derived from the distillation of coal tar. Numerous PAHs have been identified in coal tar, coal tar pitch, and creosote. Coal tar pitch volatiles are the volatile matter emitted into the air when coal tar, coal tar pitch, or their products are heated, and they may contain several PAHs.

The major use for coal tar pitch is as the binder for aluminum smelting electrodes; other uses include roofing material, surface coatings, pipe-coating enamels, and as a binder for briquettes and foundry cores. Creosote is used almost exclusively as a wood preservative.

Occupational exposure to PAHs in coal tar and pitches may occur in gas and coke works, aluminum reduction plants, iron and steel foundries, and coal gasification facilities and during roof and pavement tarring and the application of coal tar paints.

B. Carbon Black

Carbon black is derived from the partial combustion (pyrolysis) of natural gas or petroleum. It is used primarily in pigmenting and reinforcing rubber products and in inks, paints, and paper.

C. Bitumens

Bitumens are viscous solids or liquids derived from refining processes of petroleum. They are used principally for road construction when mixed with asphalt, in roofing felt manufacture, in pipe coatings, and as binders in briquettes. Occupational exposure may occur in these operations.

D. Soots

Soots are mixtures of particulate carbon, organic tars, resins, and inorganic material produced during incomplete combustion of carbon-containing material. Occupational exposure is primarily to chimney soot; potential exposure occurs to chimney sweeps, brick masons, and heating-unit service personnel.

E. Diesel Exhaust

Exposure to PAHs (methylated naphthalenes and phenanthrenes) has been documented among several occupational groups exposed to diesel exhaust, including truck drivers, underground miners, and railroad workers.

Environmental Exposure

PAHs occur in the air primarily as a result of coal burning and settle on soil, where they may leach into water. They are found in smoked fish and meats and form during the broiling and grilling of foods. They are inhaled in cigarette smoke from the burning of tobacco.

Metabolism & Mechanism of Action

PAHs are absorbed readily by the skin, lungs, and gastrointestinal tract of experimental animals and are metabolized rapidly and excreted in the feces. In humans, they are largely absorbed from carrier particles via the respiratory route. They are activated by aryl hydrocarbon hydroxylase to a reactive epoxide intermediate and then conjugated for excretion in urine or bile. The reactive epoxide may bind covalently with DNA and probably accounts for the carcinogenic activity.

Clinical Findings

A. Symptoms and Signs

1. Acute exposure—Acute inhalation exposure to naphthalene may cause headache, nausea, diaphoresis, and vomiting. Accidental ingestion has caused hemolytic anemia. Naphthalene also may cause erythema and dermatitis on repeated skin contact. Exposure to coal tar products may cause phototoxicity, with skin erythema, burning, and itching, and eye burning and lacrimation.

2. Chronic exposure—The PAHs are genotoxic, as demonstrated by increased DNA adducts, micronuclei, and chromosomal aberrations among exposed workers. Many PAHs are carcinogenic in animals. Often Bap is measured to indicate the presence of PAHs where exposure to carcinogens is suspected.

Evidence for human carcinogenicity was described initially by Percivall Pott in 1775, when he associated scrotal cancer in chimney sweeps with prolonged exposure to tar and soot. Subsequently, scrotal cancer has been reported among mule spinners exposed to shale oil and among workers exposed to pitch.

Excess cancer mortality has been found among coke oven workers (lung and prostate), foundry workers (lung), aluminum smelter workers (lung and bladder), and roofers (lung and stomach). Workers exposed to diesel exhaust have an increased risk of lung and bladder cancer. In one study, exposure to carbon black experienced by dockyard workers was associated with a twofold increased risk of bladder cancer. Road-paving workers may have a slightly higher rate of lung cancer and a moderately higher rate of stomach cancer than their nonexposed counterparts. A case-control study has suggested that prolonged occupational exposure to PAH may increase breast cancer risk, especially among women with a family history of breast cancer. Multiple studies of wildland firefighters have demonstrated excessive exposure to particulate matter (including PAHs) with an increased

risk of lung cancer and cardiovascular disease. Occupational creosote exposure is a risk for squamous papilloma and carcinoma of the skin.

The IARC considers coal tar pitch volatiles to be carcinogenic to humans (group 1), BaP and creosote possibly carcinogenic to humans (group 2A), and carbon black possibly carcinogenic to humans (group 2B). NIOSH considers that coal tar products, carbon black, and anthracene are carcinogenic and recommends that exposures be limited to the lowest feasible level. There is evidence that extracts of refined bitumens are carcinogenic in animals. There are insufficient data to assess cancer risk among workers exposed to bitumens (such as highway maintenance workers and road pavers).

Exposure-related respiratory effects in carbon black–exposed workers have included reduction in airflow, symptoms of chronic bronchitis, and small opacities on chest radiograph. There is a significant association between urinary monohydroxy polycyclic aromatic hydrocarbons (OH-PAHs) and decreased lung function, possibly related to oxidative DNA damage. Elevated liver enzymes have been found in a group of coke oven workers heavily exposed to PAHs, and excess mortality from cirrhosis of the liver has been observed in a cohort of workers heavily exposed to chlorinated naphthalenes. Some studies have indicated that occupational PAH exposure causes fatal ischemic heart disease with a consistent exposure-response relationship. Maternal occupational exposure to PAHs may increase the risk of congenital defects among offspring.

B. Laboratory Findings

Photopatch testing may demonstrate photodermatitis in workers with occupational exposure to coal tar pitch and fumes.

Differential Diagnosis

Exposure to other known or potential carcinogens in the work environment should be investigated.

Prevention

A. Work Practices

Reduction of emissions from coke ovens, aluminum works, foundries, and steel works is essential. Where gaseous emissions occur during loading or transferring of heated coal tar products, fume and vapor control systems will reduce personal exposure. Skin exposure to tars, pitches, and oils containing PAHs is avoided by wearing gloves and changing contaminated work clothes. Wild land firefighters should use appropriate personal protective equipment to reduce exposure to smoke.

B. Medical Surveillance

Periodic examination of workers exposed to coal tar pitch volatiles should include a history of skin or eye irritation and physical examination with attention to the skin, upper respiratory tract, and lungs. Urinary 1-hydroxypyrene (1-OHP) has been used for biologic monitoring of many worker populations, including coal liquefaction workers, coke oven workers, foundry workers, aluminum smelter potroom workers, underground miners, electrode paste plant workers, fireproof stone manufacturing workers, graphite electrode production workers, artificial shooting target factory workers, automotive repair workers, carbon black production workers, roofers, road pavers, asphalt workers, firefighters, and policemen. Good correlation has been found between airborne PAH exposure and urinary 1-OHP, with significant contribution from dermal exposure. Urinary 1-naphthol has been used as a biomarker of PAH exposure among naphthalene oil distillation workers, foundry workers, and creosote-impregnated wood assemblers. Urinary PAHs also may be useful biomarkers of occupational exposure. Enzyme radioimmunoassay techniques to measure PAH-DNA adducts in white blood cells also have been used as a biomarker of PAH exposure among several types of PAH-exposed workers, including foundry workers, coke oven workers, fireproof material workers, aluminum smelter potroom workers, roofers, and wildland firefighters. Dietary sources of PAHs (eg, charbroiled food) and cigarette smoking contribute to PAH-DNA adduct or urinary 1-OHP levels and should be evaluated as confounding factors. Tetrahydrotetrol metabolites of BaP in urine also may prove to be useful for biomonitoring of PAH exposures.

▶ Treatment

Photodermatitis should be treated with cortisone-containing preparations, barrier creams, or removal from exposure.

STYRENE

ESSENTIALS OF DIAGNOSIS

▶ Acute effects
  • Eye, respiratory tract, and skin irritation.
▶ Chronic effects
  • Weakness, headache, fatigue, dizziness.
  • Neuropsychologic deficits, color vision loss, sensory nerve conduction slowing.

▶ General Considerations

Styrene, also known as vinyl benzene and phenylethylene, has the chemical formula $C_5H_5CH:CH_2$. It is a colorless volatile liquid at room temperature with a sweet odor at low concentrations. The odor threshold of 1 ppm is below the permissible exposure limit, and the material has adequate warning properties. Styrene monomer must be stabilized by an inhibitor to prevent exothermic polymerization, a process that may cause explosion of its container.

▶ Use

Commercial styrene was first produced in the 1920s and 1930s. During World War II, styrene was important in the manufacture of synthetic rubber. More than 90% of styrene is produced by the dehydrogenation of ethylbenzene. Styrene is used as a monomer or copolymer for polystyrenes, acrylonitrile-butadiene-styrene (ABS) resins, styrene-butadiene rubber (SBR), styrene-butadiene copolymer latexes, and styrene-acrylonitrile (SAN) resins. Styrene is also used in glass-reinforced unsaturated polyester resins employed in construction materials and boats and in the manufacture of protective coatings.

▶ Occupational & Environmental Exposure

In closed polymerization processes, worker exposure to styrene generally is low, but exposure peaks may occur during cleaning, filling, or maintenance of reaction vessels or during transport of liquid styrene. Styrene exposure during manual application of resins (hand lamination) or spraying in open molds may exceed exposure limits. The most significant exposure to styrene occurs when it is used as a solvent-reactant for unsaturated polyester products that are reinforced with fibrous glass. Reinforced plastics/composites are used in the manufacture of boats, storage tanks, wall panels, tub and shower units, and truck camper tops. In this process, alternating layers of chopped fibers or woven mats of fibrous glass are hand applied with catalyzed resin; up to 10% of the styrene may evaporate into the workplace air as the resin cures. Average styrene exposures in plants where the reinforced products are manufactured can range from 40 to 100 ppm, with short-term individual exposures of up to 150–300 ppm. In a NIOSH study of the reinforced-plastics industry, directly exposed workers engaged in the manufacture of truck parts and boats had the highest exposure to styrene, with a mean 8-hour TWA of 61 and 82 ppm, respectively. Styrene may be emitted during cured-in-place-pipe (CIPP) installations, the most popular water pipe repair method used in the United States for sanitary sewer, storm sewer, and drinking water pipe repairs. Elevated levels of urinary styrene have been observed among these workers.

▶ Metabolism & Mechanism of Action

Occupational exposure occurs mainly via inhalation, with approximately 60% of inhaled styrene retained by the lungs. The odor threshold is 0.02–0.47 ppm. Percutaneous absorption is not significant. Styrene is metabolized by the microsomal enzyme system to styrene oxide, which is hydrated to phenylethylene glycol (styrene glycol). Styrene glycol then is metabolized to mandelic acid or to benzoic acid and then hippuric acid. Mandelic acid is further metabolized to phenylglyoxylic acid. Styrene oxide is also metabolized directly to hydroxyphenylethylmercapturic acid. The styrene oxide intermediate is genotoxic and is probably the key factor in the carcinogenic effect of styrene. Genetic polymorphisms of xenobiotic-metabolizing enzymes (EPHX1,

GSTT1, GSTM1, GSTP1) appear to play an important role in styrene biotransformation.

After short-term exposure, the venous half-life of styrene is approximately 40 minutes. The half-lives of mandelic acid and phenylglyoxylic acid are about 4 and 8 hours, respectively. In the chronically exposed worker, the half-life for mandelic acid excretion may range from 6 to 9 hours.

▶ Clinical Findings

A. Symptoms and Signs

1. Acute exposure—Concentrations of styrene from 100 to 200 ppm may cause eye and upper respiratory tract irritation. Styrene is a defatting agent and a primary skin irritant, resulting in dermatitis. Experimental human exposure to several hundred parts per million causes typical organic solvent anesthetic symptoms, with listlessness, drowsiness, impaired balance, difficulty in concentrating, and decrease in reaction time. Styrene exposure acutely enhances serum pituitary hormone secretion. There are no reports of fatalities as a consequence of styrene exposure.

2. Chronic exposure—Weakness, headache, fatigue, poor memory, and dizziness can occur in workers chronically exposed to styrene in concentrations of less than 100 ppm. Mean reaction time and visuomotor performance may be decreased in exposed workers. The incidence of abnormal electroencephalographs (EEGs) is significantly greater as well.

Studies of styrene-exposed workers have shown detectable blood levels of styrene-7,8-oxide, with dose-related increases in lymphocyte DNA adduct levels, styrene-7,8-oxide hemoglobin adduct levels, single-strand DNA breaks, chromosomal aberrations, lymphocyte micronuclei, and sister chromatid exchanges. Higher hypoxanthine–guanine phosphoribosyltransferase (*HRPT*) gene mutant frequencies have been detected in styrene-exposed individuals, associated with years of employment and styrene in blood. Several studies of styrene-exposed workers have demonstrated an association between styrene exposure and degenerative disorders of the nervous system, pancreatic cancer, esophageal cancer, and lymphohematopoietic cancer (acute myeloid leukemia, T-cell lymphomas). Significant associations have been observed in large European studies between the risk of leukemia and exposure to styrene. The IARC has concluded there is *limited evidence* in humans for the carcinogenicity of styrene (group 2A), with positive associations between exposure to styrene and lymphohaematopoietic malignancies.

A number of neurotoxic effects have been observed after styrene exposure, including electroencephalographic abnormalities, sensory nerve-conduction slowing, prolonged somatosensory-evoked potentials, and neuropsychologic deficits. Neuropsychologic symptoms generally are reversible, but some deficits such as visuomotor performance and perceptual speed persist. Neuropsychologic effects may correlate with microsomal epoxide hydrolase activity. Styrene exposure among glass-reinforced-plastic workers and plastic-boat manufacturing workers has been associated with early color and contrast vision dysfunction. The effects on contrast sensitivity increase with long-term cumulative exposure, probably reflecting chronic damage to the neuropoptic pathways. An effect on hearing acuity has been observed, possibly owing to disorganization of the cochlear membranous structures.

Moderate exposure to styrene has been associated with an altered distribution of lymphocyte subsets in worker populations and may alter leukocyte adherence in experimental test systems. Results of these studies suggest that styrene may alter the cell-mediated immune response of T lymphocytes and result in leukocyte alterations in exposed workers. Styrene also has been found to increase the risk of acute ischemic heart disease mortality among the most highly exposed workers at a synthetic rubber plant. Two cases have been reported after exposure to styrene vapor with the development of acute respiratory symptoms associated with impaired gas exchange; imaging and histopathologic findings were consistent with bronchiolitis and organizing pneumonia. Nine cases of obliterative bronchiolitis have been reported after employment in industries that use styrene to make reinforced plastics; evidence suggests styrene exposure is a potential risk factor for nonmalignant respiratory disease. Styrene may be emitted from 3-D printers and with other irritants may cause work-related asthma.

Styrene may be embryotoxic or fetotoxic in animals. Human reproductive studies (spontaneous abortions, congenital malformations, low birth weight, or reduced fertility) have been inconsistent or limited by methodologic shortcomings.

B. Laboratory Findings

A dose-response relationship exists between styrene exposure and hepatic transaminase, direct bilirubin, and alkaline phosphatase concentrations. However, these tests are nonspecific and should be interpreted in light of other confounders.

The most reliable indicator of styrene exposure is mandelic acid in the urine. Postshift mandelic acid levels in urine show a good correlation with average TWA styrene exposure over the range of 5–150 ppm. Levels of 500 mg mandelic acid per liter of urine may indicate recent exposure to at least 10 ppm styrene. A concentration of 1000 mg mandelic acid per liter of urine corresponds to an average 8-hour TWA styrene exposure of 50 ppm.

▶ Differential Diagnosis

Exposure to other solvents during the production of styrene and in the manufacture of reinforced-plastic products may cause similar symptoms of central nervous system toxicity such as headache, fatigue, and memory loss.

▶ Prevention

A. Work Practices

Styrene poses a significant fire hazard, and proper handling and storage are essential to prevent ignition of the liquid and vapor and a potential explosive reaction. Exposures should be reduced through general and local ventilation systems or through the use of automated processes and closed molds. Intensive local exhaust ventilation is the best way to reduce styrene vapor concentrations during construction of large reinforced-plastic objects, although dilution ventilation is used widely to reduce styrene vapor exposure in the boat industry.

When worker exposure cannot be controlled adequately by engineering controls, protective clothing and respirators may be needed. Where workers may come into contact with liquid styrene, appropriate gloves, boots, overshoes, aprons, and face shields with goggles are recommended. Polyvinyl alcohol and polyethylene gloves and protective clothing give good protection against styrene. To prevent eye irritation at moderately low concentrations, full-facepiece respirators are recommended.

B. Medical Surveillance

Initial medical evaluation should include a history of nervous system disorders and an examination with particular attention to the nervous system, respiratory tract, and skin. Annual medical examinations should be performed on all workers with significant air exposure above the action level or with potential for significant skin exposure. The ACGIH recommended BEI is 240 mg phenylglyoxylic acid per gram of creatinine, 300 mg mandelic acid per gram of creatinine in urine, or 0.55 mg/L in venous blood at the end of the work shift. Styrene in exhaled air also has been used as an indicator of low-level styrene exposure. Measurement of monoamine oxidase type B activity in platelets and the glycophorin A assay also have been suggested as biomarkers of styrene exposure.

▶ Treatment

Hands should be washed after skin exposure, and clothing saturated with styrene should be removed immediately. In the case of eye contact, flush the eye immediately with copious amounts of water for 15 minutes. No specific treatment is recommended for acute or chronic styrene exposure.

2,3,7,8-TETRACHLORODIBENZO-*P*-DIOXIN

ESSENTIALS OF DIAGNOSIS

- ▶ Acute effects
  - Eye and respiratory tract irritation.
  - Skin rash, chloracne.
  - Fatigue, nervousness, irritability.
- ▶ Chronic effects
  - Chloracne.
  - Soft-tissue sarcoma, non-Hodgkin lymphoma, Hodgkin disease.

▶ General Considerations

Polychlorinated dibenzo-*p*-dioxins (PCDDs) and polychlorinated dibenzofurans (PCDFs) are two large series of tricyclic aromatic compounds that exhibit similar physical, chemical, and biologic properties.

PCDFs

PCDDs

However, there is a pronounced difference in potency among the different PCDD and PCDF isomers. The most extensively studied is the 2,3,7,8-tetrachlorodibenzo-*p*-dioxin isomer (2,3,7,8-TCDD). *Dioxin* is the name used for at least 75 chlorinated aromatic isomers, including 22 isomers of the tetrachlorinated dioxin. 2,3,7,8-TCDD is the specific dioxin identified as a contaminant in the production of 2,4,5-trichlorophenol (TCP), 2-(2,4,5-trichlorophenoxy) propionic acid (Silvex), and 2,4,5-trichlorophenoxyacetic acid (2,4,5-T). In its pure form, 2,3,7,8-TCDD is a colorless crystalline solid at room temperature, sparingly soluble in organic solvents, and insoluble in water. The degree of toxicity of the dioxin compounds is highly dependent on the number and position of the chlorine atoms; isomers with chlorination in the four lateral positions (2,3,7,8) have the highest acute toxicity in animals. Under laboratory conditions, 2,3,7,8-TCDD is one of the most toxic synthetic chemicals known. The chlorinated dibenzofurans are contaminants found in some PCBs used in transformers and capacitors, including the most toxic 2,3,7,8-tetrachlorinated dibenzofuran.

▶ Use

2,3,7,8-TCDD is formed as a stable by-product during the production of TCP. Normally, 2,3,7,8-TCDD persists as a contaminant in TCP in amounts ranging from 0.07 to 6.2 mg/kg. Production of 2,4,5-T and Silvex ceased in the United States in 1979, although stockpiles are still being distributed and used. Agent Orange, used in Vietnam as a defoliant during the 1960s, was a 50:50 mixture of esters of the herbicides 2,4-D and 2,4,5-T. Between 10 and 12 million gallons was sprayed over 3–4 million acres in Vietnam; in Agent Orange, the 2,3,7,8-TCDD concentration was about 2 ppm.

The combustion of 2,4,5-T can result in its conversion to small amounts of 2,3,7,8-TCDD. Polychlorinated biphenyls can be converted to PCDFs. Soot from PCB transformer fires may be contaminated with more than 2000 mcg/g PCDFs, including the most toxic 2,3,7,8 isomers. A complex mixture of PCDDs and PCDFs may occur in fly ash from municipal incinerators. 2,3,7,8-TCDD is not used commercially in the United States.

▶ Occupational & Environmental Exposure

Occupational exposure to 2,3,7,8-TCDD can occur during the production and use of 2,4,5-T and its derivatives. Since 1949, there have been numerous accidents in chemical plants manufacturing chlorinated phenols in which workers were exposed to PCDDs. The explosion of a TCP chemical plant in 1976 in Seveso, Italy, exposed some 37,000 residents of surrounding communities to 2,3,7,8-TCDD.

Workers may be exposed to PCDDs during the production of TCP, 2,4,5-T, and PCP. Herbicide sprayers using 2,4,5-T or Silvex have been exposed to 2,3,7,8-TCDD during application. Environmental contamination occurred from spraying waste oil that contained 2,3,7,8-TCDD for dust control on the ground in Missouri. Workers exposed to slag and fly ash from municipal waste incinerators may have increased blood concentrations of PCDDs and PCDFs. The EPA banned most uses of 2,4,5-T and Silvex in 1979, although their use was allowed on sugar cane and in orchards, and miscellaneous noncrop uses were permitted. It is not possible to accurately estimate the number of US workers currently exposed to 2,3,7,8-TCDD during decontamination of worksites, from waste materials contaminated with 2,3,7,8-TCDD (such as metal recycling), or from cleanup after fires in transformers containing PCBs.

▶ Metabolism & Mechanism of Action

2,3,7,8-TCDD is an extremely lipophilic substance that is absorbed readily following an oral dose in rats. It accumulates mainly in the liver and after a single dose is largely eliminated unmetabolized in the feces with a whole-body half-life of about 3 weeks. After repeated dosing in small laboratory animals, it is stored in adipose tissue. The half-life of 2,3,7,8-TCDD in humans is 9 years. Dermal absorption may be important in workers exposed to phenoxy acids and chlorophenols. Exposure to 2,3,7,8-TCDD as a vapor normally is negligible because of its low vapor pressure.

Dioxin-like compounds are characterized by high-affinity binding to the Ah receptor, and most biologic effects are thought to be mediated by the ligand-Ah receptor complex. A second protein is required for DNA-binding capability and transcriptional activation of target genes. Growth factors, free radicals, the interaction of 2,3,7,8-TCDD with the estrogen-transduction pathway or protein kinases also may play a role in signal-transduction mechanisms. Relative potency factors have been assigned to the dioxin-like compounds on the basis of a comparison of potency with that of 2,3,7,8-TCDD. Each chemical is assigned a toxic equivalency factor (TEF), some fraction of 2,3,7,8-TCDD, and the total toxic equivalency of the mixture (TEQ) is the sum of the weighted potencies. TEF values have been calculated for PCDDs, PCDFs, and dioxin-like PCBs.

▶ Clinical Findings

A. Signs and Symptoms

1. Acute exposure—In some animals, 2,3,7,8-TCDD is lethal in doses of less than 1 mcg/kg. Acute toxicity results in profound wasting, thymic atrophy, bone marrow suppression, hepatotoxicity, and microsomal enzyme induction.

In humans, the acute toxicity of 2,3,7,8-TCDD is known from accidental release caused by runaway reactions or explosions. A process accident in Nitro, West Virginia, in 1949, was followed by acute skin, eye, and respiratory tract irritation, headache, dizziness, and nausea. These symptoms subsided within 1–2 weeks and were followed by an acneiform eruption; severe muscle pain in the extremities, thorax, and shoulders; fatigue, nervousness, and irritability; dyspnea; and complaints of decreased libido and intolerance to cold. Workers exhibited severe chloracne, hepatic enlargement, peripheral neuritis, delayed prothrombin time, and increased total serum lipid levels. Long-term follow-up studies of dioxin-exposed workers have found persistence of chloracne and some evidence of liver disease. In eight surviving workers who were accidentally exposed to 2,3,7,8-tetrachlorodibenzo-p-dioxin (TCDD) during production of herbicides, neurologic examination 50 years later revealed central nervous system impairment in all individuals. Among former employees of a pesticide production plant exposed to 2,3,7,8-TCDD in the 1980s, several decades later there was an increased risk of diabetes, peripheral nervous system, immunologic, thyroid and lipid disorders system.

2. Chronic exposure—In animals, 2,3,7,8-TCDD is a teratogen and is toxic to the fetus. Two-year feeding studies in rats and mice have demonstrated an excess of liver tumors; the feeding level at which no observable effects in rats occurred was 0.001 mcg/kg per day.

Chloracne can result within several weeks after exposure to 2,3,7,8-TCDD and can persist for decades. Among production workers, the severity of chloracne is related to the degree of exposure. In some workplaces, exposed persons had chloracne but no systemic illnesses; in others, workers experienced fatigue, weight loss, myalgias, insomnia, irritability, and decreased libido. The liver becomes tender and enlarged, and sensory changes, particularly in the lower extremities, have been reported. In exposed production workers, systemic symptoms—except for chloracne—have not persisted after exposures ceased.

Immunotoxic, reproductive, and endocrine effects appear to be among the most sensitive indicators of dioxin toxicity. Research indicates that 2,3,7,8-TCDD inhibits multiple estrogen-induced responses in rodent uterus and mammary tissue and in human breast cancer cells. Antiestrogenic effects are thought to be mediated via the aryl hydrocarbon receptor. Laboratory studies in animals suggest that dioxin-like compounds cause altered development (low birth weight, spontaneous abortions, congenital malformations) and adverse changes in reproductive health (fertility, sex organ development, reproductive behavior). 2,3,7,8-TCDD may be transferred transplacentally and via breast milk, and elevated levels of 2,3,7,8-TCDD have been detected in adult children of female chemical production workers exposed to dioxins. A correlation has been found between serum dioxin levels and menstrual cycle characteristics, particularly among premenarcheal women. Epidemiologic studies suggest an association between paternal herbicide exposure and an increased risk of spina bifida in offspring. No effect on the risk of spontaneous abortion or sex ratio of the offspring has been observed.

A number of immunologic effects also have been seen in animal studies. Human studies show alteration in delayed-type hypersensitivity after exposure to dioxins. A relation between serum 2,3,7,8-TCDD concentration and a decrease in circulating CD26 cells and decreased spontaneous background proliferation has been observed. Evidence for an effect of dioxin on the humoral immune system is sparse, and no consistent cytogenetic effects have been seen from 2,3,7,8-TCDD exposure.

2,3,7,8-TCDD may inhibit uroporphyrinogen decarboxylation, and cases of porphyria cutanea tarda among exposed workers have been reported. No association has been observed among former chlorophenol production workers between 2,3,7,8-TCDD exposure and serum transaminase levels, induction of cytochrome P450 activity, peripheral neuropathy, chronic bronchitis or chronic obstructive pulmonary disease, and porphyria cutanea tarda. Serum dioxin levels have been positively associated with levels of luteinizing and follicle-stimulating hormones and inversely related to total testosterone levels. This finding is consistent with dioxin-related effects on the hypothalamic-pituitary-Leydig cell axis in animals.

An increased risk of peripheral neuropathy, heart disease, hypertension and liver disorders has been seen in studies of Vietnam veterans exposed to dioxin. No significant clinical effect on acne, hematologic parameters, immunologic function, or cognitive functioning has been observed in this population. Combined analyses of the Vietnam cohort and a NIOSH cohort of industrial workers show modest evidence that exposed workers are at higher risk than nonexposed workers of diabetes or abnormal fasting glucose levels. Increased risk of metabolic syndrome has been observed in a community exposed to dibenzo-*p*-dioxins and dibenzofurans.

Excess risk of soft-tissue sarcoma has been associated with exposure to 2,3,7,8-TCDD and phenoxy herbicides. In a reanalysis of US chemical workers with 2,3,7,8-TCDD exposure, a positive trend was found between estimated log cumulative 2,3,7,8-TCDD serum level and overall cancer mortality. Long-term follow-up studies of the Seveso population and a large international cohort show an increase in all-cancer mortality, with increases in soft-tissue sarcoma and lymphohemopoietic neoplasms. Studies of the Operation Ranch Hand cohort suggest a modest increase in the risk of prostate cancer. Serum 2,3,7,8-TCDD levels were significantly related to breast cancer incidence in a long-term follow-up of women in the Seveso Womens' Health Study. However, another study indicates that breast cancer risk does not appear to be associated with adipose levels of PCDDs. The IARC finds 2,3,7,8-TCDD to be carcinogenic to humans (group 1). NIOSH recommends that 2,3,7,8-TCDD be treated as a potential human carcinogen and that exposure be reduced to the lowest feasible concentration.

B. Laboratory Findings

Abnormalities reported most consistently are elevated liver enzymes, prolonged prothrombin time, and elevated cholesterol and triglyceride levels. Urinary porphyrins may be elevated. Following the Seveso accident, the incidence of abnormal nerve-conduction tests was significantly elevated in subjects with chloracne.

Very low levels of 2,3,7,8-TCDD (4–130 ppt) can be detected in adipose tissue of nonexposed populations. Concentration of polychlorinated compounds in plasma may be 1000-fold less than in adipose tissue. There is a high correlation between adipose and serum 2,3,7,8-TCDD levels; serum levels are a valid measure of body burden. The correlation between plasma and adipose tissue concentrations of 2,3,7,8-TCDD with signs and symptoms is uncertain. Normative PCDD and PCDF serum values among US adults have been published recently by the CDC.

▶ Differential Diagnosis

Known causes of an acneiform eruption in the workplace include petroleum cutting oils, coal tar, and the chlorinated aromatic compounds. With systemic complaints, such as weight loss, headache, myalgias, and irritability, other underlying medical illnesses should be ruled out before attributing the disorder to 2,3,7,8-TCDD.

▶ Prevention

A. Work Practices

NIOSH recommends that 2,3,7,8-TCDD be considered a potential occupational carcinogen and that exposure in all occupational settings be controlled to the fullest extent possible. Specific guidelines for safe work practices must begin with environmental sampling to determine the presence of 2,3,7,8-TCDD contamination, including sampling of air, soil, and settled dust and wipe sampling of surfaces. For site cleanup, specific decontamination procedures should be adhered to for adequate worker protection. Protective clothing and equipment should consist of both outer and inner garments, with outer coveralls, gloves, and boots made of nonwoven polyethylene fabric. Appropriate respiratory protection must be worn, ranging from an air-purifying respirator to a self-contained breathing apparatus. Follow-up sampling should be conducted after decontamination of a site to ensure adequate cleanup.

B. Medical Surveillance

Production workers exposed to compounds contaminated with 2,3,7,8-TCDD, as well as site-decontamination personnel, should undergo baseline and periodic medical examinations with special attention to the skin and nervous system. Baseline laboratory testing should include liver enzymes, cholesterol, and triglycerides, with follow-up as required. Effective safety measures for dioxin cleanup workers will prevent clinical or biochemical disease (chloracne, liver disease, peripheral neuropathy, porphyria cutanea tarda). There has been considerable progress in the use of serum 2,3,7,8-TCDD levels, with the characterization of 2,3,7,8-TCDD body burdens in the Ranch Hand cohort, Seveso residents, herbicide production employees, and Vietnamese civilians. Serum dioxin levels may be useful for research purposes or to assess health-outcome risks for exposure reconstruction, but they are not recommended for routine medical monitoring.

▶ Treatment

Skin contaminated with 2,3,7,8-TCDD should be washed immediately and any contaminated clothing removed and placed in marked containers and disposed of appropriately. Except for symptomatic treatment of chloracne, there is no treatment for acute or chronic health effects resulting from 2,3,7,8-TCDD exposure.

VINYL CHLORIDE MONOMER

ESSENTIALS OF DIAGNOSIS

- ▶ Acute effects
  - Respiratory tract irritation.
  - Lethargy, headache.
- ▶ Chronic effects
  - Acroosteolysis, Raynaud phenomenon, skin thickening.
  - Hepatosplenomegaly.
  - Hepatic angiosarcoma.

▶ General Considerations

Vinyl chloride monomer (chloroethene) is a colorless, highly flammable gas at room temperature. It is usually handled as a liquid under pressure containing a polymerization inhibitor (phenol). It is soluble in ethanol and ether. The odor threshold is variable, so odor cannot be used to prevent excess exposure.

▶ Use

The vast majority of vinyl chloride monomer is used for the production of polyvinyl chloride resins. Polyvinyl chloride is used primarily in the production of plastic piping and conduit, floor coverings, home furnishings, electrical applications, recreational products (records, toys), packaging (film, sheet, and bottles), and transportation materials (automobile tops, upholstery, and mats).

▶ Occupational & Environmental Exposure

A 1977 NIOSH survey of three vinyl chloride monomer plants found that the 8-hour TWA ranged from 0.07 to 27 ppm. Following promulgation of the OSHA standard in 1974, exposures were reduced to less than 5 ppm. The highest exposures occur in polymerization plants, particularly during reactor-vessel cleaning.

▶ Metabolism & Mechanism of Action

The chief route of exposure to vinyl chloride monomer (VCM) is through inhalation of the gas, although dermal absorption may be significant during manual reactor-vessel cleaning. Vinyl chloride is absorbed readily through the respiratory tract. Its primary metabolite is chloroethylene oxide, which forms the reactive intermediate epoxide that can bind to RNA and DNA *in vivo* and may be responsible for the carcinogenicity observed in animal and human studies. There may be increased risk of hepatic angiosarcoma in association with *p53* gene mutations. Studies have suggested that polymorphisms of *CYP 2E1, GSTT1,* and *ADH2* may be a major reason for genetic susceptibility in VCM-induced hepatic damage.

The half-life of VCM in expired air is 20–30 minutes. Thiodiglycolic acid (TdGA) is the major urinary metabolite, but it is of limited value in biomonitoring because of metabolic saturation of vinyl chloride, variable metabolism rates, and nonspecificity. One study has suggested that TdGA can be used as an exposure marker for polyvinyl chloride workers when the air VCM level to which they are exposed is greater than 5 ppm.

▶ Clinical Findings

A. Symptoms and Signs

1. Acute exposure—VCM has relatively low acute toxicity, causing respiratory irritation and central nervous system depression at high concentrations (10,000–20,000 ppm).

2. Chronic exposure—Chronic toxicity from VCM exposure can result in liver disease, osteolysis, Raynaud phenomenon, vasculitic purpura, mixed connective-tissue disease, and scleroderma-like skin lesions.

A. ACROOSTEOLYSIS—Symptoms of Raynaud phenomenon, osteolysis in the terminal phalanges of some of the fingers, and thickening or raised nodules on the hands and forearms occurred in workers employed in production and polymerization, especially in workers assigned to clean the reactors. *Vinyl chloride disease* is a syndrome consisting of Raynaud phenomenon, acroosteolysis, joint and muscle pain, enhanced collagen deposition, stiffness of the hands, and scleroderma-like skin changes. An increase in circulating immune complex levels, cryoglobulinemia, B-cell proliferation, hyperimmunoglobulinemia, and complement activation has been found in these patients. Susceptibility to this disease has been associated with the HLA-DR5 allele. Vascular changes in the digital arteries of the hand associated with acroosteolysis have been demonstrated by arteriography, and circulating immune complexes have been identified.

B. Liver disease—Hepatic fibrosis, splenomegaly, and thrombocytopenia with portal hypertension have occurred. The characteristic pattern of changes consists of hypertrophy and hyperplasia of hepatocytes and sinusoidal cells, sinusoidal dilation associated with damage to the cells lining the sinusoids, focal areas of hepatocellular degeneration, and fibrosis of portal tracts, septa, and intralobular perisinusoidal regions.

In 1974, three cases of hepatic angiosarcoma among polyvinyl chloride polymerization workers were reported at a plant in Louisville, Kentucky. Since then, many cohort mortality studies have documented an increased risk of hepatic angiosarcoma, hepatocellular carcinoma, and liver cirrhosis. There have been over 200 cases of hepatic angiosarcoma reported worldwide, with an average latency of 22 years. Vinyl chloride is genotoxic, causing increased chromosomal aberrations, sister chromatid exchanges, and lymphocyte micronuclei among exposed workers. Specific gene mutations at the *p53* locus and mutant p21 proteins have been linked to vinyl chloride angiosarcoma. These findings suggest an effect of chloroethylene oxide, a carcinogenic metabolite of vinyl chloride. The risk of hepatic angiosarcoma is related to the time since the first exposure, duration of employment, and the extent of exposure. The IARC finds that vinyl chloride is carcinogenic to humans (group 1) causing both hepatic angiosarcoma and hepatocellular carcinoma, and NIOSH recommends that vinyl chloride be regulated as a potential human carcinogen.

Only two cases of hepatic angiosarcoma have been documented in the polyvinyl chloride processing industry, suggesting a significantly lower vinyl chloride–related neoplastic risk among fabrication workers. Hemangioendothelioma also has been reported after both vinyl chloride and polyvinyl chloride exposure.

C. Pulmonary effects—Cases of pneumoconiosis have been reported in workers exposed to polyvinyl chloride dust. Some polyvinyl chloride production and fabrication workers with high (> 10 mg/m³) exposure to polyvinyl chloride dust have reduced pulmonary function and an increased incidence of chest radiograph abnormalities. Cumulative polyvinyl chloride dust exposure is associated with mild obstructive airway disease and a higher prevalence of small opacities on chest radiograph. One case of pneumoconiosis and systemic sclerosis following a 10-year exposure to polyvinyl chloride dust has been reported.

D. Reproductive effects—Decreased androgen levels and complaints of impotence and decreased libido and sexual

function have been found among male vinyl chloride–exposed workers. Few studies have evaluated the effects of vinyl chloride exposure on the reproductive function of female workers. A significant increase in congenital abnormalities has been found in communities located near a vinyl chloride processing plant, although other studies have failed to report significant development toxicity in association with parental exposure to vinyl chloride or proximity to vinyl chloride facilities.

B. Laboratory Findings

There may be elevated levels of liver enzymes and alkaline phosphatase in workers with vinyl chloride exposure, although in some workers with hepatic angiosarcoma the liver enzymes remain normal until the final stages of disease. Fasting levels of serum bile acids and urinary coproporphyrins have been suggested as clinically useful indicators of early chemical injury in VCM-exposed worker populations with asymptomatic liver dysfunction.

▶ Differential Diagnosis

Hepatic angiosarcoma has been associated with a history of arsenic exposure and thorium dioxide (Thorotrast) ingestion. The VCM-associated sclerotic changes in skin, with skin nodules, Raynaud phenomenon, and osteolysis, are clinically very similar to idiopathic scleroderma; however, sclerodactyly, calcinosis, and digital pitting scars are unusual in VCM disease.

▶ Prevention

The risk of hepatic angiosarcoma should be greatly reduced if the 8-hour TWA is less than 1 ppm.

A. Work Practices

Worker isolation is achieved in most polyvinyl chloride plants through the use of isolated process control rooms. For operators, cleaners, and utility employees, extensive engineering controls in polyvinyl chloride polymerization plants are required to reduce 8-hour TWA worker exposures to less than 1 ppm. Preventing worker exposure during routine maintenance and cleanup operations by adequate degassing of autoclaves and reaction vessels is essential. Online gas chromatographic VCM-specific detectors can identify leaks before large emissions develop.

Employees should be required to wear half-face supplied-air respirators when the concentration of VCM exceeds 1 ppm. A full-face supplied-air respirator is required for reactor cleaning or other maintenance. Where skin contact is possible, protective uniforms, gloves, head coverings, and impervious boots are necessary.

B. Medical Surveillance

Preplacement medical examination should evaluate the presence of liver disease. Concurrent viral hepatitis and alcohol consumption should be evaluated because these factors increase the risk of liver disease in vinyl chloride-exposed workers. Preplacement and periodic measurements of liver enzymes are recommended by NIOSH, although the specificity and sensitivity of these tests are poor. An increased g-glutamyl transpeptidase level is associated with vinyl chloride exposure and may offer greater specificity for medical surveillance. However, a recent study concluded that liver function assessment only including liver function tests is not able to detect VCM-induced liver damage and only revealed alterations owing to nonoccupational factors, such as dietary and/or metabolic dysfunction. Fasting levels of serum bile acids or plasma clearance of technetium-labeled iminodiacetate have been suggested as a sensitive measure of liver dysfunction among vinyl chloride–exposed workers. Liver ultrasonography is a useful diagnostic test for medical surveillance of vinyl chloride workers, with an increased incidence of periportal fibrosis among more highly exposed workers. Surveillance using biomarkers such as *p53* gene mutations and DNA adducts are under investigation but have not yet been proven as useful screening tools.

▶ Treatment

The mean survival after diagnosis of hepatic angiosarcoma is several months. Computed tomography with intravenous contrast dynamic scanning shows a characteristic isodense appearance on delayed postcontrast scans. Chemotherapy may slightly improve the duration and quality of survival. Acroosteolysis appears to be irreversible after cessation of exposure.

REFERENCES

Acids and Alkalis

Jolly K, Douglas JA, Hamnett N, Natalwala I, van Niekerk WJ: Ongoing effects of burns. BMJ 2016;352:i1104 [PMID: 26979783].

Mahdinia M, Adeli SH, Mohammadbeigi A, Heidari H, Ghamari F, Soltanzadeh A: Respiratory disorders resulting from exposure to low concentrations of ammonia: a 5-year historical cohort study. J Occup Environ Med 2020;62(8):e431-e435 [PMID: 32541623].

Saeed O et al: Inhalation injury and toxic industrial chemical exposure. Mil Med 2018;183(suppl_2):130-132 [PMID: 30189064].

Tustin AW, Jones A, Lopez GP, Ketcham GR, Hodgson MJ: Occupational chemical exposures: a collaboration between the Georgia Poison Center and the Occupational Safety and Health Administration. Clin Toxicol (Phila) 2018;56(1):55-62 [PMID: 28650713].

Wightman RS, Read KB, Hoffman RS: Evidence-based management of caustic exposures in the emergency department. Emerg Med Pract 2016;18(5):1-20 [PMID: 27074641].

Zhang J et al: Clinical significance of urinary fluoride levels in patients with hydrofluoric acid burns. Burns 2018;44(8):2074-2079 [PMID: 30170773].

Acrylamide

Faure S, Noisel N, Werry K, Karthikeyan S, Aylward LL, St-Amand A: Evaluation of human biomonitoring data in a health risk based context: an updated analysis of population level data from the Canadian Health Measures Survey. Int J Hyg Environ Health 2020;223(1):267-280 [PMID: 31523017].

Kim H, Lee SG, Rhie J: Dermal and neural toxicity caused by acrylamide exposure in two Korean grouting workers: a case report. Ann Occup Environ Med 2017;29:50 [PMID: 29043089].

Pelucchi C et al: Dietary acrylamide and the risk of pancreatic cancer in the International Pancreatic Cancer Case-Control Consortium (PanC4). Ann Oncol 2017;28(2):408-414 [PMID: 27836886].

Acrylonitrile

Colenbie S et al: Biomarkers in patients admitted to the emergency department after exposure to acrylonitrile in a major railway incident involving bulk chemical material. Int J Hyg Environ Health 2017;220(2 Pt A):261-270 [PMID: 28110842].

Koutros S et al: Extended mortality follow-up of a cohort of 25,460 workers exposed to acrylonitrile. Am J Epidemiol 2019;188(8):1484-1492 [PMID: 30927363].

Simons K, et al: Short-term health effects in the general population following a major train accident with acrylonitrile in Belgium. Environ Res 2016;148:256-263 [PMID: 27085497].

Aromatic Amines

Cumberbatch MG, Cox A, Teare D, Catto JW: Contemporary occupational carcinogen exposure and bladder cancer: a systematic review and meta-analysis [published correction appears in JAMA Oncol 2015 Dec;1(9):1224]. JAMA Oncol 2015;1(9):1282-1290 [PMID: 26448641].

IARC Monographs Vol 127 group. Carcinogenicity of some aromatic amines and related compounds. Lancet Oncol 2020;21(8):1017-1018. [PMID: 32593317].

Mastrangelo G, Carta A, Arici C, Pavanello S, Porru S: An etiologic prediction model incorporating biomarkers to predict the bladder cancer risk associated with occupational exposure to aromatic amines: a pilot study. J Occup Med Toxicol 2017;12:23 [PMID: 28804505].

Nakano M, Omae K, Takebayashi T, Tanaka S, Koda S: An epidemic of bladder cancer: ten cases of bladder cancer in male Japanese workers exposed to ortho-toluidine. J Occup Health 2018;60(4):307-311 [PMID: 29743389].

Stojanovic J, Milovanovic S, Pastorino R, Iavicoli I, Boccia S: Occupational exposures and genetic susceptibility to urinary tract cancers: a systematic review and meta-analysis. Eur J Cancer Prev 2018;27(5):468-476 [PMID: 28403014].

Tomioka K, Saeki K, Obayashi K, Kurumatani N: Risk of lung cancer in workers exposed to benzidine and/or beta-naphthylamine: a systematic review and meta-analysis. J Epidemiol 2016;26(9):447-458 [PMID: 26947956].

Carbon Disulfide

Blanc, Paul David: *Fake Silk: The Lethal History of Viscose Rayon.* New Haven; London: Yale University Press, 2016.

Chalansonnet M et al: Combined exposure to carbon disulfide and low-frequency noise reversibly affects vestibular function. Neurotoxicology 2018;67:270-278 [PMID: 29928918].

Chung H, Youn K, Kim K, Park K: Carbon disulfide exposure estimate and prevalence of chronic diseases after carbon disulfide poisoning-related occupational diseases. Ann Occup Environ Med 2017;29:52 [PMID: 29093821].

Yoshioka N et al: Changes of median nerve conduction velocity in rayon manufacturing workers: a 6-year cohort study [published correction appears in J Occup Health. 2017;59(3):e2]. J Occup Health 2017;59(2):187-193 [PMID: 28111416].

Chloromethyl Ethers

Marant Micallef C et al: Occupational exposures and cancer: a review of agents and relative risk estimates. Occup Environ Med 2018;75(8):604-614 [PMID: 29735747].

Dibromochloropropane

Boix V, Bohme SR: Secrecy and justice in the ongoing saga of DBCP litigation. Int J Occup Environ Health 2012;18(2):154-161 [PMID: 22762496].

Ethylene Oxide

Marsh GM, Keeton KA, Riordan AS, Best EA, Benson SM: Ethylene oxide and risk of lympho-hematopoietic cancer and breast cancer: a systematic literature review and meta-analysis. Int Arch Occup Environ Health 2019;92(7):919-939 [PMID: 31111206].

Park RM: Associations between exposure to ethylene oxide, job termination, and cause-specific mortality risk. Am J Ind Med 2020;63(7):577-588 [PMID: 32378753].

Formaldehyde

Catalani S et al: Occupational exposure to formaldehyde and risk of non-hodgkin lymphoma: a meta-analysis. BMC Cancer 2019;19(1):1245 [PMID: 31870335].

Dumas O et al: Association of occupational exposure to disinfectants with incidence of chronic obstructive pulmonary disease among US female nurses. JAMA Netw Open 2019;2(10):e1913563 [PMID: 31626315].

Kwak K, Paek D, Park JT: Occupational exposure to formaldehyde and risk of lung cancer: a systematic review and meta-analysis. Am J Ind Med 2020;63(4):312-327 [PMID: 32003024].

Pexe ME et al: Hairdressers are exposed to high concentrations of formaldehyde during the hair straightening procedure. Environ Sci Pollut Res Int 2019;26(26):27319-27329 [PMID: 31321727].

Seals RM, Kioumourtzoglou MA, Gredal O, Hansen J, Weisskopf MG: Occupational formaldehyde and amyotrophic lateral sclerosis. Eur J Epidemiol 2017;32(10):893-899 [PMID: 28585120].

Warshaw EM et al: Occupational contact dermatitis in North American production workers referred for patch testing: retrospective analysis of cross-sectional data from the North American contact dermatitis group 1998 to 2014. Dermatitis 2017;28(3):183-194 [PMID: 28394773].

Nitrosamines

Díez-Izquierdo A, Cassanello-Peñarroya P, Lidón-Moyano C, Matilla-Santander N, Balaguer A, Martínez-Sánchez JM: Update on thirdhand smoke: a comprehensive systematic review. Environ Res 2018;167:341-371 [PMID: 30096604].

Fritschi L et al: Occupational exposure to N-nitrosamines and pesticides and risk of pancreatic cancer. Occup Environ Med 2015;72(9):678-683 [PMID: 25780030].

Hidajat M et al: Lifetime cumulative exposure to rubber dust, fumes and N-nitrosamines and non-cancer mortality: a 49-year follow-up of UK rubber factory workers. Occup Environ Med 2020;77(5):316-323 [PMID: 31974293].

Pentachlorophenol

IARC Working Group on the Evaluation of Carcinogenic Risks to Humans. *Pentachlorophenol and Some Related Compounds.* Lyon (FR): International Agency for Research on Cancer; 2019.

Polychlorinated Biphenyls

Catalani S, Donato F, Tomasi C, Pira E, Apostoli P, Boffetta P: Occupational and environmental exposure to polychlorinated biphenyls and risk of non-Hodgkin lymphoma: a systematic review and meta-analysis of epidemiology studies. Eur J Cancer Prev 2019;28(5):441-450 [PMID: 30234686].

Forns J et al: Prenatal and postnatal exposure to persistent organic pollutants and attention-deficit and hyperactivity disorder: a pooled analysis of seven European birth cohort studies. Int J Epidemiol 2018;47(4):1082-1097 [PMID: 29912347].

Markowitz G, Rosner D: Monsanto, PCBs, and the creation of a "world-wide ecological problem." J Public Health Policy 2018;39(4):463-540 [PMID: 30401808].

Raffetti E, Donato F, Speziani F, Scarcella C, Gaia A, Magoni M: Polychlorinated biphenyls (PCBs) exposure and cardiovascular, endocrine and metabolic diseases: a population-based cohort study in a North Italian highly polluted area. Environ Int 2018;120:215-222 [PMID: 30103120].

Polycyclic Aromatic Hydrocarbons

Koh DH et al: Comparison of polycyclic aromatic hydrocarbons exposure across occupations using urinary metabolite 1-hydroxypyrene. Ann Work Expo Health 2020;64(4):445-454 [PMID: 32064494].

Lee DG et al: Women's occupational exposure to polycyclic aromatic hydrocarbons and risk of breast cancer. Occup Environ Med 2019;76(1):22-29 [PMID: 30541747].

Navarro KM et al: Wildland firefighter smoke exposure and risk of lung cancer and cardiovascular disease mortality. Environ Res 2019;173:462-468 [PMID: 30981117].

Styrene

Bertke SJ, Yiin JH, Daniels RD: Cancer mortality update with an exposure response analysis among styrene-exposed workers in the reinforced plastics boatbuilding industry. Am J Ind Med 2018;61(7):566-571 [PMID: 29638005].

House R, Rajaram N, Tarlo SM: Case report of asthma associated with 3D printing. Occup Med (Lond) 2017;67(8):652-654 [PMID: 29016991].

IARC Working Group on the Evaluation of Carcinogenic Risks to Humans. *Styrene, Styrene-7,8-oxide, and Quinoline.* Lyon (FR): International Agency for Research on Cancer; 2019.

Li X et al. Outdoor manufacture of UV-Cured plastic linings for storm water culvert repair: chemical emissions and residual. Environ Pollut 2019;245:1031-1040 [PMID: 30682737].

Meyer KC, Sharma B, Kaufmann B, Kupper A, Hodgson M: Lung disease associated with occupational styrene exposure [published online ahead of print, 2018 Jun 13]. Am J Ind Med 2018;10.1002/ajim.22867 [PMID: 29900554].

Nett RJ et al: Non-malignant respiratory disease among workers in industries using styrene-A review of the evidence. Am J Ind Med 2017;60(2):163-180 [PMID: 28079275].

Ruder AM, Bertke SJ: Cancer incidence among boat-building workers exposed to styrene. Am J Ind Med 2017;60(7):651-657 [PMID: 28616886].

2,3,7,8-Tetrachlorodibenzo-*p*-dioxin

Cypel YS, Kress AM, Eber SM, Schneiderman AI, Davey VJ: Herbicide exposure, Vietnam service, and hypertension risk in Army Chemical Corps veterans. J Occup Environ Med 2016;58(11):1127-1136 [PMID: 27820763].

Pelclova D et al: Neurological and neurophysiological findings in workers with chronic 2,3,7,8-tetrachlorodibenzo-p-dioxin intoxication 50 years after exposure. Basic Clin Pharmacol Toxicol 2018;122(2):271-277 [PMID: 28862800].

't Mannetje A et al: Morbidity in New Zealand pesticide producers exposed to 2,3,7,8-tetrachlorodibenzo-p-dioxin (TCDD). Environ Int 2018;110:22-31 [PMID: 29031942].

Tornevi A et al: Chlorinated persistent organic pollutants and type 2 diabetes—A population-based study with pre- and post-diagnostic plasma samples. Environ Res 2019;174:35-45 [PMID: 31029940].

Vinyl Chloride

Fedeli U et al: Mortality from liver angiosarcoma, hepatocellular carcinoma, and cirrhosis among vinyl chloride workers. Am J Ind Med 2019;62(1):14-20 [PMID: 30474170].

Mundt KA, Dell LD, Crawford L, Gallagher AE: Quantitative estimated exposure to vinyl chloride and risk of angiosarcoma of the liver and hepatocellular cancer in the US industry-wide vinyl chloride cohort: mortality update through 2013. Occup Environ Med 2017;74(10):709-716 [PMID: 28490663].

■ SELF-ASSESSMENT QUESTIONS

Select the one correct answer for each question.

Question 1: Hydrofluoric acid (hydrogen fluoride)
a. occupational exposure can occur both by direct skin contact and by inhalation of fumes
b. treatment is aimed at deactivation of the fluoride ion in blood and tissue
c. burns may cause vesicles and bullae, but they should not be debrided
d. systemic effects from absorption occur only from skin burns

Question 2: Formaldehyde
a. is a colorless, nonflammable gas with an irritating odor
b. is no longer found in wood industry products
c. is primarily a by-product of the incomplete combustion of heavy metals
d. is found in small amounts in automobile exhaust and cigarette smoke

Question 3: Nitroglycerine
a. acute illness symptoms include loss of consciousness, severe headache, difficulty breathing, weak pulse, and pallor
b. symptoms increase in dynamite production with continued exposure
c. headache (powder headache) frequently begins in the occipital region
d. headache is relieved by alcohol ingestion

Question 4: Pentachlorophenol
a. is used as a wood preservative, herbicide, defoliant, and fungicide
b. may explode if used in pressure treatment of lumber
c. is usually applied to wood products as a 50% solution in mineral spirits, fuel oil, or kerosene
d. is registered by the FDA as a disinfectant and as an ingredient in antifouling paint

Question 5: Polychlorinated biphenyls
   a. causes acute symptoms of nasal and pharyngeal irritation
   b. chronic workplace exposure predictably always results in chloracne
   c. have an efficient transplacental transfer
   d. prenatal exposure predicts accelerated cognitive abilities

Question 6: Styrene
   a. exposure acutely diminishes serum pituitary hormone secretion
   b. chronic exposure may cause weakness, headache, fatigue, poor memory, and dizziness
   c. may increase mean reaction time and visuomotor performance in exposed workers
   d. exposure produces no abnormal electroencephalographs (EEGs) effects

Question 7: Vinyl chloride disease
   a. is a syndrome consisting of Raynaud phenomenon, acroosteolysis, joint and muscle pain, enhanced collagen deposition, stiffness of the hands, and scleroderma-like skin changes
   b. has a decrease in circulating immune complex levels, cryoglobulinemia, B-cell proliferation, hyperimmunoglobulinemia, and complement activation
   c. resistance has been associated with the HLA-DR5 allele
   d. is ruled out by a finding of circulating immune complexes

Solvents

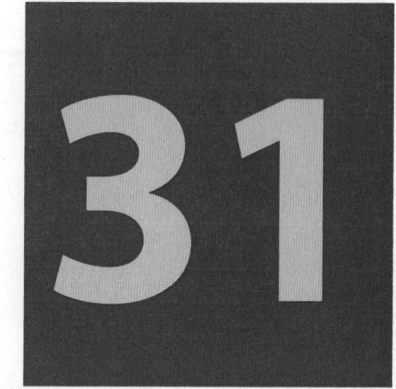

Robert J. Harrison, MD, MPH

Rahmat Balogun, DO, MS, MPH

GENERAL PROPERTIES & USE OF SOLVENTS

A solvent is any substance—usually a liquid at room temperature—that dissolves another substance, resulting in a solution (uniformly dispersed mixture). Solvents may be classified as aqueous (water based) or organic (hydrocarbon based). Most industrial solvents are organic chemicals because most of the industrial substances they are used to dissolve are organic. Solvents are used commonly for cleaning, degreasing, thinning, and extraction.

Many solvent chemicals are also used as chemical intermediates in the manufacture and formulation of chemical products. More workers are exposed to high levels of solvents during use of the substances as cleaners and thinners and in pesticide formulations.

Hundreds of individual chemicals are used to make more than 30,000 industrial solvents. There are physical, chemical, and toxicologic properties that help to classify this large group of chemicals into families with shared or distinguishing features. These features are discussed first, followed by a brief summary of the commonly used industrial solvents according to their chemical families.

PHYSICAL & CHEMICAL PROPERTIES OF SOLVENTS

▶ Solubility

Lipid solubility is an important determinant of the efficiency of a substance as an industrial solvent and a major determinant of a number of health effects. The potency of solvents as general anesthetics and as defatting agents is directly proportionate to their lipid solubility.

Dermal absorption is related to both lipid solubility and water solubility (because the skin behaves like a lipid-water sandwich), so solvents such as dimethyl sulfoxide, dimethylformamide, and glycol ethers, which are highly soluble in both (amphipathic), are well absorbed through the skin. All organic solvents are lipid-soluble, but the extent of solubility may differ to a significant degree.

▶ Flammability & Explosiveness

Flammability and explosiveness are the properties of a substance that allow it to burn or ignite, respectively. Some organic solvents are flammable enough to be used as fuels, whereas others (eg, halogenated hydrocarbons) are so nonflammable that they are used as fire-extinguishing agents. Flash point, ignition temperature, and flammable and explosive limits are measures of flammability and explosiveness. The National Fire Prevention Association (NFPA) rates flammability hazards by a numerical code from 0 (no hazard) to 4 (severe hazard). Table 31–1 lists flash points and NFPA codes. These properties are important to consider when selecting a solvent or substituting one solvent for another on the basis of undesirable health effects or efficacy.

▶ Volatility

Volatility is the tendency of a liquid to evaporate (form a gas or vapor). Other conditions being equal, the greater the volatility of a substance, the greater the concentration of its vapors in air. Because the most common route of exposure to solvents is inhalation, exposure to a solvent is highly dependent on its volatility. Solvents as a class are all relatively volatile over a wide range. Vapor pressure and evaporation rate are two measures of volatility listed in Table 31–1.

▶ Chemical Structure

Solvents can be divided into families according to chemical structure and the attached functional groups. Toxicologic properties tend to be similar within a group, such as liver toxicity from chlorinated hydrocarbons and irritation from aldehydes. The basic structures are aliphatic, alicyclic, and aromatic. The functional groups include halogens, alcohols, ketones, glycols, esters, ethers, carboxylic acids, amines, and amides.

Table 31–1. Industrial solvents: Properties, odor thresholds, and exposure limits.

	CAS #	Flash Point (°F)		Vapor Pressure (mm Hg)[b]	TLV[c] (ppm)	Odor Threshold Range[d] (ppm)	Biological Exposure Indices[e] (BEI)	General Hazard of Chemical Family and Unique Hazard of Specific Compounds
Aliphatic Hydrocarbons								Anesthetic > irritant.
Pentane	109-66-0	−40	4	420	1000	1.27–1147	—	—
n-Hexane	110-54-3	−7	3	124	50 (S)	1.5–248	Yes	Peripheral neuropathy.
Hexane (isomers)	107-83-5 96-14-0 79-29-8 75-83-2	−54 to 19	3	150	500	0.426–20	—	—
Heptane	142-82-5	25	3	40 (at 72F)	400	0.41–732	—	—
Octane	111-65-9	56	3	10	300	0.26–235	—	—
Nonane	111-84-2	88	3	3	200	2.3–21	—	—
Alicyclic Hydrocarbons								Anesthetic > irritant.
Cyclohexane	110-82-7	0	3	78	100	0.52–748	—	
Aromatic Hydrocarbons								Anesthetic > irritant.
Benzene	71-43-2	12	3	75	0.5 (S)	0.47–313	Yes	Hematopoietic cancer
Toluene	108-88-3	40	3	21	20	0.021–157	Yes	Renal tubular acidosis, cerebellar dysfunction.
Xylene (isomers)	1330-20-7 95-47-6 106-42-3 108-38-3	81–90	3	7 to 9	100	0.0012–316	Yes	—
Ethyl benzene	100-41-4	55	3	7	20	< 0.002–18	Yes	—
Cumene	98-82-8	96	3	8	50	0.008–1.3	—	—
Styrene	100-42-5	88	3	5	20	0.0028–61	Yes	Peripheral neuropathy
Petroleum distillates				See Table 31–3				Hazard relative to aliphatic and aromatic components:
Alcohols								Irritant > Anesthetic.
Methyl alcohol	67-56-1	52	3	96	200 (S)	3.05–198,686	Yes	Acidosis, optic neuropathy.
Ethyl alcohol	64-17-5	55	3	44	1000 (STEL)	0.09–40,334	—	Reproductive toxicant
1-Propyl alcohol	71-23-8	72	3	15	100	< 0.031–10,172	—	—
Isopropyl alcohol	67-63-0	53	3	33	200	1.0–2197	Yes	—
n-Butyl alcohol	71-36-3	84	3	6	20	0.0033–990	—	Auditory, vestibular nerve injury reported.
sec-Butyl alcohol	78-92-2	75	3	12	100	0.043–94	—	—
tert-Butyl alcohol	75-65-0	52	3	42 (at 77F)	100	3.3–957	—	—

(continued)

Table 31–1. Industrial solvents: Properties, odor thresholds, and exposure limits. (Continued)

	CAS #	Flash Point (°F)		Vapor Pressure (mm Hg)[b]	TLV[c] (ppm)	Odor Threshold Range[d] (ppm)	Biological Exposure Indices[e] (BEI)	General Hazard of Chemical Family and Unique Hazard of Specific Compounds
Iso-octyl alcohol	26952-21-6	180 (open cup)	2	0.4	50 (S)	0.0092–0.049	–	–
Cyclohexanol	108-93-0	154	2	1	50 (S)	0.058–0.491	Yes (Nq, Ns)	–
Glycols								Extremely low volatility.
Ethylene glycol (vapor fraction)	107-21-1	232	1	0.06	25 (Vapor)	5.12	–	Acidosis, seizures, renal failure (ingestion).
Phenols								Irritant > Anesthetic; cytotoxic, corrosive.
Phenol	108-95-2	175	2	0.4	5 (S)	0.0045–1.95	Yes	Dermal absorption of vapors.
Cresol	1319-77-3	178–187	2	0.11–0.29 (at 77F)	20 mg/m^3 (inhalable fraction and vapor) (S)	0.00005–0.0090	–	–
Ketones								Irritant, strong odor > anesthetic.
Acetone	67-64-1	0	3	180	250	0.40–11,745	Yes	
Methyl ethyl ketone	78-93-3	16	3	78	200	0.07–339	Yes	Potentiates neurotoxicity of n-hexane and methyl n-butyl ketone.
Methyl n-butyl ketone (2-Hexanone)	591-78-6	77	3	11	5 (S)	0.024–1.15	Yes	Peripheral Neuropathy.
Methyl isobutyl ketone	108-10-1	64	3	16	20	0.03–16	Yes	–
Diacetone alcohol	123-42-2	125	2	1	50	0.27–13	–	–
Mesityl oxide	141-79-7	87	3	9	15	0.54–2.84	–	–
Cyclohexanone	108-94-1	146	2	5	20 (S)	0.052–219	Yes	–
Esters								Irritant, strong odor > anesthetic.
Methyl formate	107-31-3	–2	4	476	50 (S)	67–2809	–	Optic neuropathy from metabolism to formic acid.
Ethyl formate	109-94-4	–4	3	200	100 (STEL)	2.7–30	–	–
Methyl acetate	79-20-9	14	3	173	200	0.17–2848	–	Optic neuropathy from metabolism to methanol.
Ethyl acetate	141-78-6	24	3	73	400	0.09–190	–	–
Propyl acetate (isomers)	109-60-4 108-21-4	55	3	25	100*	0.048–87	–	–

(continued)

Table 31–1. Industrial solvents: Properties, odor thresholds, and exposure limits. (Continued)

	CAS #	Flash Point (°F)		Vapor Pressure (mm Hg)[b]	TLV[c] (ppm)	Odor Threshold Range[d] (ppm)	Biological Exposure Indices[e] (BEI)	General Hazard of Chemical Family and Unique Hazard of Specific Compounds
Butyl acetate (isomers)	123-86-4 105-46-4 110-19-0 540-88-5	72	3	10	50*	0.00013–368	–	–
Pentyl acetate (isolmers)	628-63-7 123-92-2 620-11-1 624-41-9 625-16-6 626-38-0	77	3	4	50*	0.007–43	–	Odorant ("Banana oil").
Vinyl acetate	108-05-4	83	3	18	10	0.12–0.4	–	
Ethers								
Ethyl ether	60-29-7	–49	4	440	400	0.165–1924	–	Extremely volatile, flammable, explosive.
Dioxane	123-91-1	55	3	29	20 (S)	0.8–2609	–	Carcinogenic in animals.
Methyl tert-butyl ether (MTBE)	1634-04-4	–14	3	250 (at 25C)	50	0.03–0.17	–	Reproductive, renal.
tert-Amyl methyl ether (TAME)	994-05-8	19	–	75 (at 25C)	20	NF	NF	Neurologic, reproductive.
Glycol ethers								**Skin absorption without irritation.**
2-Methoxyethanol	109-86-4	102	2	6	0.1 (S)	< 0.096–90	Yes	Reproductive toxicity.
2-Ethoxyethanol	110-80-5	110	2	4	5 (S)	0.3–49	Yes	Reproductive toxicity.
2-Butoxyethanol	111-76-2	143	2	0.8	20	0.08–0.35	Yes	Anemia.
Propylene glycol monomethyl ether	107-98-2	97	3	12	50	NF	NF	–
Dipropylene glycol monomethyl ether	34590-94-8	180	2	0.5	100 (S)	NF	NF	–
Glycidyl ethers								**Sensitizers, genetic and reproductive toxins.**
Phenyl glycidyl ether	122-60-1	248	–	0.01	0.1 (S)	NF	NF	Carcinogenic in animals.
Diglycidyl ether	2238-07-5	147	–	0.09	0.01	NF	NF	–
Amines								**Irritant > anesthetic; corneal edema, visual halos.**
Methylamine	74-89-5	14 (liquid), N/A (gas)	4	3 atm	5	0.00075–4.8	–	–

(continued)

Table 31–1. Industrial solvents: Properties, odor thresholds, and exposure limits. (Continued)

	CAS #	Flash Point (°F)		Vapor Pressure (mm Hg)ᵇ	TLVᶜ (ppm)	Odor Threshold Rangeᵈ (ppm)	Biological Exposure Indicesᵉ (BEI)	General Hazard of Chemical Family and Unique Hazard of Specific Compounds
Dimethylamine	124-40-3	20 (liquid), N/A (gas)	4	1.7 atm	5	0.0076–4.2	–	–
Trimethylamine (gas)	75-50-3	20 (liquid), N/A (gas)	4	1454 (at 77F)	5	0.00002–1.82	–	–
Ethylamine	75-04-7	1	4	874	5 (S)	0.027–3.5	–	–
Diethylamine	109-89-7	–15	3	192	5 (S)	0.0033–14.3	–	–
Triethylamine	121-44-8	20	3	54	0.5 (S)	0.005–2.9	–	–
n-Butylamine	109-73-9	10	3	82	5 (C, S)	0.08–13.9	–	–
Cyclohexylamine	108-91-8	88	3	11	10	2.42	–	–
Ethylenediamine	107-15-3	93	2	11	10 (S)	1.3–4.5	–	Allergic contact dermatitis, asthma.
Dethylenetriamine	111-40-0	208	1	0.4	1 (S)	NF	NF	–
Ethanolamine	141-43-5	186	2	0.4	3	2.6–24	–	–
Diethanolamine	111-42-2	279	1	< 0.01	1 mg/m³ (Inhalable fraction & vapor) (S)	0.279	–	–
Chlorinated hydrocarbons								Cancer in animals; liver, kidney, cardiac effects.
Methyl chloroform (1,1,1-trichloroethane)	71-55-6	–	1	100	350	0.97–715	Yes	–
Trichloroethylene	79-01-6	–	1	53	10	0.5–167	Yes	Human Carcinogen, Alcohol intolerance, "degreaser's flush."
Perchloroethylene (tetrachloroethylene)	127-18-4	–	0	14	25	0.767–71	Yes	Carcinogenic in animals.
Methylene chloride (dichloromethane)	75-09-2	–	1	350	50	1.2–440	Yes	Metabolized to carbon monoxide, suspect human carcinogen.
Carbon tetrachloride	56-23-5	–	0	91	5 (S)	1.68–720	–	Cirrhosis, liver cancer.
Chloroform	67-66-3	–	0	160	10	0.102–1413	–	Suspect human carcinogen.
Chlorofluorocarbons								Weak anesthetic, irritant; cardiac effects.
Trichlorofluoromethane (F-11)	75-69-4	–	0	690	1000 (C)	5–200,057	–	–
Dichlorodifluoromethane (F-12)	75-71-8	–	0	5.7 atm	1000	199,790	–	–
Chlorodifluoromethane (F-22)	75-45-6	–	0	9.4 atm	1000	200,192	–	–

(continued)

Table 31–1. Industrial solvents: Properties, odor thresholds, and exposure limits. (Continued)

	CAS #	Flash Point (°F)		Vapor Pressure (mm Hg)[b]	TLV[c] (ppm)	Odor Threshold Range[d] (ppm)	Biological Exposure Indices[e] (BEI)	General Hazard of Chemical Family and Unique Hazard of Specific Compounds
1,1,2,2-Tet-rachloro-1,2-difluoro-ethane (F-112)	76-12-0	_	0	40	50	NF	NF	_
1,1,2-Trichloro-1,2,2-trifluoroethane (F-113)	76-13-1	_	0	285	1000	NF	NF	_
1,2-Dichlorotetra-fluoroethane (F-114)	76-14-2	_	0	1.9 atm (at 70F)	1000	NF	NF	_
Chloropentafluoro-ethane (F-115)	76-15-3	_	0	9.9 atm (at 70F)	1000	NF	NF	_
Miscellaneous								
n-methyl-2-pyrrolidone	872-50-4	204	2	0.24	None	4.2–10	Yes	_
Turpentine & monterpenes	8006-64-2	95	3	4	20	0.00006–19	_	Irritant > anesthetic; allergic contact dermatitis.
d-Limonene	138-86-3	119	2	1 (at 57F)	None	0.0018–0.31	_	Allergic Contact Dermatitis.
Dimethyl Sulfoxide (DMSO)	67-68-5	203	2	0.42	_	NF	NF	Hepatotoxic > anesthetic; skin absorption.
Dimethylformamide	68-12-2	136	2	3	5 (S)	0.047–100	Yes	Smell in breath after exposure; skin absorption.
n, n-Dimethylacet-amide	127-19-5	151	2	9 (at 140F)	10 (S)	48	Yes	
Tetrahydrofuran	109-99-9	6	3	132	50 (S)	0.092–61	Yes	Anesthetic, irritant.
1-Bromopropane	106-94-5	78	2	111	0.1	NF	NF	Neurotoxicity, hepatotoxicity, reproductive, developmental.
2-Bromopropane	75-26-3	72	3	216 (at 25C)	None	NF	NF	_

Index.

[a]National Fire Prevention Association (NFPA) rates flammability hazards by numerical code from 0 (no hazard) to 4 (severe hazard).

[b]All vapor pressure values are in mm Hg at 68F unless otherwise indicated.

[c]Threshol Limit Values Adopted from American Conferteance of Govenmental Industrial Hygienists (ACGIH) Threshold Limit Valus (TLV), 8-hour time weighted average, 2018. All values are in ppm and represent the 8 hour TWA TLV unless otherwise indicated. STEL = Short-Term Exposure Limit; C = Ceiling Limit; S = Skin TLV.

[d]Odor Threshold Rage Adopted from ACGIH Odor Threshold for Chemicals with Established Health Standards, 2nd Edition, 2013.

[e]Information about Biological Expsure Indeices (BEI) available in ACGIH Odor Threshold for Chemicals with Established Health Standards, 2nd Edition, 2013. See Chapter 44 on Biological Monitoring.

NF = Data Not Found.

_ = no value.

* = value for all isomers.

PHARMACOKINETICS OF SOLVENTS

Absorption (Route of Exposure)

A. Pulmonary

Because organic solvents are generally volatile liquids, and because the vapors are lipid-soluble and therefore well absorbed across the alveolar-capillary membrane, inhalation is the primary route for occupational exposure. The pulmonary retention or uptake (percentage of inhaled dose that is retained and absorbed) for most organic solvents ranges from 40% to 80% at rest. Because physical labor increases pulmonary ventilation and blood flow, the amount of solvent delivered to the alveoli and the amount absorbed are likewise increased. Levels of physical exercise commonly encountered in the workplace will increase the pulmonary uptake of many solvents by a factor of 2–3 times that at rest.

B. Percutaneous

The lipid solubility of organic solvents results in most being absorbed through the skin to some degree following direct contact. However, percutaneous absorption is also determined by water solubility and volatility. Solvents that are soluble in both lipid and water are absorbed most readily through the skin. Highly volatile substances are less well absorbed because they tend to evaporate from the skin unless evaporation is prevented by occlusion by gloves or clothing. Skin absorption rates vary widely among individuals by at least a factor of 4. Factors that affect skin absorption include anatomic location, gender, age, condition (including hydration) of skin, personal hygiene, and environmental factors.

For a number of solvents, dermal absorption contributes to overall exposure sufficiently to result in a "skin" designation for the American Conference of Governmental Industrial Hygienists (ACGIH) threshold limit values (TLVs), as set forth in Table 31–1. For a few solvents, significant absorption of vapors through the skin also can occur. This is most likely to occur when solvents with a "skin" designation and low TLV are used in a situation that results in very high airborne concentrations, such as in an enclosed space with respiratory protection.

Distribution

Because organic solvents are lipophilic, they tend to be distributed to lipid-rich tissue. In addition to adipose tissue, this includes the nervous system and liver. Because distribution occurs via the blood, and because the blood–tissue membrane barriers are usually rich in lipids, solvents are also distributed to organs with large blood flows, such as cardiac and skeletal muscle. Persons with greater amounts of adipose tissue accumulate greater amounts of a solvent over time and, consequently, excrete large amounts at a slower rate after cessation of exposure. Most solvents cross the placenta and also enter breast milk.

Metabolism

Some solvents are metabolized extensively, and some not at all. The metabolism of a number of solvents plays a key role in their toxicity and, in some cases, the treatment of intoxication. The role of toxic metabolites is discussed in their respective sections for *n*-hexane, methyl *n*-butyl ketone, methyl alcohol, ethylene glycol, diethylene glycol, methyl acetate, methyl formate, and glycol ethers. A number of solvents, including trichloroethylene, are metabolized in common with ethyl alcohol (ethanol) by alcohol and aldehyde dehydrogenase. Competition for these limited enzymes accounts for synergistic effects (*alcohol intolerance* and *degreaser's flush*) and may result in reactions in workers exposed to these solvents while taking disulfiram (Antabuse) for alcoholism. Chronic ethanol ingestion may induce solvent-metabolizing enzymes and lower blood solvent concentrations. Other solvents may have acute and chronic interactions similar to those of ethanol.

Excretion

Excretion of solvents occurs primarily through exhalation of unchanged compound, elimination of metabolites in urine, or a combination of each. Solvents such as perchloroethylene that are poorly metabolized are excreted primarily through exhalation. The biologic half-life of parent compounds varies from a few minutes to several days, so some solvents accumulate to some degree over the course of the workweek, whereas others do not. However, bioaccumulation beyond a few days is not an important determinant of adverse health effects for most solvents.

Biologic Monitoring

Biologic monitoring can provide a more accurate measure of exposure than environmental monitoring for some solvents (see Table 31–1). This is particularly true for substances whose pulmonary absorption is affected to a large degree by physical work and for substances with significant dermal exposure and absorption (ie, those with ACGIH "skin" designations; see Table 31–1). Unfortunately, solvents have properties that tend to make biologic monitoring less useful or practical. First, they tend to be absorbed and excreted rapidly, so biologic levels change rapidly over time. Second, exposure over very short intervals may be a more important determinant of adverse health effects than 8-hour or longer exposures. However, biologic monitoring has been investigated for a number of solvents. The ACGIH has recommended biological exposure indices (BEIs) for the following solvents: acetone, benzene, carbon disulfide, chlorobenzene, cyclohexanol, cyclohexanone, dichloromethane (methylene chloride), dimethylformamide, 2-ethoxyethanol and 2-ethoxyethanol acetate, ethyl benzene, *n*-hexane, methanol, 2-methoxyethanol and 2-methoxyethanol acetate, methyl *n*-butyl ketone, methyl ethyl ketone, methyl isobutyl ketone, perchloroethylene (tetrachloroethylene), phenol, styrene, tetrahydrofuran, toluene, trichloroethane (methyl chloroform), trichloroethylene, and xylenes. For many solvents, significant levels may be present only in exhaled air. A number of laboratories offer whole-blood or plasma analysis of solvents. For solvents with relatively slow excretion, such as perchloroethylene and methyl chloroform, analysis of blood is a reasonable alternative to analysis of exhaled air. However, for those with relatively fast excretion (most of the rest), the timing of the sample is critical—even within minutes—and the results therefore are difficult to interpret. Most solvents distribute into several compartments in the body so that the decline in blood levels exhibits several consecutive half-times, with the first being very short, on the order of 2–10 minutes. A blood sample taken immediately after an exposure will reflect primarily peak exposure at that time. A sample taken 15–30 minutes after termination of exposure will reflect exposure over the preceding few hours, whereas a sample taken 16–20 hours after exposure (prior to the next shift) will reflect mean exposure over the preceding day. The distribution of exposure over an 8-hour shift also will affect the validity of the biologic sample.

HEALTH EFFECTS OF SOLVENTS (TABLE 31-2)

SKIN DISORDERS

Up to 20% of cases of occupational dermatitis are caused by solvents. Almost all organic solvents are primary skin irritants as a result of defatting, or the dissolution of lipids from the skin. The potency of solvents for defatting the skin is related directly to lipid solubility and inversely to percutaneous absorptivity and volatility. In addition to concentration and duration of exposure, a critical factor in the development of solvent dermatitis is occlusion of the exposed area of skin, such as by clothes and leaking protective clothing. A few industrial solvents also can cause allergic contact dermatitis. A form of contact dermatitis, contact urticaria, reportedly is caused by several specific solvents. Scleroderma has been found to be significantly associated with exposure to organic solvents in a number of case-reference studies.

The most common work practice leading to solvent dermatitis is washing the hands with solvents. The occupations most commonly associated with solvent dermatitis are painting, printing, mechanics, and dry cleaning, although workers are at risk wherever solvents are used.

▶ **Clinical Findings**

A. Symptoms and Signs

Diagnosis is based on the typical appearance of the skin and a history of direct contact with solvents. The typical appearance ranges from an acute irritant dermatitis manifested by erythema and edema to a chronic dry, cracked eczema. Areas of skin affected by solvent dermatitis are more permeable to chemicals than unaffected skin and are susceptible to secondary bacterial infection.

B. Laboratory Findings

Patch testing is rarely indicated because few solvents (principally turpentine, d-limonene, and formaldehyde) cause allergic contact dermatitis. Patch testing with actual material used in the workplace may be necessary on occasion.

▶ **Differential Diagnosis**

Consideration sometimes must be given to the possibility of other sources of irritant or allergic contact dermatitis. Use of waterless hand cleansers that contain alcohols and emollients that contain sensitizers may exacerbate or cause irritant or allergic dermatitis.

▶ **Treatment & Prevention**

Treatment of dermatitis caused by solvents is the same as for contact dermatitis from other causes: topical corticosteroids, emollients, and skin care. Prevention depends on education of workers about proper handling of solvents, use of engineering controls to minimize direct contact with solvents, provisions for alternatives to washing with solvents, and the use of solvent-resistant barrier creams or protective clothing where appropriate.

▶ **Prognosis**

The resolution of solvent dermatitis depends on elimination of direct solvent contact with involved areas of skin.

Table 31–2. Major health effects of solvents.

	Health Effect
Cancer	Hematopoietic, liver, kidney, breast, cholangiosarcoma
Cardiac	Acute arrhythmias
Dermal	Irritant dermatitis
Immunological	Systemic sclerosis
Kidney	Glomerulonephritis
Liver	Hepatitis
Neurological	Peripheral neuropathy, optic and cranial neuropathy, acute and chronic encephalopathy, headache, NIHL, seizures, loss of smell and taste, color vision loss
Pulmonary	Bronchitis, lung function decline
Reproductive	Female: adverse reproductive outcomes Male: abnormal semen quality, adverse reproductive outcomes

Noise Induced Hearing Loss

CENTRAL NERVOUS SYSTEM EFFECTS

1. Acute Central Nervous System Effects

Almost all volatile lipid-soluble organic chemicals cause general, nonspecific depression of the central nervous system, or general anesthesia. Beginning with ethyl ether, a number of industrial solvents were used historically as surgical anesthetics. There is good correlation between lipid solubility, as measured by the air–olive oil partition coefficient, and anesthetic potency. Excitable tissue is depressed at all levels of the central nervous system, both brain and spinal cord. Lipid solubility—and therefore anesthetic potency—increases with length of carbon chain, substitution with halogen or alcohol, and the presence of unsaturated (double) carbon bonds.

▶ Clinical Findings

A. Symptoms and Signs

The symptoms of central nervous system depression from acute intoxication by organic solvents are the same as those from drinking alcoholic beverages. Symptoms range from headache, nausea and vomiting, dizziness, lightheadedness, vertigo, disequilibrium, slurred speech, euphoria, fatigue, sleepiness, weakness, irritability, nervousness, depression, disorientation, and confusion to loss of consciousness and death from respiratory depression. A secondary hazard from these effects is increased risk of accidents. Excitatory manifestations of early intoxication are the result of depression of inhibitory functions and correspond to stage I anesthesia.

The acute effects are related to the concentration of the chemical in the nervous system, so resolution of symptoms correlates with the biologic half-life, which ranges from a few minutes to less than 24 hours for most industrial solvents. However, it must be kept in mind that many solvent exposures are to mixtures of solvents and that the effects of each solvent are at least additive and may be synergistic.

Tolerance to the acute effects can occur, particularly for those compounds with longer half-lives, and generally is not metabolic in nature (ie, not a result of increased rates of metabolism and excretion). The development of tolerance may be accompanied by morning "hangovers" and even frank withdrawal symptoms on weekends and during vacations, alleviated by ingestion of alcohol. Additive and synergistic effects both have been described for interactions between organic solvents and drinking alcohol.

B. Laboratory Findings

Biologic monitoring may provide an accurate assessment of exposure to some solvents, but there is little information on the correlation of biologic levels with degrees of intoxication.

▶ Differential Diagnosis

Acute solvent intoxication must be distinguished from that resulting from the use of alcohol or psychoactive drugs on the basis of exposure.

▶ Treatment

The sole treatment for acute solvent intoxication is removal from exposure to solvents or any other anesthetic or central nervous system depressant until the signs and symptoms have resolved completely. The use of alcohol or other central nervous system depressant medication should be avoided. The headache from acute solvent exposure usually resolves after several hours to days, but occasional there may be chronic migraine-type headaches even after exposure has ceased. Analgesics for the acute headache may be necessary, with longer term treatment similar to that for migraine headache.

▶ Prognosis

Most symptoms resolve in a time course parallel to the elimination of the solvent and any active metabolites, although headaches may persist for up to a week or more following acute exposure. Persistence of central nervous system dysfunction following severe overexposure with coma suggests hypoxic brain damage. The occurrence of persistent neurobehavioral dysfunction following acute overexposure has been reported, particularly impairment of memory.

2. Chronic Central Nervous System Effects

Alcohol is now well recognized as causing neurobehavioral dysfunction in chronic alcoholics. It is reasonable to assume that sufficient chronic exposure to organic solvents also could cause chronic adverse neurobehavioral effects. A number of terms have been applied to these effects when associated with solvent exposure: chronic toxic encephalopathy, chronic solvent encephalopathy, presenile dementia, chronic solvent intoxication, painter's syndrome, psychoaffective disorder, and neurasthenic syndrome.

A number of epidemiologic studies of workers chronically exposed to organic solvents have demonstrated an increased incidence of adverse neurobehavioral effects. These effects have been best demonstrated in groups of workers with relatively high exposures, such as boat builders and spray painters, and with specific types of exposure, such as carbon disulfide. Such effects include subjective symptoms, changes in personality or mood, and impaired intellectual function, as assessed by a considerable number of neurobehavioral tests. Decrements in short-term memory and psychomotor function are consistent findings. Dose-response data and correlation of chronic with acute effects are becoming more available. Correlation of symptoms with test results is often lacking, so interpretation of neurobehavioral test results in an individual must be done by experienced observers. Solvent-exposed workers are at increased risk of requiring disability pension for neuropsychiatric disorders in a number of industrialized countries.

Chronic brain damage from chronic alcoholism or drug abuse is not well understood, but similar mechanisms may be present with chronic solvent exposure. Cortical atrophy may represent the underlying pathologic change. Recent studies have found conflicting results regarding the association between Alzheimer disease and history of solvent exposure.

In addition to neuropsychologic dysfunction, there are other potential chronic central neurotoxic effects of solvents that can be considered briefly here. Acute and perhaps chronic intoxication with solvents can result in vestibulo-oculomotor disturbances, presumably because of effects on the cerebellum. A syndrome called *acquired intolerance to organic solvents*, in which there is dizziness, nausea, and weakness after exposure to minimal solvent vapor concentrations with normal vestibular test results, has been reported.

Clinical Findings

Symptoms commonly reported are headache, mood disturbance (depression, anxiety), fatigue, memory loss (primarily short-term memory), and difficulty in concentrating. Clinical examination may reveal signs of impairment in recent memory, attention span, and motor or sensory function. The Swedish Q16 questionnaire (Table 31–3) may be useful in the evaluation of workers with long-term solvent exposure.

Diagnosis

Test results associated with solvent exposure in group studies include alteration of a variety of neurobehavioral tests; electroencephalography, pneumoencephalography, computed tomographic (CT) scan, magnetic resonance imaging (MRI), positron-emission tomography (PET), and cerebral blood

flow studies showing evidence of diffuse cerebral cortical atrophy; and electroencephalographic abnormalities, particularly diffuse low-wave patterns. These tests should not be used in the evaluation of individual patients without incorporating information from other sources.

The following criteria have been used for the diagnosis of chronic neurobehavioral toxicity from solvents:

A. Verified quantitative and qualitative exposure to organic chemicals that are known to be neurotoxic.

B. Clinical picture of organic central nervous system damage:
  1. Typical subjective symptoms
  2. Pathologic findings in some of the following:
    a. Clinical neurologic status
    b. Electroencephalography
    c. Psychological tests

C. Other organic diseases reasonably well excluded.

D. Primary psychiatric diseases reasonably well excluded.

Differential Diagnosis

Primary psychiatric disease may be excluded by the presence of signs of organic brain dysfunction, but these signs are not always entirely objective or clear-cut. Drug or alcohol abuse may result in a clinical state identical to chronic solvent toxicity, distinguished only by history and other evidence of exposure. Diffuse organic brain disease—particularly Alzheimer disease or, less commonly, Creutzfeldt-Jakob disease—also must be considered.

Treatment

Removal from exposure is recommended in all suspected cases. Alcohol and other central nervous system depressants should be avoided.

Depression may respond to antidepressants or other measures. Other neuropsychologic symptoms may respond to psychological counseling. Treatment of chronic solvent-induced headaches involves empirical trials of medications, psychological counseling, and biofeedback therapy. Cognitive retraining is useful in some individuals with persistent memory loss documented on neuropsychologic testing.

Prognosis

A number of follow-up studies of workers diagnosed as having solvent-associated neurobehavioral changes have been conducted. In general, those having symptoms but no impairment of psychometric test performance improved after removal from or reduction of solvent exposure. Severe impairment of initial test performance often was associated with persistent and sometimes worsening follow-up test performance, even if exposure was eliminated. Persistent impairment often was associated with persistent disabilities and considerable adverse social consequences.

Table 31–3. Swedish Q16 questionnaire for long-term solvent exposed workers.

This questionnaire is used to help determine whether long-term overexposure to solvents has affected the central nervous system (brain)—answer "yes" or "no" to each question.*

1. Do you have a short memory?
2. Have your relatives told you that you have a short memory?
3. Do you often have to make notes about what you must remember?
4. Do you often have to go back and check things you have done (turned off the stove, locked the door, etc.)?
5. Do you generally find it hard to get the meaning from reading newspapers and books?
6. Do you have problems with concentrating?
7. Do you often feel irritated without any particular reason?
8. Do you often feel depressed without any particular reason?
9. Are you abnormally tired?
10. Are you last interested in sex and then what you think is normal?
11. Do you have heart palpitations even when you don't exert yourself?
12. Do you sometimes have a feeling of pressure in your chest?
13. Do you perspire without any particular reason?
14. Do you have a headache at least once a week?
15. Do you often have a painful tingling in some part of your body?

*If solvent-expose worker answers "yes" to six or more of these questions, referral to more in depth evaluation may be indicated.

EFFECTS ON PERIPHERAL NERVOUS SYSTEM & CRANIAL NERVES

All organic solvents may be capable of causing or contributing to peripheral neuropathies. However, only a few are specifically toxic to the peripheral nervous system, including carbon disulfide and the hexacarbons n-hexane and methyl n-butyl ketone. These three causes a symmetric, ascending, mixed sensorimotor neuropathy of the distal axonopathy type that can be replicated in animals. This may be referred to as a *central peripheral distal axonopathy* because the nerves in the spinal canal are also affected. Of the three substances, only n-hexane is currently in general use as an industrial solvent. Most industrial hexane is a mixture of isomers with 20–80% of n-hexane content. Methyl ethyl ketone, a common solvent, potentiates the neurotoxicity of the hexacarbons (n-hexane and methyl n-butyl ketone). 1-Bromopropane, recently used as a chlorofluorocarbon substitute in spray adhesives, in cleaning metal and electronic components, and as a solvent for fats, waxes, or resins, has also been found to cause a variety of central and peripheral nervous system effects.

Trichloroethylene is associated with isolated trigeminal nerve anesthesia. Other organic solvents such as methyl chloroform (1,1,1-trichloroethane) are associated with peripheral neurotoxicity in case reports of occupational exposure, following exposure to mixtures of solvents, or in persons exposed to extremely high levels from deliberate "sniffing" of solvents.

There is increasing evidence that solvent exposure can result in sensorineural hearing loss, particularly in combination with noise. Some aromatic solvents (eg, toluene, p-xylene, styrene, and ethylbenzene) show, in the rat, ototoxicity characterized by an irreversible hearing loss. The loss was measured by behavioral or electrophysiologic methods and was associated with damage to outer hair cells in the cochlea of the exposed animals.

Acquired color vision disturbances have been found in association with occupational exposure to several solvents, including toluene, styrene, carbon disulfide, n-hexane, and mixed solvents. Disturbances of olfactory function (hyposmia and parosmia) have been reported in cases of solvent-exposed individuals and anecdotally in a high percentage of long-term painters. Effects on olfaction could be a result of local destruction of olfactory nerve endings in the nasal mucosa or action at a central site.

Studies of general solvent exposure have paid little attention to the peripheral nervous system. The few that have been performed suggest that at exposures more likely to result in central nervous system effects, symptoms of peripheral neurotoxicity are uncommon, but neurophysiologic function may be altered. Analogous to the effects of chronic alcoholism, solvents may be only weakly toxic to the peripheral nervous system but capable of acting additively or synergistically with dietary deficiencies or other neurotoxic agents.

▶ Clinical Findings

Typical symptoms of solvent-induced neuropathy are slowly ascending numbness, paresthesias, and weakness. Pain and muscle cramps are present occasionally. Physical findings include diminished sensation and strength in a symmetric pattern and, in most cases, depressed distal reflexes. Trigeminal neuropathy from trichloroethylene is restricted to loss of sensory function in the distribution of the trigeminal nerve. Complaints of hearing or vision impairment in individual workers attributed to solvent exposure have not been reported.

▶ Diagnosis

The diagnosis of solvent-induced neuropathy is based on a history of illness and exposure, clinical examination, and neurophysiologic testing. Nerve conduction velocities may be normal or slightly depressed. Sensory conduction velocities and sensory action potential amplitude are the most sensitive. Electromyography may indicate denervation (fibrillations and positive sharp waves). The use of evoked potentials (visual and somatosensory) shows promise. Symptoms and other clinical findings often are found with absent or slight neurophysiologic abnormalities. A sural nerve biopsy may be helpful and in the case of hexacarbons show accumulation of neurofilaments in the terminal axon.

Neurophysiologic testing may be helpful in screening large numbers of workers but has not been shown to be more sensitive in early detection of clinical neuropathy than are clinical examinations, although periodic monitoring of n-hexane–exposed workers with nerve conduction velocity testing has been recommended.

Hearing may be assessed using standard techniques but has not been shown to be related to individual solvent exposure. Color vision testing using various techniques has been shown to be useful in evaluating groups of workers but not in clinical evaluation of individual workers. Odor threshold testing and other tests of olfactory function should be performed in individuals with complaints of disturbances in either smell or taste.

▶ Differential Diagnosis

The primary differential diagnosis for peripheral neuropathy includes diabetes, alcoholism, drugs, familial neuropathies, and renal failure. Approximately 25–50% cases of peripheral neuropathy remain without an etiologic diagnosis after initial evaluation excludes these causes. A chemical-related cause should be considered in all such cases.

▶ Treatment

Treatment consists of removal of exposure to all substances toxic to the peripheral nervous system, including alcoholic beverages. Physical therapy should be encouraged for patients with weakness; this increases muscular strength to counteract loss of neuromuscular function, improves psychological outlook, and may even improve the ability of nerves to regenerate effectively. Careful clinical monitoring of workers exposed to substances toxic to the peripheral nervous system is important for early detection and prevention of permanent disability.

▶ Prognosis

Symptoms may worsen initially and then improve for up to 1 year or more. The rate of recovery is related to the rate of axonal regeneration, which is approximately 1 mm/d. An axon from the tip of the toe that has died back to the cell body in the spinal cord may take 1 year to recover. The degree of residual disability, if any, is usually proportionate to the degree of injury at the time of diagnosis and cessation of exposure. However, permanent disability should not be judged until at least 1 year after removal from exposure.

RESPIRATORY SYSTEM

All organic solvents irritate the respiratory tract to some degree. Irritation is a consequence of the defatting action of solvents, and so the same structure-activity relationships hold true for the respiratory tract as for the skin. Addition of functional groups to the hydrocarbon molecule also may increase the potency of the solvent as an irritant, as in the case of organic amine bases and organic acids, which are corrosives, and alcohols, ketones, and aldehydes, which denature proteins at high concentrations.

Respiratory tract irritation from solvents usually is confined to the upper airways, including the nose and sinuses. Solvents that are both highly soluble and potent irritants, such as formaldehyde, cannot reach the lower respiratory tract without intolerable irritation of the upper tract. However, it is possible for less potent irritants to reach the alveoli in sufficient concentrations following extremely high overexposures, such as in spills and in confined spaces, to cause acute pulmonary edema. Severe central nervous system depression is usually also a result of such exposure. Pulmonary edema without effects on the nervous system can result from exposure to phosgene gas produced by the extreme heating (as in welding) of chlorinated hydrocarbon solvents. Exacerbation of asthma or, less commonly, induction of reactive airways dysfunction syndrome after acute exposure can occur, as with any other airway irritant.

There are few studies of chronic pulmonary effects from exposure to organic solvents. Chronic bronchitis may occur as a result of long-term exposure to the more potent irritant compounds, such as the aldehydes.

▶ Clinical Findings

A. Symptoms and Signs

Irritation of the upper respiratory tract is marked by sore nose and throat, cough, and possibly chest pain. If the eyes are not protected by vapor goggles, irritation of the eyes possibly accompanied by tearing also may occur. A few solvents are specific lacrimators and induce pronounced tearing such that exposure may be sufficient to preclude inhalation and irritation of the respiratory tract. A productive cough

indicates chemical bronchitis or the imposition of an infectious bronchitis. Manifestations of pulmonary edema include a productive cough, dyspnea, cyanosis, and rakes.

B. Laboratory Findings

Upper airway irritation should not be associated with any laboratory abnormalities. Pulmonary edema is marked by infiltrates on chest radiograph, hypoxia, and perhaps hypocapnia on arterial blood gas analysis, and impaired diffusion, as shown by pulmonary function tests.

▶ Differential Diagnosis

Infectious bronchitis may be distinguished from chemical bronchitis by sputum analysis and possibly sputum culture, although chemical bronchitis may be followed by a superimposed infection. Solvent-induced pulmonary edema must be distinguished from infectious or aspiration pneumonitis.

▶ Treatment

Management of the acute pulmonary effects of solvents is the same as for any acute pulmonary irritant: administration of oxygen, bronchodilators, and other respiratory support as indicated.

▶ Prognosis

Upper respiratory tract irritation should resolve quickly without sequelae in the absence of infection. Once treated appropriately, patients with acute pulmonary edema from solvent overexposure should recover completely if protected from the effects of hypoxic tissue damage. Rarely, induction of reactive airways dysfunction syndrome occurs.

EFFECTS ON THE HEART

The principal effect of organic solvents on the heart is *cardiac sensitization*, a state of increased myocardial sensitivity to the arrhythmogenic effects of epinephrine. It can be demonstrated in animals—typically unanesthetized beagle dogs—by administration of epinephrine, either in fixed or multiple doses, before and after administration of a solvent and observation of the frequency of epinephrine-induced ventricular arrhythmias. Cases of sudden, otherwise unexplained death during abuse of solvents such as toluene in glue and trichloroethane in spot remover, usually associated with physical activity (*sudden sniffing deaths*), and occasional reports of sudden death in otherwise healthy workers overexposed to industrial solvents are probably a result of cardiac sensitization.

From animal studies, it appears that high—near-anesthetic or anesthetic—levels are required for this effect on an otherwise healthy heart and that all organic solvents may be capable of causing it, although potencies vary. Halogenated hydrocarbons, particularly 1,1,1-trichloroethane, trichloroethylene, and trichlorotrifluoroethane, were of higher potency in the dog, with thresholds to a particular dose of epinephrine at 0.5% (5000 ppm) of solvent vapors for 5 minutes, as compared with approximately 5% (50,000 ppm) for heptane, hexane, toluene, and xylene; 10% (100,000 ppm) for propane; and 20% (20,000 ppm) for ethyl ether. Thresholds for these effects in humans, particularly with any condition predisposing to arrhythmias, are unknown.

A few solvents appear to have specific cardiovascular effects. Carbon disulfide exposure is associated with increased risk of coronary artery disease in a number of epidemiologic studies. Methylene chloride can also affect cardiac function acutely both through direct myocardial sensitization and through its metabolism to carbon monoxide.

▶ Clinical Findings

A. Symptoms and Signs

Cardiac sensitization should be considered when a worker exposed to high concentrations of a solvent reports dizziness, palpitations, faintness, or loss of consciousness in conjunction with or in the absence of symptoms of central nervous system depression (see earlier). If the victim is examined promptly, an irregular pulse or low blood pressure may be detected.

B. Laboratory Findings

A resting electrocardiogram (ECG) may be normal or abnormal and is rarely diagnostic. For workers with symptoms suggestive of cardiac sensitization, ambulatory cardiac monitoring during exposure may be helpful.

▶ Differential Diagnosis

In the presence of high levels of exposure, the distinction between central nervous system depression alone and depression plus cardiac sensitization is difficult—and may not be important if all symptoms resolve with correction of overexposure. The need for evaluation for primary cardiac disease must be made on a case-by-case basis. The presence of cardiac disease does not preclude the possibility of solvent-related arrhythmias, which may occur at levels of solvent exposure lower than those usually associated with cardiac sensitization.

▶ Treatment

Given the high levels of exposure usually associated with cardiac sensitization, evaluation and appropriate correction of exposure are essential. If arrhythmias appear to be related to exposure and the exposure is not excessive or cannot be controlled adequately, removal from exposure is preferable to treatment with antiarrhythmic medication and continued exposure.

▶ Prognosis

Cases solely caused by excessive exposure should resolve with removal from exposure, although if acute cardiac damage occurs, longer-term cardiac complications may result.

EFFECT ON THE LIVER

Although it is possible that any organic solvent may cause hepatocellular damage in sufficient doses for a sufficient duration, some solvents, particularly those substituted with halogen or nitro groups, are particularly hepatotoxic. Others, such as the aliphatic hydrocarbons (eg, cycloparaffins, ethers, esters, aldehydes, and ketones), are only weakly, if at all, hepatotoxic. The aromatic hydrocarbons (ie, benzene, toluene, and xylene) appear to be weakly hepatotoxic, with only a few reports of liver toxicity in exposed workers. A few solvents, such as acetone, with little direct hepatotoxicity themselves are reported to potentiate the effects of alcohol on the liver.

▶ Clinical Findings

A. Symptoms and Signs

Liver injury may be symptomless or associated with right upper quadrant pain, nausea, and vomiting. Hepatic tenderness, jaundice, dark urine, and light stool may be present.

B. Laboratory Findings

Diagnosis of acute hepatic injury is based on the presence of abnormal liver function tests in a pattern consistent with hepatocellular dysfunction and a history consistent with exposure to a hepatotoxic solvent in the absence of exposure to any other known hepatotoxin. A pattern of liver enzyme abnormality different from alcohol hepatitis has been reported for a few solvents. Serum bilirubin may be elevated. Evaluation of liver injury caused by occupational exposure to solvents has been hampered by the lack of sensitivity and specificity of liver function tests. The use of serum bile acid measurements and antipyrine metabolism rates has been proposed as a sensitive screening method for solvent-related liver dysfunction. Occasionally, liver biopsy is necessary to distinguish solvent-induced hepatitis from chronic active hepatitis.

Routine monitoring of liver function tests is not recommended unless there is potential exposure to a hepatotoxic dose of a solvent. Monitoring a patient after abstinence from alcohol may be necessary to evaluate the possible role of drinking. Removal of exposure with monitoring of liver function tests may be helpful in making a diagnosis.

▶ Differential Diagnosis

The major entity that must be differentiated is alcohol-induced liver injury; if excessive use of alcohol cannot be ruled out, a diagnosis of solvent-induced liver injury often cannot be made with confidence. Viral and other infectious forms of hepatitis also must be considered.

▶ Treatment

Treatment consists of removal from exposure and correction of any workplace situation that can be identified as having caused or contributed to the condition.

EFFECT ON THE KIDNEYS

Although many organic solvents, particularly halogenated aliphatic hydrocarbons, show evidence of nephrotoxicity to animals in relatively high doses, there are few reports of renal effects in exposed workers perhaps partly because of the lack of sensitivity and specificity of renal function tests. Acute renal failure from acute tubular necrosis has been observed in workers with acute intoxication from halogenated hydrocarbons such as carbon tetrachloride.

Animal studies indicate that halogenated aliphatic hydrocarbons damage primarily the proximal renal tubular cells. Renal tubular dysfunction, particularly renal tubular acidosis of the distal type, has been reported in solvent abusers using mainly toluene but is not associated with occupational exposure. Acute renal failure from intrarenal deposition of oxalic acid can result from ingestion of ethylene glycol but has not been reported from other routes of exposure.

There are few studies of chronic renal effects in solvent-exposed workers. Cross-sectional studies have suggested that chronic exposure to a number of solvents or solvent mixtures may result in mild tubular dysfunction evidenced by enzymuria (increased excretion of muramidase, β-glucuronidase, and N-acetyl-β-glucosaminidase) and either a normal urinalysis or proteinuria. Case-control studies have suggested an association between solvent exposure and primary glomerulonephritis, particularly rapidly progressive glomerulonephritis associated with anti–glomerular basement membrane antibodies (the renal component of Goodpasture syndrome).

▶ Clinical Findings

A. Symptoms and Signs

Solvent abusers with renal tubular acidosis present with weakness and fatigue probably as a result of electrolyte abnormalities. Signs of acute intoxication (central nervous system depression) are often present. If it occurs, chronic renal tubular dysfunction as a result of chronic solvent exposure is usually subclinical.

B. Laboratory Findings

Renal tubular dysfunction from solvents may be manifested by polyuria, glycosuria, proteinuria, acidosis, and electrolyte disorders. Hypokalemia, hypophosphatemia, hyperchloremia, and hypobicarbonatemia have been seen as manifestations of renal tubular acidosis in toluene abusers. Acute renal failure from halogenated solvents is similar to that from any other cause. Routine monitoring of renal function generally is not recommended for workers exposed to solvents. However, the measurement of urinary excretion of low-molecular-weight enzymes such as N-acetyl-β-glucosaminidase, β-glucuronidase, and muramidase appears to offer promise as a monitor for evidence of early tubular dysfunction.

▶ Differential Diagnosis

Renal tubular dysfunction, including acidosis, can be a primary disease that first manifests in early adulthood or may occur secondary to a variety of metabolic and hyperglobulinemic states and exposure to toxic agents, including antibiotics and heavy metals.

▶ Treatment

If renal tubular dysfunction is found in a worker with a high level of exposure to a solvent, observation of renal tubular function during cessation and then reinstitution of exposure may be helpful in both establishing a diagnosis and determining the effectiveness of removal from exposure.

EFFECTS ON BLOOD

Benzene has been known for many decades to cause aplastic anemia after months to years of exposure that is often a precursor to leukemia. Even relatively low doses of benzene (based on parts per million years or peak exposures) may increase the risk of various hematologic malignancies such as acute myelogenous leukemia, multiple myeloma, chronic lymphocytic leukemia, and non-Hodgkin lymphoma. Some glycol ethers can cause either a hemolytic anemia because of increased osmotic fragility or a hypoplastic anemia because of bone marrow depression.

▶ Clinical Findings

A. Symptoms and Signs

Workers with anemia from solvents generally have presented with weakness and fatigue. Aplastic anemia can present with bleeding from thrombocytopenia or infections owing to neutropenia.

B. Laboratory Findings

Aplastic anemia from benzene may be manifested by reductions in any or all of the three cell lines, which may occur suddenly without preceding changes. The bone marrow may be hyperplastic or hypoplastic and does not always correlate with abnormalities in the peripheral blood. Hemolytic anemia from glycol ethers or other hemolytic agents is indicated by low red blood cell concentration and reticulocytosis. Monitoring of blood counts is recommended only for exposure to benzene and perhaps for the hematotoxic glycol ethers, but the results may not be predictive of anemia even for these agents.

▶ Differential Diagnosis

The usual causes of anemia, particularly hypoplastic anemia, must be considered.

▶ Treatment

The treatment of solvent-induced anemia is removal from exposure, transfusion if needed, and correction of the workplace situation if appropriate. Workers with aplastic anemia from benzene should not be reexposed to benzene.

▶ Prognosis

A significant percentage of workers with aplastic anemia from benzene subsequently will develop leukemia, which is frequently fatal.

EFFECTS ON REPRODUCTIVE SYSTEM (SEE CHAPTERS 27 AND 28)

Most organic solvents easily cross the lipid barrier of the placenta and, to a lesser degree, the testes, and therefore may pose a risk of reproductive toxicity among exposed workers. Multiple studies in animals and humans, as well as meta-analyses of retrospective case-control studies show significant increase in major malformations and a number of other adverse reproductive outcomes due to solvent exposure.

▼ PREVENTION OF SOLVENT TOXICITY

SELECTION & SUBSTITUTION OF SOLVENT

Selection of an initial solvent—or substitution of a less hazardous for a more hazardous solvent—must take into account both the desirable and undesirable properties of the solvents. This involves comparing not only health hazard (ie, toxicity, dermal absorptivity, and volatility) but also flammability, explosiveness, reactivity, compatibility, stability, odor properties, and environmental fates. Solvent substitution increasingly has been driven by the need to replace smog-forming and ozone-depleting chemicals.

ENGINEERING CONTROLS

The volatility of organic solvents makes engineering controls of paramount importance in many situations. Process enclosure, such as the closed-system use of trichlorotrifluoroethane for dry cleaning, is common in chemical manufacturing but not in other circumstances. Spray painting and other spray operations create large quantities of aerosols and vapors, so engineering controls such as paint spray booths are particularly critical. Effective functioning of ventilation systems depends on proper design and regular mechanical maintenance. The substitution of water-based for solvent-based paints is the most effective means of reducing solvent exposure from painting. Aqueous cleaning for metal parts shows promise for reducing solvent use in vehicle repair and parts manufacturing.

PERSONAL PROTECTION

Respiratory protection should be used only when engineering controls are not feasible, such as in construction, confined space, and emergency-response situations. The employer must conduct a comprehensive respiratory protection program. Frequently, there is improper fitting, selection, and maintenance of respirators for solvent work, resulting in poor or inconsistent protection. Knowledge of the odor threshold of a substance (see Table 31–1) is useful before using a respirator for levels above the TLV for that substance. If the average odor threshold is well below the TLV (eg, at least tenfold), the odor will serve as an adequate warning to signal breakthrough or other failure of the respirator to provide adequate protection. A decrease in the ability to detect odors (hyposmia) has been reported from chronic exposure to solvents, and a history of hyposmia should be sought as part of the initial medical evaluation for ability to use a respirator. Use of a respirator with an approved end-of-service life indicator may improve respirator effectiveness in these cases. Some solvents, such as methanol, methyl chloride, and formaldehyde, are not removed by standard organic vapor filters.

Protective clothing made of the proper material should be selected on the basis of studies that show the rate of penetration of materials by the solvent used. *Guidelines for the Selection of Chemical Protective Clothing*, published by the ACGIH, is a good source of this information. Inappropriate glove material may be porous to solvents while retaining an intact appearance, leading to occlusion and increased hand exposure. Plasticizers used in polyvinyl chloride gloves are vulnerable to solvents. Glove selection for mixed solvents is difficult; multilayer materials or costly specialty products may be required. Some workers, such as mechanics, may be unable to use gloves and adequately perform their work. Barrier creams are not recommended as substitutes for gloves. Protective (barrier) creams can correct or prevent loss of oils from the skin and may provide very limited protection against percutaneous absorption of solvents.

▼ SPECIFIC SOLVENTS & THEIR EFFECTS

ALIPHATIC HYDROCARBONS

ESSENTIALS OF DIAGNOSIS

▶ Acute effects

- Anesthesia: dizziness, headache, nausea, vomiting, sleepiness, fatigue, "drunkenness," slurred speech, disequilibrium, disorientation, depression, and loss of consciousness, and death.

- Respiratory tract irritation: cough and sore nose and throat.

▶ Chronic effects

- Dermatitis: dry, cracked, and erythematous skin.

- Neurobehavioral dysfunction: headache, mood lability, fatigue, short-term memory loss, difficulty concentrating, decreased attention span, neurobehavioral test abnormalities, CT scan (cerebral atrophy), electroencephalography (EEG) (diffuse slow waves).

- Peripheral neuropathy (*n*-hexane): slowly ascending numbness, paresthesias, and weakness; normal or slightly depressed nerve conduction velocity and electromyography (denervation).

General Considerations

Aliphatic hydrocarbons consist of carbon and hydrogen molecules in straight or branched chains. They are further divided into alkanes, alkenes, and alkynes.

1. Alkanes (Paraffins)

Alkanes are aliphatic hydrocarbons with single-bonded (saturated) carbons:

The physical state of an alkane depends on its number of carbons:

with the empirical formula C_nH_{2n+2}

The gases are essentially odorless, whereas the vapors of the liquids have a slight "hydrocarbon" odor.

Use

A number of liquid alkanes are used in relatively pure form as solvents and also are the major constituents of a number of petroleum distillate solvents (see later). The liquid alkanes are important ingredients in gasoline, which accounts for most of the pentane and hexane used in the United States. Hexane (generally a mixture of isomers including *n*-hexane) is an inexpensive general-use solvent in solvent glues, quick-drying rubber cements, varnishes, inks, and extraction of oils from seeds. The alkane gases are used as fuels, whereas paraffin wax (solid alkanes) is used for candles and other wax products.

Occupational & Environmental Exposure

The Agency for Toxic Substances and Disease Registry reports that *n*-hexane exposure can occur among refinery workers, shoe and footwear assembly workers, laboratory technicians, workers operating or repairing typesetting and printing machinery, construction workers, carpet layers, carpenters, auto mechanics and gas station employees, workers in plants manufacturing tires or inner tubes, and workers in air transport and air freight operations. NIOSH has recently reported that workers in the upstream oil and gas extraction industry may be exposed to lethal concentrations of the alkanes during manual tank gauging at oil and gas well sites.

Pharmacokinetics

The alkanes are well absorbed by inhalation and, to a lesser but still significant extent, through the skin. Approximately 75% of most inhaled alkanes are absorbed at rest, decreasing to 50% with moderate physical labor. Unbranched hydrocarbons such as *n*-hexane and *n*-heptane are metabolized by microsomal cytochrome P450 enzymes to alcohols, diols, ketones, and diketones, which are further metabolized to carbon monoxide or conjugated with glucuronic acid and excreted in urine.

Health Effects

The alkanes generally are of low toxicity. The first three gases (methane, ethane, and propane) are simple inert asphyxiants whose toxicity is related only to the amount of available oxygen remaining in the environment and to their flammability and explosiveness. The vapors of the lighter, more volatile liquids (pentane through nonane) are irritants and anesthetics, whereas the heavier liquids (known as liquid paraffins) are primarily defatting agents. They cause anesthesia, respiratory tract irritation, and dermatitis and are associated with neurobehavioral dysfunction, and the associated clinical findings, differential diagnosis, treatment, and prognosis are not different from those of other solvents (see earlier). In 2016, NIOSH reported nine worker fatalities that occurred while workers manually gauged or sampled production tanks. Exposures to hydrocarbon gases and vapors and/or oxygen-deficient atmospheres are believed to be primary or contributory factors to the workers' deaths.

One isomer of hexane, *n*-hexane, causes peripheral neuropathy. A number of outbreaks of peripheral neuropathy have been described, particularly in industries such as shoe and sandal making, where glues have been used containing *n*-hexane as a solvent. More recently, *n*-hexane in brake-cleaning aerosol products has been associated with neuropathy in auto mechanics.

The proximate neurotoxin is the metabolite 2,5-hexanedione. Other diketones with the same spacing between ketone (carbonyl) groups, such as 3,6-hexanedione, also can cause peripheral neuropathy. A metabolite of *n*-heptane, 2,5-heptanedione, causes peripheral neuropathy in laboratory animal studies, but *n*-heptane has not been implicated in human peripheral neuropathy in the absence of concomitant exposure to *n*-hexane. The clinical and neurophysiologic findings of *n*-hexane–induced peripheral neuropathy are typical of distal axonopathies (see above). Nerve biopsies are notable for swollen axons that contain increased numbers of neurofilaments. Methyl ethyl ketone and possibly methyl isobutyl ketone potentiate the neurotoxicity of *n*-hexane.

Exposure to *n*-hexane can be assessed by measuring 2,5-hexanedione in the urine or *n*-hexane in end-exhaled air. A concentration of 2,5-hexanedione in urine of 5 mg/L measured at the end of a work shift corresponds to exposure to a time-weighted average (TWA) of 50 ppm.

2. Alkenes (Olefins) & Alkynes

Alkenes are aliphatic hydrocarbons with double (unsaturated) carbon bonds:

with the empirical formula C_nH_{2n}

Dienes are alkenes with two double bonds. Alkynes are aliphatic hydrocarbons with triple carbon bonds. The physical state of alkenes and alkynes is determined by the number of carbons, as for alkanes.

Use

The liquid alkenes are not used widely as solvents but are common chemical intermediates. The alkenes are more reactive than alkanes, a property that leads to their use as monomers in the production of polymers such as polyethylenes from ethylene, polypropylene from propylene, and synthetic rubber and resin copolymers from 1,3-butadiene.

Occupational & Environmental Exposure

Occupational exposure estimates are not available for most alkenes and alkynes. Occupational exposure to ethylene, propylene, and 1,3-butadiene occurs primarily through inhalation during monomer and polymer production. Propylene is a common air pollutant as a result of engine exhaust emissions and industrial activity, with urban atmospheric concentrations ranging from 2.6 to 23.3 ppb in the United States and Europe. Occupational exposure to 1,3-butadiene may occur in the rubber, plastics, and resins industries. Butadiene has been detected in urban atmospheres in the United States at concentrations ranging from 1 to 5 ppb, whereas other alkenes and alkynes have been detected at comparable concentrations.

Pharmacokinetics

There is little information on absorption or metabolism of alkenes and alkynes. Absorption of these compounds should be similar to their corresponding alkanes.

Health Effects

The alkenes are similar in toxicity to the alkanes. The unsaturated carbon bonds increase lipid solubility to some extent, and therefore, irritant and anesthetic potencies as compared with corresponding alkanes. *n*-Hexene does not cause peripheral neuropathy, unlike *n*-hexane.

The presence of double bonds makes the alkenes more reactive than alkanes and dienes more reactive than alkenes. This reactivity is used in the production of polymers but in some cases also may result in additional health hazards. 1,3-Butadiene is carcinogenic in animals, whereas propylene and ethylene are not.

1,3-Butadiene is a human and animal carcinogen; elevated rates of leukemia and lymphosarcoma are associated with occupational exposure. Because of the carcinogenicity of 1,3-butadiene, the Occupational Safety and Health Administration (OSHA) has instituted a comprehensive standard with a permissible exposure level (PEL) of 1 ppm (TWA), medical surveillance, and other provisions. Both in utero embryo toxicity and male-mediated reproductive toxicity have been shown in animals. Biologic monitoring can be accomplished by urinary sampling for the product of epoxybutene hydrolysis followed by glutathione conjugation.

ALICYCLIC HYDROCARBONS (CYCLIC HYDROCARBONS, CYCLOPARAFFINS, NAPHTHENES)

ESSENTIALS OF DIAGNOSIS

▶ Acute effects
- Anesthesia: dizziness, headache, nausea, vomiting, sleepiness, fatigue, "drunkenness," slurred speech, disequilibrium, disorientation, depression, and loss of consciousness.
- Respiratory tract irritation: sore nose and throat and cough.

▶ Chronic effects
- Dermatitis: dry, cracked, and erythematous skin.
- Neurobehavioral dysfunction: headache, mood lability, fatigue, short-term memory loss, difficulty concentrating, decreased attention span, neurobehavioral test abnormalities, CT scan (cerebral atrophy), EEG (diffuse slow waves).

General Considerations

Alicyclic hydrocarbons consist of alkanes or alkenes arranged into cyclic or ring structures:

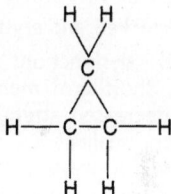

They have a slight "hydrocarbon" odor.

Use

Cyclohexane is the only alicyclic hydrocarbon that is widely used as an industrial solvent. Most of the US production is used in the synthesis of nylon. Cyclopropane is used as a general anesthetic, but this is limited by its flammability and explosiveness.

Occupational & Environmental Exposure

The use of cyclohexane in nylon production results in only limited occupational exposure. The alicyclic hydrocarbons are not reported as common environmental contaminants.

Pharmacokinetics

Similar to their corresponding alkanes and alkenes, the alicyclic hydrocarbons are well absorbed by inhalation, whereas percutaneous absorption is less important. Approximately

70% of cyclohexane that is inhaled is absorbed and excreted unchanged in urine and exhaled air and as cyclohexanol in urine.

▶ Health Effects

The alicyclic hydrocarbons are similar in toxicity to their alkane or alkene counterparts in causing irritation and central nervous system depression. They cause anesthesia, respiratory tract irritation, and dermatitis and are associated with neurobehavioral dysfunction. The associated clinical findings, differential diagnosis, treatment, and prognosis are not different from those of other solvents (see earlier). Cyclohexane does not cause peripheral neuropathy.

AROMATIC HYDROCARBONS

ESSENTIALS OF DIAGNOSIS

- ▶ Acute effects
  - • Anesthesia: dizziness, headache, nausea, vomiting, sleepiness, fatigue, "drunkenness," slurred speech, disequilibrium, disorientation, depression, and loss of consciousness.
  - • Respiratory tract irritation: cough and sore nose and throat.
- ▶ Chronic effects
  - • Dermatitis: dry, cracked, and erythematous skin.
  - • Neurobehavioral dysfunction: headache, mood lability, fatigue, short-term memory loss, difficulty concentrating, decreased attention span, neurobehavioral test abnormalities, CT scan (cerebral atrophy), EEG (diffuse slow waves).
  - • Peripheral neuropathy (styrene).

▶ General Considerations

Aromatic hydrocarbons are compounds that contain one or more benzene rings:

They are produced—directly or indirectly—chiefly from crude petroleum and to a lesser extent from coal tar. Aromatics used as solvents include benzene and the alkylbenzenes toluene (methyl benzene), xylenes (o-, m-, and p- isomers of dimethyl benzenes), ethyl benzene, cumene (isopropyl benzene), and styrene (vinyl benzene). They have a characteristic "aromatic" sweet odor.

▶ Use

Although benzene currently has only limited use as a general industrial solvent, it is still used widely in manufacturing, for extraction in chemical analyses, and as a specialty solvent. Approximately half the benzene produced is used to synthesize ethyl benzene for the production of styrene. In the United States, gasoline contains approximately 2–3% benzene and 30–50% other aromatics. Aromatics constitute a significant percentage of a number of petroleum distillate solvents (see later). Toluene and xylenes are two of the most widely used industrial solvents—principally in paints, adhesives, and the formulation of pesticides—although about a third of the toluene used goes to produce benzene and only about one-sixth of the toluene produced is used as a solvent. The solvent uses of toluene and xylenes have been decreasing owing to environmental regulations because of their photochemical reactivity. Aqueous metal-cleaning methods are now available for cleaning metal parts as a substitute for xylene. Ethyl benzene is used chiefly as an intermediate in the manufacture of styrene and to a lesser extent as a solvent. Styrene is used chiefly as a monomer in the manufacture of plastics and rubber. Most of the cumene produced is used to manufacture phenol and acetone. Other aromatic compounds have a wide variety of uses but are not used commonly as solvents and so are not discussed here.

▶ Occupational & Environmental Exposure

NIOSH states that workers at risk of being exposed to toluene include workers in locations where there are leaking underground gasoline storage tanks; technicians who work in nail salons; construction workers who use paint, adhesives or solvents; and workers involved with the production of gasoline. Toluene exposure may also occur in indoor air from the use of common household products (paints, paint thinners, adhesives, synthetic fragrances, and nail polish) and cigarette smoke. Exposure to xylene can occur among painters and furniture refinishers who use paint thinners, solvents, lacquers and paint removers; biomedical laboratory workers who use it as a solvent to fix tissue specimens and rinse stains; workers involved in distillation and purification of xylene; workers employed in industries who use xylene as a raw material; and gas station and automobile garage workers through exposure to petroleum products. Exposure to styrene can occur among workers in the reinforced plastics industry; workers involved in styrene polymerization; factory workers in rubber manufacturing; workers in industries that use styrene polyester resin; and employees of photocopy centers.

▶ Pharmacokinetics

The pulmonary absorption values for aromatic hydrocarbons do not vary significantly as a group, ranging from approximately 50–70% at rest and decreasing to 40–60% with light to moderate work and to 30–50% with moderate to heavy work. Percutaneous absorption of aromatic hydrocarbons can be significant.

All the aromatic hydrocarbons are metabolized extensively, their metabolic profiles varying with the substituents on the benzene ring. Benzene is metabolized mainly to phenol and excreted in urine as conjugated phenol and dihydroxyphenols, with a slow elimination-phase half-time of about 28 hours. Approximately 10% of benzene is excreted unchanged in exhaled air. Toluene is metabolized primarily to benzoic acid and excreted in urine as the glycine conjugate hippuric acid with a half-time of about 1–2 hours. Approximately 15–20% of toluene is excreted unchanged in expired air. Xylene is metabolized almost entirely to the *o*-, *m*-, and *p*-methylbenzoic acids and excreted in urine as the glycine conjugates *o*-, *m*-, and *p*-methylhippuric acids with a slow elimination-phase half-time of about 30 hours. Approximately 64% of absorbed ethyl benzene is excreted in urine as mandelic acid and approximately 25% as phenylglyoxylic acid. The principal metabolites of the aromatic hydrocarbons are used for biologic monitoring, as indicated in the following discussion.

▶ Health Effects

The aromatic hydrocarbons generally are stronger irritants and anesthetics than the aliphatics. Substitution on benzene (toluene, xylene, ethyl benzene, and styrene) increases lipid solubility and these toxicities slightly. Aromatic hydrocarbons cause acute anesthetic effects, respiratory tract irritation, dermatitis, neurobehavioral dysfunction, and peripheral neuropathy (styrene).

Like the petroleum distillates (see later), aromatic hydrocarbons may contain benzene in small percentages and pose a risk of hematopoietic cancer due to inhalation and dermal exposure to the benzene fraction. The concentration of benzene in aromatic hydrocarbon solvents has generally declined since the 1980s (after the passage of the US OSHA standard for benzene), but these solvents still poses a long-term risk due to the latency period for hematopoietic cancer after benzene exposure (> 30 years).

There are a few reports of liver function abnormalities in workers exposed to aromatic hydrocarbons. Renal tubular acidosis of the distal type, with serious but reversible electrolyte abnormalities, has been reported in solvent abusers exposed primarily to toluene. A syndrome of persistent cerebellar ataxia has been reported after exposure to toluene, chiefly in solvent abusers but also occasionally in workers. Toluene and xylenes have been reported to raise auditory thresholds in laboratory animals at relatively low levels of exposure.

Exposure to benzene, ethyl benzene, toluene, xylene, and styrene can be assessed by a variety of biologic monitoring techniques. Although extensive research has been conducted on the use of these techniques, given the short half-lives and acute effects of these compounds, the utility of biologic monitoring for the routine assessment of exposure is limited. Little information is available on the use of biologic levels in the diagnosis of acute intoxication from aromatic hydrocarbons.

PETROLEUM DISTILLATES (REFINED PETROLEUM SOLVENTS)

ESSENTIALS OF DIAGNOSIS

▶ Acute effects
- Anesthesia: dizziness, headache, nausea, vomiting, sleepiness, fatigue, "drunkenness," slurred speech, disequilibrium, disorientation, depression, and loss of consciousness.
- Respiratory tract irritation: cough and sore nose and throat.

▶ Chronic effects
- Dermatitis: dry, cracked, and erythematous skin.
- Neurobehavioral dysfunction: headache, mood lability, fatigue, short-term memory loss, difficulty concentrating, decreased attention span, neurobehavioral test abnormalities, CT scan (cerebral atrophy), EEG (diffuse slow waves).
- Hematopoietic cancers (due to benzene fraction).

▶ General Considerations

Petroleum distillate solvents are mixtures of petroleum derivatives distilled from crude petroleum at a particular range of boiling points. Each is a mixture of aliphatic (primarily alkane), alicyclic, and aromatic hydrocarbons, the relative concentration of each depending on the particular petroleum distillate fraction. They have a "hydrocarbon" or "aromatic" odor depending on the relative concentrations of aliphatic or aromatic hydrocarbons.

Table 31–4 lists the major petroleum distillate solvents, with the number of carbon atoms, typical percentages of components, and range of boiling points of each.

▶ Use

Petroleum distillates are among the most common general-use solvents because they are available at low cost in large quantities. Petroleum ether (petroleum naphtha) represents an estimated 60% of the total industrial solvent usage. Approximately 1.4 billion gallons of petroleum solvents (see Table 31–4) were produced in the United States. Kerosene is used as a fuel, as well as a cleaning and thinning agent; about 2.3 billion gallons are produced in the United States each year.

▶ Occupational & Environmental Exposure

A wide variety of occupations may be exposed to the petroleum distillates including printers, mechanics, painters, and workers in petroleum extraction, distribution and refining operations.

Table 31–4. Petroleum distillate solvents.

	CAS #	Synonyms (Consider Removing and replacing with CAS # instead)	Flash Point (°F)	Vapor Pressure (@ 68F)[a]	Boiling Point (F)	TLV[b] (ppm)	Carbon Number	Class Components	Percentage (%)	General Hazard of Chemical Family and Unique Hazard of Specific Compounds
Petroleum Ether	8032-32-4	Petroleum, naphtha, ligroin, benzene	NF	NF	30 to 60	—	C5-6	Alkanes (pentanes, hexanes)	100	100% aliphatic, extremely volatile, flammable.
Rubber Solvent	8002-05-9	Aliphatic Petroleum napthta	−40 to −86	40	86 to 460	—	C5-7	Aliphatic Alicyclic Aromatic	60 35 5	Mostly aliphatic, extremely volatile, flammable.
Petroleum ether, high boiling-point	64742-89-8	Light aliphatic solvent naphtha	NF	NF	95 to 320	—	C7-8	Aliphatic Alicyclic Aromatic	...	
VM&P naphtha (also Called Petroleum ether in NIOSH Handbook)	8032-32-4	Ligroin, Painters Naphtha, Varnish Makers and Painter's Naphtha, Petroleum ether	20 to 55	2 to 20	203 to 320	—	C5-11	Aliphatic Aromatic	> 80 < 20	Mostly aliphatic.
Mineral Spirits I	8052-41-3 (Stoddard Solvent)	Stoddard Solvent I, white spirits, petroleum distillate	102 to 110	—	309 to 396	100	C7-12	Aliphatic Alicyclic Aromatic	30-50 30-40 10-20	
Mineral Spirits II	NF	Stoddard Solvent II, high-flash naphtha, 140-flash naphtha	102 to 110	NF	175 to 200	—	C8-13	Aliphatic Alicyclic Aromatic	40-60 30-40 5-15	
Aromatic Petroleum naphtha (DOES NOT COME UP IN A SEARCH)	NF	Coal tar naphtha (DOES NOT COME UP AS A SYNONYM)	NF	NF	95 to 315	—	C8-13	Aliphatic Aromatic	<10 >90	Mostly aromatic.
Kerosene	8008-20-6	Kerosene, Stove Oil	100 to 162	5 (at 100F)	347 to 617	200 mg/m³	C10-16	Aliphatic Alicyclic Aromatic	...	

From Current OEM 5th Edition.
From NIOSH Handbook.
Index.

[a]All values are at 68F unless otherwise indicated.

[b]Threshol Limit Values Adopted from American Conference of Govenmental Industrial Hygienists (ACGIH) Threshold Limit Valus (TLV), 8-hour time weighted average, 2018. All values are in ppm and represent the 8 hour TWA TLV unless otherwise indicated. STEL = Short Term Exposure Limit; C = Ceiling Limit.

NF = Not Found.

— = no value.

Pharmacokinetics

The pharmacokinetics of petroleum distillate solvents are those of the individual aliphatic, alicyclic, and aromatic constituents.

Health Effects

The hazard of a particular petroleum distillate fraction is related to concentrations of the various classes of hydrocarbons it contains (see Table 31–4). Petroleum distillate solvents cause anesthetic effects, respiratory tract irritation, and dermatitis and are associated with neurobehavioral dysfunction; the clinical findings, differential diagnosis, treatment, and prognosis are not different from those of other solvents (discussed earlier).

Most of the aliphatic fractions are alkanes, including *n*-hexane. Therefore, the risk of peripheral neuropathy must be considered, particularly with exposure to petroleum ether, which may contain a significant percentage of *n*-hexane. Many petroleum distillates contain benzene in small percentages and pose a risk of hematopoietic cancer due to inhalation and dermal exposure to the benzene fraction. The concentration of benzene in aliphatic hydrocarbon solvents has generally declined since the 1980s (after the passage of the US OSHA standard for benzene), but these solvents still poses a long-term risk due to the latency period for hematopoietic cancer after benzene exposure (> 30 years).

ALCOHOLS

ESSENTIALS OF DIAGNOSIS

► Acute effects
  • Respiratory tract irritation: cough and sore nose and throat.
  • Anesthesia: dizziness, headache, nausea, vomiting, sleepiness, fatigue, "drunkenness," slurred speech, disequilibrium, disorientation, depression, and loss of consciousness.
► Chronic effects
  • Dermatitis: dry, cracked, and erythematous skin.
  • Optic neuropathy (methyl alcohol): blurred vision, blindness, hyperemic optic disk, and dilated pupil.

General Considerations

Alcohols are hydrocarbons substituted with a single hydroxyl group:

$$—C—C—OH$$

They have a characteristic pungent odor. Examples of alcohols used as solvents are ethyl alcohol, methyl alcohol, and isopropyl alcohol (see Table 31–1).

Use

Alcohols are used widely as cleaning agents, thinners, and diluents; as vehicles for paints, pesticides, and pharmaceuticals; as extracting agents; and as chemical intermediates. Methyl alcohol is used widely as an industrial solvent—one-fourth of its production—and as an adulterant to denature ethanol to prevent its abuse when used as an industrial solvent. Approximately one-third of methyl alcohol used is in the production of formaldehyde. More than half the isopropyl alcohol produced is used to manufacture acetone and the rest in a variety of solvent and chemical formulation uses. Approximately 90% of cyclohexanol is used to produce adipic acid for nylon and the rest for esters for plasticizers. Alkyl alcohol is used solely as a chemical intermediate. The higher alcohols (> 5 carbons) are divided into the plasticizer range (6–11 carbons) and the detergent range (≥ 12 carbons). About 500 kilotons of plasticizer-range alcohols are produced annually in the United States to make esters for plasticizers and lubricants, and about 260 kilotons of detergent-range alcohols are produced to make sulfate deionizers for detergents.

Occupational & Environmental Exposure

NIOSH reports that methyl alcohol is used in solvents, deicers, and the manufacturing of plastics, polyesters, and other chemicals. Workers at risk of exposure to methyl alcohol include factory workers in plants that manufacture plastics; transportation workers exposed to the deicing of vehicles; workers who work in alternative fuel industries; and workers exposed to certain solvents or cleaning agents.

Pharmacokinetics

The pharmacokinetics of the simple (primary) alcohols are similar. Approximately 50% of inhaled alcohol is absorbed at rest, decreasing to 40% with light to moderate workloads. Some alcohols are sufficiently absorbed percutaneously to be given skin TLV designations.

The primary alcohols are metabolized by hepatic alcohol dehydrogenase to aldehydes and by aldehyde dehydrogenase to carboxylic acids. The metabolic acidosis and optic neuropathy caused by methyl alcohol have been attributed to its metabolism to formic acid. Metabolic interactions of ethanol with other organic solvents, such as *degreasers' flush* in workers exposed to trichloroethylene and other chlorinated hydrocarbons, frequently are due to competition for alcohol and aldehyde dehydrogenases, with subsequent accumulation of the alcohol and aldehyde and resulting reaction. Secondary alcohols are metabolized primarily to ketones.

Health Effects

The alcohols are more potent central nervous system depressants and irritants than the corresponding aliphatic hydrocarbons, but they are weaker skin and respiratory tract irritants than aldehydes or ketones. Respiratory tract and eye irritation usually occurs at lower concentrations than central nervous system depression and thus serves as a useful warning property. This may explain why occupational exposure to alcohols has not been implicated as causing chronic neurobehavioral effects. The TLVs for most alcohols are based on prevention of irritation.

Methyl alcohol is toxicologically distinct owing to its toxicity to the optic nerve, which can result in blindness. An extensive literature is available on this effect, which occurs primarily as a result of ingestion of methanol as an ethanol substitute or adulterant. A few cases of blindness have been reported as a result of occupational inhalation exposure in confined spaces. The minimum oral dose causing blindness in an adult male has been estimated to be about 8–10 g; the minimum lethal dose is estimated to be 75–100 g. These amounts correspond to 8-hour exposure concentrations in air of approximately 1600–2000 and 15,000–20,000 ppm, respectively. Blurred vision and other visual disturbances have been reported occasionally as a result of exposure to levels slightly above the TLV of 200 ppm. Methanol in urine can be used for biologic monitoring, with 15 mg/L at the end of a work shift corresponding to an 8-hour exposure at 200 ppm.

Inhalation exposure to ethanol and propanol results in simple irritation and central nervous system depression, although propanol may be absorbed significantly through the skin. There are a few reports of auditory and vestibular nerve injury in workers exposed to n-butyl alcohol. Isooctyl alcohol is the most industrially important of the higher alcohols, but little toxicologic information about it is available.

GLYCOLS (DIOLS)

ESSENTIALS OF DIAGNOSIS

► Acute effects
  • Anesthesia (unusual because of low vapor pressure): dizziness, headache, nausea, vomiting, sleepiness, fatigue, "drunkenness," slurred speech, disequilibrium, disorientation, depression, and loss of consciousness.
► Chronic effects
  • Dermatitis: dry, cracked, and erythematous skin.

General Considerations

Glycols are hydrocarbons with two hydroxyl (alcohol) groups attached to separate carbon atoms in an aliphatic chain:

Examples include ethylene glycol, diethylene glycol, triethylene glycol, and propylene glycol (see Table 31–1). They have a slightly sweet odor.

Use

Glycols are used as anti-freezing agents and as solvent carriers and vehicles in a variety of chemical formulations. Only ethylene glycol is in common general industrial use as a solvent, but large volumes of the other glycols are used as vehicles and chemical intermediates. Approximately 40% of ethylene glycol is used as antifreeze, 35% to make polyesters, and 25% as solvent carriers. Glycols, for example, propylene glycol, are also used to generate artificial smoke or fog in entertainment and for emergency training.

Occupational & Environmental Exposure

NIOSH reports that ethylene glycol used as an antifreeze, in making polyester plastics, and for some manufacturing. Workers at risk of being exposed to ethylene glycol include factory workers involved in the manufacture of polyester; workers who use certain solvents; employees working with heating and cooling systems; and factory workers exposed to certain manufacturing processes.

Pharmacokinetics

The glycols have such low vapor pressures that inhalation is only of moderate concern unless heated or aerosolized. Ethylene glycol does not have a skin TLV designation. Ethylene glycol and diethylene glycol are metabolized to glycol aldehyde, glycolic acid, glyoxylic acid, oxalic acid, formic acid, glycine, and carbon dioxide. Oxalic acid is the cause of the acute renal failure and metabolic acidosis that occur following ingestion of ethylene glycol. The first two steps in this metabolism use alcohol and aldehyde dehydrogenase and may be competitively blocked by administration of ethyl alcohol.

Health Effects

The low vapor pressures of the glycols result in little hazard in their customary industrial use. They are not significantly irritating to the skin or respiratory tract but can produce a chronic dermatitis from defatting of the skin. The systemic toxicity of ethylene glycol commonly seen after ingestion of commercial antifreeze compounds as an alcohol substitute—seizures, central nervous system depression, metabolic acidosis, and acute renal failure—have not been reported as a result of occupational exposure. When used to generate artificial smoke or fog, they may cause acute eye and upper airway irritation and decreased lung function from long-term exposure.

PHENOLS

ESSENTIALS OF DIAGNOSIS

▶ Acute effects

- Respiratory tract irritation: cough and sore nose and throat.
- Tissue destruction (eg, hepatic necrosis with abdominal pain, jaundice, abnormal liver function tests), kidney necrosis with acute renal failure, skin necrosis with blisters and burns.
- Anesthesia: dizziness, headache, nausea, vomiting, sleepiness, fatigue, "drunkenness," slurred speech, disequilibrium, disorientation, depression, and loss of consciousness.

▶ Chronic effects

- Dermatitis: dry, cracked, and erythematous skin.

▶ General Considerations

Phenols are aromatic alcohols:

Examples include phenol, cresol (methyl phenol), catechol (1,2,-benzenediol, 1,2-dihydroxybenzene), resorcinol (1,3-benzenediol, 1,3-dihydroxybenzene), and hydroquinone (1,4-benzenediol, 1,4-hydroxybenzene).

▶ Use

The industrial use of phenols as solvents is limited by their acute toxicity. Phenol is used as a cleaning agent, paint stripper, and disinfectant, but its chief use is as a chemical intermediate for phenolic resins, bisphenol A for epoxy resins, and other chemicals and drugs. Cresol is used as a disinfectant and chemical intermediate. Catechol is used in photography, fur dyeing, and leather tanning and as a chemical intermediate. Resorcinol is used as a chemical intermediate for adhesives, dyes, and pharmaceuticals. Hydroquinone is used in photography, as a polymerization inhibitor, and as an antioxidant.

▶ Occupational & Environmental Exposure

NIOSH reports that phenol is used in many industries as a slimicide, antiseptic, and disinfectant and to manufacture a number of products. Workers at risk of being exposed to phenol include workers in the petroleum industry; workers in plants where nylon is manufactured; workers in plants that manufacture epoxy resins; and workers in plants that manufacture herbicides.

▶ Pharmacokinetics

Phenol is well absorbed both by inhalation of vapors and by dermal penetration of vapors and liquids. Phenol and cresols have skin TLV designations. Phenol is eliminated rapidly within 16 hours, almost entirely as conjugated phenol in urine.

▶ Health Effects

Phenol and related compounds are potent irritants that can be corrosive at high concentrations. As a result of their ability to complex with, denature, and precipitate proteins, they can be cytotoxic to all cells at sufficient concentrations. Direct contact with concentrated phenol can result in burns, local tissue necrosis, systemic absorption, and tissue necrosis in the liver, kidneys, urinary tract, and heart. Central nervous system depression occurs, as it does with all volatile organic solvents. A concentration of total phenol in urine of 250 mg/g of creatinine at the end of a work shift corresponds to an 8-hour exposure to the TLV of 5 ppm.

KETONES

ESSENTIALS OF DIAGNOSIS

▶ Acute effects

- Respiratory tract irritation: cough and sore nose and throat.
- Anesthesia: dizziness, headache, nausea, vomiting, sleepiness, fatigue, "drunkenness," slurred speech, disequilibrium, disorientation, depression, and loss of consciousness.

▶ Chronic effects

- Dermatitis: dry, cracked, and erythematous skin.
- Peripheral neuropathy (methyl n-butyl ketone).

▶ General Considerations

Ketones are hydrocarbons with a carbonyl group that is attached to two hydrocarbon groups (the carbonyl is nonterminal):

They are produced by the dehydroxylation or oxidation of alcohols. A great many ketones are in use; Table 31–1 lists some of the ketones that are used as industrial solvents.

Acetone and methyl ethyl ketone (2-butanone) are in most common use. The ketones have a characteristic minty odor that some people find pleasant and others offensive.

 Use

Ketones are used widely as solvents for surface coatings with natural and synthetic resins; in the formulation of inks, adhesives, and dyes; in chemical extraction and manufacture; and to a lesser extent, as cleaning agents. About one-fourth of the acetone produced is used in the manufacture of methacrylates and one-third as solvent. Almost all cyclohexanone is used to make caprolactam for nylon, but small amounts are used as solvents.

▶ **Occupational & Environmental Exposure**

NIOSH reports that exposure to methyl ethyl ketone may occur among workers who work in printing plants; employees exposed to certain paints, coatings, or glues; workers who work in shoe and sporting goods factories; manufacturing workers involved in making synthetic rubber products.

▶ **Pharmacokinetics**

Ketones are well absorbed by inhalation of vapors and to a lesser extent after skin contact with liquid. Only cyclohexanone has a skin TLV designation. The pulmonary retention of acetone at rest has been estimated to be approximately 45%. Most ketones are eliminated rapidly unchanged in urine and exhaled air and by reduction to their respective alcohols, which are conjugated and excreted or further metabolized to a variety of compounds, including carbon monoxide. Acetone is excreted in the expired air of normal, healthy individuals at approximately 120 ng/L.

▶ **Health Effects**

Ketones have good warning properties in that irritation or a strong odor usually occurs at levels below those that cause central nervous system depression. Headaches and nausea as a result of the odor have been mistaken for central nervous system depression. The TLVs for most ketones are set to prevent irritation. Methyl *n*-butyl ketone causes the same type of peripheral neuropathy as *n*-hexane. It is metabolized to the neurotoxic diketone 2,5-hexanedione to even a greater extent than *n*-hexane and therefore poses even a greater hazard. The neurotoxic potential of methyl *n*-butyl ketone was discovered following the occurrence of a large number of cases of peripheral neuropathy in a plastics manufacturing plant in Ohio in 1974. A large volume of research has been published since, from animal neurotoxicity and metabolism studies to cell culture and mechanistic studies. However, human exposure to this substance no longer occurs because the sole manufacturer ceased production. Other ketones used as solvents have not been shown to cause peripheral neuropathy, but methyl ethyl ketone potentiates the neurotoxicity of *n*-hexane and methyl *n*-butyl ketone probably

through a metabolic interaction. Concentrations of methyl ethyl ketone and methyl isobutyl ketone of 2 mg/L at the end of a work shift correspond to 8-hour exposures to the TLVs of 200 and 50 ppm, respectively.

ESTERS

ESSENTIALS OF DIAGNOSIS

▶ Acute effects
- Anesthesia: dizziness, headache, nausea, vomiting, sleepiness, fatigue, "drunkenness," slurred speech, disequilibrium, disorientation, depression, and loss of consciousness.
- Respiratory tract irritation: cough and sore nose and throat.

▶ Chronic effects
- Dermatitis: dry, cracked, and erythematous skin.

▶ **General Considerations**

Esters are hydrocarbons that are derivatives of an organic acid and an alcohol:

$$-\text{C}=\text{O}$$
$$\diagdown\text{O}-\text{C}-$$

They are named after their parent alcohols and acids, respectively (eg, methyl acetate for the ester of methyl alcohol and acetic acid). Table 31–1 lists examples of some of the many esters used as solvents. They have characteristic odors that range from sweet to pungent.

▶ **Use**

Esters—particularly the lower esters—are commonly used as solvents for surface coatings. Vinyl acetate is used primarily in the production of polyvinyl acetate and polyvinyl alcohol. Other lower esters are used to make polymeric acrylates and methacrylates. Higher esters are used as plasticizers.

▶ **Occupational & Environmental Exposure**

Workers are exposed to vinyl acetate via inhalation or dermal contact during the manufacture or use.

▶ **Pharmacokinetics**

Esters are metabolized very rapidly by plasma esterases to their parent organic acids and alcohols.

▶ **Health Effects**

Many esters have extremely low odor thresholds, their distinctive sweet smells serving as good warning properties.

Because of this property, *n*-amyl acetate (banana oil) is used as an odorant for qualitative fit testing of respirators. Esters are more potent anesthetics than corresponding alcohols, aldehydes, or ketones but are also strong irritants. Odor and irritation usually occur at levels below central nervous system depression. Their systemic toxicity is determined to a large extent by the toxicity of the corresponding alcohol. There is one report of optic nerve damage from exposure to methyl acetate as a result of metabolism to methanol and hence to formic acid (see discussion on "Alcohols"). Similarly, methyl formate may cause optic neuropathy following metabolism directly to formic acid.

ETHERS

ESSENTIALS OF DIAGNOSIS

▶ Acute effects
  • Anesthesia: dizziness, headache, nausea, vomiting, sleepiness, fatigue, "drunkenness," slurred speech, disequilibrium, disorientation, depression, and loss of consciousness.
  • Respiratory tract irritation: cough and sore nose and throat.
▶ Chronic effects
  • Dermatitis: dry, cracked, and erythematous skin.

▶ General Considerations

Ethers consist of two hydrocarbon groups joined by an oxygen linkage:

$$—C—O—C—$$

Examples include ethyl ether and dioxane (see Table 31–1). They have a characteristic sweet odor often described as "ethereal."

▶ Use

Ethyl ether was used extensively in the past as an anesthetic but has been replaced by agents less flammable and explosive. It is too volatile for most solvent uses except analytic extraction. It is used as a solvent for waxes, fats, oils, and gums. Dioxane (1,4-diethylene dioxide) is used as a solvent for a wide range of organic products, including cellulose esters, rubber, and coatings; in the preparation of histologic slides; and as a stabilizer in chlorinated solvents. Methyl *tert*-butyl ether (MTBE) has been used widely as an oxygenated fuel additive to reduce carbon monoxide emissions.

▶ Occupational & Environmental Exposure

NIOSH reports that 1,4-dioxane is used as an industrial solvent, a laboratory reagent, and in the manufacture of other chemicals. Workers at risk of being exposed to 1,4-dioxane include employees working in scientific laboratories; workers exposed to certain types of industrial solvents; factory workers involved in producing some cosmetics; and workers in paper pulping industries.

▶ Pharmacokinetics

Ethyl ether is well absorbed by inhalation of vapors; its volatility limits percutaneous absorption. More than 90% of absorbed ethyl ether is excreted unchanged in exhaled air; the rest may be metabolized by enzymatic cleavage of the ether link to acetaldehyde and acetic acid. Dioxane is well absorbed by inhalation of vapors and through skin contact with liquid and has a skin TLV designation. It is metabolized almost entirely to β-hydroxyethoxyacetic acid and excreted in urine with a half-life of about 1 hour.

▶ Health Effects

Ethyl ether is a potent anesthetic and a less-potent irritant. Higher ethers are relatively more potent irritants. Dioxane is also an anesthetic and irritant but also has caused acute kidney and liver necrosis in workers exposed to uncertain amounts. The US EPA has established that 1,4-dioxane is likely to be carcinogenic to humans; and the International Agency for Research on Cancer (IARC) has determined that 1,4-dioxane is possibly carcinogenic to humans. Exposure to gasoline containing MTBE is associated with headache, nausea, eye irritation, dizziness, vomiting, sedation, and nosebleeds. The Department of Health and Human Services (DHSS), the IARC, and the EPA have not classified MTBE for its ability to cause cancer.

GLYCOL ETHERS

ESSENTIALS OF DIAGNOSIS

▶ Acute effects
  • Anesthesia: dizziness, headache, nausea, vomiting, sleepiness, fatigue, "drunkenness," slurred speech, disequilibrium, disorientation, depression, and loss of consciousness.
▶ Chronic effects
  • Dermatitis: dry, cracked, and erythematous skin.
  • Anemia: low erythrocyte count or pancytopenia and evidence of hemolysis or bone marrow suppression.
  • Encephalopathy: confusion and disorientation.
  • Reproductive toxicity: major malformations and fetal death with maternal exposure; low sperm count, testicular atrophy, and infertility with male exposure; there is evidence of human reproductive effects.

▶ General Considerations

The glycol ethers are alkyl ether derivatives of ethylene, diethylene, triethylene, and propylene glycol (an alkyl group linked to the glycol by substitution). The acetate derivatives of glycol ethers are included in and are considered toxicologically identical to their precursors. They are known by formal chemical names (eg, ethylene glycol methyl ether [EGME]), common chemical names (2-methoxyethanol [2-ME]) as used here, and trade names (eg, Methyl Cellosolve).

▶ Use

The glycol ethers are widely used solvents because of their solubility or miscibility in water and most organic liquids. They are used as diluents in paints, lacquers, enamels, inks, and dyes; as cleaning agents in liquid soaps, dry-cleaning fluids, and glass cleaners; as surfactants, fixatives, desiccants, antifreeze compounds, and deicers; and in extraction and chemical synthesis. They are used extensively in the semiconductor industry. Because 2-methoxyethanol and 2-ethoxyethanol were found to be potent reproductive toxins in laboratory animals (and their TLVs were lowered on this basis), there has been a shift in use to 2-butoxyethanol and other longer-chained ethylene glycol ethers (EGEs) and to diethylene and propylene glycol ethers.

▶ Occupational & Environmental Exposure

The most important exposures may occur as a result of skin contact with liquids, inhalation of vapors in enclosed spaces, and spraying or heating of the liquids to generate aerosols or vapors. Skin absorption of vapors also can be a significant route of exposure. Although glycol ethers have relatively low vapor pressures, some of their saturation vapor concentrations at room temperatures can greatly exceed TLVs. Exposures easily can exceed the doses of 2-methoxyethanol and 2-ethoxyethanol that cause reproductive toxicity in laboratory animals. Consumer and worker exposure to 2-butoxyethanol in glass cleaners is widespread; this glycol ether is apparently of lower toxicity.

▶ Pharmacokinetics

The glycol ethers are well absorbed by all routes of exposure owing to their universal solubility. They have relatively low vapor pressures, so dermal exposure is often of primary importance. The acetate derivatives are hydrolyzed rapidly by plasma esterases to their corresponding monoalkyl ethers. The ethylene glycol monoalkyl ethers maintain their ether linkages and are metabolized by hepatic alcohol and aldehyde dehydrogenases to their respective aldehyde and acid metabolites. The acid metabolites 2-methoxyacetic acid and 2-ethoxyacetic acid are responsible for the reproductive toxicities of 2-methoxyethanol and 2-ethoxyethanol. These metabolites are excreted in urine unchanged or conjugated to glycine and can be used as biologic indicators of exposure; this is important because skin exposure easily can constitute the bulk of exposure.

▶ Health Effects

Acute central nervous system depression has not been reported as an effect of occupational exposure. However, a number of cases of encephalopathy have been reported in workers exposed to 2-methoxyethanol over periods of weeks to months. Manifestations include personality changes, memory loss, difficulty in concentrating, lethargy, fatigue, loss of appetite, weight loss, tremor, gait disturbances, and slurred speech.

Bone marrow toxicity usually manifested as pancytopenia has been reported in workers and laboratory animals exposed to 2-methoxyethanol and 2-ethoxyethanol. The longer-chain ethylene glycol monoalkyl ethers cause hemolysis by increasing osmotic fragility in laboratory animals, an effect that has not been reported to date in humans.

Male reproductive toxicity has been demonstrated in experimental animals for 2-methoxyethanol, 2-ethoxyethanol, and their acetate derivatives. Acute or chronic exposure of mice, rats, and rabbits to low levels of these compounds by inhalation or dermal or oral routes resulted in reductions in sperm count, impaired sperm motility, increased numbers of abnormal forms, and infertility. These effects began about 4 weeks after the onset of exposure and—in the absence of testicular atrophy—were reversible following cessation of exposure.

The testicular toxicity of the glycol ethers decreases sharply with lengthening of the alkyl group such that beginning with and proceeding through *n*-propyl, isopropyl, and butyl, they are nearly or completely inactive. The acetic acid derivatives (alkoxy acids) appear to be the active testicular toxins. In limited testing, the dimethyl ethers of ethylene glycol and diethylene glycol—but not the monomethyl ether of diethylene glycol—show some evidence of causing testicular toxicity. Ethylene glycol hexyl ether, ethylene glycol phenyl ether, and the propylene glycol ethers do not appear to be toxic to either the male or female reproductive system.

The same glycol ethers that are testicular toxins have been shown to be teratogenic in the same and additional species of laboratory animals at comparable doses. The structure-activity relationships also appear to be similar; the alkoxy acid metabolites are apparently the proximate teratogens. Major defects of the skeleton, kidneys, and cardiovascular system have been observed, with some variation in their nature and severity with species, dose, and route of administration. The ethylene glycol monoalkyl ethers with longer alkyl chains and other glycol (propylene and dipropylene) ethers have not been shown to be teratogenic with the exception of the diethylene glycol ethers, which produced typical malformations.

Several studies of occupationally exposed men and women provide evidence that the effects in humans are the same as those in animals. A comprehensive study documented 44 cases of a birth-defect syndrome in children of mothers employed at a capacitor factory in Matamoros, Mexico. The case-control study component found that all case mothers, but none of the control mothers, had heavy or continuous hand immersion in both 2-methoxyethanol and ethylene glycol during their pregnancies. Frank maternal toxicity was reported in many workers. The syndrome resembled fetal alcohol syndrome but was distinct from it.

Maternal exposure to glycol ethers was associated with various major structural birth defects in a large European case-control study incorporating all occupations. Female workers exposed to EGEs in the semiconductor industry have been reported to have higher risks of spontaneous abortion, subfertility, and menstrual disturbances and prolonged waiting time to pregnancy.

Studies of male workers exposed to 2-methoxyethanol or 2-ethoxyethanol found evidence of spermatotoxicity.

Because reproductive effects have been produced consistently in all species tested and their metabolism and other health effects appear to be similar in humans and laboratory animals, those compounds with reproductive effects in animals should be assumed to be testicular toxins and teratogens in humans. Substitution of one glycol ether for another should be approached cautiously. Not all the compounds have been tested thoroughly, and not all propylene derivatives are safe (eg, the beta isomer of propylene glycol methyl ether is a teratogen).

GLYCIDYL ETHERS

ESSENTIALS OF DIAGNOSIS

▶ Acute effects
- Dermatitis (primary irritant): irritation, erythema, and first- and second-degree burns of skin.
▶ Chronic effects
- Dermatitis (allergic contact): itching, erythema, and vesicles.

▶ General Considerations

The glycidyl ethers consist of a 2,3-epoxypropyl group with an ether linkage to another hydrocarbon group:

They are synthesized from epichlorohydrin and an alcohol. Only the monoglycidyl ethers are in common use and discussed here.

▶ Use

The epoxide or oxirane ring of glycidyl ethers makes these compounds very reactive, so their use is confined to processes that use this property, such as reactive diluents in epoxy resin systems. Epoxy resins have a wide range of applications in industry and consumer use.

▶ Occupational & Environmental Exposure

The primary exposure of workers and consumers is in the application of uncured epoxy resins. The epoxide groups of the ethers react to form cross-linkages within epoxy resins so that glycidyl ethers no longer exist in a completely cured resin. However, workers may be exposed to the ethers in their manufacture and in the formulation and application of the resin system.

▶ Pharmacokinetics

The glycidyl ethers have low vapor pressures, so inhalation at normal air temperatures usually is not a concern. However, the curing of epoxy resins often generates heat, which may vaporize some glycidyl ether. A number of uses such as epoxy paint require spraying and the generation of an aerosol. Although quantitative data are lacking, the glycidyl ethers should be well absorbed by all routes. They have a short biologic half-life owing to their reactivity. Three metabolic reactions have been proposed: reduction to diols by epoxide hydrase, conjugation with glutathione, and covalent bonding with proteins, RNA, and DNA.

▶ Health Effects

Reported effects of glycidyl ethers from occupational exposure have been confined to dermatitis of both the primary irritant and allergic contact types. Dermatitis can be severe and may result in second-degree burns. Asthma in workers exposed to epoxy resins may be a result of exposure to glycidyl ethers.

Glycidyl ethers are positive in a number of short-term tests of genotoxicity, including mutagenicity, but none has been tested adequately for carcinogenicity. They are testicular toxins in laboratory animals, but few have been tested for teratogenicity.

ALIPHATIC AMINES

ESSENTIALS OF DIAGNOSIS

▶ Acute effects
- Eye irritation, corneal edema, and visual halos.
- Respiratory tract irritation: sore nose and throat and cough.
- Dermatitis (irritant): erythema and irritation of skin.
▶ Chronic effects
- Dermatitis (allergic contact): erythema, vesicles, and itching of skin.
- Asthma (ethyleneamines): cough, wheezing, shortness of breath, dyspnea on exertion, and decreased FVC on pulmonary function testing with response to bronchodilators.

General Considerations

Aliphatic amines are derivatives of ammonia in which one or more hydrogen atoms are replaced by an alkyl or alkanol group:

$$C—C—NH_2 \qquad —C—\overset{\displaystyle OH}{C}—NH_2$$

(primary amine)   (alkanolamine)

They can be classified as primary, secondary, and tertiary monoamines according to the number of substitutions on the nitrogen atom; as polyamines, if more than one amine group is present; and as alkanolamines, if a hydroxyl group is present on the alkyl group (an alcohol). They have a characteristic odor like that of fish and are strongly alkaline.

Use

There are a large number of aliphatic amines that have a number of uses. They are used to some extent as solvents but to a greater degree as chemical intermediates. They are also used as catalysts for polymerization reactions, preservatives (bactericides), corrosion inhibitors, drugs, and herbicides.

Occupational & Environmental Exposure

Given the diversity of their uses, accurate estimates of the number of workers exposed to aliphatic amines are not possible. They are not common environmental pollutants.

Pharmacokinetics

Little is known of the pharmacokinetics of the aliphatic amines in industrial use. They are well absorbed by inhalation, and some have skin designations as a result of their percutaneous absorption (see Table 31–1). Metabolism probably is primarily deamination to ammonia by monoamine oxidase and diamine oxidase.

Health Effects

The vapors of the volatile amines cause eye irritation and a characteristic corneal edema, with visual changes of halos around lights, that is reversible. Irritation will occur wherever contact with the vapors occurs, including the respiratory tract and skin. Direct contact with the liquid can produce serious eye or skin burns. Allergic contact dermatitis has been reported primarily from ethyleneamines, as has asthma.

CHLORINATED HYDROCARBONS

ESSENTIALS OF DIAGNOSIS

▸ Acute effects
- Anesthesia: dizziness, headache, nausea, vomiting, sleepiness, fatigue, "drunkenness," slurred speech, disequilibrium, disorientation, depression, loss of consciousness, death.

- Respiratory tract irritation: cough and sore nose and throat.

▸ Chronic effects
- Dermatitis: dry, cracked, and erythematous skin.
- Neurobehavioral dysfunction: headache, mood lability, fatigue, short-term memory loss, difficulty in concentrating, decreased attention span, neurobehavioral test abnormalities, CT scan (cerebral atrophy), EEG (diffuse slow waves).
- Hepatocellular injury: abdominal pain, nausea, jaundice, and abnormal liver function tests.
- Renal tubular dysfunction: weakness, fatigue, polyuria, glycosuria, electrolyte abnormalities (acidosis, hypokalemia, hypophosphatemia, hypochloremia, and hypocarbonatemia), glycosuria, and proteinuria.

General Considerations

The addition of chlorine to carbon and hydrogen

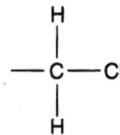

increases the stability and decreases the flammability of the resulting compounds. They have characteristic slightly pungent odors. Six chlorinated aliphatic hydrocarbons are used commonly as solvents: trichloroethylene, perchloroethylene (tetrachloroethylene), 1,1,1-trichloroethane (methyl chloroform), methylene chloride (dichloromethane), carbon tetrachloride, and chloroform. Other chlorinated aliphatic hydrocarbons, such as ethylene dichloride and chlorinated aromatics such as chlorobenzenes, are used rarely as general industrial solvents and are not discussed here. Abbreviations such as TCE and TCA will not be used because they are not standardized and can lead to errors in identification.

Use

The chlorinated hydrocarbons are used extensively as cleaning, degreasing, and thinning agents and less so as chemical intermediates. Historically, trichloroethylene was the principal solvent used in vapor degreasers, but it has been largely replaced. Perchloroethylene has replaced mineral spirits and carbon tetrachloride as the primary dry-cleaning solvent in two-thirds of facilities because of the flammability of the former and the toxicity of the latter. In turn, efforts are in progress to replace solvent cleaning of fabrics with liquid carbon dioxide. As of 2019, as a result of the acute fatalities that have resulted from the use of methylene chloride, the US EPA has prohibited the manufacture (including import), processing, and distribution of methylene chloride in all paint removers for consumer use. This followed a similar ban on the sale of methylene chloride in the European Union in 2012.

▶ Occupational & Environmental Exposure

NIOSH reports that trichloroethylene is mostly used as a solvent to remove grease from metal parts, and also as an ingredient in adhesives, paint removers, typewriter correction fluids, and spot removers. Workers at risk of being exposed to trichloroethylene include workers who use this substance for metal degreasing; workers who use it as an extraction solvent for greases, oils, fats, waxes, and tars; factory workers in the textile processing industry who use it to scour cotton, wool, and other fabrics; dry cleaning workers who use it to remove spots; factory workers in plants that manufacture pharmaceuticals; and chemical workers who use it to make other chemicals. According to the US EPA, the uses of perchloroethylene include the production of fluorinated compounds, dry cleaning and vapor degreasing, as well as a number of smaller uses. Nearly 65% of the production volume of perchloroethylene is used to produce fluorinated compounds, such as hydrofluorocarbons (HFCs) and hydrochlorofluorocarbons (HCFCs). The second largest use of perchloroethylene is as a solvent in dry cleaning facilities, with approximately 60% of dry cleaning machines now using perchloroethylene as a solvent. The third most prevalent use of perchloroethylene is as a vapor degreasing solvent. Workers at risk of being exposed to tetrachloroethylene include workers in dry cleaning industries; workers who use it to degrease metals; and workers in industries who use it to make other chemicals. According to the US EPA, methylene chloride has been used for decades in paint and coating removal in products intended for both consumer and commercial uses. Paint and coating removal, also referred to as paint stripping, is the process of removing paint or other coatings from a surface. Coatings can include paint, varnish, lacquer, graffiti, polyurethane, or other high-performance or specialty coatings. Occupational exposure to methyl chloroform can occur during the use of metal degreasing agents, paints, glues, and cleaning products.

▶ Pharmacokinetics

The chlorinated hydrocarbon solvents are all relatively volatile and moderately well absorbed by inhalation. Pulmonary uptake ranges from 60% to 80% at rest and decreases to 40–50% during activity. Percutaneous absorption of vapors is usually insignificant, but dermal absorption following prolonged or extensive contact of the skin with liquid can be significant.

Biologic monitoring of the chlorinated hydrocarbons is based on their pattern of metabolism and excretion, which varies with their structure. 1,1,1-Trichloroethane and perchloroethylene are excreted mainly unchanged in exhaled air and metabolized and excreted only slightly as trichloroethanol and trichloroacetic acid. Consequently, biologic monitoring is conducted chiefly with exhaled air and, to a lesser extent, with the parent compound in blood and metabolites in urine. Accumulation of both compounds occurs to some degree with daily exposure.

In contrast, less than 10% of trichloroethylene is excreted unchanged in exhaled air. The remainder is metabolized rapidly by alcohol and aldehyde dehydrogenases via chloral hydrate to trichloroethanol and trichloroacetic acid or to unidentified metabolites. Although the biologic half-life of the parent compound is very short, trichloroethanol is an active anesthetic and, with a half-life of 10–15 hours, accumulates to some extent over the course of a workweek. Trichloroacetic acid, though inactive, has a much longer half-life of 50–100 hours and has been recommended for use in biological monitoring. A value of 100 mg/L in urine voided at the end of the workweek corresponds to exposure to a TWA of 50 ppm trichloroethylene. However, because of large individual variability, this value can be used only to assess groups of workers and not individuals.

Methylene chloride is both excreted unchanged in exhaled air and metabolized to carbon monoxide in a dose-dependent fashion. An 8-hour exposure to methylene chloride at its prior TLV of 100 ppm results in a carboxyhemoglobin level of approximately 3–5% in a nonsmoker, whereas with exposure at its current TLV, carboxyhemoglobin levels are indistinguishable from background (1–2%). Methylene chloride in blood and exhaled air also can be used as a biologic indicator of exposure.

Chloroform and carbon tetrachloride are each approximately 50% excreted unchanged in exhaled air and 50% metabolized. Both can be measured in blood and exhaled air, but little information is available on biological monitoring for either.

▶ Health Effects

As a class, the chlorinated hydrocarbons are more potent anesthetics, hepatotoxins, and nephrotoxins than other organic solvents. Most have been found to cause hepatocarcinomas in laboratory mice following oral administration. Evidence for carcinogenicity following inhalation has been demonstrated for methylene chloride, trichloroethylene, and perchloroethylene.

A. Trichloroethylene

The TLV of 10 ppm is based on prevention of central nervous system depression, which occurs at levels below those causing evidence of hepatic dysfunction. The National Toxicology Program (NTP) Report on Carcinogens (14th edition) reports trichloroethylene is known to be a human carcinogen based on epidemiologic studies. Two recent meta-analyses found a statistically significant increased risk of kidney cancer in workers who had ever been exposed to trichloroethylene with the highest exposure having the highest overall risk. Evidence indicates that the mechanism for causing kidney cancer is likely that trichloroethylene causes genotoxicity or cytotoxicity as a result of it being metabolized (glutathione conjugation) into products that lead to damage of DNA or cells. There is also limited epidemiologic evidence for trichloroethylene having a positive association and increased risk of non-Hodgkin lymphoma (NHL) in several studies and two meta analyses, although the evidence is less consistent than for kidney cancer. There is inadequate data to evaluate the relationship between trichloroethylene exposure and liver cancer. In animal studies, trichloroethylene has caused tumors in mice and rats at different sites (kidney, liver, testicles, lung, and lymph nodes) by exposure via both inhalation and stomach tube.

B. Perchloroethylene

Evidence in humans and animals show that chronic exposure to perchloroethylene can cause neurotoxicity, resulting in decrements in color vision, visuospatial memory, and possibly other aspects of cognition and neuropsychologic function. Animal and epidemiologic evidence supports an association between perchloroethylene exposure and chronic kidney disease. Liver toxicity (ie, necrosis, vacuolation, etc.) has been reported in multiple animal species by inhalation and oral exposures to perchloroethylene. Data from animal studies have identified various manifestations of developmental toxicity including, increased mortality and decreased body weight in the offspring of rodents exposed via inhalation. The US EPA has concluded that perchloroethylene is likely to be carcinogenic in humans by all routes of exposure.

C. Trichloroethane

1,1,1-Trichloroethane is only weakly hepatotoxic, with minor injury reported following massive overexposure. It is the weakest anesthetic of this group; its TLV of 350 ppm is established to prevent this effect. Sudden deaths in situations indicative of acute overexposure have been attributed to cardiac arrhythmias as a result of cardiac sensitization. The compound is weakly positive for mutagenicity in *Salmonella*, but it has not been tested adequately for carcinogenicity or reproductive toxicity. Several case reports suggest the possibility of peripheral neuropathy associated with 1,1,1-trichloroethane.

D. Carbon Tetrachloride

Carbon tetrachloride is a potent anesthetic. Both acute and chronic effects on the liver and kidneys have been reported at levels not much higher than those causing central nervous system depression. The TLV of 5 ppm (skin) was established to prevent fatty infiltration of the liver demonstrated in animals. A case series showed that acute effects are potentiated by heavy alcohol ingestion. Deaths have occurred from both hepatic and renal necrosis, and liver cancer has been reported in workers following acute liver damage from acute overexposure. The TLV has a group A2 (suspected human carcinogen) designation. There is evidence that carbon tetrachloride is fetotoxic but not teratogenic, and it causes testicular and ovarian damage in animals at toxic doses—but there is no evidence about effects at nontoxic doses.

E. Chloroform

Chloroform is only slightly less potent than carbon tetrachloride as an anesthetic and liver toxin. The ACGIH set its TLV to 10 ppm, and it is considered a suspected human carcinogen (group A2).

F. Methylene Chloride

Methylene chloride is similar to perchloroethylene and trichloroethylene in potency as an anesthetic and liver toxin. It is unique in that it is metabolized to carbon monoxide, with formation of carboxyhemoglobin. At methylene chloride exposure levels of 100 ppm and above, carboxyhemoglobin levels can exceed 10%, so the presence of anoxia in addition to anesthesia must be considered. Methylene chloride can cause acute deaths in enclosed spaces such as bathrooms when vapors rapidly build to high levels. The OSHA PEL was lowered from 500 to 25 ppm in 1997 as part of a new comprehensive standard that acknowledges methylene chloride as a potential occupational carcinogen. The standard includes an action limit of 12.5 ppm, exposure monitoring, medical surveillance, respiratory protection, and other requirements. Methylene chloride was not teratogenic to rats and mice exposed to 1225 ppm, although it was fetotoxic, causing delayed skeletal development typically seen with exposures that stress the maternal animal.

CHLOROFLUOROCARBONS

ESSENTIALS OF DIAGNOSIS

▶ Acute effects
  - Respiratory tract irritation: cough and sore nose and throat.
  - Anesthesia: dizziness, headache, nausea, vomiting, sleepiness, fatigue, "drunkenness," slurred speech, disequilibrium, disorientation, depression, and loss of consciousness.
  - Cardiac sensitization: dizziness, palpitations, faintness, loss of consciousness, and arrhythmia on ambulatory cardiac monitoring.
▶ Chronic effects
  - Dermatitis: dry, cracked, and erythematous skin.

▶ General Considerations

Chlorofluorocarbon (CFC) solvents are aliphatic hydrocarbons (methane or ethane) that contain one or more atoms each of chlorine and fluorine. Table 31–1 lists the commonly used CFC solvents. The numbering system for chlorofluorocarbons offers a convenient method of determining their chemical formulas. The "units" digit is the number of fluorine atoms (with CFC-113, this would be 3); the "tens" digit is the number of hydrogen atoms plus 1; and the "hundreds" digit is the number of carbon atoms minus 1. (Thus, CFC-113 would contain three fluorine atoms, no hydrogen atoms, and two carbon atoms, thereby requiring three chlorine atoms to make trichlorotrifluoroethane.)

CFCs are often referred to as *Freons*, which is the trade name of CFCs manufactured by Dupont. A CFC may be formulated with another organic solvent, such as methanol or methylene chloride, in a proprietary solvent mixture.

▶ Use

CFC production now has been largely phased out because of the depletion of stratospheric ozone. The completely halogenated CFCs are those implicated in this effect; note that HCFCs are still permitted (see following discussion). Reservoirs of CFCs persist in refrigeration and air-conditioning machinery; thus, there is still occupational exposure potential. This machinery requires maintenance, and at the end of its service life, the CFC is removed and may be reused. CFCs eventually will be phased out of "essential" medical uses such as metered-dose inhalers, but many are still in use.

▶ Occupational & Environmental Exposures

The widespread use of CFCs in industry and in consumer products in the past has resulted in exposure of large numbers of workers and consumers and in global contamination of the environment. Workers who service or dispose of refrigeration equipment, vehicle air conditioners, or building air-conditioning systems are still exposed. These workers are also exposed to numerous substitutes for CFCs, such as HCFCs.

▶ Pharmacokinetics

Very little information is available on the pharmacokinetics of CFCs. Most probably are resistant to metabolism and are excreted rapidly unchanged in exhaled air. Correlations undoubtedly exist between exposure and concentrations in exhaled air, but the information is too limited to recommend biological monitoring.

▶ Health Effects

The CFCs are of relatively low toxicity. All are anesthetics but require exposure to concentrations above 500–1000 ppm before this effect is manifested. Such levels most commonly are encountered in enclosed spaces (eg, cleaning out a degreasing tank) or when the CFC is heated (eg, using a heated-vapor degreaser) or sprayed (eg, when used as a propellant). They are not associated with chronic neurobehavioral effects, nor are they strong irritants.

Prolonged or frequent skin contact can cause a typical solvent dermatitis. Cardiac sensitization was first demonstrated for CFCs after a number of cases of sudden death of persons abusing CFC-11 and CFC-12 beginning in the late

1960s. A National Cancer Institute bioassay of CFC-11 was negative for mice and inconclusive for rats, whereas CFC-22 may have caused a slight increase in salivary gland tumors in male rats. Two rarely used chlorofluorocarbons, CFC-31 and CFC-133a, were carcinogenic in a limited gavage assay in rats. CFC-22, CFC-31, CFC-142b, CFC-143, and CFC-143a are positive in one or more short-term genotoxicity tests. CFC-22, the only one of the genotoxic CFCs in common use, is a weak bacterial mutagen. A number of CFCs have been tested for teratogenicity, including CFC-11, CFC-12, CFC-21, CFC-22, CFC-31, CFC-114, CFC-123b, and CFC-142b, but because of either inadequate design or inadequate reporting, no conclusions about effects can be reached. Unpublished studies report that CFC-22 is teratogenic in rats but not rabbits, producing microphthalmia and anophthalmia at inhalation levels of 50,000 ppm.

HYDROCHLOROFLUOROCARBONS & HYDROFLUOROCARBONS

HCFCs and HFCs share useful properties with CFCs but generally have much less environmental impact. Development of these alternatives has been rapid as CFCs are removed from use, so their toxicity is relatively untested. Most are sold as refrigerants, blowing agents for plastic foams, and fire-suppression agents. A few have been used as cleaning solvents (HCFC 141b, HCFC 225ca, and HCFC 225cb) or medical aerosol propellants (HCFC-134a and HFC 227ea).

The HCFCs and HFCs vary widely in toxicity, with some apparently quite benign, whereas others are toxic to the liver or heart. Some are suspected carcinogens or teratogens. It is advisable to monitor exposed workers to detect early signs of toxic effects.

HCFC-123 (2,2-dichloro-1,1,1-trifluoroethane) has evidence of significant human liver toxicity. A group of 17 workers suffered liver damage in a 1997 outbreak. They were involved in containerizing this liquid. HCFC-123 is chemically similar to halothane and has the same toxic metabolite. HCFC-123 exposure also was implicated as the cause of liver disease in nine industrial workers who had repeated exposure because of a leaking air-conditioning system in 1996; the refrigerant also contained HCFC-124.

MISCELLANEOUS SOLVENTS

N-Methyl-2-Pyrrolidone

N-methyl-2-pyrrolidone (NMP) is a colorless liquid with a mild odor and low volatility. NMP is widely used in the manufacture and production of electronics, petroleum products, pharmaceuticals, polymers, and other specialty chemicals. NMP is used in paint removers, and as a solvent/reagent for the electronics and pharmaceutical industries. It is also used as a solvent for hydrocarbon recovery in the petrochemical processing industry and for the desulfurization of natural gas. NMP is a key cleaning component for the manufacture of semiconductors used in electronics, and for the manufacture of printed circuit boards. The US EPA found in 2019 that based on animal studies, there is clear and consistent evidence for adverse reproductive and developmental effects following NMP exposure across oral, inhalation, and dermal exposure routes.

1-Bromopropane (*n*-Propyl Bromide)

1-BP is a colorless liquid with a sweet odor. It is a brominated hydrocarbon that is slightly soluble in water. 1-BP is a volatile organic compound (VOC) that exhibits high volatility, a low boiling point, low flammability, and no explosivity. The primary use of 1-BP is as a degreaser, dry cleaning solvent, spot cleaner, stain remover; in arts, crafts and hobby materials, and adhesive accelerant. In December 2019, the US EPA found the weight of the scientific evidence for reproductive and developmental toxicity, with impaired fetal development across species with evidence of a causative association between 1-BP exposure and developmental toxicity; peripheral neurotoxicity, impaired peripheral nerve function (sensory and motor) and adverse neuromuscular impacts; and evidence from chronic cancer bioassays in rats and mice that 1-BP may pose a carcinogenic hazard to humans.

Turpentine & *d*-Limonene

Turpentine is a mixture of substances called *terpenes*, primarily pinene. Gum turpentine is extracted from pine pitch; wood turpentine, from wood chips. It has had greater home than industrial use as a solvent. It is irritating and anesthetic and is one of the few solvents that causes allergic contact dermatitis. The incidence of sensitization varies with the type of pine, being generally higher with European than American pines. Owing to the frequency of allergic dermatitis, the availability of turpentine is now more limited. One recent study suggested that occupational paternal exposure to turpentine was associated with neuroblastoma in offspring.

d-Limonene is a terpene used as a solvent for printing, art paints, and janitorial cleaning; it is usually derived from citrus peel oils. Air exposure transforms it into an oxide that causes allergic contact dermatitis. Containers should be kept tightly closed; skin protection is advised.

Dimethylformamide

Dimethylformamide (DMF) is a widely used solvent because of its solubility in both aqueous and lipid media. However, these properties also result in its being well absorbed by all routes of exposure. DMF is a potent hepatotoxin and has been associated with both hepatitis and pancreatitis following occupational exposure. DMF has recently been reported in China to cause several cases of death due to exposure in fabric production. DMF exposure has been associated with alterations of sperm function and testicular cancer. Exposure can be monitored biologically by measuring

monomethylformamide and related metabolites in urine. Alcohol intolerance, in the form of flushing of the face and upper body, develops in some exposed workers.

n,n-Dimethylacetamide

Dimethylacetamide (DMAc) is a colorless industrial solvent which is used in the manufacture of films and fibers and the production of adhesives, plasticizers, and pharmaceuticals. Like DMF, DMAc is a hepatotoxin and is known to cause hepatocellular injury that is dose dependent. It has been found to cause hepatocellular injury in 34 workers at an elastane fiber facility. Another study found that DMAc-induced apoptosis in human hepatic cells in a dose dependent pattern.

Dimethyl Sulfoxide

Like DMF, dimethyl sulfoxide is soluble in a variety of media and is well absorbed by all routes of exposure. It appears to potentiate the absorption of other substances through the skin. Its use has not been associated with significant toxicity, but it has been subjected to little scientific study. It has a characteristic garlic-like or oyster-like odor that is present in the exhaled air of exposed persons. Its use as a dermally applied anti-inflammatory agent is not approved by the Federal Drug Administration, although it is used in that way in veterinary medicine.

REFERENCES

Alif SM et al: Occupational exposure to solvents and lung function decline: a population based study. Thorax 2019;74(7):650-658 [PMID: 31028237].

Genter MB, Doty RL: Toxic exposures and the senses of taste and smell. Handb Clin Neurol 2019;164:389-408 [PMID: 31604559].

Ianos O, Sari-Minodier I, Villes V, Lehucher-Michel MP, Loundou A, Perrin J: Meta-analysis reveals the association between male occupational exposure to solvents and impairment of semen parameters. J Occup Environ Med 2018;60(10):e533-e542 [PMID: 30095585].

Sainio MA Sr: Neurotoxicity of solvents. Handb Clin Neurol 2015;131:93–110. doi:10.1016/B978-0-444-62627-1.00007-X. [PMID: 26563785].

Spinder N et al: Congenital anomalies in the offspring of occupationally exposed mothers: a systematic review and meta-analysis of studies using expert assessment for occupational exposures. Hum Reprod 2019;34(5):903-919 [PMID: 30927411].

Staudt AM, Whitworth KW, Chien LC, Whitehead LW, Gimeno Ruiz de Porras D: Association of organic solvents and occupational noise on hearing loss and tinnitus among adults in the U.S., 1999-2004. Int Arch Occup Environ Health 2019;92(3):403-413 [PMID: 30806784].

Videnros C et al: Postmenopausal breast cancer and occupational exposure to chemicals. Scand J Work Environ Health 2019;45(6):642-650 [PMID: 30958561].

■ SELF-ASSESSMENT QUESTIONS

Select the one correct answer for each question.

Question 1: Solvents
 a. are unstable liquids at room temperature
 b. dissolve other substances resulting in a layered mixture
 c. may be classified as aqueous (water-based) or organic (hydrocarbon-based)
 d. are usually inorganic chemicals because most of the industrial substances they are used to dissolve are inorganic

Question 2: Percutaneous absorption of solvents
 a. is determined solely by their lipid solubility
 b. varies widely among individuals
 c. is independent of water solubility and volatility
 d. may be enhanced with highly volatile substances

Question 3: One isomer of hexane, *n*-hexane,
 a. causes peripheral neuropathy
 b. is found in household aerosol products
 c. is less toxic when coupled with methyl ethyl ketone and methyl isobutyl ketone exposure
 d. exposure can be assessed by measuring 2,5-hexanedione in the urine or hair samples

Question 4: The aromatic hydrocarbons
 a. generally are weaker irritants and anesthetics than the aliphatics
 b. cause only subclinical anesthetic effects

 c. cause only respiratory tract irritation and dermatitis
 d. are associated with neurobehavioral dysfunction

Question 5: The alcohols
 a. are more potent central nervous system depressants and irritants than the corresponding aliphatic hydrocarbons
 b. are more potent skin and respiratory tract irritants than aldehydes or ketones
 c. irritate the respiratory tract and eye at lower concentrations than central nervous system depression
 d. have profound chronic neurobehavioral effects in many industries

Question 6: Methylene chloride
 a. is more potent than perchloroethylene and trichloroethylene as an anesthetic
 b. is less potent than perchloroethylene and trichloroethylene as a liver toxin
 c. is unique in that it is metabolized to carbon monoxide, with formation of carboxyhemoglobin
 d. exposure levels of 100 ppm are considered acceptable

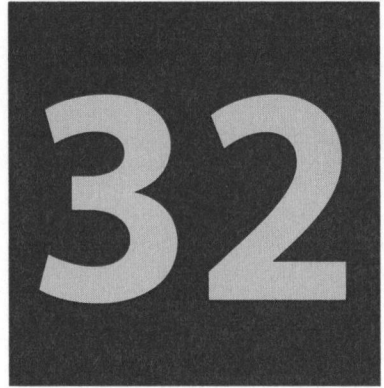

Gases & Other Airborne Toxicants

Ware G. Kuschner, MD
Paul D. Blanc, MD, MSPH

Potentially hazardous substances may be encountered as airborne toxicants across occupational, vocational, indoor environmental, and ambient exposure scenarios. These substances can exist in one or more of several physicochemical states, including gases, fumes, mists, aerosols, vapors, and smoke. Table 32–1 lists common definitions of these terms. The physicochemical distinctions among categories of airborne toxicants are of limited clinical application, but may be relevant for industrial hygiene monitoring and in interpreting workplace exposure limits. Airborne toxicants cause respiratory tract injury and/or systemic injury beyond any local effects on the airways or lungs. Either group of toxic responses can be mediated through a wide variety of mechanisms.

Victims of airborne toxicant exposure may be evaluated and treated across a professional mix of health care providers, including occupational physician or nurse specialists, primary outpatient or inpatient providers, or various subspecialists such as pulmonologists or allergists. Victims of high-intensity exposures are more likely to be managed initially by first responders (eg, paramedics, firefighters, or integrated hazmat teams) and subsequently by emergency department physicians and nurses. Other disciplines (eg, toxicology, otolaryngology, speech therapy, psychiatry, and neurology) may also become involved in the assessment and care of airborne toxicant associated illness, depending on the nature of the exposure, the acuity of the presentation, the constellation of signs and symptoms involved, and forensic or medico-legal considerations.

ROUTE OF EXPOSURE & TARGET ORGAN TOXICITY

The respiratory tract may be the toxicant's route of exposure, the toxicant's target organ for injury, or both. All of the toxicants discussed in this chapter enter the body principally, if not exclusively, through inhalation (although there are uncommon scenarios where lung injury can occur through ingestion of certain substances not covered here, such as the herbicide paraquat). In addition to being the primary route of exposure, the respiratory tract is also the target organ for many of these airborne toxicants. For example, irritant toxicants such as ammonia can cause the abrupt onset of a constellation of respiratory tract symptoms, including rhinorrhea, cough, chest tightness, wheeze, and breathlessness. In contrast, carbon monoxide is a nonirritating chemical asphyxiant that exerts its most prominent toxic effects on the central nervous and cardiovascular systems and may be acutely lethal even though causing virtually no respiratory symptoms.

DOSE-RESPONSE & TIME COURSE OF EFFECT

High-intensity exposure to toxic gases and other airborne toxicants may result in clinical findings within seconds, minutes, or hours. These scenarios represent an intensity that is at the far end of the dose-response curve, where most, if not all, exposed individuals will manifest at least some adverse effects.

Some short-term, high-intensity exposures can also cause longer-term sequelae. Examples include anoxic brain injury (eg, caused by carbon monoxide), irritant-induced asthma or reactive airways dysfunction syndrome ("RADS") (eg, caused by chlorine gas), and bronchiolitis obliterans (BO) (eg, caused by nitrogen dioxide).

Chronic health effects caused by repeated subclinical exposures to airborne toxicants are being recognized increasingly as a significant adverse health outcome. Severe bronchiolitis obliterans has been described in microwave popcorn plant workers (called "Popcorn Workers Lung" in that group) as well as in others exposed by inhalation to the chemical diacetyl, a chemical artificial butter flavorant. An earlier outbreak of severe lung disease marked by organizing pneumonia was reported among workers in Europe and North Africa indolently exposed to a textile coating agent (Ardystil). As another example, repeated *intentional* (ie, recreational) exposure to volatile solvents, nitrites, and other inhalants can cause a spectrum of chronic health effects that includes liver disease, cognitive disorders, and bone marrow toxicity.

Table 32–1. Definition of terms.

Aerosol	A dispersion of solid or liquid particles in a gaseous medium, most commonly air.
Gas	A fluid at room temperature and pressure that occupies the space of enclosure; capable of being changed into the solid or liquid phase by both an increase in pressure and a decrease in temperature.
Vapor	The gaseous phase of a substance normally in the solid or liquid state; capable of being changed to liquid or solid either by increasing pressure or decreasing temperature.
Mist	An aerosol of liquid particles that may be visible and is generated by condensation from the gaseous to liquid state or by mechanical dispersion of a liquid.
Fume	An aerosol of solid particles generated by the condensation of vaporized materials, especially molten metals, often accompanied by oxidation.
Dust	Solid particles generated by disintegration of organic or inorganic materials such as rocks and minerals, wood and grain; capable of temporary suspension in a gaseous medium such as air.
Smoke	A complex, typically visible mixture of airborne substances including particulates and gases resulting from the incomplete combustion of one or more materials.
Particulate matter	Airborne matter that varies in size and composition and which may consist of solid particles and liquid droplets (aerosols). Particulates are commonly classified by size (aerodynamic diameter in micrometers) and include coarse particles or PM10 (between 2.5 and 10 μm), fine particles or PM 2.5 (< 2.5 μm) and ultrafine particles (< 0.1 μm).

Table 32–2. Common asphyxiant gases.

Simple asphyxiants	
Acetylene	Methane
Argon	Neon
Carbon dioxide	Nitrogen
Ethane	Nitrous oxide
Ethylene	Propane
Helium	Propylene
Hydrogen	
Chemical asphyxiants	
Carbon monoxide	
Hydrogen cyanide	
Hydrogen sulfide	

▶ General Considerations

Physical asphyxiant gases displace oxygen and are toxicants insofar as they reduce the fractional inspiratory concentration of oxygen (Table 32–2). These otherwise "inert" gases contrast with toxic asphyxiants (see later) that exert their adverse effects by interfering with the delivery of oxygen to tissues or by disrupting the utilization of delivered oxygen at the cellular level.

▶ Occupational & Environmental Exposure

Simple asphyxiants are health hazards most commonly when encountered in confined spaces (eg, inside storage tanks or underground mines). Asphyxiant gases that are heavier than air also may be hazardous in low-lying semi-enclosed areas with little air movement to promote dispersion. Morbidity and death may occur if the exposure is overwhelming and rapid, insidious and occult, or if the victim is unable to flee a confined space. Although any inert gas could act as a simple asphyxiant, the substances of practical importance account for a fairly short list.

Methane gas is most commonly encountered in coal mining, where, because it is lighter than air, it may accumulate in poorly ventilated upper pockets. Methane is also released in other fossil fuel extraction settings and in the presence of organic material breakdown (including landfills). In addition to the danger from asphyxia, methane is also hazardous as an explosive gas, a characteristic shared by several other asphyxiants (eg, propane and acetylene).

Carbon dioxide is a clear and odorless gas used in food preservation. It also may be encountered in: beer and wine fermentation; settings where it is used as a refrigerant, including frozen carbon dioxide (dry ice), especially if a large amount is allowed to sublimate within an enclosed space; and mines, including off-gassing from abandoned mine sites. Carbon dioxide is also used in the leather and textile industries, water treatment, carbonated beverage manufacturing, and in purging pipes and tanks. Natural release of carbon dioxide from a volcanic lake at Lake Nyos, Cameroon, Africa, in 1986, resulted in the death of 1700 people and

SIMPLE ASPHYXIANTS: METHANE, CARBON DIOXIDE, NITROGEN, NITROUS OXIDE, ETHANE, PROPANE, ACETYLENE, NOBLE GASES

ESSENTIALS OF DIAGNOSIS

▶ Acute effects
  • Headache.
  • Nausea.
  • Confusion.
  • Loss of consciousness.
  • Coma.
  • Anoxic brain injury.
  • Cardiac arrest.
▶ Chronic effects
  • Residual anoxic injury.

3500 livestock in surrounding villages. The carbon dioxide is 1.5 times as dense as air, which allowed a dense layer of the gas to accumulate in population centers at the bottom of the hillsides surrounding Lake Nyos. This natural environmental calamity was an exception to the general rule that simple asphyxiants are only hazardous in small, confined spaces.

Nitrogen may be encountered in hazardous concentrations in a variety of work settings, including underwater work, mining, metallurgic operations, and pressurization of oil wells. In hyperbaric settings such as tunnels or in deep-sea diving occupations, nitrogen may cause narcosis, leading to behavioral changes and impaired judgment (as well as the complications of decompression; see Chapter 13).

Propane, argon, and other asphyxiant agents may be associated with exposure in high concentrations while filling tanks or when there is a leak from a tank or fuel-delivery system. NIOSH has reported nine fatalities among workers who manually gauge and sample tanks at oil and gas extraction sites. Whether the substance is heavier or lighter than air, as noted previously, may drive exposure risk in the microenvironment. Intentional exposure to bulk asphyxiant inhalants, including noble gases, can occur as a means of suicide.

► Metabolism & Mechanism of Action

By definition, the simple asphyxiants act nonspecifically by displacing oxygen from inspired air. The reduction in the fractional inspired concentration of oxygen results in hypoxia and ultimately frank anoxia. The central nervous and cardiovascular systems are the organ systems most severely affected by hypoxia.

Although carbon dioxide is considered a simple asphyxiant, at high concentrations it also acts as a potent central nervous system depressant (analogous to many solvent vapors that are not considered here as simple asphyxiants). Carbon dioxide also is a direct acute stimulant to respiration at intermediate concentrations. Tachypnea and dyspnea may be noted with carbon dioxide concentrations greater than 2–3%. Exposure to carbon dioxide in concentrations greater than 10% may be lethal within minutes.

► Clinical Findings

A. Symptoms and Signs

Responses to decreased concentrations of inspired oxygen are variable. Important predictors of clinical response include the concentration of the simple asphyxiant (ie, the magnitude of the reduction in fractional inspired concentration of oxygen), the level of physical activity (ie, metabolic activity), and the underlying health status (including the oxygen carrying capacity) of an exposed individual. The normal ambient air oxygen concentration is 21% at sea level (and not < 19.5% as noted above). Moderate oxygen deprivation (oxygen concentrations of 10–16%) may cause tachycardia, tachypnea, and exercise intolerance. As the concentration of oxygen decreases to 6–10%, the victim may experience nausea, prostration, and coma. At oxygen concentrations of less than 6%, rapid loss of consciousness and death are typical.

B. Laboratory Findings

There are no specific findings other than the reduction of blood oxygen and associated metabolic derangements (eg, lactic acidosis).

► Differential Diagnosis

A brief occupational history may quickly identify a simple asphyxiant as the likely cause of anoxic injury, especially in the context of a confined-space injury. On clinical grounds alone, it may be difficult to differentiate simple physical as opposed to toxic asphyxia (as will be discussed later). Specific laboratory findings may suggest exposure to a chemical (toxic) asphyxiant. Other causes of collapse, such as a primary cardiac or central nervous system event, may need to be excluded depending on the clinical context. Syndromes related to reduced oxygen tension due to hypobaric conditions have a different clinical presentation that is not relevant to displacement of oxygen by simple asphyxiants, although both may occur simultaneously, most notably under conditions of mining at high altitude.

► Prevention

Confined-space work should have engineering controls to ensure an adequate air supply. It is important to confirm that the air supply intake does not itself entrain other toxins (eg, carbon monoxide from a compressor). Confined-space injury often occurs in the setting of inadequate safety training, equipment, and procedures (eg, a buddy system).

► Treatment

Immediate removal from the exposure can be lifesaving; however, rescuers themselves often are in equal danger without an adequate air supply. Postexposure treatment is supportive and nonspecific, but should include the administration of supplemental oxygen.

► Prognosis

Although anoxic brain injury can occur, many survivors of simple asphyxiant gas inhalation make a complete and rapid recovery.

▼ TOXIC ASPHYXIANTS

CARBON MONOXIDE

ESSENTIALS OF DIAGNOSIS

► Acute and subacute effects
- Headache.
- Nausea.
- Confusion.

- Cardiac ischemia.
- Coma.
- Anoxic brain injury.
▶ Chronic effects
- Residual anoxic injury.

▶ General Considerations

Carbon monoxide intoxication is the leading cause of death by gas inhalation. Most fatalities are a result of environmental rather than occupational exposures. In addition to unintentional exposures, carbon monoxide inhalation remains a common method of intentional self-poisoning.

▶ Occupational & Environmental Exposure

Carbon monoxide is a by-product of the incomplete combustion of carbon-based fuels. Significant exposure can occur wherever there is any kind of incomplete combustion of such fuels and inadequate ventilation. The incomplete combustion of biomass fuel, gasoline, kerosene, and propane all result in the generation of carbon monoxide. The internal combustion engine is an important occupational and environmental source of carbon monoxide. Nonelectric forklifts and other vehicles and gas-powered compressors and generators, especially when used indoors, also represent important exposure sources. Carbon monoxide exposures are relevant among firefighters, petroleum refinery workers, indoor garage attendants, mine workers, forklift operators, and furnace operators. Home heating unit malfunction or misuse, structural fires, automobile exhaust, gas-powered recreation equipment, and cigarette smoke are the most common sources of significant nonoccupational environmental carbon monoxide exposure. Exposure also can occur after exposure to methylene chloride because metabolism of this solvent releases carbon monoxide. Massive hemolysis, which can be caused by selected toxins (see discussion on arsine gas) also can be associated with the generation of carboxyhemoglobin (COHb) through metabolism.

▶ Metabolism & Mechanism of Action

Carbon monoxide acts by avidly binding to hemoglobin to form COHb. This has two important effects. First, carbon monoxide competes with oxygen for binding sites on hemoglobin, thereby reducing the oxygen-carrying capacity of the blood. Second, the COHb unit interferes with heme-heme interactions such that the oxygen-hemoglobin dissociation curve is shifted to the left, resulting in decreased release of oxygen from hemoglobin carrier sites to the tissues where the oxygen is required. Carbon monoxide also may bind to other heme-containing moieties besides hemoglobin and also may affect the mitochondrial cytochrome oxidase system, thus compromising cellular respiration.

▶ Clinical Findings

A. Symptoms and Signs

Acute carbon monoxide toxicity may be nonspecific or, with higher intensity exposures, the neurological or cardiovascular effects may be obvious. The brain and heart are the organs most vulnerable to hypoxia, as noted previously. At high exposures, rapid loss of consciousness, coma, and death occur as with other asphyxiants. In subacute carbon monoxide exposure, symptoms are less marked and can be quite nonspecific, including headache, malaise, nausea, and vomiting. Cardiac ischemia may result from carbon monoxide exposure, particularly in individuals with underlying coronary artery disease. Chronic lower-level exposure to carbon monoxide has been associated with an increase in the incidence of dysrhythmias and, epidemiologically, with the development of atherosclerosis.

B. Laboratory Findings

Elevated COHb is confirmed through co-oximeter blood gas (venous or arterial) analysis. Some newer pulse oximetry devices also estimate COHb. Routine pulse oximetry inaccurately misreads this form of hemoglobin as oxygenated, underestimating impairment. A routine blood gas analysis (not done by co-oximetry) reports a calculated rather than measured oxygen saturation that will be falsely preserved in the setting of carbon monoxide intoxication. COHb is increased in active cigarette smoking but should not exceed 10% on this account and usually is less than that (typically 4–7% in a two-pack-per-day cigarette smoker). COHb levels above 30% are associated with moderate to severe symptoms including headache, nausea, vomiting, impaired manual dexterity, and impaired judgment. Levels of 50% can result in seizure, coma, and death. There is a great deal of symptomatic heterogeneity, however, in relation to the absolute COHb level associated with specific findings. In pregnancy, a higher fetal level may be reached than that reflected by the maternal COHb level. Electrocardiographic and biochemical monitoring (eg, serial troponin assays) can be useful because myocardial infarction can occur in carbon monoxide intoxication, even in the absence of typical chest pain symptoms.

▶ Differential Diagnosis

With severe exposure, the differential diagnosis is that of any anoxic injury. For fire victims, it is often difficult to rule out concomitant cyanide intoxication. The differential diagnosis of subacute carbon monoxide intoxication leading to nonspecific symptoms is quite wide and it is likely that many cases go undiagnosed. A high index of suspicion is needed, particularly in winter months when space-heater malfunction is common. Group exposures can be misdiagnosed as food poisoning, for example.

▶ Prevention

Carbon monoxide is odorless and has no warning properties. Internal combustion engines should not be used in indoor environments or near the intake of air supplies. Heating units should be well maintained to ensure proper venting and to avoid partial combustion. Household carbon monoxide alarms now are employed widely. Properly used, these may serve to reduce home heating mishaps. Misuse of gas-powered generators in the face of natural disasters is another source of outbreaks that warrant vigilance in the context of public health protection.

▶ **Treatment**

Immediate removal from exposure together with supplemental oxygen (100% by nonrebreathing face mask or, in the comatose patient, by endotracheal tube) are the mainstays of initial treatment for carbon monoxide intoxication. On 100% oxygen, the half-life of COHb is reduced to approximately 60–90 minutes from 5 to 6 hours on room air alone. The role of hyperbaric treatment remains controversial in low-level poisoning. It can be clearly indicated in high-level intoxication, presuming that technical access to a hyperbaric chamber is logistically feasible, especially if the chamber allows health care personnel to be in contact with the patient (ie, a multiplace device). In one controlled study, such treatment was found to reduce the risk of selected long-term cognitive deficits following acute carbon monoxide poisoning.

▶ **Prognosis**

Anoxic brain injury can occur after severe carbon monoxide exposure (ie, intoxication to the point of loss of consciousness). Injury can be nonfocal and subtle, including neurobehavioral abnormalities. Parkinsonian deficits have been documented as a sequela of severe carbon monoxide poisoning.

HYDROGEN CYANIDE

ESSENTIALS OF DIAGNOSIS

▶ Acute and subacute effects
  • Dyspnea.
  • Headache.
  • Gastrointestinal distress.
  • Dizziness.
  • Loss of consciousness.
  • Anoxic brain injury.
▶ Chronic effects
  • Residual anoxic injury.

▶ **General Considerations**

Hydrogen cyanide is a colorless gas under standard atmospheric conditions. It can be encountered in a wide array of

industrial applications. In addition to gas inhalation, exposures occur through ingestion and skin absorption of cyanide salts in solution (eg, potassium cyanide) or ingestion of such liquids. The classic "bitter almond" odor of cyanide cannot be appreciated by a substantial proportion of the population, apparently on a genetic basis. Because of its potency and rapidity of action, cyanide has long been important to forensic as well as occupational toxicology.

▶ **Occupational & Environmental Exposure**

The major current industrial uses of cyanide are in metal plating operations and in the extraction of silver and gold salts from ores. This can be an environmental contamination problem as well as occupational exposure scenario. Hydrogen cyanide is also used as an insecticide and rodenticide and in the manufacturing of adiponitrile (for nylon). As with carbon monoxide, cyanide release is a potential hazard in structural fires, primarily as a thermolysis by-product of both natural and synthetic polymers. Toxicity also can occur after exposure to acrylonitrile (see Chapter 31) because metabolism of this solvent releases hydrogen cyanide. Cyanogenic glycosides are an environmental dietary exposure source in much of the developing world, principally from cassava.

▶ **Metabolism & Mechanism of Action**

Cyanide is quickly absorbed through inhalation and skin exposures. Cyanide exerts its toxicity by binding to ferrous (F^{++}) iron in cytochrome oxidase in the mitochondrial respiratory chain, blocking oxygen utilization. As aerobic metabolism is compromised, anaerobic metabolism ensues, resulting in lactic acidosis.

▶ **Clinical Findings**

A. Symptoms and Signs

Low-level exposure leads to dyspnea, dizziness, headache, confusion, and gastrointestinal distress. Higher exposures cause rapid loss of consciousness, cardiovascular collapse, seizures, and death.

B. Laboratory Findings

Tests of blood cyanide levels are used in forensic examinations but generally are not available in a timely enough fashion to guide acute medical management. Thiocyanate levels, reflecting cyanide metabolism, do not accurately reflect the intensity of cyanide intoxication and should not be used as a proxy.

▶ **Differential Diagnosis**

The differential diagnosis includes other asphyxiants, especially hydrogen sulfide and, in fire victims, carbon monoxide. Cyanide exposure should be suspected when collapse is very sudden after inhalation, skin contact with contaminated liquids, or ingestion. Profound lactic acidosis raises the suspicion of cyanide intoxication in the appropriate clinical setting.

Prevention

Cyanide gas is released from cyanide salt solutions if the pH falls, such as will occur, for example, from inadvertent mixing of solutions with an acid. As noted, absorption following skin contact with salt solutions also leads to the same toxicity as inhaling cyanide gas.

Treatment

The most widely promoted treatment for cyanide intoxication in the United States had long been the induction of methemoglobin with nitrites (purportedly to compete for cyanide binding, sparing the cytochrome oxidase) and the administration of thiosulfate to promote detoxification of cyanide to thiocyanate. More recently an alternative treatment using hydroxycobalamin has become available. Hydroxycobalamin binds to cyanide, forming Vitamin B_{12}. Because of its challenges, the medical management of cyanide toxicity typically involves consultation with a Poison Control Center.

Prognosis

As with other asphyxiants, anoxic brain injury can occur in survivors of severe acute exposure.

HYDROGEN SULFIDE

ESSENTIALS OF DIAGNOSIS

- Acute effects
  - Mucous membrane and respiratory tract irritation.
  - Loss of consciousness.
  - Anoxic brain injury.
- Chronic effects
  - Residual anoxic injury.

General Considerations

Hydrogen sulfide is a naturally occurring toxicant generated from the breakdown of organic materials. For this reason, it is also sometimes called "sewer gas." It is associated with a pungent odor of rotten eggs and is detectable by smell in concentrations as low as 0.02 ppm, although this warning property may be lost through olfactory fatigue.

Occupational & Environmental Exposure

Geothermal and fossil-fuel energy extraction are the two major occupational sources of industrial hydrogen sulfide exposure, but other occupational risk groups include

farmers (manure processing), sewage workers, fish processors, and roofers or surfacers who work with heated tar and asphalt. Hydrogen sulfide is a particular hazard in confined spaces such as fishing-ship holds, manure pits, and sewers. It is heavier than air and therefore accumulates in low-lying areas.

Metabolism & Mechanism of Action

Like cyanide, hydrogen sulfide exerts its toxicity by blocking oxygen utilization through the cytochrome oxidase pathway. Hydrogen sulfide also has irritant properties and can cause mucous membrane and respiratory tract irritation.

Clinical Findings

A. Symptoms and Signs

High exposure leads to rapid loss of consciousness and death. Intermediate exposures may lead to pulmonary edema and acute lung injury. At lower levels, irritant effects may predominate, including airway irritation and burning eyes. Other findings may include headache, dizziness, nausea, and vomiting.

B. Laboratory Findings

Blood sulfide level measurements generally are not available in clinical laboratories. Industrial hygiene area sampling (eg, with quick-reading sampling tubes) may indicate that exposure has occurred.

Differential Diagnosis

The differential diagnosis includes other asphyxiants, the most important of which is cyanide. Signs or symptoms of mucous membrane or respiratory tract irritation would support the diagnosis because the other toxic asphyxiants are not potent irritants.

Prevention

Confined-space precautions are particularly relevant to the prevention of hydrogen sulfide injury. The odor warning properties of hydrogen sulfide are not reliable as a protective factor.

Treatment

As with cyanide, the specific management of an acutely ill hydrogen sulfide-exposed individual should utilize Poison Control Center consultation.

Prognosis

Anoxic brain injury may result from severe intoxication. In addition, the sequelae of acute irritant inhalant injury represent a potential adverse outcome (see "Irritant Inhalants" below).

IRRITANT AIRBORNE TOXICANTS

ESSENTIALS OF DIAGNOSIS

▶ Acute effects
- Mucous membrane irritation.
- Cough.
- Stridor.
- Dyspnea.
- Noncardiogenic pulmonary edema.

▶ Chronic effects
- Irritant-induced asthma (reactive airways dysfunction syndrome).
- Bronchiolitis obliterans.
- Bronchiectasis.
- Chronic respiratory insufficiency.

▶ General Considerations

Irritant airborne toxicants are a heterogeneous group of substances linked by common target-organ effects. The majority of these compounds (but importantly, not all) are moderately to highly *water soluble* and cause the abrupt onset of irritation of all mucous membranes with which they come in contact, including the eyes, nose, mouth, and throat. Exposure to water-soluble irritants, such as chlorine, ammonia, sulfur dioxide, and the acid aerosols leads to tearing, rhinorrhea, and burning of the mouth and throat. Higher-dose exposures that may occur in confined-space mishaps (which can include bathroom cleaning hypochlorite misadventure) or in large ambient releases can lead to lower respiratory tract injury as well. Water-*insoluble* irritants do not produce marked mucous membrane symptomatology but nonetheless do cause lower respiratory tract injury, including noncardiogenic pulmonary edema and BO (an obstructive airways disease characterized by scarring of the small airways). The most important of these water-insoluble toxicants are: nitrogen dioxide which is the toxicant linked to BO), phosgene, and ozone.

▶ Occupational & Environmental Exposure

A. Water-Soluble Airborne Toxicants

Chlorine gas (which is of intermediate solubility) exposures occur through industrial leaks, especially in textile and pulp bleaching (where a related and even more potent irritant, chlorine dioxide, is also common) and in the production of plastics and resins. Other releases occur primarily in transportation accidents, water-purification mishaps, swimming pool disinfectant accidents, and household cleaning product misadventures (when chlorine is released from hypochlorite up-mixing with an acid; chloramine is a related irritant released from ammonia and hypochlorite combinations). Chlorine gas was used as a chemical weapon in World War I and, more recently, in Syria.

Acid aerosol exposure is widespread in a variety of industrial processes. Important compounds include hydrochloric, sulfuric, chromic, and hydrofluoric acids. The anhydrous acid analogues (eg, hydrogen chloride) quickly form acid aerosols in normal atmospheric conditions where humidity is present.

Ammonia exposures result from refrigeration gas leaks, in the manufacture of plastics, and in petroleum refining. High-level exposures also occur when anhydrous ammonia is handled in fertilizer applications.

Other important but less widely encountered water-soluble irritant gases include: diborane (microelectronics manufacture), bromine (chemical synthesis, including flame retardants and in water treatment, including in home spas), and methyl isocyanate (pesticide manufacture; a related irritant, methyl isothiocyanate, is a breakdown product of the pesticide fumigant metam sodium). Formaldehyde, a gas in pure form that also vaporizes easily from solutions (formalin) or off-gasses as residual monomer from polymers (urea-formaldehyde resins), is an irritant that may be encountered in plastics, textiles, and paper industries, as well as in smoke and photochemical smog. Acrolein, structurally related to formaldehyde but a more potent irritant, is one of the most important combustion by-product irritants in fire smoke.

B. Water-Insoluble Airborne Toxicants

Nitrogen dioxide inhalation occurs through exposure to gas-shielded electric arc welding, combustion engine exhaust, the manufacture and use of explosives, in the manufacture of fertilizers and dyes, in reactions of nitric acid with various materials, and in silage decomposition (the cause of "silo filler's disease").

Phosgene, like chlorine, was important historically as a chemical weapon in World War I. It is still encountered when certain volatile chlorinated hydrocarbons are exposed to heat or ultraviolet light, as in arc welding on or near solvent contaminated (eg, degreased) metals. Phosgene is also used in the production of certain pesticides and in other chemical processes.

Ozone is becoming increasingly important as an alternative to chlorine in pulp paper bleaching and water disinfection. Ozone exposure in the paper industry in Sweden has been shown to be a risk factor for asthma.

▶ Metabolism & Mechanism of Action

The irritants cause tissue injury through heterogeneous mechanisms that may include free-radical or oxidant pathways. In general, these are not substances that require metabolic activation (eg, mixed function oxidase modification) in order to exert their toxic effect.

Clinical Findings

A. Symptoms and Signs

Low to moderate exposure to *water-soluble airborne toxicants* causes mucous membrane irritation marked by lacrimation, rhinorrhea, and burning of the mouth and face. These toxicants have good warning properties, prompting the victim to flee if possible. Higher exposure is associated with hoarseness, cough, and respiratory irritation and also can lead to laryngospasm and tracheal and lower respiratory tract injury. Lower respiratory tract injury may range from mild pulmonary edema to severe injury that manifests clinically as acute respiratory distress syndrome (ARDS). Lower respiratory tract injury becomes evident in the hours immediately following exposure.

The *water-insoluble airborne toxicants* typically spare the mucous membranes and upper respiratory tract. These toxicants have poor warning properties, permitting significant exposure to occur before symptoms are manifest. In contrast with the immediate onset of symptoms following exposure to water-soluble toxicants, symptoms may be delayed for hours following inhalation of water-insoluble toxicants.

B. Laboratory Findings

After significant symptomatic exposure, laboratory evaluation should include assessment of oxygenation, plain chest radiography or other imaging (eg, CT scanning), and pulmonary function testing.

Differential Diagnosis

The exposure history usually is sufficient to identify irritant inhalation as the cause of respiratory compromise. Nitrogen dioxide or phosgene exposure, however, sometimes may present as an occult cause of ARDS, for which pneumonia and sepsis typically would be the leading alternative etiology. Lower respiratory tract injury without antecedent mucous membrane irritant symptoms is *inconsistent* with exposure to a water-soluble irritant such as ammonia or chlorine.

Prevention

Precautions in the storage and transport of irritant gases are critical to prevention. Household cleaning product misadventures can be prevented by avoiding hypochlorite mixing with other products, especially acid- or ammonia-containing cleaners. Nitrogen dioxide injury in agriculture can be prevented by proper silo ventilation. Precautions against nitrogen dioxide overexposure also are important during continuous-feed (high-volume) gas-shielded welding operations (eg, tungsten inert gas [TIG] welding), especially in confined or poorly ventilated spaces.

Treatment

The treatment of irritant injury is supportive and nonspecific and includes supplemental oxygen and bronchodilator therapy. Although corticosteroids are used frequently in the treatment of irritant injury in clinical practice, this has not been supported by controlled clinical trial data. There is no proven role for prophylactic antibiotic use following such exposures.

Prognosis

In severe exposures leading to ARDS, mortality can be high, but injury of lesser severity resolves without sequelae in most cases. However, irritant-induced asthma (including reactive airways dysfunction syndrome) or, more rarely, BO or bronchiectasis may result from acute irritant inhalation.

SMOKE & OTHER COMBUSTION BY-PRODUCTS

ESSENTIALS OF DIAGNOSIS

- Acute effects
  - Mucous membrane irritation and cough.
  - Stridor and dyspnea.
  - Noncardiogenic pulmonary edema.
  - Loss of consciousness.

General Considerations

Combustion smoke is a complex mixture of gases and particulates (Table 32–3). The components of smoke depend on the material consumed, the temperature of combustion, and the amount of oxygen present. The principal relevant components of smoke include carbon monoxide, hydrogen cyanide, irritant gases, and aerosols as discussed earlier (particularly hydrogen chloride, formaldehyde, nitric oxide, and acrolein), and carbonaceous particulates (ie, soot). The by-products of internal combustion engines are similarly complex and include many of the same key constituents that can vary by engine type and other environmental factors, in particular the oxygen enrichment of the process. Diesel engine exhaust is particularly noteworthy for the fine particulate that it can produce and the relationship this may have to diesel-associated adverse health effects. Incense is made of wood and other plant matter and is impregnated with fragrances and is a source of aromatic chemical aerosols mixed with particulates. Secondhand cigarette smoke is another important source of combustion by-products.

Occupational & Environmental Exposure

Firefighters (urban and wildland) are the largest salaried occupational risk group for smoke inhalation. Home cooking and heating with biomass materials are ubiquitous sources of unsalaried occupational/environmental smoke exposure in the developing world. Residential wood fireplaces are also used widely in industrialized nations for heating and

Table 32–3. Common components of smoke from structural fires.

Substance	Exposure Limits (ppm, except where noted)	
	OSHA PEL	NIOSH REL
Carbon monoxide	TWA 50	TWA 35; C 200
Acrolein	TWA 0.1	TWA 0.1, STEL 0.3
Formaldehyde	TWA 0.75; STEL 2	TWA 0.016; C 0.1 (15 min)
Hydrogen chloride	C 5	C 5
Hydrogen cyanide	TWA 10	STEL 4.7
Nitric oxide	TWA 25	TWA 25
Nitrogen dioxide	C 5	STEL 1
Particulates (total; respirable)	TWA 15 mg/m^3 (total) TWA 5 mg/m^3 (respirable range)	Not specified

C, ceiling; min, minute exposure; PEL, permissible exposure limit; ppm, parts per million; REL, recommended exposure limit; STEL, short-term exposure limit; TWA, time-weighted average.

ambiance. Diesel exhaust sources include mobile sources (eg, motor vehicles), stationary area sources (eg, oil- and gas-production facilities, stationary engines, and shipyards), and stationary point sources (eg, chemical-manufacturing facilities and electric utilities). Incense is used worldwide for ceremonial purposes. It represents a source of intentional smoke exposure and is used commonly in confined indoor spaces.

▶ **Metabolism & Mechanism of Action**

Smoke can exert its toxicity through asphyxia (see "Carbon Monoxide" and "Cyanide" discussed earlier) or irritant effects. In addition, combustion-related oxidants can cause methemoglobinemia. Direct thermal injury typically is not a major sequela of smoke inhalation, in contrast with steam inhalation or flame inhalation in street performers (so called "fire-eaters lung"), where this can be an important cause of respiratory tract injury. The combustion products of biomass fuels such as wood, charcoal, and animal dung contribute to the development of chronic obstructive pulmonary disease, while preexisting asthma and COPD may be exacerbated in indoor environments where biomass fuel smoke is encountered in high concentrations. The precise mechanisms of action, however, are not well delineated.

▶ **Clinical Findings**

A. Symptoms and Signs

Clinical findings in smoke inhalation injury can include features of both asphyxiant and irritant injury. Carbonaceous

sputum and evidence of smoke tainted nares (as well as singed hair) represent findings specific to smoke inhalation.

B. Laboratory Findings

Blood co-oximetry should establish the COHb level and document oxygenation status. After significant symptomatic exposure, laboratory evaluation also should include pulmonary function testing and chest radiography. Profound lactic acidosis may suggest concomitant cyanide exposure.

▶ **Differential Diagnosis**

The differential diagnostic questions following smoke exposure often center on identifying the potential toxicants of greatest concern, especially following chemical fires. Very acrid smoke suggests the presence of hydrochloric acid or other acid aerosols. These are frequently released when polyvinyl chloride and other halogenated polymers are burned. Other synthetic or natural polymers ranging from polyurethanes to wool can be sources of hydrogen cyanide release through combustion.

▶ **Prevention**

Appropriate use of a self-contained breathing apparatus is the principal preventive measure used for firefighters combating structural fires, including during clean-up. The use of a breathing apparatus appears to be effective in preventing the development of pulmonary symptoms and in reducing both the deterioration in forced expiratory volume in one second (FEV$_1$) and the increase in airway responsiveness caused by smoke inhalation. Limiting exercise in the afternoon on days with poor ambient air quality is one way to limit exposure to ambient-air pollution from combustion releases (eg, wildland fires).

▶ **Treatment**

The treatment of smoke inhalation includes supplemental oxygen, empirical bronchodilator therapy, and supportive care. As with other irritant exposures, corticosteroids sometimes are used but this is supported by controlled clinical studies. Tracheal intubation and mechanical ventilation may be necessary.

▶ **Prognosis**

Temporary deterioration in pulmonary function and increases in nonspecific airway reactivity have been well documented in persons exposed to smoke, including firefighters and bystanders. In many states, firefighters can receive workers' compensation on a presumptive basis for lung cancer because of chronic fire smoke exposure. Community environmental exposures following conflagrations can lead to widespread concern over possible chronic effects. Acute respiratory symptoms, including aggravation of preexisting asthma and chronic obstructive pulmonary disease, can be anticipated. Long-term sequelae in the absence of clear-cut acute effects, however, would not be anticipated. High-intensity exposure to toxic combustion products can result in chronic respiratory health effects in previously healthy individuals including most commonly irritant-induced asthma. Other respiratory complications could be potentially relevant to those who survive hospitalization requiring intensive care for inhalation injury.

▼ OTHER AIRBORNE RESPIRATORY TOXICANTS

ARSINE

ESSENTIALS OF DIAGNOSIS

▶ Acute effects
  • Malaise and weakness.
  • Gastrointestinal distress and dyspnea.
  • Hemolysis.
  • Hemoglobinuria and hematuria.
▶ Chronic effects
  • Renal damage.

▶ General Considerations

Acute hemolytic anemia is the most consistent clinical finding. Other findings may include multi-organ-system dysfunction. Arsine gas is colorless, nonirritating, and in high concentrations has a mild garlic odor.

▶ Occupational & Environmental Exposure

Arsine gas can be produced *de novo* in metal refining and other metal-working processes when arsenic reacts with an acid in the appropriate environment. Preformed arsine gas, often stored under pressure in large quantities, has been used widely as a dopant in the microelectronics industry. In addition to a potential occupational hazard, this also presents an environmental risk to surrounding communities. Certain fungi can generate arsine in sewage.

▶ Metabolism & Mechanism of Action

Arsine is toxic to red blood cells, leading to hemolysis. Damage to other tissues may result from secondary damage from hemolysis (eg, kidney deposition of hemoglobin) or from direct toxic effects. Heme metabolism, as noted previously, can be a source of CO leading to elevated COHb levels.

▶ Clinical Findings

A. Symptoms and Signs

The signs and symptoms of arsine toxicity reflect both hemolysis with its sequelae and other systemic toxic manifestations. A triad of abdominal pain, hematuria, and jaundice is characteristic. Clinical findings also may include malaise,

headache, renal failure, cerebral edema, intracerebral hemorrhage, dyspnea, cardiovascular collapse, and death.

B. Laboratory Findings

The laboratory findings are those of intravascular hemolysis. Hemolysis may continue up to 4 days after removal from exposure. The blood arsenic level may be elevated, although this is unlikely to be available rapidly enough to aid in early diagnosis. The free hemoglobin level may help to guide management; exchange transfusion has been advocated for free hemoglobin levels greater than 1.2–1.5 g/dL.

▶ Differential Diagnosis

The principal differential diagnosis includes hemolysis as a consequence of other causes. Although chemical oxidant exposures also can cause hemolysis, this would occur in the context of significant methemoglobinemia, which is not present in arsine poisoning. Stibine (antimony hydride) exposure also can cause massive hemolysis, although it is rarely encountered industrially or environmentally.

▶ Prevention

Meticulous control measures and backup procedures should be in place whenever arsine gas is used. This should include hazardous materials (HAZMAT) incident planning relevant to community protection.

▶ Treatment

There is no specific antidote for arsine poisoning. Treatment consists of measures to support vascular, renal, hematologic, and respiratory function. Treatment of massive arsine-caused hemolysis has required exchange transfusion. Alkalinization may reduce hemoglobin precipitation in the kidneys. Interim dialysis may be required if renal failure develops. As with severe carbon monoxide and cyanide, Poison Control Center consultation should be sought in the management of clinically significant arsine exposure.

▶ Prognosis

Severe arsine exposure is life-threatening. If adequate acute supportive care and transfusion are available, fatalities may be avoidable.

PHOSPHINE

ESSENTIALS OF DIAGNOSIS

▶ Acute effects
  • Respiratory distress.
  • Headache and dizziness.
  • Gastrointestinal distress.
  • Coma.

General Considerations

Phosphine is a systemic toxicant of high potency. It is colorless and has a strong odor that is described either as "fishy" or "garlicky."

Occupational & Environmental Exposure

Like arsine, phosphine gas is used in the microelectronics industry. Phosphine is also generated from the hydrolysis of aluminum phosphide and zinc phosphide (which occurs spontaneously from contact with air moisture or when ingested), both of which are employed as rodenticides and insecticides, especially in agricultural settings (including grain fumigation), but also in home pest eradication. Phosphine gas exposure has also been reported in the setting of illegal methamphetamine synthesis. Airborne phosphine exposure among veterinary personnel can occur when treating pet animals that have ingested phosphine-containing rodenticide.

Metabolism & Mechanism of Action

When phosphine is inhaled, it can react with moisture to form phosphoric acid, which is an irritant. The systemic toxic mechanisms of phosphine are incompletely understood. A number of end organs are adversely affected, including the central nervous, cardiac, respiratory, hepatic, and renal systems.

Clinical Findings

A. Symptoms and Signs

Multi-organ-system dysfunction can be anticipated following phosphine exposure, with pulmonary, cardiovascular, and central nervous system morbidity most prominent. With lower-level exposure, pulmonary toxicity may be the primary manifestation, marked by dyspnea, cough, chest pain, and delayed-onset pulmonary edema in the hours following exposure.

B. Laboratory Findings

There are no specific laboratory findings in phosphine poisoning. Phosphorus levels are not followed in routine practice in the management of phosphine intoxication.

Differential Diagnosis

Without a history of exposure, it may be difficult to identify phosphine as the cause of the acute multisystem injury this toxicant can induce. Exposure to silos or railroad cars that may have been fumigated should raise the index of suspicion for phosphine exposure.

Prevention

Adequate post-use ventilation and other appropriate reentry restrictions should prevent overexposure in agricultural settings. In industry, strict engineering controls must be enforced. Veterinary and medical personnel should take precautions when handling poisoned animals or humans if phosphine-containing pesticide ingestion exposure is within the differential diagnosis.

Treatment

There is no specific treatment for phosphine toxicity other than general supportive care. The potential for delayed onset of pulmonary edema should be recognized. Hemodialysis is recommended only if renal failure develops. The effectiveness of exchange transfusions is questionable. The value of steroids for phosphine-exposed patients who develop acute pulmonary edema has not been established.

Prognosis

Potential sequelae related to acute lung injury are a possible problem. There are no data on other chronic effects of phosphine poisoning.

METHYL BROMIDE

ESSENTIALS OF DIAGNOSIS

▶ Acute effects
  • Dyspnea and respiratory distress.
  • Seizures.
  • Coma.
▶ Chronic effects
  • Genotoxicity.

General Considerations

Methyl bromide is a fumigant that has been used widely in agriculture. Its use has become increasingly restricted, however, because of its ozone depleting properties (rather than its well-established human toxicity). In the past, it has been used frequently in structural pest control in the urban environment as well. Methyl bromide, which is heavier than air, is a gas at room temperature but does condense at colder temperatures (< 3.3°C [38°F]).

Occupational & Environmental Exposure

Pesticide applicators have been the principal occupational risk group. Inadvertent environmental exposure occurs following misapplication or inappropriate reentry to areas treated with methyl bromide. Methyl bromide dissipates rapidly to the atmosphere, so it is most dangerous at or near the fumigation site or at a distance if inadvertently carried through enclosed connections such as piping.

Metabolism & Mechanism of Action

Methyl bromide has multiple toxic actions, including alkylation and enzyme inhibition. It has two principal target-organ effects in humans: acute lung injury and central nervous system toxicity.

► Clinical Findings

A. Symptoms and Signs

Dyspnea and pulmonary edema may coincide with neurologic compromise marked by visual disturbance, tremor, altered mental status, and seizure. In severe cases, status epilepticus ensues.

B. Laboratory Findings

Serum bromide may be elevated, but the actual level correlates poorly with symptoms. In some assays, the serum chloride may be falsely elevated because of bromine.

► Differential Diagnosis

The exposure history is critical. The combination of neurotoxicity and pulmonary injury represents an unusual constellation of symptoms that should suggest methyl bromide inhalation. Bromine airborne exposure, as opposed to methyl bromide (which can occur in the context of chemical industrial production, experimental laboratory applications, or water disinfection as an alternative to chlorine, especially in home spas) can also cause acute lung injury as well as chemical skin burns, but does not have prominent neurologic effects.

► Prevention

Methyl bromide has few warning properties. For this reason, chloropicrin, which is a mucous membrane irritant even at low concentrations, frequently is added to the fumigant. The phasing out of methyl bromide use is the definitive prevention measure. Methyl iodide, an even more toxic chemical fumigant that is not an ozone depleting agent, has been promoted as one potential substitute but is not currently licensed in the United States.

► Treatment

Treatment is nonspecific. Control of status epilepticus is usually the primary focus of care. Dimercaprol and acetylcysteine have been suggested as antidotes based on the postulated mechanism of methyl bromide toxicity. However, no adequate studies have tested the efficacy of these therapies. Accordingly, they cannot be recommended for routine use.

► Prognosis

Neurologic compromise that resolves very slowly or that may be persistent has been well documented following methyl bromide intoxication.

MILITARY & CROWD-CONTROL AGENTS & SELECTED AIRBORNE TOXICANTS WITH TERRORISM USE POTENTIAL

ESSENTIALS OF DIAGNOSIS

► Acute effects of irritant agents used in crowd-control
  • Lacrimation.
    • Mucous membrane irritation.
  • Dyspnea.
► Acute effects of selected incapacitants
  • Opioids, benzodiazepines, general anesthetics.
    • Stupor.
  • Sedation.
  • Respiratory depression.
  • Anticholinergics.
    • Altered consciousness.
  • Seizures.
  • Dry mouth.
  • Constipation.

► General Considerations

Tear gases are actually well-dispersed aerosols, not actual gases. Another military agent, the "smoke bomb," releases zinc chloride aerosol. In October 2002, the Russian military used an incapacitating agent or mixture of incapacitating agents prior to a siege of a theater in Moscow where Chechen terrorists held 800 hostages. Carfentanil, a derivative of the opioid fentanyl, and halothane, a general anesthetic gas, are believed to have been the incapacitants used in that operation. 3-Quinuclidinyl benzylate (BZ) is an anticholinergic agent that has been weaponized and has a spectrum of effects including paranoid hallucinations and other responses typical for anticholinergic toxicity (see Chapter 39).

► Occupational & Environmental Exposure

Occupationally, both military and police personnel can be exposed through accidental releases, in training exercises, and in the field. In the latter context, "environmental" exposure may be widespread.

► Clinical Findings
A. Symptoms and Signs

The tear gases, principally chloroacetophenone (CN, Mace) and *ortho*-chlorobenzylidenemalononitrile (CS), are designed to be lacrimators and mucous membrane irritants. Rarely, with severe exposure, lower respiratory injury also can occur. Capsaicin "pepper" spray is a lacrimator used for personal protection and self-defense and as a riot control agent. Pepper spray causes severe irritation to the eyes, including temporary blindness. It also has respiratory tract irritant effects and may produce cough and dyspnea. Depending on the exposure, temporary blindness may last from 15 to 30 minutes, a burning sensation of the skin may last up to 1 hour, and intense coughing with dyspnea may persist for 3–15 minutes. Zinc chloride, the principal component of smoke bombs, is a severe respiratory irritant that can cause lung injury and ARDS. Non-irritant incapacitants cause a spectrum of effects, of which the most important is alterations in mental status.

B. Laboratory Findings

There are no specific laboratory findings.

▶ Differential Diagnosis

The lacrimators (eg, CS and CN) would be anticipated to have similar effects. Involvement of other organs or systemic toxicity suggests other chemical exposures. Capsaicin can trigger severe laryngospasm and, especially in persons with asthma, life threatening bronchoconstriction. Other chemical warfare agents, especially the modern "nerve gases," cause an entirely different presentation, with systemic illness marked by severe cholinesterase inhibition. The effects of cholinesterase inhibitors are addressed elsewhere in the agricultural chemical context. Severe respiratory distress following smoke in a military exercise or other "planned" release should suggest zinc chloride toxicity. This from of zinc inhalation exposure should not be confused with zinc oxide-caused fume fever. Another warfare agent, sulfur mustard, although commonly referred to as "mustard gas," is a vesicant aerosol that leads to skin blistering and bone marrow depression in addition to respiratory injury. Opioid incapacitants may induce respiratory failure, whereas anticholinergic incapacitants may cause systemic symptoms that include altered mental status, hypertension, dry mouth, constipation, and seizures.

▶ Prevention

Confined-space exposures to any of these agents can be associated with adverse outcomes and should be avoided.

▶ Treatment

There are no specific treatments for irritant gases or other lacrimators. After removal from exposure, treatment is supportive. Physostigmine may be used as an antidote for the anticholinergic incapacitants. Flumazenil and naloxone are antidotes for benzodiazepines and opioids, respectively. In any serious illness suspected to be associated with the agents above consultation with a Poison Control Center is warranted for treatment guidance and as a public health notification step.

▶ Prognosis

There are .no commonly observed chronic residual health effects of the lacrimators, although case reports of irritant-induced asthma have been reported. Smoke bomb inhalation may lead to the sequelae of acute lung injury. Many of the chemical warfare agents are extremely and rapidly lethal.

INHALANT ABUSE ("RECREATIONAL" INHALANTS)

ESSENTIALS OF DIAGNOSIS

▶ Acute effects
- Alcohol intoxication-like effects.
- Excitation.
- Euphoria.
- Drowsiness.
- Light-headedness.
- Agitation.
- Slurred speech.
- Unconsciousness.

▶ Chronic effects
- Weight loss.
- Inattentiveness.
- Depression.
- Impaired cognition.
- Motor abnormalities.
- Liver toxicity.

▶ General Consideration

Common household products that contain volatile solvents, propellants, gases, nitrites, and aerosols are widely abused to induce psychoactive effects. Products include glues, nail polish remover, lighter fluids, spray paints, deodorants, hair sprays, canned whipped cream, and cleaning fluids. The specific inhalants include amyl nitrite ("poppers"), butyl nitrite (found in video head cleaners), butane (found in lighter fluid), methylene chloride (found in paint thinners), nitrous oxide ("laughing gas"), n-hexane (found in glue), and toluene (found in correction fluid and glue). Inhalants may be sniffed from containers, sprayed into the mouth as aerosols, introduced into a bag as a vapor or aerosol and then inhaled, or inhaled from a soaked rag.

▶ Occupational & Environmental Exposure

Recreational inhalant use refers to intentional inhalational exposure to chemicals in order to produce desired psychoactive and physical effects that may, in turn, have important acute and chronic adverse health consequences. Abuse of common consumer products may be viewed as a form of environmental toxicant exposure, particularly among young adults, adolescents, and children. It also may be viewed as a substance-abuse disorder. It is estimated that over 12 million Americans have abused inhalants at least once in their lives. According to the National Institute on Drug Abuse, 20% of eighth-grade students have engaged in recreational inhalant use. Hair stylists, wood refinishers, and anesthesiologists are occupations that may be at increased risk of experiencing *unintentional* exposure to some of the same inhalants that have abuse potential.

Metabolism & Mechanism of Action

Inhaled chemicals are absorbed rapidly from the respiratory tract into the bloodstream and delivered quickly to the brain and other organ systems. Alcohol intoxication–like effects may be produced within seconds to minutes. Intoxication may only last a few minutes, which may result in repeated intentional exposures.

Clinical Findings

A. Symptoms and Signs

Recreational inhalants produce a spectrum of acute effects, including euphoria, dizziness, slurred speech, hallucinations, headache, delusions, and loss of consciousness. A single session of inhalant abuse may cause a lethal cardiac dysrhythmia, a sequela termed *sudden sniffing death*. This can be related to the primary substance inhaled or to carrier propellants, especially if they are halogenated hydrocarbons that can sensitize the myocardium to catecholamine-related dysrhythmia. Long-term health effects from compulsive use include neurotoxicities such as cognitive abnormalities and movement disorders, as well as injury to the heart, liver, bone marrow, and kidneys.

B. Laboratory Findings

There are few specific laboratory findings. Macrocytic anemia has been described in chronic nitrous oxide abuse. Nitrates and oxidants induce methemoglobinemia. Forensic analysis may detect solvents in cases of acute mortality and very high-level exposure. Although various solvent metabolites can be detected in urine and are the basis of biological monitoring in industrial exposure settings, they are generally not relevant to clinical management (but can play a role forensically). Pathologic findings in chronic solvent exposure include brain atrophy (ie, toluene), nerve demyelination (ie, *n*-hexane), and cirrhosis (ie, hepatotoxic chlorinated solvents).

Differential Diagnosis

An exposure history typically is sufficient to make a diagnosis of acute recreational inhalant use. A spectrum of recreational drugs with psychoactive effects may produce euphoria and other neurologic effects similar to those produced by abused inhalants. The clinical presentation of sudden sniffing death is indistinguishable from sudden cardiac death as a result of congenital or acquired heart disease unless a post-mortem examination is performed (that includes forensic testing). Chronic recreational inhalant use (especially solvents) may produce clinical and pathologic-neurologic syndromes difficult to distinguishable from multiple sclerosis and cirrhosis caused by alcohol.

Prevention & Treatment

The general strategies used to prevent and treat substance abuse are relevant to the public health problem of recreational inhalant abuse.

Prognosis

Intensity, duration, and frequency of exposure and, presumably, host factors are important determinants of prognosis. Chronic neurologic, cardiac, and liver disease may result from long-term abuse.

WATERPROOFING COMPOUNDS

ESSENTIALS OF DIAGNOSIS

▶ Acute effects
- Cough.
- Dyspnea.
- Chest pain.
- Fever.
- Acute respiratory distress syndrome.
- Rigors.
- Myalgias.
- Euphoria.
- Headache.
- Loss of consciousness.
- Eye or throat burning.
▶ Chronic effects
- Pulmonary fibrosis.

General Consideration

Waterproofing sprays contain fluorinated relatively short-length polymers that, following inhalational exposure, can produce a constellation of pulmonary and systemic health effects, including acute lung injury. This fluoropolymer associated syndrome can share some clinical features with illness caused by the inhalation of fluorocarbon thermal degradation products, if the temperature of breakdown yields toxicants capable of causing acute lung injury. This should not be confused with "polymer fume fever" in which the inhalation of fluoropolymer breakdown products from somewhat lower temperatures causes a self-limited flu-like syndrome. Waterproofing spray associated illness does not require the thermal degradation of the parent compound and occurs with direct use of fluoropolymer containing products in occupational (eg, construction) or consumer applications. An outbreak of severe lung injury among consumers in Korea due to inhalation of a chemically different polymer used as a disinfectant in home humidifiers further underscores the potential toxicity of polymer inhalants.

Occupational & Environmental Exposure

Waterproofing sprays containing fluorocarbon aerosols are widely available to consumers. These products are intended to be applied to fabrics and leather in order to repel water or stains. There have also been reports of occupational illness following the use of a fluorocarbon produces on walls, flooring, and other surfaces.

Metabolism & Mechanism of Action

It has been hypothesized that waterproofing sprays modify the alveolar surface tension and disrupt surfactant causing impaired gas exchange and alveolar collapse. Direct cellular injury has also been theorized as a possible mechanism of action.

Clinical Findings

A. Symptoms and Signs

Exposure may result in constellation of pulmonary and systemic features. Rapidly evolving respiratory symptoms dominate, including cough, dyspnea, and tachypnea. Other features of toxic exposure include fever, rigors, and myalgias. Eye and throat irritation, and gastrointestinal complaints, including nausea, vomiting, and abdominal pain have also been reported.

B. Laboratory Findings

There are no specific laboratory findings. Clinical-radiographic features of acute lung injury may be observed including bilateral, diffuse interstitial opacities without pleural fluid, and hypoxemia. Bronchoalveolar lavage fluid neutrophilia has been reported. A peripheral blood leukocytosis is typical.

Differential Diagnosis

An exposure history is essential in making the diagnosis of a waterproofing spray-related adverse health effect. Systemic features may resemble an influenza-like illness and pulmonary features may be mistaken for a myriad of cardiopulmonary conditions that cause respiratory insufficiency and multi-lobar interstitial opacities. Bronchoscopy with lavage cultures may be useful in helping rule out infectious etiologies.

Prevention & Treatment

Measures to minimize inhalational exposure to waterproofing sprays include avoiding use in indoor (especially poorly ventilated) environments and employing standard measures to reduce exposure to aerosols. Removal of the offending polymers from waterproofing formulations is the cornerstone of prevention, but reintroduction of similar compounds has led to continued sporadic outbreaks of disease. Treatment consists of supportive care. It is unclear if systemic corticosteroids have a disease-moidfying effect.

Prognosis

Symptoms range from mild to severe, including respiratory failure. Recovery with supportive care is typical. Pulmonary fibrosis and persistent pulmonary function abnormalities have been described following severe injury.

REFERENCES

Henretig FM, Kirk MA, McKay CA Jr: Hazardous chemical emergencies and poisonings. N Engl J Med 2019;380(17):1638-1655 [PMID: 31018070].

Ng PC et al: Hydrogen sulfide toxicity: Mechanism of action, clinical presentation, and countermeasure development. J Med Toxicol 2019;15(4):287-294 [PMID: 31062177].

Rose JJ et al: Carbon monoxide poisoning: pathogenesis, management, and future directions of therapy [published correction appears in Am J Respir Crit Care Med. 2017;196(3):398-399]. Am J Respir Crit Care Med 2017;195(5):596-606 [PMID: 27753502].

Saeed O: Inhalation injury and toxic industrial chemical exposure. Mil Med 2018;183(suppl_2):130-132 [PMID: 30189064].

Scheepers PTJ et al: Pulmonary injury associated with spray of a water-based nano-sized waterproofing product: a case study. J Occup Med Toxicol 2017;12:33 [PMID: 29234454].

Spinou A: Current clinical management of smoke inhalation injuries: a reality check. Eur Respir J 2018;52(6). pii: 1802163 [PMID: 30523210].

■ SELF-ASSESSMENT QUESTIONS

Select the one correct answer for each question.

Question 1: High-intensity exposure to toxic gases and other airborne toxicants
   a. may result in clinical findings that develop abruptly or in a delayed manner
   b. affects only genetically susceptible individuals
   c. characteristically produces only minor adverse effects when victims are able to flee
   d. does not cause longer-term sequelae

Question 2: Simple asphyxiants
   a. are health hazards solely when encountered in confined spaces
   b. are of less concern when they are heavier than air
   c. are harmful even when encountered in low concentrations in well-ventilated spaces
   d. include methane gas, argon, carbon dioxide, and nitrogen

Question 3: Methane gas is
   a. heavier than air
   b. not explosive
   c. released in the presence of organic material breakdown
   d. not encountered in coal mining

Question 4: Carbon dioxide is
   a. lighter than air
   b. not a direct acute stimulant to respiration at intermediate concentrations
   c. not lethal at any concentration
   d. a potent central nervous system depressant at high concentrations

Question 5: Carbon monoxide
   a. competes with oxygen for binding sites on hemoglobin
   b. increases the oxygen-carrying capacity of the blood
   c. causes acute lung injury
   d. is not treated if brain injury has occurred

Question 6: Hydrogen cyanide is
   a. encountered in metal plating operations
   b. slowly absorbed through inhalation and skin exposures
   c. recognized universally by its "bitter almond" odor
   d. released to a greater degree from cyanide salt solutions if the pH increases to the alkaline range

Question 7: Hydrogen sulfide
   a. exerts its toxicity by blocking oxygen utilization through the cytochrome oxidase pathway
   b. has good warning properties through smell
   c. does not cause mucous membrane and respiratory tract irritation
   d. is not associated with burning eyes, headache, dizziness, nausea, and vomiting

Question 8: Smoke inhalation
   a. only exerts toxicity through irritant effects
   b. results in direct thermal injury
   c. does not cause methemoglobinemia
   d. produces clinical findings of both asphyxiant and irritant injury

Question 9: Arsine gas
   a. has been used as a dopant in the microelectronics industry
   b. exposure may present as a characteristic triad of abdominal pain, hematuria, and cough
   c. may cause headache, renal failure, and purple staining of urine and feces
   d. exposure with massive hemolysis does not benefit from exchange transfusion

Question 10: Phosphine gas
   a. is not used in agriculture
   b. is generated from the hydrolysis of aluminum phosphide and sodium chloride
   c. is not associated with chest pain
   d. toxicity is marked by delayed-onset pulmonary edema

Pesticides

Michael O'Malley, MD, MPH

GENERAL CONSIDERATIONS

Pesticides include chemicals, as well as biological and physical agents, used to control a diverse array of pests. The products used have evolved since the 1930s when arsenic was the principal insecticide used. During and after World War II (WWII), organochlorines and cholinesterase inhibitors supplanted many common uses of arsenic, along with the use of synthetic pyrethrins (pyrethroids). Pesticides currently registered in the United States include 1055 active ingredients formulated into 13,413 separate products.

Typified by cholinesterase-inhibiting insecticides and fumigants, older agents have biologically nonselective mechanisms, accounting for their effects on nontarget as well as target organisms. Agents with selective mechanisms occur as incidental materials in some illness investigations, but less often appear as the primary cause of reported illnesses. As discussed in the chapter subsections for individual use categories, the availability of agents with new modes of action has accompanied a gradual elimination of some compounds used for decades.

PESTICIDE USE

A comprehensive database of the 20 most used pesticide active ingredients on six dominant crops and four aggregated crop classes (PEST-CHEMGRIDS) show the global projection between 2015 and 2025 to be the herbicides glyphosate and metam potassium (about 700,000 tons per year), metam and dichloropropene (about 450,000 tons per year), and 2,4-D (about 150,000 tons per year). The most commonly used insecticides are metam potassium and metam, calcium polysulfide (about 50,000 tons per year), and chlorpyrifos (about 20,000 tons per year). Finally, the most used fungicides are metam potassium, petroleum oil (about 150,000 tons per year), and chlorothalonil (about 120,000 tons per year).

California Sales Data

California pesticide sales data from 2016 reflect the use of both agricultural compounds and antimicrobials. Some agricultural processing operations use antimicrobials, and some compounds listed as antimicrobials were also used as agricultural fungicides.

Reported sales for 2016 totaled 1,806,473,576.17 lb, with 1,516,820,420.66 lb (84%) attributable to antimicrobials. Other pesticides accounted for 289,652,862.51 lb use, with reported agricultural use amounting to 209 million pounds (details provided as follows for the most frequently used compounds). The remaining 80 million pounds represented pesticides used for nonagricultural pest control. Cumulative acreage treated totaled 101 million acres, an average treatment frequency of 3.7 times per year; on average 7.7 lb of active ingredient was used for each of the 27 million cultivated acres of cropland in California.

Most frequently used categories of compounds included chlorine, bromine, and iodine compounds; aldehydes; quaternary ammonium compounds; organic alcohols and glycols; organic acids; and isothiazoline compounds (Table 33–1).

Mandatory Agricultural Use Reporting

A review of the 100 pesticides most frequently reported provides a useful snapshot of California agricultural use. Table 33–2 summarizes the 100 most heavily used pesticide agents. This group of compounds accounted for 24 million pounds applied, about 11.5% of total reported agricultural use. The ranking, by number of acres treated, accounts for the difference in application rates between older compounds (eg, sulfur, applied at an average rate of 7.8 lb/acre) and the newer compounds (eg, conazole fungicides, applied at an average rate of 0.13 lb/acre). The fumigant compounds did not reach the top 100 by the acres treated measure, but the halogenated fumigants (1,3-dichloropropene, methyl bromide, and chloropicrin) and the methyl isothiocyanate (MITC) releasing n-methyl thiocarbamates were among the top 100 ranked by lb applied. Used data for these compounds are included because of their toxicologic importance. The insecticide/miticide propargite is also included because of its

Table 33–1. Antimicrobials.

Category	Compound List	Lb Sold 2016	% Total
Multiple Sites of Action			
Halide (bromine, chlorine, iodine) compounds—multisite mode of action	Sodium hypochlorite, chlorine, 1,3-dichloro-5,5-dimethylhydantoin, sodium dichloro-s-triazinetrione	1,377,472,717.43	91.38
Inorganic acids and bases	Phosphoric acid, orthophosphoric acid	37,632,998.98	2.50
Alcohols; glycols; alcohol amines	Isopropyl butyl, ethyl, isodecyl, and lauryl alcohols; propylene glycol; triethanolamine, triethanolamine oleate	20,799,932.18	1.38
Organic acids and organic peroxides	Glycolic acid, acetic acid, capric acid, caprylic acid, citric acid, formic acid, lactic acid, lauric acid, phenylethyl propionate, propionic acid, diethanolamine, potassium peroxymonosulfate, sodium carbonate peroxyhydrate, butoxy polypropoxy polyethoxy ethanol—iodine complex. tetraglycine hydroperiodide, sodium persulfate	15,906,777.41	1.06
Copper compounds	Copper sulfate (pentahydrate), copper ethanolamine complexes, mixed, copper hydroxide, copper ammonium carbonate, copper sulfate (basic), copper oxide (ous), copper oxychloride, copper oxide (ic), copper carbonate, basic, copper naphthenate	15,364,355.50	1.02
Quaternary ammonium compounds, amine salts, amine derivatives	8 to 18 carbon alkyl ammonium mixtures,1,3-propylenediamine, ammonium sulfate, etc.	13,607,334.16	0.90
Carbonate buffers	Potassium/sodium carbonate	12,555,358.45	0.83
Sulfur dioxide and thiocarbamate compounds—multisite	Sulfur dioxide; sodium, potassium dimethyl-dithiocarbamates, 3-iodo-2-propynyl butylcarbamate, carbendazim	5,638,403.32	0.37
Isothiazoline compounds	1,2-benzisothiazolin-3-one, octhilinone, etc.	1,602,671.59	0.11
Aldehyde	Acrolein, glutaraldehyde, formaldehyde	4,120,831.06	0.27
Hydantoin compounds	1,3-dichloro-5-ethyl-5-methylhydantoin, etc.	2,362,777.63	0.16
Membrane Effects			
Quaternary ammonium compounds, amine salts, amine derivatives	Alkyl (42% c12, 26% c18, 15% c14, 8% c16, 5% c10, 4% c8) 1,3-propylenediamine, ammonium sulfate, etc.	13,607,334.16	0.90
Phenols	ortho-phenylphenol, para-tert-amylphenol, ortho-phenylphenol, sodium salt 18, 5-chloro-2-(2,4-dichlorophenoxy) phenol, ortho-benzyl-para-chlorophenol, sodium para-tert-amylphenate, ortho-benzyl-para-chlorophenol, potassium salt, phenol, etc.	246,295.8946	0.02
Peroxides	Hydrogen peroxide, peroxyacetic acid, peroxyoctanoic acid	11,997,816	0.8
Antibiotics and bacterials; biological resins and oils	Streptomycin sulfate, Streptomyces griseoviridis strain k61, Streptomyces lydicus wyec 108; capsicum oleoresin; oils of pine, cedarwood, citronella, geranium, and lemongrass	107,526.20	0.01

Table 33–2. Mandated agricultural use reporting in California, 2016.[a]

Mode of Action	Chemical Class	Typical Compounds	lb applied	# Applications	Acres treated[a]	% of total acreage[a]
Adjuvants						
Spreading agents, surfactants	Synthetic organic polymers, organo-silicons, petroleum distillates, vegetable oils	Dimethyl alkyl tertiary amines; fatty acids, c16-c18 and c18-unsaturated, methyl esters, etc.; polyalkene oxide modified heptamethyl trisiloxane, etc.; petroleum oil, paraffin based, etc.; methylated soybean oil, etc.	9,763,849	1,326,464	47,815,897[a]	177.1
pH modulators	Inorganic base, inorganic acid, organic acid	Potassium hydroxide, benzoic acid, phosphoric acid, propionic acid, citric acid	331,493	162,907	6,032,454	22.3
Formulation aids, solubility agents	Alcohols, glycols	Diethylene glycol, propylene glycol, glycerol, butyl alcohol, isopropyl alcohol	434,005	162,739	5,252,765	19.5
Nitrogen growth adjuvant	Ammonium salt, urea salt	Ammonium sulfate, ammonium propionate, ammonium nitrate, urea dihydrogen sulfate	1,103,169	107,512	4,106,373	15.2
Insecticides						
Sodium channel modulators, blockers	Pyrethroids, indoxacarb, DDT-like organochlorines	λ-cyhalothrin, (s)-cypermethrin, esfenvalerate, permethrin, β-cyfluthrin, bifenthrin; indoxacarb	861,911	191,068	5,675,790	21.0
Mechanically disrupts gas exchange (respiration), cell membrane function or structure	Petroleum distillates	Mineral oil, petroleum oil	35,189,382	96,446	3,334,468	12.3
ACHR-nicotine competitive agonist; allosteric modulator	Neonicotinoids, spinosyns, nereistoxin analogues	IMIDACLOPRID, etc., Spinosad	723,804	126,869c	3,165,704	11.7
Glutamate-gated chloride channel agonists, stimulating GABA pathways	Avermectins, Milbemectins	Abamectin; Emamectin, Milbemectin	48,991	73039	2,430,384	9.0
Glutamate-gated chloride channel antagonists, suppressing GABA pathways	Phenylpyrazoles (antagonist); Cyclodiene organochlorines (antagonist)	Fipronil	273,134.01	1	NA	NA
Ryanodine receptor modulator, disrupting the Ca^{2+} balance	Diamide	Flubendiamide, Chlorantraniliprole, Cyantraniliprole	164,471	53,499	2,026,205	7.5
ChE inhibitors	Organophosphates, carbamates	Methomyl, chlorpyrifos, etc.	1,406,813	42,779	1,603,429	5.9

(continued)

Table 33–2. Mandated agricultural use reporting in California, 2016.[a] (Continued)

Mode of Action	Chemical Class	Typical Compounds	lb applied	# Applications	Acres treated[a]	% of total acreage[a]
Inhibitors of acetyl CoA car-boxylase, lipid synthesis, growth regulation	Tetronic acid derivatives	Spirotetramat, spiromesifen, spirodiclofen	103,368 + 20,446.93 + 42,278.07	52,333	970,964	3.6
Inhibitors of mitochondrial ATP synthase	Organotins, Propargite	Propargite, Fenbutatin oxide	213205	2208	92814.68	3.4
Chitin synthesis inhibitors	Benzoylphenyl urea compounds	Diflubenzuron, Novaluron	37331.67	45787	332,492	1.2
Fungicides						
Multisite activity	Copper salts, dinitroani-lines, inorganic element, thiocarbamate	Copper sulfate (basic), copper hydroxide, copper oxychloride, chlorothalonil, elemental sulfur, mancozeb	55,104,541	252,516	8,721,990	32.3
Inhibit mitochondrial res-piration, blocking the cytochrome bc1 complex, complex III	Strobilurins	Trifloxystrobin, azoxystrobin, pyraclostrobin	428,246	91,328	3,155,969	11.7
Ergosterol synthesis inhibitor	Triazoles, conazoles	Propiconazole, tebuconazole, difenoconazole, metconazole, myclobutanil	388,253	79,490	2,965,926	11.0
SDHI (succinate dehydroge-nase inhibitors), blocking cellular respiration	pyrazole-carboximide, pyridinyl-ethylbenzamides	Fluxapyroxad, boscalid, fluopyram	312,044	56,035	1,942,267	7.2
Inhibition intercellular mycelial growth, amino acid synthesis	Aminopyrimidine	Cyprodinil	178,317	19,677	648,850	2.4
Signal transduction— disrupts fungi specific cell-signaling events	Aza-naphthalenes, aryloxyquinoline	Quinoxyfen	51,781	17,232	569,434	2.1
Herbicides						
EPSP synthase inhibitors, blocking synthesis of aromatic amino acids	Glycine derivative	Glyphosate, potassium salt, isopro-pylamine salt	11,725,218	167,430	5,555,179	20.6
Protoporphyrinogen oxidase (PPO) inhibitors, photo-synthesis pathway	Diphenylether	Oxyfluorfen	906,293	65,534	2,222,793	8.2
	Phenylpyrazole, triazol, pyrimidinedione	Pyraflufen-ethyl, carfentrazone-ethyl, saflufenacil	51,809	50,228	2,108,734	7.8
Photosystem-I-electron diversion	Bipyridyl	Paraquat dichloride, Diquat dibromide	1,431,901	34,965	1,371,785	5.1

(continued)

Table 33–2. Mandated agricultural use reporting in California, 2016.[a] (Continued)

Mode of Action	Chemical Class	Typical Compounds	lb applied	# Applications	Acres treated[a]	% of total acreage[a]
Microtubule assembly inhibition	Dinitroaniline	Pendimethalin	2,367,872	29,662	1,137,114	4.2
Inhibition of glutamine synthetase	Phosphonoglycine, phosphinate	Glufosinate	1,040,736	38,648	1,081,173	4.0
Inhibition of acetolactate synthase ALS, branched chain amino acid synthesis	Sulfonyl urea	Rimsulfuron	24,928	19,434	583,473	2.2
Regulates stem elongation, germination, dormancy, flowering, flower development, and senescence of leaves and fruit	Multiring lactone	Gibberellins	23,116	16,634	543,927	2.0
Cellulose-biosynthesis inhibitor (CBI)	Triazine-diamine	Indaziflam	30,611	19,851	521,076	1.9
Liberation of ethylene, absorbed by the plant and interferes in the growth	Phosphonic acid	Ethephon	399,036	9,061	452,865	1.7
Photosynthesis inhibition at photosystem II	Amide	Propanil	2,269,943	5,670	418,789	1.6
Fumigants						
Multisite activity, electrophile	Halogenated hydrocarbon	1,3-dichloropropene	14,126,938	3,145	75,725	0.3
Multisite activity, electrophile	Halogenated hydrocarbon	Methyl bromide	2,602,823	728	11,031	0.04
Multisite activity, electrophile	Halogenated hydrocarbon	Chloropicrin	8,641,552	2,542	49,149	0.2
Multisite activity	Inorganic fluoride	Sulfuryl fluoride	3,296,298	5	0	
Multisite activity, releases MITC	n-methylthiocarbamate	Metam potassium	9,343,192	3,380	49,022	0.2
Multisite activity, releases MITC	n-methylthiocarbamate	Metam sodium	3,297,827	461	19,437	0.1
Multisite activity	Phosphide	Aluminum phosphide	160,799.32	2,090	Not applicable	
Multisite activity	Phosphide	Zinc phosphide	3,656.48	887	Not applicable	

[a]100 most frequently used adjuvants and active ingredients, based on acres treated.
Cumulative acres treated may exceed actual planted acres because of multiple applications/year for some materials, for example, sulfur can be applied monthly during vineyard growing season; the California Department of Agriculture estimates 27 million acres of cropland statewide.

Table 33–3. U.S. EPA data requirements for pesticide registration.

Test category	Details
Product chemistry	Production composition, physical and chemical characteristics, residue chemistry
Environmental fate	Degradation studies (hydrolysis/photolysis studies); metabolism studies; mobility studies (leaching, adsorption/desorption, and volatility of pesticides); dissipation studies (used to assess potential environmental hazards related to reentry, conditionally required foliar residue dissipation studies; hazards from residues in rotational crop and other food sources, the loss of land as well as surface and ground water resources); accumulation studies (to evaluate tendency for bioaccumulation in ecosystems)
Hazards to humans and domestic animals	**Acute studies** Oral LD50: rat Dermal LD: usually rabbit; inhalation LC: rat; primary eye irritation: rabbit; primary dermal irritation: rabbit Dermal sensitization Acute delayed neurotoxicity: organophosphates subchronic studies: required depending on nature of exposure 90-day feeding: rodent, nonrodent 21-day dermal, 90-day dermal 90-day inhalation: rat 90-rat neurotoxicity: if acute studies positive **Chronic studies:** Required for pesticides with allowable food residues (tolerances), or "significant" worker exposure chronic feeding: two-species, rodent and nonrodent carcinogenicity: two-species, rat and mouse preferred Teratogenicity: two species Reproduction: two generations Mutagenicity studies: a battery to include: Gene mutations Structural chromosomal aberrations Other genotoxic effects as appropriate Metabolism studies (pharmacokinetics)
Hazard to nontarget organisms	Short-term studies, long-term and field studies, avian and mammalian testing, aquatic organism testing, plant protection, nontarget insect

Notes
From U.S. Environmental Protection Agency, 2006.
Abbreviations: LC50 = lethal concentration affecting 50% of test population; LDso = lethal dose affecting 50% of test population.

long association with irritant dermatitis in field workers and applicators (see section on Insecticides later).

Pesticide Regulation

Regulation of pesticides differs by jurisdiction and a complete review of the topic exceeds the scope of this chapter. Extensive requirements for toxicity testing form an essential element in most countries. Table 33–3 summarizes required testing in the United States, including product chemistry, environmental fate, acute and chronic toxicity testing, and evaluation of hazards to nontarget organisms. Although pharmaceuticals receive extensive testing, including human treatment trials, no comparable system exists for requiring testing of industrial chemicals or consumer products.

The required testing permits categorization of acute toxicity for individual formulations according to four broad categories (Table 33–4) designated by Roman numerals and signal words on product labels—Danger (Category I), Warning (Category II), and Caution (Category III and Category IV).

A product may have relatively low acute systemic toxicity but still receive a Danger (Category I) label because it causes severe skin or eye irritation.

Changes in scientific knowledge and perceptions have led to difficulty in categorizing chronic effects in a similar fashion. Table 33–5 shows variations in categories used over time for categorizing the results of human and animal studies. Terms used for "probable carcinogen," for example, have changed from "B2" (used in the 1980s) to "likely human carcinogen" used currently. The International Agency for Research on Cancer (IARC) uses a different terminology that in most respects parallels that used by the U.S. Environmental Protection Agency (EPA).

Pesticide use regulations attempt to address the wide variety of pesticide categories, modes of application, and circumstances of exposure (Table 33–6). Rules for pesticide handlers include product-by-product requirements for use of protective equipment to prevent eye, skin, respiratory or systemic effects, typically listed on product labels. Some products present hazards sufficient to necessitate engineering

Table 33–4. Environmental Protection Agency toxicity labeling categories.

Hazard Indicator	Toxicity Category			
	I	II	III	IV
Oral LD$_{50}$				
Inhalation LD$_{50}$	0.2 mg/L	0.2–2 mg/L	2–20 mg/L	
Dermal LD$_{50}$	200 mg/kg	200–2000 mg/kg	2000–20,000 mg/kg	> 20,000 mg/kg
Eye effects	Corrosive; corneal opacity not reversible within 21 days	Corneal irritation or opacity clearing between 8–21 days	No corneal injury irritation reversible within 7 days	Minimal irritation, clearing less than 24 hours
Skin effects in Draize dermal irritation (rabbits)	Corrosive	Severe irritation	Moderate irritation at 72 hours	Mild or slight irritation at 72 hours
Signal word	"Danger"	"Warning"	"Caution"	"Caution"
Precautionary statements regarding systemic toxicity	Fatal (poisonous) if swallowed, inhaled, absorbed through skin. Do not breathe vapor, dust, or spray mist. Do not get in eyes or on skin or clothing.	May be fatal if swallowed, inhaled, absorbed through skin. Do not breathe vapor, dust, or spray mist. Do not get in eyes or on skin or clothing.	Harmful if swallowed, inhaled or absorbed through skin. Avoid breathing vapor, dust, or spray mist. Avoid contact with skin, eyes, or clothing.	No precautionary statements
Precautionary statements regarding topical effects on eye and skin	Corrosive, causes eye and skin damage or skin irritation.	Do not get in eyes, on skin, or on clothing. Wear goggles or face shield and rubber gloves when handling. Harmful or fatal if swallowed. (Appropriate first aid statement required.)	Causes eye and skin irritation. Do not get in eyes, on skin, or on clothing. In case of contact, wash eyes with plenty of water. Get medical attention if irritation persists.	No precautionary statements required.

From: US Environmental Protection 40 CFR Part 156.; see also https://www.epa.gov/sites/production/files/2015-03/documents/chap-07-jul-2014.pdf.

controls, such as enclosed mixing and loading systems or enclosed tractor cabs used at the time of application. Protections for field workers include restricted field reentry intervals, a form of administrative control that requires a specified waiting period before workers enter treated fields after applications. Intervals vary from waiting until sprays settle and dry after application to several weeks, usually specified on product labels. California has detailed rules for some hazardous products based primarily on past poisoning episodes (Table 33–7). Pesticides used for indoor pests overlap those used in agricultural environments, but usually employ relatively dilute formulations. Safe use depends on minimizing direct contact through label instructions. This poses no difficulty with baits, traps, and other encapsulated formulations or for "crack and crevice" applications. For indoor broadcast applications with foggers, sometimes known as "bug bombs," postapplication reentry instructions may state a specified period or "wait until spray dries." For the pyrethroid cyfluthrin, the manufacturer conducted a small-scale experimental study with human volunteers that determined the inhalation irritation threshold to be 10 mcg/m^3. Complaints of asthma aggravation following indoor pesticide applications suggest that the respiratory irritation threshold may vary considerably in the population at large. Inhalation irritation studies are not a registration requirement for indoor use materials.

Because legally applied formulations are presumed to be safe after the spray has settled and dried, postapplication studies are not usually conducted. Predicting the postapplication dissipation of illegally applied materials poses additional difficulties. These include (1) concentrated formulations applied without discrimination, (2) lack records documenting the date and site of application, and (3) application to porous materials that retard dissipation.

OCCUPATIONAL & ENVIRONMENTAL PESTICIDE EXPOSURE

Most pesticide inhalation exposures derive from aerosols generated at the time of application or from pesticide adsorbed to household or environmental dust. With

Table 33–5. EPA versus IARC schemes for classification of carcinogens.

Group	1986 Classifications	1999 Classification	IARC Classification
A	Human carcinogen	Carcinogenic to humans	Group 1: The agent (mixture) is carcinogenic to humans
B	Probable human carcinogen	Likely to be carcinogenic to humans	Group 2A: The agent (mixture) is probably carcinogenic to humans
B1	Agents for which there is limited evidence of carcinogenicity from epidemiologic studies		
B2	Agents for which there is sufficient evidence from animal studies and for which there is inadequate or no evidence of carcinogenicity from epidemiologic studies		
C	Possible human carcinogen	Likely to be carcinogenic	Group 2B: The agent (mixture) is possibly carcinogenic to humans
D	Not classifiable as to human carcinogenicity	Data are inadequate for an assessment of human	Group 3: The agent (mixture, exposure circumstance) is not classified
E	Evidence of noncarcinogenicity for humans	Not likely to be carcinogenic to humans	Group 4: The agent (mixture, exposure circumstance) is probably not carcinogenic to humans

List of chemicals evaluated for carcinogenic potential, 2006, available online at: https://cfpub.epa.gov/ncea/risk/recordisplay.cfm?deid=54932—Draft Revised Guidelines for Carcinogen Risk Assessment (External Draft, July 1999), http://npic.orst.edu/chemicals_evaluated.pdf—Chemicals Evaluated for Carcinogenic Potential Annual Cancer Report 2019, and http://monographs.iarc.fr/

Table 33–6. Occupational and environmental pesticide exposure situations.

Occupational Exposures	
Category	**Exposure**
Research and development	Accidental release of materials during synthesis or during analytical measurements
Manufacturing	Technical grade material produced in enclosed and semienclosed operations; exposures during leaks/spill and process repairs—packaging operations vary in degree of enclosure
Formulation	Technical grade material mixed with "inert" ingredients such as solvents and adjuvants
Transportation	Small to moderate volume spills associated with highway transport, potentially large volume spills associated with bulk rail transport. Fumigation in transit: rail or shipping
Pest control	Mixing: commercial material diluted with water or other material. Loading: into tanks in planes, ground rigs, backpacks, or hand-held sprayers. Closed versus open mix/loading systems. Flagging: standing at the end of fields to mark the rows to be sprayed by crop-dusting aircraft. Flagging is currently being replaced by Global Positioning System flagging in some operations
Farm work	Field workers, pickers, sorters, packers, and others who come into contact with pesticide residues on leaves and fruit. High contact work tasks include hand labor in grapes; picking row crops, such as lettuce or strawberries, results in markedly less contact—as described in results of residue transfer studies
Emergency response and medical workers	Exposed to contaminated persons and equipment in the process of responding to spills, accidents, and poisonings
Environmental and consumer exposures	Accidents and spills, especially ingestion by children (floor level materials—ant traps, etc.). Suicide and homicide. Home use: house and garden. Structural use: residents and occupants of buildings bystanders, early reentry into or failure to clear fumigated buildings. Contamination: food, water, air. Agriculture-urban interface

Table 33–7. California restricted intervals, active ingredients with currently registered formulations.

	Crops					
Pesticide	Apples	Citrus	Corn	Grapes	Peaches/Nectarines	Other Crops
Chlorpyriphos		2				
Diazinon		5		5	5	
Malathion		1		1	1	
Methomyl (Lannate)				7(i)		
Phorate (Thimet)			7			
Phosmet (Imidan)				5	5	
Propargite (Omite/Comite)	21	42	7	30	21	21(ii)
Sulfur				3(iii)		

Adapted from https://www.cdpr.ca.gov/docs/legbills/calcode/030303.htm.

(i) Applications of methomyl made after August 15 have a 21-day restricted entry interval. This interval may be terminated after 10 days if leaf samples tested pursuant to Section 6774 (c)(4) show 0.1 micrograms per square centimeter or less of dislodgeable foliar residue of methomyl.

(ii) The restricted entry interval for strawberries and field-grown roses treated with propargite is 3 days. The restricted entry interval for cotton fields treated with propargite is 7 days. However, from the end of the restricted entry interval until the beginning of harvest, the employer shall assure that employees entering propargite treated cotton fields wear work clothing with long sleeves and legs and gloves.

(iii) This restricted entry interval for sulfur applies from May 15 through harvest in the counties of: Fresno, Kern, Kings, Madera, Merced, San Joaquin, Stanislaus, and Tulare; and during March and April in Riverside County.

fumigants and a few insecticidal compounds, exposures to vapors are also a significant issue.

Skin contact accounts for most occupational exposures. Compounds absorbed across intact human skin possess a combination of relatively low molecular weight and high-lipid solubility. This correlates with the requirement of many compounds to be absorbed through the protective coverings of insects or plants. Table 33–8 lists typical occupational and nonoccupational pesticide exposure situations. The nature, extent, and route of exposure may vary among these different circumstances and the physical properties—particularly the vapor pressure—of individual pesticides.

The nature of exposure depends on whether exposure is to the commercial formulation of a pesticide, as applied in a field or structure, or to the highly concentrated technical grade active ingredient, as might occur in a manufacturing or formulating facility. A pesticide, as applied, consists of the technical-grade chemical ("active" ingredient), diluents (often organic solvents), additives ("adjuvants"), and other "inert" ingredients (see following discussion). The pesticide then is applied mixed or unmixed as sprays, dusts, aerosols, granular, impregnated preparations, fumigants, or bait.

Pesticides used by consumers for home and garden resemble those used by commercial applicators, with reduced concentration of active ingredient. The most serious home exposures occur from accidental or deliberate ingestions.

Although pesticides account for a relatively small percentage of the total childhood ingestions, childhood ingestions of organophosphates (OPs), carbamates, and dipyridyl herbicides (diquat and paraquat) may result in serious illness or death. Children also frequently attempt to ingest pesticides used at floor or ground level, such as anticoagulant rodenticides, snail baits, and ant traps, but these less often cause serious poisonings. Because of high ventilation rates compared to adults, children have proved vulnerable in serious residential fumigation incidents.

▶ High-Risk Groups

The highest exposures and incidences of poisoning occur in individuals involved in agricultural pest-control operations: mixing, loading, applying, and flagging. Mixers and loaders handle concentrated pesticides and large volumes. The use of closed systems for mixing and loading reduces these exposures and poisonings considerably. The exposure to applicators varies with the type of application, from backpack sprayers to enclosed-cab vehicles with filtered cooled air. Leaking or poorly maintained equipment may fail and produce large overexposures with any type of application device, including closed mixing/loading systems. Exposures in most manufacturing facilities are low owing to the use of automated closed systems, but exposures that require

Table 33–8. Vapor pressures of common pesticides.

Pesticide, use or structural category	Vapor pressure—mm Hg
Fumigants/nematicides	
Phosphine	23,369
Sulfuryl fluoride	$1.16 \times 10^{+4}$, 20°C
Methyl bromide	1725
Chloropicrin	17
Metam-sodium	Not measurable
Metam-sodium by-products	
Methyl isothiocyanate	16.0
Methyl isocyanate	348
Carbon disulfide	334.3
Hydrogen sulfide	15,981
Methylamine	2324.3
Common solvents	
Water	24
Toluene	30
1,1-dichloroethane	234
Organophosphate, potential contaminants	
Methyl mercaptan	1261
Ethyl mercaptan	467
N-butyl mercaptan	83
Organophosphates	
Ethoprop	3.8×10^{-4}
Phorate	6.4×10^{-4}
Malathion	1.2×10^{-4}
Chlorpyrifos	2.02×10^{-5}
Dichlorvos	1.58×10^{-2}
Dimethoate	8×10^{-6}
Phosalone	$< 1 \times 10^{-9}$
Carbamates	
Methomyl	5.0×10^{-5}
Herbicides and plant growth regulators	
2,4-dichlorophenoxyacetic acid	1.4×10^{-7}
Cyanazine	1.6×10^{-9}
Alachlor	2.2×10^{-5}
Glyphosate	7.5×10^{-8}
Hydrogen cyanamide	3.75×10^{-3}
Gibberellic acid	2.6×10^{-13}
Ethephon	9.8×10^{-8}
Fungicides	
Naphthenic acid	1.1×10^{-7} to 7.1×10^{-6}
Zinc bisdithiocarbamate (ziram)	$< 7.5 \times 10^{-8}$
Benomyl	$< 3.7 \times 10^{-9}$
Chlorothalonil	5.72×10^{-7}
Triadimefon	1.5×10^{-7}

unscheduled maintenance occur during development of new processes and process breakdowns or leaks. Exposures in formulating facilities may be much higher, particularly with the production of dusty formulations (ie, dusts, powders, and granules) in open systems.

Communities with minimal zoning and mixed agricultural and urban or suburban land use may be at risk for environmental exposure to pesticides. In recent years, most problems have been the result of high-volume applications of volatile, soil fumigation products with low environmental effect levels.

▶ Illegal Pesticide Use

Illegal pesticide use can pose high risk of pesticide poisoning in unexpected circumstances. These may include use of hazardous agricultural materials for home pest control, illegal cultivation of marijuana, and deliberate or accidental adulteration of food products. The use of nerve agents fits at the far end of this spectrum.

RECOGNITION & TREATMENT OF SYNDROMES COMMON TO MULTIPLE GROUPS OF PESTICIDES

▶ Nonspecific Systemic Effects

Many pesticide incidents require evaluation of symptoms of headache, nausea, or other nonspecific symptoms that could come from individual active ingredients, solvents, adjuvants, low-molecular-weight contaminants causing odors, or common nonoccupational illnesses.

Providers can best evaluate these complaints by history, physical examination, and follow-up. Persistent symptoms merit much greater concern than short-term symptoms. Effective communication with affected patients depends on sometimes difficult to obtain detailed knowledge of the circumstances of the reported exposure.

▶ Irritation

Many antimicrobials and other pesticides cause irritation of the eyes, skin, or respiratory tract, frequently occurring after direct contact. These may occur as the principal effect for some compounds (see discussion of the insecticide/miticide propargite) or as an incidental finding in cases of systemic poisoning (see fumigants, antimicrobials, and other compounds that react with multiple biological targets).

Irritation is also a common side effect of several classes of adjuvant compounds, including petroleum distillates, fatty acids, and organosilicon compounds.

Most skin reactions are secondary to allergic or irritant contact dermatitis. Recognition depends on careful evaluation of the pattern of exposure and its relation to the distribution and character of subsequent skin lesions. This task may be especially difficult in cases of dermatitis in field workers who may not know the pesticides used on the fields where they are working.

In addition to pesticides, skin reactions may occur when workers handle crops or pull weeds known to cause primary irritant or allergic contact dermatitis. Definitive diagnosis of irritant dermatitis depends on recognizing the irritant properties of the suspected materials as well as noting the correspondence between pattern of exposure and pattern of skin reaction.

Allergic Reactions

Allergic dermatitis can be confirmed only by diagnostic patch testing (type IV allergy), open dermal applications, or prick testing (type I allergy). Patch tests are unfortunately available only for a small number of pesticides and plants known to be sensitizers. Developing tests for new materials requires preliminary testing of control subjects to identify the maximum nonirritating concentration.

The distinction between irritant and allergic dermatitis is important from an exposure/management standpoint. Irritant dermatitis often can be prevented by reducing exposure through use of personal protective equipment or administrative measures such as reentry intervals. Prevention of allergic contact dermatitis (ACD) requires complete removal from exposure.

Individual pesticides or weeds generally are simple to avoid, given a cooperative employer, but allergy to crop plants presents a greater problem. This is an infrequent problem with most food crops but may be relatively frequent in workers handling *Alstroemeria* (Peruvian lily), carnations, primrose, chrysanthemums, and other allergenic nursery crops.

A few pesticides have been reported to cause systemic dermal reactions such as urticaria, erythema multiforme, chloracne, vitiligo, porphyria cutanea tarda, or a drug eruptionlike rash caused by inhibition of alcohol metabolism. The alcohol dehydrogenase inhibitors include the thiocarbamate fungicides (related to the pharmacologic agent disulfiram) and the plant growth regulator cyanamide.

COMMON TREATMENT MODALITIES

Nonspecific Systemic Symptoms

After brief environmental or occupational exposures, nonspecific systemic symptoms will likely resolve without treatment. If necessary, symptoms of headache can be treated with simple analgesics. For nausea, a nonsedating antinausea medication (eg, ondansetron) can be used, but should be avoided if a coexposure included an organophosphate compound (possibly affecting the cardiac QT interval—see later) or if a preexisting cardiac problem exists.

In cases of ingestion, it may be appropriate to obtain a chest x-ray to evaluate for aspiration; this is probably unnecessary in occupational cases with contact exposure to the eyes or skin.

Decontamination

Decontamination, including bathing of skin, shampooing of hair, or emptying of stomach, is essential as dictated by the route of exposure. It is important to provide privacy for conducting decontamination where possible and remember that skin decontamination may not be helpful for inhalation (eg, fumigant) exposures.

Eye Irritation

A minimum of 15-minute eye wash is recommended for direct splashes to the eye. It is problematic whether this has any benefit for exposures to irritant vapors (eg, see sections on chloropicrin and the metam-sodium by-product MITC).

Artificial tears or anti-inflammatory eye drops (eg, containing ketoprofen or ketorolac) may be useful in treating mild cases of chemical conjunctivitis where no corneal injury occurs. With possibly more complicated injuries, initial ophthalmologic referral or phone consultation may prevent persistent symptoms or patient concerns.

Where promptly available, ophthalmologic consultation often provides reassurance to patients with more severe or persistent symptoms, but may prove unnecessary where a careful slit examination with fluorescein staining is done at the time of emergency care.

Skin Irritation

Decontamination of the skin should be attempted where possible, but may not completely remove material that has already penetrated into the lower layers of skin.

Topical moisturizers may partially relieve mild irritation symptoms and prevent patients from exacerbating skin damage by excoriation. Steroid creams may provide additional symptomatic relief. For severe irritation or burns, systemic analgesics may be necessary.

PESTICIDES BY USE CATEGORY

The following sections discuss important individual pesticides for the main use categories—antimicrobials, insecticides, herbicides, fungicides, and fumigants. Each category differs in the mix of active ingredients with selective and nonselective modes of action.

The selectivity of a given mode of action is relative rather than absolute. Both OPs and pyrethroids affect well-defined molecular targets, but do not act selectively in biological terms. Chitin synthesis inhibitors and chordotonal organ agents do not affect mammalian species, but may affect multiple categories of invertebrate organisms. Neonicotinoids and ryanodine receptor modulators act at similar sites in insects and mammals, but have much greater toxicity in insects. Nicotine acts at the same cholinergic receptor site as the neonicotinoids but is toxic to both insects and mammals. Most occupational illnesses associated with nicotine probably occur in tobacco production rather than from its limited current use as a pesticide.

Some compounds cross over between use categories; for example, many isothiazoline (Kathon) compounds have antibacterial and antifungal activities. Both antibacterials and antifungals can be considered antimicrobials, but antifungals are only labeled as antibacterials when they are used in water treatment operations. The same reasoning applies to herbicides used as algaecides—they are termed antimicrobials when used in water treatment, but otherwise simply described as herbicides. Streptomycin sulfate acts by inhibiting protein synthesis; it is considered an antibacterial in human medicine, but as both a fungicide and antibacterial in agricultural use.

Compounds registered as active ingredients in some formulations may be classified as inert in others; examples include antimicrobials used in low concentrations as preservatives in fungicide, insecticide, or herbicide formulations. Petroleum oils has insecticidal properties, but when used at lower concentrations it may serve as an inert ingredient in a formulation or added to a tank mix as an adjuvant. Fumigants have broad biological activity, targeting insects, nematodes, weed seeds, and some fungi. Professional groups studying target organism resistance classify them by their mode of action as insecticides,

herbicides, or fungicides. They most clearly differ from other use categories by the combination of (1) multiple molecular targets (multisite activity) and (2) the high vapor pressures of the parent compounds (or their byproducts) compared to other most other pesticides (Table 33–9).

Adjuvants and Inert Ingredients

Adjuvants include compounds that (1) disperse the application tank mix over treated leaf surfaces, (2) increase droplet size to minimize spray drift, (3) increase penetration of the active ingredient into target plants and pest species, (4) sequester Ca^+ and Mg^+ hard water ions to minimize wear on application equipment, (5) stabilize pH in a preselected range, (6) attract target insect pests to traps containing

Table 33–9. Human and animal episodes resulting from illegal use of pesticides, identified from medical journal reports or press reports.

Year	Compound	Circumstances	Narrative
2019	Lead arsenate	Animal feed contamination	70 beef cattle exposed lead arsenate residue when contaminated storage shed converted to pasture. 14 animals had severe illness (diarrhea, paresis, ataxia, seizures); 10 of the 14 ill animals died.
2017	Aluminum phosphide	Illegal home use	Four pediatric deaths, Amarillo Texas
2008	Carbofuran, Aldicarb, Methamidophos, Chlorpyrifos	Repackaged agricultural pesticides sold in urban South Africa	Nine children poisoned between May and July 2008 associated with illegal pesticides sold in Capetown for control of rodents and other pests
2014	Carbofuran	Illegal use in marijuana cultivation	Five law enforcement officers exposed to carbofuran residue during eradication of illegal marijuana operation in Shasta County, California
2013, 2018	Sarin	Chemical agent used on civilian populations, Syria	
2000–2016	Carbofuran, methomyl, potassium cyanide	Illegal use of poison animal bait	1015 incidents, 3248 animal deaths in Greece
1998–1999	Methomyl	Methomyl contaminated salt in a commercial restaurant	107 cases 1998–1999
2000–2010	Deltamethrin	Miraculous insecticidal chalk	188 pediatric exposures reported to, Texas poison centers 2000–2010
2000–2012	Tetramine	Illegal rodenticide sold by street vendors, used in deliberate poisoning episodes	148 events, 3526 victims, including 225 fatalities.
2002	Tetramine	Illegally imported rodenticide from China	Seizures in pediatric poisoning case, residual neurological impairment
1990s	Methyl parathion	Use for home pest control in southern and midwestern United States	Scattered illnesses, extensive property damage from persistent residues resistant to decontamination
1994–1995	Sarin	Attack by cult group, Matsumoto and Tokyo	Hundreds of illnesses and scattered fatalities, exposures to medical personnel and emergency responders

pesticides, and (7) stimulate growth of pest plants to make them more vulnerable to herbicides.

Adjuvant spreading agents (fatty acid derivatives, organosilicons, and organic polymers) were the most frequently used pesticide category in California in 2016, applied an average 1.8 times annually to each acre of California cropland. Other heavily used adjuvant categories included pH modulators (acid and base compounds), glycols, and organic alcohols, acting as solubility agents called "formulation aids," and ammonium salts acting as "growth adjuvants" for herbicides.

Surfactant and Spreading Agents

The compounds that act as surfactants include petroleum distillates, vegetable oils and other plant extracts, medium chain fatty acids, fatty acid esters, and organosilicon compounds. These compounds have in common an ability to lower the surface tension of tank mixes. In concentrated form, most cause some level of irritation, akin to the model compound used in dermal irritation studies, lauryl sulfate, registered as an insect repellent active ingredient. Sodium lauryl sulfate is an ingredient in many registered adjuvant formulations.

Buffers and pH Modulators

pH modulators include organic acids and concentrated forms of sodium or calcium hydroxide. Concentrated hydrochloric acid acts as a pH modulator in chlorine water treatment systems and swimming pools. The strong inorganic acids and bases have irritant or corrosive properties, depending on the concentration and duration of contact. The organic acids are less likely to cause corrosion but may provoke irritation with prolonged exposures.

Mixer/loaders have the greatest opportunity for exposure to adjuvant active ingredients, carrier solvents, and adjuvants in concentrated form; applicators encounter the compounds in more dilute forms; and mixer/loaders handle both concentrated and dilute materials.

Although investigations typically focus principally on active ingredients, adjuvants may play a role in drift episodes where bystanders experience irritant symptoms.

Possible effect of adjuvants on toxicity or dissipation of active ingredients remains unexplored. This may prove more significant for environmental effects on invertebrates and other nontarget organisms. Slowing of dissipation for neonicotinoids, for example, might have significant effects on bees and other sensitive species.

Inert Ingredients

The U.S. EPA published a list of approved inert ingredients that can be used in pesticide formulations, replacing the list of ingredients of toxic concern and "generally recognized as safe lists" established in 1987.

Inert ingredients may include solvents and compounds with surfactant properties that overlap with the adjuvant list. As discussed earlier, many surfactants have irritant properties comparable to the "positive control" compound, lauryl sulfate, also

listed as an adjuvant ingredient. The approved list contains several organosilicon compounds commonly used in agricultural adjuvant mixtures to prevent loss of active ingredient to rain.

Other inert components include emulsifiers, solvents, carriers, aerosol propellants, fragrances, and dyes. For dry formulations, inerts can include dusts or solid carriers (eg, starch, corn cobs, citrus pulp, cracked wheat, egg solids, egg shells, walnut shells, potassium aluminum silicate, anhydrous, Fuller's earth, etc.).

Some formulations may contain isothiazoline compounds, quaternary ammonium, or other antibacterials as preservatives, typically in a concentrations that do not contribute to the intended pesticidal activity of the product (eg, below 1%). The U.S. EPA does not require disclosure of these preservative ingredients and has instituted a voluntary program for listing of fragrance ingredients. This program does not include food products used as inerts that may present concerns to sensitive individuals, including peanut oil, peanut butter, wheat gluten, alfalfa meal, and egg products.

Synergists

▶ Piperonyl Butoxide (PBO)

PBO functions by blocking insect metabolism of pyrethrin, pyrethroids, *n*-methyl carbamates, and some OPs. The California pounds sold database reports 250,086 lb of PBO for 2016, with 40,498.35 lb calculated as used for agriculture. The 502 currently registered products include technical PBO, a concentrated formulation to be used in agricultural tank mixes (PBO-8 synergist 89459- 33-aa, 91.3% of PBO [486] 8.7% of inert ingredients), and a slightly less concentrated form of PBO, pet shampoos, and other formulations for control of ectoparasites, foggers, and many ready-to-use (RTU) aerosol sprays.

PBO did not cause deaths in oral and dermal LD50 testing at the maximum doses tested, consistent with low inherent toxicity and limited absorption. Dermal absorption studies in two studies of human volunteers ranged from 2–4%. There are no reports of clinical illness occurring as a result of isolated exposure to PBO. Any illness occurring in an individual exposed to a formulation containing PBO probably is caused by another ingredient, such as allergy to pyrethrum, an effect of a carbamate or OP, or something other than the pesticide synergist.

▶ N-Octyl Bicycloheptene Dicarboximide (NOBD) (MGK 264)

NOBD functions as a synergist in a manner similar to PBO, inhibiting a different set of insects P450 metabolic enzymes. There are 508 currently registered products containing NOBD. California reported 139,921.4672 lb of NOBD sold in 2016, with calculated agricultural use of approximately 89 lb.

NOBD has low mammalian toxicity, evidenced by an oral LD50 of 2800 mg/kg in the rat, and a dermal LD50 of 470 mg/kg (HSDB).

ACTIVE INGREDIENTS BY USE CATEGORY

A complete review of all the active ingredients in each pesticide use category is beyond the scope of this chapter. The sections below focus on the most heavily used compounds, grouped by mode-of-action. Each use category contains subsections on specific laboratory measures, and compound-specific treatment measures, where appropriate. A discussion of chronic effects, including results of relevant animal tests and human case reports, case series, and epidemiologic studies is included in each section.

1. Antimicrobials

Antimicrobial pesticides include compounds used in water treatment systems and institutional and home cleaning/disinfectant products, but do not include medical or veterinary antibiotic compounds. Many have mixed uses, typified by chlorine products, commonly used as bleach and as disinfectants. Antimicrobial adjuvants include acids, bases, and other pH modifiers that also have multiple uses. To classify cases for the purpose of illness surveillance, assessment of intended product use is often necessary.

Antimicrobial sales accounted for approximately 1.5 billion pounds of active ingredient according to 2016 pesticide sales data in California. For 2015 illnesses associated with antimicrobials occurring at residences and work sites accounted for 27% of reported cases in California.

Pesticidal antimicrobials show less variation than medical antibiotics and most other pesticide use categories in terms of mode of action (as discussed below). Many have multiple biological targets and others primarily target antimicrobial membrane stability.

Antimicrobials With Nonselective Modes of Action

Halide compounds accounted for 91% of the antimicrobial sales, with sites of use ranging from industrial water systems, swimming pools, and health care institutions, to home residences. Chlorine and other halides have multiple biological sites of action targets and were frequent causes of illness related to eye, skin, or respiratory illness (see following case summary). Other compounds with multiple sites of action include alcohols, aldehydes, halides, alkyl epoxides, thiocarbamates, metal ions, and organotin compounds.

The nonselective antimicrobials have moderate to low acute systemic toxicity despite their chemical reactivity, the most toxic being the quaternary ammonium compounds (Table 33–10). Most antimicrobials have the capacity to cause acute irritant symptoms of the eyes, skin, and respiratory tract.

Other nonselective antimicrobial categories included inorganic acids and bases, phenols, and peroxides. Per literature reports, isothiazolone compounds used as industrial preservatives have been among the most problematic, causing both irritant and allergic symptoms.

Table 33–10. Mammalian toxicity for selected antimicrobial compounds.

Compounds	Oral LD50 mg/kg, species	Dermal LD50 mg/kg, species
Nonselective Mode of Action		
Sodium hypochlorite	5800	Not found
Sodium dichloro-s-triazinetrione	1670	> 10,000
Isopropyl alcohol	4710	12,870
Membrane effects—membrane destabilizers		
Quaternary ammonium–didecyl dimethyl ammonium chloride	84–331	4350
Ortho-phenylphenol	591	> 5000

Antibacterials That Affect Membrane Stability

Partially selective compounds targeting bacterial membranes (quaternary ammonium, biguanides, phenols, and peroxides) also provoke irritant symptoms. They have low systemic toxicity. Some biologicals (eg, the bacterial phage used to treat Pseudomonas syringae pv. tomato infection) have biologic specific effects on membranes. Biological oils containing abietic acid (pine oil or tall oil) also have membrane effects, acting like surfactants or soaps to disrupt bacterial membranes. Based on available information they cause a limited degree of irritation but do have the potential to cause sensitization.

Streptomycin sulfate salt acts on both fungi and bacteria by binding to ribosomes, blocking protein synthesis. It thus differs in mechanism from both the multisite and membrane-active disinfectants.

Both the membrane-active and the multisite activity compounds have been used for many years. Compared to the insecticides, herbicides, and fungicides, relatively few new antimicrobial active ingredients have been registered in recent years.

Potential Persistent Sequelae of Antimicrobial Exposure

Respiratory reactions to antibacterials occur commonly in workers doing janitorial and housekeeping work, most commonly as the result of prolonged respiratory irritation.

Isothiazolone compounds may cause sensitization as well as irritation. Concerns include their use as preservative "inerts"; as well their use in high concentrations as industrial preservatives. Multiple case reports have documented the association of isothiazolines with ACD from cutting oils. More recent reports have documented allergy with isothiazolines used as preservatives in cosmetics (in concentrations similar to those used in pesticide formulations).

Aromatic phenols, including para-tert-amylphenol, have been associated with cases of leukoderma, also known as occupational vitiligo. This may be a secondary effect of sensitization, given the low incidence of reported cases, and the observation that localized depigmentation sometimes occurs as the sequalae of a positive dermal patch test.

2. Insecticides

Sodium Channel Modulators & Blockers

▶ **Pyrethroids**

Among agricultural insecticides, pyrethroids accounted for the greatest number of acres treated, approximately 20% of California cropland. However, because of comparatively low application rates, they ranked behind the petroleum distillates and cholinesterase inhibitors in pounds used.

Pyrethroids and other insecticides have also supplanted the use of cholinesterase inhibitors for structural and residential pest control. In RTU home mixtures, pyrethroids or synthetic pyrethroids may accompany newer compounds—neo-nicotinoids or compounds that affect lipid synthesis, insect development, or energy metabolism. Many also contain PBO, a synergist that blocks the metabolism of pyrethroids and other insecticides, as discussed below.

Pyrethrum is a partially refined extract of the chrysanthemum flower, containing active compounds known *as pyrethrins* (pyrethrin I and pyrethrin II) and sesquiterpene lactone contaminants, long been recognized to cause allergies. It has not been used in a registered product in California since 1988, while 488 current products contained refined pyrethrins.

Synthetic pyrethroids differ from natural pyrethroids in their resistance to metabolism and their comparatively long physiologic and environmental half-lives.

A. Acute Toxicity

In rodent acute toxicity tests, pyrethrin mixtures demonstrate remarkable variability in effect, but most mixtures have oral $LD_{50}S$ greater than 1000 mg/kg. Pyrethrum and pyrethrin mixtures do not cause systemic toxicity on dermal application (Table 33–11).

Synthetic pyrethroids structurally resemble pyrethrins, with modifications that increase both toxicity and stability. Between two subtypes of synthetic pyrethroids, designated as type I and type II (cyanohalogen) compounds, the latter generally demonstrate greater toxicity. Animal studies also demonstrate some differential age-related toxicity of type II pyrethroids.

Deltamethrin, for example, has an LD_{50} of 5.1 for 11-day-old male rats versus 81 mg/kg for 72-day-old male rats. Because of this possible increased susceptibility, illegally imported pyrethroid chalk products (containing deltamethrin), resembling a form of hard candy, pose a risk of systemic poisoning in children. A published case report describes poisoning of a 4-year-old child with a deltamethrin chalk at an estimated dose of 2 mg/kg.

The pyrethrins and pyrethroids are absorbed from the gastrointestinal (GI) tract and hydrolyzed in the gut and tissues, and excreted rapidly. They are very slowly absorbed from the skin.

Pyrethroids function principally by excitation of the sodium channels in the nervous system. Because they stimulate superficial nerves in the dermis and upper respiratory tract, they produce symptoms at the site of contact. Data on acute toxicity in animals show moderate oral toxicity and very low systemic toxicity following skin contact (Table 33–11).

Skin contact with pyrethrins or synthetic pyrethroids produces paresthesia at the site of contact, often without visible rash. A transient rash may occur in some instances, possibly related to petroleum distillates present in RTU formulation.

Respiratory symptoms include irritation in the upper respiratory tract and stimulation of nasal secretions, resembling allergic rhinitis. In patients with preexisting asthma, lower respiratory symptoms may be significant.

Nonspecific systemic symptoms, such as nausea, headache, or dizziness, may be present in some cases. Because the metabolic half-life of absorbed pyrethroids is short, the time of course of systemic and respiratory effects resembles carbamate poisoning—it is expected to resolve in hours or days. Skin symptoms may be unpredictably persistent. It may be difficult to distinguish the effects of reexposure to surface residues of active ingredient from the effect of partially absorbed pyrethroid in the dermis.

Treatment of ingestions may require a period of hospital observation depending on the quantity ingested. In a pediatric ingestion case involving deltamethrin, transient central nervous system (CNS) symptoms occurred, but recovery was rapid following gastric decontamination. As stated above, the overall time course is comparable with that of acute carbamate intoxication.

B. Differential Diagnosis

Amphetamine, cocaine, and other stimulants may produce paresthesias similar to those associated with pyrethroids. Some common chronic diseases may have a similar effect, including Parkinson's disease, diabetic neuropathy, shingles, anxiety, fibromyalgia, and schizophrenia. With a history of recent contact with pyrethroids, the diagnosis is not complex. The sodium channel blockers, such as indoxacarb, produce numbness rather than the paresthesia associated with the sodium channel modulators. Some patients describe numbness after contact with pyrethroids, possibly related to nerve fatigue after the initial symptoms produced by nerve stimulation.

Paresthesias may also occur with common peripheral neuropathies; these occur regionally in the distribution of the affected nerve. Paresthesias from pyrethroids occur at the site of contact, although systemic paresthesias may occur in ingestion cases.

Hypersecretion from the nose caused by pyrethroids may strongly resemble that associated with allergic rhinitis or upper respiratory infections.

Systemic symptoms are nonspecific and not readily recognized as due to pyrethroids without a history of exposure.

Table 33–11. Insecticide mammalian toxicity values.

Compounds	CAS	Oral LD50 mg/kg, species	Dermal LD50 mg/kg, species
Pyrethrins, Type I and Type II Pyrethroids, and Other Sodium Channel Modulators			
Natural pyrethrins	121-21-1	260–960, rat	Very low
Type I Pyrethroids			
Permethrin	52645-53-1	430–4000	> 4000
Resmethrin	10453-86-8	1244–2500	> 3000
Cypermethrin	52315-07-8	250	< 2000
Type II (cyano-pyrethroids)			
Esfenvalerate	66230–04-4	458	2500
Cyfluthrin	68359-37-5, 85782-82-7	869–1271	> 5000
Deltamethrin	52918-63-5	128	> 2000
DDT-like Organochlorines			
DDT	50-29-3	113– 800 in rats	2500–3000 female rats
Methoxychlor	72-43-5	5000–6000 rats	> 28000 rats
Dicofol	115-32-2	575–960 rats	1000–5000 rats
Voltage-Dependent Sodium Channel Blocker			
Indoxacarb	173584-44-6	1732 male rats, 268 female rats	> 5000
Metaflumizone	139968-49-3	> 5000	> 5000
Synergist for Pyrethrins, Pyrethroids, *N*-Methyl Carbamates, and Organophosphates			
Piperonyl butoxide	51-03-6	> 4 g/kg male; > 7g/kg (female)	> 2g/kg
Neonicotinoids			
Acetamiprid	135410-20-7	146	146
Clothianidin	205510-53-8 210880-92-5	389, ♂mouse	> 2000
Imidacloprid	105827-78-9	410 (rat) 35 (mouse)	> 5000
Thiamethoxam	153719-23-4	1563	> 2000
Flonicamid	158062-67-0	884, ♂ rat	> 5000
Dinotefuran	165252-70-0	2000, ♀ rat	> 2000
Ryanodine Receptor Compounds			
Chlorantraniliprole	500008-45-7	3738	> 2000
Flubendiamide	272451-65-7	> 5000	> 2000
Cyantraniliprole	736994-63-1	> 5000	> 5000
Category I: Organophosphates and Carbamates			
Phorate	298-02-2	20–30	400
Ethoprop	13194-48-4	30–56	60

(continued)

Table 33–11. Insecticide mammalian toxicity values. (Continued)

Compounds	CAS	Oral LD50 mg/kg, species	Dermal LD50 mg/kg, species
Methomyl*	16752-77-5	15–25	1000
Dichlorvos (DDVP)	62-73-7	20–30	50–100
Category II: Organophosphates			
Chlorpyrifos	2921-88-2	50–150	2000
Diazinon	333-41-5	50–150	400
Phosmet	732-11-6	50–150	3000
Propoxur	114-26-1	100	1000
Dimethoate	60-51-5	150–500	150
Naled	300-76-5	150–500	1000
Acephate	30560-19-1	500–1000	2000
Carbaryl	63-25-2	300–600	2000
Categories III and IV Organophosphates			
Malathion	121-75-5	500–1000	4000
Tetrachlorvinphos	22248-79-9	1000–5000	5000
Spinosyns, AChR Compounds			
Spinosad A	131929-60-7	3738	> 2000
Spinetoram	187166-40-1, 187166-15-0	> 5000	> 2000
Avermectins, Glutamate Chloride Channel Compounds			
Avermectin B1a, B1b (agonist); abamectin	71751-41-2	Rat, 10; Mouse 13.6	> 2000
Fipronil (antagonist)	120068-37-3	92, 97	> 5000
Acetyl CoA Carboxylase Inhibitors, Lipid Synthesis, Growth Regulation, Tetronic Acid Derivatives			
Spirotetramat	203313-25-1	> 2000	Not found
Spirodiclofen	148477-71-8	> 2500	> 2000
Spiromesifen	283594-90-1	> 2500	> 2000
Inhibitors of Mitochondrial ATP Synthase			
Propargite	2312-35-8	2636	> 2000
Fenbutatin oxide	13356-08-6	2631	> 2000
Chitin Synthesis Inhibitors			
Diflubenzuron	35367-38-5	4640	> 2000
Novaluron	116714-46-6	> 5000	> 2000

C. Safety Issues

Foggers containing pyrethroid and pyrethrin mixtu... commonly used to control widespread household in... infestations. Sold as RTU devices, the products are ofte... used by renters or homeowners.

Propellants in the devices are typically propane or another form of flammable gas. Application or overapplication of foggers without extinguishing pilot lights or other home ignition sources can result in fires or explosions. Most do not result in pyrethroid illnesses in either householders or first responders. This may relate to decomposition of the active ingredients in the fires caused by the flammable propellants. Most of these events consequently do not appear in pesticide illness reports, but can be easily tracked from online press reports.

▶ Other Compounds Affecting the Sodium Channel

A. Indoxacarb

Indoxacarb, an active ingredient first registered in 2001, blocks voltage-dependent sodium channels, poisoning insects following ingestion or external contact. It has 30 active registrations, principally for home use, but including concentrated formulations intended for agricultural use. Total reported sales in California for 2016 amounted to 72,446 lb, with an estimated 32,050 lb reported as agricultural use. Crops treated with more than 1000 lb of indoxacarb included alfalfa (18,060 lb), broccoli (1619 lb), cotton (3763 lb), nectarine (1109 lb), and peaches (1446 lb).

1. Mammalian toxicity

Table 33–11 shows category II toxicity in a feeding study for female rats and category III toxicity for male rats. The dermal LD50, based on a limit test, was reported as more than 5000 mg/kg (the highest dose tested).

2. Illness Data

Between 1992 and 2015, the California pesticide illness surveillance program showed 13 reports with indoxacarb identified as the only implicated pesticide. These included a 2005 Fresno County drift episode associated with five cases (with a mixture of numbness or itching at the apparent site of contact, and nonspecific systemic symptoms [nausea, headache, and dizziness]).

Eye or skin irritation and nonspecific systemic symptoms occurred in several of the eight noncluster illnesses. One noncluster illness had symptoms (bloody diarrhea) suggesting a possible misclassified case of bacterial gastroenteritis.

3. Ingestion cases

Published reports from India and China described ingestion of indoxacarb associated with methemoglobinemia, seizures, renal failure, adult respiratory distress syndrome (ARDS), and peripheral neuropathy.

B. Metaflumizone

...etaflumizone shares a common mechanism with indoxa... blocking the sodium channel modulated by the pyre... s and the DDT-like organochlorine compounds.

Th...rmation

mizo... California...rrently registered formulations of metaflu... on 237,18...baits. 2016 sales data showed 498 lb sold in accounted fo...UR data reported 219 lb, 3,342 applications 227180.28 treat...agricultural land. Application to almonds mizone as the only... (95%), 3,000 applications (90%), and California illness surv...ed (96%). No illnesses with metaflu... 2015, the most recent yea...e pesticide were reported to the ...reprogram between 1992 and ... available information.

5. Ingestion cases

A 2014 report also described a cas...f methemoglobinemia associated with metaflumizone, re...mbling ingestion of indoxacarb case described above.

▶ DDT-like Organochlorines

DDT and the 2 hydroxy-substituted organochlorines dicofol and methoxychlor have low to moderate oral toxicity in mammals and very low dermal toxicity (Table 33–11). They interact with the same sodium channel receptor affected by the pyrethroids, but have different pharmacokinetic, metabolic, and environmental properties. The commonly used dust formulations of DDT, for example, did not produce topical paresthesias, but facial paresthesia could occur as a prominent feature of systemic poisonings. It is unknown whether DDT dissolved in organic solvents could penetrate the skin sufficiently to produce pyrethroid-like topical symptoms.

Most notably, they persist in the environment and accumulate in many food chains. Dicofol has a soil half-life of 16 days, methoxychlor a soil half-life of more than 6 months, and DDT a soil half-life of 2–15 years.

None of the three compounds have current registered formulations. DDT has no formulations listed in current registration databases in California; methoxychlor (135 inactive formulations) was last registered 12/31/2000; and dicofol (130 inactive formulations), was last registered 12/31/2010.

Current health concerns for DDT and related compounds focus on chronic health effects (discussed later).

Active Ingredients Acting as Mechanical Asphyxiants—Insecticidal Petroleum Oils & Biological Oils

Oils used as pesticides have a long history, acting as alternatives to synthetic insecticides and fungicides. Petroleum oils rank second to pyrethroids in number of agricultural acres treated, applied to 3,334,468 acres, approximately 12% of California crop land. Related to their suspected mode of action (thought to act by mechanically disrupting gas exchan coating treated surfaces) petroleum oils have an app rate of more than 10 lb/acre. Consequently, they among insecticides in terms of pounds applied; 3,3 2016 for petroleum oil and mineral oil combined

▶ Symptom Pattern

Crop oils used as insecticides have ir~ ~erties like other petroleum distillates. It may pr~ ~at produced by guish the irritation crop oils produc~ ~nd irritation pro- petroleum distillates used as adj~ ~same tank mixture. duced by other active ingredients

▶ Illness Data

In the 583 cases reported~ ~the California illness registry between 1992 and 2015~ ~ated exposure to petroleum oils, petroleum distillates, ~etroleum hydrocarbon accounted for 14 cases. Mixed ~posures with petroleum compounds and other active i~redients accounted for 583 cases. The other active in~edients in mixed exposure cases included OP and carbamate ChE inhibitors, pyrethroids, boric acid, abamectin, and occasionally fungicides (copper salts, chloro-thalonil, and azoxystrobin).

Common symptom patterns for the 13 cases with a petro-leum product as the only implicated pesticide included skin irritation and conjunctivitis, occurring after direct accidental exposure in pesticide handlers. Nausea, headache, and respi-ratory irritation abdominal pain occurred in some cases.

CASE EXAMPLES

1. Using a closed loading system, a worker loaded dormant oil into a spray tank. Air in the oil metering device hose line caused the oil to squirt into the worker's unprotected right eye.

   Reported medical findings: injected conjunctiva of right eye.

2. A mixer/loader contaminated his right hand and arm while measuring oil in a 5-gallon bucket. He developed itching that began in the exposed area, then spread over his body; he first noticed a rash in the evening after work.

   Reported medical findings: scattered itchy hives on the arms, legs, chest, and back.

Acetylcholine Receptor (ACHR) Competitive Agonists—Neonicotinoid Insecticides, Spinosyns, & Nereistoxin Analogues

▶ Mode of Action

ACHR-nicotine competitive agonists and allosteric modulators include neonicotinoid compounds and nereistoxin analogues (both somewhat closely resembling the natural insecticide nico-tine) and the complex multiring lactone/macrolide spinosyn compounds. Based on studies with radiolabeled ligands, each

~ne three groups of compounds affect distinct bindings sites. ~heir differential toxicity depends on their selectivity for bind-ing to insect (as opposed to mammalian) nicotinic receptors.

A. Neonicotinoid Insecticides and Spinosyns

Neonicotinoids and spinosyns affect a broad variety of pests; for spinosads these include coleoptera (beetles), lepidoptera (moths and butterflies), homoptera (aphids, psyllids, white fly, scale), and true insects. Neonicotinoids affect coleoptera, homoptera, thysanoptera, true insects, and diptera (flies). The nereistoxin analogues selectively target aphids and other sucking insects.

1. Use data

The neonicotinoids and spinosyns were applied to slightly more than 20% of California cropland in 2016. There was no reported use of the nereistoxin analogues in 2016.

2. Mammalian toxicity studies

Many neonicotinoids have oral LD_{50}s in category 2 or cat-egory 3 range, but have very low dermal toxicity and inhala-tion toxicity.

3. Illness data

Texas 2014 poison center neonicotinoid data included 1142 reports from the use of imidacloprid and dinotefuran (in pet care products and in agriculture). Ninety-seven percent were unintentional, although ingestions accounted for slightly more than half of the cases; the remaining cases involved skin or eye exposures. Few cases required referral for medi-cal treatment.

Between 1996 and 2015, 36 neonicotinoid cases (imida-cloprid, acetamiprid, and dinotefuran) were reported to the California illness registry, including episodes of drift, dermal and eye exposure, and ingestion. The outcomes resembled those described in a 2014 Texas poison control series.

Recently reported 68 cases from Sri Lanka included 61 deliberate ingestion cases and 7 dermal exposures. Typical patients developed mild symptoms (nausea, vomiting, head-ache, and diarrhea), but one case required mechanical ven-tilation and another experienced a long period of sedation. Median blood imidacloprid level at admission was 10.58 ng/L.

In a series of 70 cases reported from China, 60 had mild to moderate symptoms, 8 had severe nonfatal poisonings, and 2 patients died. In a 2001 nonfatal imidacloprid ingestion case, symptoms included drowsiness, disorientation, dizziness, oral and gastroesophageal erosions, hemorrhagic gastritis, produc-tive cough, fever, leukocytosis, and hyperglycemia. The for-mulation solvent could have provoked the sedation and the surfactant component might have caused the GI irritation.

D. Environmental fate, dissipation

Neonicotinoids have low vapor pressures and do not dis-sipate by evaporation, potentially resulting in long environ-mental dissipation times. Imidacloprid, for example, has a soil half-life of 26.5–229 days, depending on temperature, pH, environmental moisture, and incorporation into layers of soil where no photolysis occurs. For acetamiprid the reported soil half-life is 1–8 days in soil and 34 days in aqueous solution when degradation takes place solely by photolysis. The soil half-life of clothianidin is extraordinarily long, more than 1000 days, but residues close to surface have a photolysis half-life of 34 days. The aqueous anaerobic half-life is 27 days.

B. Spinosyns

The gram-positive soil bacterium *Saccharopolyspora spinosa* (an *Actinomycetes* species) produces a macrolide (multiring lactone) compound called spinosad, a mixture of spinosyn A, spinosyn D, and smaller amounts of other compounds. It has a complex mode of action: It interacts with the insect nicotinic receptors, but also interacts with gamma-aminobutyric acid (GABA) receptors similar to abamectin. The effect is relatively specific to insects and its mammalian toxicity is low by both the oral and dermal routes.

A. Illnesses related to spinosyns

In rodent toxicity testing, both spinosad and spinetoram show minimal toxicity. Eye irritation has been identified as the most common side effect.

The California illness registry showed three cases involving direct exposure to Spinosad between 1992 and 2015, two involving eye irritation after a direct exposure to an applicator and a field worker. Another involved an accidental ingestion of Spinosad containing liquid stored in a water bottle, associated with transient numbness in the face.

No fatal human ingestions could be found searching medical literature databases. Ingestion of a mixture of spinosamid and flonicamid (LD 50 1768 mg/kg in female rats, 884 mg/kg in male rats) in an 80-year-old woman caused altered consciousness, shock, respiratory failure, pneumonitis, and urinary retention. Endoscopy showed a corrosive esophageal injury. The authors attributed the patient illness to the spinosad, but acknowledged the possible role of flonicamid and undisclosed formulation solvents.

Glutamate-Gated Chloride Channel Agonists, Stimulating GABA Pathways

The glutamate-gated chloride channel agonists stimulate the inhibitory GABA pathways in the nervous system. They include the biologically derived avermectin, the phenylpyrazole compound fipronil, and the no-longer-registered cyclodiene organochlorine compounds.

Fipronil is principally used for structural pest control; the avermectins have use in home use products, and both veterinary and human medicine. Their agricultural use encompassed 9.0% of California cropland.

▶ Avermectins

Abamectin is a mixture of two complex compounds, byproducts of a bacterium found in soil called *Streptomyces avermitilis*. The two avermectin compounds B1a and B1b differ very slightly from each other in chemical structure, an ethyl group in B1a versus a methyl group in B1b at the substituent labeled R in the complex molecule of a class described as a macrocyclic lactone. Its molecular weight is 873, 50% larger than the aminoglycoside antibiotic streptomycin produced by the species *Streptomyces griseus*. It consequently has a very low solubility in both water and organic solvents. Avermectins act by stimulation of GABA receptors in the insect nervous system.

Avermectin's oral LD50 demonstrates its potentially high mammalian toxicity once absorbed. It has a low dermal toxicity, probably related to slow absorption. Cases of accidental direct exposure to abamectin typically involved eye or skin irritation. Ingestion of abamectin can produce overt systemic poisoning with symptoms of altered mental status, respiratory failure, and hypotension.

▶ Fipronil

Fipronil is a phenylpyrazole compound, an antagonist that binds to the GABA channel, and produced overstimulation of the nervous system because of the absence of the GABA-associated inhibitory activity.

A. Mammalian Toxicity

It has moderate mammalian oral toxicity, but its dermal absorption is very slow.

There are 75 currently registered fipronil products, including multiple products for control of ectoparasites on pets. Fipronil has been used extensively in Europe, Asia, and elsewhere as an agricultural insecticide, with applications as a seed treatment for corn, cotton, wheat, and other crops.

B. Ecological Effects

Fipronil has high toxicity for termites, bees, ants, and other colony insects, typified by the very low LD_{50} for bees (LD_{50} = 0.004 mcg/bee). This has led to concerns about fipronil's use as an agricultural insecticide. Regulatory action to date has included a temporary ban in France after hive losses in the southwest region of the country in 2003, and a limited ban in China in 2009. In Madagascar, two species of lizard and an endemic mammal declined because termites form part of their food chain.

C. Illness Data

Acute illness cases reported in the United States mostly occurred in residential settings (ant or roach baits or treatments for pets). One occupational case suffered a brief seizure, blurred vision, and dizziness after doing an application with minimal protective equipment. Another applicator required 7 days of hospitalization for dyspnea, diaphoresis, tremor, paresthesia, and slurred speech while applying the 80% termite control formulation of fipronil.

Ryanodine Receptor Modulators

Ryanodine receptor insecticides stimulate a calcium channel in the sarcoplasmic reticulum of muscle cells and a similar channel in the endoplasmic reticulum of other cells. The model compound is ryanodine, an insecticidal compound found in the South American plant *Ryania speciosa*. At low ryanodine concentrations the calcium channel is partially open, stimulating muscle action, but the channel is closed at high concentrations. Ryanodine receptors are present in cardiac muscle and in the cardiac conduction pathways, suggest possible mammalian cardiac effects, at least at high doses. The ryanodine receptor antagonist dantrolene, used to treat malignant hyperthermia, for example, has a dose-dependent negative inotropic effect in animal studies.

▶ Use Data

Use of the three currently registered ryanodine receptor modulators (flubendiamide, chlorantraniliprole, and cyantraniliprole) encompassed 7.5% of California agricultural acreage. The ryanodine receptor compounds particularly target lepidopteran sucking pests.

▶ Mammalian Toxicity

The ryanodine receptor is present in mammals, but the insecticidal ryanodine compounds are highly selective for insect ryanodine receptors. This is reflected in the low systemic toxicity of the synthetic ryanodine compounds. A 2014 study of the subacute effects of flubendiamide showed minor changes in hematologic indices but no other systemic effects.

▶ Illness Data

The California illness registry did not contain any reports of illness associated with any ryanodine receptor compound identified as the only implicated pesticide between 1992 and 2015.

▶ Published Reports

A 2016 report from India described an intentional overdose in a 26-year-old woman who ingested 10 cc of a chlorantraniliprole containing insecticide. She initially had normal vital signs and a normal physical examination and normal laboratory findings. During observation she developed intermittently dropped P waves on her ECG (with a rate of 58/min).

While complaining of dizziness, her systolic blood pressure subsequently dropped from 120 to 90 mm Hg. Her ECG showed a Mobitz Type I atrioventricular (AV) block—a progressively prolonged PR interval—followed by a dropped P wave. The rhythm disturbance responded to atropine and placement of a temporary pacemaker. At 48 hours, she had a completely normal cardiogram and it was possible to remove the pacemaker.

Organophosphate & Carbamate Cholinesterase-Inhibiting Insecticides

OPs are esters of phosphoric acid that exist in two forms: thion and oxon. Potency depends on the three-dimensional shape of individual compounds and their ability to bind with the cholinesterase molecule. Irreversible binding occurs with a serine molecule in the heart of the enzyme's active site and the nonphosphate portion of the molecule (leaving group) cleaved by hydrolysis. Under most circumstances, the inhibition becomes irreversible after 24–48 hours.

Carbamates are esters of carbamic acid. The OPs and *N*-methyl carbamates are considered here a single class because they share a common mechanism of acute toxicity cholinesterase inhibition, with similar signs and symptoms of acute poisoning. Carbamates differ in causing reversible rather than irreversible cholinesterase inhibition and typically have a short clinical course. The thiocarbamates and dithiocarbamates do not inhibit cholinesterase, but many have activity against plants and fungi.

OPs and carbamates are absorbed easily by inhalation, skin contact, and ingestion; the primary route of occupational exposure is dermal. They differ from one another in lipid solubility and therefore distribution in the body, particularly to the CNS.

Many commercial OPs are applied in the thion (sulfur-containing) form but readily undergo conversion to the oxon (oxygen-containing) form. Most of the oxon forms have much greater toxicity than their corresponding thion analogues. The conversion occurs in the environment, so the residues to which crop field workers are exposed may be more toxic than the pesticide that was applied. Some of the sulfur is released in the form of mercaptans, which produce the typical odor of the thion form of OPs. The mercaptans have very low odor thresholds, and the reactions to their noxious odor, including headache, nausea, and vomiting, often are mistaken for acute OP poisoning.

▶ Use Information

Organophosphate pesticides began replacing arsenic and other inorganic pesticides and organochlorines as the principal insecticides used in agriculture in the 1950s and 1960s. Mevinphos and ethyl parathion, two of the most toxic organophosphates, were prohibited from use in the United States during the 1990s. Subsequent to passage of the Food Quality Protection Act (FQPA), organophosphates have been replaced by pyrethroids for termiticide applications and for crops destined to be used in processed foods. Registrations of many category I (signal word "Danger") organophosphates have lapsed. Phorate and ethoprop, used as nematicides, still have active registrations. The number of active formulated products for still-registered active ingredients has also decreased. Malathion, for example, has 15 currently registered formulations and 469 formulations with inactive registrations; diazinon currently has 8 active and 934 inactive registered formulations.

California 2016 use reporting showed 4,336,145 lb used on 3,261,474 acres (12% of California cropland).

▶ Application Methods

Organophosphates and carbamates are applied by a variety of techniques from aerial spraying to hand application.

Granular and bait formulations significantly reduce exposure so that even highly toxic compounds such as aldicarb (0.5 mg/kg) can be used safely given proper precautions.

▶ Residue Dissipation

Organophosphate compounds show variable dissipation times. Compounds with high vapor pressures, including dichlorvos, naled, and mevinphos, have environmental half-lives measured in hours and may dissipate completely in less than 24 hours. Residues of dimethoate (LD_{50} 180–330 mg/kg) have an environmental half-life ranging from 24 to 48 hours. Phosalone (LD_{50} 82–205 mg/kg) residues, by contrast, have half-lives of 30 days or longer. Many organophosphates degrade rapidly in wet coastal environments but may be persistent for prolonged periods in hot, dry climates. Consequently, long reentry intervals (eg, 90 days or more for ethyl parathion on citrus crops) have proved necessary to prevent acute poisoning of field workers.

The risk posed by a given level of residue depends on the crop and work activity. Residues of 7 mcg/cm² of phosalone, for example, cause no cholinesterase inhibition in workers picking citrus and peaches. Levels less than 1 mcg/cm² are associated with poisoning of workers harvesting wine and raisin grapes. A dermal residue transfer coefficient (in units of cm²/h) is used to summarize the relative levels of exposure associated with various agricultural tasks. Among various hand-harvested crops, transfer factors ranged from 5000 to 9000 cm²/h for row crops to 10,000 cm²/h for orchard crops and up to 130,000 cm²/h for hand-labor tasks (cane turning) in production of table grapes. The concept of a transfer coefficient is a useful generalization, but in practice the rate of transfer may vary considerably between fields planted with the same crop.

The available literature contains comparatively few studies on dissipation of carbamate compounds. Environmental fate data required by the U.S. EPA include basic physical and chemical properties such as the Henry law constant, vapor pressure, water solubility, ultraviolet spectra, and residue data at the time of harvest but not residue dissipation studies.

For propoxur, residual systemic activity has been reported for up to 1 month. Data on carbaryl do not give a half-life but indicate that residues generally dissipate in less than 2 weeks. The half-life of carbofuran leaf residue is reported as longer than 4 days. Aldicarb presents a complicated picture because of its tendency to leach into groundwater. Plants convert aldicarb to systemic sulfoxide and sulfone transformation products, previously associated with episodes of consumer poisoning from watermelons and cucumbers.

Variability in dissipation observed in extensive studies on methomyl suggests the need for caution in generalizing from limited data. A study in California established a 0.1 mcg/cm² safe-level for hand labor in methomyl-treated vineyards after an illness episode. Residue monitoring later revealed much longer dissipation times. It was therefore necessary to adjust the hand labor reentry interval from 7 to 21 days.

▶ Mammalian Toxicity

Table 33–11 lists currently commonly used compounds according to acute toxicity. They vary widely in their cholinesterase-inhibiting potency, as reflected in their LD_{50} values. The remaining category I compounds include two compounds with specialized use as a nematicides (ethoprop and phorate).

▶ Acute Effects

Recognition of acute cholinergic symptoms remains essential to recognizing unexpected exposure to cholinesterase inhibitors. The distinctive pattern of symptoms has allowed recognition of intentional self-poisoning, forensic poisoning cases, attacks of nerve gas exposures, and acute occupational illnesses. Laboratory testing serves to confirm diagnosis, usually after the fact, with a cholinesterase test sent to a reference lab, unless the treating facility has a lab capable of doing a "stat" test.

The commonly used mnemonic, Miosis Urination Diaphoresis Diarrhea Lacrimation Excitation (of skeletal muscle or Central Nervous System) and Salivation (MUDDLES), principally describes overstimulation of the muscarinic subset of the cholinergic nervous system, reversible following administration of atropine. Nonmuscarinic signs in the mnemonic are nicotinic muscle fasciculations and CNS excitation; bradycardia is a key muscarinic sign not included in MUDDLES mnemonic.

Table 33–12 shows in detail the distribution of cholinergic receptors in the sympathetic, parasympathetic, musculoskeletal system, and peripheral nervous systems.

In cases of gradual onset occupational poisoning, only nonspecific symptoms occur. Coworkers with similar exposures may have asymptomatic cholinesterase inhibition.

▶ Cardiac Rhythm Disturbances

Cardiac arrhythmias, such as bradycardia and heart block and cardiac arrest, are less common causes of death. Ventricular arrhythmias have been observed in some of these cases, including torsade de pointes arrhythmias, associated with prolongation of the QT interval. Medications affecting the QT interval (eg, use of ondansetron for treatment of nausea) should probably therefore be avoided.

Atrial fibrillation has been reported in cases of both carbamate and organophosphate poisoning.

During the 1995 terrorist attack on Tokyo using the OP nerve agent sarin, a case of coronary spasm was observed in the precordial ECG leads, attributed to the direct effect of acetylcholine on coronary nicotinic receptors. Atherosclerotic compromise of the coronary circulation was excluded by a thallium exercise study after successful treatment of the acute poisoning.

▶ Skin Effects

Organophosphates generally have high octanol/water partition coefficients and high dermal absorption rates, but most

Table 33–12. Signs and symptoms of acute organophosphate poisoning by site of acetylcholine neurotransmitter activity.

System	Receptor Type	Organ	Action	Sign or Symptom
Para-sympathetic	Muscarinic	Eye, iris muscle, ciliary muscle	Contraction	Miosis, blurred vision
		Respiratory	Smooth muscle contraction, increased respiratory secretion	Wheezing, dyspnea
		Cardiac	Stimulation of vagus nerve	Bradycardia, arrhythmias, heart block
		Intestinal tract	Smooth muscle contraction, increased intestinal secretion	Vomiting, diarrhea, muscle cramps
		Glands: lacrimal, salivary	Secretion	Tearing, salivation, bronchorrhea, pulmonary edema, nausea, vomiting
		Bladder, fundus, sphincter	Contraction, relaxation	Urination, incontinence
Neuromuscular	Nicotinic	Skeletal	Excitation	Fasciculations, cramps, followed by weakness, loss of reflexes, paralysis
Central nervous		Brain	Excitation (early)	Headache, dizziness, malaise, apprehension, confusion, hallucinations, manic or bizarre behavior, convulsions
			Depression (late)	Depression of, then loss of, consciousness; respiratory depression

cause minimal skin irritation. Skin effects are derived from the reactivity of the nonphosphate portion (termed the *leaving group*) of individual compounds. For example, the irritant compounds dichlorvos and naled both have reactive halogen atoms in their leaving groups. Dichlorvos also has an unconjugated carbon-carbon bond. Some organophosphate formulations produce transient irritation in the Draize assay, including acephate, diazinon, dimethoate, malathion, methamidophos, methidathion, oxydemeton-methyl, phosmet, and sulfotep; many cause mild primary irritation in the challenge (epicutaneous) phase of the guinea pig maximization test. Clinically, acute irritation with these compounds occurs most frequently with accidental direct exposure to pesticide handlers (mixer/loader/applicators). These types of exposures also may provoke systemic effects; in cases of organophosphate-associated dermatitis reported from Japan, approximately 25% had at least mild coincident symptoms of systemic poisoning. Systemic poisoning also was reported in a US case of irritant dermatitis caused by dichlorvos.

Buehler (epicutaneous) sensitization assays show negative findings for acephate, chlorpyrifos, dimethoate, malathion, methamidophos, methidathion, and phosmet. Nevertheless, several are sensitizers in the guinea pig maximization test (induction of allergy by subcutaneous injection), including diazinon, fenitrothion, and methidathion. Cases of possible contact sensitivity to organophosphates have been reported for omethoate and dimethoate. A case-control study of dermatitis in farmers identified allergic reactions to malathion

and oxydemeton-methyl, as well as the carbamate compounds carbofuran and carbaryl. Further studies identified ACD caused by malathion and naled, but the patch testing conducted did not meet current standards, especially with regard to identifying nonirritant concentrations for the patch procedure.

A case report from Australia identified an isomer and contaminant of diazinon called *isodiazinon* (2-isopropyl-6-methyl-4-*S*-pyrimidinyl diethylthiophosphate) as a possible cause of porphyria cutanea tarda in a sheep rancher. Investigation in a rat study showed that isodiazinon affected porphyrin synthesis by inhibiting the liver enzyme ferrochelatase.

Other noncontact reactions include a case of erythema multiforme associated with indoor use of methyl parathion; a contact reaction to ethyl parathion resembling Erysipeloid; and a case of systemic organophosphate poisoning.

▶ **Differential Diagnosis**

Mild acute poisoning from organophosphates or carbamates most closely resembles acute viral influenza, respiratory infections, gastroenteritis, asthma, or psychological dysfunction. The most significant differential diagnosis is between severe organophosphate poisoning and acute cerebrovascular accident; unequal pupils caused by the local effect of a direct-inhibiting (oxon) organophosphate or *n*-methyl carbamate in one eye of a comatose patient is a potential source of misdiagnosis. Other conditions to be distinguished from acute organophosphate poisoning include heat stroke, heat exhaustion, and infections.

The major disorder to be distinguished from organophosphate-induced delayed neuropathy is idiopathic acute symmetric polyneuropathy. Other toxic and disease-related neuropathies generally are insidious in onset and slowly progressive in course.

Laboratory evaluation, treatment, and chronic effects of the cholinesterase inhibitors are discussed below.

Inhibitors of Acetyl CoA Carboxylase, Lipid Synthesis, Growth Regulation, Tetronic Acid Derivatives

The tetronic acid derivatives (spirotetramat, spirodiclofen, spiromesifen) function by inhibiting insect lipid synthesis and the development of the respiratory system. They are effective against mites and a variety of insect pests. The mammalian toxicity of all four compounds is low and they do not cause prolonged eye or skin irritation in Draize test.

▶ Use Information

According to California agricultural use reporting, applications of the tetronic acid derivatives encompassed 3.6% of available cropland.

▶ Mammalian Toxicity

All of the tetronic acid compounds have low mammalian toxicity. Spirotetramat can also cause moderate eye irritation in animal tests.

▶ Illness Data

California illness registry data show two cases associated with exposure to tetronic acid derivatives as the only implicated pesticide. These included a mixer/loader with eye irritation following a direct accidental exposure to spirodiclofen in 2010 and a nursery worker who reported facial tingling, nausea, and headache in 2013 after entering a nursery during a spirotetramat application.

Inhibitors of Mitochondrial ATP Synthase

The ATP synthase inhibitors include the miticides propargite, cyhexatin, and fenbutatin-oxide.

▶ Use Data

The California use data showed a total of 206,164 lb, 1973 applications, and 87,222 acres treated, with heaviest use on corn (34,571 acres) and walnuts (23,604 acres). Use of fenbutatin-oxide also changed over the same period.

▶ Propargite Illness Patterns & Illness Data

The acute systemic toxicity of propargite is low, similar to the organotin ATP synthase inhibitor fenbutatin-oxide. With sufficient contact, propargite can causes severe irritation of the eyes and the skin. Fenbutatin-oxide can also cause skin and eye irritation.

▶ Illness Data

California illness registry data showed 173 cases associated with propargite as the only implicated pesticide between 1992 and 2015. These included 28 applicator cases and 18 involving other pesticide handlers, and 123 involving field workers exposed to pesticide residue. These included a single episode that occurred after a probable overapplication, that accounted for 65 cases. Other field workers and other outdoor workers experienced symptoms during drift episodes.

▶ Published Reports

Beginning in 1974, California surveillance reports documented problems in mixer/loaders arising from use of propargite, partially resolved by the introduction of a formulation distributed in a water-soluble packaging that allowed placement in a mix tank without puncturing the bag. A large-scale field residue episode resulted from the introduction of a new formulation with a markedly higher deposition rate than the conventional wettable powder. A 1988 dermatitis outbreak among stone-fruit harvesters and concerns about possible reproductive effects found in animal studies led to adoption of a 21-day reentry period on stone fruit, a 30-day reentry for hand labor tasks in vineyards, and a 40-day reentry period on citrus. These long reentry intervals initially led to changes in the order of work, scheduling hand labor tasks before, rather than after propargite applications. The comparatively low propargite use rate may have resulted principally from introduction of alternative active ingredients.

The California illness registry showed two cases associated with fenbutatin-oxide as the only implicated pesticide between 1992 and 2015. One case involved a mixer/loader who used the contaminated sleeve of his shirt to wipe his eye resulting in severe eye pain, with conjunctivitis, a corneal abrasion, and iritis documented on examination; another involved a field worker exposed to fenbutatin-oxide drift episode (documented by residue testing), who developed a headache and upper respiratory irritation.

A. Chitin Synthesis Inhibitors

Many chitin synthesis inhibitors primarily target fungi, but this group of compounds includes the benzoylphenyl urea insecticides diflubenzuron (20,270.22 lb, 41,330 applications, and 103251.7 acres treated—most frequently on almonds, artichoke, orchard fruit), hexaflumuron (0.04 lb), novaluron (17,061.45 lb of agricultural use, 4457 applications, and 229,240.0765 acres, most frequently on strawberries, cotton, alfalfa), and noviflumuron (106.19 lb for non-agricultural pest control).

Mammalian toxicity

Both diflubenzuron and novaluron have low mammalian toxicity and cause minimal eye and skin irritation in animal testing.

Illness data

A single case was reported between 1992 and 2015 involving an applicator who attempted to apply a diflubenzuron insecticide to a mixture of coconut husk and soil using a fire hose attached to a mix tank. When he turned the hose on, he lost control of the nozzle and sprayed his face, eyes, mouth and soaked his body. He had symptoms of nausea, headache, blurred vision, wheezing, dyspnea, fatigue, tearing eyes, and decreased appetite.

CASE REPORTS

A 2015 CDC publication described a drift episode involving 20 farmworkers in a cherry orchard reporting neurologic, gastrointestinal, ocular, and respiratory symptoms after an application of pyridaben, novaluron, and triflumizole on an adjacent property. Clothing and residue sampling were positive. The report did not describe whether the tank mix involved any adjuvants or inert ingredients that might have contributed to the reported symptoms.

Biological Agents

The biologic insecticides include compounds that interfere with mating called pheromones, plant extracts, insect toxins produced by microorganisms such as *Bacillus thuringiensis* (Bt), and compounds that interfere with regulation of insect growth. In recent years the number of biologic insecticides has increased, perhaps because of the simplified data requirements promulgated by the EPA. The extensive chronic toxicity testing required for most pesticides is not required for the biologic materials. Each agent typically targets a single pest or narrow group of pests, so that few individual compounds meet the criteria for "frequently applied pesticides." These compounds have in common low systemic toxicity and most do not cause significant eye, skin, or respiratory irritation.

▶ Microbial Insecticides

Currently registered microbial insecticides include 12 Bt variants, *Bacillus sphaericus*, 2 strains of the fungus *Beauveria bassiana*, *Chromobacterium subtsugae*, spores of *Nosema*, locustate, *Paecilomyces fumosoroseus*, *Metarhizium anisopliae* strain F52, Apopka strain 97, codling moth granulosis virus, and polyhedral occlusion bodies (OBs) of the nuclear polyhedrosis virus of *Helicoverpa zea* (corn earworm).

The prototype bacterial agent is *B thuringiensis* (Bt). Bt insecticides produce delta-endotoxin, also called Crystal (Cry) and Cytolitic (Cyt) proteins with activity against several insect orders—Lepidoptera (moths and butterflies), Coleoptera (beetles), Diptera (flies)—and also against nematodes. These proteins bind to epithelial cells in the insect midgut, creating cell membranes pores, leading to cell lysis. After cell lysis, bacterial spores germinate, leading to a lethal

blood poisoning. *Bacillus sphaericus* produces insecticidal toxins with a mode of action very similar to Bt.

CYD-X contains a naturally occurring host-specific granulovirus that infects codling moth larvae (*Cydia pomonella*) after the ingestion of occlusion bodies or granules, before or during initial entry into fruit. The virus degrades quickly by the action of ultraviolet light, a property that limits its residual effect after application. It does not infect beneficial insects, fish, wildlife, livestock, or humans.

Chromobacterium subtsugae strain PRAA4-1(T), a motile, gram-negative, violet-pigmented bacterium, is toxic to Colorado potato beetle larvae and other insects. It has specific action to control the black pecan aphid *Melanocallis caryaefoliae* and coddling moth on walnuts. The product label states it is toxic to bees present at the time of treatment or exposed to residues on weeds and blooming crops.

The fungal insect pathogen (entomopathogen) *P fumosoroseus* spores germinate on the body of the target pest (Diptera such as the Mediterranean fruit fly). It penetrates the cuticle and grows within the hemolymph and other tissues of the infected insects. Sporulation from dead pests leads to infections of other insects.

Beauveria bassiana is a fungal pathogen of insects (entomopathogen). The fungal active ingredient kills the adult housefly pest by growing on the insect's exoskeleton and secreting enzymes into the pest's soft body parts to kill it.

Insect Growth Regulators

Humans do not make or use the hormones of insects in molting, egg production, or chitin synthesis. Therefore, insect growth regulators are considered to have little human toxicity. Agents include azadirachtin and neem oil and inhibitors or analogues of juvenile growth hormone.

Insect juvenile growth hormone refers to a complex of hormones that regulate development, reproduction, dormancy, and expression of genetic traits in between insect molts. It has become a common biochemical target for control of insects. Other compounds affect development by interrupting egg production. Fenoxycarb and pyriproxyfen both act as juvenile hormonal agonists that produce an overload of hormonal activity. Both have low mammalian toxicity.

Methoprene, hydroprene, and kinoprene interfere with the development of insect eggs by inhibiting the production of the egg yolk glycolipoprotein vitellogenin. The acute mammalian toxicity of all the compounds is low. None cause prolonged reactions in the Draize eye and skin irritation assays.

Cyromazine and hexythiazox are both insect growth regulators but do not have completely defined mechanisms of action. Cyromazine belongs to the s-triazine class of chemicals, but lacks herbicidal activity. It is effective against fly larvae and leaf miners. The exact mode of action of the mite growth regulator hexythiazox is not well understood. Hexythiazox kills the eggs before the mites hatch and also some immature mites. Adult mites are not killed, although adults exposed to residues may lay eggs that are not viable.

Insecticidal Soaps

Insecticidal soaps can help control soft-bodied insects including aphids, leafhoppers, spider mites, and whiteflies. The soaps act by disrupting cell membranes, requiring direct contact at the time of application to be effective. Residuals of the soaps on plant foliage do not have insecticidal activity.

Acute toxicity data for insecticidal soaps demonstrate very low mammalian toxicity, but Draize testing shows a clear tendency to cause eye and skin irritation. There are a few cases of systemic illness reported, along with eye irritation following direct accidental contact with soap, with skin irritation, and infrequently with respiratory irritation.

Insect Repellents

Frequently used insect repellents include biological oils and products containing diethyl-toluamide (DEET). Concentrated formulations of DEET (34.3–98.1%) provide 10–12 hours of protection but lower concentrations (7.15%) may provide only 2 hours of protection. Adverse effects of DEET have been described extensively. Repeated use of high-dose formulations have been associated with irritant dermatitis. Allergic reactions have also been reported including contact urticaria and anaphylaxis.

Because DEET is easily absorbed through skin, concerns have been raised about possible systemic effects, especially neurologic effects on children. Encephalopathy in adults has also been reported. A 27-year-old previously healthy man applied 25% DEET to his arms, neck, and legs repeatedly during a fishing trip on a hot and humid afternoon. He initially reported paresthesias of the limbs and face, then auditory hallucinations, progressive confusion, disorientation, and agitation He did not return to normal mental function until the third hospital day.

Natural products that have some efficacy as insect repellents include pyrethrum and oils extracted from neem, garlic, aniseed, thyme, geranium, bergamot, eucalyptus, lavender, bergamot, pyrethrum, lavender oil, coconut oil, birchwood tar, soybean, nutmeg, pine, orange blossom, clove, cinnamon, pennyroyal, and peppermint.

Compounds Used Principally as Structural Insecticides

▶ Borates and Sulfluramid

Active ingredients containing boron include boric acid, also known as orthoboric acid, sodium tetraborate (pentahydrate), barium metaborate, perboric acid sodium salt, and other compounds. There are currently 59 household insect control formulations registered in addition to a 100% boric acid dust intended for manufacturing use. There are 10 additional registered formulations containing sodium tetraborate (pentahydrate) and 3 fungicidal formulations containing barium metaborate.

Boric acid functions by disrupting water balance in insects, but the detailed mechanism has not been identified. It has low acute toxicity in mammals and minimal irritant effects. Acute accidental ingestion of boric acid causes no symptoms in more than 75% of cases. However, fatal adult and pediatric poisonings have been reported. Borate urine or blood concentrations are useful primarily for documentation of exposure. Unusual conditions associated with chronic exposure include alopecia associated with both ingestion and topical exposure. Chronic pediatric boron poisoning has also been reported following repeated use of a boric acid formulation for diaper rash.

Sulfluramid is classified as a halogenated alkyl sulphonamide; it has potent metabolites that inhibits energy production by uncoupling oxidative phosphorylation. It does not produce the same effect in mammals because of differences in metabolism. It has moderate oral toxicity but low dermal toxicity in mammals.

3. Physical Agents

Because of concerns about chemical agents, some structural pest control companies have promoted the use of physical agents.

A system using liquid nitrogen to freeze termites in wall spaces raised safety concerns about traditional termite control methods. In terms of efficacy, the method appeared to be comparable to a chemical spot treatment, but was not the equivalent of tenting a structure and applying a traditional fumigant. A California illness surveillance report described an applicator who died applying liquid nitrogen in a narrow crawl space adjacent to a bath tub. Postmortem evaluation was negative for drugs of abuse and structural heart disease, and the final diagnosis was simple asphyxia.

The effects of "heat treatment" devices are poorly documented in illness surveillance data. Press reports occasionally describe fires associated with use of the devices to treat bed bugs.

LABORATORY FINDINGS, TREATMENT, & PROGNOSIS FOR INSECTICIDE POISONING

▶ Laboratory & Hygiene Evaluation

A. Pyrethroids

There are no biologic monitoring methods for exposure to pyrethrum or pyrethroids routinely available from commercial laboratories. The metabolites measured in published exposure studies or poisoning cases probably represent a small percentage of the absorbed parent compound. Reference values published by the CDC offer the most useful comparison; levels markedly above the reference values confirm exposure, but consensus does not exist regarding specific levels representing toxic thresholds.

B. OPs and Carbamates

Samples include blood tests for cholinesterase, metabolite studies, and environmental and clothing samples of active ingredients. Samples must be sent for cholinesterase measurement before administration of pralidoxime, which will regenerate cholinesterase in red cells and plasma as well as nerves. Atropine has no effect on cholinesterase levels.

▶ Treatment

A. Pyrethroids

Treatment for occupational pyrethroid exposures and intentional poisoning is covered by standard protocols for decontamination and supportive therapy.

As demonstrated in a 1984 study with human volunteers, skin paresthesias related to pyrethroids respond to topical vitamin E cream (eg, available currently in "antiaging" products), if applied within a few hours of exposure. In practice this remedy is rarely employed.

B. OPs and Carbamates

Assessment of the severity of poisoning serves as the best guide to treat possible exposure to cholinesterase inhibitors.

Although samples should be collected at the time of initial evaluation, treatment that is otherwise indicated should not wait on the results of cholinesterase levels.

For most severe poisonings, history and clinical evaluation provides enough information to guide treatment. For patients with bradycardia or lung congestion, a test dose of atropine should be administered. Atropine blocks the effects of acetylcholine at muscarinic receptors, but does not affect nicotinic or CNS symptoms. Assessment of severity should always include the respiratory system—it is affected by all three types of cholinergic sites, predicts serious morbidity, and is critical for survival. A reasonable severity rating defines mild toxicity as involving only muscarinic signs and symptoms, moderate toxicity as involving more than one system, but not requiring assisted breathing, and severe toxicity as requiring ventilatory assistance.

A dose of atropine sulfate (0.5 mg intravenously) produces signs of mild atropinization (ie, dry mouth, dry eyes, increased heart rate, and large pupils) in a normal adult, but usually has no effect on an individual with organophosphate poisoning. A dose of 1–2 mg intravenously will produce marked signs of atropinization in a nonpoisoned adult and may reverse the signs of cholinergic excess in a case of poisoning.

For some occupational poisonings, removal from further exposure to cholinesterase-inhibiting insecticides may prove to be the only treatment necessary. Treatment with specific antidotes should be reserved for patients observed in the hospital setting.

Specific antidotes include atropine sulfate (for muscarinic symptoms) and pralidoxime to reverse cholinesterase inhibition from acute organophosphate poisoning.

If no hypoxia is present, recommended atropine doses include 1–2 mg intravenously for mild to moderate poisoning, 2–4 mg intravenously for severe poisoning, as often as every 15 minutes. The reported blood half-life is 2–3 hours. There is no maximum dosage.

It is recommended that atropine be withheld until emergency support measures (ventilatory assistance, oxygen, and clearance of secretions) are completed because of the risk of arrhythmias in the presence of hypoxia.

Patients without evidence of muscle weakness or respiratory depression may be treated with atropine alone until one or more signs of mild atropinization appear (ie, tachycardia, flushing, dry mucous membranes, or dilated pupils). Multiple doses may need to be administered over a prolonged time.

For organophosphate poisoning only, give pralidoxime chloride (2-PAM, Protopam) slowly, 1 g intravenously (no more than 0.5 g/min), repeated once in 1–2 hours and then at 10- to 12-hour intervals, if needed. Obidoxime is commonly used in other parts of the world; recommended dosage is 250 mg bolus, with subsequent continuous infusion at 750 mg/d up to 1 week. Pralidoxime acts by breaking the bond between acetylcholinesterase and organophosphate, reactivating the enzyme and restoring acetylcholine activity to normal. Its advantages over atropine include acting at the neuromuscular junction to reverse muscular paralysis. Pralidoxime does not normally cross the blood-brain barrier, although the barrier itself may be altered in severe poisoning. Overdosage is not a problem if the drug is administered slowly to avoid inducing hypotension.

The decision to use pralidoxime should occur soon after diagnosis because it is ineffective once aging (covalent binding of the organophosphate inhibitor to cholinesterase) has occurred. Post pralidoxime samples of cholinesterase can serve to document its clinical effectiveness, and, if needed, help document poisoning.

The use of pralidoxime for carbamate poisoning is controversial, but seldom necessary because the carbamate-binding to cholinesterase resolves spontaneously. Morphine, aminophylline, phenothiazines, and ondansetron are contraindicated because of the increased risk of cardiac arrhythmias. Diuretics for pulmonary edema and fluids for hypotension are also contraindicated.

▶ Prognosis

Some of the recent decrease in occupational poisonings with cholinesterase inhibitors is probably attributable to the changes brought about by regulation of the more toxic compounds. The number of hospitalized occupational poisoning cases has declined markedly and the prognosis of gradual onset poisoning is very favorable.

Intentional ingestions of category II and category III organophosphates (malathion, diazinon, and others) account for most of the hospitalized poisonings that still occur. If treatment for organophosphate or carbamate poisoning is initiated before hypoxia results in tissue damage, antidotal therapy and respiratory support should ensure complete recovery, even in the most severe cases. Persistence of manifestations beyond 24 hours indicates the possibility of continued absorption of pesticide and the need to carefully consider and examine the skin, fingernails, eyes, and GI tract as possible reservoirs.

A. Laboratory

Cholinesterase—Changes in cholinesterase activity, along with the typical signs and symptoms, provide sufficient information for the diagnosis and management of most cases. Red cell cholinesterase is called "true" cholinesterase because it is the same enzyme present in nerve endings and because its activity more closely parallels that in the nervous system than does plasma cholinesterase.

Organophosphates and carbamates may differentially inhibit one enzyme relative to the other. For example, the commonly used organophosphate chlorpyrifos (Dursban, Lorsban) preferentially depresses plasma cholinesterase, causing illness without significant depression of red cell cholinesterase.

A number of analytic methods are used to measure both red cell and plasma cholinesterase. Results obtained by one method usually cannot be compared with results from another, even if the units expressed by each are the same. There is considerable variability in cholinesterase activity in unexposed persons, so reports of results relative to "normal" do not reflect the true level of inhibition present.

Individuals with a genetic trait for atypical plasma cholinesterase have lowered plasma but not red cell cholinesterase. They have prolonged muscular paralysis after administration of succinyl choline and other neuromuscular blocking agents that are normally metabolized by plasma cholinesterase, but they are not more susceptible to cholinesterase-inhibiting pesticides. Unlike red cell cholinesterase, plasma cholinesterase is not a reliable indicator of exposure or poisoning in these individuals.

Plasma cholinesterase production may be lowered as a result of liver disease extensive enough to impair the production of proteins such as albumin. Albumin-losing conditions, such as nephrotic syndrome, may be accompanied by elevated levels of plasma cholinesterase as a result of increased hepatic protein synthesis. The only medical conditions known to influence red cell cholinesterase activity are those associated with reticulocytosis, such as recovery from hemorrhage, pernicious anemia, and some other anemias.

Two circumstances in which cholinesterase determinations may be useful are (1) routine biologic monitoring of exposure to organophosphates and (2) diagnosis of acute poisoning. In assessing exposure to carbamates, cholinesterase depression may prove difficult to document unless treatment facilities can perform cholinesterase assays on-site shortly after phlebotomy.

Severe poisoning usually is accompanied by cholinesterase levels well below normal for the laboratory. However, patients with mild to moderate poisoning often have cholinesterase levels reported as equivocal, normal, and even above normal. The diagnosis can be confirmed retrospectively by periodic (ie, weekly or biweekly) determinations of cholinesterase until levels fluctuate by no more than 30%. If the average level at this time—the retrospective baseline—is more than 30% higher than the level at the time of illness, exposure to cholinesterase-inhibiting pesticides almost certainly was present, and the illness may have been due to that exposure. The rate of recovery of red cell cholinesterase, in the absence of treatment with pralidoxime and of further exposure, depends on the rate of formation of new red cells, which is approximately 1% per day. Red blood cell cholinesterase levels will reach a plateau in about 60–70 days and plasma cholinesterase in 30–50 days.

B. Intact Pesticides and Metabolites

Measurement of the parent organophosphate or carbamate, or their metabolites, in blood or urine has been employed in field investigations. No such measurements are currently likely to be helpful in the diagnosis of acute intoxication, but may serve to document exposures that do not cause cholinesterase inhibition. The metabolite urine samples can be collected at any medical laboratory and are usually performed at a national toxicology reference laboratory.

Measurement of alkyl phosphate metabolites in urine has not been of use in biologic monitoring of exposure because of its lack of specificity and instability. Measurement of p-nitrophenol in urine can be useful for monitoring exposure to parathion; 0.5 mg/L in a sample collected at the end of an exposure interval corresponds to exposure to parathion at the current threshold limit value (TLV). Measurement of 1-naphthol in urine is used to monitor exposure to carbaryl.

Metabolite assays have also been conducted for pyrethroid insecticides, but are not usually available in clinical laboratories. Background levels for pyrethroid metabolites have been published for some populations.

Application records can prove useful in evaluating exposures to pesticide handlers, field workers, and occasionally individuals away from the site of the application. This depends on distance from the field and detailed weather information. Exposure monitoring and modeling studies both indicate very limited exposure occurs upwind of application sites.

CHRONIC EFFECTS OF INSECTICIDES & SEQUELAE OF ACUTE POISONING

Table 33–13 shows insecticides classified as probable carcinogens, teratogens, reproductive toxins, or, have significant post illness sequelae.

Carcinogenity of Insecticides

Most pyrethroids are classified as category C or "possible carcinogens" (eg, s-bioallethrin, zeta-cypermethrin, and tetramethrin), but resmethrin is classified as a likely carcinogen. Several of the synthetic pyrethroids cause cancer at maximum tolerated doses in animals, including bifenthrin, cypermethrin, permethrin, and tetramethrin; however, none are classified as probable human carcinogens. Dichlorvos, an organophosphate with reactive leaving group side chain, was classified as probable (B2 or "likely") carcinogen in the 1990s. Currently it is classified as "suggestive

Table 33–13. Animal and human studies evaluating chronic effects and sequelae of insecticides.

Chemical	Cancer, reproductive or neurobehavioral effect	EPA Potency Factor—Q*	Class
Pyrethroids			
Pyrethroids	Possible neurodevelopmental effect identified from human studies (details in text)		C
Resmethrin	Increased incidences of benign and malignant liver tumors in female rats and male mice	5.621×10^{-2}	Likely
Organophosphates			
Chlorpyriphos	Noncarcinogen; Possible neurodevelopmental effects per animal and human studies (details in text); case report of peripheral neuropathy 2 weeks after intentional ingestion, Sri Lanka; positive for neuropathy in hen test at maximum tolerated dose (100 mg/kg), negative at 10 mg/kg		E
Dichlorvos	Rat: 0, 4, 8 mg/kg/d, 5 d/wk; pancreatic adenomas, leukemias in males; 0, 10, or 20 mg/kg/d (M). Mice: 0, 20, 40 mg/kg/d (F), 5 d/wk, corn oil gavage; forestomach papillomas at high-dose males/females Suicide attempt, 2004 India, documented delayed neuropathy, axonal degeneration	2.9×10^{-1}	B2
Ethoprop	F344 rats, 0, 1, 10, or 100 ppm × 24 mo; thyroid C-cell carcinomas increased slightly —in high dose males; B6C3F1 mice/sex/group for 104 wk at 0, 0.2, 2.0, or 30 ppm, thyroid cancer in high dose; Crl:CD rats 0, 1, 60, or 600 ppm for 105 wk—adrenal pheochromocytomas in multiple dose groups; also thyroid cancer males		Likely to be carcinogenic to humans
Malathion	Combined oncogenicity/chronic feeding study rat: 100, 6000, 12,000 ppm; increase in female liver adenomas, male nasal adenomas at > 6000 ppm Negative NTE study in chicken at 1000 mg/kg; + study in rats Case report, suicide attempt 100 cc 50% malathion, Japan, 1991		D
Methamidophos	No treatment effect 1.5, 4.5 mg/kg/d hens; ChE effects at 1.5 mg/kg/d, DPR tox summary; also negative rat study 16-year-old boy developed OPIDN after acute poisoning with methamidophos, 1999 report		
Merphos (Folex)	Inhibition of lymphocyte NTE in monitored workers; Single-dose merphos between 200–2000 mg/kg in hen NTE model; no documented case of delayed neuropathy		
Propargite	Propargite caused sarcomas of the jejunum in both male and female Sprague-Dawley rats. In other studies on mice and Wistar rats, propargite did not exhibit carcinogenicity or mutagenicity. CDPR evaluated possibility of a threshold mechanism for jejunal tumors (presumably stimulation of cell proliferation by irritation). Rabbit developmental study: Reduced body weight gain; increased resorption; reduced body weight; delayed ossification; NOEL 2 mg/kg low-effect level—6 mg/kg for maternal and fetotoxicity		B2
Tribufos; S,S,S-Tributyl Phosphoro-trithioate (DEF)	Inhibition of lymphocyte NTE in monitored workers; neuropathy in hens 42 mg/kg/d dosed for 90 days, no neuropathic effect at 0, 2.6, 11 mg/kg; LOAEL for ChE inhibition 2.6 mg/kg; no documented		E
Trichlorfon	Myelopathy at high-dose exposures in rat studies 100 ppm dose; hen studies negative; 1984 Romania 4 cases, 1986 Hungary 12 cases, neuropathy following suicide attempts		

(continued)

Table 33–13. Animal and human studies evaluating chronic effects and sequelae of insecticides. (Continued)

Chemical	Cancer, reproductive or neurobehavioral effect	EPA Potency Factor—Q*	Class
Carbamate compounds			
Carbaryl	Male reproductive: spermatotoxin in rodents; study in manufacturing and formulating workers indicating no effect at relatively low levels of exposure Teratogenicity: 3.1–50 mg/kg were fed to beagle dogs during pregnancy. At levels of 6.25 and above the defect rate was increased in the offspring. Midline abdominal wall defects skeletal defects were the most common type. Negative studies reported for rodent species		
Baygon/Propoxur	Male and female rat bladder, hepatocellular adenomas mice	3.70 E-3	B2
Organochlorine (none still registered)			
Chlordane	Mouse liver	1.3	B2
DDT, DDE, DDD	Female mouse stomach; male rat leukemia	0.24–0.34	B2
Dieldrin		16	B2
Heptachlor	Mice: hepatomas at 10 ppm dose; rats: 40, 80, 160 ppm—thyroid adenomas at low/high dose	4.5	B2
Lindane	Liver tumors in mice and rats (NTP summary)	1.3	B2/C
Methoxychlor	Published studies show testicular tumors in some mouse strains 100 ppm in diet; carcinomas both sexes of rats 2000 ppm in diet		B2
Mirex	Hepatomas in mouse and rat at maximum tolerated dose and 50% MTD	1.8	B2
Toxaphene	Rat liver/thyroid	1.1	B2
Tetronic acid derivatives			
Spirodiclofen	Hepatocellular adenomas & carcinomas, CD-1 mice; testicular interstitial cell adenomas and hyperplastic foci, uterine adenocarcinomas Wistar rats, per CDPR toxicology summary		Likely to be carcinogenic to humans

evidence of carcinogenicity" by U.S. EPA and as a possible carcinogen by IARC (sufficient evidence in animals and inadequate evidence from available human studies). Other organophosphates are rated as possible carcinogens or as noncarcinogens.

The organochlorines DDT, chlordane, dieldrin, heptachlor, lindane, methoxychlor, mirex, and toxaphene are classified, based on animal bioassays, as probable human carcinogens.

Studies evaluating the relation between DDT/DDE and breast cancer, initially suggested by a 1993 study, have been inconsistent. For example, in a review of 26 studies published between 2000 and 2006, employing a variety of comparison points, most odds ratios overlapped one. Studies showing elevated risk included a 2003 study describing elevated risk in European whites with detectable DDT (> 0.5 ng/g lipid vs < 0.5 ng/g) (odds ratio [OR] ¼ 5.64; 95% confidence interval [CI], 1.81–17.65) or DDE (OR ¼ 2.21; 95% CI, 1.41–3.48). A 2000 study from Mexico City (highest quintile (> 3490 ng/g

lipid) compared with lowest quintile (< 1170) (OR ¼ 3.81; 95% CI, 1.14–12.8). The remaining studies did not show a link between DDE and breast cancer and stratification by menopausal status, tumor hormone receptor status, parity, breastfeeding, or body mass index did not reveal consistent associations.

Apart from DDT/DDE, positive associations between other organochlorines and breast cancer have been reported. In a Danish case-control study serum levels of dieldrin were associated with increasing risk from the lowest exposure group (< 6.9 ng/g lipid) to the highest (> 36.0 ng/g lipid): odds ratio = 4.6 (1.8–11.5). The observed increased breast cancer risk associated with exposure to dieldrin derived from women who developed an estrogen receptor negative (ERN) tumor (OR I vs IV quartile, 7.6, 95% CI 1.4–46.1, p-value for linear trend 0.01). Because the compounds evaluated differed from study to study, it was not possible to check for consistency of results across multiple studies.

Animal testing data identify propargite as a potential carcinogen. In an oncogenicity study conducted with Sprague Dawley rats, technical propargite (87.2% purity) was fed to albino rats for 104 weeks at concentrations of 0, 80, 400, and 800 ppm. The no-effect-level for general chronic toxicity was 80 ppm (reduced bodyweights in males at 400 [slight] and for females at 800 ppm). Jejunal sarcomas occurred in both females and males in the 400 and 800 ppm groups. Based on the known irritant effects of propargite, the sarcomas may have been related to hyperplasia caused by acute epithelial irritation (a threshold effect) rather than genotoxic effects of propargite (a nonthreshold or stochastic effect).

A 2002 report linked propargite applications, recorded on the agricultural pesticide use reporting system within a mile of a child's residence, to the occurrence of leukemia. The authors acknowledged some of the multiple limitations of the exposure information in the study. In addition, the study evaluated multiple outcomes and multiple exposures without an a priori hypothesis. It is likely that some positive associations occurred simply by chance.

Novel Pesticide Agents

No human epidemiologic studies of occupational or environmental cancer have been conducted for many of the newer agents. The most recent list of 169 compounds classified for carcinogenic potential was published by the U.S. EPA in 2006 including formerly registered compounds such as parathion and chlordimeform. Based on animal bioassays, the EPA did classify the miticide/insecticide spirodiclofen, a tetronic acid derivative initially registered in 2007, as a likely human carcinogen. Testing showed liver adenomas and carcinomas, testicular interstitial cell adenomas and hyperplastic foci, and uterine adenocarcinomas in CD-1 mice.

Reproductive Effectives: Teratogenicity & Neurodevelopmental Effects

Case reports and a few epidemiologic studies have described either teratogenicity or fetotoxicity at doses that also cause maternal toxicity. For example, in a 1989 report from Salinas, California, workers developed acute organophosphate poisoning after entering a cauliflower field contaminated with residues of oxydemeton-methyl, mevinphos, and methomyl. A crew member, 4-weeks pregnant at the time of the poisoning, subsequently gave birth to a child with multiple cardiac defects, bilateral optic nerve coloboma microphthalmia of the left eye, cerebral and cerebella atrophy, and facial anomalies. The authors considered oxydemeton-methyl the most likely cause of the birth defects because of animal studies submitted for pesticide registration. These included an inhalation study with the developmental anomalies associated with concentrations of 0.0007 mg/kg throughout the entire pregnancy; and an oral teratogenicity for Long-Evans rats fed 3 mg/kg/day for 10 days during pregnancy. Positive findings included reduction in maternal weight gain, stunted fetal growth, and hypoplasia of cerebral hemispheres.

Between 1989 and 1990, 11 (73%) of 15 births in a Hungarian village had congenital abnormalities; four children had Down syndrome and six (40%) were twins. No previously recognized genetic or teratogenic factor was found. The mean maternal age of the cases was 27.6 years. A case control study showed 9 out of 11 case mothers had consumed fish from local fish farms using the organophosphorus compound trichlorfon. Five of the nine reported very heavy fish consumption. A comparison group from the area had comparable maternal age and minimal history of fish consumption. Investigation showed tissue levels in the fish of 100 mg/kg trichlorfon; farm managers and workers reported using excessive amounts of the product, with no dilution prior to treatment.

A cohort study in Salinas, California and a separate study in New York evaluated prenatal and early childhood environmental exposure to organophosphates. Exposures were evaluated by sampling cord blood and urinary metabolites. The principal exposure to the urban cohort was chlorpyrifos, diazinon, and permethrin used for structural pest control, with occasional exposures to illegal, unregistered insecticides. The agricultural cohort had exposures to both chlorpyrifos and other organophosphates.

In two prenatal and one postpartum sample, the frequency of detectable levels of all alkyl phosphates combined ranged from 88.5% to 100.0% compared to 92.8% for pregnant women in the NHANES sample. The geometric mean level was 113 nmol/L in both of the prenatal samples and 229.5 nmol/L in the postpartum sample. The geometric mean level in the comparable NHANES sample was 70.5 nmol/L. The total dialkyl phosphates (DAP) concentration in the Salinas samples ranged from 6.5 to 34,438 nmol/L and from 6.0 to 2,610.5 in the NHANES sample.

The specific metabolite for chlorpyrifos, trichloropyridinol (TCPy), was present at a median level of 2.1 and 7.1 mcg/L in the two prenatal samples from the Salinas cohort compared to a median level of 1.6 mcg/L in the NHANES sample. The levels of the metabolite malathion dicarboxylic acid (MDA) and diazinon metabolite 2-isopropyl-4-methyl-6-hydroxypyrimidinol (IMPY) were comparable in the Salinas and NHANES samples. It was unclear how much of the exposure to Salinas cohort was occupational or "para-occupational" or related to dietary sources common to the general population.

The New York cohort study included measures of multiple environmental exposures, including PAHs and environmental tobacco smoke. At the time of interviews, 85% of subjects reported exposure during pregnancy to pesticides used for structural pest control that some form of pest control, usually for cockroaches or rodents, was used during pregnancy, with about one-third employing commercial pest control services. Use of RTU spray cans or insecticide foggers was also common and 10% used illegally registered. Using personal backpacks, 48-hour air samples collected showed detectable levels of chlorpyrifos (0.7–193 ng/m^3), propoxur, and the disinfectant *o*-phenyl phenol in all 72 subjects monitored. Diazinon (2.0–6010 ng/m^3) was identified in 71 samples, the synergist PBO (ND–11.1) in 59, and the pyrethroid permethrin in 29 (ND–7.0). The air sampling predicted the compounds found in prenatal plasma samples, which included chlorpyrifos (4.8 pg/g), diazinon (1.2 pg/g), dichloran (3.1 pg/g), and phthalimide (29.2 pg/g).

Over time, positive findings from the New York in 2003 cohort included decreased birth weight and birth length. A 2007 report correlated high OP metabolite levels with abnormal reflexes (plantar grasp, hand grasp, Babinski, Moro, placing, automatic walking, and others) recorded during administration of the Brazelton Neonatal Behavioral Assessment Scale. Blood PCB levels showed a similar relationship with the reflex findings. A related study evaluated development at 12, 24, and 36 months, finding that children with prenatal plasma chlorpyrifos above the median level scored 6.5 points lower on the Bayley Psychomotor Development Index and 3.3 points lower on the Bayley Mental Development Index at 3 years of age. On an average they showed a greater tendency to developmental delays and attention deficit disorder. At 7 years the most highly exposed children had lower scores on the Wechsler Intelligence Scale for Children, declining approximately 3% for each standard deviation (4.6 pg/g) increase in the levels of chlorpyrifos. A subsequent study employed quantitative magnetic resonance imaging (MRI) imaging to describe anatomical changes associated with the previously described functional changes.

For the Salinas cohort, the initial positive findings, published in 2004, included increase in body length and head circumference associated with some exposure measure (eg, urinary dimethyl phosphate metabolites and umbilical cord cholinesterase). Similar to the New York cohort, 381 infants, 2 months old or younger, from the Salinas cohort, were examined using the BNBAS instrument. There was a significant association between prenatal urinary metabolites and the number of abnormal reflexes and the percentage of infants with more than three abnormal reflexes. At age 7, averaged maternal DAP concentrations were associated with poorer scores for working memory, processing speed, verbal comprehension, perceptual reasoning, and full-scale intelligence quotient (IQ) when tested with the Wechsler Intelligence Scale for Children. There was an average deficit of 7.0 IQ for children in the highest 20% of maternal DAP concentrations compared with the lowest 20% those in the lowest quintile.

The documentation of the neurobehavioral effects and changes in humans also correlates with the neurodevelopmental markers in adult mice following single neonatal doses of chlorpyrifos and carbaryl.

Pyrethroids—Neonatal Susceptibility, Neurobehavioral Effects

A 2015 report from France described a cohort study evaluating exposure to pyrethroid employing prenatal monitoring

of urinary metabolites (five pyrethroid and two organophosphate insecticide metabolites), akin to the New York and Salinas cohorts exposed to organophosphates. Urinary metabolites in children were also measured. Maternal prenatal pyrethroid metabolite concentrations were not consistently associated with any children's cognitive scores. By contrast, childhood 3-PBA and cis-DBCA concentrations were both negatively associated with verbal comprehension scores and with working memory scores.

Investigations to date on pyrethroids remain incomplete in comparison with those on organophosphates. Multiple issues remain regarding dose and mechanism of reported developmental effects of both groups of compounds.

Sequelae of Acute Poisoning & Other Chronic Effects

Numerous studies have documented subclinical neurobehavioral deficits relative to control subjects in previously poisoned workers and to a lesser extent in workers with applicators with long-term exposures who never experienced acute poisoning. The recorded deficits include vibrotactile sensitivity, decreased sustained attention, and decreased speed of information processing, memory and abstraction, and cognitive tests.

Poisoning by the organophosphate nerve agent sarin produced persistent neurobehavioral deficits, including significant amnesia in some victims of the 1995 terrorist attack on the Tokyo subway. The most severe deficits were seen in patients who experienced prolonged hypoxia. Cases of posttraumatic stress also occurred. Findings in less severely poisoned cases more closely resembled those seen in studies of applicators poisoned by organophosphate insecticides.

Studies of workers who handled organophosphates without a history of overt poisoning show less consistent findings of subclinical neurobehavioral impairment. A study of sheep dippers handling organophosphates showed findings similar to the studies of overtly poisoned workers. Other studies of nonpoisoned organophosphate handlers demonstrated equivocal or negative findings.

Organophosphate Delayed Neuropathy

Organophosphate-induced delayed neuropathy (OPIDN), a health effect of organophosphate pesticides unrelated to cholinesterase inhibition, is caused by inhibition of an enzyme known as neurotoxic esterase (NTE). It occurs in the central and peripheral nervous systems of various species, and it is an indicator of neurotoxic potential and a potential tool for biologic monitoring. Animal studies indicate that 75% irreversible inhibition of NTE initial activity will be followed 10–14 days later by a progressive ascending peripheral neuropathy. The potent NTE inhibitors no longer have active registration, typified by mipafox, methamidophos, and EPN. Recently reported cases of OPIDN occurred after ingestion of weak NTE inhibitors (malathion, diazinon, chlorpyrifos, etc. [see Table 33–13]).

▶ Ecological Toxicity

Pyrethroids can be highly toxic to fish and aquatic invertebrates in the laboratory and are highly toxic to bees and other beneficial insects. The 96-hour LC50 of deltamethrin for fish, for example, ranges between 0.048 and 5.13 mcg/L. Although pyrethroids dissipate rapidly through photolysis or hydrolysis, they may persist in aquatic sediments. Pyrethroids are also highly toxic to bees and other nontarget arthropods in the laboratory. Ecologic effects may be mitigated by dissipation of residues, allowing recovery of affected populations.

▶ Neonicotinoid Effect on Nontarget Insects

An urban park used imidacloprid to control foreign pests (two alien wood-boring beetles, the Asian longhorned beetle, *Anoplophora glabripennis*, and the emerald ash borer, *Agrilus planipennis*) causing loss of native conifers. The imidacloprid treatment successfully eliminated the exotic borer beetles. Subsequent to the treatment, elm trees in the park experienced outbreaks of spider mites (*Tetranychus schoenei*). Laboratory experiments showed that imidacloprid debilitated insect predators of spider mites, promoting the nontarget *Tetranychus* species to pest status.

Honeybees appear to be uniquely sensitive to the effects of neonicotinoids compared to birds, fish, mammals, and other insects (Table 33–14). Neonicotinoids metabolites may be even more toxic to the bees than the active ingredients. Although this suggests that neonicotinoids contribute to hive collapse or other problems with bee colonies, other factors may also prove important.

A 2013 review of the hive collapse disorder problem by a committee of U.S. Department of Agriculture and U.S. EPA scientists indicated a consensus that multiple factors underlie the disorder: viral infections, the parasitic mite *Varroa destructor,* the bacterial disease European foulbrood, nutrition, changes in gut microbial flora, and acute and cumulative effects of pesticides.

A 2017 study described a field study in the United Kingdom, Germany, and Hungary, evaluating the effects of neonicotinoid treated seed on bee populations. Negative effects occurred for honeybee populations in Hungary and United Kingdom and positive effects in Germany. Reproduction in wild bees (*Bombus terrestris* and *Osmia bicornis*), correlated negative reproduction with neonicotinoid residues.

FUNGICIDES

The following section discusses fungicides grouped by their mode of action and ranked by frequency of use (Table 33–15). The most frequently used active ingredients including compounds with multisite activity.

Elemental Sulfur

Elemental sulfur is one of the most heavily used crop agricultural chemicals in California, applied as a dust to control mildew and other fungal pathogens.

Although sulfur is an inorganic substance, it can legally be applied on "organic" farms in California and is an important component of integrated pest management (IPM) systems. California data for 2016 show 46,888,158 lb of reported agricultural use, 125,639 applications, and 5,587,422 acres treated (21% of California crop land).

Sulfur has a low potency when compared with many organic fungicides. The average annual application rate per acre on all crops was 8.4 lb/acre and 5.8 lb/acre on table grapes. For comparison, the average application rate for the strobilurin fungicide azoxystrobin was 0.19 lb/acre.

▶ Mammalian Toxicity

Animal tests indicate that inorganic sulfur is basically nonreactive. It has low acute toxicity. It produces no irritation in the Draize dermal irritation assay and is negative in predictive allergy tests submitted for pesticide registration. Nevertheless, sulfur is among the most frequently reported sources of illness in agricultural workers, a discrepancy likely explained by transformation of elemental sulfur to various sulfur oxide

Table 33–14. Ecotoxicity of neonicotinoids.

Chemical	Oral or contact LD50, mcg/bee Honeybee	Other Insect species, Oral or contact LD50	Oral LD50, mg/kg Bobwhite quail	Fish LC50
Acetamiprid	7.1	NA	180	Carp > 100 mg/L 48 h
Clothianidin	0.022	NA	> 2000	117 ppm/96 hr, bluegill sunfish
Dinotefuran	0.032–0.061	NA	> 2000	(Rainbow trout) > 99.5 mg/L (96 h);
Imidacloprid	0.078, contact; 0.0039, oral	NA	152	(211 mg/L), rainbow trout
Thiacloprid	24.2	NA	2716	(Rainbow trout) 30.5 mg/L/96 h
Thiamethoxam	0.0299, contact	NA	> 5200	> 100 mg/L for 96 h, rainbow trout

Table 33–15. Mammalian toxicity for selected fungicides.

Compound	CAS #	Oral LD50, mg/kg	Dermal LD50, mg/kg
Multisite activity			
Elemental sulfur	7704-34-9	> 5000	> 2000
Copper hydroxide	20427-59-2	1000	Not found
Copper sulfate	7758-99-8, 1344-73-6	Rat 300, mouse 43	> 2000
Copper oxychloride	1332-40-7	299	Not found
Copper naphthenate	1338-02-9	2000	> 2000 mg/kg
Naphthenic acid	1338-24-5	3000	Not found
Chlorothalonil	1897-45-6	3700 mouse	> 2500, rat; > 5000, rabbit
Mancozeb	8018-01-7	5000 rat	> 10,000 rat
Thiram	137-26-8	560	> 1,000 rat
Ziram	137-30-4	320	> 6,000 rat
Inhibitors of mitochondrial respiration, cytochrome bc1 complex, complex III, Strobilurins			
Trifloxystrobin	141517-21-7	> 4000–5000	> 2,000 rabbit
Azoxystrobin	131860-33-8	> 5000	> 2,000 rat
Pyraclostrobin	175013-18-0	> 5000	> 2,000 rat
Ergosterol synthesis inhibitors			
Difenoconazole	119446-68-3	1453	> 2010 mg/kg rabbit; Rat 2010 mg/kg
Imazalil (Enilconazole)	35554-44-0	227	4200
Metconazole	125116-23-6	566 mouse, 660 rat	> 2000
Myclobutanil	88671-89-0	1600	> 2000
Propiconazole	60207-90-1	1517	> 4000
Tebuconazole	107534-96-3	> 5000	> 1000
Triadimefon	43121-43-3	90	310 rat; > 2000 rabbit
SDHI (Succinate dehydrogenase inhibitors), block cellular respiration			
Fluxapyroxad	907204-31-3	> 2000	> 2000
Boscalid	188425-85-6	> 5,000 (Technical boscalid)	> 2,000
Fluopyram	658066-35-4	> 2000	> 2,000
Methionine (amino acid) synthesis inhibitors			
Cyprodinil	658066-35-4	> 2000	> 2000
Pyrimethanil	53112-28-0	4150	>5000
Signal transduction disruptors			
Quinoxyfen	124495-18-7	> 5000	> 2000
Other fungicides			
PCNB	82-68-8	1700	> 5000
Benomyl	17804-35-2	> 10,000	> 1000

Source: https://chem.nlm.nih.gov/chemidplus/name/imazalil, imazalil tab.

compounds. Some, such as sulfur dioxide and sulfuric acid, are known to cause irritation, and others, notably the sulfite compounds, are recognized causes of allergic reactions.

Sulfur may also oxidize spontaneously at elevated temperatures or in contact with perspiration on the skin.

▶ Drift & Respiratory Irritation

The respiratory effects of sulfur include exacerbation of asthma and allergic reactions. It is not possible to evaluate the possible allergic reactions by immunologic blood tests or challenge testing.

A 2018 epidemiologic study evaluated the community risk of exposure to sulfur based on California pesticide use reporting data. The study reported a statistical association between reported applications of sulfur within a mile of individual residences and decreased pulmonary function. The exposure definition did not include location of residents at the time of reported applications or whether the residence was upwind or downwind of the application site.

Copper Salts

Most copper salts can be used as wood preservatives or as antimicrobials in water treatment operations. Compounds with predominantly agricultural use include elemental copper, copper sulfate, copper hydroxide, copper oxychloride, and copper octanoate. Copper naphthenate has unique use in structural pest control for control of fungal rot for exterior wood products (eg, fence and roofing material).

▶ Mammalian Toxicity

Copper salts have moderate acute toxicity and cause significant irritation of the eyes and skin. In human ingestion cases, irritation of the GI tract is significant and acute corrosion may occur with concentrated formulations.

A. Ingestion

In ingestion cases, copper salts can cause a variety of physiologic effects, including GI bleeding, methemoglobinemia, hemolysis, and renal failure.

Copper Naphthenate

Naphthenic acid is a butyric acid derivative of pentane, extracted from petroleum distillates ("naptha"). Copper naphthenate is a viscous mixture of naphthenic acid and its cyclohexane analogue, with an unpleasant odor and an affinity for "fibrous substrates." It has a low vapor pressure, drastically limiting dissipation by evaporation. No data exist to predict a specific rate of dissipation after application, but its odor may generate complaints in months after application. Nine products for use on exterior wood products have active registrations, with concentrations between 10% and 91% active ingredient. Most list insects as well as fungi as target pests.

Copper naphthenate has low systemic toxicity. Predictive irritation testing in animals showed moderate to severe irritation or corrosion (for the most concentrated formulations). The Buehler predictive test for ACD was negative.

Cases demonstrate contact irritation associated with application of copper naphthenate and cluster illness following its indoor use. Indoor applications are prohibited on current labels but misuse still occurs intermittently.

A 1992 case report described the possible association between elevated serum copper and the indoor use of copper naphthenate (25 gallons of 6% copper naphthenate was used to build the foundation of a house in Tennessee). Family noted symptoms of nausea, vomiting, burning of the eyes, dizziness, and headache within 1 hour after entering the home. Serum copper, initially tested in the index case 14 months after exposure, was approximately 215 mcg/dL (normal range 75–145 mcg/dL), with persistent neurocognitive symptoms 35 months after exposure.

Dithiocarbamate, Thiocarbamate Compounds

The thiocarbamates have broad-spectrum activity, affecting the squalene-epoxidase in sterol biosynthesis (pyributicarb), and metal-dependent and sulfhydryl enzyme systems (dithiocarbamates). The Disulfiram (Antabuse), used to treat alcoholism because of its ability to produce an adverse reaction in the presence of alcohol, is a dithiocarbamate and shares a number of properties with other compounds in the class. Several dithiocarbamates, including the ethylene-bis-dithiocarbamates (EBDCs), are used as accelerators in the vulcanization of rubber. Compounds currently registered include mancozeb, thiram, and ziram.

▶ Toxicity

The thiocarbamate fungicides have low acute toxicity, but can cause irritant and allergic contact dermatitis. However, thiocarbamates are also associated with short-term systemic effects. Similar to disulfiram (also known under the trade name Antabuse), thiocarbamates can inhibit the enzyme alcohol dehydrogenase. Workers who consume alcohol after hours may experience a reaction marked by skin rash, headache, nausea, vomiting, flushing, dizziness, confusion, and disorientation.

Phthalimide Compounds

Captan is the only phthalimide fungicide still in use, with 23 currently registered formulations. The related compounds captafol (difolitan) have not been used since the last compound registered in January 1998. Captafol and plondrel have low systemic toxicity but can cause immediate and delayed allergic reactions. Skin irritation also may occur given sufficient exposure.

The phthalimido compounds act as reactive electrophiles. This property also accounts for the carcinogenicity of the compounds in rodent bioassays. Both captan and folpet cause intestinal tumors in rodent species. Captafol causes lymphosarcoma in feeding studies with mice. The EPA ranking system designates all three compounds as probable human carcinogens.

Structural analogies with the drug thalidomide have raised concerns that the phthalimido compounds could cause teratogenicity in agricultural workers. Studies of teratogenic effects of captan show positive effects in chick embryos but negative effects in Syrian hamsters, rabbits, and nonhuman primates.

Chlorothalonil

Chlorothalonil is an electrophile that affects multiple cellular targets, including enzymes important for fungal spore germination and fungal respiration. California 2016 use data showed 1,124,450 lb applied to 541,201 acres of California cropland. Most frequently treated crops included almonds and pistachios, landscape maintenance, onions, potatoes, and prunes.

Chlorothalonil has low mammalian oral and dermal toxicity, but causes significant irritation to the eyes and skin. Predictive allergy testing with the Buehler test and guinea pig maximization test proved negative, but chlorothalonil provoked a positive reaction in the local lymph node assay at a concentration of 0.002%.

Both irritation and allergy symptoms appear in cases reported in California and in the published literature.

An outbreak of irritant dermatitis and conjunctivitis in a Portuguese tent manufacturing operation that used chlorothalonil-impregnated fabric has been described. Of 11 workers employed in the operation, 3 resigned prior to the investigation. The remaining eight workers reported erythema, pruritus, and scaling of the eyelids, face, and arms; conjunctivitis; and pharyngitis after handling batches of treated fabric. The authors considered cumulative irritation from aorne exposure to chlorothalonil to be the cause of the outbreak.

Contact dermatitis has been reported in vegetable growers, woodworkers, and flower growers.

Investigations in Panama reported chlorothalonil as a possible cause of erythema dyschromicum perstans (ashy dermatitis), a form of contact dermatitis affecting the basement layer of the epidermis. Positive patch test reactions to chlorothalonil (0.001% in acetone) were observed in 34 of 39 banana farm workers presented with erythema dyschromicum perstans-like dermatitis. Biopsies from all the patients were compatible with a chronic pigmented dermatitis or erythema dyschromicum perstans-like dermatitis.

Cases reported from Japan include a case of photoallergic contact dermatitis and a case of contact allergy. Related cases of chlorothalonil skin allergy were accompanied by cases of asthma.

Asthma was a primary endpoint in an employee of a fungicide formulating operation reported from England. There was no history of skin reactions, but an inhalation challenge with 12.5 g chlorothalonil in 250 g lactose mixture (for 30 min) resulted in a 20% decline in forced expiratory volume beginning 3 hours after exposure. It was not possible to confirm that the mechanism was allergic rather than irritant by testing a specific chlorothalonil IgE by RAST, by skin testing for either delayed or immediate allergy, or by testing controls using the same inhalation challenge administered to the patient.

Other Multisite Activity Compounds

Fungicides with multisite activity include formerly registered mercury compounds (phenylmercuric oleate, chloromethoxy propyl mercuric acetamide, and phenylmercuric acetate) used in paint and seed treatments.

Inhibitors of Mitochondrial Respiration, Cytochrome bc1 Complex III (Strobilurin Fungicides)

The strobilurin fungicides function by inhibiting mitochondrial respiration targeting cytochrome bc1 complex (complex III). Frequently used compounds include trifloxystrobin, azoxystrobin, and pyraclostrobin, used on approximately 12% of California cropland.

The acute mammalian toxicity for the strobilurin compounds is low but can cause skin and eye irritation in animal tests.

California illness data showed 11 cases associated with either azoxystrobin or trifloxystrobin between 1992 and 2015 without a consistent pattern of illness, most with nonspecific systemic symptoms. The 11 cases included 6 cases of indirect exposure of field workers to either residue or drift. One possible case of facial dermatitis occurred in an applicator.

In a 2007 episode reported from Iowa, 27 workers detasseling from corn field developed symptoms contact with drift from a nearby application of pyraclostrobin. Symptoms included upper respiratory irritation and skin and eye irritation; several had nonspecific systemic symptoms. The same report described three separate drift episodes involving five additional patients and the case of a crop-duster who suffered chemical burns attributed to pyraclostrobin after a crash on takeoff.

Ergosterol Synthesis Inhibitors

Commonly used group names for the ergosterol synthesis inhibitor (ESI) compounds include triazoles, azoles, and imidazoles. Important individual compounds include difnoonazole, metconazole, myclobutanil, propiconazole, tebuconazole, and triadimefon.

Inhibition sites for fungal ergosterol biosynthesis include $C^{14}\alpha$-demethylase in the Cytochrome P450 complex, 3-keto reductase, and C^{14}-α demethylase, squalene epoxidase, and Δ^{14}-reductase and $\Delta^{7}\rightarrow\Delta^{8}$ isomerase. The conazole C^{14}-α demethylase inhibitors group structurally resembles ketoconazole, miconazole, fluconazole, and other compounds used in human medicine.

Notable secondary effects of the triazole medications include delayed contact dermatitis and fixed drug eruptions. In addition to affecting the P450 complex demethylase enzyme, the triazoles have the capacity to affect other cytochrome complex enzymes. This may affect the metabolism of other medications.

▶ Skin, Eye, & Respiratory Irritation & Predictive Allergy Testing

Triadimefon, a triazole with long use history, has high to moderate toxicity on ingestion. Secondary effects of residue contact are probably limited by a maximum application rate of only 8 oz/acre. Imazalil (also known as enilconazole) has moderate acute toxicity. Other triazoles have low to moderate toxicity.

Predictive irritation tests show moderate or severe irritation for some triazole formulations, but the degree of irritation does not always increase and appears to correspond to the concentration of principal active ingredient, suggesting an effect related to formulation solvents or other inerts.

▶ Illness Data

Between 1992 and 2015, 31 illness reports in California involved one of the ergosterol synthesis inhibitors (difenoconazole, myclobutanil, propiconazole, tebuconazole, triadimefon) as the only implicated pesticide. Resulting from accidental direct exposures, residue contact or drift, 23 cases occurred in an agricultural setting. Myclobutanil accounted for 14 cases, many involving eye and skin irritation, but including some cases of nonspecific systemic symptoms (headache, nausea, or vomiting).

A 2002 report from Panama described confirmed ACD in eight workers who had one to three plus reactions to 1% imazalil, compared to 0 of 48 control subjects. The circumstances of exposure and the similarity of the symptoms strongly resembles those of the citrus packing workers and other California farmworkers exposed to conazole fungicides.

Succinate Dehydrogenase Inhibitors, Amino Acid Synthesis Inhibitors, & Signal Transduction Inhibitors

Three relatively new groups of agents are used on slightly more than 11% of California cropland. **These include three** succinate dehydrogenase inhibitors (SDHI) compounds, blocking cellular respiration, **amino acid synthesis inhibitors blocking intercellular mycelial** growth (cyprodinil), and cellular signal transduction disruptors.

Available information indicates the SDHI compounds have very low systemic toxicity in mammals and cause minimal eye and skin irritation. A search of the California illness registry did not identify any reported illness associated with either Boscalid (first registered in 2003), fluopyroxam (first registered in 2012), or fluxapyroxad (first registered in 2014) identified as the only implicated active ingredient. Succinate dehydrogenase also functions in mammalian mitochondria; it is not certain whether the apparent differential toxicity of the SDHI compounds is based on selective affinity for the fungal enzyme, differential metabolism, or some other mechanism.

Cyprodinil functions by blocking synthesis of the amino acid methionine at the cystathionine β-lyase step—inhibiting production of homocysteine from cystathionine. The principal California crops treated in 2016 included almonds, grapes, strawberries, and pistachios. The related compound pyrimethanil also inhibits methionine synthesis and is used on the same array of crops.

Both cystathionine β-lyase inhibitors have low mammalian toxicity and cause minimal skin-eye irritation in predictive animal tests. A search of the California illness registry did not identify any reported illness associated with either cystathionine β-lyase inhibitors as the sole implicated pesticide.

Quinoxyfen interferes with cellular function by interfering with physiologic signaling. The related compound Proquinazid functions by the same mechanism but does not have an active registration. Both compounds have low systemic toxicity in animal testing. A search of the California illness registry did not identify any reported illness associated with either quinoline compound. Nevertheless, both compounds appear as potential skin sensitizers in predictive allergy models. A cases series published in 2001 described three employees (a research chemist, a supervisor, and a process worker) of a UK manufacturing operation who developed sensitization on repeated contact with quinoxyfen.

Other Fungicides

Pentachloronitrobenzene (PCNB) belongs to a group of aromatic hydrocarbons, believed to inhibit lipid peroxidation, changing the concentration of lipid signaling compounds (eg, malondialdehyde [MDA]) and, in particular, 4-hydroxy-2-nonenal (4-HNE). It was formerly used as a seed treatment but currently registered products are designated for either soil or ground application. Broccoli, brussel sprouts, landscape maintenance, golf course, and turf applications account for approximately 98% of use, according to California data. Small quantities are used on nursery and ornamental plants.

PCNB has low systemic toxicity in animal tests but some formulations caused skin irritation in predictive testing.

Predictive testing using the Buehler test (induction period applications done topically, rather than by subcutaneous injection, as used in the guinea pig maximization test) was negative with a 23.8% emulsifiable concentrate and also with a 95% technical material. However, reports of possible PCNB secondary effects include suspected sensitization. Currently registered products carry a warning about sensitization.

▶ Illness Data

A search of the California illness registry (1992–2015) identified four cases associated with PCNB as the sole implicated pesticide. A patch test survey of California published in 1994 showed positive reactions to PCNB in 2 out of 39 nursery workers tested and 0 out of 21 control subjects. Although PCNB was commonly used in the nursery industry in the 1990s, it was not possible to confirm prior exposure in either case.

▶ Laboratory Tests & Treatment of Fungicide Poisoning

A. Copper

Severe intoxication is associated with serum copper levels greater than 500 mcg/dL. The significance of levels slightly above reference values in the context of exposure to copper naphthenate remains uncertain. For copper poisoning, chelation is possible with D-penicillamine (300 mg every 6 hours) if the patient is able to take oral medication. Alternatives include intramuscular injection of Dimercaprol (British anti-lewisite; 3 mg/kg every 6 hours) or intravenous injection of ethylenediaminetetraacetic acid (EDTA, 1 g twice a day).

D-penicillamine therapy and EDTA should be used with caution if nephrotoxicity from copper hemolysis occurs. The value of chelation in treatment of copper ingestion remains to be established.

▶ Allergic Reactions

Documentation of cutaneous allergic reactions to fungicides should be performed with patch testing involving three visits for each patient scheduled over 96 hours. There are no validated blood tests for allergies to fungicides.

▶ Treatment

Standard protocols for decontamination and poison center consultation apply to cases of fungicides ingestion. Removal from exposure or product substitution is the most successful remedy for cases of suspected allergy.

▶ Chronic Effects of Fungicide Exposures

Many fungicides with multiple sites of activity are reactive electrophiles or have electrophilic metabolites. Electrophiles have a tendency to react with skin proteins and cause delayed or immediate contact dermatitis. Since the 1970s electrophilic reactions with DNA and other biological targets have been recognized as human or animal carcinogens.

Table 33–16 shows fungicides identified as category B2 (probable) carcinogens, including the thiocarbamate compound mancozeb, the phthalimido compound captan, the triazole compound terrazole, the chloronitrile compound chlorothalonil, and the midazolidine compound iprodione. Coal tar creosote, used as a fungicide and wood preservative (last registered in 2000), is a recognized human carcinogen, based chiefly on a large volume of individual case reports of skin cancer.

▶ Formerly Registered Compounds

The fungicide hexachlorobenzene (HCB—last registered in 1988, a mixture with 10% HCB and 50% maneb) was associated with a prolonged epidemic of porphyria cutanea tarda in Turkey from 1955 to 1961. The source of the epidemic proved to be HCB-treated wheat seed used in the production of flour. An estimated 3000–4000 cases occurred, with a reported mortality rate of 10%. Many survivors had prolonged after-effects, documented in follow-up studies published during the 1980s.

Phenylmercuric acetate (last registered in 12/31/91) was a common ingredient of interior latex paints used until the early 1990s. A 1990 case reported described acrodynia (pain in the fingers and hands) that developed in a 4-year-old boy 10 days after the interior of his residence was painted with 17 gallons of an interior latex paint. Other symptoms included leg cramps, a generalized rash, pruritus, sweating, tachycardia, an intermittent low-grade fever, marked personality change, erythema and desquamation of the hands, feet, and nose, weakness of the pelvic and pectoral girdles, and lower-extremity neuropathy. A 24-hour urine sample contained 324 nmol of mercury per liter (normal < 100) and other family members also had elevated urine mercury. Registrations of organic mercury compounds for use in paint lapsed after 1991.

FUMIGANTS & NEMATOCIDES

California use data show that fumigants are applied to less than 1% of California cropland. However, application rates calculated from use data range from 170 to 236 lb/acre; 1-3 dichloropropene, metam sodium/potassium and chloropicrin all rank among the top 10 pesticides in pounds used. Considering the small percentage of cropland treated, the fumigants have a large environmental impact for the following reasons.

Fumigants and/or their by-products have high vapor pressures and a high degree of chemical and biological reactivity. Recorded effects include respiratory and eye irritation, CNS injury, hepatic and renal injury, as well as carcinogenicity and reproductive effects in animal studies. Use of insecticides has gradually shifted to a diverse group of low-toxicity compounds. The reactivity and toxicity of prospective fumigants, by contrast, tends to present barriers to registration and widespread use (discussed in the section on alternatives to methyl bromide).

Applications for fumigants include structural pest control, treatment of stored commodities, and control of soil pests. Structural and commodity fumigations usually target insects, but soil fumigation also assists in control of nematodes, weed, and some soil fungi.

Equipment used for soil fumigation includes shank injection equipment, broadcast sprinklers on risers, and drip irrigation lines. Structures such as houses, warehouses, grain elevators, and greenhouses may be sealed, fumigated, and then aerated before being reoccupied. Tarps made of impermeable material are also used to cover fields treated with halogenated hydrocarbon fumigants (dichloropropene and methyl bromide). To limit off-gassing of highly water soluble by-products of metam sodium and other fumigants that release MITC, postapplication water treatments are employed. Phosphide compounds are applied in solid formulations, as pellets of aluminum, magnesium, or zinc phosphide, which liberate

Table 33–16. Animal studies evaluating chronic effects of fungicides.

Chemical, use category or structural class	Cancer or reproductive effect	EPA Potency Factor-Q* (mg/kg/d)$^{-1}$	Classification
Thiocarbamates & ETU			
Mancozeb; Maneb	Thyroid follicular cell adenomas and carcinomas, combined thyroid follicular cell adenomas and/or carcinomas in male and female rats.		B2
Ethylene thiourea	Cancer: rat thyroid; mouse liver Reproductive: ETU produces neural tube and brain malformations in rats; other species not affected except at high-dose levels.	1.1 E-1	B2
Phthalimido compounds			
Captan	Intestinal tumors occurred in multiple strains of male and female mice; renal and cortical/tubular cell neoplasms occurred in rats. Female rats developed uterine sarcomas. Reproductive: Positive studies in chick embryos reported in public literature; incomplete ossification observed in rabbit study reported to Cal-EPA at 30 and 100 mg/kg/d; study in hamsters negative; literature report on teratogenicity on nonhuman primates negative.	3.6 E-3	B2
Triazoles			
Terrazole (etridazole—fungicide)	Cancer: male and female rats dose-related lung adenomas Male reproductive: chronic rat study showed testicular atrophy at mid and high doses	7.2 E-2 male 5.4 E-3 f. rare tumor	B2
Substituted aromatics			
Chlorothalonil	Cancer: kidney and forestomach tumors in male/female rats at and below MTD	1.1E-2	B2
Miscellaneous fungicides			
Benomyl and MBC (Benomyl and thiophanate methyl breakdown product)	Reproductive: Encephalocele, hydrocephalus, microphthalmia, and anophthalmia in animal model systems over doses ranging from 15.6 mg/kg to 125 mg/kg. Male reproductive: Dose-dependent decreases in mean testis weight and mean seminiferous tubular diameter and occlusions in efferent ductules in rodents dosed with 400 mg/kg of benomyl metabolite carbendazim (MBC).		
Iprodione—Imidazolidine	Male and female mouse liver at 4000 ppm in diet; rat testes-testicular adenomas at 1600 ppm in diet (CDPR)	4.39 E-2	Likely
Coal tar creosote	Human/animal skin carcinogen, last registered 2000		A

phosphine gas when in contact with water in the environment or after ingestion by pests such as rodents. The mixture of phosphine gas and carbon dioxide is used for commodity fumigation and pumped under pressure from tanks into commodity containers or warehouse storage spaces.

Newly Registered Compounds & Methyl Bromide Alternatives

Since 2000 newly registered fumigants have included a phosphine/carbon dioxide (CO_2) gas mixture, intended as a safer variation of the phosphide salts that release phosphine gas.

Safety issues with the phosphide fumigants are discussed as follows, but do not apply to the gas formulation because of the CO_2 content. Although the phosphine gas/CO_2 formulation is gradually increasing in use, its application is relatively complex compared to the use of aluminum phosphide tablets.

Methyl bromide alternatives that have not been registered include propargyl bromide. Its use is limited by both toxicity and safety concerns because of its tendency to decompose with mild shock. Methyl iodide was registered in 2010 but had limited use prior to voluntary cancellation by the registrant in 2012.

Dimethyl disulfide has also been evaluated, as well as a mixture of allyl isothiocyanate and furfural. Allyl isothiocyanate is currently only registered as an animal repellant. Dimethadione is structurally similar to furfural, a natural compound that targets nematode cuticles. The relatively selective mechanism of action thus distinguishes it from the broad biocidal activity of most other fumigants.

Halogenated Hydrocarbons, Methyl Bromide, Methyl Iodide, 1,3-Dichloropropene, & Chloropicrin

Halogenated fumigants, including chloropicrin, are electrophilic chemicals, reacting with nucleophilic amino acids (glutamine, asparagines, cysteine, and serine) at or near the active sites of enzymes in target pathogens or target pests.

Most halogenated fumigants and nematicides are well absorbed by all routes of exposure and are excreted rapidly without significant bioaccumulation. Both methyl bromide and 1,3-dichloropropene fit this pattern. Inhalation of vapors is the most common route of exposure, although dermal absorption of vapors or liquid also can occur. The vapors and liquids usually are primary irritants and in some cases are quite potent. At sufficient concentrations, acute CNS depression may occur. The halogenated hydrocarbon fumigants share many of the effects of the halogenated hydrocarbon solvents, including cardiac sensitization, direct cellular toxicity to the liver and kidneys, and carcinogenicity in laboratory animals. Table 33–17 shows acute systemic toxicity for currently used fumigants.

Chloropicrin

▶ Use Data

Currently chloropicrin, used by itself, or in mixtures with methyl bromide or dichloropropene, is used on 0.2% of California cropland. Chloropicrin best serves to control fungi and has less activity against nematodes and weeds than other soil fumigants. Many applications occur as part of mixtures with methyl bromide and dichloropropene, but some applications were made using formulations containing only chloropicrin. It cannot be mixed with nucleophilic compounds such as metam sodium.

Chloropicrin has high acute toxicity relative to other fumigants on inhalation and both oral and topical (dermal) administration. Nevertheless, its most noteworthy effect is eye irritation, noticeable at levels below the threshold of respiratory and skin irritation and systemic toxicity.

In a human volunteer study sponsored by a consortium of chloropicrin registrants, the threshold for irritant effects was evaluated. For exposures lasting 20 minutes, the minimum concentration detectable by 50% of the subjects was 75 ppb. The no observed effect level (NOEL) for this portion of the study was 50 ppb. For 1-hour exposures concentrations of 100 and 150 ppb produced subjective eye irritation in most subjects and lower concentrations were not tested. Using a standard 10-fold uncertainty factor 20, an estimated NOEL for a 1-hour exposure to chloropicrin (calculated from the 100 ppb lowest observed effect level [LOEL]) would be 10 ppb.

▶ Sample Community Episode

In the agricultural community of Salinas, California, residents downwind of a preplant drip application of chloropicrin in

Table 33–17. Selected fumigants and nematocides. Mammalian toxicity for selected fumigants.

Fumigant or nematicide	CAS #	LC50 ppm	Duration, hours	LD50 mg/kg
1, 3-Dichloropropene	542-75-6	855–1035 ppm (male) 904 ppm (female)	4	300 (male); 224 (female)
Methyl bromide	74-83-9	1158	1	214
Methyl iodide	74-88-4	3.9 mg/L (691 ppm)	4	80–214
Chloropicrin	76-06-2	14.4	4	
Sulfuryl Fluoride	2699-79-8	1000	4	Not given
Aluminum phosphide	20859-73-8	See values for phosphine	NA	11.5 mg/kg
Phosphine-CO$_2$	7803-51-2	11	4	Not given
Metam-sodium, potassium	137-42-8, 137-41-7	NA	NA	450 mg/kg
Methyl-isothiocyanate	556-61-6	440	4	2780 mg/kg

2005 reported eye irritation and other symptoms. A total of 439 residents of the 142 households in affected neighborhoods and 1 emergency responder were interviewed. Ocular symptoms were present in 302 (93.2%) of the symptomatic cases. Nonocular (usually systemic or respiratory) symptoms occurred in 170 cases (52.5%), but occurred significantly more frequently in residents who lived within 0.46 miles of the application site. Air-modeling showed a plume of chloropicrin in the affected neighborhoods, with estimated 1-hour TWA (time-weighted average) air concentrations between 0.15 and 0.025 ppm. Ocular, respiratory, and systemic symptoms corresponded to a plume of chloropicrin, with estimated concentrations as high as 0.15 ppm. Cases occurred between 0.36 and 2.89 miles from the application site.

Methyl Bromide

▶ Indoor Exposure

Poisoning with methyl bromide and other halogenated hydrocarbon fumigants may occur gradually over hours of inhalation exposure, even at the high levels present inside of tarped buildings.

For individuals impaired by alcohol, drugs, or mental illness, the eye and respiratory irritation provoked by chloropicrin (present as a warning agent) may not be sufficient to make them leave a treated building.

Symptoms may be nonspecific and difficult for victims to recognize as poisoning, including headache, nausea, vomiting and dizziness, drowsiness, fatigue, slurred speech, loss of balance, and disorientation. Tremors, myoclonus, and generalized seizures may occur. If such cases survive until hospitalization, death may occur after several days due to simultaneous liver and renal failure, possibly complicated by adult respiratory distress syndrome.

Acute and chronic poisoning from methyl bromide may be followed by prolonged and, in some cases, permanent organic brain damage marked by personality changes and cognitive dysfunction. Workers have been diagnosed as suffering from severe psychological disorders until a source of methyl bromide exposure was recognized.

▶ Direct Accidental Exposures

Direct contact with liquid halogenated hydrocarbons may result in erythema and blisters. Severe damage to the skin can occur if liquid is spilled on clothing and shoes, which retard evaporation. Many current agricultural formulations contain 20–50% chloropicrin, adding to the potential problems with irritation.

Topical exposures frequently lead to skin burns, eye irritation, or respiratory irritation, but may also show systemic effects. Since serious systemic poisoning sometimes occurs following dermal exposure, these cases deserve careful evaluation.

▶ Use in Structural Pest Control

Serious systemic poisonings and fatalities commonly occurred after exposure in confined spaces, usually associated with structural pest control applications. Many occurred after deliberate violations of tented structures, but failure to properly clear a treated apartment building caused two fatalities in a 1991 case in California.

▶ Agricultural Fatalities

Fatal exposures associated with agricultural use of methyl bromide occur infrequently. A 1989 fatality in a shoveler (covering the edges of a field tarp with dirt) from a methyl bromide application crew had no measured serum bromide at autopsy. Gross examination of the heart showed a well-defined coronary infarction.

In 2009, however, a worker in a methyl bromide formulation facility died following explosion of a canister containing a mixture of methyl bromide and chloropicrin. Initial findings on hospital admission included burns of the back and extremities. Ambulance crew members who attended the patient en route to the hospital complained of headache and irritation of the eyes and respiratory tract.

▶ Other Reports

Two noteworthy occupational poisonings occurred in the California cold storage industry over a period of several weeks. Two produce inspectors unknowingly inhaled methyl bromide off-gassing from produce treated on entry to the United States after shipment from Chile. Both had transient ataxia, cognitive impairment, and elevated levels of serum bromide. A subsequent industrial hygiene survey of the cold storage industry showed elevated methyl bromide air concentrations in enclosed locations in other facilities. These ranged as high as 20 ppm, 20 times the California 1-ppm 8-hour exposure standard.

A 2015 report from France described severe poisoning in a previously healthy 74-year-old man who required 2 months intensive hospital treatment. He presented with neurologic symptoms, initially thought to be a hemorrhagic stroke. The cause was determined to be poisoning after the patient's son found he had used an old fire extinguisher containing methyl bromide to unclog a sink. Testing showed a serum bromide level more than 120 mg/mL.

Another 2015 case report, from Turkey, described a severe nonfatal poisoning case in a 44-year-old man associated with the use of a mixture of 98% methyl bromide and 2% chloropicrin used for bed bug control. The patient survived after 48 days of treatment in the hospital. After rehabilitation he had a residual speech disorder and spasticity in the right quadriceps muscle, but was able to walk independently. Brain MRI showed axial fluid-attenuated inversion recovery (FLAIR) in the cerebral peduncles and corpus. A 2013 review suggested that FLAIR imaging was semi-diagnostic for methyl bromide poisoning but did not support the conclusion with population data or studies using MRI readers blinded to exposure status.

Dichloropropene

The level of dichloropropene use has decreased drastically because of regulatory concerns related to its carcinogenicity. A cancer bioassay evaluated the response of mice to lifetime inhalation exposure of 1,3-dichloropropene. There was a positive trend of increase with dose in pulmonary adenomas in male mice. The compound is currently used in mixtures with varying amounts of chloropicrin in order to decrease community air concentrations of dichloropropene.

▶ Illness Data

Between 1992 and 2015, the California illness registry received 198 reports regarding cases associated with exposure to dichloropropene. All but five cases involved mixtures with chloropicrin, with frequent eye and upper respiratory irritation symptoms resembling the sample episode described above for chloropicrin.

▶ Other Reports

A 2002 report from Italy described a typical case of dichloropropene poisoning causing a serious skin reaction following a workplace accident: A 28-year-old farmer developed dermatitis of the hands, abdomen, and flanks after direct contact with 1,3-dichloropropene, leaking from a fumigation device. Although the rash disappeared in a few days, he had residual postinflammatory hyperpigmentation. Three weeks later he handled dichloropropene and developed erythema, vesicles, and itching on the sites affected by the initial exposure. He received treatment for suspected ACD with topical and systemic corticosteroids. A closed patch test with 1% dichloropropene in petrolatum produced a ++ reaction at 48 and 72 hours. Control patch tests on five healthy volunteers produced no reaction.

Methyl Iodide

Similar to methyl bromide, methyl iodide is used for control of nematodes, fungi, and weeds. Methyl iodide was briefly registered in the United States in 2010, but withdrawn by the registrant in 2012, after very limited use.

The acute effects of methyl iodide are similar to those produced by methyl bromide, but occur at somewhat lower doses and include thyroid effects. In addition to neurotoxicity, skin burns can be significant problems. Experience with methyl iodide is limited to case reports, each involving neurologic symptoms very similar to those produced by methyl bromide.

▶ Case Reports

A recent report described substantial dermal exposure and contact burns requiring extensive full thickness grafting during a 17-day hospitalization. Neurobehavioral symptoms developed after discharge from the hospital, with difficulty with memory and concentration. Neurobehavioral testing showed abnormalities in measures of attention, memory, information processing, and performance of simultaneous tasks.

An English chemical worker suffered a burn on the extensor surface of his right wrist while handling methyl iodide a week before presenting to the hospital with symptoms that resembled a right-sided stroke, with abnormal neurologic examination findings including bilateral nystagmus, slurred speech, an ataxic gait, and past pointing on the right side.

Sulfuryl Fluoride

Sulfuryl fluoride has been the main replacement for methyl bromide in structural pest control. Of the four currently registered formulations of sulfuryl fluoride, three are registered for applications to structures, shipping containers, boats, and industrial areas. One formulation is registered for fumigation of commodities (nuts, beans grains, and food processing operations). Chloropicrin is added for structural applications, within an intended concentration of 0.25%. Because chloropicrin is not added at the time of sulfuryl fluoride manufacture, its application at the time of treatment does not insure uniform concentrations throughout the structure. The vapor pressure of chloropicrin is markedly lower than that of sulfuryl fluoride and it likely dissipates from treated structures more slowly than sulfuryl fluoride. Post aeration sulfuryl fluoride levels must be 1 ppm or lower.

▶ Acute Toxicity

Sulfuryl fluoride has a lower acute toxicity than methyl bromide. In animal studies with sulfuryl fluoride, the interval between initial exposure and death depends on the concentration of sulfuryl fluoride present, as indicated by the series of acute inhalation toxicity (LC50) studies and time-to-incapacitation studies.

For sulfuryl fluoride concentrations similar to those present during typical fumigations (800–4000 ppm), animal studies demonstrate a poisoning syndrome with an exposure-fatality interval of several hours. At concentrations of 20–40,000 ppm, incapacity and death occurs in a very short amount of time.

Ocular, dermal, and respiratory irritant symptoms produced by sulfuryl fluoride overlap with those produced by chloropicrin and may accompany accidental exposures. Systemic symptoms may include acute delirium and seizures. Most severe human poisoning occurs after violation of tarped structures or failure to properly conduct posttreatment aeration in a fashion similar to methyl bromide.

A 2008 case report described a fatal poisoning in a 37-year-old woman exposed to sulfuryl fluoride after the start of home fumigation. She developed symptoms of abdominal pain and shortness of breath; despite aggressive treatment with calcium gluconate, the patient deteriorated approximately 2 hours after arrival. Autopsy findings included acute tracheitis with pulmonary congestion and edema. Testing for fluoride showed an antemortem blood concentration of 24 mg/L and a postmortem urine concentration of more than 100 mg/L.

MITC-RELEASING FUMIGANTS

The soil fumigants metam sodium, metam potassium, and dazomet, all function as profumigants, releasing the active fumigant MITC after reacting with air or water. Dazomet is used in small quantities for landscape maintenance and for fumigating soil mixtures used to grow ornamental plants.

The principal degradation product (or by-product) of metam (either the sodium or potassium salt) is MITC, but can include a complex mixture of irritant compounds (methylamine, carbon disulfide, hydrogen sulfide, and low levels of methyl isocyanate [MIC]), depending on the soil pH and other environmental conditions.

Metam Sodium

The degradation products of metam sodium include a complex mixture of irritant compounds: the primary pesticidal agent MITC, MIC (approximately 4% of the level of MITC), carbon disulfide, hydrogen sulfide, and methyl amine. The toxicologic effects of the mixture have not been characterized.

Exposure to airborne MITC for 1 hour produces burning eyes and other irritant symptoms at concentrations of 800 ppb. Exposure for 4 minutes may produce similar symptoms at concentrations of 1900 ppb. Those with asthma or smoking-related pulmonary disease may experience respiratory problems at concentrations that only produce eye symptoms in others.

In community exposures, nonspecific systemic symptoms such as nausea, headache, and diarrhea accompany the irritant symptoms in a portion of those exposed. The symptoms produced by hydrogen sulfide, carbon disulfide, and methyl amine have a high degree of overlap with those produced by MIC and MITC, but quantitative experimental data on dose-response for these compounds do not exist.

Irritant dermatitis is associated initially with direct skin contact in metam sodium applicators. However, dermatitis has not been a frequent problem in community exposure to airborne metam-sodium by-products.

Dazomet

Use of dazomet is much lower than use of metam sodium and it causes far fewer episodes of illness. However, the comparatively small volumes of dazomet incorporated in soil can pose a risk to gardeners and landscapers.

A report from England in 1982 described contact dermatitis from use of dazomet as a biocide in a paper mill. The affected worker had a 3-month history of eyelid dermatitis that began after work shifts. Patch testing showed a ++ reaction to 0.01% and 0.1% of the formulated product containing 24% active ingredient. A report from Wales in 1993 described contact dermatitis from dazomet used as an antimicrobial in a rubber cushion.

A 67-year-old male farmer presented with an acute onset of itchy bullae and erythema on his feet, confirmed on examination. The severe pruritus and extensive bullae resolved with administration of prednisolone 20 mg/day for 3 days. Gas chromatography demonstrated the presence of MITC in the boots. The allergic nature of the dermatitis was confirmed by testing with rubber from the contaminated boots and negative results with patches made from new boots of the same type. Patch tests with the contaminated boots were negative in 10 control subjects.

Phosphide Fumigants

Phosphide fumigants generate phosphine (PH_3) gas on contact with either moisture in the environment or acid in the intestinal tract. It is relatively more toxic than other fumigants, but is generally applied in far smaller quantities (as a commodity fumigant and as a rodenticide) than the soil fumigants. Phosphine functions by inhibiting mitochondrial complex IV electron transport, a mechanism similar to sodium cyanide.

Aluminum phosphide is the model compound, but there is gradually increasing use of a new product containing phosphine and carbon dioxide that does not present a risk of uncontrolled oxidation. Most fatal cases of poisoning occur in cases of aluminum phosphide ingestion, most frequently in countries that do not restrict the sale to professional applicators.

▶ Acute Toxicity

Cases of acute aluminum phosphide ingestion result in death from pulmonary edema, seizures, and respiratory depression. Nonfatal cases have been marked by liver injury with abdominal pain, nausea, vomiting, jaundice, elevated hepatic enzymes, and coagulopathy with bleeding. Occupational cases infrequently cause fatal outcomes but may result in symptoms severe enough to require hospitalization. Severe poisoning and fatal outcomes have occurred during fumigation in transit by either ship or rail.

Aluminum phosphide reacts with water to generate phosphine gas. In concentrations of 2% or more, phosphine may combust spontaneously. Improper disposal of aluminum phosphide residue can lead to spontaneous ignition when it comes in contact with water (see following discussion).

▶ Illness Data

Between 1992 and 2015, 215 cases associated with exposure to phosphine or phosphine generating fumigants were reported in California. These included cluster episodes associated with inappropriate disposal of aluminum phosphide residue in dumpsters, exposures to grain inspectors, and packing plant workers required to work in warehouses near commodities under fumigation.

▶ Case Reports

A 2008 report from France described poisoning aboard a freighter carrying a cargo of peas fumigated in transit with aluminum phosphide tablets. Because the hold carrying the peas was not airtight, gas from the hold leaked into spaces used by the crew. One crew member died after developing abdominal pain and dizziness; by the time he reached a hospital ashore he had chest pain suggesting a possible myocardial infarction, then abruptly developed respiratory distress and had a seizure. It was not possible to measure tissue levels of phosphine despite multiple attempts; after a second mariner became ill, measurements aboard ship with colorimetric tubes confirmed the presence of phosphine gas in the holds and cabins. The circumstances of exposure resembled poisonings reported by CDC investigators in 1980. In that episode 1 of 2 children on board the vessel died, and 29 crew members aboard a grain freighter became acutely ill with headache, fatigue, nausea, vomiting, cough, and shortness of breath after inhaling phosphine generated by aluminum phosphide used to treat the cargo.

In 2009, a fumigation stack containing aluminum phosphide became soaked with rain water and caught fire at a pistachio processing plant in California. The trained applicator in charge of the fumigation did not get time to respond to the fire before untrained temporary workers began dousing the burning pallets with water. Those responding to the fire had exposure to pyrolysis by-products, particulates, and extinguisher ingredients. Ten workers taken for medical evaluation had respiratory and nonspecific systemic symptoms consistent with exposure to phosphine gas. Six of the 10 workers had respiratory distress, indicated by chest pain, shortness of breath, elevated respiratory rate, or decreased oxygen saturation.

A 2011 publication from a children's hospital reported that a family with six members was exposed to phosphine gas after their yard was treated with aluminum phosphide for a rodent infestation. Burrows in the yard apparently communicated with an open space under steps leading to the front door and seeped into the home. The inhalation of phosphine gas initially caused symptoms of abdominal distress in all of the family members. Within 36 hours of exposure, the 4-year-old sibling died of cardiopulmonary failure in a local emergency department. After an initial presentation of respiratory distress, the 15-month-old toddler progressed to complete cardiopulmonary collapse and did not survive despite aggressive life support.

An agricultural formulation of aluminum phosphide used for residential pest control in Texas in 2017 caused the evolution of phosphine gas. A 45-year-old woman previously in good health initially presented to an emergency room with nausea, vomiting, diarrhea, and dyspnea, accompanied by four children with similar symptoms, assumed to be acute gastroenteritis. Because of worsening respiratory distress, family again presented to the emergency room; although the woman survived with aggressive hospital care, all four children died in the emergency room.

Fumigant Laboratory & Industrial Hygiene Measures

Exposure to sulfuryl fluoride can be evaluated by measuring fluoride levels in serum. Reference values range from 0.01 to 0.2 mg fluoride per milliliter of serum. The elimination half-life for serum fluoride (varying from 3 to 7 hours, based on exposure of cryolite workers and 3 hours based on exposures to rabbits) necessitates measurement within 1–2 days of exposure. High-dose sulfuryl fluoride exposure may also result in low serum calcium levels.

No specific clinical tool exists for monitoring exposure to MITC metam-sodium by-products. Measurement of environmental levels of MITC in excess of the 0.8-ppm irritation threshold clearly would suggest the cause of concurrent ocular or upper respiratory symptoms. Pulmonary function studies and methacholine challenge tests may prove of value in cases of residual airway reactivity.

During the 1990s, permit conditions and the metam-sodium applicators trade association encouraged the use of odor monitoring to detect offsite movement of MITC. Odor monitoring is a poor means of detecting MITC because the average odor threshold (1700 ppb) is approximately twice the 800-ppb 1-hour ocular irritation threshold (based on a registrant conducted experiment with human volunteers).

Following inhalation exposure to phosphine, no specific tests are available in most laboratories to aid in diagnosis. However, in cases of phosphide ingestion, aluminum may be elevated in serum and other tissues. Phosphine can be measured in expired air in either inhalation or ingestion. It may prove possible to use colorimetric tubes or direct-reading industrial hygiene instruments.

The current 0.3 ppm TLV, calculated as an 8-hour TWA, is intended to prevent systemic phosphine poisoning. The short-term exposure limit is 1 ppm. These standards are based primarily on a study reported in 1964 describing phosphine exposures to Australian grain terminal workers. Most of the phosphine measurements reported were area samples, making it difficult to identify the level of exposure associated with individual cases of illness. It was consequently difficult to identify levels of exposure that were tolerated without symptoms.

In 1998, the reregistration eligibility document (RED) for aluminum phosphide and magnesium phosphide published by the U.S. EPA suggested an 8-hour limit of 0.1 ppm, based on risk assessment from animal studies. In 2018, California posted possible changes to its occupational exposure limits, suggesting an 8-hour limit of 0.05 ppm and a short-term-exposure-limit (STEL) of 0.15 ppm.

Treatment for Fumigant Poisonings

Most fumigant poisonings require supportive therapy for eye irritation, contact dermatitis or skin burns, and respiratory irritation that may possibly progress to pulmonary edema. Neurologic symptoms ranges from headache to altered consciousness or seizures. Survivors of severe poisoning may require prolonged rehabilitation care.

Sulfuryl fluoride poisonings may present with severe and difficult to treat hypocalcemia.

Chronic Effects & Sequelae of Acute Poisonings for Fumigants

Table 33–18 summarizes human and animal studies documenting chronic effects of fumigants, including cancer, reproductive effects, and persistent effects of acute poisoning.

Table 33–18. Animal and human studies evaluating chronic effects of fumigants and nematocides.

Chemical, use category or structural class	Cancer or reproductive effect	EPA Potency Factor-Q* (mg/kg/d)$^{-1}$	Cancer classification
Dichloropropene (Telone II)	Forestomach/liver tumors in male rats; forestomach tumors female rats; forestomach, lung, urinary bladder in female mice-tox summary, combined rat	Oral 1.8 E-1; inhalation 9.66 E-2	B2
Methyl bromide	Reproductive: Omphalocele, misrouting of subclavian artery, gallbladder agenesis in studies reported to CDPR		
Methyl iodide	Inseminated New Zealand white female rabbits (24/group) exposed to MeI 0, 2, 10, and 20 ppm) for 6 hours per day, 7 days per week by whole-body inhalation, exposure from GD 6 through 28, and sacrificed on day 29. Developmental NOEL was 2 ppm (1.5 mg/kg/d) for the effects on reduced fetal weight and viability; and increased late resorption and fetal death at 10 ppm and 20 ppm Cancer: thyroid tumors—rated as unlikely to cause cancer at doses that do not affect rat thyroid hormone homeostasis		
Ethylene oxide	Cancer: Leukemia in rats and monkeys; mice show lung cancers, and lymphomas; human cancer in case reports; NIOSH study showed increased risk of leukemia in US cohort. IARC classification: limited evidence for human carcinogenicity Reproductive: Dominant lethal mutations produced when male mice injected with single 150 mg/kg dose of ethylene oxide. Similar effect produced by inhalation of 1000 ppm. Aberrations in cervical vertebrae in mice treated intravenously with 75–150 mg/kg Male: Decreased sperm count and motility in monkeys inhaling 50–100 ppm.; currently registered https://apps.cdpr.ca.gov/cgi-bin/label/labq.pl?p_chem=277&activeonly=on 11 registered products; limited reported agricultural use chmrpt16 – p 26/933; 8,570,537.02717 lb sold 2016		IARC classification category 1
Propylene oxide	Sprague-Dawley rats receiving propylene oxide by stomach tube in doses of 15 or 60 mg/kg of body weight twice weekly for 109.5 weeks exhibited a dose-dependent increase in forestomach tumors. Additional rat study showed pheochromocytomas and mesotheliomas. Mouse inhalation study showed hemangiomas and hemangiosarcomas.		B2
Dazomet	Male reproductive: 150 ppm in CDPR dog chronic study—testicular tubular atrophy		
Metam-sodium	CDPR cancer: mouse liver masses at 240 ppm (high dose) in females Cancer CDPR: angiosarcomas in combined rat study at concentrations >= 0.056/mL Fetotoxicity: in feeding studies; principal by-product methyl-isothiocyanate negative in similar studies; other by-products include carbon disulfide and hydrogen sulfide. The former is noted to produce malformations in feeding studies.	1.98 E-1	B2

▶ Cancer

Fumigants identified as probable or definite carcinogens include dichloropropene, ethylene oxide, propylene oxide, and metam sodium.

▶ Reproductive Effects

A rabbit teratogenicity study of methyl bromide described abdominal wall defects. Maternal toxicity limited most of the other rabbit and rodent teratogenicity studies on methyl bromide.

Sequelae of Fumigant Poisonings

▶ Methyl Bromide

A 1969 report described 10 patients with methyl bromide poisoning evaluated in California, apparently as medical-legal or workers' compensation cases, related to commodity fumigation. Apart from four fatalities, five cases had residual symptoms and all symptoms resolved in one patient after observation for 18 months. Fatigue and malaise described as "neurasthenia" (a vague term that may roughly translate as "weakness" or "fatigue") was the most common residual symptom. Other symptoms included nausea, vertigo, slow cognition, muscle pain, and a residual central scotoma.

A 2015 report described severe accidental methyl bromide in a family vacationing in the US Virgin Islands. The downstairs unit of their rented condominium had been fumigated with methyl bromide 2 days before they sought treatment. Symptoms included generalized weakness, severe myoclonus, fasciculations, altered sensorium, and word-finding difficulty. Three required mechanical ventilation and treatment with the neuromuscular blocker rocuronium because of difficulty controlling seizures. Three of the four patients received inpatient physical rehabilitation for significant neurologic dysfunction, although the report did not describe the specific residual deficits.

▶ Sulfuryl Fluoride, Post-aeration Poisoning

A 2016 CDC report described a Florida poisoning episode apparently related to failure to properly aerate the structure and failure to conduct post aeration testing. Four family members reentered the home 48 hours after the fumigation began; the mother and the 9-year-old son became ill within hours, with symptoms of nausea and vomiting. All four family members had symptoms the next morning and three sought treatment at a local emergency room. The 9-year-old had altered mental status, accompanied by dysarthria, dystonia, rigidity, and hyperreflexia. He required calcium gluconate in order to correct hypocalcemia. He developed choreoathetosis 4 days after hospitalization, consistent with a subsequent brain MRI showing an injury of the basal ganglia. The symptoms persisted throughout treatment for the next several weeks at a rehabilitation facility.

HERBICIDES

Herbicides are pesticides used to prevent or control the growth of unwanted plants or kill them once they have appeared. They have largely replaced mechanical methods of weed control and are currently the largest category of pesticides used in agriculture. Included here are plant growth regulators that alter plant development, defoliants that cause leaves to drop prematurely, and desiccants that accelerate the drying of plant parts. With the exception of the bipyridyls (paraquat and diquat), most frequently used herbicides have modes of action specific to plant biochemistry, resulting in relatively low mammalian toxicity.

EPSP Synthase Inhibitors

Glyphosate and its various salts function by inhibiting enolpyruvylshikimate-3-phosphate synthase (EPSP), blocking the synthesis of aromatic amino acids (eg, tyrosine and phenylalanine). Their use encompasses more than 20% of California cropland. From California 2016 sales data, an estimated 11 million additional pounds is used on nonagricultural landscapes and gardens.

Separate 2019 publications from the United Kingdom and Japan described the complexity of identifying the surfactants in various formulations containing glyphosate, based on laboratory analysis. Compounds found include polyoxyethylene alkylamine (POEA or Polyethoxylated tallow amine). This mixture contains a fatty acid with a terminal amine linked to a polymer formed by chaining 8–19 molecules of ethylene oxide. Other surfactants identified in analysis of the formulations included the cationic alkyl bis (2-hydroxyethyl)methylammonium and a nonionic alkyl glucoside compound.

A 1997 report for the U.S. Department of Agriculture reviewed ingredients listed for adjuvant compounds recommended for use for agricultural formulations of the isopropyl amine salt of glyphosate. A typical commercial recommended adjuvant contained a blend of polyoxyethylated polyol fatty acid ester, polyol fatty acid ester, and paraffin base petroleum oil. It is uncertain how such tank-mix surfactants affect the symptoms of pesticide handlers or field workers accidentally exposed to drift.

▶ Acute Mammalian Toxicity

As discussed earlier, glyphosate formulations typically contain surfactants, the likely cause of eye or skin irritation, that commonly affect applicators and other pesticide handlers. Animal tests for glyphosate show low mammalian toxicity.

▶ Illness Data

California illness registry data for the period 1992–2015 included 449 cases associated with glyphosate as the only implicated pesticide, with typical cases involving eye or skin irritation to pesticide handlers. Serious illnesses from glyphosate sometimes occur after ingestion, with symptoms also likely related to the surfactant content. Newer formulations that contain mixtures of glyphosate and diquat have toxicity in proportion to the concentration of diquat, especially in cases of deliberate or accidental ingestion.

An additional 40 cases involved mixtures of glyphosate and the bipyridyl compound diquat (discussed later). Some of these involved tank mixes with more than two pesticides and some involved a RTU "fast-acting" mixture of glyphosate and diquat.

Twelve ingestion cases involving mixtures of glyphosate and diquat often required hospitalization, although some received only brief emergency care. Five resulted in death and one additional case required treatment for renal failure.

▶ Acute Case Reports

A 1984 case report from England described allergic photo contact dermatitis associated with handling a glyphosate formulation (provocation testing done using 1% formulated product). The herbicide registrant disclosed to the authors that the formulation contained benzisothiazolone as a preservative. Additional testing, published in a separate 1986 brief report, showed no reaction to 1% glyphosate (active ingredient) and a positive reaction to 1% benzisothiazolone.

A 2008 case report from Spain described a 37-year-old gardener who developed an irritant reaction after applying a dilute glyphosate solution from a leaking back-pack sprayer. She reported having redness on the arms her first day working with the herbicide, resembling eczema by the second day. She developed reddish-purple papules at the site of the initial reaction and erythema-multiforme-like target lesions on the abdomen, axillae, and groin 5 days later. On a skin biopsy the reaction showed histologic characteristics of an auto-eczematous (ID) reaction.

A 2019 report from French poison centers analyzed the severity of glyphosate ingestion cases in relation to presence of POEA surfactants. The authors noted that more severe cases occurred among 235 formulations containing POEA (7.8%), compared to the 105 cases involving other surfactants (1.9%). The authors reported the two groups had similar demographic characteristics and comparable volumes of ingested liquid. All five fatalities occurred in the POEA group.

Protoporphyrinogen Oxidase Inhibitors, Photosynthesis Pathway

The diphenyl ether compound oxyfluorfen, the phenylpyrazole pyraflufen-ethyl, the triazol carfentrazone-ethyl, and the pyrimidinedione saflufenacil function by inhibiting protoporphyrinogen oxidase (PPO) in the photosynthesis pathway. As a group their use encompassed slightly more than 8% of agricultural cropland in California.

▶ Acute Mammalian Toxicity

Acute mortality studies in rodents show low mammalian toxicity. They cause minimal irritation in predictive animal testing and are nonsensitizers.

▶ Illness Data

California illness registry data showed 53 cases associated with PPO inhibiting herbicides, with 52 cases involving oxyfluorfen and 1 involving carfentrazone-ethyl. Most involved contact reactions to the eyes or skin, but some demonstrated nonspecific systemic symptoms. These included a group of 9 (of 15) workers who reported nausea, lightheadedness, and headache after contact with residue of oxyfluorfen 30 minutes after its application to a field where they were transplanting cauliflower.

Bipyridyls

The bipyridyl compounds diquat and paraquat have a specific mechanism (altering electron transport in the photosystem I pathway in the presence of sunlight). However, both compounds are so chemically reactive (generating oxygen free radicals) that they have many adverse effects on nontarget organisms.

Reported use for 2016 for the bipyridyls encompassed slightly more than 5% of California agricultural land, although the total treated acres reported included some non-agricultural acreage (landscape maintenance land and highway rights-of-way).

▶ Clinical Syndromes, Pharmacokinetics

Bipyridyls are absorbed following ingestion and less frequently following inhalation or skin contact. They damage epithelial tissues such as skin, nails, cornea, GI tract, and respiratory tract, as well as the liver and kidneys.

Paraquat is more toxic to humans than diquat. A small sip of the liquid concentrate can kill an adult, which accounts for the hundreds of deaths reported worldwide from accidental and deliberate ingestion of this herbicide. An experimental trial that consisted of adding an emetic to formulations of paraquat was instituted recently in an attempt to reduce the frequency of fatal ingestions.

Pulmonary injury from paraquat ingestion has been well described in numerous case reports and series. Neither paraquat nor diquat has been adequately tested for carcinogenicity.

▶ Topical Effects

Direct contact with concentrated liquid dipyridyls results in skin irritation and fissuring and in cracking, discoloration, and sometimes loss of the fingernails. Liquid splashed in the eye can cause conjunctivitis and opacification of the cornea. Inhalation of spray mist can irritate the nose and throat, causing nosebleeds and sore throat.

▶ Illness Data

California illness data showed 207 cases associated with the bipyridyl compounds between 1992 and 2015. Most cases involved workplace, skin, eye, or respiratory irritation, without signs of systemic illness. The ingestion cases involved RTU mixtures of glyphosate and diquat, or workers with access to restricted formulations of bipyridyls. A handful of ingestion cases involved diquat or paraquat placed in unlabeled containers.

Other Herbicides

Table 33–19 shows other frequently used herbicide compounds, noteworthy for their selective modes of action and low acute mammalian toxicity. These include dinitroaniline microtubule assembly inhibitors (pendimethalin), two categories of amino acid synthesis inhibitors (the phosphinate compound glufosinate that blocks glutamine synthesis and the sulfonyl urea compounds that block synthesis of branched chain amino acids). The gibberellins have a broad impact on plant development from germination to stem elongation, flowering, and senescence. Other important groups of compounds include the cellulose biosynthesis inhibitors (the triazine-diamine compound indaziflam) and photosynthesis system II inhibitors (the amide compound

Table 33–19. Mammalian toxicity of selected herbicides and plant growth regulators.

Mode of Action	Chemical Class	Compounds	Oral LD50	Dermal LD50
EPSP synthase inhibitors, blocking synthesis of aromatic amino acids	Glycine derivative	Glyphosate, potassium salt, isopropylamine salt	4300	
Protoporphyrinogen oxidase (PPO) inhibitors, blocking photosynthesis pathway	Diphenylether	Oxyfluorfen	5000	
	Phenylpyrazole, pyrimidinedione	Pyraflufen-ethyl, carfentrazone-ethyl, saflufenacil	5143 > 5000 5000	> 4000 > 400 > 2000
Photosystem-I-electron diversion	Bipyridyl	Paraquat dichloride, diquat dibromide	112–344	> 2000
Microtubule assembly inhibition	Dinitroaniline	Pendimethalin	1050	> 5000
Inhibition of glutamine synthetase	Phosphonoglycine, phosphinate	Glufosinate	2000	> 4000
Inhibition of acetolactate synthase ALS, branched chain amino acid synthesis	Sulfonyl urea	Rimsulfuron	> 5000	> 2000
Regulate various developmental processes, including stem elongation, germination, dormancy, flowering, flower development, and leaf and fruit senescence.	Multiring lactone	Gibberellins	> 5000	> 2000
Cellulose-biosynthesis inhibitor (CBI)	Triazine-diamine	Indaziflam	> 2000	> 200
		Hydrogen cyanamide		
Liberation of ethylene, which is absorbed by the plant and interferes in the growth	Phosphonic acid	Ethephon	1600	5000
Inhibition of photosynthesis at photosystem II	Amide	Propanil	367	4830
Plant auxin analogues	Phenoxy compounds	2,4-D and derivatives Triclopyr and derivatives	2140	> 2000
Plant dormancy disruptors		Hydrogen cyanamide	125	84
Plant growth regulator		Gibberellic acid	6300	> 2000

propanil). Compounds causing unusual acute poisoning or possible chronic effects are as follows.

▶ Phenoxy and Pyridine Auxin Analogues

The phenoxy and pyridine auxin analogues have chemical shapes similar to the natural plant auxin 3-indole-acetic acid. The compounds have a differential detrimental effect on broadleaf weeds.

The principal herbicidal derivatives of phenoxy acetic acid include 2,4-dichlorophenoxyacetic acid (2,4-D), 2,4,5-trichlorophenoxyacetic acid (2,4,5-T), 2-methyl-4-chlorophenoxyacetic acid (MCPA), and their salts and ester derivatives. 2,4,5-T and its homologues are no longer manufactured or used in the United States because of contamination with

2,3,7,8-tetrachlorodibenzo-p-dioxin (TCDD). Dioxin contamination arose from difficulties precisely controlling production of the 2,4,5-T intermediate 2,4,5-trichlorophenol, causing low to moderate level contamination during routine operations and intermittent catastrophic process accidents.

A. Use Data

California 2016 pesticide use data show the greatest use for 2,4-D dimethylamine salt (364,378.50, 9,367 agricultural applications), 2,4-D, 2-ethylhexyl ester (31,887.35 lb, 332 agricultural applications), 2,4-D (9,666.98 lb, 438 applications). Most frequently reported application sites included landscape maintenance and rights of way, but some use was reported for nursery crops and citrus. Common uses not covered by the agricultural use reports included home and garden products—concentrates, RTU sprays, and "weed and feed" mixtures. Sales data for these compounds were not reported for 2016 to allow an estimate of the total pounds used outside of agriculture.

B. Mammalian Toxicity, Irritation studies, & Sensitization Studies

Phenoxy compounds have low acute mammalian toxicity.

The phenoxy and pyridine auxin analogues have chemical shapes similar to the natural plant auxin 3-indole-acetic acid. The compounds have a differential detrimental effect on broadleaf weeds. Some liquid formulations of 2,4-D demonstrate moderate irritation to the skin in predictive animal tests. One 20% liquid caused sensitization in the Buehler (epicutaneous) test, but four other products did not. This variation in the skin reactivity could relate to differing "nonactive" or "inert" components between the formulations or differences in test procedures between labs.

C. California Illness Data

California illness data for 2,4-D as the only implicated pesticide showed 11 cases reported between 1992 and 2015. These typically involved eye, respiratory, and/or skin irritation following accidental exposure during application. Four cases had principally nonspecific systemic symptoms (eg, nausea or headache).

▶ Case Reports

A 1970 case report described the accidental ingestion of 30 cc chlorophenoxyacetic acid by a man driving a tractor. He initially experienced facial flushing and diaphoresis and upper GI irritation accompanied by vomiting. After vomiting subsided, he developed intense aching in his chest, painful and tender muscles, tender abdomen, and a fever of 103°F. Although the fever subsided in 48 hours, he had residual muscle pain, then began passing dark-colored urine. This resolved by the fifth hospital day, but he continued to have muscle pain, accompanied by elevation of muscle enzymes.

Three cases of peripheral neuropathy have been reported in a single case series (1959) following relatively large dermal exposures to 2,4-D over the course of a few days. Clinically, these resembled idiopathic acute symmetric polyneuropathy (Guillain-Barré syndrome) and OPIDN in their symptoms, also preceded by an initial influenza-like illness associated with nausea, vomiting, diarrhea, and myalgias, followed by an asymptomatic interval and then, 7–10 days later, by rapidly ascending loss of both motor and sensory nerve function. Respiratory function was spared in most cases. A 1963 case report of primarily sensory neuropathy described symptoms 4 days after spraying 2,4-D. Investigations failed to establish whether the neuropathy described resulted from an inert ingredient, a contaminant, or an unrelated cause.

Triclopyr & Its Derivative Salts

Triclopyr functions as an analogue of the natural auxin indole-3-acetic acid. Currently registered compounds include a butoxyethyl ester and a triethylamine salt.

▶ Use Data

Frequent sites of application included forest timberlands, landscape and golf course maintenance, and on orchard floors.

▶ Mammalian Toxicity & Illness Data

Triclopyr has low acute mammalian systemic toxicity but is irritating to the eyes and skin in predictive animal tests. The California illness registry contained 17 cases reported between 1992 and 2015 with triclopyr as the only implicated pesticide. Recorded application sites included ornamental plants, lawns, forest trees and forest lands, and uncultivated nonagricultural areas. Symptoms included eye, respiratory, and skin irritation with some cases demonstrating nonspecific systemic symptoms.

Ethephon

Ethephon is a simple chloride derivative of phosphonic acid that functions by altering plant production of ethylene and subsequent maturation and development. Cotton, tobacco, peppers, grapes, walnut, and tomatoes accounted for 98.5% of reported agricultural use in California.

▶ Mammalian Toxicity & Irritation in Predictive Animal Tests

Ethephon has moderate to low toxicity in rodent oral acute toxicity tests, and very low acute systemic toxicity when applied dermally, but a strong tendency to cause corrosion on eye or skin contact.

▶ Illness Data

The California illness registry included reports of seven cases involving ethephon as the principal implicated pesticide between 1992 and 2015. Five cases involved applicators who suffered eye irritation (four cases) and one who suffered skin irritation after direct accidental exposure. Two cases involved drift exposure to field workers.

Hydrogen Cyanamide

Inhibition of catalase and other enzymes by hydrogen cyanamide applied to dormant grapes, cherries, and other woody fruits stimulates uniform budding, applied 30–40 days prior to the desired time of budding. In warm climates, it compensates for lack of winter chilling necessary to produce natural springtime budding and also increases fruit production if supported by appropriate amounts of water and fertilizer.

In 50% aqueous solutions, cyanamide also serves as an effective biocide. Hydrogen cyanamide also inhibits the liver enzyme alcohol dehydrogenase. In some countries hydrogen cyanamide is also used as medication to treat alcoholism, similar to the way disulfiram is used in the United States.

Use Data

There are three active formulations of hydrogen cyanamide currently registered, all 50% aqueous solutions for use on grapes, cherries, figs, kiwis, and blueberries accounting for almost all of the use.

A related compound, calcium cyanamide, can be confused with hydrogen cyanamide. Agricultural formulations of calcium cyanide degenerate into urea when applied to soil and are used as fertilizers rather than as plant growth regulators.

Acute Mammalian Toxicity

Hydrogen cyanamide has high systemic mammalian toxicity compared to other herbicides and plant growth regulators. It is corrosive or markedly irritating depending on the concentration. It has a markedly higher vapor pressure than other herbicides and plant growth regulators, and inhalation can be a significant route of exposure.

Illness Data

The California illness registry contains five reports identifying hydrogen cyanamide as the only implicated pesticide. These included applications to cherries in three cases, applications to kiwis in one case, and applications to blueberries in one case.

Case Reports

A 2001 report from Italy summarized illness surveillance data documenting 23 cases associated with exposure to hydrogen cyanamide, including 22 occupational cases and 1 case associated with accidental ingestion. Eighteen cases had skin rashes (maculopapular rashes, erythema or contact irritation, and two had eye irritation. Twelve cases required hospitalization. A 2005 follow up report described five additional cases. In 2009 two similar cases were reported from France, both involving "Antabuse"-like reactions between hydrogen cyanamide exposure and subsequent alcohol use.

A report from India in 2007 described four cases of skin reactions resembling erythema multiforme in two cases and toxic epidermal necrolysis (Stevens-Johnson Syndrome) in two cases. A 2011 report from India described poisoning after intentional ingestion of hydrogen cyanamide, with signs and symptoms including metabolic acidosis, pleural effusion, sinus tachycardia, confusion, and drowsiness.

A 2005 report from Spain described a 67-year-old man admitted to the hospital because of fever and pancytopenia, who had taken 120 mg of cyanamide daily for 6 months as aversive therapy for alcohol dependence. A bone-marrow biopsy showed severe aplastic anemia. Treatment included the bone marrow stimulant filgrastim, cyclosporin, and methyl prednisolone for 2 months. At that point, discontinuing cyanamide aversion therapy was the only necessary

long-term treatment. A literature review described additional aplastic anemia cases associated with cyanamide aversion therapy, as well as previously reported cases of peripheral neuropathy and cyanamide-associated liver injury.

Laboratory Evaluation & Treatment Following Herbicide Poisoning

Most acute herbicide exposures only require supportive treatment and do not have specific laboratory tests available. Exceptions include the bipyridyls and phenoxy herbicides, where laboratory measurements principally assist in documenting exposure and evaluating prognosis.

Bipyridyls

In the early phase of acute poisoning, the findings are nonspecific and usually are related to dehydration from nausea and diarrhea. In the later phase, liver injury is indicated by elevated bilirubin and hepatocellular enzymes. Renal injury, primarily tubular, is indicated by proteinuria, hematuria, pyuria, and elevated serum urea nitrogen and creatinine. Oliguric renal failure typical of acute tubular necrosis may occur. Laboratory evidence of pulmonary fibrosis from paraquat in the form of a progressive decline in arterial oxygen tension and diffusion capacity for carbon monoxide commonly precedes the appearance of pulmonary symptoms. Later, pulmonary function findings are typical of restrictive lung disease. The diagnosis of acute intoxication from paraquat or diquat can be confirmed by analysis of either compound in blood and urine.

The primary treatment during any phase of intoxication from paraquat or diquat is supportive, particularly during periods of organ failure. Bentonite and Fuller's earth are possibly more effective absorbents for dipyridyls in the GI tract than activated charcoal. If available, they should be administered as a 7 g/dL suspension in normal saline in quantities of at least 2 L to any patient suspected of ingesting any quantity of a dipyridyl within the preceding several days. If neither bentonite nor Fuller's earth is available, activated charcoal should be administered.

Hemoperfusion with coated charcoal may be effective in removing paraquat from the blood if it is performed before the chemical has been distributed to tissues. However, few patients have a confirmed diagnosis and can be placed in a facility where the procedure can be performed early (24–48 hours after ingestion).

Supplemental oxygen should be administered only as necessary to maintain minimally acceptable levels of oxygenation. Early experimental results with the free-radical scavenger superoxide dismutase have been disappointing. Corticosteroids and cytotoxic agents such as azathioprine have been tried with uncertain results.

Phenoxy Herbicides

Treatment of 2,4-D is supportive, with emphasis on hydration, and evaluation for rhabdomyolysis and other complications of myotonia. Alkalinization of urine should be considered to increase clearance of 2,4-D. As 1977 European report showed the plasma half-life of 2,4-D decreased from 219 hours for urine pH values from 5.10-6.5 to 4.7 hours for urine pH values from 7.55 to 8.8. Consideration of dialysis may prove useful in some compromised patients where high-volume fluid treatment and alkalinization of urine may prove harmful.

Herbicides & Cancer

Table 33–20 shows herbicides and growth regulators classified as probable carcinogens, including the growth regulator daminozide, and the acetanilide herbicides (alachlor, butachlor, and acetochlor) used in the production of corn. The chlorophenoxy compound 2,4-D is associated with astrocytomas in male rats, with a statistically significant test for trend (high dose 6/50 vs 1/50 in controls). Several epidemiologic studies demonstrate a significant association with non-Hodgkin lymphoma (NHL).

▶ Glyphosate

A pooled analysis of North American and Canadian studies, the North American Pooled Project (NAPP), reported an elevated risk of all NHL with any glyphosate use (OR = 1.51, 95% CI 1.18–1.95) with a dose-response effect with greater use (> 2 days/year, OR = 2.66, 1.61–4.40). Increases were observed for small lymphocytic lymphoma (SLL; 2.58, 95% CI 1.03–6.48, among those using for more than 5 years), and for follicular lymphoma (OR = 2.36, 95% CI 1.06–5.29), diffuse large B-cell lymphoma (DLBCL; OR = 3.11, 95% CI 1.61–6.00), and other subtypes (OR = 2.99, 95% CI 1.10–8.09) for use more than 2 days per year.

Three meta-analyses have been conducted on glyphosate and NHL that demonstrate significant increases in NHL risk with any glyphosate exposure, with particularly stronger increases reported for B-cell lymphoma. The IARC Working Group also conducted their own meta-analysis and has reported a meta risk-ratio of 1.3 (95% CI 1.03–1.65), with consistent findings across studies (low heterogeneity). The Agricultural Health Study (2017) found no association between glyphosate and NHL, but nondifferential exposure misclassification may have accounted for this finding.

RODENTICIDES

Poisoning with rodenticides is used for control of rats, mice, and other small mammals that interfere with human activities.

Rodenticides typically have delayed action if used as bait, because rats will avoid returning to feed where another rat has died after eating. Unfortunately, what is attractive, edible, and ultimately lethal to a rat also appeals to pets and other animals and small children.

Because application of baits results in negligible exposure to applicators, the primary human health hazard from most rodenticides is childhood poisoning from ingestion, although serious poisoning from single pediatric ingestions of warfarin is rare.

▶ Use Information

The rodenticides do not appear in the list of most frequently used agricultural compounds because most use is nonagricultural (Table 33–21). Zinc phosphide (discussed in the section on fumigants) is the most widely used compound. The anticoagulants include short- and intermediate-acting compounds, represented by warfarin, chlorophacinone and diphacinone, and the long-acting compounds ("superwarfarins"), represented by brodifacoum, bromadiolone, difenacoum; and the indandione derivative. California data shows 12 active product registrations, including 10 with the word "gopher" in the title. However, all products simply list "rodents" as the target pest. Sales and use data show limited use compared to the anticoagulant compounds.

▶ Anticoagulant Compounds

There are few reports of harmful exposure from the manufacture, formulation, or application of dry anticoagulant rodenticides. There is one report of bleeding in a farmer following extensive and prolonged skin contact with a liquid warfarin solution.

Childhood ingestion of anticoagulants occurs with some frequency, although bleeding as a result occurs in a small portion of cases with first-generation anticoagulants. The long-acting anticoagulants require fewer doses to cause bleeding.

All the anticoagulants act through inhibition of hepatic synthesis of prothrombin (factor II) and factors VII, IX, and X. In humans and rats, the half-lives of these factors are longer than the half-life of warfarin, so repeated doses are necessary before significant depression and bleeding occur. Resistance to warfarin in humans and rats appears to be genetic and may be a result of rapid metabolism.

The anticoagulants also produce capillary damage through an uncertain mechanism, although this, too, is reversed by administration of vitamin K. Skin necrosis and dermatitis have been reported as rare. Complications of therapeutic use of warfarin may occur, but have not been reported as a result of exposure to rodenticides. The indanediones cause neurologic and cardiovascular toxicity in some animal species, but these effects have not been reported in humans.

▶ Acute Toxicity (Table 33–21)

Most cases of accidental ingestion do not result in evidence of toxicity even without treatment because doses usually are single and relatively small. Repeated doses could be followed by bleeding, primarily from the mucous membranes such as the gums and nasal passages and into the skin, joints, and GI tract. Abdominal, flank, back, and joint pain reflect bleeding into those areas.

▶ Illness Data

California illness registry data show 78 cases associated with warfarin (1 case), second-generation anticoagulants (44 cases),

Table 33–20. Cancer and reproductive effects related to herbicides.

Chemical, use category or structural class	Cancer or reproductive effect	EPA Potency Factor-Q* $(mg/kg/d)^{-1}$	Classification
Growth regulator			
Daminozide	Rat: uterine sarcomas; UDMH contaminant—female liver tumors Mouse: liver angiosarcomas at 10,000 ppm in diet; lung adenomas and adenomacarci- nomas, angiosarcomas in mouse drinking water study 3000 mg/kg/d (CDPR)	8.70E-03	B2
Herbicide			
Acetanilides			
Acetochlor	rat nasal adenomas at 1000 ppm, maximum tolerated dose	1.69E-02	B2
Alachlor	rat nasal—tumors in mice and rats at multiple sites and doses	8.0E-2	B2
Butachlor	Sprague-Dawley rats administered butachlor in the diet—100, 1000, and 3000 ppm for 26 mo, showed neoplasia in the olfactory epithelium of the nasal turbinate, glandular stomach mucosa, thyroid follicular epithelium. Stomach tumors observed only at the 3000 ppm level. Increased incidence of nasal and thyroid tumors occurred only at levels of 1000 ppm and above.		Known/likely
Aniline and nitroaniline derivatives			
Asulam	In a 2 year rats feeding study 0, 1000, 5000, and 25000 ppm for 108 wk showed statistically significant increase in thyroid gland c-cell carcinomas, adenomas and carcinomas in both low- and mid-dose males; also showed significant increase in benign adrenal medullary pheochromocytomas in high-dose males.		C
Bipiridyls			
Paraquat	Controversy based on similarity of structure to acute substantia nigra poison PPP+, a CNS derivative of MPTP, cause of "frozen addict" syndrome. Paraquat poisons sub-stantia nigra on injection into the brain, but does not easily cross the blood-brain barrier after oral or dermal contact.		
Phenoxy and phenol compounds and related contaminants			
2,4-D	Astrocytomas male rats, statistically significant test for trend, high dose 6/50 vs 1/50 in controls; several completely negative studies; epidemiologic association with non-Hodgkin lymphoma in several studies		C
2,3,7,8-Tetrachlorod-ibenzo-para-dioxin (TCDD); contami-nated of banned 2,4,5-trichlorophe-nol related phenoxy compounds, not 2,4-D	Cancer: By gavage, TCDD increased thyroid follicular cell adenomas in male rats and neoplastic nodules of the liver in female rats, hepatocellular carcinomas in mice of both sexes and thyroid follicular cell adenomas in female mice. Also positive feed-ing and positive skin application studies. Other studies indicate that TCDD is most effective as a promoter, rather than an initiator of cancer. Reproductive: Cleft palate, kidney anomalies mice/rats; feto toxic to variety of experi-mental animals; mouse NOEL = 0.1 mcg/kg/d; male toxin at doses above those producing above effects		B2
Thiocarbamates			
Molinate (Ordram)	Testicular damage in rats 1 week after treatment with 200, 400 mg/kg molinate; At 3 wk after administration of the two higher-dose levels, germ cells in the seminiferous tubules were almost completely absent. NOEL: 100 mg/kg		
Other compounds			
Glyphosate	Non-Hodgkin lymphoma		IARC 2A; U.S. EPA not likely carcinogenic in humans
Oryzalin	Increase in mammary gland tumors in females and skin and thyroid tumors in both sexes		Likely carcinogenic in humans
Oxadiazon	Liver tumors in two species (mice and rats) following chronic exposure to oxadiazon		Likely carcinogenic in humans

Table 33–21. Rodenticide acute toxicity and use data.

Rodenticide	Single Dose	Oral LD50 (mg/kg)	Elimination half-life	Pounds USED, California 2016	# Agricultural Applications	SOLD 2016
First-generation anticoagulant						
Warfarin	No	180		0.32	67	9.10434
Second-generation anticoagulant						
Bromadiolone	Yes	1.7	3.5 days initial phase, then 24 days	72.99	257	44.95714
Chlorophacinone	No	1	6–23 days	5.71	5.71	13.92732
Diphacinone	No	3	15–20 days	108.67	4220	209.809
Difethialone	Yes	0.56	2.3 days	7.77	113	6.89745
Induction of hypervitaminosis, hypercalcemia						
Cholecalciferol (Vitamin D)		42		2868.95	11	25.50525
Uncoupler of mitochondrial oxidative phosphorylation						
Bromethalin	Yes	0.57	2.3 days	3.37	101	85.51948
Mitochondrial complex IV electron transport inhibitors						
Zinc phosphide	Yes	50		3656.48	887	19898.05
Sodium cyanide	Yes	4.3		2868.95		3079.65
Antagonist of glycine and acetylcholine receptors						
Strychnine	Yes	1–30		108.67	4220	825.3239

and 23 cases involving exposure to strychnine (most involving deliberate ingestion). All but five cases involved nonagricultural settings.

Laboratory Findings

Prolonged prothrombin time may appear 24–48 hours after ingestion of an anticoagulant and is often the only evidence of toxicity following a single exposure. Coagulation time will be increased in cases of significant poisoning, but bleeding time may be normal. Specific factors other than prothrombin may be depressed. Warfarin can be measured in plasma and its metabolites in urine, but these measurements have little utility.

Treatment

Treatment of single acute ingestions is usually unnecessary, but patients should be observed (at home) for 4–5 days following ingestion. Vitamin K may be administered orally in a dosage of 15–25 mg for adults and 5–10 mg for children with a history of ingestion, or intramuscularly in a dosage of 5–10 mg for adults and 1–5 mg (up to 0.6 mg/kg) for children

with prolonged prothrombin time or bleeding. Following treatment, prothrombin times should be determined every 6–12 hours and used as the basis for further treatment.

Treatment of warfarin poisoning is usually effective within 3–6 hours. The prognosis is determined by the extent and location of bleeding, but most treated cases do well. Poisoning with second-generation anticoagulants requires prolonged treatment, depending on the dose ingested.

Chronic Effects & Sequelae of Rodenticides

Neither the U.S. EPA list of probable carcinogens or the IARC carcinogen list contains currently registered rodenticides. Reproductive studies of bromadiolone show maternal toxicity rather than teratogenicity. Chlorophacinone also showed principally maternal toxicity, but hydroureter occurred more frequently in treated animals than controls.

Sequelae of Chronic Poisoning (Table 33–22)

Most cases of strychnine poisoning and anticoagulant ingestion recover with no after effects.

Table 33–22. Rodenticide chronic effects, reproductive effects, and sequelae of acute poisoning.

Chemical, Use Category or Structural Class	Cancer or Reproductive Effect	EPA Potency Factor -Q* (mg/kg/d)$^{-1}$	Classification
Anticoagulants			
Chlorophacinone	A combined reproductive/teratogenicity tested the effect of 0, 12.5, 25, 50, or 100 mcg chlorphacinone/kg/d on pregnant CD7 mice. NOEL for maternal toxicity was 50 ug/kg. Hydroureter appeared as a possible effect in the study, with a dose-related upward trend, but also occurred in control animals.		
Neurotoxins			
Strychnine	Administering strychnine, a potent antagonist of glycine receptors, to pregnant rats caused marked toxic effects on the ensuing embryos. Abnormalities included anencephaly, general aplasia (embryos with a decrease in craneo–caudal length of 40% or more, as well as a decrease in the number of somites) and absence of cerebral vesicles.		
Alpha-Naphthyl thiourea (ANTU)	Intentional ingestions reported between 1978 and 1980 resulted in autonomic neuropathy and death of pancreatic islet (Beta) cells, causing brittle insulin-dependent diabetes.		

A 2017 publication, for example, reported accidental poisoning in a 40 year old who ingested a reported Southeast Asian herbal supplement that proved to contain strychnine. Clinical symptoms included dizziness, headache, and nausea, motor dysfunction, with full recovery reported.

Alpha-naphthylthiourea (ANTU, Vacor)

California data show the most recent registration for an ANTU seed protectant rodenticide in 1989 that functioned by antagonizing metabolism of nicotinamide. Although few problems occurred with normal handling of the compound, intentional poisoning cases reported between 1978 and 1980 showed unusual residual effects. These included autonomic neuropathy and death of pancreatic islet (Beta) cells, causing brittle insulin-dependent diabetes. The authors of the initial 1978 drew an analogy with the antimetabolite streptozotocin, used to treat pancreatic cancer, that has a similar effect on Beta cells.

REFERENCES

Agricultural land loss and conservation. https://www.cdfa.ca.gov/agvision/docs/Agricultural_Loss_and_Conservation.pdf.

Calvert GM, Rodriguez L, Prado JB; Centers for Disease Control and Prevention (CDC). Worker illness related to newly marketed pesticides–Douglas County, Washington, 2014. MMWR Morb Mortal Wkly Rep. 2015 Jan 23;64(2):42-4. PMID: 25611169; PMCID: PMC4584598.

Centers for Disease Control and Prevention (CDC). Acute pesticide poisoning associated with pyraclostrobin fungicide–Iowa, 2007. MMWR Morb Mortal Wkly Rep. 2008 Jan 4;56(51-52):1343-5. PMID: 18172421.

Cimino AM, Boyles AL, Thayer KA, Perry MJ: Effects of neonicotinoid pesticide exposure on human health: A systematic review. Environ Health Perspect 2017;125(2):155-162 [PMID: 27385285].

Hertz-Picciotto I et al: Organophosphate exposures during pregnancy and child neurodevelopment: Recommendations for essential policy reforms. PLoS Med 2018;15(10):e1002671 [PMID: 30356230].

Kim KH, Kabir E, Jahan SA: Exposure to pesticides and the associated human health effects. Sci Total Environ 2017;575:525-535 [PMID: 27614863].

Naughton SX, Terry AV Jr.: Neurotoxicity in acute and repeated organophosphate exposure. Toxicology 2018;408:101-112 [PMID: 30144465].

O'Malley MA, Fong H, Mehler L, Farnsworth G, Edmiston S, Schneider F, Runge MJ, Pina R, and Calvert GM. Illness associated with exposure to methyl bromide-fumigated produce–California, 2010. MMWR Morb Mortal Wkly Rep.2011 60: 923-6, erratum in MMWR 2011 Jul 22;60(28):959.

Pourhassan B, Meysamie A, Alizadeh S, Habibian A, Beigzadeh Z: Risk of obstructive pulmonary diseases and occupational exposure to pesticides: a systematic review and meta-analysis. Public Health 2019;174:31-41 [PMID: 31306887].

Richardson JR, Fitsanakis V, Westerink RHS, Kanthasamy AG: Neurotoxicity of pesticides. Acta Neuropathol 2019;138(3):343-362 [PMID: 31197504].

Ritz BR, Paul KC, Bronstein JM: Of Pesticides and Men: A California story of genes and environment in Parkinson's disease. Curr Environ Health Rep 2016;3(1):40-52 [PMID: 26857251].

Schneir A, Clark RF, Kene M, Betten D. Systemic fluoride poisoning and death from inhalational exposure to sulfuryl fluoride. Clin Toxicol (Phila). 2008 Nov;46(9):850-4. doi: 10.1080/15563650801938662. PMID: 18608259.

Vainio H: Public health and evidence-informed policy-making: The case of a commonly used herbicide. Scand J Work Environ Health 2020;46(1):105-109 [PMID: 31486846].

■ SELF-ASSESSMENT QUESTIONS

Select the one correct answer for each question.

Question 1: In the United States, the Environmental Protection Agency (EPA)
   a. regulates the registration, sale, and conditions of use of all pesticides
   b. defers to "Occupational Safety and Health Administration (OSHA)" the responsibility for the protection of agricultural workers exposed to pesticides
   c. narrowly defines pesticides for registration for sale and use
   d. ignores studies of hazards to nontarget organisms

Question 2: Organophosphates
   a. are esters of phosphoric acid that exist in any number of forms
   b. bind with the cholinesterase molecule
   c. bind with the phosphate portion of the serine molecule
   d. have no irreversible effects

Question 3: Carbamates
   a. share a common mechanism of chronic toxicity with organophosphates
   b. present unique signs and symptoms of acute poisoning

   c. differ from organophosphates in causing reversible rather than irreversible cholinesterase inhibition
   d. typically have a longer clinical course than organophosphate poisoning

Question 4: Treatment of organophosphate poisoning
   a. should be instituted on clinical grounds alone
   b. should be delayed pending determination of cholinesterase levels
   c. may follow a test dose of atropine with marked signs of atropinization
   d. may follow a test dose of atropine with no signs of atropinization

Question 5: Fumigants
   a. have innately high vapor pressures or by-products with high vapor pressure
   b. have a low degree of chemical and biological reactivity
   c. cause respiratory and eye irritation, CNS injury, and retinal injury
   d. have no measurable carcinogenicity and reproductive effects in animal studies

The Changing Nature of Work

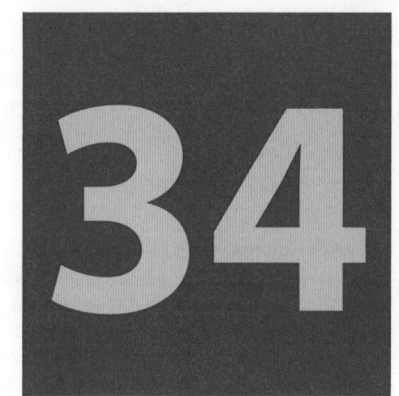

John Howard, MD, JD

Changes in the nature of work, where work is conducted, the demographics of the workforce, and in the ways employment is arranged pose new challenges for the practice of occupational health and safety. While employment in the manufacturing and energy sectors has declined, employment in the services and health care, and social assistance sectors has increased. New technological advancements like nanotechnology, automation, sensor technology, machine learning, data analytics, and robotics are changing the nature of work.

Changes in the age, gender, and racial/ethnic composition of the workforce are also occurring. Up to five generations are now working alongside each other in the workplace—traditionalists, baby boomers, Gen X, Gen Y ("millennials"), and Gen Z. Each generation has different attitudes about the role of work in their lives, different ways of communicating, and different perspectives on how workers should be managed.

Work arrangements are also changing. The "standard" employer–employee relationship, which provided a "safety net" of federal and state law protections (including safety and health protections) for those workers deemed by law to be "employees," now exists alongside alternative work arrangements that lack the same labor law protections. These alternative arrangements include co-employment, or "temporary" worker arrangements, independent contractor, or "entrepreneurial" arrangements, and newer arrangements often called "gig" or "platform" arrangements, which are intermediated by an online digital platform rather than by a traditional employer.

CHANGING NATURE OF THE WORKFORCE

▶ Age Composition

The share of the US population aged 55 or older is rising rapidly. In 2000, the 55-year-and-older cohort made up 13% of the workforce. By 2020, this group had increased to 20% of the workforce, and by 2050, older workers will still constitute 19% of the workforce. However, millennials (those born between 1981 and 1997) have caught up with the baby boomers (those born between 1946 and 1964). In April of 2016, population estimates from the U.S. Census Bureau showed that millennials were estimated to number 75.4 million individuals, surpassing the 74.9 million baby boomers.

Age-related changes in the workforce require practitioners to engage in a type of demographic risk management. Older workers bring value to the firm because of their experience, but older workers have more chronic medical conditions that may affect their work performance. The most common chronic medical conditions seen in older workers, such as hypertension, arthritis, and respiratory and cardiovascular disease, may lead to more absences and a diminished physical tolerance. Physically demanding tasks may pose both a productivity risk and a safety risk for the firm with an aging workforce. Occupational safety and health practitioners need to be wary of emphasizing the frailties and limitations associated with age without evaluation of each worker on an individual level. Mature workers can often function at a similar physical and cognitive level than younger workers. In addition, the organization may benefit from a mature worker's experience with the particular process, condition, or task. An emphasis on positive outcomes for both aging workers and their organizations can support the safety and health actions that lead to productive aging for all workers.

▶ Diversity

A. Generational Diversity

Multiple generations in the same workplace may have different attitudes about work, loyalty toward the employer, respect for authority, learning styles and training needs, supervision, how work-life balance should be considered, and how attached a worker should be to a particular workplace or to one's work associates. Generational diversity can also pose a challenge to achieving organizational coherence as well as creating a consistent safety and health culture. Perceptions about how to achieve safety culture may vary across individuals and generations and can create stress among workers. Creating a constructive organizational culture in a diverse workforce depends on occupational safety and health leadership. Managers and occupational safety and health practitioners need to understand generational values and work styles, find commonalities among generations, encourage employees to share their perceptions of other generations, and promote exchange of safety ideas across generations to ensure good mental health in the workplace.

1. Gender diversity—The increased share of women in the workforce has led to a greater emphasis on gender-specific issues such as adverse health effects of work on women, equal pay, prevention of gender-specific discrimination, and maternal and child leave policies. Gender diversity has become a business asset. The Gallup Organization found that in the retail and hospitality industries, gender-diverse business units have 14% higher revenue than less diverse business units. Gender-diverse teams perform better than single-gender teams largely because different viewpoints and approaches assist a firm in tailoring goods and services to an increasingly gender-diverse customer base.

2. Racial and ethnic diversity—The workforce has become more racially and ethnically diverse over the past century. Immigration, higher fertility rates, and higher labor force participation rates among minority populations such as Hispanics, Asians, and African Americans have led to an expanded minority share of the American workforce. By 2050, there will be no single racial or ethnic majority in the United States.

▶ Diversity Management

Workplace diversity can be thought of as the process of understanding, acknowledging, accepting, and valuing the age, gender, racial/ethnic, varying abilities, and cultural differences among workers. Diversity management entails avoiding stereotyping people based on age, gender, sexual orientation, and racial or ethnic status, emphasizing cross-cultural communication strategies, encouraging diverse teamwork, and treating all workers equally based on objective performance criteria. Organizations that fail to invest in managing the diversity inherent in the changing workforce demographics risk higher employee turnover rates, higher absenteeism rates, and invite lawsuits based on sex, race/ethnic, and age discrimination. A strong business case can be made for firms that engage in effective diversity management, successful talent recruitment and retention, improved market understanding, and enhanced worker creativity and innovation.

At the same time when safety professionals promote the demographic diversity in their workforce, they must be careful to make safety-related decisions based on a worker's ability to get the job done. Making safety-related decisions based on age, gender, or race may constitute employment discrimination. Diversity management benefits the organization and its workers by creating a fair and safe environment where everyone has access to the opportunity to succeed. Safety

managers must also use a balanced approach to changing organizational culture. In addition to providing information and training on rules and regulations, safety managers should aim for more permanent changes by emphasizing the importance of organizational values.

CHANGING NATURE OF THE WORKSPACE

The traditional workplace owned or rented by an employer at which employees conduct their jobs still exists, but the virtual workplace—spatially and temporally distributed across geography and time zones—is on the rise. The increasing use of digital means to connect workers by video or audio capabilities is rapidly transforming what we consider to be a workplace. The home, automobile, coffee shop, all of these can serve as digitally connected workspaces. Loosening the controls that employers have over the physical surroundings for a worker also lessens their responsibilities for ensuring a safe space for workers and places the onus on the worker. Smart devices serve as electronic leashes, tethering the worker to the organization. As a result, the traditional 8-hour workday and 40-hour work week have been considerably lengthened. The greater use of dispersed workgroups—often global—may impair developing trust among coworkers because of a lack of face-to-face interactions.

Even the traditional workspace is seeing smaller individual workspaces and more common meeting areas to accommodate the increasing use of teams. These changes can increase workspace noise levels, increase distractions from work, and can led to longer work hours to get individual assignments completed. All these changing nature of the workplace may contribute to increase work-related stress. These "work organization" exposures can lead to employee anxiety and depression, degrade cardiovascular health, and increase mortality.

CHANGING NATURE OF WORK

The physical and digital worlds are converging across all industry sectors leading to the 4th Industrial Revolution that is merging the physical and cyber worlds. The Internet of Things (IoT)—the convergence of industrial machines, sensors, data, and the Internet—is unleashing new ways to optimize the functionality, efficiency, and reliability of physical systems. Advanced robotics, artificial intelligence, and machine learning are making it possible to automate more and more worker tasks, opening the possibility of both productivity gains and labor market disruption. Applied physics, materials science, and chemistry are interacting to develop advanced materials with radically useful attributes, including incredible strength, conductivity, or the ability to "remember" previous states. Next-generation genomics is bringing low-cost genetic analysis and "editing" to improve medical diagnostics, accelerate drug discovery, and develop drought- and pest-resistant crops.

In all industry sectors, the nature of work is changing. Prominent among the emerging physical and chemical hazards facing workers are nanomaterials and powerful lasers being used in new additive manufacturing or 3D techniques. Collaborative robots ("cobots") that work in the same workspace as human workers are also increasingly used in manufacturing, increasing the risk profile of the workspace. Unmanned aerial vehicles, or drones, are being used in construction for monitoring projects and for inspecting compliance with permit requirements. Drones can also perform operations hazardous to workers, for example, climbing at heights and spray painting the sides of tall buildings.

The increasing use of sensor technology as a new tool of exposure assessment challenges existing models of risk assessment and risk management. Sensors—located on functional fabrics worn by workers, distributed in the work environment, or placed on or inside a worker—will generate large amounts of data that will need to be analyzed to determine their relevance to protecting worker health and their utility in developing and implementing effective control mechanisms. Sensors are at the heart of the new industrial Internet. Sensors can become intelligent assets—devices equipped with sensors and connected to one another—that produce massive amounts of sensor-based analytics turning occupational health practitioners into occupational data scientists.

In addition to these physical changes to the nature of work, new organizational methods can also present psychosocial hazards to workers. Work is becoming more cognitively complex, more dependent on social or "soft" skills, and more dependent on technical competence. Management methods often emphasize continual reorganization to maintain competitive advantage that may increases pressures on workers to be more agile and responsive to rapid changes. These social changes to the nature of work may lead to adverse mental and physical health effects for the employee and lead to poor performance by the organization.

CHANGING STRUCTURE OF WORK ARRANGEMENTS

The structure of work arrangements is changing dramatically. The relationship between entities offering jobs and individuals accepting those jobs comes in several different forms. In addition to the use of the more traditional one employer-one employee relationship ("standard employment relationship"), greater use of the co-employment arrangement ("temporary") and new forms of the independent contract ("entrepreneurial") arrangements are becoming more prevalent. Firms benefit economically from these new "flexible" work arrangements, but the new work arrangements are often "precarious" and detrimental to worker health, an important consideration for occupational health and safety practitioners.

▶ Types of Work Arrangements

A. Standard Employment

The standard employment relationship is an arrangement in which an employer exerts directive control over how a worker provides services to that employer. The twentieth century industrial model of the standard relationship predominately involved an individual who provided services exclusively to one employer on a predictable workweek schedule (usually 40 hours per week) at the employer's place of business with the mutual expectation of long-term career development. In exchange for submitting to an employer's control, a worker was given protections under numerous federal and state labor laws. Chief among these is protection under the Occupational Safety and Health Act (OSHAct). Employees can file a complaint with the federal Occupational Safety and Health Administration (OSHA), or with their state occupational safety and health plan, and their employer can be cited for their failure to comply with occupational safety and health standards. Workers who are classified as independent contractors are not covered by the OSHAct.

B. Co-employment

Following World War II, women war factory workers started being hired by a labor supplier for time-limited work assignments at the premises of another employer. This type of temporary help services model is also known as a co-employment or joint employment arrangement. The agency pays wages and unemployment and workers' compensation premiums, and assigns their employee to the client employer who directs the agency employee's work. Historically, temporary agency workers were assigned office administrative support tasks, but the use of temporary workers by firms is now expanding out of the low-wage sector into the legal services, business and financial operations, information technology, manufacturing, health care delivery, and education occupations.

1. Independent contractor—A worker is an independent contractor if the payer has the right to control or direct only the result of the work and not what will be done and how it will be done. An independent contractor provides services as part of an entrepreneurial business relationship, and not as part of an employment relationship. Independent contractors are excluded from protection by federal or state occupational safety and health laws, including occupational safety and health laws.

C. Gig or Platform Work

Workers who are connected to their customers by a digital platform on the Internet for short-term assignments are known as "gig" or "platform" workers, on-demand workers, new economy workers, or "app-based" workers. The Internet platform considers itself merely a facilitating intermediary, not an employer. However, there is continuing litigation about the legal status of "gig" workers in many states—are they independent contractors as some digital platform companies assert, or are they traditional employees? Employers or digital platform intermediaries can intentionally (as an integral part of their business model), or inadvertently, misclassify workers as independent contractors when they should have been classified as employees. Determining whether a platform worker is an independent contractor or an employee can be a complex legal classification task. If an employer misclassifies workers as contractors when they are really employees, the employer can be liable to the **Internal Revenue Service (IRS) for civil penalties or fines**. The continuing controversy over the legal status of gig workers has led to new proposals. These include creating a new category of worker—the independent worker—between the employee and the independent contractor—who may be able to buy benefits that are portable from job to job, for example, workers' compensation insurance coverage.

▶ Prevalence of Nonstandard Work Arrangements

Uncertainty exists about the number of workers involved in various alternative work arrangements. Much of the uncertainty arises from the lack of definitional clarity around what is a nonstandard work arrangement. The Bureau of Labor Statistics (BLS) uses the terms *contingent* and *alternative* workers to cover many who are in nonstandard work arrangements. Although the two terms are a bit overlapping, BLS defines a contingent worker as someone who does not have an implicit or explicit contract for ongoing employment, and an alternative worker as composed of four groups: independent contractors, on-call workers, temporary workers, and workers provided by contract firms. Using these definitions, BLS reported that in 2018 contingent workers represented 6.7%, and alternative workers in alternative arrangements represented 10.2% of the total employed workforce. Electronically mediated workers (ie, gig or platform workers) accounted for 1.0% of total employment, that is, approximately 1.6 million workers.

▶ Management Advantages Under Alternative Work Arrangements

A. Organizational Flexibility

Firms want to maximize their organizational flexibility to meet changes in customer demand. Greater operational flexibility allows firms to more easily adjust to up-and-down fluctuations in the business cycle. Firms that want to shed labor during a downturn can more easily do so if they are using nonstandard workers. When demand returns, resupplying the firm with nonstandard workers can help position firms more quickly than can the hiring process for standard workers. Acquiring workers through nonstandard arrangements is also more efficient when a firm needs workers with highly specialized skills for short-term projects such as information technology initiatives or manufacturing turnarounds.

B. Labor Cost Reduction

Nonstandard workers free the firm from the high costs of hiring and firing permanent workers. The labor cost differential between a full-time employee with benefits and an independent contractor or gig worker can be 30% or more. Given the narrow operating margins many firms operate under, reducing health insurance, pension, unemployment insurance, and other regulatory costs associated with permanent employees can be a strong financial incentive leading to the greater use of nonstandard workers.

C. Institutional Factors

Firms are under financial pressure to externalize or contract out all but their "core" activities. Unlike activities that improve customer value and generate profits, "noncore" activities are routine tasks that add little value or profit to the firm's income statement. To secure financing from capital markets, enhance investor confidence, and compete better globally with firms with lower labor costs, firms are looking for ways to shed noncore workers by greater use of nonstandard work arrangements.

D. Concern About Collective Action

A firm's concern about, or experience with, labor-management conflicts may also be an incentive for the use of arrangements lacking collective bargaining rights. Characterizing themselves as mere intermediaries, and workers as microentrepreneurs, digital platforms can avoid collective action efforts.

E. Worker Preferences

Some workers seek flexible scheduling jobs that provide them with more work-life balance than a standard employment job would. Temporary help services employees, independent contractors, and gig workers prefer nonstandard work arrangements over standard arrangements. However, some temporary and gig workers do agency or contract work as a way to get a permanent job.

F. Recruitment Through Crowdsourcing

Firms interested in avoiding the costs of recruitment, hiring, mentoring, monitoring, career development, and retention rely on a labor market supplier to provide them with workers. Platform intermediaries even eliminate the labor supplier step by outsourcing recruitment to an undefined, generally large group of people in the form of an open call through an Internet application.

▶ Safety Management Issues in Alternative Work Arrangements

The increased use of alternative arrangements alongside the standard arrangement leads to a "blended" workforce. In a blended workforce, workers in standard and alternative arrangements work together on the same project, often doing the same type of work. A blended workforce can present various organizational management challenges for a firm. Working alongside temporary workers can negatively affect standard workers' attitudes toward the firm and their temporary coworkers. In addition, the use of temporary workers can adversely affect a standard employee's perception of their own job security.

Blended workforces also present challenges to safety management. The agency-client relationship that governs the assignment of temporary workers may result in differences in the safety training that temporary and permanent employees receive for hazardous jobs, differences in personal protective equipment provided, and differences in workers' perception of safety practices. Managers may have difficulty in creating an organizational culture in which all workers, regardless of their employment status, can participate. Safety managers need to develop ways to overcome the heterogeneity of employment relationships that hinder building a strong organizational culture of safety at the workplace.

Determining responsibility for safety in a blended workforce can also be challenging. Both agency and client employers can become confused about which of them bears particular safety responsibilities for temporary agency workers in the host employer's workplaces. Reacting to tragic fatalities and serious injuries involving temporary workers, OSHA and the National Institute for Occupational Safety and Health (NIOSH) jointly developed in 2015 a set of recommendations aimed at how agency and client/host employers can better understand their mutual responsibilities to safeguard temporary agency workers at hazardous workplaces.

OSHA and NIOSH recommend that prior to accepting a new host employer as a client, or a new project from a current client/host employer, the temporary staffing agency and the client employer review all task assignments and job hazard analyses to ensure that the temporary workers receive appropriate site- and job-specific training and any needed personal protective equipment. Agency staff should be trained to recognize safety and health hazards at the employer's workplace. Host or client employers should be knowledgeable about the safety training and training certifications of the temporary workers who will be assigned to their workplace. The agreement between the temporary staffing agency and the client employer should specify safety responsibilities to eliminate any confusion about which employer is responsible for the safety and health of assigned workers. Staffing agencies and their client employers should inform each other of worker injuries and illnesses when they learn of them. Finally, maintaining contact with workers assigned by the temporary staffing agency to a client can help ensure that the host employer is fulfilling all required safety responsibilities.

Health & Safety Implications of Alternative Work Arrangements

The way work is organized can be a potential workplace hazard. Work organization studies have taken their place alongside studies of physical, chemical, and biological

Table 34–1. Exposures seen in nonstandard work arrangements.

Temporariness What is the duration of your current job? How many months in the previous year did you work steadily?
Disempowerment Do you have power to settle your own wages or are they determined solely by your hirer?
Vulnerability Are you afraid to demand better working conditions or fairer treatment?
Wages Do your wages cover basic needs? Do your wages allow for unexpected expenses?
Worker rights Do you have sick time or medical or family leave? Do you have paid holidays? Do you have wage and hour protection? Are you covered by a workers' compensation policy?
Exercise of worker rights Are you able to exercise any of the rights workers in standard employment relationships have?

hazards in the workplace. For nearly 20 years, how work is organized has been recognized as a dedicated area in the field of occupational health and safety research. Work organization studies focus on the ways work is arranged, scheduled, and managed as a potential risk factor for adverse health outcomes. Early studies demonstrated that adverse mental health outcomes can result from (1) major organizational restructuring changes; (2) downsizing of the workforce; or (3) sudden termination. By the beginning of the 21st century, attention turned to the study of work arrangements as hazardous "exposures" affecting worker health (Table 34–1). By 2005, a review of 27 studies published indicated an association between adverse psychological health effects and temporary employment.

A. Injury

Beginning in the 1990s, studies began to demonstrate higher physical injury rates among temporary agency workers than standard employment workers. For example, temporary nurses had higher rates of sharps injuries than standard employment nurses did. Temporary workers in the petrochemical industry had higher rates of injury, especially when they were engaged in maintenance and turnaround procedures. Temporary workers had twice the injury rate than their standard employment coworkers in the plastics manufacturing industry. In 2005, a systematic review of international studies indicated that 7 of 13 reports showed an increased risk of work-related injuries among temporary workers. In 2006, a study of temporary and contract workers reported that such workers had two times the rate of fatal and nonfatal work-related injuries than standard employment workers.

A study of the workers' compensation claims rates found the temporary worker injury rate to be double that of standard employment workers. Temporary workers reported lower hazard exposures, but less ability to cope with the hazards to which they were exposed because of a lack of experience screening, safety training, and schedule control.

B. Illness

Illness outcomes were also found to occur at a higher frequency in alternative arrangement workers. Increased illness morbidity may be related to the lack of paid sick leave benefits for nonstandard workers. Working while sick can increase the risk of injury. Workers with paid sick leave benefits were less likely than workers without access to paid sick leave to sustain a work-related injury. Practitioners should review their client firms' sick leave policies to enhance their utility as a tool for illness prevention, especially to stem infectious disease outbreaks.

C. Mortality

In general, studies have shown that differences in life expectancy across various demographic groups can be explained by different job conditions. Specifically, shortened life spans can be related to the type of work arrangement. A study using longitudinal data showed that the overall mortality rate for temporary workers was 1.2–1.6 times greater than the rate for permanent employees, chiefly from alcohol-related and smoking-related cancer. Workers who moved from temporary to permanent employment experienced a lowering of their mortality risk over those who remained in the temporary employment arrangement.

D. Reasons for Differential Health Risks

The differences in injury, illness, and fatality rates between workers in standard employment arrangements and alternative arrangements are not entirely clear. Working people who live below the poverty line are particularly vulnerable to these unusual schedules. A majority of US retail workers do not have regular schedules. They are on call when the employer wants them, and unable to predict how much they will earn from week to week or even day to day.

Temporary workers in various industries are often assigned the most hazardous work. The reasons for this may be multiple. First, employers may find that their liability if a worker sustains an injury in the course of doing hazardous work is reduced if the worker is a temporary worker as opposed to a worker in a standard employment relationship with the employer. Second, nonstandard workers may be less likely to raise objections to doing a hazardous job because of a fear of losing their job if they complain. This is understandable as temporary workers employment is precarious; they

can be easily replaced by another worker from the temporary staffing agency. Gig workers can be easily deleted from the Internet platform from which they are receiving their work assignments. Third, workers who are subjected to frequent short-term temporary assignments may lack sufficient site-specific safety training or lack access to appropriate personal protective equipment to do the job assigned to them without risk of injury or death. The lack of coordination between the temporary staffing agency and the client/host employer about who bears the safety responsibilities for a particular worker may result in neither employer taking responsibility for worker safety. Fourth, serial-temporary workers lack a social connection to the permanent workers at each workplace since their work is often of a short-term nature. This work pattern may deprive them of personal relationships that could protect them from worksite-specific hazards. Longevity in a job creates social relationships between workers that can protect a worker from an unsafe act. And, fifth, workers may also be reluctant to ask for additional training or file a complaint with OSHA because of their precarious job status.

E. The COVID-19 Pandemic

The COVID-19 pandemic resulted in a historic change in the nature of work for highly educated workers. More than one third of American workers took on some freelance work in the first year of an accelerating gig economy. A major portion of white-collar work was transferred to home offices, and video meetings have become the principal means of interaction. Many employers have observed with satisfaction that most remote workers feel more productive working away from the office and say they would like to continue working remotely. Remote work offers savings on office space for the employer, and saves the worker commuting costs. A significant benefit to remote workers is that their choice of employers is greatly expanded if they are not required to return to the workplace.

The pandemic has exposed and exacerbated a range of social inequalities and injustices. The requirements for computer literacy and graduate education to be eligible for white-collar remote work have excluded a preponderance of disadvantage and minority workers from opportunities. Immigrants remain on the margins of US society. Nearly three-quarters of undocumented immigrants work in sectors officially deemed essential to the nation's "critical infrastructure", yet they receive virtually no government assistance with their work or with job losses.

CONCLUSION

The changing nature of work presents both challenges and opportunities for the occupational health practitioner. Ensuring the prevention of worker health and safety incidents has always been the focus of occupational health practice. Recently, such incidents have become the leading cause of financial loss for businesses around the globe, outpacing the costs of high-profile incidents like cyber-attacks of IT outages. The financial threat posed to organizations by worker injury and illness provides an enhanced opportunity for occupational health practitioners to provide their expertise to enhance worker health and safety in the changing world of work.

REFERENCES

Benach A, et al: What should we know about precarious employment and health in 2025? Framing the agenda for the next decade of research. Int J Epidemiol 2016;45:232 [PMID: 26744486].

Bureau of Labor Statistics: Contingent and Alternative Employment Arrangements—May 2017. Washington, DC: U.S. Department of Labor, June 7, 2018. file:///C:/Users/zkz1/Desktop/BLS.Con.Alt.Employment.pdf.

Bureau of Labor Statistics: Electronically mediated work: new questions in the contingent worker supplement—September 2018. Washington, DC: U.S. Department of Labor. https://www.bls.gov/opub/mlr/2018/article/electronically-mediated-work-new-questions-in-the-contingent-worker-supplement.htm.

Foley M: Factors underlying observed injury rate differences between temporary workers and permanent peers. Am J Ind Med 2017;60:841 [PMID: 28869311].

Howard J: Nonstandard work arrangements and worker health. Am J Ind Med 2017;60:1-10 [PMID: 27779787].

Koranyi I, Jonsson J, Rönnblad T, Stockfelt L, Bodin T: Precarious employment and occupational accidents and injuries—a systematic review. Scand J Work Environ Health 2018;44(4):341-350 [PMID: 29443355].

Occupational Safety and Health Administration (OSHA)/National Institute for Occupational Safety and Health (NIOSH): Protecting Temporary Workers, 2015. http://www.cdc.gov/niosh/docs/2014-139/pdfs/2014-139.pdf.

Rönnblad T, Grönholm E, Jonsson J, et al: Precarious employment and mental health: a systematic review and meta-analysis of longitudinal studies. Scand J Work Environ Health 2019;45(5):429-443. [PMID: 31165899].

Schulte PA, Grosch J, Scholl JC, et al: Framework for considering productive aging and work. J Occup Environ Med 2018;60:440 [PMID: 29420331].

■ SELF-ASSESSMENT QUESTION

Select the one correct answer for each question.

Question 1: A crucial aspect of diversity management involves
- a. creating a more homogeneous workforce based according to age
- b. avoidance of stereotyping workers based on age, gender, sexual orientation, and racial or ethnic status
- c. making placement decisions for work assignments based on gender
- d. none of the above

Question 2. A significant benefit to remote workers
- a. Is diminished by video meetings.
- b. can be measured in lower workers' compensation costs.
- c. will take many years to discern.
- d. is that their choice of employers is greatly expanded.

Total Worker Health

Natalie V. Schwatka, PhD

Lee Newman, MD, MA

Total Worker Health (TWH) is defined by National Institute for Occupational Safety and Health (NIOSH) as policies, programs, and practices that integrate protection from work-related safety and health hazards with promotion of injury and illness prevention efforts to advance worker well-being. It is a holistic approach that integrates frameworks and practices from several disciplines to identify and control exposures to hazards that impact workers' safety, health, and well-being. These exposures may be overt, such as chemical exposures or physical hazards. Alternatively, they may be more insidious, such as exposure to a stressful work environment. TWH also promotes the creation of a healthy work environment, for example, by considering workplace ergonomics and work design, the impact of health care and other organization benefits on worker health and well-being, and factors contributing to a supportive work environment. The goal of TWH is to provide a safe workplace where all workers can also improve their overall health and well-being.

In 2009, the American College of Occupational and Environmental Medicine (ACOEM) issued a guidance statement stating that occupational and environmental medicine (OEM) physicians are prominent players in the field of workforce health and productivity. While they did not use the term *TWH* in their statement, they did call for more OEM attention and resources for health promotion services, in addition to health protection services, to ensure that our workforce is able to continue working productively. OEM physicians understand the consequences of injuries and illnesses. They also have the medical knowledge to understand the importance of managing chronic illness. They have seen how work-related injuries and illnesses as well as chronic illness can interact during the injury recovery and return to work process. In contrast to conventional worksite wellness programs, the TWH approach prioritizes safety first, followed by organizational and individual behaviors that contribute to overall health.

To address national priorities for the future of TWH, NIOSH published two national agendas. First, the National TWH Agenda (2016–2026) represented the first TWH-focused national effort to coalesce TWH research, practice, policy, and capacity building goals. Second, NIOSH developed its latest National Occupational Research Agenda (NORA) that includes a new cross-sector program called *Healthy Work Design and Well-Being* (HWD). HWD seeks to improve the design of work, work environments, and management practices to improve worker safety, health, and well-being. For example, their current goal for the construction industry is to reduce the impact that nonstandard work arrangements have on respiratory diseases, musculoskeletal disorders, fatal and nonfatal injuries from falls, and hearing loss. In the construction industry independent contracting, in particular, is a form of temporary work where employers improperly classify workers as sole proprietors. The implications are that workers do not have access to employer-based benefits, such as health care or workers' compensation insurance, and employers are less accountable to Occupational Safety and Health Administration (OSHA) rules and regulations intended to protect workers.

THE CASE FOR TWH

Effective TWH approaches benefit employers, employees, families, and can have local and nationwide impact. Employers may benefit from a happier, healthier, and more productive and committed workforce with less burnout and lower rates of turnover. For workers, TWH practices protect them from work-related injuries, illnesses, and fatalities *and* facilitate improved health, wellness, and productivity. Workers' families and communities benefits from healthier members who can contribute physically, mentally, and financially to their welfare. TWH benefits the nation by helping to reduce the burden of work-related injury and disability as well as chronic disease. Concerns have been voiced about this approach potentially diluting the employer's focus on ensuring worker safety and possibly shifting responsibility onto the individual worker. However, current TWH frameworks and approaches address this concern, by focusing on safety first-and-foremost, and on the organizational level behaviors that, if modified, can address policies, programs and practices that can promote better health and mitigate work practices that are detrimental to health and well-being.

From an OEM practitioner perspective, the case for TWH is apparent. In clinic, when we treat injured workers, we must not only address the medical needs of the patient but must also confront social and structural factors that will impact that patient's care and likelihood of recovery. For example, consider how often workers recover from an injury or illness only to be returned to the same hazardous conditions, placing them at risk for reinjury or new injury. As another example, consider patients who have delayed recovery. It is not unusual for the delay to be related, in part, to underlying manager-worker conflict, unfair working conditions such as mandatory overtime, or relentless workplace, financial, and/or home stress. TWH approaches are used to address these and other challenges by engaging employers to modify conditions of work that contribute to such issues, as discussed below.

COMPONENTS OF TWH

There are two key frameworks that guide current TWH research and practice. The first framework is a systems approach to worker health, safety, and well-being. This approach looks to the worker's environment, rather than the worker's behaviors, to better understand how to protect and promote health. Environmental factors include management and leadership practices, safety and wellness programs, organization of work, exposure to physical and psychosocial hazards, supervisory and social supports, job demands and control over job demands, among others. The second is a participatory approach to involving workers in TWH policies, programs, and practices. Workers can provide valuable insights into the conditions of work that affect their health, safety, and well-being. Without their input, worker engagement in TWH initiatives will lag and the initiatives will fail. Thus, organizations seeking to implement a TWH approach must focus on developing the systems that protect and promote employee health, safety, and well-being in a collaborative manner.

Businesses can utilize a variety of policies and programs to protect and promote employee health. First and foremost, a TWH system must include provisions to protect workers from hazards created on the job. These provisions will depend on the type of work being performed, but it generally should include processes for hazard identification, prevention, and control as well as training. To promote health and well-being, businesses should first address working conditions. This includes psychosocial conditions, such as poor social support, work/family conflict, and work organization and behavioral factors, such as harassment, high job demands and low job control, and job insecurity. Employees should also be given fair wages, access to health care benefits, paid time off, employee assistance programs, and health promoting policies and programs, such as tobacco cessation programs and chronic disease prevention programs.

Beyond these policies and programs, businesses must garner leadership and worker support and take steps to evaluate program processes and outcomes, identifying achievable organizational level goals. Businesses should evaluate program goals and objectives against employee interests and needs. Company leadership should spearhead TWH initiatives by communicating their value for them and allocating resources, including personnel, time, money, space, etc. Along the way, they need to ask for worker's input to make sure all relevant concerns are addressed. Any policy a company creates should be transparent and developed with input from workers. It must also address the importance of worker's privacy and protections against discrimination. This will increase the trust of workers and the sustainability of the policies. The final key component of TWH is program evaluation.

IMPLEMENTING TWH PRACTICES

As illustrated in Table 35–1, there are many potential avenues by which occupational medicine physicians and other occupational health professionals can assist organizations in advancing worker well-being through a TWH approach. The issues range from contributing to mitigation of workplace hazards and exposures—including workplace stress, for example, to consideration of the organization of work itself, the built environment in which work is performed, education of leadership on precepts of TWH and culture of health and safety, how workforce demographics affect health and productivity, and policies around compensation, benefits, return-to-work, harassment, and accommodation for an aging workforce. TWH, like occupational safety and health, aligns with the so-called hierarchy of controls. Figure 35–1 illustrates the application of the hierarchy to TWH.

According to NIOSH, the first step in implementing a TWH approach is the elimination of workplace conditions that cause or contribute to worker illness and injury. Next, substitute unsafe and unhealthy workplace conditions or practices with safer policies, programs, and management practices that promote a culture of safety and health in the workplace. This includes offering employees comprehensive employer-sponsored benefits and flexible work schedules, as well as increasing employees' knowledge and access to resources about safety and health. Finally, employers should encourage and support employees to improve their health, safety and well-being.

NIOSH's "Fundamentals of Total Worker Health Approaches: Essential Elements for Advancing Worker Safety, Health, and Well-Being" provides a five-step framework for organizations that would like to implement TWH practices.

1. *Leadership commitment* to TWH is the most critical step. Organizational leadership is responsible for designing the policies, programs, and practices that protect and promote employee health. They must also actively support and demonstrate a commitment to these initiatives via allocation of resources, communication, accountability, and recognition. This support must be demonstrated

Table 35–1. Potential roles for occupational health care professionals in consulting, research, health promotion, health protection.

Core Content Areas	Examples of Considerations When Advising Employers, Designing Interventions, Conducting TWH Research
Control of hazards and exposures	• Chemicals • Physical agents • Biological agents • Psychosocial factors • Human factors
Organization of work	• Fatigue and stress prevention • Work intensification program • Safe staffing • Overtime and shift work management • Flexible work arrangements • Adequate meal and rest breaks
Built environment supports	• Healthy air quality • Access to healthy, affordable food options • Safe and clean restroom and eating facilities • Safe access to the workplace • Environments designed to accommodate worker diversity
Leadership	• Shared commitment to safety, health, and well-being • Supportive managers, supervisors, and executives • Responsible business decision making • Meaningful work and engagement • Worker recognition and respect
Compensation and benefits	• Adequate wages and prevention of wage theft • Equitable performance appraisals and promotion • Work-life programs • Paid time off • Disability insurance • Workers' compensation benefits • Affordable, comprehensive health care, and life insurance • Retirement planning and benefits • Chronic disease prevention and disease management • Access to confidential, quality health care services • Career and skills development
Community supports	• Healthy community design • Safe, healthy affordable housing, and transportation options • Safe and clean environment (air and water quality, noise levels, tobacco-free policies) • Access to safe green spaces, outdoor utilization • Access to affordable, quality health care and well-being resources
Changing workforce demographics	• Multigenerational and diverse workforce • Aging workforce and older workers • Vulnerable worker populations • Workers with disabilities • Health disparities • Employees in small enterprises • Global and multinational workforce

(continued)

Table 35–1. Potential roles for occupational health care professionals in consulting, research, health promotion, health protection. (Continued)

Core Content Areas	Examples of Considerations When Advising Employers, Designing Interventions, Conducting TWH Research
Policy issues	• Health information privacy • Reasonable accommodations • Return-to-work • Equal employment opportunity • Family and medical leave • Address bullying, violence, harassment, and discrimination • Policies for prevention and monitoring of job stress • Promoting productive aging
New employment patterns	• Contracting and subcontracting • Precarious and contingent employment • Multiemployer worksites • Organizational restructuring, downsizing and mergers • Financial and job security

Adapted from "Issues Relevant to Advancing Worker Well-Being Through Total Worker Health®." CDC/National Institute for Occupational Safety and Health.

at the top by owners and executives as well as in the middle by midlevel managers and supervisors.

2. *Elimination of hazards and promotion of well-being in the workplace* is a core feature of TWH. Businesses must first and foremost identify and control hazardous exposures that can lead to work-related injuries, illnesses,

and fatalities. They must also identify and control hazards that inhibit workers from taking care of their own health and well-being, such as poor supervision, lack of health care or leave benefits, and lack of employee assistance programs. Businesses can use the TWH Hierarchy of Controls to make decisions about how to protect and

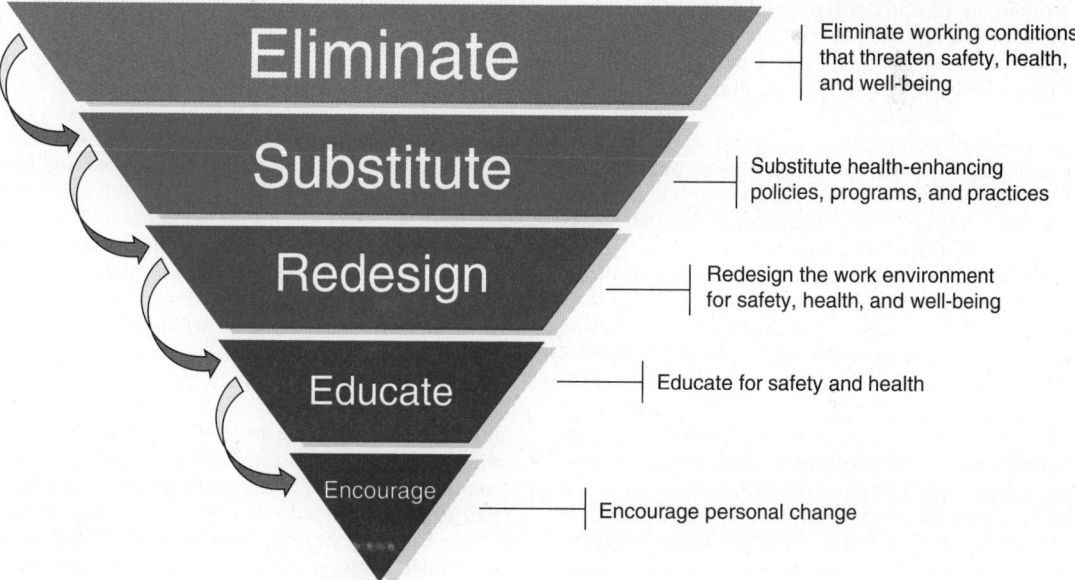

▲ **Figure 35–1.** Total Worker Health, like occupational safety and health, takes a "hierarchy of controls" approach to developing preventive strategies to benefit worker health, safety, and well-being. (Source: CDC/NIOSH.)

promote health. As in the traditional Hierarchy of Controls, the elimination of work conditions that threaten worker safety or well-being is the most effective method of increasing TWH, followed by substitution of current workplace designs with safer and healthier options. The redesign of the work environment is next, followed by worker education, and last, encouragement of workers to implement healthy personal change. All of these TWH initiatives must be regularly evaluated for relevance, quality, effectiveness, and assurance of being nondiscriminatory.

3. *Engagement of workers in the program design and delivery*, as mentioned previously, is key to ensuring program relevance to worker needs as well as program success.

4. *Protection of confidentiality and privacy of workers* is needed to ensure that all sensitive data collected is securely maintained to comply with relevant laws and to maintain employee trust.

5. *Effective integration of systems* includes identifying opportunities for collaboration across organizational units that touch workforce health, safety, and well-being—safety department, risk management, wellness programs, human resources, and benefits management, among others.

The University of Massachusetts Lowell's TWH Center of Excellence, Center for the Promotion of Health in the New England Workplace, emphasizes the third step in their TWH implementation guide—"The healthy workplace participatory program." Their guide centers on the engagement of workers in the process of identifying working conditions that harm workers' health and developing solutions to prevent or mitigate these hazards. The seven-step process includes a steering committee of managerial level employees as well as a design team consisting of line level, nonmanagerial employees. In a program evaluation of this process, they stressed the importance of training team members on TWH principles, providing adequate time and resources to the teams, and planning for team turnover. Their guide can be found at this website: https://www.uml.edu/Research/CPH-NEW/Healthy-Work-Participatory-Program/.

The Harvard TWH Center of Excellence, Center for Work, Health and Well-Being, emphasizes step number five in their TWH implementation guide—"Implementing an integrated approach: Weaving worker health, safety, and well-being into the Fabric of Your Organization." The guide discusses how to collaborate with key stakeholders, identify goals and objectives for an integrated initiative, target working conditions, implement changes that sustain positive working conditions, and evaluate and continually improve these efforts.

There are a several assessments that may aid businesses in implementing a TWH approach. OEM physicians who have consulting practices may choose to rely on some of these instruments.

The ACOEM Corporate Health Achievement Award has a history of providing businesses with a comprehensive assessment of their leadership and management, workers' health, environmental conditions, and organizational benefits, health promotion, absence and disability, and productivity programs. Although such "award programs" tend to be self-selective and at times self-promoting, they can help raise awareness of the most important elements needed for a successful TWH program.

The Harvard TWH Center of Excellence developed the Workplace Integrated Safety and Health Assessment (WISH) to help businesses understand how well they are implementing an integrated approach to protecting and promoting worker health. At the worker level, NIOSH maintains a compilation of surveys on work organizations topics such as flexibility, job control, and social supports. All survey instruments can be found at this website: https://www.cdc.gov/niosh/topics/workorg/.

The University of Colorado TWH Center of Excellence, Center for Health, Work & Environment has developed mentoring and educational programs for businesses, especially small- and medium-sized enterprises to become certified as TWH-compliant businesses. In 2013, Health Links (www.healthlinkscertified.org) was founded as a nonprofit, academic, community-based program focused on helping businesses build a culture of health, safety, and well-being. Health Links helps businesses implement a TWH approach through assessment, advising, connection to other businesses and to local resources, and certification.

TWH PRINCIPLES IN PRACTICES

▶ Small Business

Small businesses face unique opportunities and challenges when it comes to managing traditional occupational safety and health, as well as in implementing TWH practices. Smaller organizations typically have fewer resources to draw upon when implementing TWH practices. Health outcome data show that employees in smaller organizations have higher rates of occupational injuries, illnesses, and fatalities, as well as a greater burden of chronic health conditions and lifestyle health risks, compared to employees in larger businesses. However, when it comes to implementing a TWH approach, their small size can often be an asset. We find that there is a strong correlation between micro-business's (< 10 employees) safety programs and health promotion programs. In other words, if a small business has safety programming, they are also likely to have health promotion programming. The same cannot be said for medium- and larger-sized organizations, where businesses tend to either have integrated programs or they have strong safety programs but poor health promotion programs. Many small organizations are motivated to implement a TWH approach because of the value to their company (ie, employee recruitment and retention) and to their employees (ie, morale). Larger organizations tell us their main motivation is the return on investment, such as through reduced health care costs, and secondarily employee engagement, and lower absenteeism and presenteeism.

The CDC/NIOSH-funded Small+Safe+Well (SSWell) study is an example of a small business TWH intervention. The intervention attends to both the transactional and transformational aspects of organizational change. First, businesses participate in Health Links (see above) to assess their TWH business strategy. Second, a senior leader at the business participates in a TWH Leadership Training Program to understand how to ensure that their TWH business strategy is effective. Preliminary analyses suggest that with organizational and leadership engagement in fostering a culture of health *and* safety come improvements in TWH policies, programs, and practices; changes in employee perceptions of these practices (ie, safety and health climates), and ultimately, change in employee motivation, practices, health, and productivity.

▶ International Agrobusiness

International interest in TWH has paralleled that of NIOSH, as reflected in the work of the World Health Organization (WHO). The WHO Health Workplace Framework and Model provides an outline for avenues of influence, a process, and core principles that are essential to changing organizational and individual behaviors in support of worker safety and well-being. Utilizing a combination of core concepts from the WHO framework, the University of Colorado's model, and tools such as Health Links, we have been demonstrating the feasibility of introducing TWH even in complex, multinational agribusiness. Since 2016, a TWH Center has collaborated with a large sugar producer with mills in Guatemala, Nicaragua, and Mexico, to help reduce workplace injuries, illnesses, and fatalities, and promote improvements in health and well-being. The challenges are significant, including a workforce with a large proportion of seasonal migrant workers, management teams based at the mills and city-based corporate management, as well as a host of contractors providing transportation and other services. The workforce suffers from structural and social challenges including endemic poverty, malnutrition, infectious diseases, as well as rising rates of chronic health conditions such as cardiovascular disease, hypertension, and diabetes. At the beginning, occupational injuries, illnesses, and fatalities had begun to decrease due to the development of an occupational safety system that included leadership training on safety culture. Through surveys of the senior leadership team, managers, supervisors, and workers, TWH programs build on their success in safety. For example, the leadership and management teams are now trained on their role in promoting health and well-being in addition to safety, recognizing the strong interconnection between sleep, fatigue, injury risks, and productivity. They have identified workplace, as well as family and financial stress, as contributors to strain, occupational injuries, and other health outcomes. Steps are being taken to change organizational policies and practices to reduce the employer's contribution to workplace stress, fatigue, effects of shift work, heat stress, and hearing loss, as well as introduction of educational programs to help with

tobacco cessation, nutrition, among others. By applying core principles of TWH, it is possible to enhance ongoing efforts in occupational safety. Leadership commitment to worker well-being has been a critical component in the program's success.

▶ Construction Industry

The Oregon Healthy Workforce Center developed the "Be Super Toolkit" to help construction supervisors improve their TWH supervisory skills by including online training for supervisors on communication, employee supports, and team building; behavior tracking of supervisor goals; "get healthier" scripted cards for supervisors to discuss TWH topics with their crews; and "take home activities" that supervisors can use with family or friends outside of work.

The Harvard Center for Work, Health & Well-being also developed a construction industry. TWH intervention may focus on ergonomics and health promotion. One intervention had two components. First, the crews on site participated in a soft tissue injury prevention program focused on improving musculoskeletal health. This included safety manager feedback to supervisors on ergonomic audits of the job site, supervisor training, and a worker ergonomics tool box talk. Second, the intervention included a health week with daily key messages about psychosocial factors and individual health behaviors (eg, diet) that impact health in tool box talk format.

FUTURE WORKFORCE NEEDS AND TWH

Work is changing to include more nontraditional forms of employment, such as contract and temporary work. These precarious workers often do not have the same workplace protections as traditional employees, including lacking access to workers' compensation and health care benefits. Vulnerable populations, such as older workers, nonwhite workers, and immigrant workers, are at increased risk of poor health outcomes. Relatedly, the rise in globalization will create supply chains that span across multiple countries and increase the amount of labor migration and immigrant workers. Work, environment, and communities are all key social determinants of health. Climate change, decline of unions, declining federal funding for OSH, health care, and other policy changes, and emerging technologies bring with them uncertain new exposures and hazards as well as the potential for improved health protection and the contribution of work to worsening health disparities. Clearly, more transdisciplinary approaches that take a more holistic approach to the safety and well-being of the workforce are needed.

OEM physicians and other clinical occupational health care providers will play a critical role in addressing these future workforce needs and are uniquely positioned to research, practice, and lead the field of TWH. Additional training opportunities are available. Major occupational safety and health training programs and professional societies have begun to develop TWH tracks, sessions, and symposia on the subject at their conferences.

Occupational health care professionals bring to TWH an understanding of public health, occupational illness and injury prevention, workplace hazards, administrative medicine, and chronic illness. With additional training in areas such as occupational health psychology, organizational behavior change, consulting, health promotion, communication, intervention design, and evaluation, they can be effective in helping employers develop a TWH climate and adopt sustainable programs that offer a higher level of health protection and health promotion.

REFERENCES

Gómez MAL, Sparer-Fine E, Sorensen G, Wagner G: Literature review of policy implications from findings of the center for work, health, and well-being. J Occup Environ Med 2019;61(11):868-876 [PMID: 31453894].

NIOSH: *Fundamentals of Total Worker Health Approaches: Essential Elements for Advancing Worker Safety, Health, and Well-Being, 2017.* https://www.cdc.gov/niosh/docs/2017-112/pdfs/2017_112.pdf.

Peckham TK, Baker MG, Camp JE, Kaufman JD, Seixas NS: Creating a future for occupational health. Ann Work Expo Health 2017;61(1):3-15 [PMID: 28395315].

Punnett L, Cavallari JM, Henning RA, Nobrega S, Dugan AG, Cherniack MG: Defining 'Integration' for Total Worker Health®: a new proposal. Ann Work Expo Health 2020;64(3):223-235 [PMID: 32003780].

Schill AL, Chosewood LC: The NIOSH Total Worker Health" program. J Occup Environ Med 2013;55:S8-S11 [PMID: 24284752].

Schulte PA, Delclos G, Felknor SA, Chosewood LC: Toward an expanded focus for occupational safety and health: a commentary. Int J Environ Res Public Health 2019;16(24):4946 [PMID: 31817587].

Schwatka NV, Dally M, Tenney L, Shore E, Brown CE, Newman LS: Total worker health leadership and business strategies are related to safety and health climates in small business. Int J Environ Res Public Health 2020;17(6):2142 [PMID: 32213806].

Sorensen G et al: Integrating worksite health protection and health promotion: a conceptual model for intervention and research. Prev Medicine 2016;91:188-196 [PMID: 27527576].

Tamers SL, Chosewood LC, Childress A, Hudson H, Nigam J, Chang CC: Total Worker Health® 2014–2018: the novel approach to worker safety, health, and well-being evolves. Int J Environ Res Public Health 2019;16(3):321 [PMID: 30682773].

■ SELF-ASSESSMENT QUESTIONS

Select the one correct answer for each question.

Question 1: Total Worker Health (TWH)
- a. seeks to identify and control exposures to hazards that impact worker safety
- b. lacks definition other than worker well-being
- c. ignores exposure to stressful work
- d. addresses preventive health over safety in the workplace

Question 2: The first step in implementing a TWH approach is the
- a. development of a committee of health and safety professionals
- b. institution of a dietary program for obese workers
- c. report to management of the success of the program
- d. elimination of workplace conditions that cause or contribute to worker illness and injury

Occupational Mental Health & Substance Use Disorders

Caitlin Costello, MD

John Chamberlain, MD

Occupational mental health is increasingly recognized as an important focus of an effective occupational health and safety program. Unaddressed mental health issues, including substance use disorders, are significant occupational health problems and causes of considerable economic loss. Both diagnosed and undiagnosed psychiatric disorders and substance use disorders can contribute to poor performance or quality of work, absenteeism, decreased function while in the workplace (ie, presenteeism), strain in work relationships, and potential safety issues (including fatalities). Rates of absenteeism and presenteeism are higher for mental health disorders than other chronic medical conditions, and stress and anxiety account for more work absences than physical injuries or illnesses.

Although some workers may conceal their psychiatric disorders and substance use disorders out of fear of stigma and the possibility of termination, these mental health issues are commonly encountered in the workplace. The amount of time a person spends at work and the structured nature of work make it an ideal place to detect mental health and substance use disorders. Some mental health conditions can be ascribed to occupational stressors. For these reasons, occupational physicians are in a pivotal position to recognize, assess, and manage mental health conditions.

COMMON MENTAL HEALTH CONDITIONS IN THE WORKPLACE

Though more than 200 psychiatric disorders, including substance use disorders, are included in the *Diagnostic and Statistical Manual of Mental Disorders*, only the conditions that are most likely to present in today's work environment will be discussed in this chapter. Practitioners familiar with these mental health conditions will be able to facilitate the evaluation, treatment, and management of employees with psychopathology.

MAJOR DEPRESSIVE DISORDER

ESSENTIALS OF DIAGNOSIS

▶ Feelings of worthlessness, hopelessness, and sometimes guilt.

▶ Loss of energy or fatigue, daily.

▶ Difficulty concentrating and making decisions.

▶ Loss of interest or pleasure in activities; withdrawal from activities.

▶ Disturbed sleep (insomnia, hypersomnia).

▶ Reduced appetite and sex drive.

▶ Thoughts of death and suicide.

▶ General Considerations

Depression is one of the most prevalent mental health disorders, affecting 16 million Americans every year, with women being at a significant increased risk compared to men. Given the rate of occurrence, the personal pain, and the cost to employers associated with major depression, effective employee health policy and clinical intervention should be the goals for health planning regarding this all too common mental disorder.

▶ Clinical Findings

The hallmark of major depression is a severely depressed mood lasting at least 2 weeks. Symptoms most frequently include anhedonia, decreased energy, reduced participation in activities, and feelings of guilt or worthlessness. Other signs include impairment in concentration or cognitive functioning, sleep disturbance, changes in appetite (usually decreased), somatic complaints such as body aches and constipation, and thoughts of death.

Initial episodes of depression are more likely to be preceded by a recognizable stressor than recurrent episodes. Clinical depression regularly presents with other psychiatric and medical conditions. Anxiety, posttraumatic stress disorder (PTSD), and substance abuse are often comorbid disorders accompanying major depression. Chronic pain is routinely associated with depression.

▶ Differential Diagnosis

- Depressive disorder due to another medical condition (eg, hypothyroidism)
- Adjustment disorder with depressed mood
- Bipolar disorder
- Persistent depressive disorder (dysthymia)
- Substance- or medication-induced depressive disorder
- Nonpathological sadness

▶ Treatment

Cognitive behavioral therapy for depression instructs patients to confront self-defeating thoughts and change negativistic behaviors. Selective serotonin reuptake inhibitors (SSRIs) are the most commonly used medical intervention for major depression. Combined treatment involving psychotherapy and antidepressant medication is more effective than either intervention alone. It should be noted that untreated clinical depression frequently remits within 3–12 months. The effectiveness of antidepressants in mild cases of depression is minimal. Cases of refractory depression are those that do not respond to at least two adequate trials of antidepressants. While controversial, electroconvulsive therapy (ECT) is used in treatment resistant cases.

BIPOLAR DISORDER

ESSENTIALS OF DIAGNOSIS

Manic episodes
- ▶ Euphoric and/or irritable mood.
- ▶ Increased involvement in goal-directed activities.
- ▶ Racing thoughts and flight of ideas.
- ▶ Decreased need for sleep.
- ▶ Difficulty focusing, distractibility.
- ▶ Self-inflation and grandiosity.
- ▶ In some cases, delusions, hallucinations, and/or paranoia.

Depressive episodes
- ▶ See Essentials of Diagnosis in Major Depressive Disorder.

▶ General Considerations

Formerly known as manic depressive illness, bipolar disorder is a mood disorder that can cause tremendous disruption in the lives of afflicted individuals. The lifetime prevalence for bipolar disorder in US adults is approximately 4.4%. Employees with bipolar disorder, when not in a manic episode, can be creative and productive. In the midst of mania, those same people can be a profound source of disruption in the work setting and elsewhere.

▶ Clinical Findings

Bipolar disorder is a cyclical mood disorder involving at least one episode of abnormally elevated energy level and mood that usually alternates with one or more episodes of depression. Manic episodes usually begin abruptly and most commonly occur during spring and summer. Less severe than overt mania is hypomania that does not cause serious impairment in occupational functioning or involve psychotic symptoms.

Mania is a period of elevated mood lasting 1 week or more with accompanying decreased sleep, pressured speech, racing thoughts, impulsivity, and poor judgment. Irritability, aggression, and recklessness usually create problems in relationships and work functioning. Persons in the midst of a manic episode can engage in spending sprees, take on risky business deals, and demonstrate a degree of hypersexuality. Grandiosity can reach delusional levels.

▶ Differential Diagnosis

- Schizophrenia spectrum and other psychotic disorders
- Substance-induced manic episode
- Major depressive disorder (MDD)
- Anxiety disorder
- Attention-deficit/hyperactivity disorder

▶ Treatment

Therapeutic counseling is effective in bringing attention to situations that may trigger manic episodes and in increasing recognition of warning signs of an emerging recurrence. Mood stabilizers including lithium, carbamazepine, and lamotrigine have demonstrated efficacy in treating bipolar disorder. Atypical antipsychotics such as olanzapine are used to treat mania with agitation and psychotic symptoms.

GENERALIZED ANXIETY DISORDER

ESSENTIALS OF DIAGNOSIS

- ▶ Overt anxiety or fear.
- ▶ Excessive apprehension or worry.
- ▶ Difficulty concentrating.
- ▶ Insomnia.
- ▶ Irritability and agitation.
- ▶ Feelings of impending doom.

▶ Autonomic hyperarousal symptoms such as sweating, tachycardia, tremulousness.

▶ Somatic symptoms such as headaches, nausea, dizziness, muscle tension.

▶ General Considerations

Anxiety disorders are the most common mental health diagnosis in the United States. Approximately 31% of the adult population experiences any anxiety disorder during their life. Benzodiazepines, which are commonly prescribed for anxiety disorders, can cause cognitive impairment, even at prescribed doses. Intoxication can result in lethargy, sedation, and impaired coordination, posing a risk for workers with safety-sensitive jobs.

▶ Clinical Findings

Excessive anxiety or worry about everyday situations such as money, family, work, or social relations is the hallmark of generalized anxiety disorder. Afflicted individuals have difficulty stopping or controlling worrisome thoughts, which can lead to impairment in work performance. These worries are usually pervasive, long-standing, disproportional to the actual likelihood of feared event, and occur without precipitants. In addition to excessive worry, symptoms may include restlessness, difficulty concentrating, agitation, somatic symptoms, fatigue, and disturbed sleep.

▶ Differential Diagnosis

- Anxiety disorder due to another medical condition (eg, hyperthyroidism or pheochromocytoma)
- Substance-induced anxiety disorder
- PTSD or adjustment disorder
- Depressive, bipolar, or psychotic disorder
- Obsessive-compulsive disorder
- Social anxiety disorder
- Nonpathological anxiety (controllable, shorter duration, precipitants, less interference with daily functioning, and usually not accompanied by physical symptoms)

▶ Treatment

Management of acute symptoms of generalized anxiety usually includes benzodiazepines. Rather than prolonged treatment with benzodiazepines, the symptoms of restlessness, difficulty concentrating, irritability, muscle tension, fatigue, and sleep disturbance respond well to cognitive behavioral therapy. Pharmacotherapy includes the use of SSRIs. Other psychotropic drugs demonstrating efficacy are buspirone and imipramine. Nonpsychotropic alternatives include the β-blocker propranolol and the calcium channel agent pregabalin.

POSTTRAUMATIC STRESS DISORDER

ESSENTIALS OF DIAGNOSIS

▶ Exposure to an extreme traumatic event.

▶ Intrusive recollections, disturbing dreams.

▶ Hypervigilance, startle responses, difficulty sleeping.

▶ Avoidance of external reminders of trauma.

▶ Persistent and exaggerated negative beliefs and emotions.

▶ Social withdrawal.

▶ General Considerations

The lifetime prevalence for PTSD in US adults is 6.8%. Employees involved in critical incidents can sometimes develop PTSD. Additionally, employment in certain industries increases the likelihood of involvement in violence, which can induce PTSD symptoms. Law enforcement officers, security guards, and bartenders experience the highest rates of workplace violence and are therefore at risk for developing PTSD.

▶ Clinical Findings

The hallmark of PTSD is exposure to an actual or threatened stressor (death, serious injury, or sexual violence) followed by indicative emotional and behavioral symptoms. Examples of stressors are armed robbery, personal assault, or a serious motor vehicle accident. The traumatic event is reexperienced through flashbacks, dreams, or exposure to stimuli that are associated with the event. Behavioral symptoms include increased states of arousal such as hypervigilance, irritability, startle reactions, difficulty concentrating, and sleep difficulties. Other diagnostic criteria include avoidance of people and activities associated with the traumatic event, negative thoughts about oneself or the world, detachment from others, and persistent negative moods such as fear, anger, or guilt.

▶ Differential Diagnosis

- Adjustment disorder
- Acute stress disorder (less chronic form of PTSD)
- Depressive, anxiety, or psychotic disorder
- Obsessive-compulsive disorder
- Traumatic brain injury

▶ Treatment

Early clinical intervention is effective in reducing morbidity and disability. Propranolol instituted soon after the traumatic incident can reduce autonomic arousal and improve long-term outcome. Cognitive behavioral therapy and SSRI antidepressants are effective in reducing nightmares, sleep disturbance, reexperiencing, and avoidance. Where available, group therapy involving employees from the same class of workers, such as public safety workers, can be an effective form of clinical intervention as well.

SUBSTANCE USE DISORDERS

Alcohol Use Disorder

ESSENTIALS OF DIAGNOSIS

▶ High tolerance of alcohol.

▶ Craving for alcohol and inability to control use.

▶ Withdrawal symptoms.

▶ Poor functioning at work.

▶ Recurrent use despite awareness of medical and social issues caused by alcohol use.

▶ General Considerations

Alcoholism is by far the most serious chemical dependency problem encountered in the workplace. An estimated 1 in 13 working adults meets the diagnostic criteria for alcohol use disorder. Intoxication, withdrawal, and chronic use cause various cognitive and physiologic symptoms. The occupational physician must be able to recognize the early signs of alcohol-induced impairment and direct employees to appropriate treatment to minimize the economic impact that untreated alcoholics can have on themselves, coworkers, employers, and the public.

Early identification of the alcoholic patient in the occupational setting can be facilitated by focused history taking, a carefully focused physical examination, and use of selective laboratory studies. An effective method for obtaining an alcohol history is to use a structured interview and to obtain history from independent sources. Inquiring about the patient's relationship, occupational, and financial history is important because problems in these areas often are associated with substance abuse.

The physical examination can yield subtle clues to alcohol abuse. In many cases, employees abruptly cease alcohol use when asked to present for a medical evaluation, precipitating signs of mild withdrawal. In addition, signs of trauma, particularly in the lower extremities, associated with falls while intoxicated can be helpful clues. Fractures, particularly of the ribs, have been associated with alcohol abuse. Signs of frank organ injury such as spider angiomas and organomegaly are also helpful for diagnosis when present, but these injuries represent end-organ damage, usually seen only in cases of advanced alcoholism.

Questions about quantity of alcohol, time period of drinking, and choice of beverage usually are not fruitful because alcoholics tend to minimize and/or deny their alcohol intake. The CAGE questionnaire ("cut-annoyed-guilty-eye") is a highly effective tool in establishing a diagnosis of alcohol use disorder:

1. Have you ever felt you should **cut** down on your drinking?
2. Have people **annoyed** you by criticizing your drinking?
3. Have you ever felt bad or **guilty** about your drinking?
4. Have you ever had a drink first thing in the morning to steady your nerves or get rid of a hangover (**eye-opener**)?

Patients who answer two of four CAGE questions positively have a score that correlates in excess of 90% with the diagnosis of alcohol use disorder. The CAGE questionnaire is easy to administer in the context of a workplace medical evaluation. The importance of obtaining independent reports of an employee's alcohol use from coworkers, supervisors, and family members should not be underestimated. Reports from supervisors and coworkers on changes in work performance, absenteeism, and observed use of alcohol and drugs can be obtained during a workplace evaluation. Contacting a patient's family or friends outside the workplace, however, needs to be done with the patient's permission.

▶ Clinical Findings

Tolerance, withdrawal, and craving are the primary diagnostic criteria for alcohol use disorder. Other diagnostic criteria include impairment in fulfilling responsibilities at home, school, or work; continued use despite psychological, physiologic, social, and occupational issues; inability to control use despite desire to reduce or stop; and significant time spent acquiring, using, and recovering from the effects of alcohol.

Alcohol intoxication identifiers include impaired motor skills, slurred speech, drowsiness, lack of inhibition, nystagmus, and stupor. Alcohol withdrawal symptoms include diaphoresis, tachycardia, mild hypertension, upper extremity symmetric tremor, and seizure. Chronic alcohol abuse is a major risk factor for stroke, liver disease, and neurologic impairment.

▶ Differential Diagnosis

• Sedative use disorder

• MDD or bipolar disorder

• Dementia

• Nonpathologic use of alcohol

Cannabis Use Disorder

ESSENTIALS OF DIAGNOSIS

▶ High tolerance of cannabis.

▶ Craving for cannabis and inability to control use.

▶ Withdrawal symptoms.

▶ Poor functioning at work.

▶ Recurrent use despite awareness of medical and social issues caused by cannabis use.

General Considerations

Tetrahydrocannabinol (THC), the active ingredient of cannabis, creates a feeling of euphoria and relaxation but also causes impairment in judgment and motor coordination. Cannabis intoxication, therefore, can create a dangerous work environment.

Cannabis is the substance most commonly detected in workplace urine testing. Cannabis is usually smoked and is absorbed readily from the respiratory and intestinal mucosa. THC is lipid soluble and tends to remain in body tissues for days to weeks. It can appear in the urine for weeks after chronic use.

Clinical Findings

Tolerance, withdrawal, and craving are the primary diagnostic criteria for cannabis use disorder. Other diagnostic criteria include impairment in fulfilling responsibilities at home, school, or work; continued use despite psychological, physiologic, social, and occupational issues; inability to control use despite desire to reduce or stop; and significant time spent acquiring, using, and recovering from the effects of cannabis.

Cannabis intoxication produces a state of emotional and muscular relaxation and euphoria but may also cause impaired cognition and motor skills, dysphoria, paranoia, and depersonalization. Signs of intoxication include dry mouth, bloodshot eyes, and tachycardia. Cannabis withdrawal can cause anxiety, depression, irritability, anger, aggression, insomnia, weight loss, and other physiologic and psychological symptoms. Impairment in occupational and relational functioning is particularly common in cannabis use disorder.

In susceptible individuals, cannabis use can produce depression, anxiety, or even psychosis. Chronic use is associated with apathy and decreased short-term memory as well as impaired judgment and problem-solving ability. Chronic use also can lead to respiratory complications, including bronchitis and permanent lung injury.

Differential Diagnosis

- Other substance use disorder
- MDD or bipolar disorder
- Generalized anxiety disorder
- Schizophrenia
- Delirium

Stimulant Use Disorder

ESSENTIALS OF DIAGNOSIS

- ▶ High tolerance of stimulants.
- ▶ Craving for stimulants and inability to control use.
- ▶ Withdrawal symptoms.

- ▶ Poor functioning at work.
- ▶ Recurrent use despite awareness of medical and social issues caused by stimulants.

General Considerations

The central nervous system (CNS) stimulants include cocaine and amphetamines. Amphetamines differ from cocaine in that their half-life is longer, and they produce a prolonged period of intoxication.

Cocaine is produced as an extract from the coca leaf in the form of pure alkaloid, or "free base," and crystalline hydrochloride salt, which is water-soluble and absorbed rapidly by the respiratory and enteric mucosa. The crystalline version usually is insufflated into the nose or taken orally. Free base cocaine is volatile and usually is smoked with a pipe. This form of ingestion results in rapid absorption, leading to an intense euphoria that lasts about 30–45 minutes. This intense but short-lived effect makes cocaine popular for users who do not desire a prolonged effect. This feature has implications for the workplace, where impairment may be short-lived and intermittent but quite severe.

Amphetamines often are used as appetite suppressants and to boost energy. They are absorbed rapidly via the respiratory and gastrointestinal (GI) tracts and are usually taken orally or intranasally. Methamphetamine is smoked in the same way as "crack" cocaine and is relatively volatile. Methamphetamine also is more potent and faster acting than other forms of amphetamine.

Clinical Findings

Tolerance, withdrawal, and craving are the primary diagnostic criteria for stimulant use disorder. Other diagnostic criteria include impairment in fulfilling responsibilities at home, school, or work; continued use despite psychological, physiologic, social, and occupational issues; inability to control use despite desire to reduce or stop; and significant time spent acquiring, using, and recovering from the effects of stimulants.

Cocaine intoxication increases energy and decreases appetite and the need for sleep. Unintended effects may include mania, panic attacks, paranoia, psychotic symptoms, and impulsive violent behavior. Cocaine produces an intense adrenergic discharge, resulting in tachycardia, hypertension, and mydriasis. These syndromes, in turn, can produce acute cardiovascular complications, including myocardial infarction, seizures, cerebral vascular accidents, and cardiac arrhythmias. The physical symptoms of cocaine intoxication resolve within days of removal of the drug, but psychiatric complications of cocaine use can create an acute psychiatric emergency. Withdrawal symptoms include dysphoria, fatigue, irritability, and psychomotor retardation. Chronic use can lead to cognitive impairment, intense depression, suicidal ideation, and paranoid psychosis.

Amphetamine-abusing workers are more likely to show acute autonomic signs of intoxication such as tachycardia, hyperemia, and mydriasis. Acute amphetamine intoxication is associated with severe toxic psychosis characterized by motor agitation, intense paranoia, and violence. Withdrawal symptoms include dysphoria, irritability, extreme fatigue, psychomotor agitation, increased appetite, and vivid dreams. Initially, amphetamines have positive effects for many individuals (weight loss and increased energy); long-term use, however, leads to personality changes and psychiatric symptoms, including insomnia, depression, paranoia, and psychosis.

▶ Differential Diagnosis

- Bipolar disorder
- Anxiety disorders
- Attention-deficit/hyperactivity disorder
- Schizophrenia spectrum and other psychotic disorders
- Other substance use disorder

Opioid Use Disorder

ESSENTIALS OF DIAGNOSIS

- ▶ High tolerance of opioids.
- ▶ Craving for opioids and inability to control use.
- ▶ Withdrawal symptoms.
- ▶ Poor functioning at work.
- ▶ Recurrent use despite awareness of medical and social issues caused by opioids.

▶ General Considerations

The use and abuse of opioids, in the form of prescription analgesics, is one of the fastest growing illicit drug problems in the United States. Opioid problems in the workplace take two forms. The first type is the worker who is prescribed opioids for a medical reason, including medication prescribed for an industrial injury. Such patients can develop opioid use disorder in the course of their medical treatment and can present a special challenge to the occupational physician. The challenge is to first diagnose the pattern of abuse or dependence, then work with the treating physician to develop a shared understanding of the problem. These patients need simultaneous treatment both for their medical condition and for the opioid dependence. Often these patients need a multidisciplinary approach to detoxification, rehabilitation, and workplace reentry.

The second type of opioid abuse is the worker with an opioid use disorder not associated with a medical condition. These patients are more likely to engage in intravenous drug use and usually obtain their drugs from illegal sources. These two factors place these patients at high risk for a variety of serious medical complications, including hepatitis B and C, human immunodeficiency virus (HIV) infection, endocarditis, and infections at the injection site (phlebitis and cellulitis).

Naturally occurring narcotics (opiates) and synthetic agents (opioids) act as CNS depressants. Opiates and opioids produce intense euphoria and feelings of emotional tranquility and sedation. The duration of these effects varies by route of administration and type of opioid used. The opioids with low protein binding, such as heroin, move into the CNS quickly but are absorbed slowly from the GI tract. This is the reason why addicts, in an attempt to achieve rapid euphoria, tend to use these drugs intravenously.

Opioids produce profound mental and psychomotor slowing that will interfere with almost any work task. Depression of cardiopulmonary function is a particular risk for workers in special environments that require the use of respirators or breathing apparatus. The varying concentration (drug versus filler) of street drugs poses the risk of accidental overdose on and off the worksite. Opioids differ in their half-life and potency. All are excreted in the urine and are readily detectable with urine drug testing. It is important to note that both heroin and codeine are metabolized by the body to morphine. Therefore, patients using either of these agents will test positive only for morphine on urine drug testing.

Detection of opioid abuse, particularly in the nonprescription addict, can be somewhat challenging. Addicts also can be quite covert in their drug use. Careful history taking, with particular attention to the presence of apathy, depression, and sedation, can be helpful. Needle tracks, miosis, signs of constipation, weight loss, and infectious complications of intravenous drug use seen on physical examination all can alert the physician to a covert opioid addiction problem. Urine drug testing can be helpful in supporting such a diagnosis.

▶ Clinical Findings

Tolerance, withdrawal, and craving are the primary diagnostic criteria for opioid use disorder. Other diagnostic criteria include impairment in fulfilling responsibilities at home, school, or work; continued use despite psychological, physiologic, social, and occupational issues; inability to control use despite desire to reduce or stop; and significant time spent acquiring, using, and recovering from the effects of opioids.

Opioid intoxication usually starts with an experience of euphoria, followed by apathy, decreased alertness, slurred speech, impairment in judgment and psychomotor ability, miosis, and other behavioral and physiologic symptoms. Opioid withdrawal symptoms include agitation, anxiety, mydriasis, insomnia, nausea, vomiting, and diarrhea. Chronic opioid use can cause dysphoria, opioid-induced hyperalgesia, and decreased immune system functioning.

▶ Differential Diagnosis

- Other substance use disorder
- MDD
- Anxiety disorders
- Other medical conditions

Sedative Use Disorder

ESSENTIALS OF DIAGNOSIS

- ▶ High tolerance of sedatives.
- ▶ Craving for sedatives and inability to control use.
- ▶ Withdrawal symptoms.
- ▶ Poor functioning at work.
- ▶ Recurrent use despite awareness of medical and social issues caused by sedatives use.

▶ General Considerations

Sedatives, most commonly benzodiazepines, are used to treat anxiety disorders and insomnia. They are generally safe; however, they can cause cognitive impairment, even at therapeutic doses. If intoxicated by these drugs, an individual may become lethargic, very sedated, and have impaired coordination. Legally prescribed and used widely, sedative use poses a serious risk in the workplace, particularly with safety-sensitive jobs. Many individuals using benzodiazepines combine them with alcohol, which may aggravate the negative effects. The combination of sedatives and alcohol is a common cause of accidental overdose.

The occupational physician should work with management to establish a program to screen employees taking benzodiazepines, even for appropriate conditions and in therapeutic dosages. These employees may need to be excluded from duties that require a high degree of concentration and motor skills. Patients with a dependence on these drugs may require detoxification and stabilization before workplace reentry. Consultation with the patient's prescribing physician is extremely helpful to determine benzodiazepine dependency and to formulate a return-to-work treatment plan.

▶ Clinical Findings

Tolerance, withdrawal, and craving are the primary diagnostic criteria for sedative use disorder. Other diagnostic criteria include impairment in fulfilling responsibilities at home, school, or work; continued use despite psychological, physiologic, social, and occupational issues; inability to control use despite desire to reduce or stop; and significant time spent acquiring, using, and recovering from the effects of sedatives.

Sedative intoxication symptoms include labile mood, impaired judgment and cognition, hostility or aggression,

slurred speech, lack of coordination, and nystagmus. Symptoms associated with sedative withdrawal include agitation and irritability, autonomic hyperarousal, anxiety, insomnia, nausea, vomiting, and hallucinations. Symptoms of chronic sedative use can include depression and impaired cognitive functioning.

▶ Differential Diagnosis

- MDD
- Anxiety disorders
- Alcohol or other substance use disorder
- Neurocognitive disorders

▶ Prevention for Substance Use Disorders

Employers should make standards for acceptable use of alcohol and drugs explicit to employees through manuals, trainings, and directives. A written policy, tailored to the particular workplace, is the starting point for a company when setting a strategy to prevent substance abuse in the workplace. Policies should make clear that alcohol and drug abuses are unacceptable in the workplace and include a description of what constitute violations of the policy, consequences for violations, expectation that employees are responsible for seeking treatment and complying with treatment recommendations, the circumstances for drug testing (preplacement, for cause, random), and the consequences for a positive drug test. Drug monitoring programs also can be effective tools for prevention.

▶ Treatment for Substance Use Disorders

The treatment of choice for most patients with a substance use disorder is an outpatient substance abuse treatment program followed by a longer course of aftercare. Those patients with medical complications or requiring detoxification first may need a brief hospitalization. Effective treatment programs involve pharmacotherapy for comorbid psychiatric illnesses, substance abuse education, cognitive behavioral therapy, motivational enhancement therapy, stress and relationship management, and recovery programs such as AA and NA. Substance use disorders are chronic medical problems with a high risk of relapse; therefore, these patients require ongoing treatment that continues long after they complete an outpatient treatment program. Active involvement in 12-step programs, including working with a sponsor and continuing involvement in AA or NA, will greatly strengthen the chances for sustained recovery.

▼ OCCUPATIONAL STRESS

In addition to psychiatric disorders identified in the *Diagnostic and Statistical Manual of Mental Disorders*, occupational stress also impacts the health and productivity of workers. There is substantial evidence that stress caused by the work environment represents a risk factor for the development of mental health problems. Employees undergoing occupational stress are at greater risk of coping through alcohol use (regular drinking and binge drinking) and other substance use. Further, chronic exposure to work-related stress can result in greater morbidity and prevalence of medical problems. Work-related factors that induce stress include quantitative as well as qualitative job requirements, environment in the workplace, organization of work processes and working time, emotional demands, social relationships, compatibility of the individual's family and occupational requirements, communication culture, workplace managerial structure, leadership style in the workplace, and individual risk of workers.

THE IMPACT OF SPECIFIC DISORDERS IN THE WORKPLACE

DEPRESSION

Depression is a serious, and one of the leading causes of global disability, problem in adults of working age. Depression may have a greater adverse effect on work outcomes (eg, work limits, absenteeism, and work productivity) than other medical conditions. People with depression require more sickness absences than other people, including individuals with debilitating physical conditions (eg, rheumatoid arthritis and heart disease).

Even subthreshold or subsyndromal depression, also known as minor depression, adversely impacts work function and health. This condition, characterized by depressive symptoms that do not meet the full diagnostic criteria for MDD, has an estimated prevalence of about 5–20% in both primary care and community populations. Although the symptoms of subthreshold depression do not meet the full criteria for MDD, this condition has significant adverse outcomes for those afflicted by it (eg, decreased quality of life, mental suffering, and impaired function) and is a risk factor for the development of MDD. Individuals suffering from this disorder report greater absenteeism from the workplace as well as more presenteeism (decreased productivity when at work).

BIPOLAR DISORDER

Bipolar disorder is characterized by impairments in psychosocial functioning, with occupational disability being one of the most significant. Depression and neurocognitive deficits (eg, attention, executive functioning, and verbal memory) are the bipolar disorder features most often correlated with impaired occupational functioning. In the United States, with the annual cost of lost productivity attributable to bipolar disorder is $14.1 billion.

POSTTRAUMATIC STRESS DISORDER

The incidence of PTSD is greater among injured workers than among victims of other traumatic incidents. In order to minimize medical and mental health expenses, lost wages and productivity, and disability payments, it is important to identify PTSD symptoms early and institute appropriate treatment strategies. Practitioners should keep in mind that recovery from physical injury and mental preparation to return to work do not necessarily occur in the same timeframe. As such, mental/emotional and physical recovery following a work-related injury must be separately evaluated. Individuals might experience trouble resuming work where the injury occurred.

SUBSTANCE USE DISORDERS

Nearly 11 million adult US workers meet the diagnostic criteria for substance use disorders. Among employed adults, alcohol is the most commonly used substance, and misuse of alcohol is correlated with negative occupational outcomes (eg, turnover, accidents, absenteeism, as well as other causes of lost productivity). Most of the costs related to substance use disorders are due to lost productivity. Workers with substance use disorders arc absent from work almost 50% more days than those without substance use disorders. The average employee is absent from work 2 days a year due to hangovers from alcohol. Additionally, a large majority of people with substance abuse problems bring their substance abuse into the workplace in a variety of ways. In addition to a small percentage of workers who are under the influence of alcohol or other drugs while at work, employees who come to work with hangovers from alcohol are less productive and more likely to be involved in conflict at work.

Substance use disorders usually are accompanied by a decline in social and occupational functioning, making the workplace a good place to observe this decline in an individual's functioning and to direct the worker to appropriate treatment.

RESPONDING TO MENTAL HEALTH AND SUBSTANCE USE DISORDERS IN THE WORKPLACE

A substantial proportion of depressed employees in the United States do not participate in treatment or are not adequately treated. Further, the average delay in receiving appropriate treatment is 6–7 years. There are multiple potential obstacles to engaging in treatment. For example, the employee may not recognize the need for assistance or they may fear the stigma associated with mental illness and its treatment. In addition, financial issues, availability of treatment, and convenience of engaging in treatment represent structural factors that may be barriers to treatment. However, removing these barriers can significantly diminish lost productivity. Because the duration of untreated illness represents a predictive factor related to treatment outcome, early identification of employees suffering from depression is crucial to reducing cost and improving treatment outcome.

Psychiatric Consultation

There are a number of circumstances involving mental health matters in the workplace that require specialty consultation. The rationale for psychiatric consultation regarding workplace mental health issues includes the need for diagnostic clarification, mental health treatment planning, fitness-for-duty psychiatric evaluation, psychiatric disability evaluation, threat assessment, psychopharmacologic medication adjustment, psychotherapy, and psychometric testing.

The initial clinical impression in cases involving an employee with psychopathologic symptoms should be confirmed or amended based on input from an experienced mental health practitioner. Similarly, the treatment plan should be developed with assistance of a psychiatrist or psychologist once the diagnosis has been established. Evaluation of an employee's fitness or impairment can require specialty consultation to identify recommended accommodations for behavior that may allow for a return to some form of work. The potentially dangerous employee warrants an assessment of the threat level posed. Employees returning to work who are taking psychotropic medication should also have the benefit of a psychiatric consult on whether the drug(s) used should be amended. Counseling or psychotherapy beyond basic supportive coaching is yet another intervention best left to mental health professionals. Finally, concern over mood instability, interpersonal conflict, or a history of head injury should give consideration for standardized psychometric testing directed toward assessing the specific concern.

The American Psychiatric Association recommends the initial psychiatric assessment include assessment of many areas, such as history of present illness; reasons the person is presenting for examination; a psychiatric review of systems (anxiety and panic symptoms, past or current sleep abnormalities, impulsivity); history of psychiatric diagnoses; previous aggressive or psychotic ideas; history of aggressive behaviors; history of suicide attempts, suicide plans, and suicidal ideas; details of each attempt; and history of intentional self-injury. In addition, the assessment should include a review of the psychiatric treatment history (psychiatric hospitalization as well as emergency department visits related to psychiatric issues), prior psychiatric treatments, responses to prior treatments, and history of adherence to pharmacological as well as nonpharmacologic treatments. The initial examination should further address the person's substance use history including tobacco, cocaine, marijuana, alcohol, hallucinogens, heroin, opioids, and other substances. Moreover, the evaluation should include evaluation for the misuse of prescription medicines, supplements, and over-the-counter (OTC) medicines. The examiner should also assess for recent or present substance use disorders as well as changes in the pattern of using alcohol and other substances.

Organizational Response to Substance Abuse

By taking certain steps, organizations will be ready to address substance abuse problems when they occur. Components necessary to respond to drug and alcohol problems include drug testing, an Employee Assistance Program (EAP), and access to a psychiatrist for fitness-for-duty exams and treatment referrals.

Workplace drug testing is particularly important in industries high in health and safety risks, such as transportation and heavy manufacturing. Drug testing can be used by employers to detect drug use by employees or job candidates and as a tool for prevention. It can identify recent use of alcohol, prescription drugs, and illicit drugs as a screening tool for potential health and safety and performance measures.

EAP professionals are a useful resource for occupational physicians. They provide workers with confidential screening for substance use and mental health disorders, provide brief counseling, refer individuals to appropriate treatment resources, and follow up on treatment progress. The goal is to motivate the employee to seek assistance with the EAP, resolve the problem, and return to acceptable job performance.

When an employee is felt to have such an impairment due to substance abuse, the company should put the employee on administrative or medical leave and directly request a psychiatric fitness-for-duty exam or ask a psychiatrist, EAP professional, or occupational physician to determine if one is necessary. Removing an impaired employee from the workplace is clearly in a company's best interest. Such an employee generally is not allowed back to work until he or she has been seen for the fitness exam by a psychiatrist, completed appropriate treatment, and been reevaluated by a psychiatrist to ensure that he or she can perform his or her normal job functions in a safe manner.

Psychiatric Fitness-for-Duty Examinations

The psychiatric fitness-for-duty examinations should be reserved for mental health records, which are typically more highly protected than general medical records. They are governed by federal law and also state statutes in which mental health treatment and evaluation records have special provisions protecting confidentiality, as is often seen with substance abuse treatment and HIV medical records. Situations requiring the use of a psychiatric fitness-for-duty exam include preemployment psychological screening, a disruptive employee, impairment due to substance use, requests for mental-based leaves, failed attempts at return to work following psychiatric care, and threat assessment. Employees who repeatedly create disruption in a work group may do so as a result of mental illness. A fitness exam can provide valuable information for treatment referral and case management by the employer. A brief psychiatric exam may support an employee taking time away from work when that individual is in need of stress reduction and clinical intervention.

There are occasions when a treating doctor releases an employee to resume full duties prematurely following a leave of absence for treatment of a mental disorder. Safety concerns in employees treated for depression and anxiety may represent a basis for a psychiatric examination prior to workforce reentry. A bus driver may or may not be safe to resume responsibility for transporting patrons on public transit after experiencing a psychotic break. A machine operator may need to be weaned off benzodiazepines before returning to full duty after treatment for anxiety. Police officers involved in shootings routinely undergo psychiatric consultation before regaining access to their weapon.

The psychiatric fitness-for-duty exam must address the employee's functionality, with the examiner being aware of the essential and nonessential job functions as detailed in a written job description. Pertinent information should be communicated timely. Delays in conducting the exam and producing a report can cause disruption not only to the identified employee but also to the work group awaiting direction.

WORKPLACE STRATEGIES FOR ADDRESSING MENTAL HEALTH

Although mental illness is the leading reason for both work incapacity and sickness absence, most workplace health systems have tended to ignore mental illness. However, with increasing understanding of the negative consequences of mental health problems in work settings, there has been corresponding growth in workplace strategies to deal with common mental health issues. In particular, there has been a focus on detection, prevention, and management of anxiety and depression. The strategies to address common mental disorders at work have developed from three major disciplines: psychology, medicine, and public health.

Interventions to enhance workplace mental health are cost-effective for employers. Unfortunately, there is not a simple, universal answer to enhancing mental health in the workplace. Best practices emphasize the importance of using a multifaceted method to address issues at the organizational, team, and individual levels. Factors to be considered include good management, work design, organizational culture, supporting recovery, promoting and enabling early intervention, promoting and enabling help-seeking, as well as encouraging programs for returning employees to work. Programs focusing on mental illness treatment or prevention likely result in a favorable return on investment.

A review of the efficacy of workplace mental health strategies identified moderate evidence to support two primary prevention approaches: increasing worker control and encouraging physical activity. Cognitive behavioral therapy-based stress management had stronger evidence than other secondary prevention approaches (eg, counseling). Tertiary prevention approaches focusing on work (eg, CBT-based and problem-focused programs for returning employees to work) demonstrated moderate evidence for improving occupational outcomes and strong evidence for improving symptoms.

REFERENCES

American Psychiatric Association Foundation, Center for Workplace Mental Health: http://workplacementalhealth.org/.

Barrech A, Kilian R, Rottler E, et al: Do working conditions of patients in psychotherapeutic consultation in the workplace differ from those in outpatient care? Results from an observational study. Int J Environ Res Public Health 2018;15:227 [PMID: 29385714].

Centers for Disease Control and Prevention: Mental health in the workplace. https://www.cdc.gov/workplacehealthpromotion/tools-resources/workplace-health/mental-health/index.html.

Goetzel RZ: Mental health in the workplace. J Occup Enviro Med 2018;60:322 [PMID: 29280775].

Joyce S: Workplace interventions for common mental disorders: a systematic meta-review. Psychol Med 2016;46:683 [PMID: 26620157].

Junne F: The role of work-related factors in the development of psychological distress and associated mental disorders: differential views of human resource managers, occupational physicians, primary care physicians and psychotherapists in Germany. Int J Environ Res Public Health 2018;15:559 [PMID: 29558427].

National Institute of Mental Health: https://www.nimh.nih.gov/health/statistics/mental-illness.shtml.

National Institute on Drug Abuse. https://www.drugabuse.gov/.

O'Donnell L: Social aspects of the workplace among individuals with bipolar disorder. J Soc Social Work Res 2017;8:379 [PMID: 2941659].

U.S. Department of Health and Human Services Substance Abuse and Mental Health Services Administration: Key substance use and mental health indicators in the United States: results from the 2017 National Survey on Drug Use and Health.

■ SELF-ASSESSMENT QUESTIONS

Select the one correct answer for each question.

Question 1: The hallmark of major depression is
a. the inability to get out of bed
b. diminished productivity
c. irritable mood
d. a severely depressed mood lasting at least 2 weeks

c. three or more episodes of mania
d. at least one episode of anxiety and one episode of major depression

Question 2: Bipolar disorder is a cyclical mood disorder involving
a. at least one episode of abnormally elevated energy level and mood which usually alternate with one or more episodes of depression
b. at least one episode of depression followed by an episode of abnormally elevated energy level and mood

Fatigue, Shiftwork, & Sleep Disorders

Robert Kosnik, MD, DIH

David Claman, MD

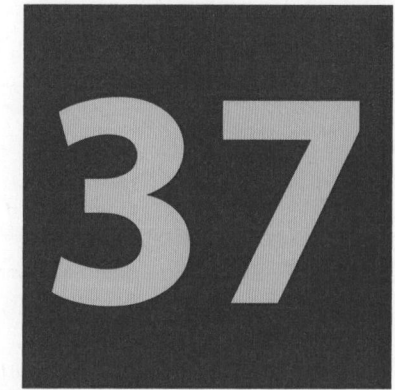

FATIGUE

Fatigue is defined as a biological drive for recuperative rest. It affects a large majority of workers. The major cause of fatigue is insufficient or disrupted sleep. Fatigue occurs as a function of the length of time awake, the time of day, workload, general health, and lifestyle outside of work. It is a function of the homeostatic drive for sleep and the circadian rhythm of sleep/wakefulness. Fatigue and excessive daytime sleepiness (EDS) are also consequences of disorders of the central or peripheral nervous systems and/or other disease states, including common illnesses such as infections, asthma, gastrointestinal disorders, and metabolic abnormalities. Attention to fatigue in workers is important, not only because it affects work and safety but because of the negative impacts of fatigue on overall health.

Fatigue and workplace sleepiness are found in all work settings. Excessive sleepiness in the workplace and on highways is a serious safety hazard. Insufficient or disrupted sleep may result in accidents and injuries and may have adverse effects on mental and physical health. Workers are at a higher risk of fatigue when their work causes sleep deprivation and sleep deficit. Physical workload affects fatigue-related performance and safety outcomes. Intense mental workload can also contribute significantly to fatigue development. Most workers in service economies are assigned to alternative work schedules, many of which result in fatigue. For safety critical tasks, the consequences of a mistake or error in judgment may result in serious injury or death. Identifying and preventing fatigue is particularly important in the transportation sector, health care sector, and among first responders.

Work is organized into a variety of different work schedules which can be fixed or flexible. Shiftwork is a working time arrangement in which workers succeed one another at the workplace so that the establishment can operate longer than the hours of a normal workday. The basic categories of shift systems are fixed shift systems in which workers always work the same shift, and rotating shift systems, in which workers are assigned to work shifts that vary regularly over time, typically often through the night shift. Night work has additional implications for fatigue because it requires work in opposition to the biological clock.

CIRCADIAN RHYTHM

The circadian rhythm (body clock) is an internally generated biological rhythm of behavioral and physiological functions over approximately a 24-hour cycle. Humans are diurnal, awake, and active during daylight, and resting and sleeping at night. This sleep-wake behavior is determined by the regular oscillation of circadian rhythms. The most important circadian rhythm is core body temperature that reaches a nadir during sleep and a peak during the early afternoon. The production and release of nearly all hormones exhibits a circadian pattern.

The sleep-wake cycle is an essential circadian rhythm that serves as the foundation for daily well-being. Work efficiency at night is not the same as during the day. Work safety is impaired with the severe circadian disruption of shiftwork and night-shift work. When considering health, safety, and productivity, the time when sleep occurs is as important as the duration. Sleep quality suffers when sleep is obtained during the diurnal period when an individual is normally active. The sleep drive (the urge to sleep) increases late at night and reaches a peak in the early morning hours. There is also a small increase in sleepiness in the early to mid-afternoon.

Circadian rhythms persist in the absence of time cues. They can be affected by cues such as light or dark, and by the time when these cues occur. Light early in the normal day reinforces one's circadian rhythm. Work that shifts from day to evening seldom disrupts the core body temperature and sleep/wakefulness circadian rhythms. Night-shift workers, on the other hand, have fatigue from both sleep deprivation and circadian rhythm disruption. Some workers assigned to night work are able to adjust to some degree; others are not and may develop a shiftwork sleep disorder.

Table 37–1. Signs and symptoms of fatigue-related performance impairment.

Sign	Symptom
Inability to concentrate	• Unable to organize a series of activities • Preoccupation with a single task • Focus on a trivial problem, neglecting more important ones
Diminished decision-making ability	• Misjudges distance, speed, time, etc • Fails to appreciate the gravity of the situation • Fails to anticipate danger • Fails to observe and obey warning signs • Overlooks items that should be included • Chooses risky options • Has difficulty with simple arithmetic, geometry, etc
Poor memory	• Fails to remember the sequence of task or task elements • Has difficulty remembering events or procedures • Forgets to complete a task or part of a task
Slow response	• Responds slowly (if at all) to normal, abnormal, or emergency situations
Mood change	• Quieter, less talkative than usual • Unusually irritable
Attitude change	• Unaware of own poor performance • Too willing to take risks • Ignores normal checks and procedures • Displays a "don't care" attitude

SHIFTWORK

ESSENTIALS OF DIAGNOSIS

▶ Fatigue with work shift assignment.

▶ Diminished work performance.

▶ Sleep alterations.

▶ Aggravation of other diseases.

▶ Changes in behavior.

▶ Increased drug use.

▶ General Considerations

Between 20% and 25% of the US workforce is assigned to an alternative work schedule—some form of rotating shiftwork, evening work, or night work. Rotating shifts usually involve regularly changing work hours. Employees' shifts change periodically (eg, every 2–30 days), so that times spent working day, evening, and night shifts are shared by the workforce. These schedule changes have consequences for mental

and physical well-being, and may influence performance and safety.

▶ Pathogenesis

Many physiologic systems operate within a regular circadian rhythm. The circadian pacemakers, which time the approximately 24-hour rhythms in sleep and wakefulness, resynchronize slowly after an abrupt phase shift in environmental time cues. Examples of circadian physiologies include body temperature, glucocorticoid secretion, cognitive function, gastric emptying, pulmonary function, effects on metabolism of medications, and many psychological processes. While the symptoms of jet lag are transient, the repeated shifts in the activity/sleep schedule experienced by night-shift workers on rotating or permanent schedules are often associated with chronic sleep deprivation and, over a number of years, with increased risk for various medical disorders.

▶ Differential Diagnosis

• Chronic insomnia.

• Bipolar disorder, persistent depressive disorder (dysthymia), or cyclothymia disorder.

• Major depressive disorder with seasonal pattern (seasonal affective disorder).

• Substance use disorder.

▶ Prevention

A key issue with shiftwork schedules is the readjustment, or entrainment, of these physiologic rhythms. With change from a day to a night work schedule, or as a result of travel over time zones, the normal synchronization of the various circadian physiologic rhythms is disrupted. Because each physiologic rhythm readjusts at its own rate, this internal desynchrony may last for long periods. There is seldom complete reentrainment to night-shift work. Additionally, there is significant individual variation in the ability to adapt and, for some, deterioration of tolerance to shiftwork with ageing.

A significant portion of the shiftwork population has some level of desynchronosis at any given time. Poor adapters may develop a constellation of characteristic pathologic manifestations of shiftwork intolerance, sometimes referred to as shiftwork-maladaptation syndrome. Clinical intolerance to shiftwork has been defined by the presence of sleep alterations, persisting fatigue (not disappearing with normal time off periods), changes in behavior, digestive disturbances, and the regular use of sleeping pills.

▶ Clinical Findings

In addition to disrupting biological rhythms, shiftwork, particularly that including night work, disrupts social and family life, potentially negatively affecting performance efficiency, health, and social relations. Proper alignment between sleep-wakefulness and internal circadian time is crucial for cognitive performance. Individuals with shiftwork sleep disorder are at risk for significant behavioral and health-related morbidity associated with their sleep-wake symptoms. Adverse effects can manifest themselves in the short term as sleep disturbances, psychosomatic troubles, mistakes at work, and accidents. Rotating shifts and night work aggravate many preexisting chronic disorders as a result of the disruption of circadian functions. In the long term, there is an increased risk for metabolic, psychoneurotic, cardiovascular, and gastrointestinal diseases. Women shift workers are vulnerable to negative reproductive outcomes.

▶ Complications

Medical surveillance programs have been recommended for shift workers and are mandatory in some countries. Rotating shifts and night work may aggravate some preexisting chronic disorders as a result of the disruption of circadian functions. Shiftwork may complicate management of chronic diseases for which timing and adjustment of medications are important. The implications for clinical case management are relevant and, in several instances, critical.

Shiftwork can interfere with mechanisms regulating drug kinetics and actions at selective brain sites, either directly or through effects on the gastrointestinal/hormonal cycles. Insulin-dependent diabetes mellitus may be more difficult to control. The alteration of the sleep cycle may increase seizure frequency in epileptics due to sleep deprivation or disturbance of medication regulation. Asthmatics may also experience difficulty with medication adjustments.

The risk of cardiovascular disease in shift workers is significantly increased. Some studies have indicated increases in hypertension in shift workers. Other studies show an increased mortality among shift workers. Obesity, high triglycerides, and low concentrations of high-density lipoprotein (HDL) cholesterol occur together more often in shift workers than in day workers, which might indicate an association between shiftwork and metabolic syndrome. Shiftwork may be associated with insulin-resistance syndrome in workers younger than 50.

There is a potential reproductive risk from shiftwork. Reproductive outcomes among women shift workers include increased spontaneous abortions, preterm births, and intrauterine growth retardation. Night-shift work is being studied for increases in the risk of cancer at several sites among men and increases in the risk for breast cancer among women. There is a tendency of increased risk of breast cancer either after over 20 years of night shift or after a shorter period of rotating shifts.

Workers assigned to shiftwork schedules, and 12-hour working days, are significantly prone to a variety of mental health disorders. There is a common disturbance of mood in dysrhythmic workers, with a disturbing tendency toward depression as the condition becomes chronic. The majority of individuals subject to shiftwork or jet travel–related time shifts in their sleep-wake schedules commonly report some degree of depressive symptoms.

Extensive disruption in circadian function is known to occur among patients with bipolar disorder. It is plausible that circadian dysfunction underlies pathogenesis of this common abnormality. An estimated 2.6% people have lifetime bipolar I disorder. Subtle disturbances of short-cycle rhythms such as the rapid eye movement (REM)/non-REM sleep cycle could contribute to the ultra-rapid cycles of mood, energy, sleep, and activity that characterize early-onset bipolar disorder. Some studies demonstrate that licit and illicit drug use increases significantly in this group of workers, with no benefit to worker health or safety, and possibly adding to the chronicity of the problem.

▶ Treatment

There is substantial evidence that appropriately timed, bright-light treatments can successfully overcome the circadian misalignments associated with desynchronosis. The mood elevation and increased alertness that would result from this intervention might remove the influence that desynchronosis has in aggravating depression, drug abuse, and a variety of other mental health disturbances.

SLEEP DISORDERS

Sleep disorders may complicate adjustment to any work assignment, and especially to more demanding work schedules such as rotating shifts and night shifts. Sleep disorders become additive to sleep debt brought on by any sleep deprivation. There are a number of screening questionnaires for the identification of sleep disorders. The Stanford Sleepiness Scale, Epworth Sleepiness Scale, Insomnia Sleep Questionnaire Packet, and StopBang questionnaire (all available on websites) are widely used. There are also questionnaires for vigilance and self-perceived fatigue and a variety of other performance measurements.

Sleep Apnea

Obstructive sleep apnea (OSA) is a common, important, and treatable medical condition affecting 2–4% of the middle-aged adults, with prevalence increasing with the worsening obesity epidemic. Obstructive apnea is cessation of breathing due to airway collapse, accompanied by respiratory effort. Hypopneas are shallow breathing events that cause similar oxygen desaturation and electroencephalogram (EEG) arousals to apneas. Repetitive episodes of airway closure interrupt sleep quality, and resulting awakenings with adrenergic surges can affect blood pressure, cardiac function, and cardiovascular health. EDS caused by frequent sleep interruption is detrimental to the patient's qualify of life and is a safety concern in the workplace.

Risk factors for OSA include obesity, snoring, witnessed apnea, age, male gender, anatomic obstruction (especially tonsillar hypertrophy), and abnormal airway anatomy. Many patients report symptoms of daytime sleepiness. Obesity is the most common risk factor, but thinner patients can also have

OSA, particularly younger patients with enlarged tonsils, or patients with craniofacial abnormalities such as retrognathia.

Diagnostic evaluation requires a sleep study, optimally a formal polysomnogram (PSG) in the sleep lab, to calculate the AHI (AHI is the number of apneas and hypopneas per hour of sleep). Normal AHI is < 5, mild OSA is AHI 5–14, moderate OSA is AHI 15–30, and severe OSA is AHI > 30. Home sleep apnea testing (HSAT) can also be performed, but the AHI may be underestimated since HSAT does not accurately quantify the hours of sleep time. HSAT is best performed when supervised by an experienced sleep specialist who is managing the patient's care.

Cardiovascular morbidity and mortality are strongly associated with severe OSA (Apnea-Hypopnea Index > 30). Cardiovascular manifestations of OSA include hypertension, arrhythmias, atrial fibrillation, stroke, and congestive heart failure (CHF). Observational studies have shown improved cardiovascular outcomes with continuous positive airway pressure (CPAP) treatment. A CPAP machine provides a constant airway pressure to ensure that the airway remains open during sleep.

Treatment depends on the severity of apnea, clinical symptoms, and comorbidities such as hypertension, atrial fibrillation, stroke, and CHF. Conservative measures include weight loss, sleeping in lateral position, avoiding alcohol and sedatives for 3 hours before bed, and treating nasal congestion. Additional treatments are CPAP (most commonly) and bilevel (positive airway pressure machines that allow a higher pressure with inspiration, and a lower pressure with exhalation), oral appliances, and ENT surgery.

For patients with moderate to severe apnea and those with significant symptoms, CPAP is generally first-line therapy, because it has the highest success rate, and CPAP effectiveness can be objectively monitored with memory data from the CPAP machine. Oral appliances (which hold the jaw in a more forward position to pull the tongue forward) and ENT surgery (a range of available options can be considered) usually have a lower chance of therapeutic success but may be reasonable to consider in mild OSA, and also in patients who are noncompliant with CPAP.

CPAP titration with mask fitting is done during the PSG in the sleep lab, to optimize leak issues and provide a positive initial CPAP experience. Auto-CPAP can also be used as initial therapy, but fitting the patient for mask or nasal pillows is done in the daytime by the equipment company. Patients have to make mask adjustments on their own at home.

When morbid obesity is present (body mass index [BMI] ≥ 40), the prevalence of obesity hypoventilation syndrome (OHS) is increased to 20% or more. OHS is characterized by BMI ≥ 30 with Pco_2 > 45. Clinical symptoms of snoring, apnea, fatigue, and daytime sleepiness are similar to OSA, but daytime hypoxemia may be present and morning headaches may be more prominent. When morbid obesity is present, serum bicarbonate is usually > 27, and sleep studies usually show persistent hypoxemia. In these cases, sleep study usually shows persistent hypoxemia and more aggressive treatment with bilevel and/or oxygen may be necessary.

Sleep deprivation from any cause can impact performance, so medical intervention in the area of sleep duration is appropriate. Since OSA is an important cause of daytime sleepiness, it is important to ask appropriate screening questions to determine if diagnostic evaluation is indicated. This is especially true when sleepiness could affect driver or pilot safety. Practitioners should check with appropriate regulatory agency (Federal Motor Carrier Safety Administration [FMCSA], Federal Railroad Administration [FRA], Federal Aviation Administration [FAA], Coast Guard, and National Transportation Safety Board [NTSB]) for current specific recommendations and requirements.

Central sleep apnea (CSA) is characterized by cessations in airflow (apnea) in the absence of respiratory effort. It is less common in adults, accounting for approximately 5% of sleep apnea. CSA is considered to be the primary diagnosis when ≥ 50% of apneas are scored as central in origin (cessation of breathing in the absence of respiratory effort). Symptoms of snoring, apnea, and disrupted sleep may be similar to OSA. Patients with CSA tend to complain more of insomnia than of hypersomnolence, which may be a helpful distinguishing feature from OSA.

Potential causes of CSA include high altitude, CHF, hypoventilation (from chest wall, neuromuscular, neurodegenerative disease or congenital central hypoventilation), nasal obstruction, postnasal drip, gastroesophageal reflux disease (GERD), opiate medications, and treatment-emergent CSA occurring on CPAP. The term "complex" sleep apnea has been used to describe OSA patients who develop central hypoventilation apnea when they are treated with CPAP (treatment-emergent). Complex sleep apnea has been estimated to occur in 6–15% of OSA patients treated with CPAP but usually resolves over time with continued CPAP treatment. If necessary, both opiate CSA and "complex" sleep apnea can be treated with a bilevel device.

In patients suspected of having hypoventilation, daytime hypoxemia may be present, and arterial blood gas to measure Pco_2 is often necessary. Treatment with bilevel is generally recommended, which addresses both CSA and hypoventilation. Opiates can also cause CSA, and the risk appears to be dose related. Patients with CHF, more commonly systolic dysfunction, may show a waxing and waning pattern of CSA termed Cheyne-Stokes respiration (CSR). CSA is associated with a higher mortality risk, and treatment should always focus on basic cardiology treatments for CHF with a treating specialist. Additional options include standard bilevel, CPAP, and nocturnal oxygen.

Insomnia

Insomnia is the most common sleep symptom, with up to 33% of the US population reporting occasional difficulty sleeping and up to 10% reporting chronic insomnia. It can occur at the beginning, middle, and/or end of the night. Insomnia has a wide range of potential causes, including medical illness, psychiatric illness, circadian rhythm disorders, and sleep disorders. If medical issues (such as chronic obstructive pulmonary disease [COPD], asthma, CHF, GERD, sinus drainage, or pain) are causing symptoms that disturb sleep, specific treatment should be instituted. If psychiatric illness is a factor, obtaining appropriate management by a specialist is advisable.

Insomnia can often be caused by stress, which may be focused on life or health issues, or develop into anxiety about sleeping. Unhelpful sleeping habits, often described as poor sleep hygiene, frequently contribute to insomnia. Examples of poor sleep hygiene include irregular sleep schedule (going to bed at variable times), napping in afternoon or evening, and caffeine late in the day. When anxiety becomes focused on bedtime, causing muscle tension, the term *psychophysiological insomnia* is used, and relaxation techniques at bedtime are an important aspect of treatment.

Cognitive Behavioral Therapy for Insomnia (CBTI) is the optimal behavioral approach to chronic insomnia. It incorporates sleep restriction, stimulus control, sleep hygiene, mindfulness and cognitive therapy. CBTI, either in individual or group sessions, has been shown to improve both insomnia and depression over a 6- to 8-week course of weekly sessions.

Restless Legs Syndrome

Restless legs syndrome (RLS) presents with symptoms of insomnia. Prevalence is estimated at 3–10% of adults and is more common in women than men. Difficulty falling asleep due to the restless need to move is the most common presenting symptom, and sedentary activities can worsen symptoms. The vast majority of patients with RLS will also have periodic limb movements during sleep (PLMS). To diagnose PLMS in a patient with leg kicking during sleep, PSG is indicated to see if PLMS is causing frequent EEG arousals. RLS often occurs in families, showing an autosomal dominant inheritance pattern, and is also more common in patients with renal failure and Parkinson disease. RLS symptoms increase with iron deficiency. Women are at higher risk during pregnancy and from menstrual blood loss. If ferritin is < 75 mcg/L, iron supplementation for 3–6 months is indicated with a therapeutic goal of > 100 mcg/L.

Narcolepsy

Narcolepsy is a sleep disorder characterized by EDS, often irresistible sleepiness described as "sleep attacks." Narcolepsy is a rare condition, with reported prevalence of 0.05% of adults, and peak incidence at age 15–25. The tetrad of symptoms include EDS, cataplexy (muscle weakness associated with emotions such as laughter or anger), sleep paralysis (transient inability to move usually upon awakening), and hypnogogic hallucinations (dreaming at sleep onset or

when waking up). Many patients also report disrupted sleep patterns at night. EDS is present in 100% of patients, and cataplexy in is present 60–70%. Narcolepsy is a lifelong condition, and symptoms tend to be stable over time. Naps, even brief naps of 10–20 minutes, are typically restorative, which can be a clinical clue and also part of a treatment plan.

REFERENCES

Bokenberger K, Sjölander A, Dahl Aslan AK, Karlsson IK, Åkerstedt T, Pedersen NL: Shift work and risk of incident dementia: a study of two population-based cohorts. Eur J Epidemiol 2018;33(10):977-987 [PMID: 30076495].

Caldwell JA, Caldwell JL, Thompson LA, Lieberman HR: Fatigue and its management in the workplace. Neurosci Biobehav Rev 2019;96:272-289 [PMID: 30391406].

Cowie MR: Sleep apnea: state of the art. Trends Cardiovasc Med 2017;27(4):280-289 [PMID: 28143688].

Drager LF, McEvoy RD, Barbe F, Lorenzi-Filho G, Redline S, INCOSACT Initiative (International Collaboration of Sleep Apnea Cardiovascular Trialists): Sleep apnea and cardiovascular disease: lessons from recent trials and need for team science. Circulation 2017;136(19):1840-1850 [PMID: 29109195].

Farrell PC, Richards G: Recognition and treatment of sleep-disordered breathing: an important component of chronic disease management. J Transl Med 2017;15(1):114 [PMID: 28545542].

Fischer FM, Silva-Costa A, Griep RH, Smolensky MH, Bohle P, Rotenberg L: Working Time Society consensus statements: psychosocial stressors relevant to the health and wellbeing of night and shift workers. Ind Health 2019;57(2):175-183 [PMID: 30700668].

Krystal AD, Sorscher AJ: Recognizing and managing insomnia in primary care and specialty settings. J Clin Psychiatry 2016;77(4):e471 [PMID: 27137433].

Leso V, Vetrani I, Sicignano A, Romano R, Iavicoli I: The impact of shift-work and night shift-work on thyroid: a systematic review. Int J Environ Res Public Health 2020;17(5):1527 [PMID: 32120919].

Li W, Chen Z, Ruan W, Yi G, Wang D, Lu Z: A meta-analysis of cohort studies including dose-response relationship between shift work and the risk of diabetes mellitus. Eur J Epidemiol. 2019;34(11):1013-1024 [PMID: 31512118].

Moreno CRC, Marqueze EC, Sargent C, Wright Jr KP Jr, Ferguson SA, Tucker P: Working Time Society consensus statements: evidence-based effects of shift work on physical and mental health. Ind Health 2019;57(2):139-157 [PMID: 30700667].

Pahwa M, Labrèche F, Demers PA: Night shift work and breast cancer risk: what do the meta-analyses tell us?. Scand J Work Environ Health 2018;44(4):432-435 [PMID: 29790566].

Swanson CM, et al: The importance of the circadian system & sleep for bone health. Metabolism 2018;84:28-43 [PMID: 29229227].

Wickwire EM, Geiger-Brown J, Scharf SM, Drake CL: Shift work and shift work sleep disorder: clinical and organizational perspectives. Chest 2017;151(5):1156-1172 [PMID: 28012806].

■ SELF-ASSESSMENT QUESTIONS

Select the one correct answer for each question.

Question 1: The majority of individuals subject to shiftwork or jet travel–related time shifts in their sleep–wake schedules commonly report some degree of
a. anxiety
b. manic symptoms
c. depressive symptoms
d. job dissatisfaction

Question 2: Extensive disruption in circadian function is known to occur among patients with
a. aerobic exercise regimens
b. bipolar disorder
c. high levels of productivity
d. chemical dependency withdrawal

Workplace Violence Prevention

Jane Lipscomb, PhD, RN

Kathleen McPhaul, PhD, MPH, RN

Matt London, MS

Workers in a great variety of industries and occupations face the serious problem of workplace violence (WV). A basic definition of workplace violence is any physical assault or threat that a worker experiences associated with their job. The perpetrator of such violence may be a stranger, a client/patient, a coworker, or an intimate partner. The probability of a worker experiencing workplace violence at the hands of one of these classes of perpetrators varies by industry and occupation. Workplace violence directed at health care and social assistance workers are at high risk of workplace violence, in part due to the fact that they are often required to provide care to anyone seeking such services, including those patients or clients who have or develop behavioral problems that place workers at risk of violence. However, many of the risk factors and prevention strategies for these workers can be applied across industry sectors.

The occupational health provider has a role in evaluating and preventing injuries arising from physical assaults and threats of assaults. These clinical encounters may occur in employee health clinics, primary care settings, urgent/emergent care, injury compensation clinics, and in settings evaluating return to work and ability to work. Occupational health providers often provide consultation and oversight to large workplaces and health systems and may not clinically evaluate the employee. Evaluating the work environment and employer safety program, as with any other hazardous exposure, is critical to determine if other employees are at risk and to evaluate the effectiveness of prevention programs, security activities and safety services for returning the injured employee to the work environment.

Victims of workplace violence must be treated with considerable care and concern for their long-term well-being and ability to return to work. Particularly for victims of severe assaults, sexual assaults, or repeat victimizations, serious psychological problems often result.

Occupational health providers should have the expertise to ensure that these injured workers do not return to the same unmitigated hazards when they return to work. As with other occupational diseases and injuries, the clinician must assess whether the patient can return to the work environment. This is a decision based both on their fitness to return and on whether the same risk factors remain at the workplace. Similarly, the clinician should consider whether coworkers are at similar risk to the presenting patient/worker.

WORKPLACE VIOLENCE—MAGNITUDE OF THE PROBLEM & RISK FACTORS

WV is any act or threat of physical violence, harassment, intimidation, or other threatening disruptive behavior that occurs at the work site, or during the course of work. It ranges from threats and verbal abuse to physical assaults and even homicide. As with most occupational injuries and illness, less severe injuries are under-reported, so the best data by industry exist for homicides, followed by Occupational Safety and Health Administration (OSHA) recordable incidents and data from the Department of Justice's National Crime Victimization Survey (NCVS).

Homicide is currently the fourth-leading cause of fatal occupational injuries in the United States. According to the Bureau of Labor Statistics Census of Fatal Occupational Injuries (CFOI), of the 5147 fatal workplace injuries that occurred in the United States in 2017, 458 (8.8%) were workplace homicides. By comparison, the numbers of homicides were 417 and 500 in 2015 and 2016, respectively. Eighty-five percent of workplace homicide victims (n = 356) in 2015 were men and 61 were women, yet homicides represented 18% of fatal occupational injuries to women in 2015, compared with 8% of fatal occupational injuries to men. First-line supervisors of retail sales workers (40 fatalities), cashiers (35 fatalities), police and sheriff's patrol officers (34 fatalities), and taxi drivers (27 fatalities) were the occupations with the greatest number of homicides in 2015. In contrast to the public perception that most workers are killed at the hands of disgruntled coworkers, the most common types of assailant in workplace homicides in 2015 were robbers, responsible for 128 workplace homicides. Coworkers were the assailants in 50 workplace homicides, and spouses or domestic partners were responsible for another 25 workplace homicides (BLS.gov, 2018).

Incidents of nonfatal workplace violence are much more common and are distributed in different industry sectors when compared with homicides. In the United States, estimates of the number of victims of workplace violence range from nearly 600,000 to 2 million workers each year. Since underreporting of workplace violence is prevalent, even the higher estimate is likely to underestimate the true magnitude of the problem. According to the most recently published data from the Department of Justice's National Crime Victimization Survey, from 1993 to 2009, 572,00 *violent victimizations*, such as simple and aggravated assaults, rape, sexual assault, robbery, occurred annually at work against persons age 16 or older. Among all victims, 12% reported physical injuries, half of them requiring medical treatment. Less than half of incidents were reported to the police.

In 2017, the incidence rate of violence-related injuries in health care and social assistance sector was over three times the rate in all of private industry (14.7 vs 4.0 per 10,000 workers). The rates among high-risk settings within the overall sector were 181.1 per 10,000 workers for psychiatric and substance abuse hospitals, 78.0 per 10,000 within residential mental health facilities, and 34.8 per 10,000 in nursing and residential facilities, respectively. Other high-risk subsectors include elementary and secondary education (21.2 per 10,000) and transit and ground passenger transportation (10.8 per 10,000) (BLS, 2018).

Across industry sectors, the risk is increased for workers who handle/exchange money with the public and those who work with volatile, unstable people. Working alone or in isolated areas may also contribute to the potential for violence. This risk factor certainly increases the likelihood that an assault, should it occur, will result in serious injury, including potentially death.

Providing services and care and working where alcohol is served may also impact the likelihood of violence. Additionally, time of day and location of work, such as working late at night or in areas with high crime rates, are also risk factors that should be considered when addressing issues of workplace violence. As noted above, at higher risk are workers who exchange money with the public, delivery drivers, health care professionals, public service workers, customer service agents, law enforcement personnel, and those who work alone or in small groups.

The risk of WV varies greatly based on a number of factors. Logically, prevention measures also vary depending on the setting and the risk factors that are present. To help address this variation, researchers in the 1990s developed a Typology of Workplace Violence, based on the relationship of the perpetrator to the target (worker). According to this scheme, workplace violence is classified into four types based on the perpetrator and victim/worker relationship: type I (stranger/criminal intent), type II (customer/client), type III (worker-on-worker), and type IV (personal relationship) (Iowa Report).

TYPOLOGY OF WORKPLACE VIOLENCE

▶ Type Description

I. Criminal intent—The perpetrator has no legitimate relationship to the business or its employee and is usually committing a crime in conjunction with the violence. These crimes can include robbery, shoplifting, trespassing, and terrorism. The vast majority of workplace homicides (85%) fall into this category.

II. Customer/client—The perpetrator has a legitimate relationship with the business and becomes violent while being served by the business. This category includes customers, clients, patients, students, inmates, and any other group for which the business provides services. A large portion of customer/client incidents occur in the health care industry, in settings such as nursing homes or psychiatric facilities; the victims are often caregivers. Police officers, prison staff, flight attendants, and teachers are some other examples of workers who may be exposed to this kind of WV, which accounts for approximately 3% of all workplace homicides.

III. Worker-on-worker—The perpetrator is an employee or past employee of the business who attacks or threatens another employee(s) or past employee(s) in the workplace. This may be a supervisor, peer, or even a subordinate. Worker-on-worker fatalities account for approximately 7% of all workplace homicides.

IV. Personal relationship—The perpetrator usually does not have a relationship with the business but has a personal relationship with the intended victim. This category includes victims of domestic violence who are assaulted or threatened while at work and accounts for about 5% of all workplace homicides.

Type I violence is prevalent among late night retail workers and taxi drivers, who are at risk of injury from violence committed during an attempted robbery. Type II violence, on the other hand, results when perpetrators have a legitimate reason to be in the establishment such as patients receiving health care or community residents receiving services. Perhaps most well-known but far less prevalent is type III violence that occurs among coworkers. This includes those disturbed and/or disgruntled employees who bring firearms to work and murder fellow employees and supervisors. The US Postal Service experienced several high-profile incidents of this type of workplace violence in the 1970s and 1980s; hence the term "going postal." However, these incidents can occur periodically in any workplace. Finally, intimate partner violence also known as domestic violence can also occur in the workplace. In fact, the workplace is the location where a perpetrator of intimate partner violence can often locate a partner who has fled the abuse. The US Office of Personnel

Management (OPM) requires federal employers to provide policies and programmatic support to employees who experience intimate partner violence at work (US OPM, 2013).

A workplace at risk for patient-on-worker violence is also at increased risk for other types of violence, in part because of the lack of a comprehensive violence prevention program that should address all types of workplace violence. Regardless of the industry sector, workplace violence prevention measures need to be tailored to the specific setting and workforce. The principles of a comprehensive occupational health and safety injury prevention program are outlined by the US OSHA. The American National Standards Institute (ANSI) describes similar principles necessary for developing an effective health and safety management system focused on the risk of violence.

HEALTH CARE & SOCIAL ASSISTANCE SECTORS & WORKPLACE VIOLENCE

Workplace violence is one of the most significant occupational hazards facing health care workers, in particular in the behavioral health setting. This is in part because of the failure to recognize violence as a public health problem amenable to an occupational health approach to prevention and the view that violence toward those working with or in the presence of individuals with cognitive impairment, mental illness or a tendency toward violent acts "is part of the job."

Health care leads other sectors in the incidence of nonfatal workplace assaults. Of all nonfatal assaults against workers resulting in lost workdays, approximately one-third are in the health care sector. Patients cause the majority of these assault injuries. According to BLS data, reported cases of nonfatal workplace violence against health care workers have increased approximately 6% per year in recent years.

Social assistance occupations face similar rates of workplace assault as health care. Within both fields the incidence rates vary significantly, based on setting. Community-based care for the developmentally disabled, the chronically mentally ill, care for the elderly with dementia and cognitive impairment, as well as social services that address child abuse in the home may be high risk for assault and injury to employees. These services are typically chronically underfunded, workers have less formal training (except for social workers), and workplaces themselves may be homes or community settings without security. Often employees work alone without the infrastructure and security features of large workplaces, such as hospitals. Residential facilities and hospitals for the acutely mentally ill, whether forensic or civil, pose a very high risk of widespread and serious incidents of assault.

According to the most recently published data from the Department of Justice's National Crime Victimization Survey, from 1993 to 2009, the groups within health care with the highest average annual rate of workplace violence were mental health workers (20.5 assaults per 1000 workers) and custodial-care workers in mental health (37.6 assaults per 1000 workers). An average of 77% of psychiatric nurses surveyed reported experiencing physical violence during the previous year.

Emergency department workers face a high risk of injuries from assaults by patients or patients' family members. Public safety officers and others carrying weapons in emergency departments create opportunities for severe or fatal injuries. Since no department in a health care setting is immune from workplace violence, all departments should have violence prevention programs.

Organizational factors have been associated with patient assaults, including understaffing (especially during times of increased activity such as meal times), lack of training, insufficient communication within and between work shifts, poor workplace security, long wait times for patients, unrestricted movement by the public around the facility, and the transport of patients. Environmental factors also may be important, including working alone or with poor visibility, and the presence of materials that can be used as weapons. The presence of trained security personnel reduces the rate of assault, so does a system for identifying the charts of patients who have a history of violence. The rate of assault is increased when (a) administrators consider assault to be part of the job, (b) there is a high patient-to-worker ratio, and (c) work is primarily with patients with psychiatric disorders or with patients who have long hospital stays.

Communication and treatment philosophy among and between health care professionals and direct care staff play a critical role in reducing the hazard of workplace violence. Conflicting philosophies of care often exist within a workplace, resulting in inconsistent boundaries and treatment of patients by staff, and of staff by supervisors. Poor and inadequate communication can lead to inconsistent approaches to client behaviors.

A respectful and effective therapeutic relationship is the foundation for caring for the mentally ill. The ability to form and sustain therapeutic relationships is compromised by high caseloads, burdensome paperwork, and highly stressful work environments. Home visits are generally done alone (ie, not in pairs), but visiting in pairs is considered much safer. Clients are more acutely ill, more often have co-occurring substance abuse disorders, and are much more likely to be violent. Direct care workers experience a lot a violence, including verbal hostility, threats, and physical assaults. This is partly because it is difficult and sometimes impossible to obtain relevant information pertaining to a client's past history of aggression, assault, and criminal behavior. Staff safety training is critical, but the content of safety training is not standardized across the system, and the safety training is often inconsistent. Knowledgeable and supportive supervisors and upper management are extremely important to staff safety.

PREVENTING WORKPLACE VIOLENCE

Health care workplaces can be made safer for workers, patients, and visitors alike through the development and implementation of a comprehensive workplace violence prevention program (WVPP) that includes strong employee involvement; comprehensive and ongoing risk analyses; use of engineering and administrative controls, such as security alarm systems; adequate staffing; and training and ongoing evaluation.

The US OSHA outlines the principles of a comprehensive occupational health and safety injury prevention program. In 1996, OSHA published "Guidelines for Preventing Workplace Violence for Health Care and Social Service Workers." In 2015, OSHA updated and published a revised set of guidelines to delineate hazard control measures across settings. Both the 1996 and 2015 federal guidelines describe a comprehensive WVPP that provides a framework for addressing the hazard via the basic elements of a health and safety program. A WVPP is synonymous with a health and

safety management system focused on the risk of workplace violence.

The program must have as its foundation strong management commitment and worker involvement. These foundational elements then support the other program elements, namely, comprehensive risk analysis, effective control of hazards, training, recordkeeping, and regular program evaluation. Worker involvement is important in any comprehensive illness and injury prevention program, but particularly in developing a WVPP. Frontline health care workers are skilled at recognizing patients who may be at risk of violence. Additionally, those workers are key to identifying prevention strategies that are effective and that do not have unintended negative consequences, either to staff or patient safety or to patient care (Table 38–1).

TABLE 38–1. Preventing workplace violence.

A. **Management commitment and employee involvement**—Management commitment must be evident in the form of high-level management involvement and support for a written workplace violence prevention policy and its implementation. Meaningful employee involvement in policy development, risk assessment, joint management-worker violence prevention committees, postassault counseling and critical incidence debriefing, and follow-up are all important program components. This should include frontline workers and, where a union exists, union representatives. Without both management commitment and employee involvement, it is unlikely that an effective program will be developed.

B. **Worksite analysis**—A worksite analysis is the foundation on which an effective program exists. This analysis should utilize all available "data" sources and be repeated, at least in part, on a periodic basis. "Data" sources include OSHA logs, first reports of injuries, other incident reports, and workers compensation data. This information can be invaluable in identifying trends and risk factors. These data are often supplemented by staff surveys and focus groups. Regular walk-through surveys of all areas of the facility should be conducted and should include staff from each area and from all shifts. Special attention should be paid to those areas where assaults have occurred. A safety committee has an important role in ensuring a robust worksite analysis. Such a committee should review and track incidents by organizational, environmental, patient, unit, and staff-level factors. A safety committee or a violence prevention committee is an ideal forum for direct care and management review and analysis of incidents and identification and evaluation of prevention strategies.

C. **Hazard prevention and control**—Hazard prevention and control measures should be designed based on the risk factors identified above. The classic industrial hygiene hierarchy of controls should be followed. To the extent possible, exposure to the potential violence should be eliminated. An example is transferring an unstable, violent patient to a different facility, one that is better equipped to provide care to such a high-risk patient. The next priorities for prevention are engineering and administrative controls. Engineering controls to be considered include modifying the layout of admissions areas, nurses' stations, medication rooms, lounges, patient rooms, or offices; limiting access to certain areas; and evaluating all furnishings to ensure that they are not used as weapons. Administrative controls include developing and implementing appropriate policies and procedures, code procedures, staffing levels and providing regular training are important administrative controls. Finally, personal protective devices may be warranted, such as issuing cell phones and personal alarm devices to workers. Staff involvement is just as important in designing effective controls as it is in conducting a thorough risk assessment. Frontline staff can help identify unintended consequences of various prevention measures and can provide feedback as to whether implemented changes have been effective. Additionally, programs need to be in place to provide support to assault victims and to their coworkers. These can include easy access to medical and mental health services, assistance with the workers' compensation system, and support in accessing the criminal justice system, when appropriate.

D. **Training and education**—At the time of hiring and periodically thereafter, worksite- and job-specific training should be provided covering the risk factors, prevention measures, and relevant policies and procedures. This should not be a generic training. For direct care staff, training should include skills in aggressive behavior identification and management. Violence prevention training should also include information on the prevalence of violence in mental health work, risk factors for staff assault, a description of the written violence prevention program, how to report an incidents, and participation in committees addressing patient on staff violence.

E. **Recordkeeping and program evaluation**—Recordkeeping and program evaluation are inextricably linked and should focus not only on incidents of physical and verbal assaults but also on near misses. Reporting should be something that staff are actively encouraged to do. Reports should be followed up and investigated promptly, with the results reported to the individual who made the report. Obviously, employees should not be retaliated against for filling out an incident report or filing a workers' compensation claim. The reporting and investigation of incidents is a critical means of evaluating the effectiveness of the WVPP and of identifying control measures which need to be modified or implemented. Staff should be encouraged to report all incidents, regardless of their severity. The reporting and review of incidents should be a critical aspect of the risk assessment and hazard control process. The number and severity of incidents should be tracked to evaluate the impact of organizational, unit, and staff-level changes such as enhanced security procedures, renovations to units, as well as changes in the patient population.

▶ Initial Evaluation & History Taking

The care of a traumatic injury from an assault represents the entry point to the health care system for an employee exposed to violence at work. Even in instances of less complex bruises and contusions that are treated locally with "first aid" (and not reportable on the OSHA 301 Log), occupational health providers who conduct the initial evaluation have the responsibility to assess the factors that contributed to the injury. It is critical that the occupational medicine provider recognize the substantial emotional and psychological trauma associated with the event. Never send an employee who appears uninjured back to work without an assessment of the emotional impact of the incident and of their knowledge of how to prevent another assault. Best practice also includes a referral to the employee assistance program (EAP) or an assaulted staff action program (ASAP), if available, and informing the collective bargaining units, if present.

Questions to ask at the initial clinical evaluation include the following:

1. What are your job responsibilities? And what were you doing at the time of the assault? Were you alone with the client/patient? Did you know the client, their history of and triggers for violence?
   a. This question allows the provider to understand the many possible factors, including assisting with bathing, such as in geriatric care, providing medications, counseling a patient while in an office, attending to an injury such as in emergency room, or simply walking down a poorly lit corridor. This question should also illicit whether the assault was spontaneous or in the course of restraining a patient.
2. How often in the course of your job do you work with unstable, volatile individuals who have a history or prior violence or agitate behavior?
   a. This question helps the provider assess the risk for assault. This will drive a further assessment of the robustness of the safety program as well as the timing and ability of the employee returning to work.
3. Describe the response to your assault/injury. How did you get help? Is there a formal security system such as video surveillance, panic buttons, other staff nearby? Does your employer provide training in verbal de-escalation and physical maneuvers to avoid injury?
   a. This may be the point at which the provider obtains preliminary details of the WVPP, if there is one, and the nature of the management commitment to workplace violence prevention.

▶ Employee Resources & Referrals

A worker assaulted by a patient/client may experience guilt, emotional distress, depression, anxiety, and posttraumatic stress disorder (PTSD) following the incident. Formal programs need to be in place to provide support to assault victims and to their coworkers. These should include easy access to medical and mental health services, assistance with the workers' compensation system, and support in accessing the criminal justice system, when appropriate.

An evaluation of 14 empirical studies of ASAP, a voluntary, system-wide, peer-help, crisis intervention program for staff victims of patient assaults found a 25–62% reduction in staff assaults associated with the programs. The studies found the presence of significant numbers of females as both assailants and victims in several categories of assaults.

The postincident debrief process will contribute to the root-cause analysis as it will inform corrective actions needed to prevention future staff injuries and therefore materially reduce the risk of the hazard. Staff will have the necessary expertise to work directly with individual clients and groups of clients. This expertise should be tapped following any incident in order to improve working conditions and client care.

Many health care organizations provide confidential employee counseling services as part of their overall employee benefits package. These EAPs are intended to help employees deal with personal problems that might adversely impact their job performance, health, and well-being. EAPs generally include short-term counseling and referral services for employees and their household members. Supervisors may also refer employees based on unacceptable performance or conduct issues. Many organizations and workers view their EAP as a valuable resource for employees following a violent incident. In our experience, we have found EAP programs and professionals have a limited focus, namely individual-level strategies to manage the emotional and psychological effects of a violent incident. They often do not have the skills to place the individual response in the context of the larger problem of workplace violence and therefore are of limited value.

Returning to work often carries with it the risk of further psychological trauma by having to come in contact with and/ or care for the individual who perpetrated the assault. For many injured workers, the emotional trauma is much more debilitating than the physical injury. These workers need to be referred to a mental health provider to begin to address the emotional trauma associated with the assault. Care needs to be exercised in referrals for mental health services.

Injured workers may also need assistance navigating the worker's compensation system. Workers seeking compensation for the emotional impact of an assault, with or without physical injury, may prove very challenging. In applying for compensation, they will need the support of a provider to confirm that their injury is work-related. Although work-relatedness of workplace violence is widely recognized, having a claim accepted may still be a challenge in many jurisdictions.

Injured workers may also choose to press charges against the patient/perpetrator of the assault. In doing so, they may need the support of an occupational health physician to support their case and potentially testify in any hearing held on the charge.

FACTORS TO CONSIDER WHEN RETURNING THE EMPLOYEE TO WORK

When returning an employee to work after an assault, consider the employee's perspective. What concerns them the most? There is a range of responses that the employer may take to ensure the employee's safety upon return to the workplace. An employer who aims for a best practice WVPP will have been in touch with the employee during the recovery and rehabilitation from the injury offering empathy, concern and optimism for getting the employee back to work. This is generally the supervisor's role, but it is even more effective when higher leadership reaches out with concern and commitment to evaluate the safety program. Another best practice is an employer that reevaluates the WVPP in light of a serious injury due to assault and communicates the review to worker and to the employee's provider. What did the review find? Was there a failure of assessing the risk, that is, knowing the nature of the patient's history of violence and behavioral triggers? Was there a failure of communication? Was there a failure of training? Staffing? Supervision? Lighting? Were there clinical issues with the patient? How are these being addressed? Are other staff at risk? Is there the possibility of "light duty" or return to work in a different capacity for the injured employee?

Workplace violence is an occupational hazard with clear implications for the clinical care of injured individuals, as well as clear and evidence-based responsibilities for assessing the effectiveness of the employer's violence prevention efforts. By obtaining the initial critical history of the injury, elucidating the risk factors, and maintaining contact with the employee and employer, the occupational health provider plays the pivotal role in ensuring that the injured employee receives appropriate clinical care for their injuries, and, as important, does not return to a high-risk workplace without assurance of an effective safety and violence prevention program.

▶ Lessons Learned From the Field

Field work and focus groups with groups of workers suggest many common themes and suggestions that go beyond what can be addressed by formal policies and procedures. Many of these issues address the critical role of communications and treatment philosophy among and between professional and direct care staff.

- Staff note that conflicting philosophies of care often exist within a workplace, resulting in inconsistent boundaries and treatment of patients by staff and of staff by supervisors. Poor and inadequate communication can lead to inconsistent approaches to client behaviors. Examples of such communication include poor communication of pending program changes and not enough communication among staff about patients' risks. Treatment team are often removed and separate from day-to-day patient behavior and direct care staff experience. Workers also report that poor communication resulted from lack of trust between professional and direct care staff and even within professional disciplines.

- A respectful and effective therapeutic relationship is the foundation for caring for the mentally ill. The ability to form and sustain therapeutic relationships is compromised by high caseloads, burdensome paperwork, and highly stressful work environments.

- Caseloads have increased, and many case managers believe that excessive caseloads diminish the effectiveness of case management and other services by causing staff burnout, reduced ability to develop trusting and therapeutic relationships with patients, less knowledge of patient history, and pressure to cut corners or conduct home visits alone.

- Home visits are generally done alone (ie, not in pairs), but visiting in pairs is considered much safer. When there is worker and supervisor discretion about paired visits (especially in the context of high caseloads and fiscal constraints), there will be pressure for staff to go out alone.

- Clients are more acutely ill, more often have co-occurring substance abuse disorders, and are much more likely to be violent. In this context, direct care workers experience violence including verbal hostility, threats, and physical assaults.

- It is difficult and sometimes impossible to obtain relevant information pertaining to a client's past history of aggression, assault, and criminal behavior.

- Staff safety training is critical, but staff report receiving little or no safety training, inconsistent safety policies, or no regularity in training.

  Knowledgeable and supportive supervisors and upper management are seen as extremely important to staff safety.

REFERENCES

Byon HD, Lee M, Choi M, Sagherian K, Crandall M, Lipscomb J: Prevalence of type II workplace violence among home healthcare workers: a meta-analysis. Am J Ind Med 2020;63(5):442-455 [PMID: 32052510].

Liu J, Gan Y, Jiang H, et al: Prevalence of workplace violence against healthcare workers: a systematic review and meta-analysis. Occup Environ Med 2019;76(12):927-937 [PMID: 31611310].

Phillips JP: Workplace violence against health care workers in the United States. N Engl J Med 2016;374(17):1661-1669 [PMID: 27119238].

Rudkjoebing LA, et al: Work-related exposure to violence or threats and risk of mental disorders and symptoms: a systematic review and meta-analysis. Scand J Work Environ Health 2020;3877 [PMID: 31909816].

Saragoza P, White SG: Workplace violence: practical considerations for mental health professionals in consultation, assessment, and management of risk. Psychiatr Clin North Am 2016;39(4):599-610 [PMID: 27836154].

Spelten E, Thomas B, O'Meara PF, Maguire BJ, FitzGerald D, Begg SJ: Organisational interventions for preventing and minimising aggression directed towards healthcare workers by patients and patient advocates. Cochrane Database Syst Rev 2020;4:CD012662 [PMID: 32352565].

Wyatt R, Anderson-Drevs K, Van Male LM: Workplace violence in health care: a critical issue with a promising solution. JAMA 2016;316(10):1037-1038 [PMID: 27429201].

■ SELF-ASSESSMENT QUESTIONS

Select the one correct answer for each question.

Question 1. OSHA
  a. requires the reporting of all violence in the workplace to state agencies
  b. offers guidelines to state agencies designed to enhance recognition of workplace violence
  c. provides the principles of a comprehensive occupational health and safety injury prevention program
  d. has a legislative mandate to prevent workplace violence

Question 2. Type I violence
  a. is prevalent among late night retail workers and taxi drivers, who are at risk of injury from violence committed during an attempted robbery
  b. results when perpetrators have a legitimate reason to be in the establishment such as patients receiving health care or community residents receiving services

  c. occurs between co-workers
  d. is a problem of US Postal Service workers

Question 3. Determining whether or not an employee may become violent
  a. has less to do with a static profile of that person than a series of dynamic variables (behaviors)
  b. is impossible to predict and a waste of time to consider
  c. has less to do with personality than job satisfaction
  d. requires training in violence assessment

Occupational Safety

Nina Townsend, MPH, CSP, CIH

Worldwide, nearly 3 million people are killed as a result of workplace safety incidents or illnesses each year. Roughly 4000 workers are killed at work each year in the United States, where Hispanic workers are disproportionately more likely to die at work. The most common causes of workplace deaths are transportation incidents, workplace violence, falls, and being struck by an object.

Occupational safety is the science and practice of anticipating, identifying, evaluating, and controlling hazards for the potential to cause injury or illness to people or harm to property or the environment. Safety professionals focus on a wide variety of workplace hazards, including electrical hazards; machinery with potential to cut, crush, or pull in a person or body part; work at heights; confined spaces; excavations and trenches; explosive or flammable materials or environments; and moving equipment, such as motor vehicles, forklifts, or heavy construction equipment, with the potential to hit or run someone over. Workplace health hazards are primarily addressed by industrial hygiene, which is covered in the following chapter.

Safety professionals are trained to recognize that all occupational "accidents" can be anticipated from and be attributed to operational deficiencies or unsafe or unhealthy work conditions or practices. Safety professionals strive to identify and correct the underlying enabling factors that may lead to safety incidents in order to prevent them from occurring.

The occupational physician—whether employed directly by a company, retained on a consulting basis, or working in a clinic or hospital serving the industrial community—will be called on to work with safety professionals. In very large organizations, the physician and the safety professional may be part of a health and safety, loss-control, or risk-management team, or even may work in the same department. In smaller organizations, the safety professional often will be the point of contact for the company with the consultant occupational physician.

The physician's interactions with the safety professional generally occur while:

- Providing emergency and nonemergency medical services
- Performing medical monitoring of workers potentially exposed to hazards
- Implementing worker health maintenance programs
- Participating in worker training programs on health hazards
- Serving on management oversight committees reviewing the safety program
- Assisting in incident investigations or reviews
- Interpreting the medical aspects of hazard assessments or regulatory standards

PROFESSIONAL QUALIFICATIONS

In the United States, the Occupational Safety and Health Act of 1970 (OSHAct) created the Occupational Safety and Health Administration (OSHA), an administrative agency within the Department of Labor, and made it responsible for the promulgation and enforcement of safety standards applicable to employers. Some OSHA standards recognize certified safety professionals (CSP), as well as certified industrial hygienists (CIH) and physicians, as "qualified" and "competent" to evaluate and control regulated hazards.

Several universities offer baccalaureate, masters, and even doctoral degrees specifically in occupational safety and health or safety management. Some state and community colleges offer associate degrees or technical certification in safety. The Board of Certified Safety Professionals (BCSP) certifies practitioners in the safety profession in the United States. About 17,500 currently hold the CSP, and 28,000 retain a related occupational safety certification administered by the BCSP. The importance of safety certification continues to grow. In the United States, some laws, regulations, and standards cite it. More importantly, many companies list it as a job requirement, government agencies rely on it, and contracts for safety services require it.

Certifications in Safety

CSP is the highest professional designation for safety professionals given by the BCSP. It is held by safety professionals who have met education and experience standards, have demonstrated by examination the knowledge that applies to professional safety practice, and continue to meet recertification requirements established by the BCSP.

BCSP offers a number of certifications available to individuals with varying levels of experience and formal training, including the

- Associate Safety Professional (ASP)
- Graduate Safety Practitioner (GSP)
- Construction Health and Safety Technician (CHST)
- Occupational Health and Safety Technologist (OHST)
- Safety Trained Supervisor (STS)
- Certified Environmental, Safety and Health Trainer (CET)

RESPONSIBILITIES OF SAFETY PROFESSIONALS

The responsibilities of safety professionals vary widely depending on the size and type of organization, the degree of inherent risks within the workplace, and the level of safety management expertise. In a small service organization, for example, the "safety coordinator" may be someone without formal safety training, whose responsibilities are limited to ensuring that the organization complies with applicable OSHA regulations. In a medium-sized manufacturing company, the safety practitioner may be a trained professional with a wide range of safety and as well as some health and environmental responsibilities. In large, complex organizations, a staff of certified professionals from among several different departments usually covers the full scope of safety, health, and environmental responsibilities. The staff may include safety professionals, industrial hygienists, occupational physicians and nurses, engineers, environmental specialists, ergonomists, insurance personnel, security officers, and fire-protection professionals.

Safety professionals may take on many roles within a company. Depending on their role, safety professionals may be engineers, systematically analyzing equipment, tasks, and processes to identify inherent hazards and failure modes, and designing controls. They may be managers applying management principles and methods to establish, facilitate, coordinate, and achieve safety goals and objectives. Many serve as inspectors observing and evaluating worksites, job tasks, and policies and procedures for deficiencies or lack of regulatory compliance; as well as, educators and trainers of workers, supervisors, and managers. The most common role is some combination of the above.

SAFETY & HEALTH MANAGEMENT SYSTEM

A principal responsibility of a safety professional in any organization is to facilitate and coordinate the development and implementation of an effective safety and health management system. The elements of this system are the related policies, goals, plans, programs, procedures, and standards. Their collective purpose is to systematically guide the organization to (1) prevent work-related injuries and illnesses, (2) comply with applicable health and safety regulations, and (3) minimize injury/illness, regulatory and compliance costs, and violations.

Safety professionals seek to make the occupational safety and health management system a self-regulating process by incorporating performance monitoring, feedback, and correction capabilities. Some administrative and hazard-control elements may be required by government regulation. The safety professional is usually responsible for ensuring that the safety and health management system includes these required elements (Table 39–1).

ELEMENTS OF THE SAFETY SYSTEM

Injury and Illness Prevention Programs (IIPP) are commonly used with the goal of reducing the number and severity of workplace injuries and alleviating the associated financial burdens of these injuries. Worker participation is an important element to an effective IIPP. Many states have requirements or voluntary guidelines for workplace IIPPs. Many employers in the United States already manage safety using IIPPs. Most successful IIPPs are based on a common set of key elements. These include management leadership/assignment of responsibility, ensuring worker participation and compliance, hazard identification, hazard prevention and control, education and training, accident investigation, and program evaluation and improvement.

Elements of an IIPP

Responsibility—the employer's written IIPP should provide the name and/or job title of the person(s) with the authority and responsibility for its implementation. Workers should be able to give the name of the individual designated as responsible for the IIPP.

Compliance—a system should be set forth in writing to ensure that workers comply with safe and healthful work practices. These can be recognition programs for workers who comply or disciplinary or retraining programs for those who do not.

Communication—a system should be established and documented for communicating with workers about safety and health matters—in a form and language easily understood such as meetings, training programs, and posted or written notifications. Workers should be encouraged to inform their employer of hazards at the worksite without fear of reprisal.

Hazard assessment—procedures should be included for identifying and evaluating workplace hazards, such as periodic inspections performed by both workers and management (Table 39–2).

Table 39–1. Elements of a safety and health management system.

Administrative Elements	Hazard Control Elements
Safety and Health (S&H) Policy Statement	Code of Safe Practices[a]
Statement of S&H Responsibilities	Hazard Identification and Control Program
Procedure for Communicating S&H Information[a]	Job Safety Analysis Program
Process & Criteria for Setting S&H Performance Goals & Indicators	Hazardous Energy Control Procedure[a] (Lockout/Tagout)
S&H Program Audit, Feedback, and Correction Program	Hazardous Substance Control and Communication Program (Haz/Com)[a]
S&H Education and Training Procedure[a]	Confined Space Safety Program[a]
Procedure for Development of Annual S&H Plan and Budget	Trenching and Shoring Safety Program[a]
Procedure for Establishing and Operating S&H Committees	Vehicle Operation Safety Program
S&H Procedure and Standards for Engineering Designs	Laboratory Hygiene Program[a]
Contractor S&H Procedure	Ergonomic Hazard Control Program[b]
OSHA Compliance Procedure	Indoor Air Quality Program
Program for Employee S&H Participation	Personal Protective Equipment Standards[a]
Medical Management Program[a]	Respiratory Protection Program[a]
S&H Performance Evaluation Criteria Accountability Process	Hearing Conservation Program[a]
	Housekeeping Standards
	Accident/Incident Investigation Procedure[a]

[a]OSHA required program, procedure, or activity.

Incident/exposure investigation—a procedure to investigate workplace incidents that have led to or could lead to injuries or illnesses should be provided in the IIPP.

Hazard correction—methods and procedures for correcting all existing workplace hazards, and unsafe or unhealthful work conditions or work practices in a timely manner should be provided in the IIPP, and specific methods to correct the hazard should also be included.

Training and instruction—an effective program of instructing workers on general safe work practices and hazards specific to each job assignment must be provided in the IIPP, and the required training must be given.

Table 39–2. Hazard assessment: Focuses on the relationship between the worker, the task, the tools, and the work environment.

Common Tasks	Possible Hazards	Hazard Type
Chipping, grinding, machining, masonry work, wood working, sawing, drilling, chiseling, powered fastening, riveting, and sanding	Flying objects such as large chips, fragments, particles, sand, and dirt	Impact
Furnace operations, pouring, casting, hot dipping, and welding	Anything emitting extreme heat	Heat
Acid and chemical handling, degreasing, plating, and working with blood	Splash, fumes, vapors, and irritating mists	Chemicals
Woodworking, buffing, and general dusty conditions	Harmful dust	Dust
Welding, torch-cutting, brazing, soldering, and laser work	Radiant energy, glare, and intense light	Optical radiation

Keeping records—there must be adequate written documentation of the steps taken to implement and maintain the employer's IIPP.

Other important elements of a safety system or IIPP include emergency action planning (EAP), fire prevention planning, access to worker exposure and medical records, implementation of a hazard communication program, provisions for personal protective equipment (PPE), auditing, and general requirements for work areas.

HAZARD IDENTIFICATION & ASSESSMENT

Safety professionals use systematic methods to identify, assess, eliminate, and control hazards. A number of tools are available for this purpose.

▶ Systems Safety Analysis

Systems safety analysis is not a single technique or process but rather a group of analytic techniques wherein operations (such as manufacturing a printed circuit board) or machines (such as punch presses) are viewed as if they were a single system. That system, in turn, should have each of its discrete parts, steps, or functions analyzed for potential hazards. All of this must be limited by practical considerations of operational effectiveness, time availability, and cost-effectiveness. Systems safety analysis is used to assess complex processes and facilities.

Some techniques utilized include fault hazard analysis, which looks at all of the ways the system can fail, why, and what the consequences would be; common cause failure analysis, which takes into account interdependencies within the system; failure modes, effects, and criticality analysis (FMECA); and, a number of other analysis techniques specific to individual hazards or industries.

▶ Human Factors Considerations

Human decisions and actions have to be considered as part of the system, and systems should be designed with humans in mind to reduce the likelihood of an incorrect decision or pressures to deviate from specified work-practices. Human factors are an established field of study with much of the earliest research coming from the aviation industry. The general concept is that humans err or may take short cuts when under pressure and that systems should be designed to eliminate or reduce the chance that a negative outcome can occur as a result of a human decision or action.

▶ Job Safety Analysis

The job safety analysis (JSA) technique was developed during World War II when large numbers of inexperienced workers had to be integrated into the workforce quickly and safely. JSAs are done by analyzing each step of a task individually to determine all potential hazards present and process failures that can occur, then recommends controls strategies. JSAs are primarily used to assess tasks and jobs of individual workers or teams.

This task can be led by supervisors or lead workers, who, in turn, gain great understanding and appreciation of the areas under their control. The workers who participate develop a better recognition of the hazards they face, therefore serving as an effective teaching tool. There are other comprehensive models that include human error rate prediction, management oversight risk tree, and technique and operation review.

HAZARD PREVENTION & CONTROL

Controlling exposures to occupational hazards is the fundamental method of protecting workers. Traditionally, the hierarchy of controls has been used as a means of determining how to implement feasible and effective controls (Figure 39–1).

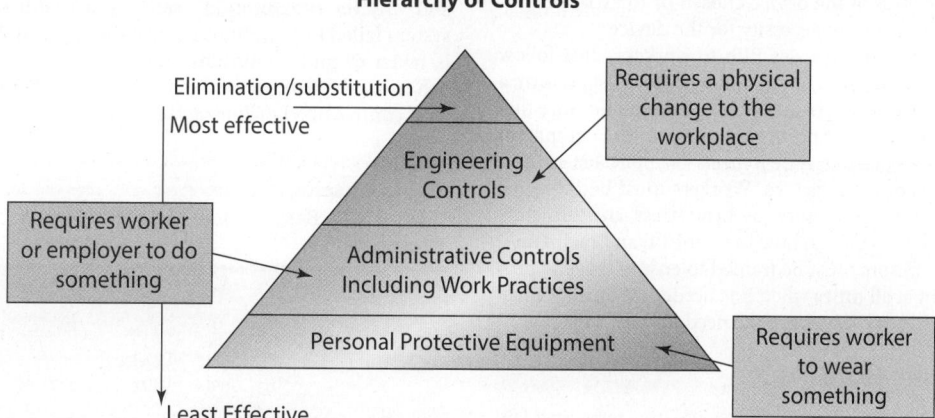

Hierarchy of Controls

Elimination/substitution
Most effective
Requires a physical change to the workplace
Engineering Controls
Requires worker or employer to do something
Administrative Controls Including Work Practices
Personal Protective Equipment
Requires worker to wear something
Least Effective

▲ **Figure 39–1.** Hierarchy of controls: The employer should first aim to eliminate the hazard altogether.

- Elimination—removal of the hazard entirely.
- Substitution—replacement of the hazard with a safe or less dangerous or toxic alternative.
- Engineering controls—methods such as ventilation or machine guarding that reduce or prevent exposure to the hazard.
- Administrative controls—includes controls such as written operating procedures or training.
- PPE—gear or clothing used by the worker to protect themselves (eg, hardhat, fall protection harness, respirator, or gloves).

The control methods at the top of the list are more effective and protective than those at the bottom. Following the hierarchy normally leads to the implementation of inherently safer systems, ones where the risk of illness or injury has been substantially reduced.

► Personal Protective Equipment

The least effective but very common method of providing for worker safety in hazardous conditions is the use of PPE. These devices are intended to protect workers in case an incident occurs (eg, fall protection such as a harness) or to insulate the worker from a hazardous condition (eg, earplugs for noise or respirators for airborne contaminants) that is part of the normal operation.

The weakness of PPE is that the effectiveness of the equipment is largely user-dependent, rather than inherent to the equipment itself. Workers must be trained to wear the protection, must wear it properly, and must maintain the device in good working condition. In situations where engineering or administrative controls are not yet effective in eliminating the hazard, protective devices must be issued as a last line of defense to prevent injury to the worker. The occupational health physician may be called on by the safety professional to evaluate a worker's fitness for safely wearing the PPE. The occupational physician may be consulted about the appropriateness of the device chosen or to assist in educating workers about the necessity for the device.

Any program that provides PPE to workers must follow the same basic procedures. First, the employer must perform a hazard assessment where hazards are evaluated to ensure that the selected PPE will be appropriate. Second, the equipment itself must be checked to ensure it meets all applicable government standards of manufacture. Workers must be informed of the hazards involved, such as heat stress and difficulty breathing, and be trained in how to wear PPE and maintain it properly. Supervisors must be trained to ensure that the protection is worn at all times when it is needed. Warnings must be posted to inform everyone of the need for protection.

INCIDENT INVESTIGATION

Many safety professionals prefer to use the term *incident* to *accident* because there is a general misconception that accidents are "freak," random occurrences that cannot be anticipated. This misconception can inhibit an organization's prevention efforts. Safety professionals regard incidents as preventable events that indicate correctable deficiencies in the organization's safety and health program.

An injury or illness incident may be acute, as in the case of contact with an unguarded rotating saw blade or with a corrosive chemical, or chronic, from such hazardous exposures as frequent repetitive body motions and long-term inhalation of toxic vapors.

Safety professionals conduct and/or coordinate incident investigations to uncover their proximate and enabling causal factors so that measures can be identified and implemented to prevent a recurrence. The investigation process involves the systematic collection, analysis, documentation, and communication of relevant information (Table 39–3).

Incidents almost never have just one cause and are the result of chains of events and circumstances. Finding the causes of an incident calls for more than simply reviewing the injured worker's actions at the scene; the physical conditions and all equipment must be scrutinized to determine what could be done to prevent recurrences. Such items as workflow patterns, environmental conditions, and stress levels also must be considered. Safety professionals often develop a written procedure to systematically guide the investigative process including the types of incidents to investigate, who is involved, how the investigation is conducted, and how findings are communicated and implemented.

► Root-Cause Analysis

Correcting hazards without eliminating their *root causes* treats only the symptoms of the problem; the hazards eventually will reappear. Root-cause analysis is a tool used by safety professionals to identify the enabling or root causal factors of hazards by systematically analyzing the events, conditions, and values that logic, experience, and training lead them to believe could have contributed to the existence of the hazard. The findings then are evaluated to determine where, how, and why the organization's safety and health management system failed to prevent or control the enabling factors. Care is taken to understand any root causes that drove human behaviors that contributed to the incident occurring. Permanent control of contributing factors is achieved by correcting

Table 39–3. Basic steps for conducting an accident investigation.

Gather information	Step 1—Secure the accident scene
	Step 2—Collect facts about what happened
Analyze the facts	Step 3—Develop the sequence of events
	Step 4—Determine the causes
Implement solutions	Step 5—Recommend improvements
	Step 6—Write the report

Table 39–4. Haddon matrix with examples of safety efforts.

	Pre-crash	Crash	Post-crash
Human factors	• Education and licensing • Driver impairment • Crash avoidance maneuvers (braking, turning, etc)	• Health at time of crash • Sitting properly in restraint • Impairment	• Response to EMS • Severity of injury • Type of injury
Vehicle/equipment factors	• Crash avoidance equipment and technology (lights, tires, collision avoidance, etc) • Vehicle design • Vehicle load	• Speed of travel • Functioning of safety equipment (seat belts, air bags, child restraints) • Energy absorption of vehicle	• Ease of extraction from vehicle • Integrity of fuel systems and battery systems
Physical environment	• Road hazards • Distractions • Weather conditions	• Roadside features • Guardrails • Type and size of object struck	• Distance of EMS personnel • Notification of EMS personnel • Accessibility to crash victims
Social/economic	• Enforcement activities • Insurance incentives • Social norming • Ability to use safety equipment appropriately	• Laws concerning use of safety equipment	• Trauma system equipment, personnel, training • Information sharing

Source: From https://one.nhtsa.gov/nhtsa/Safety1nNum3ers/june2015/S1N_June15_ChangeTrafficSafety_3.html.

identified inconsistencies, contradictions, and omissions in the organization's safety and health or operating policies, programs, and procedures. Determining that the root cause is human behavior and not changing any aspect of the procedures is not very likely to prevent similar incidents in the future.

The Haddon Matrix

The Haddon Matrix, developed in the 1970s, is one tool that can be used to assess the various contributing factors before, during, and after an incident. The matrix separates factors into human factors, equipment factors, and physical and socioeconomic environment factors. An example of a vehicle crash is shown in Table 39–4.

EMERGENCY ACTION PLANNING

OSHA and often other regulatory agencies require employers in nearly all cases to prepare and implement an emergency action plan (EAP) for emergency situations. Generally, the EAP development, implementation, and management are led by the safety professional.

Emergency Planning

Federal, state, and local authorities now require that businesses establish an EAP to assess and plan for a variety of foreseeable emergencies. They should include answers to questions such as:

1. What events might precipitate an evacuation?
2. Who needs to be notified of the emergency—medical, fire department, police, others?
3. What medical facilities are likely to be needed?
4. Will electrical and gas services be shut off?
5. Are there manufacturing processes that must be shut down in emergencies?
6. Who will do the shutdowns? How? Are they appropriately trained?
7. Who can authorize evacuation?
8. How will workers be instructed to evacuate?
9. Who will be responsible to see that evacuation is carried out safely?
10. Where should evacuated workers go?
11. How will it be determined that all employees, contractor personnel, and visitors have been evacuated?

Emergency or Chemical Response Teams

Worksites that use large quantities of toxic or hazardous materials often will form specialized teams of employees to contain or control exposures to the workers, the general public, or the environment resulting from accidental discharge. The occupational physician often will be asked to help in the planning and training stages when these teams are formed.

Fire Brigades

Industries or operations located at remote sites or with special fire hazards often require the formation of firefighting teams. These trained employees are responsible for ensuring swift reaction to the outbreak of fire and for containing the fire until professional help arrives.

▶ Emergency Medical Facilities

State regulations now require nearly all places of employment to provide a minimum level of emergency medical capability. Depending on the exposures involved, the safety professional, in concert with the occupational physician, may make the case for provision of more than the basic emergency medical capability.

For an office building with no special hazards, the Red Cross multimedia training certifications for two or three employees, perhaps with cardiopulmonary resuscitation (CPR) training added, very well might be sufficient. However, a hazardous chemical processing plant may require an emergency medical technician (EMT), or an occupational health nurse (OHN) for each shift.

HAZARD COMMUNICATION

In order to ensure chemical safety in the workplace, information about the identities and hazards of the chemicals must be available and understandable to workers. US OSHA's Hazard Communication Standard (HCS) (29 Code of Regulations, Section 1910.1200), which was largely harmonized with international standards (referred to as the Globally Harmonized System or GHS) in 2012, requires the development and dissemination of specific information. Parts of this regulation are often referred to as "Workers Right-to-Know." Chemical manufacturers and suppliers are required to evaluate the hazards of the chemicals they produce or import and prepare labels and safety data sheets to convey the hazard information to their downstream customers. Safety data sheets have a required 16-section format to organize the safety, health, transportation, and environmental information. Labels are required to contain specified pictograms, signal words, and precautionary statements unique to each type of hazard. All employers with hazardous chemicals in their workplaces must implement a hazard communications program that includes labels and safety data sheets for their exposed workers, and train them to handle the chemicals safely and appropriately.

ACCESS TO EMPLOYEE EXPOSURE & MEDICAL RECORDS

In the United States, the safety professional may be responsible for implementation of the OSHA regulation mandating access to employee exposure and medical records (29 Code of Regulations, Section 1910.1020). It requires that employers provide certain parties with access to employee exposure and medical records. Employees and their designated representative (eg, union or physician, with the employee's written consent) and OSHA have a right to examine relevant medical exposure records.

In general, these records include medical records consisting of physician and employment questionnaires or histories, laboratory results, medical opinions, diagnoses, treatments, etc.

The safety professional may seek support from or consultation with the occupational physician to obtain these data. The occupational physician should ensure that access to these records does not affect existing legal and ethical obligations concerning the maintenance and confidentiality of employee medical information, or any other aspect of the medical-care relationship.

Exposure records consist of medical records (including biological monitoring data), safety surveys, and air and exposure monitoring data.

INSPECTIONS & MONITORING

The safety professional, especially in the industrial environment, is responsible for numerous inspections. US federal and state regulations now require annual inspections of the work environment designed to recognize potential hazards. Often, this type of inspection is actually performed as part of the health and safety committee's duties so that various points of view are considered, to identify the potential for incidents (health and safety committees are discussed in the next section). However, even when this is the case, the safety professional must review the results and recommendations. Various pieces of equipment, such as gas detectors, cranes, and forklifts, also require periodic inspection to ensure that they are in place, fully functional, certified, and suitable for the intended purposes.

HEALTH & SAFETY COMMITTEES

While not always required, health and safety committees, comprised of management and workers are a best practice for ensuring workplace hazards are identified, communicated, and corrected. They may receive complaints anonymously, conduct inspections, and request outside technical expertise, if needed, in the pursuit of achieving a safe and healthy work environment. Effective safety committees hold regularly scheduled meetings, taking minutes and following up on identified hazards and, crucially, have active participation and commitment from upper management.

OTHER SAFETY PROGRAM ELEMENTS

▶ Fire Protection

Safety professionals usually are required to take charge of fire-protection activities of the organization in addition to their worker safety responsibilities. In fact, only organizations with extraordinary casualty exposure will employ a fire-protection engineer.

The primary duty is, of course, to prevent fires. The fire safety program follows much the same pattern as has been outlined for the workplace safety program, which was designed to keep injuries from occurring: (1) training, (2) communications, (3) emergency protective equipment, (4) chemical safety, and (5) incident investigation.

The safety professional should be involved in the construction and remodeling of facilities, as well as occupancy plans, in order to minimize risk to the office or plant occupants and environment. Once the facility has been constructed, fire-prevention activities usually are limited to monitoring of hazardous areas, fire emergency planning, training, and monitoring of the adequacy of fire-suppression equipment.

▶ Motor Vehicle Safety

As mentioned at the beginning of this chapter, transportation incidents account for the largest single cause of death at work in the United States. The safety professional and occupational health physician should work closely to address motor vehicle safety. Some protocols they might put in place include training, vehicle maintenance, fatigue management, medical and driver-history screening of drivers, and, increasingly, GPS monitoring of vehicles.

SAFETY PERFORMANCE GOALS & INDICATORS

Safety professionals help their organizations develop and administer safety performance goals and indicators. There are several criteria a safety professional may use to evaluate the effectiveness of the safety program and basically two types of goals and indicators, results-directed and activity-based.

Measurement criteria might include

- Incidence and severity rates
- Medical care costs
- Insurance company "experience modification or XMod rating"
- Comparison with peer companies
- Equipment and materials damage costs
- Inspection findings
- Responses to worker questionnaires
- OSHA Log (Form 300) data

The OSHA incident and severity rates (eg, total recordable incident rate [TRIR] or days away restricted transfer rate [DART] are the principal results-directed safety performance indicators of most organizations. They can be compared against the previous year's rate and the industry average to help evaluate current safety performance. An annual goal to reduce this rate below the industry average or below last year's rate would be an example of a results-directed goal.

The frequency and quality of employee safety meetings are examples of activity-based performance indicators. Greater frequency and higher-quality safety meetings can demonstrate leadership support and commitment to safety, which can encourage employee participation and compliance with safe work practices. Another activity-based goal would be to have qualified trainers hold structured safety meetings every month.

Safety professionals regularly monitor and analyze the safety performance indicators to help identify any significant trends.

REGULATORY COMPLIANCE

Overseeing the organization's efforts to comply with government (eg, OSHA) regulations is a major responsibility for all safety practitioners. This responsibility is fulfilled by analyzing and interpreting the regulations to determine their applicability to the organization and then communicating the requirements to the affected personnel. Safety practitioners also develop written programs and procedures that are required by the regulations and conduct or arrange mandated training for workers.

If industrial hygiene or medical specialists are employed within the organization, they usually have the lead responsibility for analyzing and interpreting complex health-related regulations. If these specialists are not available in the organization, the safety professional often will consult with an external industrial hygienist or occupational physician.

There are many safety and health regulations that pertain directly to occupational physicians. In the United States, OSHA specifically references medical practitioners in regulations covering such subjects as blood-borne pathogens; physical examinations for asbestos, lead, cadmium, arsenic, and other specified toxic substances; biologic monitoring; audiometric and hearing examinations; respiratory protection; pulmonary function testing; laboratory hygiene; regulated carcinogens; sanitation; and hazard communication.

CASE MANAGEMENT

Case management is often a process involving multiple parties, including the safety professional, physician, a workers' compensation specialist, and perhaps others with the goal of providing necessary information and services to manage and treat worker injuries or illnesses. Employers want their safety professional and the treating physician to ensure that injured workers receive the proper medical care necessary to return them to full health in the shortest period of time at the lowest cost. The following are ways in which safety professionals and occupational physicians can and should collaborate for better case management.

Safety professionals can provide relevant work-history and exposure information to treating physicians as soon as possible after an injury and illness is reported. If the safety practitioner fails to provide such information in a timely manner, the physician or an assistant should contact the safety practitioner for input prior to completion of the diagnosis. This can prevent both the reality and perception of an inaccurate or biased diagnosis. Information obtained by the occupational physician through annual facility visits and discussions with managers will help to preclude misdiagnoses and misperceptions and can obviate the need for case input from safety professionals except in unusual cases.

Safety professionals should provide and medical care providers should seek information on the organization's modified-duty program and available modified-duty jobs in advance of determination of a treatment protocol for an injured or ill worker. Insurance data indicate that workers with nondisabling injuries recover sooner when they are placed in a job they are able to perform than those who are kept off work. Safety professionals and occupational physicians can work together on presentations and programs to educate employers about the health and cost benefits of providing modified-duty jobs.

REFERENCES

American Society of Safety Engineers: http://www.assp.org.
Board of Certified Safety Professionals: http://www.bcsp.org.
International Labour Organization: https://www.ilo.org/global/topics/safety-and-health-at-work/lang--en/index.htm.
National Institute for Occupational Safety and Health: http://www.cdc.gov/NIOSH.
US Department of Labor: Occupational Safety and Health Administration. http://www.osha.gov.

■ SELF-ASSESSMENT QUESTIONS

Select the one correct answer for each question.

Question 1: The highest professional designation recognized by the BCSP is
   a. Site Safety Coordinator (SSC)
   b. Associate Safety Professional (ASP)
   c. Certified Safety Professional (CSP)
   d. Occupational Safety and Health Technologist (OSHT)

Question 2: The safety and health management system
   a. designates the company role in preventive health care
   b. guides the organization to prevent work-related injuries and illnesses
   c. establishes the insurer's role in health care
   d. evades compliance costs

Question 3: Injury and Illness Prevention Programs (IIPP)
   a. reduce the number and severity of workplace injuries
   b. alleviate the costs of preventive health care on workers
   c. are required by law in all states
   d. discourage worker participation and compliance

Question 4: IIPPs should include
   a. selection of insurance underwriters
   b. bonus awards for loss prevention
   c. hazard assessment
   d. medical treatment

Question 5: An emergency action plan (EAP)
   a. is required by OSHA in nearly all cases
   b. requires outside consultants
   c. centers on the availability of health care facilities
   d. ignores prevention planning

Question 6: OSHA's Hazard Communication Standard (HCS)
   a. requires chemical manufacturers to evaluate the hazards of all chemicals
   b. requires employers with hazardous chemicals to train workers to handle the chemicals safely and appropriately
   c. exempts companies from providing precautionary statements along with labels
   d. no longer requires employers to provide safety data sheets

Question 7: OSHA mandates access to employee exposure and medical records
   a. without legal and regulatory statute
   b. after approval by the employer
   c. except physician and employment questionnaires or histories, laboratory results, medical opinions, diagnoses, treatments, etc.
   d. including industrial hygiene monitoring data

Question 8: Prevention and control of workplace hazards
   a. exempts equipment maintenance
   b. should use the hierarchy of controls
   c. allows workers to decide on which PPE they want to use
   d. delegates responsibility to workers to identify and prevent workplace hazards and exposures

Question 9: A job safety analysis (JSA)
   a. entails daily observation and weekly analysis
   b. uncovers the hazards in the work environment or in a task or activity
   c. can be performed only by trained professionals
   d. is an effective teaching tool for consultants

Industrial (Occupational) Hygiene

Nina Townsend, MPH, CSP, CIH

It is unknown how many illnesses are caused or aggravated by workplace hazards across the globe, but even an outdated estimate from the World Health Organization suggests that between about 50 and 150 million new cases of occupational disease occur annually, and the International Labour Organization estimates that 2 million die from these illnesses each year. In 2015, in the United States, nearly 150,000 workplace illnesses were reported in private industry alone. This is likely an undercount as occupational illness is rarely correctly identified as work-related. Figure 40–1 shows the breakdown of these illnesses by type.

Industrial hygiene is the science of anticipating, recognizing, evaluating, and controlling workplace conditions that may cause workers' injuries or illness. Industrial hygiene and safety disciplines certainly overlap; however, generally speaking, industrial hygiene tends to focus on preventing occupational illness whereas safety tends to focus on preventing injury. Traditionally, this means that industrial hygienists focus on hazards such as exposure to chemicals, noise, heat and cold, radiation, biological hazards, and ergonomics.

Industrial hygienists use environmental monitoring and analytical methods to detect the extent of worker exposure and employ engineering controls, work practice controls, and other methods to control potential health hazards. Hazards arising from the workplace include the potential harm to the community from poorly controlled emissions and such issues as exposures to household members from contamination taken home on workers' clothing.

PROFESSIONAL QUALIFICATIONS

The American Board of Industrial Hygiene (ABIH) issues the Certified Industrial Hygiene (CIH) title in the United States. The sanctioning body for similar certifications in the United Kingdom is the British Occupational Hygiene Society (BOHS), and there are others in other countries. These certifications are common job requirements in industry and government and require continuing education to maintain them.

ANTICIPATION OF HEALTH HAZARDS IN THE WORKPLACE

Anticipation of health hazards may range from a reasonable expectation to mere speculation. This concept implies that the industrial hygienist will understand the nature of changes in the processes, products, environments, and workforces of the workplace and how those changes might affect human health or well-being. For example, installation of a new piece of equipment or process will likely introduce new or additional hazards. Industrial hygienists should be involved in all process changes from the design stage to ensure that hazards are eliminated, minimized, and controlled using the hierarchy of controls. As another example, changing weekly work schedules from five 8-hour days to three 12-hour days almost certainly will impact workers. Along with the psychosocial and physical effects of shiftwork, there may be danger of chemical intoxication if the chemical exposures lead to excessive body buildup without the usual 16-hour "rest" period.

RECOGNITION OF HEALTH HAZARDS IN THE WORKPLACE

In a workplace where the processes are well established, the recognition of health hazards by an industrial hygienist may be as simple as going through the materials and processes and noting which have the potential for causing harm to workers. In the workplace where the processes and work environment are not so well established or are rapidly changing (eg, hazardous waste site clean-up), the recognition of hazards can be more difficult.

Sources of information about health hazards include clinical data about health problems in exposed populations; historical information about former processes and activities; information in scientific journals, trade association bulletins, and government agency reports; conversations with peers; and reports from current and former workers, union representatives, supervisors, or employers.

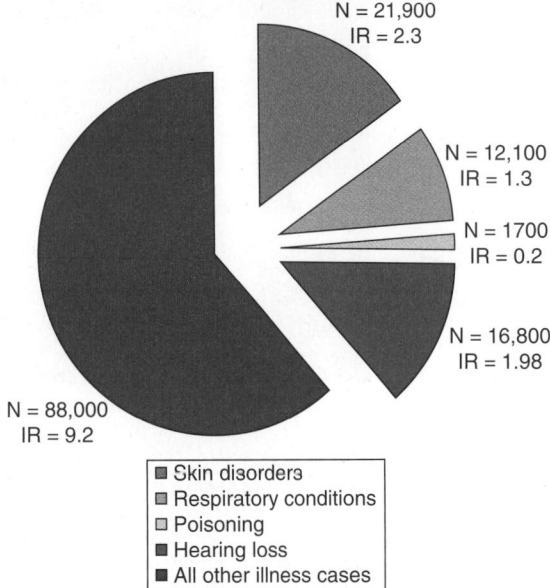

N = 21,900
IR = 2.3

N = 12,100
IR = 1.3

N = 1700
IR = 0.2

N = 16,800
IR = 1.98

N = 88,000
IR = 9.2

- ■ Skin disorders
- ■ Respiratory conditions
- □ Poisoning
- ■ Hearing loss
- ■ All other illness cases

**Incidence rate (IR) = Number of cases per 10,000 full-time workers

▲ **Figure 40–1.** The number and rate (IR)** of workplace illnesses, private industry, 2015, BLS*. (Source: https://www.cdc.gov/niosh/topics/surveillance/images/laborforce-data/chart4.jpg.)

Inspections of the workplace are the best source of directly relevant information about potential health hazards. There is no substitute for observation by an experienced observer of work practices, the use of chemical and physical agents, and the apparent effectiveness of control measures. The physician should be able to recognize major and obvious health hazards in a workplace and distinguish those hazards that may require formal evaluation by the industrial hygienist.

▶ The Walk-Through Survey

The *walk-through survey*, conducted jointly by the industrial hygienist, safety professional, and the occupational physician whenever possible, is the first and most important technique used to recognize occupational health hazards. It is also helpful to have management, or a supervisor or team lead (foreman) available to explain the processes. The survey should begin with a proper introduction to facility management, a discussion of the purpose of the survey, an inquiry about any relevant recent complaints, and a discussion of how results will be used and shared. If appropriate, a simplified process flow diagram also should be prepared at this time.

Following the process flow through the facility is usually most productive. The survey thus might begin at the loading dock, where materials entering the facility can be examined. These incoming materials then should be followed into the process flow stream, and each of the processes of interest in the facility should be observed in action. The survey should continue through to the final product produced by the facility and its packaging. The surveyors also should follow the pathway of any waste materials and determine their disposal sites. It is usually appropriate, and recommended, to discuss work practices with the workers directly involved because the perception of those practices can be very different on the shop floor from what it is in the executive offices.

On completion of the walk-through survey, the industrial hygienist will ordinarily have a closing conference with the facility management or field project manager, at which time identified and potential concerns can be discussed and follow-up measures agreed on. Where the industrial hygienist is a regulatory agency representative, follow-up surveys may require special notices and interaction with agency officials as well as facility management. In any case, a report on the walk-through survey, together with conclusions and recommendations, should be completed for recordkeeping purposes.

▶ Observations to Be Made

At each point in the facility or site process or activity, the industrial hygienist and physician should observe:

- All handling procedures (including procedures for handling unknown materials or materials about which insufficient information is available).
- Any protective measures that are employed, such as ventilation.
- Use of personnel protective equipment, such as respiratory protection and protective clothing.
- The apparent effectiveness of engineering controls, as indicated by absence of characteristic odors, visible dust accumulations, and loud noise.
- The numbers of employees at each process step.
- Any relevant demographic data on sex or age that might affect employees' sensitivity to chemical or physical hazards in the workplace.
- Obvious stigmata such as drying and roughening of the skin (eg, where exposure to solvents occurs).

▶ Data Review

An important part of the industrial hygienist's role in recognition of health hazards in the workplace is data review. Such data may include reports from physicians on clinical findings that may be related to exposures in the workplace, past exposure monitoring data, as well as a review of company records on materials coming into the workplace that may represent significant health hazards. One source of this information, in the United States, is the Occupational Safety and Health Administration (OSHA) Log 300, in which employers are required to maintain information about injuries and illnesses that result from work. Another is workers' compensation data. The current OSHA Hazard Communication Standard (portions of which are referred to as "workers right-to-know") makes explicit the duty of the employer to inform workers of the nature and hazards of materials to which they may be exposed. For materials purchased from a third party, data on their hazards are usually derived from safety data sheets (SDSs).

Materials of Uncertain Toxicity

In some cases, the industrial hygienist must assess the potential for harm of chemicals for which no reliable human toxicological data are available. This need arises most often in research and development settings but also wherever chemical intermediates are produced. If uncertainty exists, controls should be selected using the precautionary principle and take extra measures until uncertainty is resolved. Control banding is a practice used in some industries—pharmaceuticals, in particular—to protect against exposures to agents with limited toxicology data. In control banding, agents are grouped based on their basic chemical and likely toxicologic properties, and controls are implemented based on information about similar known compounds.

EVALUATION OF HEALTH HAZARDS IN THE WORKPLACE

Evaluation of health hazards within a facility or during a work activity includes measurement of exposures, comparison of those exposures with existing standards, and recommendation of controls, if needed.

Exposure Measurements

Exposure measurements are intended to be surrogates for determinations of doses delivered to the individual. The mere existence of chemicals in the workplace or even in the workplace atmosphere does not necessarily mean that the chemicals are being delivered to a sensitive organ system in a quantity sufficient to cause harm. The effective dose depends on such things as the size of contaminant particles (eg, dust or fumes) in the air, the use of protective devices (eg, respirators and protective clothing), and the existence of other contaminants in the workplace.

There are three major routes of exposure: inhalation (typically the largest contributor), ingestion, and dermal absorption. The task of determining the dose delivered to the worker may be further complicated by the existence of multiple pathways of absorption and metabolism. Some contaminants, such as lead, are absorbed through both inhalation and ingestion, and both routes of intake must be considered in evaluation of the potential for harm. Many solvents are absorbed readily through the skin, and mere determination of airborne levels may not be sufficient to determine the complete range of potential exposures.

Sampling & Analysis of Airborne Contaminants

Inhalation of airborne contaminants is the primary route of entry for systemic intoxicants in the workplace. Thus evaluation and control of airborne contaminants is an important part of any occupational health program.

Sampling and analysis of airborne contaminants is the definitive function of the industrial hygienist. Recent developments in instrumentation have made it possible to measure very low concentrations of airborne contaminants.

Occupational exposure limits (OELs), which are discussed in more detail later in this chapter, have generally been lowered in recent years, as both our ability to discern clinical effects and our expectations of no risk of health effects have increased; however, government standards have generally not kept pace. This is also discussed later in this chapter. A good example of this phenomenon is concern about disturbed or damaged asbestos in buildings. An industrial hygienist should attempt to ensure that avoidable exposure to airborne asbestos is eliminated. There is no definitive evidence that there is a threshold dose below which the asbestos-related disease mesothelioma will not occur. In addition, substantial liability may attach to the building owner who permits unnecessary exposure to building employees or tenants. Thus measurements of asbestos concentrations down to and including ambient levels have become commonplace.

General Approaches to Air Monitoring

There are two major approaches to air monitoring for determination of airborne contaminant levels: personal and area sampling. In personal sampling the industrial hygienist places a collection device near the breathing zone of a worker (Figure 40–2). The collection device may be either active, requiring that air be drawn through it, or passive, requiring no pump or other suction source. The second approach (area sampling) employs fixed or mobile sampling stations in the work area.

A. Personal Sampling

Personal sampling is usually preferred because exposures are measured at the point nearest to the worker's breathing zone, and the sampling system moves with the worker. Thus measurements are more likely to represent actual potential exposures. Figure 40–3 shows an example of a worker with a personal sampler in place.

B. Area Sampling

Area sampling is used when personal sampling devices are not available or are too intrusive or when a larger volume of air must be captured to assess very low concentrations of contaminants. In these circumstances, or when direct-reading instruments (usually larger and often requiring line power) are to be used, area monitoring by means of fixed monitoring stations may be employed. Fixed monitoring

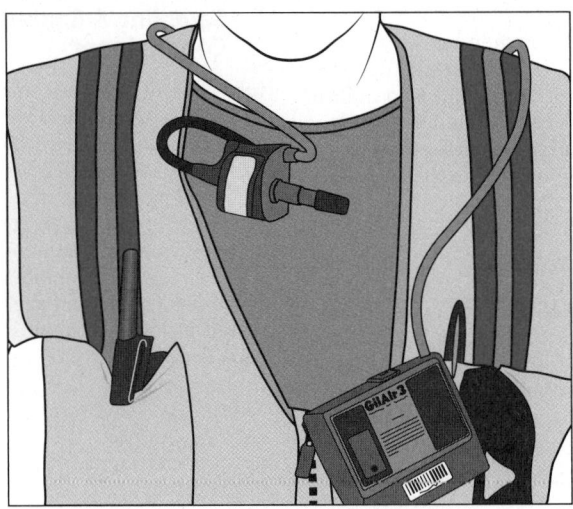

▲ **Figure 40–2.** Worker wearing an air sampling unit of pump, tubing, and cassette to capture nuisance dust for subsequent analysis to determine exposure.

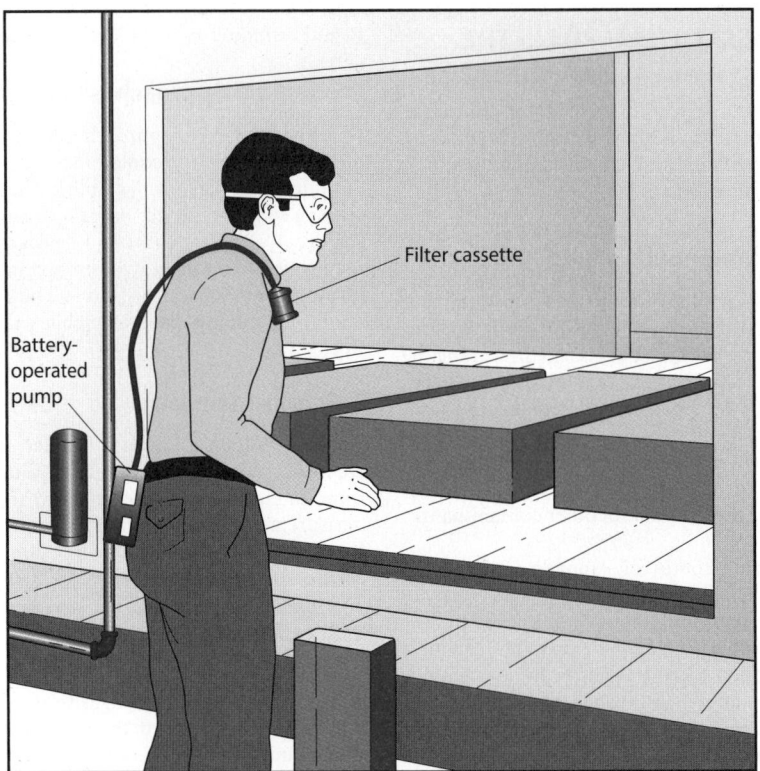

▲ **Figure 40–3.** Worker wearing personal breathing zone monitor. The monitor samples air near enough to the nose and mouth to catch the same type of air that the worker is breathing.

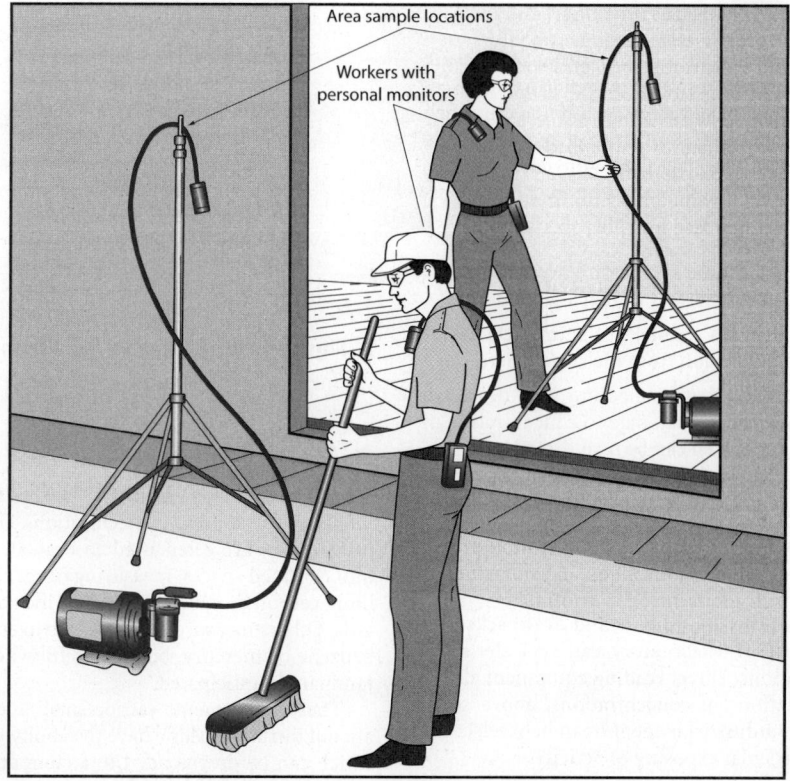

Area sample locations

Workers with personal monitors

▲ **Figure 40–4.** Worker wearing personal monitor. Industrial hygienist is gaining additional information by installing an area monitoring device.

stations also may be used to measure emissions from sources, to measure background concentrations, or to measure concentrations in several areas simultaneously in order to evaluate the effectiveness of controls. Figure 40–4 shows the application of both area sampling and personal sampling inside a work area.

DURATION & TIMING OF MONITORING

▶ Determination of Time-Weighted Average, Peak, & Short-Term Exposures

The duration and frequency of potential exposures should be identified before beginning the sampling process to determine the appropriate sampling duration. Whenever possible, time-weighted average (TWA) exposure (the exposure averaged over a specified period of time, usually 8 hours) determinations should be made for the entire period of work to be evaluated. The TWA is usually required for determination of compliance with relevant standards and also may be useful for comparison of exposures at various points within the facility.

Although chronic diseases usually are the result of long, continued exposures, high exposures over short time periods

may cause acute effects. For example, peak exposures may overwhelm such defenses as the mucociliary pathway for removal of contaminants. Peak exposures may be determined instantaneously using direct reading equipment (as discussed later in this chapter) or by taking an integrated sample for a relatively short period during the performance of a specific operation. OSHA has exposure limits for 15-minute exposures, called short-term exposure limits (STELs) and ceiling limits, which are exposure levels that shall not be exceeded at any time. It is important to measure these shorter exposures as well, since a full shift exposure may not exceed the 8-hour TWA, but a short task during that shift could exceed the STEL or ceiling.

SAMPLING FOR SPECIFIC CONTAMINANTS

The general approaches introduced earlier may be applied to determination of individual agents or groups of agents. In general, sampling and analytic methods are divided into those for gases and vapors and those for airborne particles. Sampling methods are typically specified by regulations. OSHA and the National Institute of Occupational Safety and Health (NIOSH) methods can be found in the NIOSH Pocket Guide to Chemical Hazards, available online.

1. Gas & Vapor Sampling

Some examples of gases that may be important to measure in the workplace are hydrogen sulfide (which can kill in seconds), carbon monoxide, or oxygen (too little or too much is incredibly dangerous). Vapors of interest might include benzene, hexane, methyl ethyl ketone, methylene chloride, or other solvents. Gas and vapor sampling may be accomplished by a variety of methods, including

1. Active collection, by drawing a measured volume of air through a collection system that is then analyzed.

2. Passive collection, with a dosimeter that attracts gas or vapor molecules by diffusion from the atmosphere.

3. Collection in a color-sensitive medium in a device in which color change is proportionate to concentration of the contaminant and which can be read directly.

4. Collection in an evacuated container used to carry a sample of air to a convenient site for analysis.

5. Direct evaluation by direct-reading instruments sensitive to one or several gases or vapors.

Each sampling method has benefits and drawbacks. For instance, samples sent to a laboratory can typically measure lower concentrations. Direct reading equipment allows immediate determinations of concentrations, above some level of detection. An industrial hygienist can help select the best method for a particular exposure or activity.

▶ Collection Media & Analysis

The collection media is specified in each sampling method. Common media and analysis methods are listed below.

Example Analytes	Media	Analysis Method
Low-molecular-weight hydrocarbons, inorganic gases, and vapors such as benzene, toluene, and xylene	Activated charcoal sorbent tubes (Figure 40–5) or dosimeters	Gas chromatography
Oxygenated hydrocarbon species like alcohols and aldehydes	Silica gel	Gas chromatography
Higher-molecular-weight species such as cyclohexanone, endrin, formic acid, and naphthalene	Tenax or chromosorb tubes	Gas chromatography, mass spectrometry
Various, good for trace concentrations	Evacuated canisters (area sampling)	Gas chromatography, mass spectrometry, gas-phase infrared spectrometry

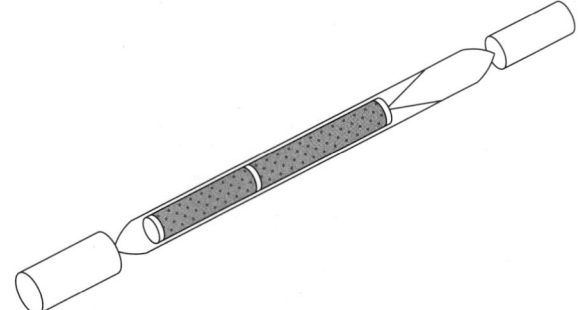

▲ **Figure 40–5.** Charcoal tube. Approximate actual size.

▶ Direct-Reading Instruments

Direct-reading instruments are used to take direct measurements of "real time" concentrations (Figure 40–6). These instruments are often used to evaluate the safety of entry into confined spaces, measuring oxygen, the lower explosive limit, carbon dioxide, hydrogen sulfide, and other acute hazards. Others measure only one or two contaminants, such as benzene or mercury, but are useful when that specific contaminant is anticipated.

These instruments can be small and carried easily, and are not intrusive. Many have the ability to log and store data, which can be downloaded to a computer and used to construct individual chemical exposure profiles over time.

Examples of direct reading instruments include

- Portable chromatographs—larger devices that are calibrated to measure a large number of compounds.

- Infrared spectrophotometers—used to measure hundreds of gases and vapors at sub-ppm levels.

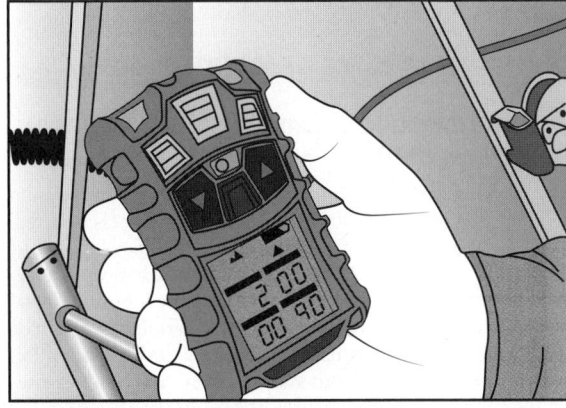

▲ **Figure 40–6.** Handheld 4-gas meter designed to measure lower explosive limit (LEL), carbon monoxide (CO), oxygen (O_2), and hydrogen sulfide (H_2S).

- Photoionization detectors—typically used to measure volatile organic compounds (VOCs) and may be adapted to measure specific hydrocarbons, such as benzene.
- Flame ionization detectors—also used to measure carbon-containing molecules in a gas stream.
- Electrochemical sensors—typically specific to a compound, such as oxygen, carbon monoxide, or hydrogen sulfide
- Colorimetric indicators

2. Particulate Material Sampling

Hazardous particulates in the workplace include asbestos, silica, lead, PM2.5, and others. Measurement of airborne particulate contamination can be done either by collection of integrated samples with subsequent laboratory analysis or by use of direct-reading instruments. Integrated sample collection and analysis is by far the more common method of evaluation both because of certain inherent difficulties associated with direct-reading measurements and because of the greater precision associated with laboratory analysis.

Each analyte has a set method or methods for analysis, which will specify the equipment needed as well as the sampling and analysis methods. As mentioned previously, in the United States, these are set by NIOSH or OSHA. Some sampling methods include

- Filter sampling—air is drawn through a filter and the filter is sent to a laboratory for analysis.
- Size-selective sampling—since smaller particles penetrate to the alveolar and lower bronchiolar (unciliated) airspaces and larger particles tend to stay in the upper respiratory system or thoracic cavity, assessing what actually penetrates to the air exchange regions of the lung is sometimes necessary. This is done using a size-selective sampling device such as a cyclone preceding the filter. Crystalline silica, PM2.5, and PM10 may be measured this way.

▶ Analysis of Particulate Material Samples

As in analysis of gases and vapors, methods are often established by regulatory or governmental bodies, such as OSHA and NIOSH, and must be properly selected to analyze the agent of interest.

A. Microscopy

For materials such as asbestos, where the numerical concentration of particles in air is the most important dose factor, the number of particles on the filter is counted by microscopic techniques.

The most common analytic procedure used for evaluation of asbestos is phase-contrast microscopy (PCM) as specified by NIOSH and OSHA. PCM is relatively simple, but not all airborne asbestos fibers are visualized or counted

(only those longer than 5 μm) and other (nonasbestos) fibers are also counted. Where more detailed information on the total airborne fiber count is needed, transmission electron microscopy (TEM) is used. This method, which is capable of visualizing all airborne asbestos fibers (and differentiating asbestos fibers from non-asbestos fibers), is more complex and costly.

B. Other Analytic Approaches

Other commonly used analytic approaches are gravimetric (weight) analysis, atomic absorption or emission spectroscopy for analysis of elements in the particles such as metals, x-ray diffraction for identification of crystalline materials, and gas chromatography where certain organic compounds exist in particulate form.

3. Surface Contamination Evaluation (Wipe Sampling)

Evaluation of surface contamination can be used to assist in assessing exposure potential and evaluating the effectiveness of control and housekeeping measures—particularly in manufacturing facilities where separation of manufacturing areas from cafeterias, offices, or dressing rooms is important. A typical program would call for the wipe sampling on a monthly or quarterly basis. Wipe sampling must be done according to a well-defined protocol if it is to have any significant utility for long-term evaluations.

Wipe sampling is useful also for identifying contaminated areas where a spill of a potentially hazardous material has occurred (Figure 40–7). As an example, wipe sampling is used routinely to evaluate the extent of contamination resulting from spills of such materials as polychlorinated biphenyls (PCBs) and pesticides for which absorption through the skin may be an important route of entry.

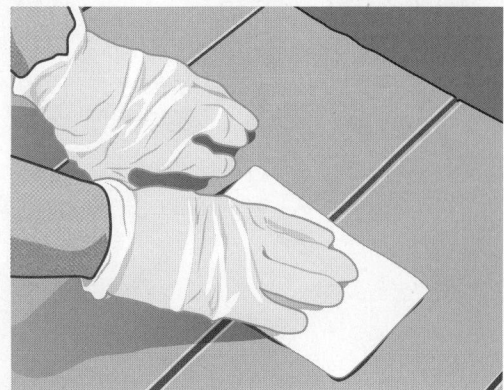

▲ **Figure 40–7.** Surface wipe sample to determine potential lead contamination.

Other methods of surface evaluation also are sometimes useful. For example, polynuclear aromatic hydrocarbons fluoresce readily when irradiated with ultraviolet light, and this characteristic can be used to make qualitative surveys of areas where contamination is feared. Another example is color-changing swab used to detect lead dust.

PHYSICAL AGENT EVALUATION

Physical agents include noise, temperature extremes (heat and cold stress), ionizing and nonionizing radiation, vibration, and lighting. Some facilities maintain their own noise measurement equipment, but since evaluation of other physical agents such as ionizing or nonionizing radiation requires specialized training and equipment, they are often addressed by consultants.

▶ Noise Exposure Evaluation

Hearing loss is the third-most common chronic physical condition among adults in the United States after hypertension and arthritis. Nearly one-quarter of the hearing problems among US workers are caused by occupational exposures. Generally, noise exceeding 85 dB is considered hazardous. There are two principal types of equipment used to assess noise levels, sound-level meters, and noise dosimeters.

A. Sound-Level Meters

Sound-level meters consist of a microphone and electronic circuitry, with a meter that gives a readout in decibels. Filtering circuits permit evaluation of noise levels weighted in accordance with their effects on hearing.

Sound-level meters also may be fitted with filtering circuits for determination of noise levels within specified bandwidths. One octave or one-third octave bandwidth circuits are often employed to isolate and identify the specific frequencies of occurrence of the noise. This identification of sources and frequencies is essential for determining appropriate controls in complex noise environments.

Figure 40–8 shows a sound-level meter in use. Note that the instrument is used to measure noise intensity in an area and thus is analogous to area sampling for chemicals.

B. Noise Dosimetry

Noise dosimeters consist of a small microphone placed close to the ear of the worker, connected to a recording circuit to record noise exposure. The devices may either give an overall integrated average exposure for the course of

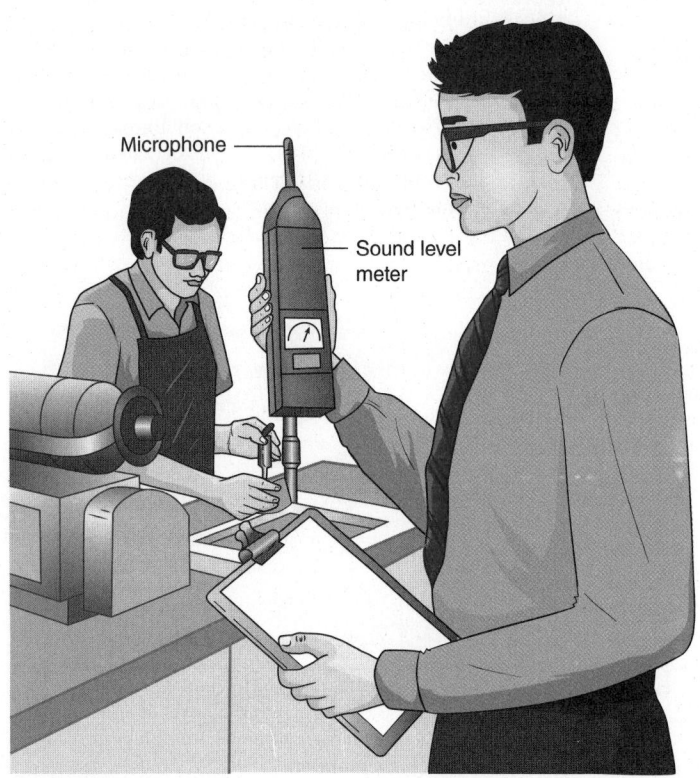

Microphone

Sound level meter

▲ **Figure 40–8.** Industrial hygienist using a sound-level meter in a work area.

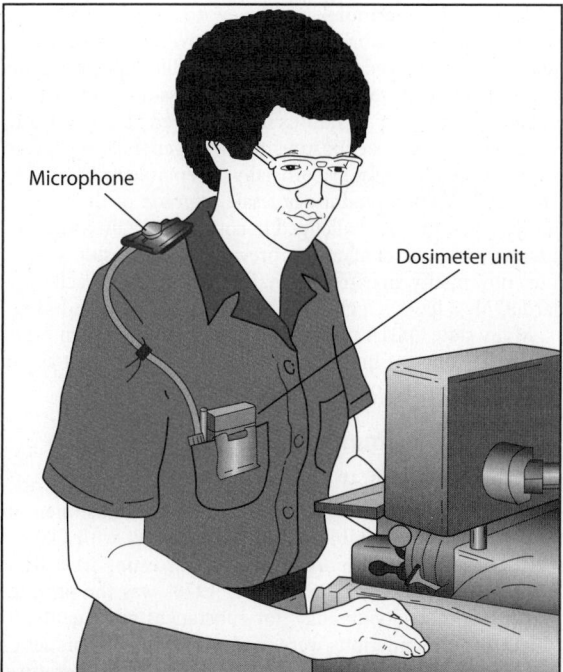

Microphone

Dosimeter unit

▲ **Figure 40–9.** Worker wearing a noise dosimeter with a microphone located close to the ear.

the measurement period or a readout showing exposure as a function of time. Dosimetry is the preferred approach because the measurement better estimate the workers' actual exposure. Figure 40–9 shows the use of a dosimeter. Note that the microphone is located close to the worker's ear.

▶ **Evaluation of Other Physical Agents**

Other physical agents ordinarily require specialized equipment for competent evaluation. However, many industrial hygienists are experienced in evaluations for such agents as electrical and magnetic fields, microwaves, heat and cold stress, ionizing radiation, ultraviolet and infrared radiation.

OBSERVATIONS OF WORK PRACTICES & PROCESS VARIABLES

Exposures often vary substantially from time to time during a day, week, month, or year. While monitoring worker exposures, the tasks they conduct should be observed and a description of the tasks and workplace should be noted. The description of the workplace must include personal protective devices so that an estimation of *true exposure* (actual intake of chemical into the worker's body) can be approximated.

Ventilation equipment and other engineering controls also must be evaluated so that sampling results are placed in a sensible context. Workers and supervisors ordinarily will be able to estimate how closely conditions during the survey period approximate "usual" conditions. General conditions in the workplace, including such things as whether windows and doors are open or closed, also must be evaluated and recorded. The ideal industrial hygiene report will be detailed enough so that another industrial hygienist entering the workplace later will be able to determine whether conditions are the same as or different from those that existed during the survey period.

COMPARISON WITH STANDARDS

▶ **Statistical Considerations**

The industrial hygienist must determine whether exposures measured are likely to cause harm to those exposed. If such harm seems likely, action must be taken to reduce exposures to tolerable levels (discussed further in the Control of Health Hazards section). In most cases, the industrial hygienist will refer to a set of standards for various individual chemical contaminants or physical agents. Exposures usually are considered to be acceptable (1) if the measured concentrations are less than the OEL and (2) if exposures are unlikely to rise above that allowable limit under reasonably foreseeable circumstances.

Certain precautions are needed in such comparisons. All industrial hygiene measurements have some level of sampling and analytic error and cannot be absolutely reflective of all possible workplace conditions. Therefore, it is prudent to construct confidence intervals about the sample means so that the range, within which the true average concentration may be expected to fall, is known. The upper 95% confidence limit should fall below the allowable exposure limit before it can be stated, with 95% certainty, that the true average concentration is below that standard, assuming that the samples taken can be presumed to be otherwise reflective of typical conditions in the workplace.

▶ **Occupational Exposure Limits**

Lists of OELs for airborne contaminants have been available for more than 70 years. The first standards were for a few widely recognized health hazards such as lead, mercury, and benzene. Currently, hundreds of chemicals and physical agents are either regulated (eg, by federal or state OSHA programs) or have recommended control limits (from NIOSH or professional associations). In the United States, the most important limits are derived from the following sources:

1. The American Conference of Governmental Industrial Hygienists (ACGIH) threshold limit values (TLVs): 2018 TLVs® and BEIs®, https://www.acgih.org/tlv-bei-guidelines/tlv-chemical-substances-introduction. (NOTE: this reference is not free and biological exposure indices (BEIs) are biological exposure indices for medical monitoring.)

2. The recommended exposure levels (RELs) of the National Institute for Occupational Safety and Health: *NIOSH Pocket Guide to Chemical Hazards (NPG)*, www.cdc.gov/niosh/npg/npg.html.

3. The permissible exposure limits (PELs) of the OSHA: *NIOSH NPG*, www.cdc.gov/niosh/npg/npg.html.

The PELs prepared by some state OSHA programs are legally enforceable by regulatory agencies. The TLVs and RELs should be considered advisory. Generally speaking, legally binding OELs are rarely updated and tend to be outdated.

These limits are typically based on TWA exposures, though they each may have some upper limit of exposure for shorter periods as well, expressed as a ceiling or as an STEL (see section on Duration & Timing of Monitoring).

▶ ACGIH Threshold Limit Values

The most important of these sets of limits, in the United States and many other countries, is the table of TLVs published annually by the Threshold Limit Values Committee of the American Conference of Governmental Industrial Hygienists (ACGIH). The TLVs are updated on a periodic basis and have been published annually since the mid-1940s. In 1970, on enactment of OSHA, the 1968 TLVs were adopted and given the status of law. In their use as OSHA regulations, they were named PELs. ACGIH also publishes a booklet with the data on which the TLVs are based.

According to the 2018 ACGIH publication of the TLVs and BEIs (biological exposure indices), the TLVs and BEIs are "health-based values… established by committees that review existing published and peer-reviewed literature… [and] represent conditions under which ACGIH believes that nearly all workers may be repeatedly exposed without adverse health effects." They are based on the "typical worker" and do not take into account economic or technical feasibility, nor do they represent "fine lines between safe and dangerous exposures."

The TLVs include values for chemical substances and physical agents (ie, heat, ionizing radiation, lasers, noise and vibration, radiofrequency and microwave radiation, ultraviolet and infrared radiation, and visible light). Another section includes biologic exposure indices for about 50 chemicals for which well-established acceptable levels of the parent chemical or its metabolites in body fluids have been documented.

▶ OSHA Permissible Exposure Limits

As mentioned, the OSHA PELs were first established in 1970, by adopting in toto the 1968 ACGIH TLVs, as well as some other voluntary standards from the American National Standards Institute. Of the approximately 500 chemicals with PELs, only about 30 have had significant updates since 1970. Industrial experience, new developments in technology, and available scientific data clearly indicate that in many instances those adopted limits are now obsolete and

inadequate. Furthermore, many new toxic materials commonly used in the workplace are not covered. These inadequacies are evidenced by the lower allowable exposure limits recommended by many technical, professional, industrial, and government organizations in the United States and elsewhere. Thus certain exposures that are generally agreed to be potentially harmful are officially acceptable to OSHA. In 1989, OSHA attempted a wholesale upgrade of their PELs, but the attempt was challenged in court by certain industrial interests, and the challengers prevailed. As a result, OSHA must now justify, in extreme detail, each change in each standard. Only a few such changes have been made since 1989.

Many state OSHA plans have established their own list of allowable exposure limits, which must be as stringent as the PELs, often relying on the TLVs.

▶ NIOSH Recommended Exposure Limits

NIOSH has established recommendations for many workplace chemical and physical agents since its establishment in 1970. NIOSH was established in the same act with OSHA, with a legal mandate to provide research to support OSHA. A major function of NIOSH in the 1970s was the production of "criteria documents" for substances and agents, in which recommendations were made for RELs. In this set of documents, NIOSH provided an evaluation of the literature, recommended control measures, and recommended upper limits for exposures.

Since the early 1980s, fewer of these documents have been produced. Many of the allowable exposure recommendations of NIOSH are lower than the recommended TLVs or PELs for the same chemicals. In part, this is a result of NIOSH's practice of recommending exposure limits for 10-hour workdays rather than the 8-hour workdays assumed by ACGIH and OSHA.

▶ Standards Outside of the United States

Below are descriptions of some of the standards and guidelines utilized outside of the United States. The TLVs are the most widely used and adopted set of guidance limits. The International Labour Organization has an index with information on standards setting in a number of countries. A website for locating and comparing international OELs for chemicals is the GESTIS Substance Database from the Institute for Occupational Safety and Health of the German Social Accident Insurance. It should be noted that many countries have established legally binding exposure limits but lack enforcement capability.

A. European Union Community

The European Agency for Safety and Health at Work has issued a set of directives regarding occupational exposure to certain chemicals. Member states are required to establish national exposure limits based on these directives, which include a handful of binding limits and a number of recommended limits.

B. Germany

The German maximum workplace concentrations (MAK values) and biological tolerance value for occupational exposure (BAT values) are developed in a similar fashion and with similar goals to the TLVs and BEIs. They are submitted annually to the German Federal Minister of Labour and Social Affairs, which may amend or adopt them as they are.

C. United Kingdom

The United Kingdom has workplace exposure limits (WELs) for about 500 substances.

D. China

China's Ministry of Health has permissible concentrations (PC-TWA and PC-STEL) and maximum allowable concentrations (MACs) for nearly 400 gases and vapors, dusts, and biological agents.

E. Mexico

The Mexican Secretariat of Labor and Social Welfare issues the maximum permissible exposure limits (LMPEs as TWAs, STELs, and ceilings).

▶ Other Sources of Standards

Several other sources of recommended exposure limits are available to the industrial hygienist. Among these are the "Workplace Environmental Exposure Limits" formerly promulgated by the American Industrial Hygiene Association for several chemicals not listed by the TLV Committee. This list is now maintained by the Occupational Alliance for Risk Science (OARS), which is managed by Toxicology Excellence for Risk Assessment (TERA).

Where no established standards are available for guidance, in-house research may be necessary to establish guidelines. Where a chemical not previously used is being widely adopted in a particular industry, a trade association study of the effects of that chemical may be an appropriate venue for such research. Because of the potential risks associated with subtle health effects not easily foreseen, such control limits should be established with great caution.

▶ Exposure Limits for Unusual or Extended Work Shifts

As noted earlier, the usual exposure limits have been established assuming regular work shifts of 8 (ACGIH and OSHA) or 10 (NIOSH) hours. Where the work shifts differ significantly from the usual day, consideration must be given to the effects of higher overall exposures on workers. An adjustment can be made by cutting the allowable exposure limit in inverse proportion to the workday or workweek as a fraction of the usual 8-hour day or 40-hour week.

A more conservative general approach is to take into account both the increased workday and the decreased period away from exposure. Detailed physiologically based pharmacokinetic models may also be established, but these require detailed knowledge of the metabolic pathways of each substance to be so regulated, including information on the biologic half-life of each of the substances.

CONTROL OF HEALTH HAZARDS

On completion of the evaluation, the industrial hygienist should be in a position to recommend any necessary controls. Recommendations should take into account not only the conditions found during the survey but also those that may be expected to prevail in the future. Planned process modifications should be taken into account, and recommendations should be adaptable to future needs. Controls should be adequate to prevent unnecessary exposure during incidents and emergencies, as well as during normal operating conditions. Consideration must be given to fail-safe operation of controls; that is, recommended controls always should operate to protect workers regardless of process fluctuations.

The controls process must always include continuous evaluation of their effectiveness. Equipment ages, personnel changes, processes evolve, and the level of attention to control by management varies with time. All these forces act to change the effectiveness of a given control. The evaluation of effectiveness is the province of the industrial hygienist, who must involve physicians, managers, engineers, and workers in the evaluation.

▶ Elimination & Substitution

All possibilities for outright elimination of the hazard or substitution for a nontoxic or less toxic agent should be explored. Substitution, of course, can be done only if a useful substitute is available—one that is suitable for existing processes or for which the processes can be relatively easily adapted.

▶ Engineering Controls

Engineering controls on toxic exposures consist mainly of enclosure (building structures around the sources of emissions), isolation (placing hazardous process components in areas with limited human contact), and ventilation.

A. Ventilation

Ventilation for the control of health hazards may be either local exhaust ventilation or general (dilution) ventilation. Local exhaust ventilation conforms to the principle that control should be implemented as near to the source as practically possible. For example, application of a local exhaust inlet on a specific tool, such as a grinder, is inherently more desirable than performing the grinding operation in a ventilated hood, which, in turn, is more desirable than installing general ventilation in the room where the grinding is performed. In a situation where a very toxic substance is being manipulated in such a way that exposure is possible, all three ventilation systems might be reasonable to use. Thus the operator would be protected by ventilation of the specific tool, nearby workers (as well as the operator) would be protected by the hood, and the remainder of the building would be protected by the general ventilation system. Figure 40–10 is a conceptual model of a typical operation showing the three zones of control required.

On the other hand, where sources are more diffuse or dispersed, or where many people must be protected from relatively low-level contaminants, such as in indoor air quality in an office building, general ventilation alone may be appropriate.

Design of ventilation systems for contamination control ordinarily should be done by engineers with specific background and expertise. Similarly, an industrial hygienist without engineering training and experience in the processes to be controlled may produce an unsatisfactory design. The ACGIH publishes a document on industrial ventilation that provides guidance on the principles of ventilation control.

B. Other Engineering Controls

In addition to ventilation, enclosure, and isolation, some specific engineering controls may be appropriate in the specific process environment. It is, for example, often necessary to design process pipelines and valves to minimize splashes and ejection of toxic chemicals. Control systems that will permit safe and orderly shutdown of the process to avoid runaway reactions also may be of substantial benefit.

▶ Administrative and Work-Practice Controls

Preventing exposures within the process environment can be accomplished through administrative controls such as establishing controlled areas, safe walkways or paths through the work environment, and areas where smoking and eating are prohibited. Another example is prohibiting personnel who do not have adequate training from entry into spaces where health or safety hazards exist. Another includes scheduling of work in such a way that dangerous operations are carried out when the fewest workers are present.

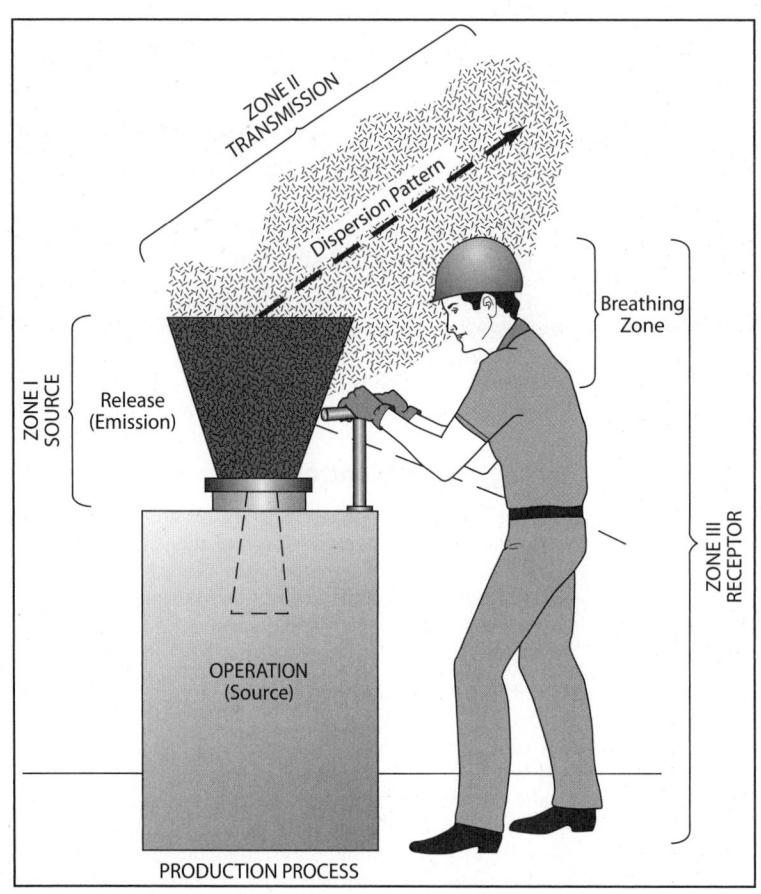

▲ **Figure 40–10.** Conceptual model of the three zones of influence to control workplace hazards.

Less desirable is the practice of worker rotation–scheduling individual workers to perform tasks for short periods, where excessive exposures would be incurred if the task were performed by a single worker for a longer period. This practice was at one time common in the nuclear power industry, where temporary employees were used to perform maintenance tasks in high-radiation environments. These "jumpers" were employed and paid by the day, although their actual work period may have been as short as 15 minutes. Such practices, where exposure to carcinogenic or genotoxic agents is spread across a larger population group, is not considered acceptable, although individual exposures are lower.

Work-practice controls include standard (sometimes referred to as "Safe") operating procedures (SOPs), which set forth protocols for the way work is done. These may include details like when and how to use engineering controls, how to handle contaminated tools, or how frequently to change respirator cartridges. Work-practice controls require that workers receive education on the hazards to be avoided and training on the desired practices and require supervision of workers to ensure compliance.

▶ Personal Protective Equipment

Personal protective equipment (frequently referred to as PPE) use is the least desirable control method. This is because of the difficulty in ensuring both that it is used and used correctly. On construction sites, PPE may consist of hard hats, high visibility vests, and safety shoes, and in laboratory environments, it may consist of protective eyewear, gloves, and protective garments such as laboratory coats. Where there is potential for inhalation of hazardous gases, vapors, or particulates, respiratory protection may be required.

Personal protective equipment must be carefully selected not to cause additional health or safety risk. A chemical protective suit, for example, can contribute to heat stress. Workers must be medically cleared to wear a respirator to ensure their lungs and cardiovascular systems can handle the additional resistance of the cartridge or filter and then must be fitted for the specific model and size of respirator they are wearing. In fact, without proper attention to selection, fitting, training, and maintenance of respirators, exposures during their use may be nearly as high as for those of unprotected workers.

Respirators often are handed out without adequate attention to any of these precautions. It is common, for example, to see workers with beards wearing tight-fitting respirators in areas where contaminants are present in the air. The devices may not protect the user sufficiently if they do not fit tightly, which is difficult if the wearer has facial hair along the respirator seal.

Similarly, gloves protect against exposure to solvents and other toxicants only if chosen with knowledge of what materials are suitable in each case. Ironically, prolonged wearing of gloves into which skin hazardous materials have either leached or leaked through holes may result in substantial exposure to the worker—sometimes higher than would occur without the gloves.

EMERGING ISSUES

Among the new workplace exposure issues is the emergence of nanotechnology, the use of extraordinarily small particles in industrial processes. It is not yet clear what the harmful effects of these small particles may be, and the prudent occupational physician and industrial hygienist will be cautious about both allowable exposures and clinical evaluation.

REFERENCES

International Labour Organization: Chemical Exposure Limits https://www.ilo.org/global/topics/safety-and-health-at-work/areasofwork/chemical-safety-and-the-environment/WCMS_151534/lang--en/index.htm.
NIOSH: *Manual of Analytical Methods*. 5th ed. https://www.cdc.gov/niosh/nmam/default.html.
NIOSH: *Pocket Guide to Chemical Hazards*. https://www.cdc.gov/niosh/npg/default.html.
NIOSH: *Worker Health Surveillance*. https://www.cdc.gov/niosh/topics/surveillance/default.html.
OSHA: *Personal Protective Equipment*. https://www.osha.gov/SLTC/personalprotectiveequipment/.

■ SELF-ASSESSMENT QUESTIONS

Select the one correct answer for each question.

Question 1: The walk-through survey
   a. is the most important technique used to recognize occupational health hazards
   b. is not necessary
   c. is needlessly delayed by preparation of a simplified process flow diagram
   d. should end at the loading dock, where materials entering the facility can be examined

Question 2: The OSHA Hazard Communication standard (workers right-to-know)
   a. requires employers to alert workers to all hazardous agents to which they may be exposed
   b. relies solely on workers reading SDSs
   c. is satisfied by walk-through surveys
   d. specifies that the employer may be subject to governmental investigation

Question 3: Sampling and analysis of airborne contaminants
  a. primarily discovers unsuspected contamination
  b. is a definitive function of the industrial hygienist
  c. is the sole responsibility of the physician
  d. is unable to measure very low concentrations of hazardous materials

Question 4: Phase-contrast microscopy (PCM)
  a. is specified by NIOSH for the analysis of all inhaled fibers
  b. is not as accurate as gravimetric methods
  c. visualizes all asbestos fibers
  d. gives an imperfect index of exposure to all asbestos fibers

Question 5: Wipe sampling
  a. would not be appropriate for a PCB spill
  b. does not detect pesticide residue
  c. is a useful measure of housekeeping effectiveness
  d. should be done on a daily basis

Question 6: Sound-level meters
  a. give a readout in decibels of hearing loss
  b. evaluate exposures to components of the noise spectrum
  c. have replaced dosimeters
  d. give primacy to the non-speech frequencies

Question 7: TLVs, PELs, and RELs
  a. represent recommended and required exposure limits
  b. fully protect workers in regulated industries
  c. ensure a risk-free workplace environment
  d. specify that the level of risk is acceptable

Disease Surveillance

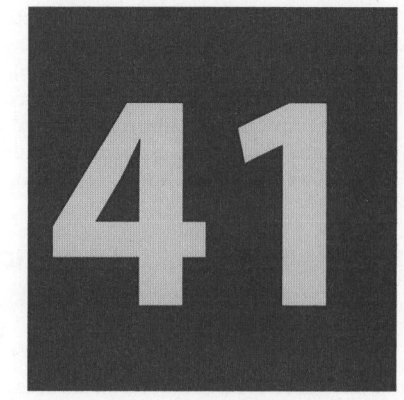

A. Scott Laney, PhD, MPH

Eileen Storey, MD, MPH

Disease surveillance in the context of occupational health focuses on acute and chronic illnesses attributable primarily to work. While fragmented and incomplete in the United States, these systems provide important information on patterns of work-related illness within occupations and/ or industries, opportunities for prevention, and measures of intervention effectiveness. There is growing interest in broader disease surveillance among working populations, focused on chronic diseases, which interfere with productivity and drive health care costs. This places less emphasis on work as a causative factor but enhances awareness of work and the workplace as an opportunity for intervention and prevention.

An important component of comprehensive occupational disease surveillance is hazard surveillance. This can include surveys of workers, qualitative assessment of workplaces, hazardous material registries, and environmental monitoring. It may also document mitigation strategies including substitution, engineering controls, and use of personal protective equipment.

Surveillance requires action in response to information acquired. This can involve providing information to workers, employers, unions, health and safety organizations, and clinicians; it can involve the development or application of interventions to reduce or eliminate exposures associated with documented outcomes; or it can involve the development of guidelines, regulations, and policy. Occupational health surveillance findings may prompt research into emerging issues related to new hazards or old hazards in new work environments.

Clinicians play critical roles in surveillance systems. The information they record regarding the health status of patients, diagnoses, functional status, and ability to work are essential to understanding the status of populations. In many states, reporting work-related illnesses and injuries is mandated, creating a system that alerts public health agencies to clusters of events and emerging hazards.

PURPOSE OF OCCUPATIONAL HEALTH SURVEILLANCE

The primary purpose of occupational health surveillance is the prevention of occupational and work-related diseases and injuries. As described in the *Technical and Ethical Guidelines for Workers' Health Surveillance*, the International Labor Office outlines five objectives of workers' health surveillance programs whose primary objectives are prevention:

1. Describe the health status of working populations and socioeconomic groups, by estimating the occurrence of occupational injuries and diseases (frequency, severity, and trends in mortality and morbidity).

2. Stimulate occupational epidemiologic studies and explain the causes of occupational injuries and diseases, by identifying the physical, behavioral, organizational, psychosocial, and occupational exposure factors that cause specific injuries and diseases or their respective risk factors.

3. Predict the occurrences of occupational injuries and diseases and their distributions in working populations, in order to determine the specific focus for prevention.

4. Prepare action-oriented research and intervention studies, to eliminate causal factors through prevention and to mitigate their consequences by curative and rehabilitative activities.

5. Assess the effectiveness of previously implemented control measures.

Public health surveillance systems seek to assess the burden and distribution of occupational diseases in the population. Unlike medical surveillance programs, which target specific groups of workers with known or possible exposures to specific risk factors, these systems survey the population at large to identify patterns and trends within industries, occupations, and workplaces. Population-based occupational health surveillance is most often conducted by federal, state, or local health authorities with statutory authority to monitor and follow-up on work-related morbidity and mortality. Medical monitoring, most commonly accomplished through medical tests and procedures, is focused on the individual worker and designed to assess an individual's risk for occupational morbidity and for early diagnosis of work-related illness.

POPULATION-BASED OCCUPATIONAL DISEASE SURVEILLANCE

▶ Mortality

In the United States, death certificates are the primary source of information available to researchers for assessing cause(s) of death. Historically, there has been a lack of uniformity related to occupation and industry coding on death certificates between states. Because of differences in how information was recorded, aggregated analyses were often not possible. Therefore, early studies of mortality by occupation using death certificates were largely individual state-based efforts. In fact, a formal survey conducted in 1979 found that only six states coded industry and occupation and that there was no uniform coding system observed. To address this lack of uniformity in coding, a large collaborative initiative was launched in the 1980s between the National Institute for Occupational Safety and Health (NIOSH), the National Center for Health Statistics (NCHS), and other federal agencies and state health departments. This effort established a number of programs aimed at the standardization and routine recording of usual industry and occupation on death certificates (Figure 41–1). An initial governmental report was produced presenting the relative risks of mortality for selected causes of death by occupation and industry from 24 states (http://www.cdc.gov/niosh/pdfs/97-114.pdf). The success of that collaboration led to the ongoing National Occupational Mortality Surveillance System (NOMS) (https://www.cdc.gov/niosh/topics/noms/default.html). NOMS data are used to evaluate trends and identify potential risks for both acute and chronic disease mortality for industrial and occupational groups. Analyses and reports from NOMS are based on data from more than 11,000,000 death records for adults, age 18 and above, that died during the years 1985–1998 in 26 US states. More recently, data have been collected, coded, and analyzed for the years 1999, 2003–2004, and 2007–2013 from about 25 contributing states, who have provided data for one or more years. The NOMS website will be updated periodically.

The National Occupational Respiratory Mortality System (NORMS) is a data storage and interactive data-retrieval system developed and maintained by NIOSH. NORMS is an extension of NOMS utilizing a compilation of national mortality data obtained annually from the NCHS multiple cause-of-death records for a number of respiratory conditions including malignant and nonmalignant workplace-associated diseases (http://webappa.cdc.gov/ords/norms.html).

Currently, data from NORMS are presented in the NIOSH Work-Related Lung Disease Surveillance Report (eWoRLD), which is an ongoing updated report available on the web. It presents mortality numbers and rates for all pneumoconiosis, hypersensitivity pneumonitis, and mesothelioma deaths by US geographic region (https://wwwn.cdc.gov/eworld).

It is important to note that there are many well-known limitations related to using death certificate data to assess temporal trends in mortality. Some of these include variability in reporting practices over time; revisions to the International Classification of Diseases (ICD) coding system; and the primary measure of effect, the proportionate mortality ratio, which does not directly derive mortality rates. However, there are many advantages in occupation-based mortality surveillance in the contemporary setting. The national vital statistics system has standardized the collection and reporting of death data. As electronic reporting has become more universally adopted, the quality and accessibility of the data have improved (http://www.cdc.gov/nchs/nvss/about_nvss.htm). These systems have been continually maintained and updated and are now largely available in up to date online reports.

▶ National Surveys

The National Health Interview Survey (NHIS), conducted by CDC's NCHS, is an ongoing cross-sectional household survey of the civilian noninstitutionalized population residing in the United States. Begun in 1957 in collaboration with the U.S. Census Bureau, NHIS is a large ongoing national survey that uses a complex multistage sampling strategy. The main objective of NHIS is to monitor the health of the US population. Interviews are conducted face-to-face in the homes of participants. With an annual sample size of over 87,000 persons and extensive demographic, health, and behavioral/emotional factors, NHIS has proven to be a valuable resource for understanding the health of the nation. Information regarding the occupation, industry, workplace, and employment conditions of currently employed sample adults as well as those who have ever worked (eg, retired persons) is available in the adult socio-demographic section and the data are publicly available for analysis. NIOSH supplemented the NHIS to ask questions specific to work in 1988, 2010, and 2015. Researchers have utilized NHIS data to assess employment-associated hearing loss, carpal tunnel syndrome, tobacco use prevalence, secondhand smoke exposure, prevalence of short sleep duration, and work-related asthma. NHIS has been linked to death certificate records to assess lung cancer mortality by occupation as well as a variety of other occupational studies. Detailed information regarding the NHIS data as well as instructions for accessing the data are available at http://www.cdc.gov/nchs/nhis.htm.

The National Health and Nutrition Examination Survey (NHANES) is a program of studies of children and adults whose primary purpose is to assess the health and nutrition status of the civilian noninstitutionalized US population. NHANES, conducted by NCHS, examines a nationally

U.S. STANDARD CERTIFICATE OF DEATH

LOCAL FILE NO.   STATE FILE NO.

NAME OF DECEDENT — For use by physician or institution

To Be Completed/Verified By: FUNERAL DIRECTOR

1. DECEDENT'S LEGAL NAME (Include AKA's if any) (First, Middle, Last)
2. SEX
3. SOCIAL SECURITY NUMBER

4a. AGE-Last Birthday (Years) | 4b. UNDER 1 YEAR (Months / Days) | 4c. UNDER 1 DAY (Hours / Minutes) | 5. DATE OF BIRTH (Mo/Day/Yr) | 6. BIRTHPLACE (City and State or Foreign Country)

7a. RESIDENCE-STATE | 7b. COUNTY | 7c. CITY OR TOWN

7d. STREET AND NUMBER | 7e. APT. NO. | 7f. ZIP CODE | 7g. INSIDE CITY LIMITS? ☐ Yes ☐ No

8. EVER IN US ARMED FORCES? ☐ Yes ☐ No
9. MARITAL STATUS AT TIME OF DEATH ☐ Married ☐ Married, but separated ☐ Widowed ☐ Divorced ☐ Never Married ☐ Unknown
10. SURVIVING SPOUSE'S NAME (If wife, give name prior to first marriage)

11. FATHER'S NAME (First, Middle, Last)
12. MOTHER'S NAME PRIOR TO FIRST MARRIAGE (First, Middle, Last)

13a. INFORMANT'S NAME | 13b. RELATIONSHIP TO DECEDENT | 13c. MAILING ADDRESS (Street and Number, City, State, Zip Code)

14. PLACE OF DEATH (Check only one: see instructions)

IF DEATH OCCURRED IN A HOSPITAL: ☐ Inpatient ☐ Emergency Room/Outpatient ☐ Dead on Arrival
IF DEATH OCCURRED SOMEWHERE OTHER THAN A HOSPITAL: ☐ Hospice facility ☐ Nursing home/Long term care facility ☐ Decedent's home ☐ Other (Specify):

15. FACILITY NAME (If not institution, give street & number) | 16. CITY OR TOWN, STATE, AND ZIP CODE | 17. COUNTY OF DEATH

18. METHOD OF DISPOSITION ☐ Burial ☐ Cremation ☐ Donation ☐ Entombment ☐ Removal from State ☐ Other (Specify)
19. PLACE OF DISPOSITION (Name of cemetery, crematory, other place)

20. LOCATION-CITY, TOWN, AND STATE | 21. NAME AND COMPLETE ADDRESS OF FUNERAL FACILITY

22. SIGNATURE OF FUNERAL SERVICE LICENSEE OR OTHER AGENT | 23. LICENSE NUMBER (Of Licensee)

To Be Completed By: MEDICAL CERTIFIER

ITEMS 24-28 MUST BE COMPLETED BY PERSON WHO PRONOUNCES OR CERTIFIES DEATH
24. DATE PRONOUNCED DEAD (Mo/Day/Yr)
25. TIME PRONOUNCED DEAD

26. SIGNATURE OF PERSON PRONOUNCING DEATH (Only when applicable) | 27. LICENSE NUMBER | 28. DATE SIGNED (Mo/Day/Yr)

29. ACTUAL OR PRESUMED DATE OF DEATH (Mo/Day/Yr) (Spell Month) | 30. ACTUAL OR PRESUMED TIME OF DEATH | 31. WAS MEDICAL EXAMINER OR CORONER CONTACTED? ☐ Yes ☐ No

CAUSE OF DEATH (See instructions and examples)

Approximate interval: Onset to death

32. PART I. Enter the chain of events—diseases, injuries, or complications—that directly caused the death. DO NOT enter terminal events such as cardiac arrest, respiratory arrest, or ventricular fibrillation without showing the etiology. DO NOT ABBREVIATE. Enter only one cause on a line. Add additional lines if necessary.

IMMEDIATE CAUSE (Final disease or condition resulting in death) → a. _____
Due to (or as a consequence of):

Sequentially list conditions, if any, leading to the cause listed on line a. Enter the UNDERLYING CAUSE (disease or injury that initiated the events resulting in death) LAST
b. _____
Due to (or as a consequence of):
c. _____
Due to (or as a consequence of):
d. _____

PART II. Enter other significant conditions contributing to death but not resulting in the underlying cause given in PART I

33. WAS AN AUTOPSY PERFORMED? ☐ Yes ☐ No
34. WERE AUTOPSY FINDINGS AVAILABLE TO COMPLETE THE CAUSE OF DEATH? ☐ Yes ☐ No

35. DID TOBACCO USE CONTRIBUTE TO DEATH? ☐ Yes ☐ Probably ☐ No ☐ Unknown

36. IF FEMALE: ☐ Not pregnant within past year ☐ Pregnant at time of death ☐ Not pregnant, but pregnant within 42 days of death ☐ Not pregnant, but pregnant 43 days to 1 year before death ☐ Unknown if pregnant within the past year

37. MANNER OF DEATH ☐ Natural ☐ Homicide ☐ Accident ☐ Pending Investigation ☐ Suicide ☐ Could not be determined

38. DATE OF INJURY (Mo/Day/Yr) (Spell Month) | 39. TIME OF INJURY | 40. PLACE OF INJURY (e.g., Decedent's home; construction site; restaurant; wooded area) | 41. INJURY AT WORK? ☐ Yes ☐ No

42. LOCATION OF INJURY: State: Street & Number: City or Town: Apartment No.: Zip Code:

43. DESCRIBE HOW INJURY OCCURRED:
44. IF TRANSPORTATION INJURY, SPECIFY: ☐ Driver/Operator ☐ Passenger ☐ Pedestrian ☐ Other (Specify)

45. CERTIFIER (Check only one):
☐ Certifying physician-To the best of my knowledge, death occurred due to the cause(s) and manner stated.
☐ Pronouncing & Certifying physician-To the best of my knowledge, death occurred at the time, date, and place, and due to the cause(s) and manner stated.
☐ Medical Examiner/Coroner-On the basis of examination, and/or investigation, in my opinion, death occurred at the time, date, and place, and due to the cause(s) and manner stated.
Signature of certifier:

46. NAME, ADDRESS, AND ZIP CODE OF PERSON COMPLETING CAUSE OF DEATH (Item 32)

47. TITLE OF CERTIFIER | 48. LICENSE NUMBER | 49. DATE CERTIFIED (Mo/Day/Yr) | 50. FOR REGISTRAR ONLY-DATE FILED (Mo/Day/Yr)

To Be Completed By: FUNERAL DIRECTOR

51. DECEDENT'S EDUCATION-Check the box that best describes the highest degree or level of school completed at the time of death.
☐ 8th grade or less
☐ 9th - 12th grade; no diploma
☐ High school graduate or GED completed
☐ Some college credit, but no degree
☐ Associate degree (e.g., AA, AS)
☐ Bachelor's degree (e.g., BA, AB, BS)
☐ Master's degree (e.g., MA, MS, MEng, MEd, MSW, MBA)
☐ Doctorate (e.g., PhD, EdD) or Professional degree (e.g., MD, DDS, DVM, LLB, JD)

52. DECEDENT OF HISPANIC ORIGIN? Check the box that best describes whether the decedent is Spanish/Hispanic/Latino. Check the "No" box if decedent is not Spanish/Hispanic/Latino.
☐ No, not Spanish/Hispanic/Latino
☐ Yes, Mexican, Mexican American, Chicano
☐ Yes, Puerto Rican
☐ Yes, Cuban
☐ Yes, other Spanish/Hispanic/Latino (Specify)

53. DECEDENT'S RACE (Check one or more races to indicate what the decedent considered himself or herself to be)
☐ White
☐ Black or African American
☐ American Indian or Alaska Native (Name of the enrolled or principal tribe) ____
☐ Asian Indian
☐ Chinese
☐ Filipino
☐ Japanese
☐ Korean
☐ Vietnamese
☐ Other Asian (Specify) ____
☐ Native Hawaiian
☐ Guamanian or Chamorro
☐ Samoan
☐ Other Pacific Islander (Specify) ____
☐ Other (Specify)

54. DECEDENT'S USUAL OCCUPATION (Indicate type of work done during most of working life. DO NOT USE RETIRED).

55. KIND OF BUSINESS/INDUSTRY

▲ **Figure 41–1.** National Center for Health Statistics. US standard death certificate. Available from http://www.cdc.gov/nchs/nvss/mortality_methods.htm.

representative sample of about 5000 persons each year. The NHANES interview includes demographic, socioeconomic, dietary, and health-related questions. The examination component consists of medical, dental, and physiologic measurements, as well as laboratory tests. Recent occupational studies using NHANES have described increased prevalence of hypertension among protective service workers, prevalence of airway obstruction by industry and occupation, and physical activity patterns in relation to employment, among other health outcomes and risks. From 2007 to 2012, questions related to exposures to pulmonary toxicants were included and pulmonary function testing was conducted. In addition, NIOSH created a Job Exposure Matrix for COPD risks that is available at the NCHS Research Data Center to use with NHANES and other data sets.

NHIS and NHANES are good sources for normative data for comparison purposes. It is often useful to use these sources as a benchmark in workplace investigations to evaluate elevated risk (http://www.cdc.gov/nchs/nhanes.htm).

▶ State-Based Systems

Many state health and/or labor departments conduct surveillance for occupational injuries, illnesses, and hazards. Data sources include the Behavioral Risk Factor Surveillance System (BRFSS), death certificates, cancer registries, hospital discharge data, workers' compensation systems, the Survey of Occupational Injuries and Illnesses (SOII), Census of Fatal Occupational Injuries (CFOI), the Adult Blood Lead Epidemiology and Surveillance program (ABLES), and physician reports. For over 30 years, NIOSH has provided technical and financial support to some of these states to establish or expand state-based surveillance activities in occupational safety and health. As of 2021, 26 states receive funding. All collect at least 15 of 24 Occupational Health Indicators (OHIs), and 7 conduct expanded surveillance and interventions in specific areas.

A. Occupational Health Indicators

The Council of State and Territorial Epidemiologists (CSTE) and NIOSH developed a set of indicators that states can use to evaluate the status of occupational health at a state level and to guide prevention priorities and intervention efforts. These include measures of specific health outcomes, exposures, populations at risk, and resources to address occupational health challenges in the state. Details regarding these indicators can be found in Table 41–1 and at http://www.cste.org/group/OHIndicators.

B. Expanded Surveillance Programs

Seven states conduct surveillance with specific emphasis on conditions including pesticides, fatality assessment, control, and evaluation (FACE), occupational respiratory disease, and musculoskeletal disorders. These targeted efforts

Table 41–1. Occupational health indicators.

1. Nonfatal injuries reported by employers
2. Work-related hospitalizations
3. Fatal work-related injuries
4. Amputations reported by employers
5. Amputations identified in state workers' compensation systems
6. Hospitalizations for work-related burns
7. Musculoskeletal disorders reported by employers
8. Carpal tunnel syndrome cases identified in state workers' compensation systems
9. Pneumoconiosis hospitalizations
10. Pneumoconiosis mortality
11. Acute work-related pesticide poisonings reported to poison control centers
12. Incidence of malignant mesothelioma
13. Elevated blood lead levels among adults
14. Workers employed in industries with high risk for occupational morbidity
15. Workers employed in occupations with high risk for occupational morbidity
16. Workers in occupations with high risk of occupational mortality
17. Occupational health and safety professionals
18. OSHA enforcement activities
19. Workers' compensation awards
20. Hospitalizations for low-back disorders
21. Asthma among adults caused or made worse by work
22. Work-related severe traumatic injury hospitalizations
23. Influenza vaccination coverage among health care personnel
24. Occupational health-related ED visits

Source: https://www.cste.org/page/OHIndicators.

tap some of the resources described below and combine sources to generate a deeper understanding of the problem. States conduct work in different areas and develop intervention strategies with partners in their jurisdictions. Resulting materials area available for broad use at https://www.cste.org/members/group.aspx?id=109057&hhSearchTerms=%22occupational+and+health%22.

C. BRFSS

The BRFSS is an annual, random-digit-dialed telephone survey collected by all 50 states, Washington, DC, and 3 US territories to assess health risk behaviors, preventive health practices, chronic health conditions, and health care access. Over 500,000 interviews are conducted each year. The BRFSS includes a standard set of core questions asked by all states, optional modules, and state-added questions. Some modules collect information related to work and health, and the system has provided important insight on work-related asthma, depression and mental distress by occupation, lifetime risk of workplace eye injury, work-related noise-induced hearing loss, binge drinking by occupation, and a variety of other health risk factors. Since 2013, an ongoing NIOSH project has supported the collection of industry and occupation as an optional module in 32 states.

D. Cancer Registries

In each US state, medical facilities (including hospitals, physicians' offices, radiation facilities, surgical centers, and pathology laboratories) are required to report incident cancers to a central cancer registry. Cancer registries manage information on all cancer cases and cancer deaths including the longest held occupation and industry of the patient. State-based cancer registries monitor cancer trends over time and are fundamental to understanding the distribution of cancer in certain populations. These systems allow for identification of clusters of concern, the ability to assess cancer types by occupation, and the ability to inform cancer control programs.

The CDC administers the National Program of Cancer Registries (NPCR), which supports central cancer registries in 46 states representing 97% of the US population (http://www.cdc.gov/cancer/npcr/). Combined with the National Cancer Institute's (NCI) Surveillance, Epidemiology and End Results (SEER) Program (http://www.seer.cancer.gov/) incident cancer and cancer mortality statistics are collected for the entire US population. The CDC and NCI have combined registry data to produce reports and provide public access to data on the latest cancer information covering the entire US population. The United States Cancer Statistics (USCS) website provides a variety of national and state-based cancer profiles, data query and visualization tools, fact sheets, publications, and public use datasets. (https://www.cdc.gov/cancer/npcr/uscs/index.htm).

E. Hospital Discharge Data

Hospitals typically maintain a diagnostic index or discharge summary that reflects the census of inpatients by presenting conditions for a particular period of time. In some cases, this information is aggregated for a broad geographic area to reflect the pattern of hospitalizations across institutions and often housed at state health departments. Information from such sources serves as a valuable planning tool for within-institution resource allocation or for characterizing some between-institution differences. This information also may serve as an indicator or early-warning sign for health outcomes of special concern. It does not, however, provide a broad view of morbidity for the population of interest. For many conditions, discharge data tend to represent the extremes or episodes of illness severe enough to require hospital admission. This information also may include multiple case reports of the same individual with recurrent episodes of illness rather than a unique hospital discharge for each patient. Unique personal identifiers for each case may not be available owing to confidentiality issues. These data may better reflect the health care needs of a subgroup than the incidence or prevalence of diseases of interest.

F. Workers' Compensation Data

Worker's compensation systems are specific to each state. Designed to provide health benefits and wage-replacement for lost work time, they are not designed as surveillance systems. They document acute injury and illness far more than chronic disease, which is rarely compensated. Case definitions and data elements vary across states, in addition to eligibility requirements. In 2012, NIOSH convened a workshop with other federal, state, and private organizations to consider how workers' compensation systems could contribute to efforts to understand the burden and risks for occupational injuries and illnesses (http://www.cdc.gov/NIOSH/docs/2013-147/pdfs/2013-147.pdf). Following that workshop NIOSH launched the Center for Workers' Compensation Studies (CWCS) designed to conduct collaborative research with a broad range of stakeholders including academic investigators and public and private insurance groups and organizations. A variety of publications and webinars are available as is an ongoing solicitation for collaborative projects and studies (https://www.cdc.gov/niosh/topics/workercomp/cwcs/about.html).

▶ Mandated Reporting of Diseases by Clinicians & Laboratories

In many states, reporting of all or specific subsets of occupational diseases, injuries, and exposures is mandated for clinicians and/or laboratories. State-based reporting builds on the concept of occupational sentinel health events, that is, "a disease, disability, or untimely death, which is occupationally related and whose occurrence may (1) provide the impetus for epidemiologic or industrial hygiene studies or (2) serve as a warning signal that materials substitution, engineering control, personal protection, or medical care may be required." These systems are not meant to provide true counts of events, but rather to stimulate reporting, often among "sentinel providers" who develop expertise in the recognition and management of occupational illnesses. Such reports provide opportunities for follow-back with employers to identify workplaces at risk and emerging hazards. These systems are independent of workers' compensation systems. In fact, analyses of the overlap between physician reports and workers' compensation reports in some states demonstrate little overlap and provide opportunities to estimate the frequency of the conditions being partially reported into both systems.

A. Laboratory-Based Surveillance

Several states require laboratory reporting of agents such as arsenic, cadmium, lead, mercury, other metals, and carbon monoxide. Some monitor indicators of exposure to substances such as cholinesterase levels. Building on this requirement, the Adult Blood Epidemiology and Surveillance system (ABLES) is a state-based laboratory-reporting program to monitor and intervene on adult lead exposure in 37 states. The objective of the program, and a Healthy People 2020 objective, has been to reduce the rate of adults who have blood lead levels (BLL) of 10 mcg/dL or greater by targeting interventions to reduce exposures at work. More recent research has demonstrated that decreased renal function is associated with BLLs at 5 mcg/dL and lower, as a result, in 2015 NIOSH designated 5 mcg/dL of whole blood as the reference blood level for adults. Currently the ABLES, CSTE, and National Notifiable Disease Surveillance System define a case of elevated BLL as greater than 5 mcg/dL. Emphasis on residential, municipal, and occupational lead abatement in the United States has led to reductions in elevated BLL in adults. Since 2000, ABLES has documented a 54% decrease in the national prevalence rates of BLLs of 25 mcg/dL or greater. More information is available at http://www.cdc.gov/niosh/topics/ABLES/description.html.

B. Clinician-Based Reporting

Many states require reports of occupational illness or injury from clinicians who make such diagnoses. Conditions such as the pneumoconioses (eg, asbestosis, coal workers' pneumoconiosis, silicosis), work-related asthma, musculoskeletal disorders, and pesticide toxicity are among those most commonly defined as reportable. Clinicians can find information on reporting cases at their state health department website. The Council of State and Territorial Epidemiologists (CSTE) maintains a website, which provides information on reporting requirements for all states and territories. This can be found at https://www.cste.org/page/SRCA?.

In addition, CSTE develops a list of nationally notifiable conditions. These conditions are reported from the states to the CDC to provide data at the national level. The list includes conditions classically considered occupational, such as silicosis and pesticide-related illness, as well as conditions such as hepatitis and anthrax, which are often associated with occupational exposures.

C. Intervention and Prevention

Surveillance systems must be tied to intervention activities to result in prevention of occupational illnesses. States have successfully used information generated through their surveillance systems to identify old hazards in new settings and emerging hazards. Examples include reduction of lead exposure to bridge workers, reduction of silica exposure among construction workers, recognition of cleaning and disinfection agents as important contributors to asthma in health care workers, and the risk of advanced silicosis in workers manufacturing or installing natural or manufactured stone countertops.

▶ Mandated Employer-Based Reporting Systems

Federal regulation (29 CFR Part 1904) requires the recording of all work-related fatalities and most work-related injuries and illnesses involving loss of consciousness, restricted work activity or job transfer, days away from work, or medical treatment beyond first aid. Most employers with more than 10 employees, and establishments not classified as a partially exempt industry must record work-related injuries and illnesses using Occupational Safety and Health Administration

(OSHA) Forms 300, 300A, and 301 (http://www.osha.gov/recordkeeping/RKforms.html). These reports include information regarding, where the event occurred, a description of the injury or illness, the number of days away from work, and other demographic and health care-related data. It is important to note that OSHA logs are maintained by the employer and are made available to OSHA upon request. OSHA logs are not publicly available information and mandated access is limited to OSHA, the Bureau of Labor Statistics (BLS) (in a modified form), employees, former employees, their personal representatives, and authorized employee representatives. In 2019, OSHA issued a final rule requiring that employers with more than 250 employees (>20 employees for designated industries) submit the annual summary report electronically to OSHA (form 300A).

The annual Survey of Occupational Injuries and Illnesses (SOII) conducted by the BLS is an ongoing survey of between 170,000 and 180,000 US establishments in the United States. From its inception in 1973 to 2008, SOII surveyed private sector establishments only. In 2008, the public sector was added. The survey directs respondents to report injury and illness information directly from the OSHA logs. Injuries are more commonly reported than illnesses, and chronic diseases are rarely reported. In 2017, BLS reported 3.5 million nonfatal injuries and illnesses. In the private sector, more than 95% were injuries (http://www.bls.gov/iif/oshsum.htm). The most common illnesses reported in 2017 were skin diseases or disorders, hearing loss, respiratory conditions, and poisonings. Even for injuries, there is concern that the SOII substantially undercounts work-related events, and there is a concerted effort underway to improve the system. A government accountability office investigation conducted in 2009 revealed that enhancing OSHA's records audit process could improve the accuracy of worker injury and illness data (http://www.gao.gov/products/GAO-10-10).

For the mining industry, a parallel system is in place under a separate mandate and administered by the Mine Safety and Health Administration (MSHA). 30 CFR Part 50 requires that all accidents, injuries, and illnesses occurring at a mining operation be documented on Form 7000-1 (https://www.msha.gov/sites/default/files/Support_Resources/Forms/7000-1.pdf) (Figure 41–2) and mailed to MSHA within 10 working days after an accident or occupational injury occurs or illness is diagnosed. The requirement of universal reporting of all work-related illnesses is the strength of this system. Annual reports by commodity are available from MSHA and access to the raw data is also publicly available (https://arlweb.msha.gov/drs/drshome.htm). Although reporting of occupational illnesses and injuries is required by law, substantial underreporting has been documented.

▶ Epidemiology Studies

Epidemiology studies often provide the basis for occupational health surveillance systems to be developed and implemented. In addition, surveillance systems themselves can provide data that can be used in epidemiologic analyses.

Mine Accident, Injury and Illness Report

U.S. Department of Labor
Mine Safety and Health Administration

- Section A - Identification D

Approved For Use Through   07/31/2014 OMB Number 1219-0007

MSHA ID Number   Contractor ID   Report Catagory

○ Metal/Nonmetal Mining   ○ Coal Mining

☐ Check here if report pertains to contractor

Mine Name   Company Name

- Section B - Complete for Each Reportable Accident Immediately Reported to MSHA

1. Accident Code (circle applicable code - see instructions)

○ 01 - Death   ○ 02 - Serious Injury   ○ 03 - Entrapment
○ 04 - Inundation   ○ 05 - Gas or Dust Ignition   ○ 06 - Mine Fire   ○ 07 - Explosives   ○ 08 - Roof Fall
○ 09 - Outburst   ○ 10 - Impounding Dam   ○ 11 - Hoisting   ○ 12 - Offsite injury

2. Name of Investigator   3. Date Investigation Started   4. Steps Taken to Prevent Recurrence of Accident

Month   Day   Year

- Section C - Complete for Each Reportable Accident, Injury or Illness

5. Circle the Codes Which Best Describe Where Accident/Injury/Illness Occurred (See instructions)

(a) Surface Location: ○ 02 Surface at Underground Mine   ○ 30 Mill, Preparation Plant, etc.   ○ 03 Strip/Open Pit Mine   ○ 04 Surface Auger Operation
○ 05 Culm Bank/Refuse Pile   ○ 06 Dredge Mining   ○ 12 Other Surface Mining   ○ 17 Independent Shops (with own MSHA ID)   ○ 99 Office Facilities

(b) Underground Location: ○ 01 Vertical Shaft   ○ 02 Slope/Inclined Shaft   ○ 03 Face   ○ 04 Intersection   ○ 05 Underground Shop/Office   ○ 06 Other

(c) Underground Mining Method: ○ 01 Longwall   ○ 02 Shortwall   ○ 03 Conventional Stoping   ○ 05 Continuous Mining   ○ 06 Hand   ○ 07 Caving   ○ 08 Other

6. Date of Accident   7. Time of Accident . am / . pm   8. Time Shift Started . am / . pm

Month   Day   Year

7 / 8

9. Describe Fully the Conditions Contributing to the Accident/Injury/Illness, and Quantify the Damage or Impaiment

10. Equipment Involved   Type   Manufacturer   Model Number

10 MAN

11. Name of Witness to Accident/Injury/Illness   12. Number of Reportable Injuries or Illnesses Resulting from This Occurrence

13. Name of Injured/Ill Employee   14. Sex · Male · Female   15. Date of Birth

Month   Day   Year

16. Last Four Digits of Social Security Number   17. Regular job Title   · 18. Check if this Injury/Illness resulted in death. ☐   · 19. Check if Injury/Illness resulted in permanent disability (include amputation, loss of use, & permanent total disability.) ☐

12 / 14 / 16 / 17 / 18 / 19 / 20 / 21 / 22 / 24

20. What Directly Inflicted Injury or Illness?   21. Nature of Injury or Illness

22. Part of Body Injured or Affected   23. Occupational illness (circle applicable code - see instructions)

○ 21 Occupational Skin Diseases
○ 22 Dust Diseases of the Lungs   ○ 23 Respiratory Conditions (toxic agents)   ○ 24 Poisoning (toxic Materials)
○ 25 Disorders (physical agents)   ○ 26 Disorders (repeated trauma)   ○ 29 Other

24. Employee's Work Activity When Injury or Illness Occurred

	Experience	Years	Weeks
	25. Experience in This Job Title		
	26. Experience at This Mine		
	27. Total Mining Experience		

For Official Use Only

Degree
Accident Type
Accident Class
Scheduled Charge
Keyword

- Section D - Return to Duty Information   Answer 30 & 31 when case is closed

- 28. Permanently Transferred or Terminated (if checked, complete items 29, 30, &31) ☐

29. Date Returned to Regular Job at Full Capacity (or item 28)

Month   Day   Year

30. Number of Days Away from Work (if none enter 0)

31. Number of Days Restricted Work Activity (if none, enter 0)

Person Completing Form (name)   Title

Date This Report Prepared (month, Day, year)   Area Code and Telephone Number

MSHA Form 7000-1,   Mar. 03 (revised)

Reset Form

▲ **Figure 41–2.** MSHA form 7000-1. Mine accident, injury, and illness reporting form.

Some longitudinal studies of health behaviors, risk factors, medication and supplement use, and health outcomes have used occupational cohorts for convenience. These studies have followed physicians, nurses, teachers, and others. Other cohorts have been constructed because of perceived risk related to work, such as the Gulf Long Term Follow-up Study (GuLF Study) and the agricultural health study. This section will describe three large ongoing longitudinal health studies of occupational cohorts: the Agricultural Health Study, the California Teachers Study, and the GuLF study.

The Agricultural Health Study is a prospective cohort of 89,656 pesticide applicators and their spouses recruited from Iowa and North Carolina. The study is jointly conducted by the NCI, the National Institute of Environmental Health Sciences (NIEHS), and the Environmental Protection Agency (EPA). The study comprises principally the main prospective cohort and assesses cancer and noncancer health outcomes through ongoing data collection. One facet of the study involves linkage to established disease surveillance systems including cancer registries, transplant registries, vital statistics, and others. Cross-sectional studies have been conducted from the cohort and have included analyses of questionnaire data, biomarker studies, and geospatial studies. Nested case-control studies, exposure studies, and validation studies have also been pursued in the Agricultural Health Study. This study has assessed numerous health outcomes among agricultural workers including neurologic risks, cancer risks, injuries, and genetic associations. A comprehensive list of publications from this large cohort can be found online at https://aghealth.nih.gov/.

The California teachers study, originally funded by cigarette taxes for the support of breast cancer research, is a large prospective cohort of 133,479 female current and former teachers and administrators. The study began in 1995 and has tracked the morbidity and mortality of the inception cohort since that time. This study found significantly higher rates of breast cancer among teachers compared to other California women. The increased risk of breast cancer among teachers appears to be robust and has since been observed in Canadian school teachers. In addition to increased breast cancer risk, California school teachers also had higher rates of reproductive cancers including endometrial and ovarian as well as increased colon/rectum cancer compared to other California women. More recently, mortality data have become available from the California teacher cohort. The leading causes of death include ischemic heart disease, stroke, breast cancer, and respiratory conditions including bronchitis/asthma and pneumonia/flu. The California teachers study has been invaluable in identifying potential health risks associated with teaching in public schools. A comprehensive list of publications from this large cohort can be found online at https://www.calteachersstudy.org/.

The GuLF study is the health study for workers involved with the cleanup of the Deepwater Horizon Gulf Oil Spill. In April of 2010, an explosion occurred on the deepwater horizon oil drilling rig leading to 11 fatalities and the release of an estimated 2.2 million gallons of crude oil into the Gulf of Mexico in the months that followed. During that time, temporary workers were deployed to clean up oil from beaches, coastline, and open water. At the peak of activity, there was an estimated 48,000 workers engaged in the response. The total number of workers involved over the course of the entire effort is unknown but likely exceeds 60,000. During the response, NIOSH developed a voluntary roster of response workers to create a record of those who participated in cleanup activities and a mechanism to contact them about possible work-related symptoms of illness or injury. The total number of workers rostered by NIOSH was 55,512. (http://www.cdc.gov/niosh/topics/oilspillresponse/worker-roster.html.)

The roster information along with company records were given to NIEHS to conduct a long-term follow-up study of those involved with response to the spill and approximately 33,000 workers participated in the initial telephone survey. Follow-up interviews were conducted from 2013 to 2016 and more than 19,000 participants completed the follow-up phone survey. A subset of the participants (>3500) completed comprehensive medical examinations including physiologic measurements, assessments of lung and neurologic function, and physical and mental health screenings. Detailed study information, including publications and reports are available at https://gulfstudy.nih.gov/en/index.html.

Large epidemiologic studies, particularly prospective cohort studies, are useful surveillance tools that can provide insights into occupational injuries and illnesses. They are especially useful for identifying risks of occupation-associated diseases of long latency and identifying risk factors of importance. Disease surveillance requires the systematic ongoing collection of health information. Epidemiology studies are often one of the more robust tools for accomplishing that purpose.

CHALLENGES & OPPORTUNITIES IN OCCUPATIONAL DISEASE SURVEILLANCE

No comprehensive national surveillance system exists for workplace-associated exposures or diseases in the United States. Occupational health data come from the numerous systems and studies described in this chapter. The result of the fragmentary nature of the data is that an accurate comprehensive picture of the incidence and prevalence of occupational diseases is difficult to obtain. Each data source (eg, annual SOII, workers compensation data, death records) is designed for a different purpose and has its own unique strengths and limitations. In addition, occupational health disparities create challenges for surveillance of contingent workers, the underemployed, and vulnerable groups such as ethnic minorities and the elderly.

▶ Underreporting in Occupational Disease Surveillance

A long identified commonality between most of the occupational disease surveillance data sources is a lack of sensitivity due primarily to underreporting and to a lesser extent mis-classification. Figure 41–3 demonstrates the key factors that must occur in physician reporting systems for a case to be included in a state-based occupational disease surveillance system. Accurate reporting relies not only on access to care but also to worker and physician perceptions related to illness and cause. In some circumstances the exposure-response relationship coupled with acute onset and increased sever-ity make the likelihood of reporting high. For example, a large chlorine spill in a confined space leading to acute and severe asthma attack will more likely be captured in a phy-sician-based reporting system than mild to moderate build-ing-related asthma due to a damp indoor environment (as highlighted in Figure 41–3), though the overall prevalence of building-related asthma is much greater than asthma associ-ated with an industrial spill. This highlights that the effects of underreporting occur for every illness but are also differen-tially reported by disease and exposure event type.

Because of the well-known and long-standing deficiencies in occupational disease surveillance, highlighted in National Academy of Science reviews, congressional oversight hear-ings, and Government Accountability Office reports, much attention has been given to improving the current surveil-lance systems and to building a comprehensive nationwide system for surveillance of occupational illnesses and injuries. The Council of State and Territorial Epidemiologists (CSTE) sponsored an occupational health surveillance work group meeting in 2009 and laid out nine specific recommendations for filling the data gaps and disseminating information to the public:

- Include an annual nationwide survey of the labor force to identify occupational injuries and illnesses among inter-viewed workers as an essential component of a compre-hensive national surveillance system.

- Expand state-based surveillance using multiple data sources and use data from selected states and on selected conditions to provide periodic estimates of the under-count in the annual employer based survey.

- Work with those establishing standards for electronic health records and advocate with policy makers to ensure that information about a patient's work and indicators of work-relatedness of health conditions are collected as standardized variables in all electronic health records.

- Routinely collect information about industry and occu-pation in all National Center for Health Statistics and National Institute of Health morbidity surveys and the BRFSS.

- Use workers' compensation data to supplement other sur-veillance systems.

- Expand the use and utility of existing national health data bases.

- Market surveillance findings in creative formats and venues.

- Provide direct and timely access to available surveillance data in user friendly formats.

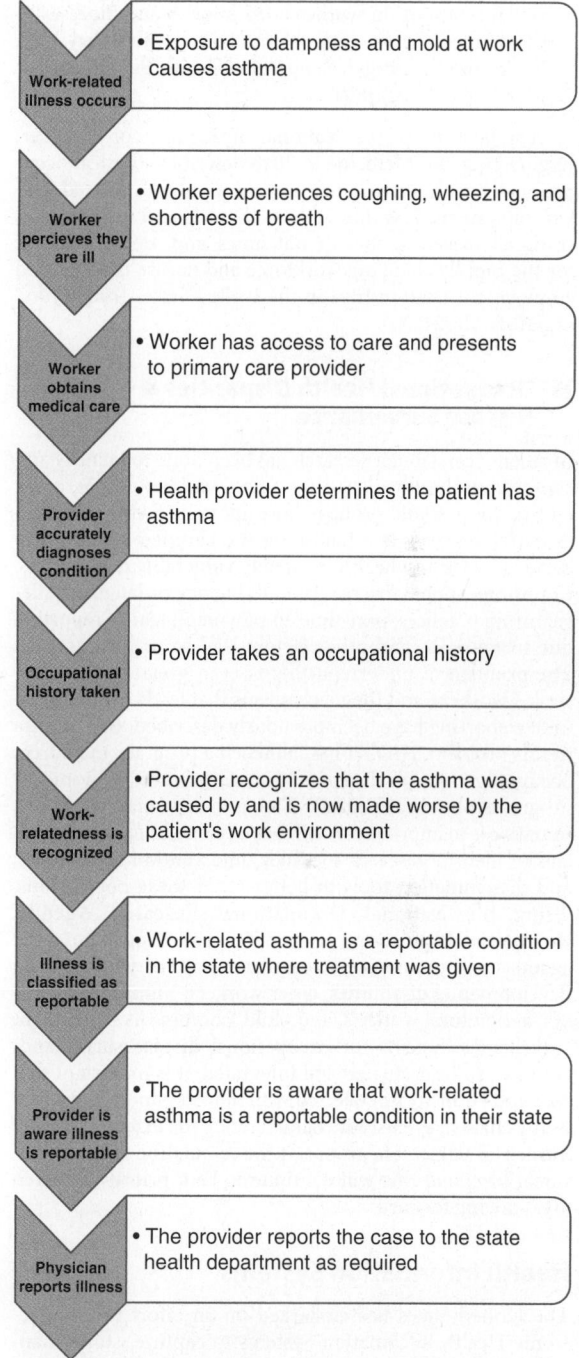

▲ **Figure 41–3.** Factors that must occur in physician-reporting systems for a case to be included in a state-based occupational disease surveillance system. Asthma exacerbation example.

- Produce and disseminate a comprehensive annual surveillance report on work-related injuries and illnesses in the United States. (http://c.ymcdn.com/sites/www.cste.org/resource/resmgr/OccupationalHealth/Surveillance-MeetingSummary.pdf).

A report from the National Academies of Sciences, Engineering and Medicine in 2018 described an ideal occupational health surveillance system as a coordinated system of systems. It would address hazards and exposures as comprehensively as health outcomes and would account for the rapidly changing workforce and nature of work and employment relationships in the United States (https://doi.org/10.17226/24835).

▶ Occupational Health Disparities & Disease Surveillance

In recent years, much research has been done to identify and characterize health disparities across various demographic and socioeconomic groups. An important factor in health disparity research is establishing the complex relationship between work and health in already vulnerable populations. Communication barriers related to literacy or language, illegal hiring practices, part-time employment, fear of reporting due to reprisals, and other factors lead to underreporting. The problem of underreporting is even greater for underserved workers, and the mechanisms that lead to differential underreporting have been previously described. In response to this problem, NIOSH has launched a program to address occupational health disparities (https://www.cdc.gov/niosh/programs/ohe/default.html). The primary mission of this initiative is to improve surveillance of vulnerable populations and to identify research methods, intervention approaches, and dissemination tools to better reach these populations. Using the National Occupational Research Agenda, the Special Populations at Risk Team developed research agendas and promoted increased funding for workers with developmental disabilities, older workers, immigrant workers, agricultural workers, and child laborers. As the current surveillance systems for occupational disease surveillance continue to be evaluated and integrated, it is important that race and ethnicity be collected with industry and occupation. Many challenges exist for characterizing the extent of disease burden in vulnerable groups at the population and occupational level and this will continue to be a priority research area moving forward.

Health Information Systems

The United States has embarked on an effort to use electronic Health Information Systems to capture, store, manage, and transmit health information developed in the clinical arena. NIOSH is developing an Occupational Data for Health Information Model to standardize content and structure of information related to the work of patients and/or household members. Incorporated into Health Level Seven International Interoperability Standards, the ODH will support clinical care, population health, and public health reporting. An example of emerging opportunities for surveillance is Electronic Case Reporting (eCR). This is the first initiative sponsored by a collaborative among public health, health care, and information technology partners called Digital Bridge. Demonstration projects are underway in several states. (https://digitalbridge.us/infoex/). The Council of State and Territorial Epidemiologists (CSTE) sponsors the Reportable Condition Knowledge Management System (RCKMS), a portal which allows public health jurisdictions to select conditions to be identified and reported from electronic health records (https://www.cste.org/members/group.aspx?code=RCKMS). In 2018, CSTE published RCKMS content for the nationally notifiable diseases which include Pesticide Related Illness and Silicosis.

CONCLUSION

Because a majority of working-age adults spend a considerable portion of their waking hours at work, the impact of work-related illness on the individual, the employer, and the overall economy is substantial. It is important to identify and ameliorate work attributable or exacerbated illnesses and injuries. To this end, occupational exposure and disease surveillance systems have and continue to be useful in monitoring worker health. These systems continue to evolve and are responsible for informing enforcement standards and employer-based health protection and promotion efforts. Because technological advances and work processes are constantly changing, occupational exposure and disease surveillance will remain an important facet of public health.

REFERENCES

Binazzi A, Levi M, Bonafede M, et al: Evaluation of the impact of heat stress on the occurrence of occupational injuries: meta-analysis of observational studies. Am J Ind Med 2019;62(3):233-243 [PMID: 30675732].

Largo TW, Rosenman KD: Surveillance of work-related amputations in Michigan using multiple data sources: results for 2006-2012. Occup Environ Med 2015;72(3):171-176 [PMID: 25391831].

Luckhaupt SE, Alterman T, Li J, Calvert GM: Job characteristics associated with self-rated fair or poor health among U.S. workers. Am J Prev Med 2017;53(2):216-224 [PMID: 28495222].

Luo H: Socioeconomic status and lifetime risk for workplace eye injury reported by a US population aged 50 years and over. Ophthalmic Epidemiol 2012;19:103 [PMID: 22364578].

Ma CC, Gu JK, Charles LE, Andrew ME, Dong RG, Burchfiel CM: Work-related upper extremity musculoskeletal disorders in the United States: 2006, 2009, and 2014 National Health Interview Survey. Work 2018;60(4):623-634 [PMID: 30124463].

Mazurek JM, Syamlal G: Prevalence of asthma, asthma attacks, and emergency department visits for asthma among working adults—National Health Interview Survey, 2011–2016. MMWR Morb Mortal Wkly Rep 2018;67(13):377-386. [PMID: 29621204].

National Academies of Sciences, Engineering, and Medicine: *A Smarter National Surveillance System for Occupational Safety and Health in the 21st Century*. Washington, DC: The National Academies Press. DOI: https://doi.org/10.17226/24835.

Rugulies R, Ando E, Ayuso-Mateos JL, et al: WHO/ILO work-related burden of disease and injury: protocol for systematic reviews of exposure to long working hours and of the effect of exposure to long working hours on depression. Environ Int 2019;125:515-528 [PMID: 30737040].

Syamlal G, Jamal A, Mazurek JM: Combustible tobacco and smokeless tobacco use among working adults—United States, 2012 to 2014. J Occup Environ Med 2016;58(12):1185-1189 [PMID: 27930476].

■ SELF-ASSESSMENT QUESTIONS

Select the one correct answer for each question.

Question 1: Public health surveillance systems
   a. seek to assess the burden and distribution of occupational diseases in the population
   b. target specific groups of workers with known or possible exposures to specific risk factors
   c. survey discrete groups of workers to identify patterns and trends within industries, occupations, and workplaces
   d. are funded by federal, state, or local health authorities without statutory authority to monitor and follow up on work-related morbidity and mortality

Question 2: Death certificates
   a. are the only source of information available to researchers for assessing cause(s) of death
   b. provide uniformity related to occupation and industry coding on death certificates between states
   c. make aggregated analyses possible between states
   d. are undergoing standardization and routine recording of industry and occupation

Question 3: The National Health and Nutrition Examination Survey
   a. examines a nationally representative sample of about 1000 persons each year
   b. is a program of studies of children and adults whose primary purpose is to assess the health and nutrition status of US residents
   c. has no physical examination component
   d. has found no increased prevalence of airway obstruction by industry

Question 4: Cancer registries
   a. accumulate data on a voluntary basis by working with hospitals
   b. manage information on select cancer cases
   c. exclude information on occupation and industry of the patient
   d. exist in 45 states representing 96% of the US population

Question 5: The annual Survey of Occupational Injuries and Illnesses
   a. is conducted by the Bureau of Labor Statistics at NIOSH
   b. surveys private sector establishments only
   c. directs workers to report injury and illness information directly to OSHA
   d. substantially undercounts work-related events

Question 6. Occupational disease surveillance
   a. excludes hazard surveillance
   b. is limited to environmental monitoring
   c. utilizes hazardous material registries
   d. replaces engineering controls.

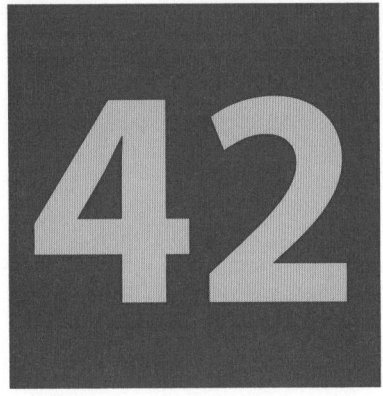

Surveillance & Screening in Occupational Health

Laura S. Welch, MD

GENERAL PRINCIPLES

Millions of workers are exposed to hazards in US workplaces, and their health can be protected with aggressive surveillance programs. Table 42–1 lists the number of workers in the United States exposed to hazards for which there is an Occupational Safety and Health Administration (OSHA) standard; many others are exposed to hazards for which no standard yet exists.

The World Health Organization defines public health surveillance as "the continuous, systematic collection, analysis and interpretation of health-related data needed for the planning, implementation, and evaluation of public health practice. Such surveillance can:

- serve as an early warning system for impending public health emergencies;
- document the impact of an intervention, or track progress towards specified goals; and
- monitor and clarify the epidemiology of health problems, to allow priorities to be set and to inform public health policy and strategies."

In occupational health specifically, surveillance is the systematic collection and interpretation of both health and exposure data. The goals of occupational safety and health surveillance across all populations include identifying populations at elevated risk of disease or injury as well as estimating the magnitude of those risks; identifying high-risk populations for purposes of resource allocation for prevention; and evaluating the impact of prevention programs. Where risks are not fully characterized, surveillance can also generate hypotheses for further study of the etiology of injuries and illnesses.

Surveillance is either population- or case-based. Case identification is a key component of medical surveillance, which should then be followed by efforts to identify other cases and other individuals at risk, and subsequently to identify the occupational factors that are responsible. Cases can

be identified through medical screening, employer reporting of cases such as is required by OSHA in some circumstances, workers' compensation data, or reporting from medical providers.

Hazard surveillance is an important part of the prevention of occupational injury and illness. It consists of the regular characterization of chemical biological and physical hazards in the workplace, such as with direct measurement of airborne contaminants or a systematic ergonomic walkthrough; it may also include assessment of work organization. In the field of occupational health, a medical surveillance program should be designed to support and integrate with hazard surveillance and exposure control programs.

Medical screening can be a component of medical surveillance, but only if the results of a screening of one individual are combined with screening results from others into a systematic analysis of trends across a working population. Medical surveillance as used in OSHA standards more accurately equates to screening.

MEDICAL SCREENING

Medical screening is the administration of an assessment to detect organ system dysfunction prior to the onset of disease or to detect disease at an early stage where an intervention can be effective. In the context of screening prevention is defined as primary, secondary, or tertiary. Primary prevention would be reduction of the exposure in the absence of medical screening, while secondary prevention includes early detection of disease, and tertiary prevention focuses on prevention of disability. When designed properly all screening tests should be evaluated for sensitivity, specificity, predictive value, and reliability or reproducibility.

Sensitivity is determined by the number of individuals with positive tests who have a disease divided by the number of individuals with the disease. A test with high sensitivity will not miss many individuals who have the disease; high sensitivity means there will be few false-negative results. Specificity is the number of individuals who have a negative test and

Table 42–1. OSHA health standards. Estimates of workers exposed to chemical or physical hazards.

1910.xxxx	Substance/Hazard	# Workers	Reference(s) and (Year)
95	Noise	30,000,000	OSHA (2009), NIOSH (2009)
120	HazWaste/HazMat	1,758,000	OSHA (1989)
134	Respirator	4,953,568	OSHA (2009), OSHA (1998)
1001	Asbestos	6,389,586	OSHA (1994)
1003	13 carcinogens		
1017	Vinyl chloride		
1018	Arsenic, inorganic	660,000	OSHA (1998)
1025	Lead	2,400,000	ATSDR 2005 (1978), OSHA (1993)
1026	Chromium, hexavalent	558,000	OSHA (2006)
1027	Cadmium	524,816	OSHA (1992)
1028	Benzene		
1029	Coke-oven emissions	6135	OSHA (1998)
1030	Blood-borne pathogens	5,576,026	OSHA (1991)
1043	Cotton dust		
1044	1,2-Dibromo-3-chloropropane		
1045	Acrylonitrile		
1047	Ethylene oxide		
1048	Formaldehyde	2,156,801	OSHA (1992)
1050	Methylenedianiline	3836	OSHA (1992)
1051	1,3-Butadiene	9703	OSHA (1996)
1052	Methylene chloride	237,496	OSHA (1997)
1450	Laboratory chemicals		
1053, (also 1926.1153)	Silica dust	2,300,000	OSHA (2017)

do not have the disease divided by the number of individuals who do not have the disease. A test with high specificity will infrequently identify patients as having a disease when they do not, that is, few false-positive tests. Sensitivity and specificity are interdependent; an increase in sensitivity is accompanied by a decrease in specificity and vice versa.

In addition to sensitivity and specificity one must consider the predictive value of the diagnostic test. Predicted value integrates the prevalence of the disease in the population with sensitivity and specificity. The positive predictive value (PPV) of the test represents the likelihood that a patient with the positive test has the disease, and conversely the negative predictive value (NPV) is the likelihood that an individual who has a negative test is free of the disease. For any given values of sensitivity and specificity, a positive test is more likely to represent a true positive if the population has a high prevalence of disease. In an occupational setting, screening is often conducted for conditions that are likely to be rare in the working population, so it is very important to understand the predictive value of a positive test. (Calculators are widely available to determine the PPV and NPV.)

In a population where the pretest probability of disease is 1%, using a test that has a sensitivity of 90% and specificity of 50%, the likelihood of disease being present with a PPV is 1.8% while the likelihood of the disease being absent with NPV is 99.8%. If the sensitivity and specificity were both

90%, these numbers would change to a PPV of 8.3% and a NPV of 99.9%. When we raise the pretest probability of disease to 10% and use a test with a 90% sensitivity and specificity, the PPV is increased to 50% and the NPV is 98.8%. One can see from these examples how much influence the population presence of disease has on the PPV of a screening test; even a test with a very high sensitivity and specificity is likely to produce mostly false positives when the prevalence of disease is low. Medical surveillance programs still need to use these tests; however, the occupational physician must understand the applications and limitations so as to be able to inform the employer about their interpretation.

When designing a screening program, one should also consider the reliability of the test itself. Will testing same person multiple times reveal the same result, and if not, what is the variation test to test?

The primary focus of medical screening in an occupational setting is the health of an individual worker, to identify toxic health effects on an earlier stage than they would have been identified without such screening. Table 42–2 identifies the process that should be used in designing a medical screening program.

As noted previously, the medical exams required under OSHA standards fit into this definition of medical screening. If the employer collects test results across a working population, these OSHA mandated tests can be used as medical surveillance as well. Table 42–3 lists the hazards for which OSHA requires medical testing and a summary of the required tests. Each standard identifies the rationale for selection of a screening test and, in some cases, mandate-specific action criteria such as medical removal. As will be described next, OSHA standards also proscribed the process of recording results to the worker to the employer. A medical provider designing a medical surveillance program to comply with OSHA standards should also follow the process outlined in Table 42–2, which may go beyond what is required by OSHA.

▶ Biological Monitoring

Screening and surveillance can include biological monitoring, which can be used to supplement the results of hazard surveillance as well as used to assess the health of an individual worker. Biomarkers are measurable indicators in a biological system or organism, such as the presence of a chemical or its metabolite within biological specimens, measured alterations in structure or function, or identifiable genetic variations. Biomarkers of exposure provide a measure of body burden of a chemical or its metabolite, while genetic biomarkers may help estimate the impact that factors of the individual can have on exposure, uptake metabolism, and/or repair. Testing such as pulmonary function measurements that assess organ system function but do not measure a specific agent, metabolite, or genetic change are generally not biomarkers.

Since biomarkers measure the actual body burden of chemical agents, they can capture the impact of all exposure routes, including through the skin. They can be used to reconstruct exposures after acute events or unexpected exposures and are very useful in evaluating the effectiveness of exposure control measures.

Selection of an appropriate biomarker for an exposure requires knowledge of the distribution, metabolism, and excretion of the agent. For example, lead remains in the blood with a half-life of about 1 month while many organic solvents have a half-life of less than 1 hour. Before using biomonitoring, one must assess whether biomonitoring could add information that is actionable and interpretable. Only three agents have biological monitoring specified in an OSHA standard. The American Conference of Governmental Industrial Hygienists (ACGIH) reviews the basis for biological monitoring and has established a specific biological exposure index (BEI) for many more agents; the BEI is the result found if individual is exposed at the threshold limit value (TLV) and is not intended to represent dermal exposures. The BEIs are invaluable in designing biomonitoring beyond the OSHA required tests (Table 42–4).

Biological monitoring may create ethical challenges for the medical provider. From the employee's point of view, collecting blood or urine outside of a strictly medical setting often provokes anxiety. Workers may worry that their tissues will be tested for illicit drugs rather than to confirm specified workplace exposures or have concerns that their health insurance may be affected after being found highly exposed. OSHA regulations provide basic protections, but even the best regulatory standard does not fully protect employees from negative outcomes when they participate in biological monitoring. To ensure the program meets highest ethical standards whenever possible, environmental monitoring should be the primary way to assess exposures, with biological monitoring as the secondary indicator of over exposure. Choose biological monitoring tests that are accurate, reliable, and have high predictive values. Employers should inform workers in writing about the risks and benefits of any planned biological monitoring, and workers should have the right to choose whether to participate (as is the case with all OSHA-mandated medical examinations).

▶ Hazard Surveillance

While direct measurement of individual exposures is considered optimal, such information rarely is available for epidemiology studies or occupational surveillance. Available sampling and workplace characterization data may be combined into a job-exposure matrix (JEM), which defines the presence or absence of specific exposures, and possibly levels of exposure, within a given industry, department, or for a specific job title.

EXAMPLES OF SURVEILLANCE PROGRAMS

Evaluation of the occupational health of a population is conducted by primarily by employers or by government agencies.

Table 42–2. OSHA 29CFR 1910 subpart Z and 29CFR 1926—toxic and hazardous substances.

1910.xxxx	Substance	Specific Questionnaire[1]	Physical Examination-Organ System Content	Body Fluid Tests	XR/Physio Tests	Medical Removal Plan?
1001	Asbestos	Yes	CV, lung, GI	FOBT	CXR, PFT	No
1002	Coal tar pitch	No	None	None	None	No
1003–1016	13 carcinogens	No	None	None	None	No
1017	Vinyl chloride	No	Liver, spleen, kidneys, skin, connective tissue, pulmonary	None	None	Yes
1018	Arsenic, inorganic	No	Nose, skin	None	CXR	No
1025	Lead	No	Dental, hematologic, GI, renal, CV, pulmonary, neuro	Hemoglobin, hematocrit, ZPP, BUN, serum creatinine, urinalysis, blood lead levels, peripheral smear morphology, red cell indices; if requested by employee, pregnancy testing and fertility testing (female/male)	None	Yes
1026	Chromium, hexavalent	No	Skin, respiratory	None	None	
1027	Cadmium	No	Respiratory, cardiovascular (BP), urinary, and for males over 40—prostate palpation	CdU, CdB, β_2M; CBC, UA, BUN/Cr	CXR, PFT	Yes
1028	Benzene	Preplacement exam requires special history	None	CBC, differential	PFT initially and every 3 years if respiratory protection used 30 days/y	Yes
1029	Coke oven emissions	No	Skin	Weight, urine cytology, urinalysis for sugar, albumin, hematuria	CXR, PFT	
1030	Bloodborne pathogens	No	None	HBV, HIV	None	
1043	Cotton dust	Yes	None	None	PFT	Yes
1044	1,2-Dibromo-3-chloropropane	Yes	Reproductive, genitourinary	Sperm count, FSH, LH, total estrogen (females)	None	No
1045	Acrylonitrile	No	Respiratory, GI,[a] thyroid, skin, neurologic (peripheral and central)	FOBT	CXR	
1047	Ethylene oxide	No	Pulmonary, skin, neurologic, hematologic, reproductive, eyes	CBC, white cell count with differential, hematocrit, hemoglobin, red cell count; if requested by employee, pregnancy testing and fertility testing (female/male)	None	

(continued)

Table 42–2. OSHA 29CFR 1910 subpart Z and 29CFR 1926—toxic and hazardous substances. (Continued)

1910.xxxx	Substance	Specific Questionnaire[1]	Physical Examination-Organ System Content	Body Fluid Tests	XR/Physio Tests	Medical Removal Plan?
1048	Formaldehyde	No	Skin, respiratory	None	PFT if required to use respirator	Yes
1050	Methylenedi-amine	No	Skin, liver	LFT, UA	None	Yes
1051	1,3-Butadiene	Yes	Liver, spleen, CV, skin	CBC	None	
1052	Methylene chloride	No	Lungs, cardiovascular (including BP and pulse), liver, nervous, skin	None	None	Yes
1053 (also 1926.1153	Silica	No	A physical exam, with special emphasis on the respiratory system	Baseline screening for TB	PFT, CXR	No

[a]Some standards specify emphasis on specific organ systems without mandating a specific form.

In the United States there are a number of national surveillance systems focused on occupational injury or disease, which are used by government agencies and independent researchers to look at the nature and extent of occupational injury and specific occupational diseases. These include the Survey of Occupational Injury and Illness (SOII) maintained by the Bureau of Labor Statistics, the National Electronic Injury Surveillance System maintained by the Consumer Product Safety Commission, and the National Biomonitoring System managed by the Centers for Disease Control and Prevention (with data on general environmental exposures). The National Institute for Occupational Safety and Health (NIOSH) maintains over 20 surveillance systems, including fatalities in specific industries, the health of coal miners, surveillance of work-related lung diseases, and the Adult Blood Lead Epidemiology and Surveillance system for lead

Table 42–3. Physician duties in conducting medical exam as part of surveillance program.

Understand the employee's job duties, work practices and conditions, and exposure controls. This may include at least one site visit to the facility and/or workplace, and/or knowledge of the particular industry, job, or occupation.
Understand the **hazard(s)** including the relevant **toxicology.**
Identify target organ toxicity for each hazard
Selection of test for each screenable health effect
Standardize the testing process
Compile and evaluate information about the individual worker by taking a detailed history, assessing specific medical conditions and symptoms, with a focus on the occupational history.
Conduct a **physical examination** focusing on the hazard and on health conditions related specifically to the patient and recording both pertinent positives and negatives.
Interpret biological monitoring (eg, blood lead and ZPP levels, or urine cadmium and β_2-microglobulin levels) and/or physiologic monitoring data (eg, pulmonary function tests, audiograms, or chest radiographs), including comparative analysis with prior tests and trends among similarly exposed groups
Review and interpret applicable **exposure monitoring (industrial hygiene) data,** and recognize its representativeness and/or level of uncertainty.
Understand applicable **laws and regulations** (eg, standards) and, if applicable, the company's internal policy and procedures regarding the hazard.
Formulate an **appropriate differential diagnosis** for symptoms (alone and in combinations, including their temporality), examination findings, and laboratory or other test findings to explain particular findings (for symptoms, examinations, and tests) as they relate to the target hazard as well as plausible nonoccupational conditions.
Synthesize and analyze this information to assess an individual worker's health status and risk, and render the physician's written opinion and recommendations (if needed).
Communicate opinions and explain findings, justification, and recommendations to the patient, employer, and any other vested parties in a disinterested yet compassionate manner that conveys credibility, confidence, and caring.
Ensure that recommendations or additional requested or required information is **followed up, reviewed, and documented.**

Table 42–4. OSHA standards that include biomarkers.

Standard	Biomarker	Trigger
Lead general industry	Blood lead and ZPP	30 days or more over action level
Lead construction	Blood lead and ZPP	Based on tasks performed
Cadmium	β_2-microglobulin, urine, and blood cadmium	30 days or more over action level
Benzene	Phenol in urine	After unplanned release

exposure. Unfortunately, the current surveillance systems for occupational health, including BLS and workers' compensation databases, do not fully capture the impact of occupational injuries and illnesses. For example, the BLS SOII derives its nonfatal workplace injury and illness data from a sample of OSHA logs kept by employers. The SOII undercounts occupational injuries and illnesses for several reasons; the survey does not cover self-employed workers or federal government employees, and disease cases with a long latency from exposure to clinical presentation are less likely to be reported. In state-based surveillance systems reporting may require identification of a health condition as work related by a medical provider, and most medical providers have little to no training in occupational medicine; in addition, workers may not suggest to their doctor that an injury or illness could be work related due to a lack of awareness or fear of retaliation. Other systems depend on case reports from state health department, hospitals, or employers, and many do not collect data from the entire United States. However, even with these limitations, these systems have provided the public health community with a wealth of information to track workers' health generally.

Other national databases contain some information on occupation and health, even not specifically designed as a medical surveillance system; these include the National Longitudinal Study of Youth, the Health and Retirement Survey, and the National Health Interview Survey. The Center for Construction Research and Training produces a periodic report on the construction industry drawn from these and other national data systems. The Construction Chart Book is a model that could be replicated for other industries using the same data sets.

Surveillance programs have been established for specific exposed populations; an excellent example is the two medical surveillance programs for individuals exposed in the collapse and remediation of the World Trade Center in 2001 in New York City. The Fire Department of New York maintains surveillance of firefighters on the scene, while the Mt. Sinai School of Medicine coordinates surveillance for other workers and community members. Both programs show the strength and importance of surveillance set up to investigate specific exposures or events. Mandated medical surveillance programs have been established by lawsuit (eg, the Fernald Medical Monitoring Program) or by statute (eg, the Former Worker Medical Surveillance Programs supported by the Department of Energy for former atomic weapons workers).

In an effort that could create a nationwide occupational medicine surveillance system, NIOSH is undertaking an effort to integrate occupation into electronic medical records. This effort was recommended by the Institute of Medicine in 2011; that report laid out specific steps such as identifying a standard coding system for occupation and developing demonstration projects which included recommendations for clinical use of occupational data. When this program is fully implemented, it will provide an important opportunity for case finding and population-based surveillance, as well as potentially improving the health of workers with work-related injury and illness

ETHICS

Occupational physicians are often asked to provide medical examinations and determine fitness for duty but may not be involved in designing or implementing a true medical surveillance program. In some circumstances the physician has a duty to report findings to a state agency and should understand his/her responsibilities as a medical provider as well as those of the employer when screening for occupational injury and illness.

Guidelines for ethical practice have been outlined by the American College of Occupational and Environmental Medicine (ACOEM) and by the International Commission on Occupational Health.

ICOH identifies three principles and then provides more specific guidance with 26 specific recommendations:

> The purpose of occupational health is to serve the health and social well-being of the workers individually and collectively. Occupational health practice must be performed according to the highest professional standards and ethical principles. Occupational health professionals must contribute to environmental and community health.

> The duties of occupational health professionals include protecting the life and the health of the worker, respecting human dignity and promoting the highest ethical principles in occupational health policies and programs. Integrity in professional conduct, impartiality and the protection of the confidentiality of health data and of the privacy of workers are part of these duties.

> Occupational health professionals are experts who must enjoy full professional independence in the execution of their functions. They must acquire and maintain the competence necessary for their duties and require conditions which allow them to carry out their tasks according to good practice and professional ethics.

The ACOEM organizes its guidelines around seven principles, similar to those from the ICOH: an obligation to enhance a safe and healthy workplace environment; an obligation to maintain ethical standards; an obligation to avoid discrimination; an obligation to maintain professional competence; an obligation to maintain patient confidentiality; an obligation to advise and report; and an obligation to address conflict of interest (ACOEM 2010).

Employer-Physician-Employee Conflicts

A medical surveillance program involves the employer, the employee, and the physician. The physician can be expected to be both a patient (employee) advocate and a consultant to (and paid by) the employer, roles that can create potential conflicts of interest. By law the employer must provide a safe and healthful workplace and has the responsibility to identify and reduce or eliminate hazardous exposures. Physicians who participate in medical surveillance may be relegated to the role of providing medical screening, while decisions about interventions on behalf of individuals or groups of employees are the employer's management's responsibility. The physician may observe situations in which identified problems are permitted to continue or recommendations incorrectly implemented, impacting employees' health and safety. The physician has a duty to inform the employer of such concerns, and to take reasonable measures to ensure that they are acknowledged. As a last resort, a physician whose opinions or recommendations have been rebuffed or ignored may have an ethical obligation to anonymously or even openly report the company to a regulatory enforcement agency. Physicians should thus carefully assess the risks involved with doing business with companies that may not act ethically when a health problem is identified.

At the same time, trust and credibility of the physician are the keys to employee cooperation and communication. The physician provides a service that is paid for by the employer—never by the employee/patient. If a physician loses the employees' trust—whether through an action or passive acceptance of a situation that endangers one or more employees—he/she may be rendered ineffective and potentially subvert the purpose for which his/her services are engaged.

Doctor-Patient Relationship

Employees in a medical surveillance program are sent to the physician as a requirement of employment. The physician is almost always not of their own choosing. Even though the physician examines the employee at the request of the employer, a doctor-patient relationship is established and the applicable standards of ethical care apply. When any type of direct clinical evaluation is involved in medical surveillance, the physician's ethical obligation is to advocate on behalf of the patient. This duty carries many implicit risks and necessitates disclosing any conflicts truthfully and completely. The physician must advise the employee of any medical condition, occupational or nonoccupational, which dictates further medical examination or treatment.

The doctor-patient relationship still exists when the physician reviews an employee's biological monitoring or other test result without actually knowing or examining the employee. If the physician detects an abnormality that could impact the employee's health, he/she has an obligation to directly inform the employee and advise him/her accordingly.

Physicians who provide preventive medical surveillance services on referral from an employer should remain objective and protect their balance of obligation between the employer and the employee-patient. It may therefore in the best interest of all for such physicians not to become a treating physician for employees. Moreover, while the medical surveillance examination affords a unique opportunity for physicians to provide counseling and information about nonoccupational conditions and lifestyle—particularly for workers who otherwise are healthy and/or do not have a personal physician or perceived need for medical care—the examination should primarily focus on workplace health issues.

Confidentiality

Physicians who perform medical surveillance services must follow standards of care for medical practice as well as the requirements of the applicable regulations. For OSHA regulations, this includes 29CFR1910.20 Access to Employee Exposure and Medical Records, as well as requirements in specific health standards. For all clinical evaluations, workers must be provided the results and interpretations of exposure and health outcome monitoring. Clinical management and follow-up are required in many circumstances, such as when blood pressure or liver function tests are abnormally increased. Reports to the employer should reflect simply that each worker has been evaluated according to the requirements of the standard and state if any modifications of the work environment are needed. Physicians who include examination results along with fitness for duty opinions are violating the employee's right to privacy and patient confidentiality. For the employer, medical information for medical surveillance should be maintained separately from employment information including drug screening results, which are not subject to the same regulations as medical surveillance exams.

The physician also has a duty to protect confidential information learned about the company and its processes and methods. Usually this information is protected in a contractual agreement between the employer and the physician or medical practice.

REFERENCES

ACOEM Code of Ethics: https://acoem.org/Guidance-and-Position-Statements/Reference-Materials-Related-OEM-Documents/ACOEM-Code-of-Ethics 2010.

ACGIH Guide to TLVs and BEIs: https://www.acgih.org/tlv-bei-guidelines/tlv-bei-introduction 2017.

Fagan KM, Hodgson MJ: Under-recording of work-related injuries and illnesses: an OSHA priority. J Safety Res 2017;60:79-83 [PMID: 28160817].

ICOH Code of Ethics: http://www.icohweb.org/site/code-of-ethics.asp 2014.

NIOSH Medical Surveillance: https://www.cdc.gov/niosh/topics/surveillance/default.html 2019.

■ SELF-ASSESSMENT QUESTIONS

Select the one correct answer for each question.

Question 1: Medical surveillance
   a. is the same as medical screening in the workplace
   b. excludes medical screening and safety surveys
   c. entails compiling and analyzing the health data from workers over a period of time
   d. is confined by law to physicians and industrial hygienists

Question 2: Medical surveillance
   a. evaluates trends of biological monitoring laboratory tests on workers to assess the effectiveness of exposure controls
   b. distinguishes between health effects from exposures and those from preexisting medical conditions or habits
   c. is not required when exposures are below permissible levels
   d. is the process of identifying, quantifying, and removing causative factors that increase the risk of occupational diseases or injuries

Question 3: Primary prevention methods
   a. are intended to minimize employee exposure to hazards and risk of injury or occupational disease
   b. must reduce risk to the point where adverse health effects attributable to that agent do not occur
   c. primarily minimize or avoid employee exposure to hazards through engineering
   d. exclude worker training and risk information

Question 4: Health-based regulations
   a. are neither exposure driven nor performance based
   b. are set by NIOSH and must be administered by both OSHA and MSHA in the United States
   c. are derived from allowable exposure levels determined by current scientific knowledge about each toxicant
   d. apply to hazardous substances such as lead, asbestos, and benzene

Question 5: The company's compliance plan
   a. requires each company or organization to test hazardous materials
   b. is optional if workers do not complain of adverse health effects
   c. must be reviewed and reevaluated at regular intervals at least annually
   d. excludes outcomes measures

Question 6: Action level (AL)
   a. is determined by OSHA for employees whose exposure to a regulated substance exceeds the PEL
   b. initiates medical surveillance
   c. triggers removal of employees with adverse effects resulting from overexposure
   d. ensures that employees will not experience any adverse effects associated with exposure to a toxicant

Question 7: OSHA and MSHA requirements for medical surveillance
   a. specify that the company determine the minimum requirements for the physician's level of training, expertise, or qualifications to conduct medical surveillance examinations
   b. require federal review of physician credentials by NIOSH
   c. require employers to be aware of the significance or complexity entailed in medical surveillance
   d. are codified as regulations such that employers may assume that all doctors are trained and knowledgeable for any problem or service that they or their facility offers

Question 8: Confidentiality of employees' health information by examining physicians
   a. is not required for information obtained during examinations provided to workers at the employers' expense
   b. is waived by OSHA for purposes of risk reduction requiring company participation
   c. prevents discussion of drug use, smoking, and alcohol consumption with the patient
   d. usually is protected in a contractual agreement between the employer and the physician or medical practice

Question 9: Most OSHA health standards
   a. require employers to analyze temporal trends and associations between exposure and health data using statistical methods to assess the efficacy of exposure control methods
   b. are updated at least every 5 years to reflect current scientific knowledge and technology
   c. are efficiently managed using standard business tools and methods such as spreadsheets, checklists, and paper files and folders
   d. require that physicians evaluate health effects and risks of employees on an individual basis, not as a group

Question 10: Temporary removal of an employee from an exposure by a physician

   a. must first be approved by the company to ensure the employee's job and pay is safeguarded

   b. is required only when the results of the employee's most recent biological monitoring or other test exceed the allowable regulatory threshold

   c. can be based on the physician's assessment of the employee's medical condition which places the employee at increased risk of adverse health effects resulting from exposure

   d. is the most effective way for the company to prevent employees from being overexposed to hazardous workplace agents

Biologic Monitoring

Rupali Das, MD, MPH

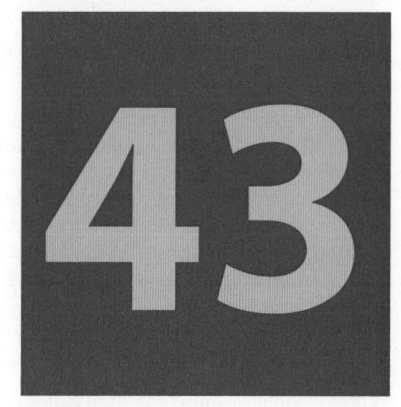

Biologic monitoring or biomonitoring is the measurement of a chemical, its metabolite, or a biochemical effect in a biologic specimen for the purpose of assessing exposure. The term biomonitoring may be used for measuring chemicals in nonhuman organisms, forensic medicine, and drug development; in this chapter it refers to human exposure monitoring. Biomonitoring is an important tool to identify the nature and amount of chemicals in the body resulting from occupational and environmental exposures. Biologic monitoring has evolved from a research tool to an essential component of exposure assessment. Although biomonitoring has been used to monitor workers for decades, it is increasingly being applied to nonoccupational settings.

While classical exposure assessment relies on the measurement of chemicals in the external environment to estimate the dose of a chemical, biomonitoring provides a more direct measure of the internal dose. Traditionally, dose estimation is accomplished with environmental monitoring, the measurement of the ambient (external) exposure using chemical samples taken from the air, water, hard surface, or other media (eg, food) in the workplace or community. Environmental monitoring provides information about exposure only from the specific external source measured. Conversely, biologic monitoring provides a measure of the quantity of a chemical absorbed from all sources and routes of exposure (eg, dermal absorption, inhalation, and/or ingestion) and does not distinguish the source of exposure or whether exposure occurred at the workplace, at home, or in other settings.

Environmental measurements do not reflect the amount of a chemical that gets into the body and may not correlate well with the biomonitored level for several reasons. The primary route of exposure may not be the environmental medium measured; for example, air measurements will not accurately indicate uptake if dermal absorption is a more significant exposure route. Moreover, individual differences in work practices, activity levels, genetics, demographic characteristics (eg, age, gender, and ethnicity), and physical factors, (eg, amount of body fat) impact the absorption, distribution, metabolism, and excretion of a chemical.

The decision to conduct biomonitoring is complex and based on multiple factors. Multidisciplinary collaboration involving toxicologists, epidemiologists, chemists, health educators, and clinicians is required for proper program implementation and interpretation of results. Basic considerations include the availability of appropriate biologic markers, the ability to properly collect relevant samples, availability of qualified laboratories, and resources to appropriately plan and conduct all phases of a program.

BIOLOGIC MARKERS

Biologic markers or biomarkers are indicators of biochemical, genetic, molecular, immunologic, or physiological signals of events in biologic systems. The ideal biomarker is sensitive, specific, biologically relevant, practical, inexpensive, and available. Seldom does a biomarker meet all these criteria; most represent a compromise. With respect to chemicals, biomarkers are defined as follows:

Biomarkers of exposure are chemicals, their metabolites, or a reaction product between a chemical and a target molecule (eg, dialkylphosphate metabolites of organophosphate pesticides or hemoglobin adducts from ethylene oxide exposure).

Biomarkers of effect are measurable biochemical, physiological, behavioral, or other alterations in an organism that are associated with potential health effects (eg, reduced acetyl cholinesterase activity as an indicator of exposure to organophosphate pesticides).

Biomarkers of susceptibility are indicators of inherited or acquired abilities to respond to the challenge of exposure to chemicals (eg, lower levels of paraoxonase-1 [PON1] are associated with increased susceptibility to organophosphate toxicity).

BIOLOGICAL MATRIX

The biological medium or matrix used for biomonitoring often determines the choice of a biomarker. Although blood and urine are most commonly analyzed, biomonitoring may be conducted in any biological matrix. The most commonly used matrices are described as follows in alphabetical order.

Adipose Tissue

Adipose tissue is rarely used today for biomonitoring due to the invasiveness of sample collection and advances in biomonitoring of other more accessible biological tissues. From 1970 to 1989, the U.S. Environmental Protection Agency's National Human Adipose Tissue Survey collected and analyzed human adipose tissue specimens for the presence of lipid-soluble chemicals.

Whole Blood & Serum

Whole blood is the most common pathway for most chemicals and their metabolites and reflects recent exposures; it is easily collected since venipuncture is considered minimally invasive. However, whole blood has limited applications for biomonitoring, for example, analyzing metals such as lead, total mercury, and cadmium. Blood can be a valuable matrix for measuring adducts of hemoglobin, albumin, or DNA. For volatile substances and others with short half-lives, there may be considerable variation in levels, depending on the timing of collection.

Serum is used to analyze lipid-soluble chemicals (persistent organic compounds) and their metabolites, such as dioxins, furans, polychlorinated biphenyls (PCBs), and organochlorine pesticides. Serum levels may be reported in two ways: per gram of total lipid, reflecting the amount of these compounds stored in body fat, and per whole weight of serum. Serum biomonitoring requires processing of whole blood, including centrifugation and analysis and correction of lipid levels. The drawbacks of using blood and serum for biomonitoring include some participants' resistance to venipuncture and the need to collect large volumes that are required for some analyses (eg, dioxins and furans).

Breast Milk

Breast milk is an ideal matrix to biomonitor levels of lipid-soluble persistent organic pollutants (POPs) in the environment; it is easy to collect and provides information on the exposures of mothers as well as infants. Since 1976, the World Health Organization has collected and evaluated information on levels of POPs in human breast milk as an important indicator of environmental contamination in the European Union. Study participants may be reluctant to breast feed due to concerns about potential adverse impacts of chemicals in breast milk. Therefore, it is critical to encourage breast-feeding and to provide education that breast-feeding reduces child mortality and has positive impacts on health that extend into adulthood. These benefits outweigh the risk of potential harm to infants through exposure to environmental pollutants by ingesting breast milk.

Exhaled Air

Measurements of chemicals in exhaled air are most appropriate for volatile organic compounds such as benzene,

methylene chloride, and toluene. A few other chemicals, such as metals, may be measured in exhaled air but this use remains largely a research tool. Additional applications include the measurement of exhaled nitric oxide (NO), a well-known method to assess airway inflammation. The benefits of exhaled breath biomonitoring are that it may be collected noninvasively and offers a direct comparison to measurements from air monitoring.

Hair

Hair is readily available and may be used to screen for heavy metals such as mercury. It has also been used as a research tool to assess exposure to POPs. Hair biomonitoring poses challenges as samples must be cleaned to reduce contamination from surface deposition, and interpretation of hair biomonitoring results is complex.

Furthermore, measurements do not readily distinguish ambient from internal exposure. Other, less readily available, analytic techniques must be used to provide this critical information.

Saliva

Saliva has been evaluated as a matrix for measuring selected nonpersistent chemicals, pesticides, and therapeutic drug levels. Highly sensitive analytical techniques are required for saliva biomonitoring, as levels of nonpersistent chemicals may be considerably lower than those in blood. Further research and refinement in technique is required before saliva can routinely be used for biomonitoring of chemical exposures.

Umbilical Cord Blood

Environmental chemicals that cross the placenta may be measured in cord blood immediately after birth. Results serve as indicators of infants' exposures prior to and during birth. Although the properties of cord blood are different than those of venous blood (eg, the lipid content is lower), in general biomonitoring using this matrix is similar to that described earlier for blood and serum.

Urine

Urine is the easiest sample to collect; typically large volumes of urine are available and there is good participant acceptance. Urine is appropriate for biomonitoring of substances that are excreted by the kidneys, such as nonlipid soluble (nonpersistent) compounds (eg, biphenol A [BPA]) and some metals (eg, arsenic, cadmium, and inorganic mercury). A 24-hour urine collection provides the most accurate assessment of exposure, but for practical reasons, usually a spot urine sample, a single sample collected at a specified time. Because significant variations in dilutions can occur throughout the day, spot urine samples should be adjusted for urine specific gravity or urine creatinine. Ideally, the analyzing laboratory should report spot urine results as both uncorrected (micrograms per liter) and corrected for creatinine (micrograms per gram). Urine specimens that are highly concentrated (specific gravity > 1.030 or creatinine > 3 g/L) or extremely dilute (specific gravity < 1.010 or creatinine < 0.3–0.5 g/L) are not suitable for biomonitoring and a new specimen should be collected. Urine monitoring may not be appropriate for individuals with advanced renal disease as results are likely to be inconsistent and cannot be reliable compared to those with normal renal function.

Other

Other matrices infrequently used for biomonitoring include amniotic fluid, meconium, nails, and teeth.

TIMING OF SAMPLE COLLECTION

POPs, including dioxins, PCBs, and organochlorine insecticides, are readily absorbed into the blood supply and distributed into the fatty portions of tissues and, in lactating women, in breast milk. Biomonitored levels of POPs indicate accumulated exposures years prior to sample collection. Metabolism and excretion of POPs are very slow, and consequently they have long half-lives in the body, usually on the order of years. An exception is lactating women, in whom the half-life of POPs is about 6 months since lipid-soluble POPs accumulate in the breast milk and are removed from the body during breastfeeding.

Unlike persistent compounds, the timing of sample collection relative to exposure is a critical determinant of the measured concentration of *nonpersistent chemicals*. Nonpersistent organic chemicals, such as cholinesterase-inhibiting and pyrethroid pesticides, phthalates, and polycyclic aromatic hydrocarbons (PAHs), are rapidly metabolized and excreted in the urine (Figure 43–1). These chemicals and their metabolites have very short half-lives in blood, on the order of hours to days and, unless samples are collected immediately after exposure, the concentrations are typically orders of magnitude lower than urinary metabolite levels.

Most individuals, whether at work or in other aspects of life, are exposed to chemicals repeatedly. Concentrations of nonpersistent chemicals may show considerable variation throughout the day due to repetitive exposure and rapid metabolism (Figure 43–2). For these chemicals, a single sample may not characterize average exposure over a period of time; instead, biomonitoring provides a snapshot in time of the levels of these chemicals in a particular tissue, rather than a stable measure of "total body burden." This variability suggests that biomonitoring of nonpersistent substances may be particularly relevant for assessing shift-related exposure in occupational settings, where time of sample collection relative to ambient concentrations of the substance being biomonitored is known. At the same time, it may pose challenges for assessing the internal dose among other populations where environmental exposures are variable and less known.

EXPOSURE & DISEASE: INTERPRETING RESULTS

For most chemicals that are biomonitored today, measured concentrations do not correlate well with clinical illness or the likelihood of disease. Table 43–1 lists examples of substances that are biomonitored in occupational and environmental settings and the suspected or known health effects. For many of these substances, biomonitoring will help to elucidate the relationship between exposure and disease.

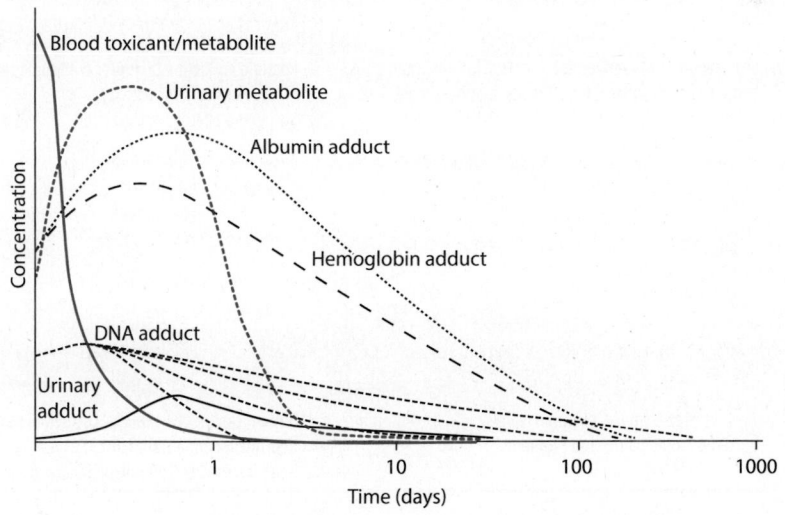

▲ **Figure 43–1.** Theoretical fate of a nonpersistent chemical and its metabolites and adducts in blood and urine.

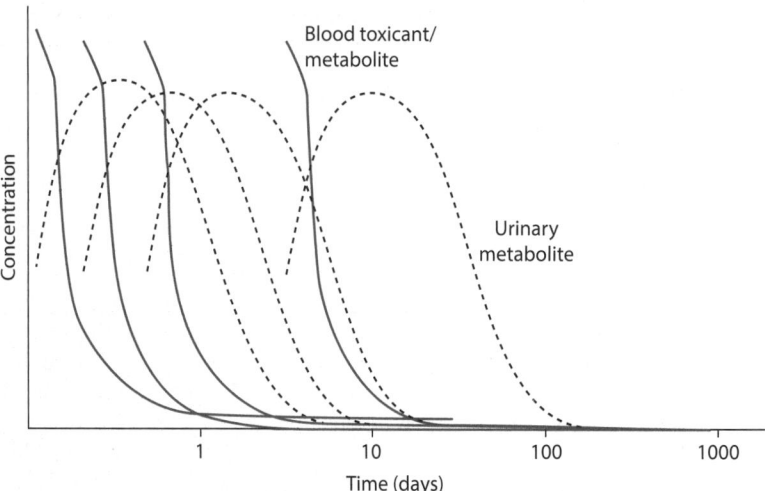

▲ **Figure 43–2.** Theoretical variation in levels of a nonpersistent chemical in blood and urine from chronic, repeated exposure.

Table 43–1. Uses and known and suspected health effects of selected chemicals that may be biomonitored in occupational and environmental settings.

Chemical Class Example Compounds in Class	Uses	Known or Suspected Health Effects
Environmental Phenols		
Benzophenone-3	Used in sunscreens and plastics to block ultraviolet radiation	Reports of photosensitization and allergy Possible endocrine disruptor: weak estrogenic and antiandrogenic activity
Bisphenol A (BPA)	Used to make protective coatings, eg, inside metal food cans to prevent rust and corrosion; building block for polycarbonate	Endocrine disruptor: possible effects on the developing nervous and immune systems; may promote obesity Prenatal period and early childhood are critical exposure windows
Parabens	Widely used as preservatives in cosmetics, lotions, shampoos, deodorants, pharmaceuticals, foods, and beverages	Possible endocrine disruptor with male reproductive effects and weak estrogenic activity Suspected allergic sensitization
Triclosan	Added to soaps, other consumer products labeled "antibacterial" or "antimicrobial"	Possible endocrine disruption and inhibitor of metabolism of other environmental phenols. Concern exists that widespread use may encourage growth of antibiotic-resistant organisms Suspected allergic sensitizer
Metals		
Arsenic	Occurs naturally in some foods and drinking water in some areas; used in semiconductors; historically used as pesticides	Inorganic: human carcinogen (lung, bladder, skin) Possible association with diabetes, hypertension, childhood neurodevelopmental effects
Cadmium	Found in cigarette smoke, costume jewelry, nickel-cadmium batteries, some paints and pigments	Human carcinogen (lung); obstructive pulmonary disease Neurodevelopmental toxin Bone fracture and diminished bone mineral density

(continued)

Table 43–1. Uses and known and suspected health effects of selected chemicals that may be biomonitored in occupational and environmental settings. (Continued)

Chemical Class Example Compounds in Class	Uses	Known or Suspected Health Effects
Lead	Formerly used in paint and gasoline; still used in many consumer products, including some pottery and plastic products; found in dust and soil in and around houses built before 1978 and at job sites, such as painting, construction, and battery recycling	Multiple health effects, including anemia, renal and neurologic toxicity; hypertension in adults; neurodevelopmental toxicant in children
Mercury	Inorganic form historically released into the environment from mining operations; found in emissions from coal-burning plants; used in silver dental fillings and fluorescent light bulbs; found in some imported skin-lightening and antiaging creams. Organic mercury builds up in certain fish and seafood	Inorganic: neurocognitive and behavioral disturbances; renal tubular necrosis; peripheral neurotoxicity Organic: central nervous system toxicity; developmental deficits; cardiovascular effects
Perfluorochemicals (PFCs)	Used to make products resistant to oil, stains, grease, and water, eg, stain-resistant carpets, wrinkle-free clothing, and grease-proof food containers	Endocrine disruption: possible reproductive and developmental toxicity at very low levels; potentially carcinogenic. Toxicity varies by individual congener in this class
Phthalates	Added to vinyl to make it soft and flexible; products include shower curtains, flooring, and plastic tubing; also found in some nail polish and scented products	Endocrine disruption: anti-androgen and possible estrogenic or anti-estrogenic activity at very low levels
Polybrominated diphenyl ether (PBDE) flame retardants	Added to products such as furniture foam, textiles, and electronics, often to meet flammability standards	Lower brominated PBDEs (< 5 bromine atoms) may be neurodevelopmental and reproductive toxicants and cause endocrine disruption at very low levels: thyroid hormone disruption; alterations in expression of estrogen-regulated genes and receptors; anti-androgen
Polycyclic aromatic hydrocarbons (PAHs)	Occurs naturally in petroleum products; found in cigarette and wood smoke and in grilled meat; sources include volcanic eruptions and fires	Fetal growth retardation, respiratory disorders, and cardiovascular disease following fine particle exposure but role of PAH vs particulates unclear; specific PAH-containing chemical mixtures (eg, soot, coke oven emissions, coal tars and coal tar pitches) have been classified as human carcinogens

The continuum from exposure to resulting health outcome is influenced by the toxicity of the chemical, the amount absorbed into the body, individual pharmacokinetics (absorption, distribution, metabolism, and excretion), and individual susceptibility. These include demographic factors (eg, age, ethnicity), genetics, environmental and behavioral stressors, nutritional and general health status, and other exposures. As a result of these factors, persons with chronic illnesses, the elderly, infants and children, and women who are pregnant or of childbearing age are among the subpopulations considered to be at increased risk for the adverse effects of exposure to chemicals.

While biomonitoring may not allow reliable prediction of adverse health effects, results may be interpreted using one of two comparison methods: health-based values or reference ranges.

Health-Based Values

Health-based values are chemical concentrations below which an individual would not be expected to develop adverse health effects, that is, symptoms or signs of disease or abnormal clinical laboratory tests. These values are based on published and unpublished scientific literature, including unpublished industry studies; may incorporate safety factors; and are commonly applied in occupational settings. Currently available guidance values for occupational exposure are summarized in Table 43–2. Exceedance of health values implies increased risk of health effects and typically triggers requirements such as medical evaluation and increased environmental and biological monitoring to evaluate the potential for adverse effects. For the general population these values are available for a limited number of substances, that is, lead and mercury; acetyl- and butyl-cholinesterase activity levels may be included in this category but are not as reliable due to intraindividual variation and require confirmation with individual baseline (ie, preexposure) values.

In the United States, the most commonly used health-based biomonitoring guidance values for occupational exposures are the proprietary biological exposure indices (BEIs) issued by the American Conference of Governmental Industrial Hygienists (ACGIH). These values are based on a

Table 43–2. Current occupational biomonitoring guidance standards.

Standard	Organization
Biological exposure index (BEI) https://www.acgih.org/tlv-bei-guidelines/biological-exposure-indices-introduction	American Conference of Government Industrial Hygienists
Biomonitoring guidance values (BMGV) https://www.hsl.gov.uk/online-ordering/analytical-services-and-assays/biological-monitoring/bm-guidance-values	UK Health and Safety Executive
Biological tolerance values (BAT) https://onlinelibrary.wiley.com/doi/book/10.1002/9783527812127	Deutsche Forschungsgemeinschaft
Exposure equivalents for carcinogenic substances (EKA) http://onlinelibrary.wiley.com/doi/10.1002/9783527666034.ch3/summary	Deutsche Forschungsgemeinschaft
Occupational exposure limit values (OELV) http://ec.europa.eu/social/main.jsp?catId=148&langId=en&intPageId=684	European Commission Scientific Committee on Occupational Exposure Limits

critical evaluation of the literature and studies submitted for review, with an emphasis on studies that address minimal or no adverse health effect levels in exposed workers and animals. When available, human studies are given preference. BEIs exist for over 40 substances, generally represent levels in healthy workers exposed at ACGIH threshold limit values (TLVs), and indicate concentrations below which adverse health effects are not expected (Table 43–3).

Of the other available occupational guidance values, the most rigorous are the biological tolerance values (BAT values) for occupational exposure to noncarcinogenic substances. BAT values are based on quantitative data and are the rough equivalent of BEIs. There are over 100 BAT values, defined as the concentration of a chemical substance, its metabolites, or an effect indicator in biological media at which the health of an employee is usually not affected, even after repeated or long-term exposure. Substances for which there is evidence of human cancer risk have no BAT values, as there is no "safe" biological level for carcinogens. Instead, exposure equivalents for carcinogenic substances (EKA values) are developed and allow the calculation of body burdens based on air levels.

Reference Ranges

Reference ranges are observed measurements for a particular population and are often expressed as the 95th percentile, that is, 95% of the observed values fall below this level. Exceedance of these values suggests that the measured concentration in an individual is statistically higher than the population range but does not indicate the likelihood of health effects occurring as a result of exposure. As chemical exposures, and therefore biomonitoring results vary by demographic, occupational, and other variables, it is imperative that reference values be obtained from a comparison population in which these factors resemble those of the participants.

The U.S. Centers for Disease Control and Prevention's (CDC's) National Biomonitoring Program conducts biomonitoring and generates reference ranges for the general US population. Similar comparisons for worker cohorts may be generated by individual employers for their own employees but are typically not publicly available. In Germany, the Human Biomonitoring Commission establishes reference values based on studies of the German population.

Regardless of the population being biomonitored and the comparison method used, sorting out occupational from nonoccupational exposures is a challenge because biomonitoring reflects exposure from all sources. The use of exposure questionnaires, environmental monitoring, and consultation with an industrial hygienist can assist the interpretation of biomonitoring results. Common "lifestyle" factors that may impact occupational biomonitoring include:

- *Cigarette smoking.* Cadmium concentrations in blood and exhaled breath may be higher in smokers.
- *Seafood consumption.* Levels of organic mercury may be elevated in individuals who regularly consume seafood; shellfish may contain an inorganic arsenic metabolite and consumption may cause spurious elevation of urinary arsenic.
- *Drinking water.* Certain groundwater sources in the United States, and to a greater extent in other countries (eg, Bangladesh, Chile, India), have elevated arsenic concentrations.

LABORATORY CONSIDERATIONS

Laboratory factors are critical to obtaining accurate, meaningful results since biomonitoring measures minute amounts of substances that may be present in the environment, using complex and sensitive instruments. Involving laboratory professionals in the design of biomonitoring studies will minimize potential errors when interpreting results. Issues that should be considered prior to initiating a biomonitoring study in partnership with a laboratory include

Table 43–3. Chemicals for which there are reference ranges or health-based values to guide biologic monitoring.[a]

Chemical *Determinant*	Media (units)	NHANES Geometric Mean[b] (95% CI)	Occupational Guidance Level[c]	Timing of Work-Related Sample[d]	Half-life	Comments
Acetone	Urine (mg/L)	—	25	EOS	3 h	
	Blood (mg/dL)	—		DS?	4–6 h	Elevated during diabetic or fasting ketoacidosis
	Alveolar air (mg/m³)	—		DS	4 h	
Aniline						
p-Aminophenol	Urine (mg/L)	—	50	EOS	—	Large individual variability
Methemoglobin	Blood (%)	—	1.5	EOS	—	Not specific
Arsenic *Total arsenic*	Urine (mcg/L)	9.28 (8.47–10.2)	35	EWW	2–4 d	No seafood for 2 days before collection
Benzene						
	Blood (ng/mL)	< LOD		EOS	8 h	
t,t-Muconic acid	Urine (mcg/g Cr)	—	500	EOS	5 h	
S-Phenylmer-capturic acid	Urine (mcg/g Cr)	—	25	EOS	9 h	
1,3-Butadiene						
N-1- and N-2(hydroxybutenyl) valine-Hb adducts	Blood (pmol/g Hb)	—	2.5	NC		
1,2 Dihydroxy-4-(N-acetylcysteinyl)-butane	Urine (mg/L)	—	2.5	EOS		
2-Butoxyethanol						
Butoxyacetic acid	Urine (mg/g Cr)		200	EOS	3–6 h	
Cadmium	Urine (mcg/g Cr)	0.238 (0.224–0.253)	5	NC	10–30 y	Reflects cumulative exposure and concentration in kidney
	Blood (mcg/L)	0.302 (0.293–0.311)	5	NC	10–15 y	Reflects recent and cumulative exposure; levels in smokers may be twice as high as nonsmokers
Carbamate pesticides *RBC cholinesterase*	Blood (% baseline)		< 80[e]	EOS	1–2 h	Nonspecific effect of this class of pesticides
Carbofuran *Carbofuranphenol*	Urine (mcg/g Cr)	< LOD			6–12 h	Example of pesticide in this class; common metabolite of several pesticides in this category
Carbon disulfide *2-Thioxo-thiazolidine-4-carboxylic acid (TTCA)*	Urine (mg/g Cr)	—	0.5	EOS	5 h	Elevated following exposure to disulfiram (Antabuse), dithiocarbamate fungicides, and brassica vegetables

(continued)

Table 43–3. Chemicals for which there are reference ranges or health-based values to guide biologic monitoring.[a] (Continued)

Chemical *Determinant*	Media (units)	NHANES Geometric Mean[b] (95% CI)	Occupational Guidance Level[c]	Timing of Work-Related Sample[d]	Half-life	Comments
Carbon monoxide	End-exhaled air (ppm)	< 7[f]	20	EOS	5 h	Elevated in smokers
Carboxyhemoglobin (COHb)	Blood (%)	2.13[g]	3.5	EOS	1–8 h	Elevated in smokers, after driving on urban highways, and after exposure to dichloromethane
Chlorobenzene	Blood (ng/mL)	< LOD			1–2 h	
4-Chlorocatechol	Urine (mg/g Cr)	—	100	EOS, EWW	3 h	
p-Chlorophenol	Urine (mg/g Cr)	—	20	EOS, EWW	7 h	
Chromium	Blood (mcg/L)	< LOD				Chromium (III) is an essential trace dietary element; chromium (VI) is a carcinogen
Total chromium	Urine (mcg/L)	—	25	EOS, EWW	7 h	Indicates cumulative and recent exposures
			10	Increase during shift		Indicates daily exposure
Cobalt	Blood (mcg/L)	0.151 (0.146–0.156)	1	EOS, EWW	29 h	
	Urine (mcg/L)	0.369 (0.341–0.398)	15	EOS, EWW	30 h	
Cyclohexanone						
1,2-Cyclohexanediol	Urine (mg/L)	—	80	EOS, EWW	14 h	
Cyclohexanol	Urine (mg/L)	—	8	EOS	14 h	
Dichloromethane (Methylene chloride)	Blood (ng/mL)	< LOD			< 1 h	
	Urine (mg/L)	—	0.3	EOS	1–8 h	
	End-exhaled air (ppm)	—		EOS	10–12 h	No guidance level. May be used as screen for exposure
Carboxyhemoglobin (COHb)	Blood (%)	2.13	3.5	EOS	1–8 h	Elevated in smokers, after driving on urban highways, and after exposure to carbon monoxide
N-Methylacetamide	Urine (mg/g Cr)	—	30	EOS, EWW	16 h	
N-Methylformamide	Urine (mg/L)	—	15	EOS	2–5 h	
N-Acetyl-S-(N-methylcarbamoyl) cysteine	Urine (mg/L)	—	15	EOS	23 h	Also a metabolite of isothiocyanates, a component of wine and cruciferous vegetables
2-Ethoxyethanol (Ethylene glycol, EGEE) and 2-Ethoxyethyl acetate (Ethylene glycol monoethyl ether acetate, EGEAA)	Urine (mg/g Cr)	—	100	EOS, EWW	22 h	

(continued)

Table 43–3. Chemicals for which there are reference ranges or health-based values to guide biologic monitoring.[a] (Continued)

Chemical *Determinant*	Media (units)	NHANES Geometric Mean[b] (95% CI)	Occupational Guidance Level[c]	Timing of Work-Related Sample[d]	Half-life	Comments
Ethyl benzene	Blood (ng/mL)	< LOD				Reflects recent exposure; elevated in smokers
	End-exhaled air	—		NC		No guidance level. May be used as screen for exposure
Mandelic acid + phenylglyoxylic acid	Urine (g/g Cr)	—	0.15	EOS, EWW	2–8 h	Also metabolites of styrene
Fluorides	Urine (mg/L)	—	2 3	PTS EOS	5 h	Exposure sources include drinking water, dental products, floor varnishes
Furfural					2 h	
Furoic acid	Urine (mg/L)		200	EOS		
n-Hexane	End-exhaled air (ppm)	—		DS	1–2 h	
2,5-Hexanedione	Urine (mg/L)	—	0.4	EOS, EWW	15 h	Major metabolite; also a metabolite of methyl n-butyl ketone
2,5-Dimethylfuran	Urine (ng/mL)	< LOD				Minor metabolite
Lead	Blood (mcg/dL)	1.12 (1.08–1.16)	30	NC	28 d, blood 5–19 y, bone	CDC recommends follow-up and management of children and pregnant women > 5 mcg/dL (reference level)
Zinc protoporphyrin (ZPP)	Blood (mcg/dL)	—		NC	2–4 wk	Indirect and insensitive biomarker for lead. Increase lags blood lead level elevation by 2–6 weeks. Iron deficiency anemia, porphyria, and inflammatory diseases may cause elevation
Mercury	Blood, total (mcg/L)	0.863 (0.792–0.941)				Due mostly to dietary intake of seafood containing organic mercury and therefore not recommended for assessment of occupational exposure
	Blood, inorganic (mcg/L)	< LOD	15	EOS, EWW		
	Blood, methyl mercury	0.413 (0.361–0.472)				Due mostly to dietary intake of seafood containing organic mercury
	Urine (mcg/g creatinine)	< LOD	20	PTS	60 d	Best indicator of inorganic mercury; higher levels with greater numbers of teeth filled with mercury-containing amalgams
Methanol	Urine (mg/L)	—	15	EOS, EWW	1–3 h	Present in aspartame and some foods
2-Methoxyethanol (EGME), 2-Methoxyethyl acetate (EGMEA)						
2-Methoxyacetic acid	Urine (mg/g Cr)	—	1	EOS, EWW	77 h	

(continued)

Table 43–3. Chemicals for which there are reference ranges or health-based values to guide biologic monitoring.[a] (Continued)

Chemical *Determinant*	Media (units)	NHANES Geometric Mean[b] (95% CI)	Occupational Guidance Level[c]	Timing of Work-Related Sample[d]	Half-life	Comments
Methyl *n*-butyl ketone (2-Henxanone)						
2,5-Hexanedione	Urine (mg/L)	—	0.4	EOS, EWW	15 h	Also a metabolite of n-hexane
Methyl chloroform (1,1,1-Trichloroethane)	End-exhaled air (ppm) Blood (ng/mL)	— < LOD	40	PLS	4 h	Nonspecific; should be used only as screening; metabolite of chloral hydrate
Trichloroacetic acid	Urine (mg/L)	—	10	EOW	7–10 h	
Trichloroethanol	Blood (mg/L) Urine (mg/L)	— —	1 30	EOS, EWW	8 h 7–10 h	
Methyl ethyl ketone	Urine (mg/L)	—	2	EOS	3.5 h	
Methyl isobutyl ketone	Urine (mg/L)	—	1	EOS	3.5 h	
N-Methyl-2-pyrrolidone						
5-Hydoxy-N-methyl-2-pyrrolidone	Urine (mg/L)	—	100	EOS	6.5 h	
Molybdenum	Urine (mcg/L)	42.7 (40.8–44.7)			Variable	Essential trace element
Nitrobenzene	Blood (ng/mL)	< LOD				
p-Nitrophenol	Urine (mg/g Cr)	< LOD	5	EOS, EWW	60 h	Not specific; also a metabolite of parathion
Methemoglobin	Blood (%)	—	1.5	EOS		Not specific
Organophosphate pesticides						
RBC cholinesterase	Blood (% baseline)	—	< 80[e]	Discretionary	20–30 d	Nonspecific effect of this class of pesticides
Chlorpyrifos						Example of pesticide in this class
RBC cholinesterase	Blood (% baseline)	—	70	Discretionary	20–30 d	Nonspecific
3,5,6-Trichloro-2-pyridinol	Urine (mcg/g Cr)	0.779 (0.706–0.859)			26 h	Also metabolite of chlorpyrifos-methyl
Parathion						
RBC cholinesterase	Blood (% baseline)	—	70	Discretionary	20–30 d	
p-Nitrophenol	Urine (mcg/L) Urine (mcg/g Cr)	0.454 (0.407–0.506) —	0.5	EOS, EWW	60 h	Also a metabolite of nitrobenzene
Pentachlorophenol	Urine (mg/L total PCP in urine)	< LOD	1	EOS	10 h	Due to short half-life several months of exposure are required to reach steady state
Perfluorochemicals						Multiple chemicals exist in this class; examples are presented
Perfluorooctanoic acid (PFOA)	Serum (mcg/L)	3.96 (3.67–4.27)				
Perfluorooctane sulfonic acid (PFOS)	Serum (mcg/L)	20.9 (19.3–22.5)				

(continued)

Table 43–3. Chemicals for which there are reference ranges or health-based values to guide biologic monitoring.[a] (Continued)

Chemical *Determinant*	Media (units)	NHANES Geometric Mean[b] (95% CI)	Occupational Guidance Level[c]	Timing of Work-Related Sample[d]	Half-life	Comments
Phenol	Urine (mg/g Cr)	—	250	EOS	3 h	Also found with high exposure to benzene; household products such as medications and cleaners may contain phenol and result in up to 10 mg/g Cr
Polybrominated Diphenyl Ethers (PBDEs)						Multiple chemicals exist in this class; examples are presented
2,2',4,4'-Tetrabromodi phenyl ether (BDE 47)	Serum (ng/g lipid)	< LOD		NC	1.8 y	
2,2',4,4',5-Penta bromodiphenyl ether (BDE 99)	Serum (ng/g lipid)	< LOD		NC	2.9 y	
2,2',4,4',6-Pentabro modiphenyl ether (BDE 100)	Serum (ng/g lipid)	< LOD			1.6 y	
Polychlorinated biphenyls (PCBs)						Multiple chemicals exist in this class; examples are presented
2,3,7,8-Tetrachlorod ibenzo-p-dioxin (TCDD)	(pg/g lipid)	< LOD			8 y	
2,3,3',4,4',5-Hexachlo robiphenyl (PCB 156)	Serum (ng/g lipid)	< LOD)			5 y	
Polycyclic aromatic hydro-carbons (PAHs)						> 100 chemicals exist in this class
2-Hydroxyfluorene	Urine (ng/g Cr)	240 (222–259)			< 10 h	Metabolite of fluorene
1-Hydroxy-naphthalene	Urine (ng/g Cr)	1.52 (1.37–1.68)			< 10 h	Metabolite of naphthalene, the most abundant PAH in cigarette smoke
1-hydroxypyrene	Urine (ng/g Cr)	79.1 (73.2–85.4)			< 10 h	Metabolite of pyrene; elevated in smokers and with some dermal medications
	Urine (mcg/l)		2.5	EOS, EWW		
2-Propanol *Acetone*	Urine (mg/L)	—	40	EOS, EWW	3 h	
Pyrethroid pesticides						
Cypermethrin, Cyfluthrin, Permethrin *cis-3-(2,2-Dichlorovinyl)-2,2-dimethylcyclo-propane carboxylic acid*	Urine (mcg/g Cr)	< LOD			6 h	
Cypermethrin, Deltame-thrin, Permethrin *3-Phenoxybenzoic acid*	Urine (mcg/g Cr)	< LOD			6–24 h	

(continued)

Table 43–3. Chemicals for which there are reference ranges or health-based values to guide biologic monitoring.[a] (Continued)

Chemical *Determinant*	Media (units)	NHANES Geometric Mean[b] (95% CI)	Occupational Guidance Level[c]	Timing of Work-Related Sample[d]	Half-life	Comments
Styrene *Mandelic acid* *Mandelic acid +* *phenylglyoxylic acid*	Blood (ng/L) Urine (mcg/L) Urine (mcg/L) Urine (mg/g Cr)	< LOD — 112 (102–123) 	 40 400	 EOS EOS	5 h 20 h	Half-life in adipose tissue is 2–4 days Nonspecific; also metabolites of ethylbenzene (used in the manufacure of styrene)

Tetrachloroethylene
  (Perchloroethylene)
	Blood (mg/L)
	End-exhaled air (ppm)
		< LOD
		—
			0.5
			3
				PTS
				PTS
					Biphasic:
					  0.5 h,
					  35 h
					8 h
						Half-life in fat is 72 h

Tetrahydrofuran	Blood (ng/mL) Urine (mg/L)	< LOD —	 2	 EOS	5 h Highly variable	
Toluene *N-Acetyl-S-(benzyl)-L-* *cysteine* *o-Cresol*	Blood (ng/L) Urine (mg/L) Urine (mcg/L) Urine (mg/g Cr)	0.092 (0.082–0.103) — 6.80 (6.43–7.20) 	20 0.03 0.3	PLS EOS EOS	1 h < 5 h	Higher levels in smokers, after gasoline refueling
Trichloroethylene *Trichloroethanol* *Trichloroethylene* *Trichloroacetic acid*	Blood (mg/L) Blood (mg/L) End-exhaled air (ppm) Urine (mg/L)	< LOD — — —	 0.5 15	 EOS, EWW EOS, EWW EOS, EWW	 12 h 30 h 41 h	Nonspecific Nonspecific; also metabolite of hexachloroethane
Trichloromethane	Blood (pg/mL)	8.60 (6.82–10.8)				
Uranium	Urine (mcg/L)	0.009 (0.008–0.011)	200	EOS	15 d	Nonoccupational sources are drinking water and root vegetables

[a]Selected chemicals are presented here. Additional biomonitoring reference data are available in the CDC National Report on Human Exposure to Environmental Chemicals. Cr = creatinine; Hb = hemoglobin; < LOD = high proportion of results below level of detection, so value could not be calculated; ---= Not measured

[b]Except where noted, this is the Geometric Mean (95% confidence interval) for age group 20 years and older as reported in the most recent data presented in CDC Fourth National Report on Human Exposure to Environmental Chemicals.

[c]Except where noted, these levels are the Biologic Exposure Index (BEI*) levels developed by ACGIH. Blank cells indicate that no US occupational exposure guidance levels exist.

[d]Timing of sample collection abbreviations defined below:

    DS   During shift
    EOS   End of shift
    EWW   End of workweek
    PTS   Prior to next shift
    PLS   Prior to last shift of work week

[e]Based on state cholinesterase monitoring guidelines (CA, WA).

[f]Health New Zealand.

[g]Agency for Toxic Substances and Disease Registry.

contamination, specimen management, and quality assurance (QA) and quality control (QC).

Contamination

Sample contamination is a much greater concern for biomonitoring studies compared to other clinical laboratory tests. Sources of contamination include

- Specimen collection instruments (eg, lead in needles or glass tubes and phthalates in urine containers)
- Materials used in the laboratory (eg, triclosan in hand soaps)
- Environmental pollutants, including ambient air in the collection facility or laboratory (eg, dust contaminated with polybrominated dibrominated ethers [PBDEs]); and external air (eg, degradates of pesticides entrained through inadequate ventilation) as well as skin surface contamination (eg, lead)

For example, both environmental degradation of the insecticides chlorpyrifos and chlorpyrifos-methyl as well as human metabolism result in the formation of the metabolite 3,5,6-trichloro-2-pyridinol (TCPy). By merely measuring TCPy in urine and not in the ambient environment, exposures to chlorpyrifos, chlorpyrifos-methyl, or TCPy itself cannot be distinguished from sample contamination.

Methods to minimize and control for contamination include using the appropriate type of containers, prescreening specimen collection materials, obtaining field blanks to control for background contamination, and conducting analyses in clean rooms. Additionally, developing detailed collection and processing protocols and training clinical and laboratory personnel on proper implementation will minimize contamination. Finally, documenting specimen collection details, such as time and location of collection, is essential to aid in assessing potential contamination sources if suspect results are obtained.

Specimen Management

Proper specimen management is necessary to ensure that chemicals of interest do not deteriorate. Examples of common errors include

- Improper mixing of blood collection tubes containing the anticoagulant EDTA resulting in blood clots which can trap heavy metals and result in erroneously low levels
- Storage or shipping temperatures that are too high resulting in degradation of acetyl cholinesterase or too low resulting in hemolysis of whole blood
- Waiting too long to centrifuge blood and process serum; the resulting blood clot impacts analysis by trapping both lipids and chemicals

Adherence to detailed and strict processing, storage, and shipping protocols will minimize errors during this phase. Both the clinic where specimen collection occurs and the analyzing laboratory must maintain and share specimen collections, storage, and shipping protocols and records.

Quality Assurance & Quality Control

Prior to initiating a biomonitoring study, it is essential to verify that the partner laboratory has a quality management system, which ensures the integrity of the samples, the analytic technique, and the data generated. Laboratories must adhere to strict QA and QC standards for consistent and meaningful results.

QA refers to the overall laboratory operation, which should include proficiency testing programs that compare measured results with those of an external laboratory or standard. For example, certification of laboratories meeting minimum standards for analysis of blood lead requires that blind samples be submitted to other laboratories and the results compared with those of a reference laboratory. Analysis of a random sample of "split" specimens by another—preferably a reference—laboratory is an alternative to an internal quality assurance program.

QC involves internal assessment of accuracy and precision, including daily instrument calibration and analysis of control specimens concurrently with study samples. Written standard operating procedures (SOPs) are expected to specify specimen collection, handling, and transport and sample processing, analysis, QC, and proper training of chemists. Laboratories certified under the Clinical Laboratory Improvement Act of 1988 (CLIA) must meet specific requirements in order to report results that may be used for diagnostic purposes (as opposed to research only).

Selecting a Laboratory

Few laboratories have demonstrated QA/QC and the ability to analyze a wide range of substances. Even the most experienced laboratories can fail to meet minimum standards and without a regular quality management program, analytic quality cannot be ensured. Laboratories should be considered based on their ability to provide documentation of validation procedures, including *sensitivity*, the minimum level of an analyte that can reliably be detected by a particular assay (limits of detection, LOD) and *specificity*, the ability to differentiate a unique analyte from other closely related structures. The analytic method must be described clearly and in sufficient detail to allow other laboratories to repeat measurements. The laboratory should have documented the analytical range, LOD, and other performance parameters, in addition to the SOPs. The laboratory and clinician should collaborate to establish the appropriateness of biomonitoring the substances of interest; sample collection, management, and shipping protocols; and details of reporting results. Protocols for managing abnormal results should be established in advance. This may include repeating the assay on the same sample, obtaining a new sample for analysis, and evaluating contamination and QA/QC methods.

IMPLEMENTING BIOLOGIC MONITORING PROGRAMS

Regardless of the setting, multidisciplinary collaboration is essential for biomonitoring studies or programs. Clinicians, laboratorians, toxicologists, epidemiologists, industrial hygienists, and ethicists are among the critical partners to include during the planning phases of any biomonitoring project or program. Unless they are clearly associated with an urgent public health response, projects or programs that involve biomonitoring must be reviewed and approved by Institutional Review Boards (IRBs) for the protection of the participants. Protocols should ensure that participants are ethically treated and fully informed of the risks and benefits, including the potential inability to assess the clinical impacts of the results and intent to store samples for future analyses, if relevant.

Biomonitoring of Workers

Biologic monitoring in the occupational setting may be a voluntary or required component of routine medical surveillance as well as worker monitoring during and after emergency response. In the United States, biomonitoring for lead and cadmium is required by OSHA medical surveillance standards; other requirements vary by state and exist for an extremely limited number of chemicals (eg, limited monitoring of cholinesterase activity for certain workers, required in California and Washington). Similarly, considerable variation in biomonitoring requirements exists internationally. During routine surveillance, environmental monitoring that identifies exceedance of a specified standard (ie, cadmium, lead) may trigger individual clinical worker evaluations, including obtaining a thorough occupational and environmental history to verify all potential sources of exposure and biomonitoring. The decision to conduct biomonitoring of workers as part of emergency or disaster response depends in large part on logistics and feasibility. Even when conducted as part of emergency response, proper protocol and technique must be followed for the results to be accurate and meaningful.

Regardless of the setting in which it is conducted, abnormal biomonitoring results should be verified by repeating the measurement on the sample collected and, if feasible, obtaining additional samples for verification. Conducting environmental monitoring simultaneously with biomonitoring and comparison to relevant standards is critical to help identify potential exposure sources and assess necessary control measures, such as engineering controls, modified work practices, appropriate protective equipment, or removal from work (Table 43–2).

Ethical and social considerations require that clinical protocols be established to ensure confidentiality of results; voluntary, not mandatory, participation; and responsible results communication. Clinicians should be available to provide consultation on test results and their clinical implications. Biomonitoring results, like other medical records, should be maintained for at least 30 years; some jurisdictions may require longer retention periods.

Biomonitoring in Public Health & Research

Research institutions have incorporated biomonitoring into their work, and increasingly governmental agencies both in the United States and internationally are beginning to apply it to address public health investigations and disease prevention efforts. As stand-alone biomonitoring programs are resource-intensive, partnering with other public programs that collect biological samples may be considered. For example, state-based mandatory disease-reporting requirements may include conditions that require the measurement of chemical biomarkers (eg, lead, pesticide, and carbon monoxide poisoning). For many such diseases, however, only the clinical diagnoses, and not the biomonitoring results, are reportable. Public health biomonitoring may also utilize "remainder samples," for example, dried blood spots from newborn screening tests or maternal screening during pregnancy. It is imperative to consider the local ethical and social concerns and legal and scientific restrictions associated with using remainder specimens. Several established public health biomonitoring programs are described in Table 43–4.

Public health biomonitoring programs are constrained by specific legislative directives. Their scope is determined by statutory authority and by restrictions imposed by funding agencies. The public health goals of biomonitoring may be broad or specific and include the following.

A. Targeted Investigations

Biomonitoring is an important adjunct to epidemiologic investigations and can help determine the extent of exposure to an individual or entire community and actions that may be warranted to reduce exposure and protect health. Examples include the following:

- Use of illegally imported mercury-containing face creams resulted in inorganic mercury toxicity in several members of a family and led to a state-wide educational campaign to raise awareness of exposure sources and health hazards of mercury.

- Levels of perfluorochemicals (PFCs) in adults living in a community with contaminated groundwater were reduced after a campaign to reduce exposure to the source of drinking water.

B. Population Surveillance

An important use of biomonitoring is to measure population exposures over time and space, identify individuals and populations at risk, and evaluate the impact of public policies. For example, CDC's National Biomonitoring Program documented the dramatic decline in the US population's blood lead levels that corresponded with the removal of lead from gasoline. Biomonitoring studies have also demonstrated that Californians have some of the highest levels of PBDE flame retardants in the world. This is most likely due to unique fire

TABLE 43–4. Selected biomonitoring programs.

Program	Populations/Substances measured	Purpose	Results Communication
Federal (US)			
CDC: National Biomonitoring Program https://www.cdc.gov/biomonitoring/index.html	Environmental chemicals in blood, serum, or urine specimens measured in a subset of the National Health and Nutrition Survey (NHANES), a nationally representative, randomized sample of US adults and children	Public health surveillance of US population Tracks trends of chemical exposures over time Data establish a reference population (or baseline) and to identify differences in the distribution of exposure across age, sex, and race/ethnicity Results are used as reference values for comparison with other biomonitoring programs/ participants.	Aggregate results published periodically in the "National Report on Human Exposure to Environmental Chemicals," http://www.cdc.gov/exposurereport/. Results include geometric mean, selected percentiles (50th, 75th, 90th, 95th) of measured levels by gender, age, and selected race/ethnicity Results with clear clinical significance and notification thresholds (eg, lead, mercury) are returned to participants
State-level[a]			
California—Biomonitoring California (California Environmental Contaminant Biomonitoring Program) https://biomonitoring.ca.gov/ **4 Corners States Biomonitoring Program (Utah, Arizona, Colorado, New Mexico)** http://www.4csbc.org/ **Massachusetts—Massachusetts Biomonitoring Program** https://www.mass.gov/biomonitoring **New Hampshire—NH Biomonitoring Program** https://www.dhhs.nh.gov/dphs/lab/biomonitoring.htm **New Jersey—Biomonitoring Program** https://www.nj.gov/health/phel/env-testing/chemical-terrorism-lab/biomonitoring.shtml **Washington—Washington State Environmental Biomonitoring Survey** https://www.doh.wa.gov/DataandStatisticalReports/EnvironmentalHealth/Biomonitoring **Other:** States may conduct limited biomonitoring as part of the CDC-funded Environmental Public Health Tracking Program https://www.cdc.gov/biomonitoring/state_grants.html	**CA:** Chemicals of public health concern in California in blood, serum, or urine specimens from the state's population and targeted subpopulations (eg, firefighters, mothers and newborn infants, at-risk communities), as recommended by an independent Scientific Guidance Panel; chemical groups include metals, environmental phenols, pesticides, PAHs, PFCs, PBDE-flame retardants **4 Corners States:** Exposure to metals from well water; exposure to herbicides, pesticides, and phthalates from consumer products **MA:** Urine and blood for heavy metals and PCBs in a sample of state residents **NH:** Urine arsenic and uranium from exposure to well water in volunteers and randomly selected households **NJ:** Contaminants in blood and urine, including heavy metals, PCBs, and PFCs in deidentified samples collected from blood banks and clinic laboratories. The State of New Jersey Biomonitoring Commission provides scientific guidance and oversight for activities. **WA:** Urine levels of arsenic, organophosphate and pyrethroid pesticides, BPA, and pthalates are measured in a representative sample of the state's general population and in targeted subpopulations (eg, residents of subsidized housing, pesticide applicators). An Advisory Committee helps prioritize biomonitoring activities	In general, state biomonitoring programs measure levels of chemicals of concern in the general or specific at-risk populations and track trends over time; assess the effects of regulations, policies, and practices on chemical exposures; and inform regulatory efforts to reduce harmful exposure.	**CA:** Publicly available information about studies and aggregate results presented at Scientific Guidance Panel meetings open to the public and in biannual data summary reports to state Legislature Individual results are returned in writing and in an understandable manner to participants. **4 Corners States:** Education and health communication is delivered in various formats throughout the biomonitoring process, including by mail, phone, and email. **MA:** Results are returned in writing to participants. **NH:** Results and assistance with interpretation are available. **NJ:** Results are not systematically returned to individuals. **WA:** Results are returned to participants.

(continued)

TABLE 43–4. Selected biomonitoring programs. (Continued)

Program	Populations/Substances measured	Purpose	Results Communication
International			
Canada: The Canadian Health Measures Survey includes national baseline data on concentrations of environmental chemicals in blood, serum, an urine https://www.canada.ca/en/health-canada/services/environmental-workplace-health/environmental-contaminants/human-biomonitoring-environmental-chemicals/canadian-health-measures-survey.html	Chemicals of public health concern in Canada in a stratified randomly selected population representing the Canadian population.	Establish reference ranges for concentrations of chemicals in Canadians, to allow for comparisons with sub-populations in Canada and comparisons with other countries; establish baseline levels of chemicals and track trends over time; assess effectiveness of regulatory and environmental risk management actions and provide information for setting priorities to reduce exposure to environmental chemicals	Aggregate data on the Canadian population's exposure to environmental chemicals are presented in publicly available reports. Individual lead, mercury, and cadmium results are reported to participants. All other test results may be received upon request to Statistics Canada.
European Union: Consortium to Perform Human Biomonitoring on a European Scale (COPHES) http://www.eu-hbm.info/cophes	A pilot study demonstrated the feasibility of a coordinated and harmonized bio-monitoring across Europe; further capacity building is needed for the program to grow. Mercury, cadmium, phthalates, and environmental tobacco smoke in hair and urine from mother-child pairs were measured in 17 countries.	Harmonize human biomonitoring activities across the European Union	Aggregate results have been disseminated to the public and individual results were communicated to study participants.
Germany: (1) The German Federal Environment Agency (Umweltbundesamt, UBA) conducts the German Environmental Survey (GerES). https://www.umweltbundesamt.de/en/topics/health/assessing-environmentally-related-health-risks/german-environmental-surveys/german-environmental-survey-2014-2017-geres-v (2) The Human Biomonitoring (HBM) Commission of the UBA develops scientifically based criteria for the interpretation of HBM. http://www.umweltbundesamt.de/gesundheit-e/monitor/index.htm https://www.umweltbundesamt.de/en/topics/health/commissions-working-groups/human-biomonitoring-commission-hbm-commission	(1) GerES conducts blood and urine bio-monitoring of several contaminants in representative samples of the general and select German population and is an important basis for developing "reference values" in blood and urine. Environmental sampling has also been conducted. (2) HBM values are based on human toxicology and epidemiology studies. HBM I: concentration of a substance in human biological matrices below which adverse health effects are not expected. HBM-II: concentration of a substance in human biological matrices above which there is an increased risk for adverse health effects.	(1) Reference values characterize the background exposure of the general population to environmental pollutants at a given time; they are used to identify individuals or groups with increased exposure. (2) The HBM-I is a "control value"; and the HBM-II value is an intervention or action level above which there is a need for exposure reduction and medical evaluation	Results are not systematically returned to participants.

[a]Several US states may be conducting feasibility studies or considering implementing biomonitoring programs. Only selected established programs are described here.

regulations in this state that had historically required the use of these substances in foam and furnishings. PBDE flame retardants were commonly added to furniture, infant products, and electronics for many years. US production of some PBDE mixtures ended in 2006, and the last PBDE mixture was phased out in 2013. Products made before these phase-outs can still contain PBDEs and result in ongoing exposures.

C. Rapid Response

Biomonitoring can be part of response to acute chemical exposures after an uncontrolled chemical release or other type of incident. Chemical exposures resulting from ingestion of contaminated food, uncontrolled releases to air and water, or chemical spills may incorporate biomonitoring to quantify exposure and as part of clinical evaluation for medical diagnosis and treatment. For example, biomonitoring conducted in response to a mercury spill in a school can provide assurance that children were not exposed at a level of health concern. Biomonitoring of emergency response workers conducted after disaster response can provide important information on chemical exposures, including combustion of by-products.

D. Resource for Research

Biomonitoring programs may begin as research; those that do not begin as research may lead to questions that result in a shift in direction. Review and approval by IRBs is imperative for research programs. If research projects are anticipated in advance, the consent form approved by IRBs must address activities, such as community preferences and standards and practices of academic institutions, public health agencies, and appropriate IRB. Federal, state, and local laws will influence decisions on whether to include in the project such research components as returning clinically indeterminate results to participants, archiving of residual specimens for future projects, use of specimens to support the development of analytical methods in the laboratory, and sharing data and specimens with external investigators.

COMMUNICATING RESULTS

Appropriately communicating results is one of the greatest challenges when conducting biomonitoring, as current laboratory capability for assaying chemicals in biological media is far ahead of the ability to determine health effects associated with measured levels. The audiences, contents of the message, and communication methods are determined by various factors, including purpose of biomonitoring, legislative mandates, informed consent agreements, and IRB determinations. Reporting results can be resource-intensive if it includes individualized reports and in-person meetings with biomonitoring participants. In spite of its challenges, results communication is an essential component of both occupational and community biomonitoring, and must be considered during study design.

A common dilemma when biomonitoring is whether results should be reported when clinical significance cannot be interpreted. In traditional clinical practice, individual test results are typically reported to participants by medical practitioners when the results are considered clinically relevant based on expert judgment that the results are associated with adverse health outcomes or when the results trigger intervention based on medical guidelines or legal mandates. This clinical model is still the norm for many occupational settings. In contrast, biomonitoring in communities and for research is more likely to consider participants as "owning" their biomonitoring data and having a right to know about it and the potential to inform individual action even when health effects are uncertain. Elements that should be considered as part of results returned during the planning stages of a biomonitoring program are listed in Table 43–5.

For the few substances with known health alert values, clinical relevance of biomonitored levels, and sources of exposure (eg, arsenic, cadmium, lead, mercury), results communication will likely follow the established clinical model. In contrast, for the majority of biomonitored substances, for which health effect and exposure information is ill-defined, the content of results communication materials may be determined by a multidisciplinary team, including health communication professionals. Representatives of the population being biomonitored should also be consulted, either as members of the results communication team or as focus groups to test the material and determine if they effectively communicate the intended message.

Results Communication in the Occupational Setting

When biomonitoring is conducted in workplaces, both workers and employers need to be notified if levels exceed occupational standards or if health effects related to exposure are suspected. Federal and state standards may specify the triggers for communicating results, the audiences, and who is responsible. Historically, workers may not have been notified about individual biomonitoring findings except where required by law. Even where mandates for reporting results do not exist, it is prudent and ethical to plan for communicating results prior to implementing a biomonitoring program.

Biomonitoring results may serve as a basis for efforts to reduce exposures or conduct health screenings to potentially

Table 43–5. Elements to include when returning results to biomonitoring participants.

Description of uses of chemical and how exposure may occur
Reasons why biomonitoring was conducted
Individual chemical concentrations measured
Range of chemical concentrations values for cohort
Relevant reference ranges or known health standards
Potential health implications of findings
Potential sources of exposures
Recommended actions for employer, community, and individual

reduce morbidity and mortality risks. Results communication materials should address the fact that biomonitoring results might be impacted by nonoccupational exposures. Industrial hygiene monitoring and additional information about exposure sources should be used to differentiate between different sources of exposures, if possible.

Biomonitoring in the workplace entails specific privacy and liability considerations. Workers may be concerned that biomonitoring is an invasion of privacy and that employers might discriminate on the basis of results. Employers may be concerned that biomonitoring findings could trigger workers' compensation claims even when health implications are uncertain and consequently may be reluctant to agree to biomonitoring unless it is mandated. Biomonitoring results should be considered equivalent to other confidential health information; employers should not be notified of individual results. Instead, employer notifications should describe observed exceedances over regulatory limits or other health standards, not individual data, as well as recommended work modifications to reduce exposure. Mandated workplace biomonitoring should be differentiated from research. Research study protocols and informed consent documents should specify that identified results from biomonitoring conducted for research purposes in work settings will be confidential, maintained separately from employee health and other medical records, and communicated to nobody but the employee without their express consent.

Results Communication in the Community Setting

There are few legislative requirements and no uniformly accepted standards for reporting results in community or research settings. Although the community-based participatory model is generally used to guide results reporting in nonoccupational settings, the approach varies greatly.

When considering whether to report results to participants, individuals' right to know and to take appropriate action to reduce exposures must be weighed against the following factors:

- Potential fear, worry, or stigma caused by levels perceived to be high but with unknown health implications

- Possible legal and economic consequences, such as effects on health insurance or property values from knowledge about levels of a chemical

- Potential unintended promotion of unnecessary or counterproductive interventions (eg, unwarranted chelation).

Biomonitoring results should be confidential and managed in the same manner as other individually protected health information. Public health and research biomonitoring information should be maintained separately from medical records.

REFERENCES

American Conference of Governmental Industrial Hygienists. Biological Exposure Indices (BEI). 2019. https://www.acgih.org/tlv-bei-guidelines/biological-exposure-indices-introduction.

Clinical and Laboratory Standards Institute: http://www.clsi.org/.

European Centre for Ecotoxicology and Toxicology of Chemicals. MAK and BAT Values 2017. http://www.ecetoc.org/mediaroom/mak-bat-values-2017-german-version-now-online/.

Haines DA, Saravanabhavan G, Werry K, Khoury C: An overview of human biomonitoring of environmental chemicals in the Canadian Health Measures Survey: 2007-2019. 2017;220:13-28 [PMID: 27601095].

National Report on Human Exposure to Environmental Chemicals. Washington DC: Department of Health and Human Services, Centers for Disease Control and Prevention; 2019. https://www.cdc.gov/exposurereport/index.html.

Office of Environmental Health Hazard Assessment. Medical Supervision (Cholinesterase Monitoring) of Agricultural Pesticide Applicators. Guidelines For Physicians. 6th ed. Office of Environmental Health Hazard Assessment, California EPA. 2017. https://oehha.ca.gov/pesticides/california-medical-supervision-program.

Umwelt Bundesamt. Human Biomonitoring Commission, 2018. https://www.umweltbundesamt.de/en/topics/health/commissions-working-groups/human-biomonitoring-commission-hbm-commission.

World Health Organization. Human biomonitoring: Facts and figures. 2015. http://www.euro.who.int/__data/assets/pdf_file/0020/276311/Human-biomonitoring-facts-figures-en.pdf.

◼ SELF-ASSESSMENT QUESTIONS

Select the one correct answer for each question.

Question 1: Biologic markers are
  a. distinct from *biomarkers*
  b. measurement of a chemical, its metabolite, or a biochemical effect in a biologic specimen
  c. reliably sensitive, specific, biologically relevant, practical, and inexpensive
  d. easily applied to a wide variety of occupational exposures

Question 2: Measurements of chemicals in whole blood
  a. are of marginal value with chemical metabolites
  b. reflect chronic more than acute exposures
  c. have unlimited applications for biomonitoring
  d. can be a valuable matrix for measuring adducts of hemoglobin, albumin, or DNA

Question 3: Biomonitoring of exhaled air
   a. is of no value for volatile organic compounds
   b. entails an invasive procedure
   c. may be used to assess airway inflammation
   d. does not offer a direct comparison to measurements from air monitoring

Question 4: Health-based values for interpreting biomonitoring results
   a. are chemical concentrations above which an individual does not develop adverse health effects
   b. may not include proprietary industry studies
   c. may incorporate safety factors
   d. are not used in occupational settings

Question 5: Biological exposure indices (BEIs) are
   a. available for over 100 substances
   b. based on studies that address minimal or no adverse health effect levels in exposed workers and animals
   c. levels that ensure healthy workers
   d. indicative of concentrations above which adverse health effects do not occur

Question 6: Biologic monitoring in the occupational setting
   a. may be a voluntary or required component of routine medical surveillance
   b. is required by OSHA standards for chromium
   c. makes it unnecessary to verify potential sources of exposure
   d. ignores logistics and feasibility

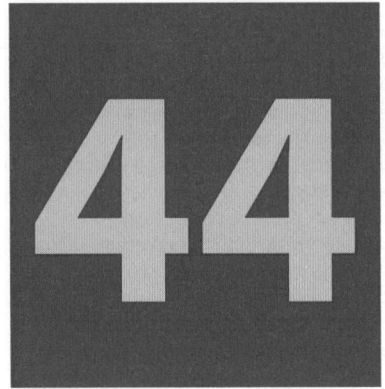

CBRNE Preparedness

Dana Thomas, MD, MPH

Camille Hawkins, MD, PA-C

INTRODUCTION

Disasters and their resultant health implications present medical professionals with challenges outside their normal practice. These events may occur naturally or be man-made. In both instances, the potential for widespread devastation is a real and ever-present danger which demands occupational health care professionals be adequately prepared to respond. Disaster preparedness for all types of emergencies from acts of nature, including pandemics, to acts of terror requires understanding of potential hazards, the ability to forecast emergencies, formulate plans, and train for response. The intent of this chapter is to outline and discuss some of the relevant chemical, biological, radiologic, nuclear, and explosive (CBRNE) events that may cause disasters at local, national, and global levels. This is not intended to be an inclusive list of all CBRNE agents, only those considered most likely to naturally occur or be purposely developed and used as weapons of mass destruction.

CBRNE release may result from natural disaster, unintentional human error, or by malignant terrorist intent. For example, in 2005 Hurricane Katrina damaged levees in New Orleans which had not been properly designed or constructed to withstand storm surges. The resultant unprecedented flooding had biological and chemical ramifications due to sewage that infected the flood waters and contaminated the local waterways with bacteria. In the 2 weeks following Katrina, *Vibrio vulnificus* caused 22 human infections and 5 deaths. Weeks later, *Escherichia coli* found in standing water was still ten times greater than the Environmental Protection Agency (EPA) permissible level for human contact requiring workers to wear protective clothing to decrease the outbreak of skin rashes. Although it took months for water distribution to be brought back on line, interim testing of potable water revealed lead and arsenic levels in excess of EPA drinking water standards. Changes in pipe ecology due to the intrusion of these same contaminants were also a threat. Additionally, homes on well water provided concern for contamination. In Houston,

where evacuees were being temporarily housed, Norovirus infections rates were nearly 20%.

When an earthquake-triggered tsunami struck Japan leading to the Fukashima Daiichi nuclear power plant disaster, nearly 16,000 deaths occurred and 160,000 people lost their homes and livelihoods. Cleanup efforts are still taking much longer than expected. Subsequent radiation exposure continues at unprecedented levels. In 2017, six years after the mishap, the Tokyo Electric Power Company reported radiation levels of 530 Sieverts per hour in the containment vessel of reactor 2, a significant distance from the melted fuel. Both of these CBRNE examples are considered complex emergencies, when a man-made disaster occurs on top of a natural disaster, or vice versa.

Increased access and exposure to CBRNE agents in the twenty-first century presents a greater threat now than ever before. Technological advances have made it easier today for potential terrorists to obtain or develop novel biological agents or highly infectious "superbugs" to be used as weapons against humanity. Global cooperative efforts have been aimed at decreasing these threats. In 2014, the United States participated in a Joint External Evaluation utilizing the Global Health Security Agenda (GHSA) Assessment Tool. The GHSA is intended to improve each country's ability to "Prevent, Detect, and Respond" to health threats by sharing best practices. The GHSA objective is early detection and effective response to infectious disease threats. Since most governments work in silos, the goal for successful prevention and preparedness is to quickly address threats and universally share information across multiple agencies, especially during a mass casualty response.

When a CBRNE event does occur, it is important to immediately recognize the signs and properly identify the cause. Anticipated effects may be direct (eg, chemicals which cause difficulty breathing, blisters, convulsions, or death) or indirect (eg, need for implementation of continuity of operations [COOP] including alternate business sites or potential disruption of public health infrastructure). The scale of the event directly determines the degree of morbidity and mortality seen.

Currently, sophisticated cyberattacks/hacking attempts pose the most significant security threats and potential compromise of critical infrastructure to the United States. The Department of Homeland Security considers critical infrastructure assets to those which provide essential services that underpin American society and serve as the backbone of our nation's economy, security, and health. This critical infrastructure is broken into 16 essential sectors: chemical, commercial facilities, communications, critical manufacturing, dams, defense industrial base, emergency services, energy, financial services, food and agriculture, government facilities, healthcare and public health, information technology, transportation, waste and wastewater, nuclear reactors/utilities and their waste. Disruption of critical infrastructure in any of these 16 essential sectors, by natural, human-caused, or accidental/technical occurrences could trigger a CBRNE event. Over 80% of this critical infrastructure exists within the private domain and is not under direct government control.

Today's national security efforts include planning and exercises, research and development, and educational outreach programs. What had been an area limited to specialized military units has evolved to include first responders, police, firefighters, emergency medical services, hazardous materials (Hazmat) response units, and bomb squads. Professionals from diverse backgrounds working in public and private partnerships have come together to address the CBRNE threats. Preparation for potential bioterrorist acts shares much in common with preparation for naturally occurring pandemics from influenza or other novel viral threats, like the SARS virus in 2004. Ultimately, a coordinated, methodical all threats, all hazards approach will result in the nation being prepared to recognize, respond, and contain a CBRNE event.

Occupational health professionals are in a unique position to contribute to the overall preparedness strategy serving as a salient part of the solution. Considering the attributes an occupational health professional brings to this challenge, our expertise and training uniquely prepares us in:

- toxicology, infectious disease, and physical trauma
- epidemiology and emergency response
- health and safety program planning and instruction
- outreach to businesses and medical facilities

▼ CHEMICAL AGENTS

Chemical agents are broken down into traditional and nontraditional categories. Traditional category chemical agents include nerve (eg, tabun and sarin), choking, blood, blister (mustards), and incapacitating types (eg, riot control). Agents in the nontraditional category include chemicals and biochemicals specifically researched and developed for warfare and are outside of the traditional compounds. Both traditional and nontraditional agents have been used

as chemical weapons, however, only those in the traditional category will be discussed in this text. So, what are chemical weapons?

Chemical weapons are agents that are normally occurring in the environment that have been modified specifically with the intent to cause harm. Chemical weapons were used during World War I (WWI) leading to extensive morbidity. The agents consisted primarily of chlorine, mustard, and phosgene. During World War II (WWII), nerve agents were developed by Germany although they were never deployed. In the 1950s and 1960s both the United States and the former Soviet Union developed large stockpiles of both nerve and mustard agents. After signing the Chemical Weapons Convention (CWC) in 1996, both nations pledged to destroy their arsenals of these compounds. As of 2018, 193 states have signed the CWC, with only three UN states (Egypt, North Korea, and South Sudan) not signing or ratifying the treaty. Currently over 96% of the world's declared chemical stockpiles have been destroyed.

Chemical weapons can be released in higher lethality gas forms such as aerosol and vapor, or in less lethal but extremely dangerous liquid and particulate forms. These weapons (nerve and mustard agents) were used in the Iran-Iraq War resulting in over 100,000 casualties. They have also been used by terrorist groups, the most notable being the 1995 release of liquid Sarin on a subway in Tokyo by a cult terrorist group. There were 12 initial casualties with one additional death occurring 14 years later when a comatose victim died. In addition, another 600 people were injured including a number of medical responders suffering effects after secondary exposure, reducing their ability to respond. In the immediate aftermath, local medical facilities were overwhelmed by the nearly 6,000 persons seeking care, many of whom had no direct evidence of exposure or toxicity. The Tokyo event demonstrated the need for preparedness at emergency medical facilities, both to protect themselves from secondary exposure and to be able to effectively triage large numbers of persons presenting after an incident. See Table 44–1 for a chemical triage table.

Table 44–2 lists chemical agents that might be used as weapons. The toxic industrial compounds listed are covered elsewhere in this text. The diagnosis and treatment of the most commonly used agents from this table are discussed in greater detail in the following sections.

NERVE AGENTS

ESSENTIALS OF DIAGNOSIS

Mild:
- ▶ Burning eyes and miosis.
- ▶ Increased salivation/drooling and rhinorrhea.
- ▶ Bronchorrhea and wheezing.
- ▶ Localized or diffuse muscle twitching.

Table 44–1. Guide for chemical agent triage.

	Immediate	Delayed	Minimal	Expectant
Agent Type	Intervention required within minutes	Intervention required, may delay minutes to hours	Survival likely, even with minimal care	Survival unlikely, even with care
Nerve	Unconscious/seizures present/or apneic. Severe airway, GI, or muscle compromise. Impending circulatory collapse	Significant but not life-threatening respiratory involvement and systemic effects. Asymptomatic liquid exposure	Walking/talking, local effects (miosis) w/o systemic involvement. Resolving effects from vapors	Unconscious, prolonged apnea > 5 min, not responsive to treatment, pulseless, brain death likely
Vesicants	Significant life threatening loss or impending loss of airway or breathing	Significant but not life-threatening respiratory involvement and systemic effects. Burns > 1% BSA or critical areas	Walking/talking, local effects such as eye irritation. Burns < 1% BSA	Unconscious, absent respirations & pulse. Not responsive to txmt, brain death, burns > 50% BSA
Pulmonary	Significant life threatening loss or impending loss of airway or breathing	Significant but not life-threatening respiratory involvement. SOB 4 hours postexposure	Walking/talking, resolving or minimal pulmonary symptoms	Unconscious, absent respirations & pulse. Not responsive to txmt, brain death, burns > 50% BSA

- Gastrointestinal symptoms (nausea, vomiting, cramping diarrhea).
- Diaphoresis.
- Urinary urgency.

Severe:

- Copious bronchorrhea and respiratory arrest.
- Disorientation.
- Seizures.
- Loss of consciousness and coma.
- Flaccid paralysis.

▶ Toxicity

Nerve agents are considered some of the most toxic materials made by man. The LCt_{50} (vapor or aerosol exposure lethal to 50% of the population exposed) of V agents is approximately 50 mg-min/m³ and that of the G agents ranges from 70 to 400 mg-min/m³. Dermal LD_{50} is estimated to be 10 mg/kg or less for V agents and for G agents ranges from 30 to 1000 mg. Exposure risk for the G agents is primarily inhalation while the V agents are primarily a dermal hazard.

▶ General Considerations

Nerve agents exert toxicity through inhibition of the enzyme acetylcholinesterase (AChE) at synaptic endings within the cholinergic nervous system, preventing the hydrolysis of acetylcholine (ACh). The accumulation of ACh at nerve endings causes repeated stimulation and continued propagation of the neurotransmitter signal and cholinergic overactivity. Acetylcholine (ACh) functions in both the central and peripheral nervous systems. Muscarinic receptors are found in the autonomic nervous system and impact internal organs such the heart, lungs, gut, and bladder, along with sweat glands in the skin. The nicotinic receptors are typically found in autonomic ganglia and skeletal muscles.

Table 44–2. Substances that may be used as agents of chemical terrorism.

Nerve agents
  GA: Tabun (ethyl *N,N*-dimethylphosphoramidocyanidate)
  GB: Sarin (isopropyl methylphosphonofluoridate)
  GD: Soman (pinacolyl methyl phosphonofluoridate)
  GF: (cyclohexylmethylphosphonofluoridate)
  VX: (*o*-ethyl-[*S*]-[2-diisopropylaminoethyl]methylphosphonothiolate)
  VR: (A 234, also known as the Novichok 7 nerve agent)
Blister agents
  Lewisite (an aliphatic arsenic compound, 2-chlorovinyldichloroarsine)
  Nitrogen and sulfur mustards
  Phosgene oxime
Pulmonary agents
  Phosgene
  Chlorine
Explosive nitro compounds and oxidizers
  Ammonium nitrate combined with fuel oil
Flammable industrial gases and liquids
  Gasoline
  Propane
Poison industrial gases, liquids, and solids
  Cyanides
  Nitriles
Corrosive industrial acids and bases
  Nitric acid
  Sulfuric acid

Use

Initially, these substances, also called organophosphates, were developed as insecticides but due to their extreme toxicity they are now only considered for use as chemical warfare or terrorism. While nerve agents were not used during WWII, Iraq used Tabun and Sarin against Iran in the 1980s. Iraq also used these weapons against a subpopulation of Kurds. In 2004, two American soldiers were exposed to Sarin while in Baghdad. More recently, the Syrian government and affiliated forces have launched more than 336 attacks using chemical agents against their own people, between 2012 and 2018 as reported by the Global Public Policy Institute. Nerve agents are considered a real threat, emphasizing the importance of early recognition of this characteristic toxidrome.

Use of chemical agents as warfare and acts of terrorism has far reaching impact which sometimes occurs long after the initial attack. On 4 March, 2018, former Russian military officer and double agent, Sergei Skripal, and his daughter were poisoned in Salisbury, England, with a Novichok nerve agent developed during the cold war. This Novichok agent is considered 5–8 times more poisonous than VX. Months later on 30 June, 2018, a similar poisoning of a British couple, Dawn Sturgess and Charlie Rowley, occurred in Amesbury, seven miles from Salisbury, with the same nerve agent. Rowley reportedly found the substance in a discarded perfume bottle which he gifted to his girlfriend, Sturgess, who died after spraying the chemical on her wrists and rubbing them together.

Absorption, Metabolism, & Excretion

Nerve agents block the normal action of AChE which is to hydrolyze (break down) the chemical messenger ACh. This creates an excess accumulation of ACh leading to a cholinergic crisis. Agents may be absorbed after inhalation, skin contact, or ingestion. The rate of absorption is fastest after inhalation and contact with mucosal surfaces or warm, moist skin surfaces. Inhalation may cause symptoms within minutes, while skin contact may result in toxicity being delayed from 4–18 hours. The agents vary in the binding to AChE, some "aging" immediately (irreversible) while others may be released. Nerve damage may be persistent, lasting more than 24 hours to days or weeks, or nonpersistent, dissipating much faster. In general, recovery requires cessation of exposure and replenishment of AChE stores.

Clinical Findings

A. Symptoms and Signs

Nerve agent toxicity may be triaged as mild, moderate, or severe based on clinical presentation. This is summarized in Tables 44–3 and 44–4. The key to clinical management is to recognize that vapor exposure results in immediate effects at the point of contact (eye, mucosa) while skin contact may present with variable effects, even delayed by hours.

Ocular effects include miosis, lacrimation, conjunctival injection, pain, blurred or dim vision, and transient blindness. Miosis may take up to 60 days to resolve. This is a prominent

Table 44–3. Nerve agent vapor exposure—clinical signs developing early or immediately.

	Clinical Findings	Actions
M I L D	No symptoms Unilateral miosis or miosis *alone* after vapor exposure Slight rhinorrhea with no other symptoms	No treatment/observe/draw RBC ChE
	Rhinorrhea with chest tightness Urinary urgency	One (1) ATNAA or One (1) Duodote repeated within 5–10 minutes if symptoms persist
M O D E R A T E	Chest tightness, cough, bronchorrhea Nausea, vomiting, diarrhea Localized or diffuse muscle twitching Muscular weakness Urinary urgency	Two (2) ATNAA or Two (2) Duodotes immediately with additional dose within 5–10 minutes if symptoms do not subside One (1) diazepam or midazolam injection after exposure to nontraditional agents Oxygen
S E V E R E	Chest tightness/dyspnea, copious secretions, respiratory distress, apnea Gastrointestinal symptoms Muscle fasciculations, flaccid paralysis Altered mental status/disorientation Seizures/LOC	Three (3) ATNAA or Three (3) Duodotes One (1) diazepam or midazolam injection Repeat every 5 minutes if seizures persist up to three (3) doses Oxygen Support airway and breathing until ready for transport

Table 44–4. Nerve agent skin exposure—clinical signs may be variable and delayed.

		Clinical Findings	Actions
N O N E		No symptoms	No treatment/observe/draw RBC AChE Provide emergency contact information
M I L D		Localized sweating/fasciculations	One (1) ATNAA or One (1) Duodote repeated within 5–10 minutes if symptoms persist Medical observation for 12–24 hours
M O D E R A T E		Localized fasciculations, muscular weakness Nausea, vomiting, diarrhea, generalized weakness, headache	Two (2) ATNAA or Two (2) Duodote immediately with additional dose within 5–10 minutes if symptoms do not subside One (1) diazepam or midazolam injection Oxygen
S E V E R E		Chest tightness/dyspnea/copious secretions, apnea Gastrointestinal symptoms Generalized muscle fasciculations/flaccid paralysis Altered mental status/disorientation Seizures/LOC	Three (3) ATNAA or Three (3) Duodote One (1) diazepam or midazolam injection. Repeat every 5 minutes if seizures persist up to three (3) doses Oxygen Support airway and breathing until ready for transport

vapor sign, but may not be seen until late after skin contact. Extreme rhinorrhea and salivation are prominent findings with both inhalational and dermal exposures. Careful and repeated respiratory assessment is critical, with wheezing and bronchorrhea being ominous signs requiring aggressive treatment and monitoring. Impact on pulse and blood pressure is variable and cannot be used as a reliable indicator of exposure. Signs and symptoms of gastrointestinal and urinary stimulation are signs of serious systemic toxicity. Sweating and localized muscle twitching may be seen at the site of liquid exposure.

As the dose increases more muscle fibers and muscle groups become involved, leading to full body fasciculations and jerking movements. Confusion and generalized seizures occur as the brain is impacted. If the victim recovers, persistent neurologic effects have been observed, such as difficulty in concentration, sleep disturbances, mood changes, and fatigue.

B. Laboratory Findings and Imaging

Nerve agents inhibit AChE measured red blood cell cholinesterase activity. In acute intoxication, especially **inhalation**, clinical signs must be immediately recognized, a diagnosis made, and life-saving treatment instituted immediately without waiting for laboratory results. After skin contact, determination of serial RBC cholinesterase activity may be useful since inhibition occurs before clinical signs. Other laboratory tests include arterial blood gases or pulse oximetry to assess respiratory status.

▶ Prevention

For research laboratory workers or at demilitarization sites appropriate chemical agent safety practices include material containment and proper respiratory and skin protection.

Antidote kits should be immediately available and emergency medical staff trained in their use. Medical responders must consider using respiratory and skin protection until they can assure victims have been adequately decontaminated.

▶ Treatment

Treatment involves elimination of exposure, decontamination, basic/advanced life support, and use of antidotes. Immediate care, administration of medication, and supportive measures can be the difference between life and death, which can occur within 5 minutes after the appearance of symptoms. Atropine is the drug of choice and will block ACh at the muscarinic sites, leading to drying of secretions. Severe cases may require large amounts of atropine. Pralidoxime is used to remove the nerve agent from AChE restoring normal enzyme activity. Benzodiazepines (diazepam and midazolam) are used as anticonvulsants. These medications are available as autoinjectors for emergency use. DuoDote is a combination of 2 mg of atropine and 600 mg of pralidoxime. Diazepam (10 mg intramuscular [IM] dose) is also available as an autoinjector. Emergency treatment recommendations are shown in Tables 44–3 and 44–4.

Prognosis

Prognosis is dependent on quick recognition, prompt decontamination, and administration of antidote. Expect full recovery for mild to moderate cases. After severe poisoning, there may be long-term neurologic sequelae present for months to years.

VESICANTS (MUSTARD)

ESSENTIALS OF DIAGNOSIS

- ▸ Ocular irritation, blurred vision.
- ▸ Erythema and skin blistering.
- ▸ Respiratory irritation/bronchospasm.
- ▸ Delayed respiratory effects (pneumonia, bronchiectasis).
- ▸ Bone marrow suppression.
- ▸ Acute pain/arsenic toxicity (with HL, Lewisite).

Toxicity

Mustard has been used as a chemical warfare agent on multiple occasions causing significant morbidity. The LCt_{50} (vapor or aerosol exposure lethal to 50% of the population exposed) is approximately 1500 mg-min/m^3. The LD_{50} of a liquid dose is estimated to be about 100.0 mg/kg. Exposure pathways are inhalational, dermal, and ingestion.

General Considerations

Mustard has a low volatility and is persistent. Mustard gas is five times denser then air, therefore, is more likely to settle in low areas and closed spaces. Volatility is increased in warmer weather making mustard a major hazard with temperatures above 100°F by increasing the rapid onset of symptoms. Colder weather retards the progression of symptoms. Mustard is an organic compound of chorine and sulfur that smells like mustard, garlic, or horseradish. Nitrogen mustards contain nitrogen and chlorine atoms. As highly reactive molecules, these chemicals act as an alkylating agent to cause tissue damage by interrupting proteins from linking, causing DNA damage and cell death. Of note, alkylating agents were one of the first drugs used to treat cancer in 1940 by using this same activity against cancer cells. Mustard also has mild cholinergic activity.

Use

Blistering agents, especially mustard, remain a high concern due to their incapacitating and lethal effects and ease of manufacturing. The potential effectiveness of mustard on the battlefield was recognized early and used by Germany, the Allies, and Italy in WWI. It was also used by Japan against the China, Egypt in Yemen, and most recently by Iraq in the Iran-Iraq war. During WWI, this agent was not used until the last year of the conflict but is considered responsible for 70% of all of the chemical casualties and for 1.5 million of the

5 million casualties. Due to the past extensive stockpiling of Mustard, it is still considered a threat.

Unexploded ordinances from this time period continue to be problematic. In August 2018, a fisherman was hospitalized in Philadelphia with extensive second degree burns and blisters after dredging up an old bomb off the NJ coast. His injuries were consistent with a mustard exposure. Fishing vessels along the Atlantic Coast routinely find munitions that were presumably dumped at sea decades before. Additional WWI artillery shells discovered in 2015 on Joint Base McGuire-Dix-Lakehurst were found to contain mustard gas. Thankfully these munitions were found and safely disposed of prior to unprotected human contact and injury.

Absorption, Metabolism, & Excretion

Mustard is highly reactive and penetrates the dermis and mucosal membranes. A mustard agent at freezing can be transported into warm environments, liquify as it warms, and slowly produce vapor. When absorbed, it rapidly reacts with cellular DNA to disrupt function and cause damage. Once reacted, it is no longer actively available and not found in fluids such as blister fluids or other biological fluids.

Clinical Findings

A. Symptoms and Signs

Clinical signs and symptoms may not be apparent for several hours; however, tissue damage occurs in as quickly as 2 minutes. The eyes are the most sensitive to mustard exposure, with effects seen at much lower doses than those required to damage the skin and airways. Conjunctivitis or injection, lacrimation, edema, and a feeling of sandy grit in the eyes have been observed.

Blepharospasm, corneal haziness, and hemorrhage may be seen as well, with blindness a potential complication. Vapor also affects warm, moist skin areas such as armpits, groin, and the antecubital fossae. Symptoms initially are similar to a painful sunburn with erythema occurring after several hours. Vesicles later develop and coalesce into large bullae over the next 24–36 hours.

Pulmonary involvement results from direct tissue injury from the upper airway through the bronchi. Symptoms include hoarseness, sneezing, rhinorrhea, sore throat, and cough. As dose increases erythema, mucosal edema, rhonchi, and crackles are observed. High levels of exposure can cause laryngospasm, chemical pneumonitis, and acute respiratory distress. Following acute symptoms, pseudomembranes may form causing mechanical obstruction. Rarely, systemic absorption may cause bone marrow suppression. Complications of less intense exposure include bacterial bronchitis and/or pneumonia.

B. Laboratory Findings and Imaging

Basic laboratory measurements include a complete blood count, arterial blood gases, and a chest x-ray. Urine, blister fluid, and plasma may be tested for thiodiglycol, SBMTE, or thiodiglycol protein adducts for postexposure confirmation.

Information on how to request this type of laboratory testing from the Centers for Disease Control and Prevention (CDC) is found at http://emergency.cdc.gov/chemical/lab.asp.

▶ Prevention

For research laboratory workers and at demilitarization sites appropriate chemical agent safety practices include containment and personal protective equipment.

▶ Treatment

Decontamination is the most important step in patient treatment. If decontamination occurs within 2 minutes of exposure, it is unlikely any damage will occur. Eye exposures are medical emergencies and require immediate irrigation with copious amounts of isotonic sterile fluids or water. A Morgan lens may be used for continuous copious irrigation. Immediate ophthalmologic consultation is warranted.

Skin contact with the mustard agents usually does not exhibit immediate symptoms. Cellular interaction can occur within 1–2 minutes with visible clinical effects 2–48 hours later (usually within 4–8 hours). Even if decontamination has not occurred within 2 minutes, decontamination still should be performed with copious amounts of soap and water. Reactive skin decontamination lotion is available for localized skin decontamination but there are no specific antidotes for mustard exposure. Over time, the area of chemical burn may require debridement or skin grafting.

▶ Prognosis

With immediate decontamination prognosis is excellent. Chemical tissue injuries from mustard are slow to heal. Severe eye injuries may take up to 2 months to heal or be permanent. Pulmonary injuries may take weeks or months to stabilize. The impact of skin injuries will depend on the extent and severity of the damage and the need for skin grafts.

▼ BIOLOGICAL AGENTS AND TOXINS

Biological organisms are bacteria, viruses, parasites, fungi, and other microorganisms naturally occurring found widely in soil, water, plants, and animals. Since many microbes rapidly reproduce, requiring minimal resources for survival, they pose a significant danger across multiple occupational settings when specifically developed to cause morbidity and mortality. Intentionally manufactured and produced to be used as weapons, they become biological weapons, pathogens, and toxins. Over 1200 weaponizable biological agents and toxins have been described and studied to date. Biological agents are classified in three categories:

1. Biological toxins—poisons from plants, animals, microorganisms

2. Biological modulators—agents that cause disruption in immune response

3. Pathogens—disease-causing microorganisms

Using biological vehicles as warfare has been practiced since ancient times with reports dating back to the sixth century BC when the Assyrians poisoned enemy wells with a fungus known to produce delirium, to Scythian archers dipping arrowheads into manure and rotten corpses to increase their deadliness, to Tatars throwing plague-infested bodies over enemy walls, and the British providing Smallpox-infected blankets to unfriendly tribes. During WWI, Germans sent diseased horses (Glanders) to rival cavalries and the Japanese in WWII deposited plague-infested fleas into Chinese cities.

Following WWII, the United States, Russia, and other nations began to investigate the potential use of biological warfare agents, including *Bacillus anthracis*, *Francisella tularensis*, as well as some toxins discussed below. While the international Biological Weapons Convention (BWC) of 1975 stated that these nations would never "develop, produce, stockpile or otherwise acquire or retain microbiological agents or toxins for hostile purposes or in armed conflict" various forms of research continued into the 1990s. The widespread availability of biological agents make them a major terrorist threat. The past several decades have seen the actual use of anthrax, ricin toxin, salmonella, and other agents by terrorist groups.

ANTHRAX (*Bacillus anthracis*)

ESSENTIALS OF DIAGNOSIS

▶ Cutaneous: serosanguinous papule that becomes necrotic.

▶ Inhalational: fever, cough, dyspnea, chest pain, widening mediastinum.

▶ Gastrointestinal: nonspecific pain, discomfort.

▶ Infectivity

- Cutaneous: estimated to be 10 or less spores
- Inhalational: median lethal dose (LD_{50}) = 2500–50,000 spores
- Person-to-person transmission is unlikely

▶ General Considerations

Anthrax, *B anthracis*, is an infectious disease that affects animals and humans. It is caused by a gram-positive, spore-forming, rod-shaped, aerobic, and/or facultative anaerobic bacterium. Spores are hardy and persist in soil and *B anthracis* has commonly infected grazing ruminants. "Wool sorters disease" was a term used to describe both cutaneous and inhalational anthrax occurring in the early twentieth century from handling contaminated hair of livestock. Infection with *B anthracis* begins when the spores are ingested by macrophage cells, become vegetative, reproduce, and release toxins. The dividing bacteria create both a protective capsule and cellular toxins, causing tissue destruction and swelling. The clinical disease takes on different characteristics based on the route of exposure.

Use

Due to their environmental persistence, *B anthracis* spores were weaponized by several nations prior to being banned by the BWC international treaties. In 1979, a release from a biological weapons facility in the former Soviet Union caused over 70 deaths from inhalational anthrax. Anthrax spores were mailed to governmental officials in the United States in 2001 causing 22 cases of disease (11 cutaneous, 11 inhalational with 5 deaths) and led to prophylactic treatment of nearly 10,000 persons. *B anthracis* is a select agent that requires CDC registration prior to possession, use, storage or transfer.

Clinical Findings

A. Signs and Symptoms

Inhalational anthrax begins with nonspecific symptoms of malaise, fatigue, myalgia, and fever. Mild chest pain/discomfort and a nonproductive cough may be present. Following 2–3 days of these symptoms, there may be a short period of improvement. This is followed by the sudden onset of increasing respiratory distress with dyspnea, stridor, cyanosis, increased chest pain, and diaphoresis. Pneumonia has not been a consistent finding but can occur in some patients. Meningitis is present in up to 50% of cases, and some patients may present with seizures.

Cutaneous anthrax first appears as a small papule that progresses to a vesicle containing serosanguinous fluid. The fluid may contain many organisms and a paucity of leukocytes. The vesicle typically ruptures leaving a necrotic ulcer. The lesion is usually painless. Edema may be present and can occasionally be massive, encompassing the entire face or limb. Patients usually have fever, malaise, and headache. There may also be local lymphadenitis (enlarged lymph glands).

Gastrointestinal anthrax is rare and occurs after ingestion. It presents with nonspecific symptoms of nausea, vomiting, and fever. This is followed in most cases by severe abdominal pain, vomiting of blood, and bloody diarrhea. Patients with oropharyngeal disease present with severe sore throat or a local oral or tonsillar ulcer, usually associated with fever, toxicity, and swelling of the neck due to cervical or submandibular lymphadenitis and edema. Dysphagia and respiratory distress may also be present.

B. Laboratory Findings and Imaging

Diagnosis depends on identification of bacteria on culture or gram stain. Lesions may also be tested for organisms using polymerase chain reaction (PCR) assays or immunofluorescence. Lymphadenopathy with a widening of the mediastinum may be present on chest x-ray.

Prevention

There is a licensed vaccine available, **BioThrax** (Anthrax vaccine adsorbed), that is effective for workers at risk of airborne exposure. It is administered intramuscularly (0.5 mL) in a primary series at 0, 1, and 6 months followed by boosters at 12 and 18 months. Annual boosters are recommended thereafter. Individuals are considered to have adequate immunity 4 weeks after the second dose of vaccine. Anthrax vaccine is not currently recommended for the general public in a pre-event setting. Pre-event chemoprophylaxis is effective with oral ciprofloxacin or doxycycline. Postevent considerations include accelerated vaccination programs and antibiotics.

For researchers, Biosafety level 2 or level 3 practices, containment, and facilities are recommended for activities using cultures, clinical materials, and potential aerosols. Sodium hypochlorite (bleach) has a high level of disinfection against *B anthracis* when used at a concentration of 0.79% with a minimum contact time of 20 minutes.

Treatment

For effective treatment, antibiotics should be given as soon as possible following suspicion of exposure. Current CDC recommendations for postexposure prophylaxis (PEP) following an inhalational exposure to *B anthracis* is 60 days of oral antibiotics using either ciprofloxacin (500 mg twice per day) or doxycycline (100 mg twice per day). Nonvaccinated persons should also receive a 3-dose series of the current anthrax vaccine. Antibiotic choice should be based on information pertaining to bacterial resistance, if known. Transition to amoxicillin is recommended in cases when the bacterium is susceptible to penicillin. This use is considered "off-label" treatment. Ciprofloxacin and doxycycline are recommended to treat uncomplicated cutaneous anthrax.

Prognosis

Untreated, inhalational anthrax is estimated to result in 100% mortality. This emphasizes the importance of containment, respiratory protection, and prompt medical treatment. Vaccination is effective in preventing disease in laboratory animals. Prompt antibiotic treatment has resulted in survival rate over 55% in the recent outbreaks reported.

CHOLERA (*Vibrio cholerae*)

ESSENTIALS OF DIAGNOSIS

- Painless, profuse diarrhea.
- Nausea.
- Thirst.
- Weakness.

Infectious Dose

CFR is only 1% if promptly treated. Without treatment, mortality can be as high as 50%. If *V cholerae* is ingested with water the infectious dose is 10^3–10^5, when ingested with food, fewer organisms 10^2–10^4 are required to produce disease.

Person-to-person: Unlikely.

General Considerations

V cholerae is an acute bacterial infection of the gastrointestinal tract. Organisms adhere to the intestinal mucosa, producing an enterotoxin that elicits a secretory diarrhea. A multitude of natural events can lead to widespread flooding and indirectly cause cholera outbreaks and other infectious disease. Cholera pandemics were more common in the early nineteenth and twentieth centuries before the widespread use of antibiotics and chemicals used to treat water supplies. When cholera is intentionally spread through sabotage of food and water supplies, it becomes a bioweapon. In 1947, the Japanese poisoned more than 1000 water wells of Chinese villages killing more than 30,000 people with epidemics that lasted for years after the Japanese had surrendered.

In Haiti, drainage from encampments housing UN Peacekeepers from Nepal inadvertently contaminated local rivers with cholera. The UN Peacekeepers support after Haiti's 2010 earthquake resulted in the endemic establishment of the disease. Almost a million Haitians have suffered from cholera infection and nearly 10,000 have perished, on an island not previously affected.

The World Health Organization estimates over a million cases of cholera occurred throughout Yemen, 2016–2017, during the war with Saudi Arabia. Fortunately, the case fatality rate has been less than 1% throughout most of the war. Cholera has occurred in waves, with 10,000 cases per week reported in September 2018. An oral cholera vaccine campaign was initiated in 2018. Although less likely to be a major threat in the United States, due to the potential for high morbidity, cholera remains a major biological threat.

Use

V cholerae is utilized as an incapacitating agent causing severe dehydration, electrolyte imbalance, hypovolemia, and sometimes death. Diarrheal illness may be self-limited or be severe and protracted lasting 3–5 days. In severe cases, death occurs within hours, if not properly identified and aggressively treated. Bioterrorists may be able to readily gain access to this agent, easily deploy it in food and water causing significant numbers of casualties.

Clinical Findings

A. Symptoms and Signs

Incubation period after ingesting contaminated food or water may be 4 hours to 5 days, the average being 2–3 days. Some cases may be mild and self-limiting after a few bouts of watery diarrhea. More severe cases produce copious "rice water" painless diarrhea with mild or moderate abdominal discomfort. Nausea, fever, malaise, increased thirst, leg cramps, and generalized weakness may occur. When diarrheal symptoms are severe, dehydration, hypotension and hypovolemic shock will rapidly follow.

B. Laboratory Findings and Imaging

It is important to properly differentiate cases of acute watery diarrhea with laboratory testing due to the potential for rapid spread and need for enteric precautions. Stool specimen is gold standard for *V cholerae* confirmation. The culture is confirmed on thiosulphate citrate bile salt sucrose (TCBS) agar, or PCR is performed. Public health officials may use the Crystal VC dipstick rapid test in areas with limited laboratory testing. However, this dipstick test has limited sensitivity and specificity.

Prevention

Ensure appropriate field sanitation, proper personal hygiene, and secure all food and water sources from potential tampering. The U.S. Food and Drug Administration (FDA) approved a single-dose oral cholera vaccine in 2016 manufactured by PaxVax. This vaccine is currently available in the United States. Antibiotic therapy is not recommended prophylactically.

Treatment

Aggressive rehydration must be instituted, either orally, or IV Ringer lactate. Oral antibiotic therapy options are doxycycline (100 mg twice daily for 3 days) or sulfamethoxazole/trimethoprim (TMP-SMX), tetracycline, or ciprofloxacin.

Prognosis

Excellent if diagnosed and promptly treated with antibiotics and hydration.

BURKHOLDERIA MALLEI & PSEUDOMALLEI

ESSENTIALS OF DIAGNOSIS

- ▶ Fever, malaise, myalgia.
- ▶ Ulcerating, granulomatous lesions of the skin and mucous membranes.
- ▶ Severe rapidly fatal pneumonia.
- ▶ Relapse and/or reactivation of disease process many years later.

Infectious Dose

Burkholderia pseudomallei:

Infective dose:	Unknown for humans (animal LD_{50} range from $< 2 \times 10^0$ to 6.3×10^6 cfu)
Person-to-person:	Rare (transmission of blood)

Burkholderia mallei:

Infective dose:	Unknown for humans (animal LD_{50} range from 1×10^0 to 5×10^4 cfu)
Person-to-person:	Unlikely (transmission through blood or nasal secretions)

General Considerations

B mallei (glanders) *and pseudomallei* (melioidosis) are very closely related zoonotic diseases with natural reservoirs in horses, mules, donkeys, and goats. *B pseudomallei* also occurs in swine, monkeys, rodents, cats, and birds. These organisms can infect humans with *B pseudomallei* being the more likely of the two to do so. Naturally occurring spread to humans occurs after inhalation, skin contact (through microabrasions), or contact with mucosal surfaces after prolonged contact with natural reservoirs. Glanders is endemic to parts of Africa, Asia, Middle East, and Central and South America. Melioidosis is a leading cause of sepsis in Northern Australia and bacterial pneumonia in Thailand. Both diseases have variable incubation periods ranging from 1 to 21 days. Treatment for either is difficult requiring multiple antibiotics, and case fatality rate is high, up to 50%, even with aggressive antimicrobial therapy. Persons with impaired immunity (diabetics, alcoholics, chronic renal disease, cystic fibrosis, and steroid use) are at increased risk.

The severe course of infection, aerosol infectivity, and worldwide availability of this pathogen has resulted in *B pseudomallei*'s inclusion as a potential agent of biological warfare or bioterrorism and is listed on the CDC list as a select agent.

Use

B mallei has been widely used as a biological warfare agent during the Civil War, WWI, WWII, and Afghanistan. The agent was used by Germany in WWI to disrupt troop transport. *B pseudomallei* infected forces during the French Indochina conflict and Vietnam War. Several countries have shown interest in these agents in biological warfare programs. The former Soviet Union developed and may have used *B mallei* in Afghanistan. Bioterrorists may be able to readily gain access to these agents and cause significant numbers of casualties.

Clinical Findings

A. Symptoms and Signs

Each disease can produce an acute localized infection, acute septicemic infection, acute pulmonary infection, and chronic suppurative infection. Disease severity depends on route of exposure, virulence, inoculum, and host health.

B pseudomallei and *B mallei* primarily cause an **acute pulmonary infection** after inhalational exposure or hematogenous spread from septicemia. Clinical presentation is nonspecific, including fever, cough, chest pain, hemoptysis, tachypnea, or pharyngitis. A more chronic form of pulmonic infection can also present with weight loss, cavitary lesions in the upper lobes, hemoptysis, and infiltrations, similar to tuberculosis.

The **acute localized infection** stems from exposure to mucous membranes, percutaneous injection, or skin contact where microabrasions might be present. The incubation period at the site is typically less than 6 days and will result in localized abscesses, cellulitis, and lymphadenitis. Fever, malaise, and septicemia may subsequently develop. The **acute septicemic infection** can include symptoms of fever, myalgia, pneumonitis, hepatosplenomegaly, and shock. A **chronic suppurative infection** can cause cutaneous lesions or internal abscesses.

With *B mallei*, an **acute pulmonary infection** can be more intense and include fever, malaise, myalgia, rigor, and chest pain. Diagnostic criteria are shown in Table 44–4. *B pseudomallei* has a more variable incubation period and is much more likely to relapse after treatment and become chronic.

B. Laboratory Findings and Imaging

Laboratory results consist of a nonspecific leukocytosis. Chest x-ray findings include infiltrates, cavitations, and/or miliary lesions. Abscesses can be seen on CT and ultrasound. The definitive diagnosis requires isolation and positive identification of the organism. While there is no validated *in vitro* diagnostic test, agglutination/complement fixation as well as PCR have been used on an experimental basis.

Prevention

Both *B mallei* and *B pseudomallei* are considered hazardous to laboratory workers with potential exposures from aerosolization or cutaneous exposures. Working with this agent requires Biosafety level 3 containment if aerosols or droplets are a risk. Respirators and skin protection are important. Decontamination using sodium hypochlorite (bleach) is effective with a concentration of 0.79% and a contact time of 20 minutes.

Given the potential for reemergence of *B mallei* (Glanders) and the high incidence of *B pseudomallei* (Melioidosis) in endemic areas development of vaccines has been studied but they are still not fully developed or available.

Treatment

Limited information exists regarding the use of antibiotics for the treatment of infected humans. The treatment of choice for oral antibiotic therapy options are TMP-SMX with or without a secondary oral medication of doxycycline. Dosing recommendations are shown in Table 44–5.

Prognosis

Due to the rarity of glanders, it is difficult to determine prognosis as opposed to the more common melioidosis. With acute pulmonary infection and sepsis case fatality rates can approach 90%. Even after treatment, case fatality rate can still approach 50%. Localized infections are typically much less severe with a case fatality rate of less than 20% with treatment. Chronic suppurative infections can last many years requiring multiple rounds of treatment.

Table 44–5. Treatment recommendations melioidosis and glanders.

Intensive IV Therapy	Oral Eradication Therapy
Imipenem 25 mg/kg up to 1 g Q6H -Or-	TMP-SMX 8/40 mg/kg up to 320 mg/1600 mg Q12H -And-
Meropenem 25 mg/kg up to 1 g Q8H -Or-	Doxycycline 2.5 mg/kg up to 100 mg Q12H -Or-
Ceftazidime 50 mg/kg up to 2 g Q6H	Amoxicillin-clavulanate 500 mg Q8H or 875 mg Q12H for adults

PLAGUE (*Yersinia Pestis*)

ESSENTIALS OF DIAGNOSIS

▶ Flea bites that lead to swollen painful nodes (bubonic).

▶ Fever, cough, rapidly progressive pneumonia, hemoptysis (pneumonic).

▶ Fever, chills, prostration, abdominal pain, shock (septicemic).

▶ Infectivity

Infective dose:	Estimated 100–500 organisms (aerosol) (some lab studies in animals have shown this to be < 100 organisms)
Person-to-person:	Respiratory droplets from pneumonic victim

▶ General Considerations

Plague is caused by the bacterium *Y pestis*, a gram-negative, nonmotile coccobacilli. This bacterium is found naturally in wild rodents (rats, mice, and squirrels) and the fleas they carry. These fleas travel from the infected host rodent to humans in search of a blood meal spreading bubonic plague. Pneumonic plague is spread by infected respiratory drops in a sick person's cough.

There have been three major historic plague pandemics. The first recorded, Justinian Plague, began in 541 AD followed by frequent outbreaks over the next 200 years killing over 25 million people. Black death, or the Great Plague, was the second pandemic originating in China in 1334. It spread rapidly along the trade routes into Europe claiming 60% of the population. The third, Modern Plague, started in China in the 1860s and moved to Hong Kong by 1894. It spread for 20 years around the world by rats on steamships. This final pandemic claimed approximately 10 million lives. During this time, the pathogen and route of infection was finally identified and contained with insecticides. Today, infection still easily spreads by ground squirrels and other small mammals in the Americas, Africa, and Asia.

Plague is endemic in many areas of the world, including the Western United States. Natural plague outbreaks remain prevalent with up to 4500 cases with 300 deaths reported to the World Health Organization annually. The most recent epidemics were reported in India in the early twentieth century and in Vietnam during wartime in the 1960s and 1970s. Plague is commonly found in sub-Saharan Africa and Madagascar accounting for over 95% of the reported cases. *Y pestis* is a Tier 1 select agent that requires CDC registration prior to possession, use, storage, or transfer.

▶ Use

Y pestis remains a biological agent of concern for terrorist use due to its wide availability and natural vectors for disease spread. Pneumonic plague may be spread from person to person with close contact. To date there has been no documented outbreak from intentional release of the organism.

Plague has had a remarkably rich history since the Roman Empire. Potentially linked back as far as 165 AD by Roman soldiers returning home from battle in the Persian Gulf. For centuries, plague has been disastrous for people living in Asia, Africa, and Europe. Prior to isolating the organism, widespread panic often ensued in areas of plague because the cause was unknown and due to the devastation from epidemics. Given the highly contagious nature and extremely high mortality rate if untreated, Plague has been used as a weapon of biological warfare for centuries. Warfare strategies are similar to that of Glanders have included hurling corpses over city walls, dropping infected fleas from airplanes, and aerosolizing the bacteria during the Cold War.

▶ Clinical Findings

A. Signs and Symptoms

Pneumonic plague presents with fever, headache, weakness, and rapidly developing pneumonia. Victims develop shortness of breath, chest pain, productive cough, and bloody or watery sputum. The pneumonia progresses for 2–4 days and may cause respiratory failure, shock, and death without treatment. Pneumonic plague may be spread from person to person due to inhalation of infectious secretions with close contacts.

Bubonic plague presents with sudden onset of fever, headache, chills, weakness, and swollen, tender lymph glands ("buboes") in the area draining the site of a bite or percutaneous exposure. Without proper treatment sepsis may develop.

Septicemic plague produces fever, chills, prostration, abdominal pain, shock, bleeding into skin and other organs, and can lead to rapid death. Disseminated intravascular coagulation may cause the skin and other tissues to blacken, especially the fingers, toes, and nose. Septicemic plague can occur as the first symptom of plague, or may develop secondary to untreated bubonic or pneumonic plague. Blood and other bodily fluids are infectious and can cause secondary exposure.

B. Laboratory Findings and Imaging

Laboratory testing will correlate with the nature and severity of the illness. Disseminated intravascular coagulation is an ominous development. Gram-negative coccobacilli may be identified on gram stain of sputum or bubo aspirate. Wayson stains reveal a light blue bacillus with dark blue polar bodies also known as a "safety pin" appearance. A definitive diagnosis is made by culturing the organism from blood, sputum, or bubo aspirates.

▶ Prevention

There are no vaccines available for plague. Wearing appropriate personal protective equipment is essential when working with the organism in the laboratory. *Y pestis* cultures, samples, and other potentially infectious specimens should be conducted in a biological safety cabinet by trained personnel wearing appropriate PPE within a BSL-3 laboratory. Sodium hypochlorite (bleach) is an effective disinfectant for *Y pestis* when used at concentrations of 0.79% with a minimum contact time of 20 minutes.

▶ Treatment

For effective treatment, broad-spectrum antibiotics must be given within 24 hours of the onset of symptoms. Streptomycin is FDA approved to treat plague, however, many antibiotics may be effective, including aminoglycosides, tetracycline, chloramphenicol, and fluoroquinolones. Prophylactic antibiotics such as doxycycline (100 mg twice daily) or ciprofloxacin (500 mg twice daily) for 10 days will protect persons who have had direct contact with infected victims, aerosols, or other materials suspected or known to contain *Y pestis*.

▶ Prognosis

Early recognition and prompt treatment should result in complete recovery. Once septicemic complications develop the fatality rate is 30–50% despite treatment.

TULAREMIA (*Francisella tularensis*)

ESSENTIALS OF DIAGNOSIS

▶ Ulcerative skin lesion, lymphadenopathy (ulceroglandular).

▶ Fever, prostration (typhoidal).

▶ Subclinical pneumonitis, respiratory distress.

▶ Infectivity

Infective dose:	10–50 organisms after inhalation or injection
Person-to-person:	No

▶ General Considerations

F tularensis causes tularemia in humans and animals. *F tularensis* is a small, aerobic, nonmotile, nonsporulating, gram-negative coccobacillus. The bacteria is harbored by a wide variety of animals including rabbits, muskrats, beavers, deerfly, mosquito, rodents, and arthropods such as ticks. *F tularensis* is also resistant to lower temperatures and is able to survive for weeks in water, soil, and carcasses. This is a select agent and any work with *F tularensis* requires special security considerations and licensing through the CDC.

▶ Use

Environmental hardiness and low infective dose have made *F tularensis* a candidate for use as a biological weapon. While outbreaks have occurred during wartime, there is no evidence this has ever been specifically used as a weapon. Prior to the institution of modern Biosafety containment practices, tularemia was one of the most common forms of laboratory-acquired infections in researchers. Approximately 100–200 cases of naturally occurring tularemia are reported in the United States each year.

▶ Clinical Findings

A. Signs and Symptoms

F tularensis can infect humans through the skin, mucous membranes, gastrointestinal tract, and lungs. The disease has an incubation period of 2–10 days. As few as 10–50 organisms will cause disease in humans by aerosol or cutaneous route. The initial tissue reaction to infection is a focal, intensely suppurative lesions and ulcers.

Ulceroglandular disease is the most common form, presenting as an ulcerative lesion accompanied by regional lymphadenopathy and systemic symptoms. **Typhoidal** tularemia presents with fever, chills, myalgias, and prostration. Subclinical pneumonitis is commonly present. An intentional release of *F tularensis* would lead to hemorrhagic inflammation of the airways early in the course of illness. This may progress to pneumonia and systemic illness. The onset of tularemia is usually abrupt, with fever, headache, chills and rigors, generalized body aches, dry cough, and sore throat. Nausea, vomiting, and diarrhea may occur. Typhoidal tularemia may have a fatality rate as high as 70% if untreated.

B. Laboratory Findings and Imaging

White blood cell counts may be normal or elevated. Lymphocytosis may be seen later in the course of disease. Chest x-rays may reveal a pneumonitis; although, lobar consolidation, effusions, cavitation, and hilar adenopathy may also occur. Diagnosis depends on isolation of the organism from blood or lesions. Clinical laboratories should be alerted if tularemia is suspected and a culture is grown using Biosafety level 3 practices. Tularemia can be diagnosed using serology by microagglutination assay or enzyme-linked immunosorbent assay (ELISA) with a rise in titer developing 2 or more weeks after infection.

Treatment

F tularensis is susceptible to aminoglycosides and other antibiotics. Streptomycin (1 g IM twice daily) or gentamicin (5 mg/kg IM or IV once daily) for 10 days are the preferred treatment for clinical disease. Doxycycline (100 mg twice daily) or ciprofloxacin (500 mg twice daily) for 14 days may be used for postexposure prophylaxis.

Prevention

Documented laboratory acquired infections have resulted from accidental inoculation with cultures or from inhalation of infectious aerosols. *F tularensis* live vaccine strain is available only as an investigational new drug from the United States Army Medical Research Institute for Infectious Diseases (USAMRIID). Laboratory work with cultures or contaminated materials should be performed using Biosafety level 3 containment practices. Sodium hypochlorite (bleach) has a high level of disinfection. Heat sterilization, autoclaving, 70% ethanol, and formaldehyde gas can also be used for decontamination.

Prognosis

With prompt treatment complete recovery should occur. Delay in diagnosis can result in a more chronic illness with symptoms that persist for months.

Toxins

Although both are produced by a living organism, toxins differ from biological organisms by mechanism of action. Toxins essentially poison their hosts rather than overwhelming their victims by replication. Therefore, infected hosts are not contagious. Toxins are characterized as neurotoxins, cell-damaging, and super-antigen which nonspecifically stimulate the immune system. There are potentially hundreds of different toxins, but few have been developed into mass-casualty weapons. Grouped according to biological source, they are bacterial, viral, algal, fungal, plant, marine, arthropod, molluscan, or vertebrate.

Some toxins are used in medicine to heal, or treat, disease. For instance, viper venom is used to lower high blood pressure and prevent clotting. Botulinum toxin is used to treat multiple maladies from migraines to wrinkles and bacterial toxins (diphtheria and pseudomonas) are used to treat cancer.

BOTULINUM TOXIN

ESSENTIALS OF DIAGNOSIS

- ▶ Diplopia and blurred vision initially.
- ▶ Weakness, lassitude, and dizziness followed by descending paralysis.
- ▶ Dysphagia and slurred speech.
- ▶ Neck weakness.
- ▶ Respiratory difficulties then paralysis.
- ▶ Full motor paralysis.

Toxicity

Oral:	1 mcg
Inhalation:	20–80 ng
Injection:	1 ng
Transmission:	No

General Considerations

Clostridium botulinum produces seven related botulinum neurotoxins (types A–G), all producing botulism. The microorganism is a gram-positive, rod-shaped, spore former and is a strict anaerobe. Botulism cases occur naturally due to ingestion of contaminated food, wound infection, and infantile consumption. All forms of botulism can be fatal and are considered medical emergencies.

Use

Botulinum toxin is one of the most toxic substances known to man. It is considered a candidate for bioterror because of the potential for contamination of food or water supplies. There have not been any reported outbreaks due to intentional poisoning.

Absorption, Metabolism, & Excretion

Botulinum toxin is readily absorbed after ingestion or inhalation. It may also be absorbed through nonintact skin or injection. Botulinum toxins attack the presynaptic terminal of the peripheral nerves blocking the release of neurotransmitters such as acetylcholine, inhibiting muscle contraction. The calculated lethal dose for humans is approximately 1 mcg by ingestion and 1 ng by injection. Lethal doses by aerosol delivery are 20–80 times greater than those measured by injection (based on animal studies). Intact skin provides an effective barrier against systemic absorption.

Clinical Findings

A. Symptoms and Signs

Symptoms begin 12–36 hours following ingestion of the toxin, but may be delayed as long as 8 days after. Weakness, lassitude, dizziness, and blurred vision are early complaints. Other symptoms are double vision, difficulty swallowing, dilated pupils, and a dry tongue. Fever is rarely observed. As the disease progresses, descending muscles weakness occurs (particularly the neck, proximal extremities, and respiratory musculature) leading to respiratory paralysis, airway obstruction, and death. Severe nausea and vomiting are frequently observed with type E intoxication.

B. Laboratory Findings and Imaging

Botulism is a life-threatening disease; therefore, rapid clinical diagnosis is in the patients best interest. *C botulinum* toxin can be isolated in feces, gastric fluid, wound and tissue swabs, and serum and will support the diagnosis. However, confirmatory tests often take 1–6 days for growth and confirmation. Treatment must not be delayed and should be started immediately based on clinical diagnosis. Tryptone-peptone-glucose-yeast (TPGY) extract medium, cooked meat medium, and *C botulinum* isolation medium are used. ELISA assay is available but takes 1–2 days to perform. Mouse bioassay is also available but also requires days to perform.

▶ Treatment

Support treatment is essential with treating botulism. Severe cases require prolonged assisted ventilation and other systemic support. Antitoxin is quite effective if given in the latent period, however, it cannot reverse paralysis so it becomes ineffective once signs and symptoms begin to appear. Heptavalent Botulinum Antitoxin (HBAT) is available as an investigational new drug from the CDC (770-488-7100). This may prevent or decrease respiratory failure and aid in recovery. Recovery may take weeks to months and is dependent on the type of toxin. Wound botulism is also treated with antitoxin and although antibiotics are unproven in clinical trials, Penicillin G, 3 million units IV every 4 hours is typically given after debridement.

▶ Prevention

An investigational vaccine was used over the past 50 years but is no longer available. Next-generation botulinum vaccines are actively being investigated. Research handling of botulinum toxin should be conducted by trained personnel in a class II cabinet in a Biosafety level 2 or 3 laboratory. Aerosol exposure or percutaneous injection are serious potential hazards for research personnel. Sodium hypochlorite (bleach) has a high level of disinfection against botulinum toxin when used at a concentration of 0.1–5% with a minimum contact time of 30 minutes.

▶ Prognosis

Persons provided ventilator support should survive and recover completely. The main risk during the illness is the development of complications during the 3–6 week period of paralysis.

RICIN

ESSENTIALS OF DIAGNOSIS

▶ Tracheobronchitis, pneumonitis, pulmonary edema.
▶ Gastrointestinal disturbances (nausea, vomiting, hemorrhage, hepatotoxicity).
▶ Systemic toxicity (liver, kidney, bone marrow, cardiac).

▶ Toxicity

The reported estimated lethal dose of ricin in humans is 1–25 mcg/kg when inhaled or injected, and 2–20 mg/kg when ingested.

▶ General Considerations

Ricin is a phytotoxic poison that is derived from processing the castor bean plant, *Ricinus communis*. Active toxin can be in the form of a powder, a mist, or a pellet and can be dissolved in water or a weak acid. It is environmentally stable and is not affected by extreme weather conditions, such as hot or cold temperatures. Ricin can be inactivated at temperatures above 176°F. Ricin is a cellular toxin that inhibits protein synthesis by binding to and catalytically modifying ribosomes. This material is highly toxic if inhaled, ingested, or injected. The clinical manifestations of ricin poisoning depend on the route of exposure. Affected individuals could be a threat to treating personnel if they are not properly decontaminated.

▶ Use

Ricin has been used in covert assassination attempts by injection. In 1978, a Bulgarian journalist and writer, Georgi Markov, living in London, died after he was intentionally injected a poison-rich pellet by a man using the tip of an umbrella. During WWII ricin was investigated as a possible warfare toxin by the United States. Subsequent research for this intent was banned in 1975. Because castor beans are readily available, this remains a potential terror agent of concern and some reports suggest it may have been used as recently in the 1980s during the Iraq conflict. Ricin is a select agent that requires CDC registration prior to possession, use, storage, or transfer of quantities greater than 100 mg.

▶ Absorption, Metabolism, & Excretion

Ricin is more toxic after inhalation or injection than ingestion. It is not absorbed through intact skin. Symptoms depend on route and dose of exposure.

▶ Clinical Findings

A. Symptoms and Signs

The toxicity, symptoms, onset, and outcome depend on both the dose and the route of exposure. After **inhalation**, symptoms occur within 4–8 hours and the primary organ system affected is the respiratory tract. Symptoms include shortness of breath, cough, and chest tightness, along with systemic symptoms. Hemoptysis and pulmonary edema may develop over the next 18–36 hours leading to respiratory failure and death.

Ingestion of ricin may cause localized symptoms of gastrointestinal discomfort but usually results in delayed symptoms of nausea, vomiting, diarrhea, and gastrointestinal bleeding within 1–3 days. Systemic absorption can lead to failure of major organs (liver, spleen, and kidneys) and death.

Topical contact with powder or mist forms of ricin could cause immediate (hours) local irritation of the eyes and skin, though should not result in systemic toxicity. **Percutaneous exposure**, however, can cause serious systemic toxicity affecting the nervous system (seizures) and cardiovascular system (hypotension) within hours. In general, if a lethal exposure has occurred, death will result within 36–72 hours from exposure. If the exposure does not result in death within 3–5 days, the victim should expect to recover.

B. Laboratory Findings and Imaging

Leukocytosis with counts as high as five times normal have been reported. Other findings will reflect organ damage based on the site of exposure. Lung damage is not a prominent feature after ingestion or injection.

There are tests available to potentially confirm the presence of ricin toxin in biological tissues. These include a time-resolved fluorescence immunoassay and a PCR assy. These are available in the United States through state health departments.

▶ Treatment

There are not any vaccines or antidotes available to prevent or treat ricin toxicity. Recognition of potential exposure, rapid decontamination of the toxin, and supportive medical interventions are the only available options. Eye or skin contact should be irrigated immediately with copious amounts of water. After ingestion, gastric lavage, catharsis, and activated charcoal may reduce absorption and systemic toxicity. Any case in which ricin exposure is considered probable should be hospitalized for observation. Supportive care would be based on the clinical findings and organ systems impacted.

▶ Prevention

For research laboratory workers, BSL-2 safety practices, containment equipment, and facilities are recommended for work with ricin. Laboratory coat, gloves, and full-face respirator should be worn if there is any potential for creating a toxin aerosol.

▶ Prognosis

If the victim can be supported for 3–5 days after poisoning there is a good chance of survival.

BIOLOGICAL PREPAREDNESS

The primary defense against a biological terror event is the ability to respond. Effective response is only possible with proper preparation and skilled training long before an actual need arises. Public health programs developed to respond to natural pandemics, such as influenza, provide many of the elements necessary to respond to a bioterrorist event. Rapid detection and diagnosis with triage and delivery of appropriate medical supplies (including mass vaccination and prophylactic medications) are critical. While training

for mass casualty events used to be exclusively the domain of military and emergency response teams, since the advent of increased terrorist activities on US soil, including but not limited to 9/11, it is incumbent on all health care providers to be ready and trained to act. A Bio-Response Report Card from the WMD Center, released in 2011, reported an evaluation of the United States capabilities that demonstrated the nation does not yet have adequate bio-response capability to meet fundamental expectations during large-scale biological event (noncontagious, contagious, drug-resistant, or global crisis). Occupational health providers have the unique training necessary to integrate into community preparedness and response planning to assist in education, response, and recovery.

RADIATION AND ENERGETICS

There are as many as 225 explosive device detonations each week in the United States which are classified as criminal in nature. Between 1983 and 2002, there were a total of 36,110 incidents causing 5,931 injuries and 699 deaths. Bullets and bombs are still the most common threat of various terrorist organizations.

The radiological threat from a "dirty bomb" is likely to be small scale but can still cause significant physical illness and death, as well as large-scale psychological illness. These devices are not technologically challenging (as compared to a nuclear device). The utilization of a radiologic device could produce major economic, social, and psychological disruptions.

The nuclear threat from a terrorist organization is difficult to assess. Three known groups, though, have actively tried to acquire these capabilities which include Aum Shinrikyo (Japan), Chechen rebels (Russia), and al Qaeda. If these or other organizations were to acquire nuclear capabilities then the result of a nuclear detonation would be catastrophic in terms of lives lost, structural damage, and social impact.

Occupational health providers should understand the acute effects of exposure as well as what to recommend for mitigation of potential ionizing radiation effects after an event. The effects of a nuclear event range from prompt effects, that occur within the first minute of the explosion, and delayed effects ("fallout") which occur over weeks.

Prompt effects, in the high-damage zone, are due to damaged and collapsed structures as well as very high radiation levels. The moderate damage zone may extend out to about a mile and include structural damage, downed utility poles, overturned vehicles, collapsed buildings, and fires. The light damage zone starts outside the moderate damage zone and consists of broken windows and damage to less stable structures.

Prompt radiation exposure can be the most hazardous. Thermal radiation will also result in those persons in "line-of-sight" exposures. Flash blindness occurs from the initial brilliant blast and can last up to several minutes. This can occur out to 12 miles from the initial blast.

Delayed effects from fallout come from contact with contaminated debris. Over a distance these particles tend

Table 44–6. Public guidelines for actions after a radiation event.

1. Shelter in the most protective building or structure possible and plan to stay there at least 12–24 hours. During this time, the fallout will dissipate greatly. Maximizing personal distance from source will minimize does. This allows for safer egress.
2. Duck and cover. Avoid windows. The blast wave can take more than 10 seconds to reach a distance of 3 miles.
3. Avoid all sources of potential radiation. Use personal protection equipment if available.
4. Tune-in to local radio stations and listen for instructions from authorities.
5. Vehicles do not offer protection. If in a vehicle, use it only to find more permanent shelter.
6. Particles of fallout come from the initial blast. Decontaminating the skin or removing the outer layer of clothing in a controlled manner will help mitigate the effects of radiation. No special solution is required for radioactive material, use of soap and water will suffice. Carefully bag all contaminated clothes/belongings.

to settle out and radiation levels tend to drop off promptly with an estimated amount of 55% within the first hour and around 80% within the first day. The pattern seen with fallout is dependent on meteorological conditions. The highest doses most dangerous to people are typically found within 20 miles downwind. The various particles, particularly gamma particles, are the most dangerous. For this reason, sheltering in place is recommended. General guidelines for the public in the event of a radiation event are shown in Table 44–6.

When a CBRNE radiation event occurs decontamination may be required. There are three types of decontamination:

1. Neutralization: Most widely used, particularly for chemical warfare agents. Neutralization is the reaction of the contaminating agent with other chemicals to render the agent less toxic or nontoxic.

2. Physical removal: The relocation of the contaminant from one area to another, less mission critical area. This removal usually leaves the agent in its original toxic form and involves neutralization at a later time.

3. Weathering: A process such as evaporation or irradiation to remove or destroy the contaminant. The agent is exposed to natural elements such as heat, sun, wind, or precipitation to dilute or destroy the toxin.

OPPORTUNITIES FOR OCCUPATIONAL HEALTH PROFESSIONALS

▶ Support for Research Operations

Research on detection, prevention, and treatment of chemical and biological terror agents remains a priority in the United States and other nations. This work invariably requires the handling of small amounts of the actual agents,

placing researchers at risk. Research work with conventional chemical weapons in the United States is under the jurisdiction of the Department of Defense, as are the continuing efforts to destroy remaining chemical weapon stockpiles. *Surety programs* insure the reliability and medical fitness of persons conducting this work, as well as work with nuclear materials and biological select agents.

Occupational health professionals must evaluate research staff for substance abuse, physical capabilities, and both medical and psychological fitness. The medical team also plays a critical role in medical response to a release or exposure incident. Unlike planning for a hypothetical community event, the occupational health professional must prepare protocols and conduct drills to react to an actual occupational mishap.

The CDC has also initiated a suitability program for researchers working with select agents. While not as defined or rigorous as the Surety program, the concepts are similar. Occupational health professionals at universities, public agencies, and private laboratories must participate in both medical and psychological fitness assessments and emergency planning. Links to program descriptions are contained in the reference section.

▶ Medical Preparedness Training

As demonstrated over the past two decades, terrorist events may occur anywhere, anytime. Emergency medicine may be on the frontlines in responding to a major chemical event; however, a more subtle biological event could present to various primary care providers across a region. Occupational health professionals can assist their communities in being prepared to identify and respond to such events.

Since the Oklahoma City bombing and 9/11, training opportunities are continuing to be developed to assist clinicians in emergency planning and preparedness. Most of these courses provide attendees with a skill set which will help them integrate into a real event. Courses are generally set up to provide an all-hazards approach and deliver basic information regarding each CBRNE or natural disaster component. Objectives are general and help promote recognition of an event, activation of appropriate response systems, and delivery of care.

CBRNE preparedness represents a new frontier for occupational physicians. The threats are very real and the need for preparedness is critical. The skill set of the occupational physician provides a solid foundation to effectively support these programs for employers, academia, and government. This should become an integral part of future training programs in occupational and environmental medicine.

In summary, neither disease nor destruction from CBRNE events respect borders; therefore, global efforts to contain disease remain relevant objectives for all nations. The likelihood of a CBRNE incident occurring during peak hours mandates a response plan that, at a minimum, will advise and protect as many people as possible. Therefore, a solid comprehension of CBRNE is the best defense against these specific hazards.

REFERENCES

CDC. Emergency preparedness and response https://www.cdc.gov/niosh/topics/emergency.html.

CDC. Biosafety in microbiological and biomedical laboratories. http://www.cdc.gov/biosafety/publications/bmbl5/.

CDC. Cholera, general information. https://www.cdc.gov/cholera/general/index.html.

CDC. History of plague. https://www.cdc.gov/plague/history/index.html.

CDC. Exposures to discarded mustard. https://www.cdc.gov/mmwr/preview/mmwrhtml/mm6216a7.htm.

CDC. Ricin toxin from Ricinus communis (castor beans). https://emergency.cdc.gov/agent/ricin/facts.asp.

Chemical Weapons Convention. https://www.opcw.org/chemical-weapons-convention.

Department of Homeland Security. Preparedness, response and recovery. http://ipv6.dhs.gov/files/prepresprecovery.shtm.

Global Public Policy Institute. https://www.gppi.net/2019/02/17/the-logic-of-chemical-weapons-use-in-syria.

NCBI. The history of biological warfare. https://www.ncbi.nlm.nih.gov/pmc/articles/PMC1326439/.

OSHA. Emergency preparedness. http://www.osha.gov/SLTC/emergencypreparedness/index.html.

USAMRIID. Occupational health manual for laboratory exposures to select (BSL-3 & BSL-4) and other biological agents, 2011. http://www.acoem.org/uploadedFiles/What_is_OEM/Occupational%20Health%20Manual%20for%20Laboratory%20Exposures.pdf.

■ SELF-ASSESSMENT QUESTIONS

Select the one correct answer for each question.

Question 1: Nerve agent
- a. vapor exposure results in immediate effects on the eye, mucosa, and skin
- b. ocular effects include miosis, lacrimation, conjunctival injection, pain, and blurred or dim vision
- c. miosis resolves rapidly
- d. effects on pulse and blood pressure are reliable indicators of exposure

Question 2: Mustard
- a. has a high volatility and is persistent
- b. is a highly reactive molecule and acts as an alkylating agent to cause cellular tissue damage
- c. has a pronounced cholinergic activity
- d. is found in fluids such as blister fluids or other biological fluids

Question 3: Anthrax
- a. is an infectious disease that affects animals and humans
- b. spores are hardy but do not persist in soil
- c. infection begins when the spores are ingested by lymphocytes and become vegetative
- d. clinical disease has the same characteristics regardless of the route of exposure

Question 4: Inhalational anthrax
- a. begins with nonspecific symptoms of malaise, fatigue, myalgia, and fever
- b. invariably causes chest pain and a nonproductive cough
- c. symptoms persist and steadily become more severe
- d. leads to pneumonia in most patients

Question 5: Cutaneous anthrax
- a. first appears as a small papule that progresses to a vesicle containing serosanguinous fluid
- b. lesions are very painful
- c. patients seldom have fever, malaise, and headache
- d. always causes local lymphadenitis

Question 6: Gastrointestinal anthrax
- a. is the most common form of infection
- b. presents with nonspecific symptoms of nausea, vomiting, and fever
- c. rarely causes severe abdominal pain, vomiting of blood, and bloody diarrhea
- d. would very likely cause dysphagia

Question 7: Botulinum toxin
- a. is considered a candidate for bioterror because of the potential for contamination of food or water supplies
- b. is slowly absorbed after ingestion or inhalation
- c. is readily absorbed through skin
- d. attacks the presynaptic terminal of the peripheral nerves blocking the release of acetylcholine and inhibiting muscle contraction

Question 8: Ricin is
  a. absorbed through the skin
  b. unstable and is affected by extreme weather
     conditions
  c. a cellular toxin that inhibits protein synthesis by
     binding to and catalytically modifying ribosomes
  d. less toxic after inhalation or injection than ingestion

Question 9: After inhalation of ricin
  a. symptoms occur immediately
  b. the primary organ affected is the central nervous
     system
  c. there are no systemic symptoms
  d. hemoptysis and pulmonary edema may develop over
     the next 18–36 hours leading to respiratory failure
     and death

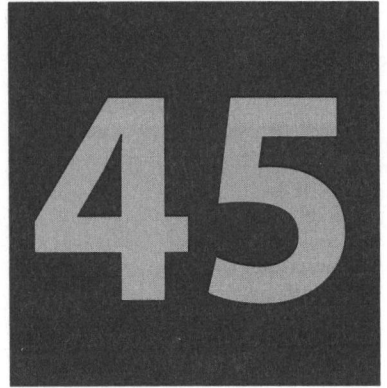

Responder Safety and Health

Sherry L. Burrer, DVM, MPH-VPH, DACVPM

Jill Shugart, MSPH, REHS, CP-FS, DAAS

Lisa J. Delaney, MS, CIH

Judith Eisenberg, MD, MS

Introduction

An increasing number and variety of workers are being called upon to respond to disasters. In 2017 alone, 16 severe weather incidents in the United States, ranging from wildfires to hurricanes, caused more than $1 billion worth of damage. Disasters are unpredictable and can be human-induced (such as a chemical spill or radiation incident) or naturally occurring (such as a flood or an emerging infectious disease outbreak)—any of which, if severe enough, can become a public health crisis.

Like the disasters that prompt them, responses can vary from large and complex to smaller-scale efforts that do not make the news. Disaster response and recovery work require a variety of workers from first responder groups such as law enforcement, firefighters, and emergency medical services to nontraditional responders such as utility workers, construction workers, other skilled support workers, relief workers, and volunteers. Ensuring the safety and health of this diverse group of responders is a vital part of any response.

After the terrorist attacks on September 11, 2001, US federal planners recognized the need for a nationwide incident management system, which led to the development of the National Incident Management System (NIMS). NIMS provides a whole-community approach for federal, state, local, tribal, and territorial government agencies as well as private sector and nongovernmental organizations to work together in planning for, responding to, and recovering from incidents.

The Incident Command System (ICS) is a component of NIMS that grew from concepts used in the United States Forest Service in the 1970s to improve interoperability with other agencies when managing wildfire incidents. This work led to the development of ICS, a system that involves a standard approach to the command, control, and coordination of on-scene incident management. Within ICS, response assets are organized in five functional areas: command, operations, finance/administration, logistics, and planning (Figure 45–1).

An Incident Commander is designated and has overall incident management authority. For small, relatively straightforward responses, Incident Commanders may retain responsibility for responder safety throughout the response, but for more complex responses they may delegate this authority to a Safety Officer. The Safety Officer ensures personnel safety, monitors hazardous and unsafe situations, and prepares a site-specific safety and health plan. Online ICS training is available on the Federal Emergency Management Agency (FEMA) Training website.

Responders work in potentially hazardous environments and can face a multitude of known and novel exposures and safety hazards through the course of their work, which might result in adverse health effects. Not all hazards present in a disaster will be immediately identified at the beginning of response operations, and the hazards can change over time as work requirements progress. Table 45–1 lists common hazards by various disaster types.

Examples of workers who commonly respond to disasters

- Traditional first responders
  - Law enforcement
  - Fire services
  - Emergency medical services
- Utility workers (such as electrical power line workers)
- Construction workers and other skilled support
- Debris removal teams
- Healthcare personnel
- Public health personnel
- Mental health teams
- Shelter workers
- Disaster relief workers
- Volunteers

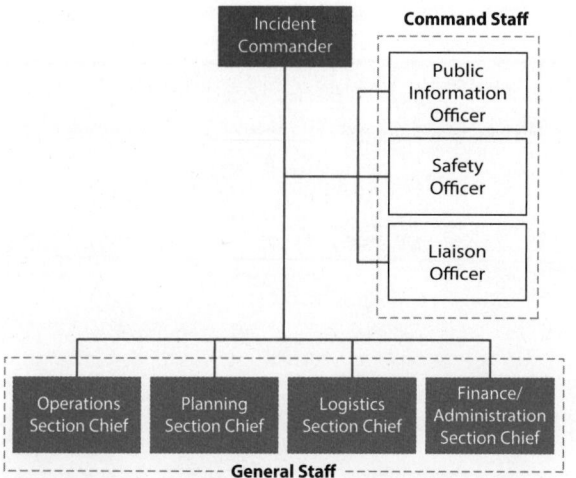

▲ **Figure 45–1.** Basic Incident Command System (ICS) structure.

Occupational safety and health (OSH) professionals (such as Safety Officers) or other designated personnel identify OSH hazards and select protective measures based on the known hazards and other OSH-related information available at the time. As more information becomes available and additional OSH hazards are identified, these recommendations can change. The use of personal protective equipment (PPE), such as respiratory protection and gloves, is the least desirable measure within the hierarchy of controls to protect responders (Figure 45–2). However, PPE is typically the most commonly used protective measure for responders, because engineering or administrative controls are often not feasible in these settings.

In addition to the risks of direct exposure to chemical, biological, or radiological hazards, responders can encounter dangers posed by many other hazards or stressors, including structurally unstable physical environments, austere conditions, long or irregular work shifts, the physical burden of working in PPE, social conflict or unrest, inclement weather, and extremes in temperature, humidity, and altitude. Psychological stressors are also recognized as a risk to responder health. These stressors include role ambiguity, fear of the unknown, and sleep deprivation, as well as psychological trauma arising from events witnessed during a response and the impact of direct loss for local responders. Even after the immediate response activities end, responders continue to face hazardous conditions as they undertake recovery efforts. Therefore, it is important for attending physicians who are treating responders and community members impacted by a disaster to recognize the many potential health hazards these groups might encounter.

Unfortunately, little is known about responder short-term and long-term health effects associated with potential exposures during emergency response and recovery activities.

After the terrorist attacks on September 11, 2001, when over 450 responders died and hundreds more were seriously injured, the World Trade Center Health Registry—one of the few, but most in-depth sources of information and support for postdisaster research studies—was created. At this time, the United States began to focus greater attention on how to protect responders before, during, and after disasters.

The National Institute for Occupational Safety and Health (NIOSH) led an interagency work group to develop the Emergency Responder Health Monitoring and Surveillance™ (ERHMS™) framework. The goal is to address the safety and health of responders across all phases of a response: predeployment, deployment, and postdeployment (Figure 45–3). The ERHMS framework, adopted by the National Response Team as a Technical Assistance Document, contains guidelines and recommendations applicable across a range of disaster types, settings, and sizes to address all aspects of protecting responders. The best way to incorporate the ERHMS framework into the ICS structure during a response is to create an ERHMS Unit. The ERHMS Unit, ideally under the purview of the Safety Officer, would comprise a group of medical and public health professionals (such as epidemiologists) who could carry out or direct responder health monitoring and surveillance for the response. The ERHMS framework and its principles will be described in this chapter.

Pre-deployment

Predeployment is the first phase of a response in the ERHMS framework. This phase occurs before anyone is deployed to any type of disaster. During predeployment, responders and organizations prepare for a successful response and establish the foundation for health monitoring and surveillance of responders. The predeployment phase consists of four key activities: (1) rostering and credentialing, (2) health screening, (3) safety and health training, and (4) data management (Table 45–2).

The purpose of conducting rostering and credentialing is to ensure all responders are properly tracked and have the appropriate training and experience to effectively accomplish the response mission. A roster should include several types of information, such as demographics (eg, age and sex), occupation, training, credentials, and licenses for each individual; it also may include background check information. Information can be self-reported or collected by authorized individuals within an organization (such as human resources personnel). This information can be collected on paper forms or electronic devices (such as tablets). Most organizations will use their own data collection systems; however, to prepare for a response involving multiple agencies, all parties involved should consider coordinating their data collection ahead of time so the information collected is in a compatible format across organizations. The ERHMS framework recommends that organizations review and update roster information for each responder on an annual basis and always verify its completeness prior to any deployment.

Table 45–1. Select disaster types and their potential hazards.

Potential Hazard[a,b]	Hurricane	Earthquake	Wildfire	Infectious Disease Outbreak	Chemical Spill	Dirty Bomb
Smoke inhalation		X	X			X
Chemical inhalation	X	X	X		X	X
Chemical dermal exposures	X	X			X	X
Carbon monoxide	X	X	X			
Bloodborne pathogens				X		X
Disease transmission	X	X	X	X		
Needlesticks	X	X		X		
Mold	X					
Radiation exposures						X
Cold stress[c]		X			X	X
Heat stress[c]	X	X	X		X	X
Noise	X	X	X			
Dangerous driving conditions	X	X	X		X	X
Safety hazards associated with debris removal	X	X	X			X
Unstable structures	X	X	X		X	X
Energized power lines/cables	X	X	X			X
Slips/trips/falls	X	X	X		X	X
Insect bites	X		X			
Stray/wild animals	X	X	X			
Stressful work conditions	X	X	X	X	X	X
Long work hours	X	X	X	X	X	X
Social unrest	X	X		X		X

[a]These lists are not exhaustive. The hazards are those most commonly seen with the listed disasters.
[b]The majority of these hazards are covered in more detail elsewhere in this book.
[c]Cold and heat stress are not results of a disaster but most often are related to the outdoor temperature where the disaster occurs. An exception would be heat stress caused by the burden of working in PPE, even in moderate temperatures.

A health screening of all responders during the predeployment phase detects and documents conditions that might negatively affect responders, including physical and behavioral health, during their response work. These health screenings are important because they ensure responders are physically and mentally fit for the job they are expected to fill during an incident. The ERHMS framework recommends that both baseline and annual health screenings be conducted by a licensed medical professional and that predeployment health screenings be conducted immediately before a deployment.

Baseline and annual health screenings are generally more complete than predeployment screenings, which can be focused for a specific incident or concentrate on recent

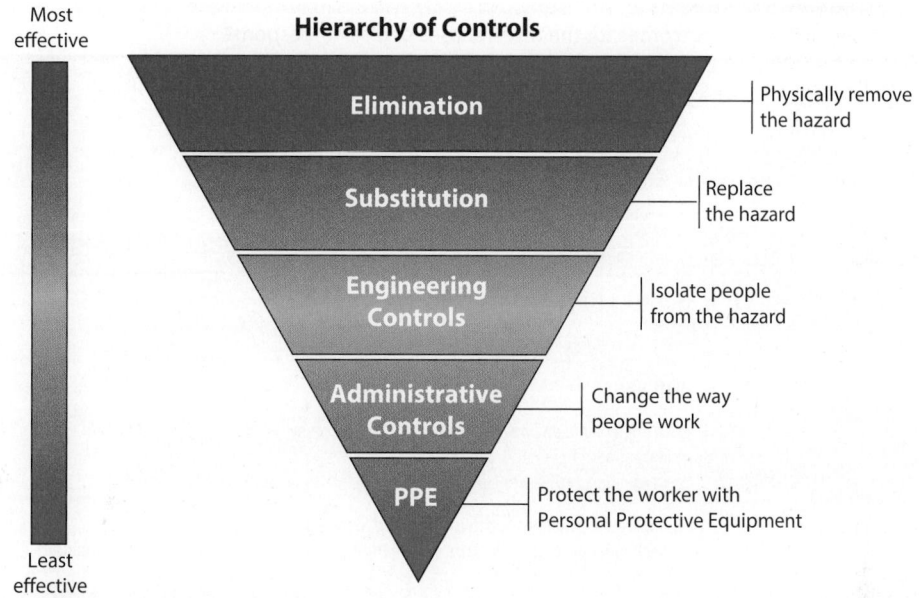

▲ **Figure 45–2.** Hierarchy of controls.

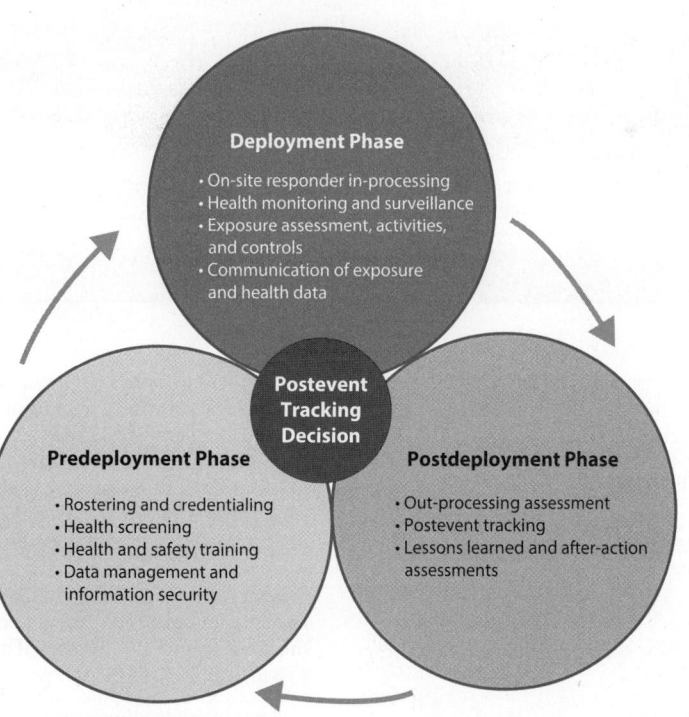

▲ **Figure 45–3.** Three phases of disaster response and associated ERHMS activities.

Table 45–2. ERHMS activities and outcomes for the three phases of disaster response.

Predeployment Phase	
Activity	**Outcome**
Rostering and credentialing	• Organization has list of qualified responders
Health screening	• Responders are physically and behaviorally fit for duty
Safety and health training	• Responders are properly trained to decrease illness and injury
Data management and security	• Data are confidential and secure
Deployment Phase	
Activity	**Outcome**
On-site responder in-processing	• Incident command has list of participating responders • Responders are identifiable by their badging • Responders receive site-specific training and personal protective equipment
Health monitoring and surveillance	• Individual responder health is monitored, if necessary • Responder population data are systematically collected and analyzed to assess trends in injury and illness
Exposure assessment, activities, and controls	• Records are created of responder exposures, tasks performed, and controls implemented for responder safety
Communication of exposure and health data	• Open lines of communication are maintained between ICS command, federal/state/local/tribal/territorial authorities, responders, media, and public
Postdeployment Phase	
Activity	**Outcome**
Responder out-processing	• Incident command has list of responders who have demobilized • Self-reported responder health and exposures are documented • Medical or behavioral health referrals are made, if necessary • Information about incident-related illnesses, injuries, and exposures is shared with responder • Short- or long-term health tracking is initiated, if necessary
Determining the need for long-term tracking	• Responders in need of long-term health tracking are identified • Type of long-term tracking is chosen
After-action review	• Successes, gaps, and lessons learned are documented and available to be applied to ERHMS activities during subsequent incidents

changes from a baseline or annual health screening. Here are examples of information that should be gathered during a predeployment health screening:

- Preexisting physical, medical, and behavioral conditions
- Allergies
- Prior toxic and traumatic exposures
- Medications
- Immunizations
- Functional or access needs, such as wheelchairs and hearing aids

At the beginning of health screening, physicians should obtain information about the responder's anticipated deployment activities, deployment setting (eg, office or field assignment), weather conditions (such as extremely hot or cold temperatures), and any other characteristics of the deployment environment that might put the responder in harm's way or cause adverse health effects. Additional medical screening can be required if a responder will be working in an area with contaminated floodwaters, infectious disease vectors, hazardous materials, or radiation; will be required to wear a respirator; or has a chronic illness or recent injury. Fitness for deployment should be determined on the basis of the most strenuous anticipated activities. Additional factors to consider include the following:

- Type of medication a responder is already taking or might need specifically for the deployment

- Sufficient supplies of medications to last throughout deployment
- Need for electricity to operate medical devices (such as a continuous positive airway pressure machine) or for refrigeration of medication
- Appropriate vaccinations required to travel to a particular location or enter a worksite

Ideally, the organization to which each responder belongs will also keep historic, incident-specific exposure, injury, and illness data for those responders. Maintaining accurate records allows tracking of repeated exposures over multiple disaster responses and facilitates monitoring of long-term health issues or surveillance for the delayed onset of illnesses within the organization's responder population. More information on monitoring and surveillance is found in the Deployment section. Organizations should document health screening information on paper or electronically in an employee's record (eg, a medical record or health questionnaire) and update it annually or as conditions change.

Safety and health training is important to ensure responders learn how to properly conduct the job tasks they will be expected to perform during a response and how to prevent injuries and illnesses. Some responders, such as law enforcement officers and firefighters, will already have specific training or certifications that are required to perform their duties during an incident. However, many new responders will not begin their career already equipped with the necessary knowledge, experience, and training for the roles and responsibilities they will be asked to perform.

Safety and health training is the responsibility of the response organization. These trainings should include fundamental topics such as preparing for disasters, understanding ICS, recognizing hazards, and practicing self-care. Training topics will also depend on specific duties and may include site operations, hazard communication, PPE, management of responder exposures, and decontamination. Conducting safety and health training not only ensures responders have the appropriate skill set but also allows managers to track which responders are trained, monitor training effectiveness by assessing illness and injury rates, and determine what training will be beneficial for future responses. Safety and health training can be conducted online or in the classroom and should be documented by the response organization at least annually.

To track the safety and health of responders, personally identifiable information (PII) will need to be collected. PII is data that can be used to determine an individual's identity, either alone or when combined with other personal or identifying information. It is critical to secure and properly maintain this information. Specifically, PII should be collected only under these circumstances:

- It can remain confidential, accurate, and complete.
- It is made available only to authorized personnel.
- It is standardized so it can be shared securely with partner response organizations when needed.

An organization should follow its internal rules and the laws of the country in which it resides to safeguard PII properly. Methods of protecting PII include limiting data collection to only the data absolutely necessary for organizational operations, deidentifying data as soon as possible (ie, removing PII), and using role-based permissions for access to data (ie, only properly trained personnel in authorized roles can access certain data).

The details of how to implement a data management system during a response and the required security components need to be established in the predeployment phase, prior to an incident. This will ensure PII and critical health data can be securely and confidentially collected during all three phases of a response and analyzed to determine if responders have developed acute, delayed, or long-term adverse health effects.

One example of an electronic data system that can be used to store data in all three phases of ERHMS is ERHMS Info Manager™ (Figure 45-4). NIOSH developed this no-cost, custom-built software as an option for emergency response organizations to use in implementing the ERHMS framework. ERHMS Info Manager uses Epi Info™, data collection and analysis software developed by the Centers for Disease Control and Prevention (CDC), to construct data collection tools, make calculations, and conduct analyses. ERHMS Info

---

Why health screening is necessary during the predeployment phase of a response

In April 2010, an explosion on the Deepwater Horizon oil rig led to the largest oil spill in US history, requiring tens of thousands of workers to support response and clean-up efforts. In reaction to concerns that exposure to the spilled crude oil or the chemical dispersants was making cleanup workers ill, British Petroleum (BP) requested that NIOSH conduct an evaluation of the responders' infirmary visit records as part of their worker health surveillance program. Review of these records by NIOSH revealed a majority of these admissions were for heat-related illnesses, medical conditions exacerbated by working in a hot and humid environment, or both. Further review of patient and contracting-employer records showed that (1) workers were not screened in the predeployment phase for medical conditions that would increase their risk for heat-related illness, (2) no acclimatization program for workers brought in from cooler geographic regions was in place, and (3) no heat stress management policies were in place at the worksites. As a result of NIOSH's findings, BP required all contracting employers to implement these important activities. A NIOSH follow-up assessment showed the efficacy of these recommendations, as cleanup worker hospitalizations dropped off sharply. For more information on the NIOSH evaluation, see Gibbins et al. (2010).

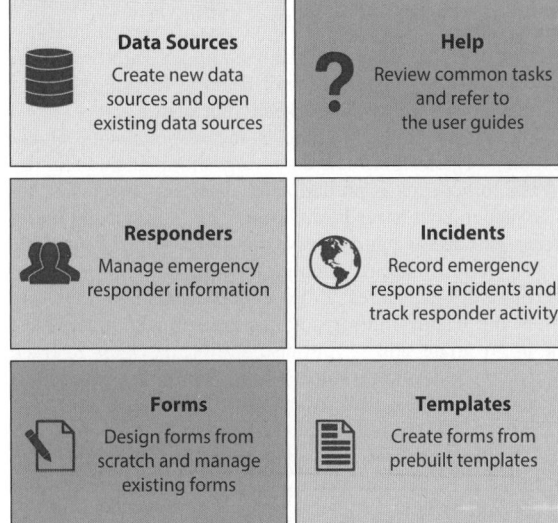

Data Sources Create new data sources and open existing data sources	**Help** Review common tasks and refer to the user guides
Responders Manage emergency responder information	**Incidents** Record emergency response incidents and track responder activity
Forms Design forms from scratch and manage existing forms	**Templates** Create forms from prebuilt templates

▲ **Figure 45–4.** ERHMS Info Manager start screen.

Manager allows users to manage responder readiness by collecting information on rostering, training, and medical screening. This information improves organizations' preparedness prior to a disaster and enables them to make decisions by analyzing exposure data collected during a response. NIOSH has also developed a user guide and training videos to accompany the software and has collaborated with Epi Info to ensure technical support is available to all users at no cost.

ERHMS Info Manager is for use by anyone involved in the deployment and protection of responders, such as incident management leadership and health, safety, and medical professionals. Data are collected on the users' computers and servers and are not collected by or available to CDC. Response organizations can also use other customizable data collection tools (such as Microsoft Excel®, Microsoft Access®, or organization-specific platforms) to store this information, as long as a data management and security plan is in place.

Deployment

Deployment is the second phase of a response in the ERHMS framework. This phase encompasses responders' safety and health while they are actively participating in an incident response. The deployment phase consists of these key activities: (1) On-site responder in-processing; (2) Responder health monitoring and surveillance; (3) Exposure assessment, activities, and controls; and (4) Communication of health and exposure data (Table 45–2).

The goal of on-site responder in-processing is to ensure there is an accurate account of all responders who are working on-site in response to a disaster. Although a roster of an organization's response personnel is created during the predeployment phase, the responders who arrive on location

may represent a subset of the entire predeployment roster. Additionally, responders from multiple organizations can deploy, as well as volunteers wanting to provide response support. Therefore, the first step in the deployment phase is to create an on-site responder roster to track the personnel who are deployed for the incident and to confirm that they were qualified to be dispatched. Ideally, each responder selected to participate in the response during predeployment was chosen to fulfill a specific role or to use their expertise to complete various tasks. The Logistics Section within the ICS structure typically checks in the arriving responders. Its staff should work with the Safety Officer and the supporting ERHMS Unit to make sure the on-site roster contains the following information for each responder:

- Anticipated role
- Education and training history
- Relevant physical or behavioral history and limitations
- Certifications (such as confined space entry or hazardous materials)
- Respirator fit testing results (if required)
- Site-specific training received
- PPE received

Additional information may be included in the on-site roster, as determined by the implementing organization. The on-site responder roster creates a repository of information from which Command Staff and the appropriate General Staff can be formally notified that additional personnel with specific training, skill sets, and subject matter expertise are now available to fulfill the roles and tasks that initially justified their selection. Policies and procedures regarding access, security, storage, and entry of new information into these deployment personnel files should have been addressed during the predeployment phase.

Once on-site responders are rostered, the second step is to issue them response ID badges. Badging provides a method to clearly identify a responder's role on-site. For small, local incidents, a badge might include only basic information, such as the responder's name and organization. More advanced badging systems are useful for complex, highly hazardous, or larger responses with hundreds or thousands of responders who might be needed for a prolonged period. These more advanced systems can more easily maintain accountability of responder movement and tasks during the response and ensure that only individuals who have the required training and security access are allowed into certain locations.

Regardless of the method, badging serves as a basis for vital deployment functions such as these:

- Tracking responder access on-site
- Rapid accounting of responders in case of emergency
- Managing responder PPE distribution
- Alerting staff about approaching PPE change-out requirements
- Tracking staff training

ID badges can be used to limit access to an area with a newly identified exposure or safety hazard until a responder's supervisor within the chain of command has received documentation that necessary training was completed and that any additional PPE necessitated by the nature of the newly identified hazard has been issued. Additionally, unique responder identification can assist in tracking completion of hazard-specific medical preexposure testing or enrollment in ongoing medical monitoring indicated by a responder's risk of exposure to the new hazard.

Site-specific training is the third step in responder in-processing. This training occurs once the responder arrives at the incident location and is often referred to as "just-in-time" or "toolbox" training. The responders receive a general response orientation on site-specific rules, logistics, and emergency procedures, in addition to hazard-specific training they might not have had the chance to receive in the predeployment phase. New or unique hazards identified during the course of an incident response also should be included in this training. Then, completion of the new hazards training and receipt of appropriate PPE before working in or around the new hazards should be documented in the responders' deployment personnel files.

On-site responder in-processing also could include information on the demobilization process, so responders are aware of the documentation they must submit prior to leaving the response and understand how all the information collected about them during the response will be protected and stored once the incident response is completed.

Responder health monitoring, surveillance, and exposure assessment are done concurrently during the deployment phase. Just as the Incident Command Staff use an iterative assessment and planning process to make adjustments in personnel and resource management as the response unfolds, repeated assessments of workers and their potential exposures are also needed. This process will identify which responders might benefit from targeted medical monitoring during their participation in a response.

Medical monitoring is the ongoing systematic assessment of an individual responder's health as it relates to actual or potential hazardous exposures (such as lead, carbon monoxide, or heat). Monitoring involves medical evaluation of the responder for signs and symptoms that could result from the hazardous exposures of interest and biological testing (when applicable). The decision to include a responder in a medical monitoring program is based on their roles, activities, and documented exposures that occurred during the response. An occupational health practitioner (such as a physician, nurse practitioner, or registered nurse) with knowledge and experience in health monitoring should perform or supervise this task. For example, if a responder is deployed to work in an environment containing pulmonary irritants or sensitizers, on-site medical staff may perform periodic monitoring of their respiratory health, including asking questions about asthma-like symptoms, conducting a physical examination with lung auscultation to listen for wheezing, or performing a pulmonary function test (PFT) to look for evidence of an obstructive pattern that is characteristic of bronchoconstriction or asthma. Ideally, the responder's home organization would have record of predeployment PFTs and biological testing to serve as a baseline for interpretation of mid- or postdeployment results.

As an incident evolves, the following data should be entered into the responder's deployment personnel records:

- Medical monitoring results
- Other medical examination and test results
- Exposures to on-site hazards
- Personal and environmental sampling results verifying on-site exposures
- Documentation of adverse health effects or traumatic injuries occurring during the response

These records should also be updated whenever new hazards are found in responders' work areas during deployment. Updates for new hazards should include the following information: environmental area sampling results that identified new hazards, additional site-specific training and PPE requirements, and documentation that the necessary responders completed the additional training and received the appropriate PPE.

When a responder is demobilized, the responsible entity within the ICS structure should provide a copy of the responder's deployment personnel file to the responder and his or her organization if requested. Responders should share these records with their healthcare providers if delayed-onset symptoms occur that could be related to exposures documented during their participation in the response. Results of medical monitoring of responders, along with their associated environmental exposure data, may also lead to their postdeployment medical monitoring. This is especially true if they had documented exposure to a substance known to have a long latency period.

Responder health surveillance is the ongoing systematic collection, analysis, interpretation, and dissemination of the responder population's illness and injury data during the deployment phase to provide objective information on which to base future OSH actions involving an incident's responders. Responder health surveillance can be either active or passive. Active surveillance involves deliberate, regular outreach to collect exposure- or illness-specific information, test results, or other healthcare encounter data. Passive surveillance relies on responders or healthcare practitioners to initiate the submission of data regarding health effects believed to be related to a responder's participation in the response.

Surveillance data sources and variables are chosen to capture information about the physical and behavioral illnesses and injuries experienced by the responder population. Response-related sources to consider include response-related records (eg, administrative injury and illness records, such as Occupational Safety and Health Administration logs) and response-run first aid stations, medical stations, and clinics. Local area clinics, urgent cares, emergency departments, and hospitals should also be considered. Additionally, periodic surveys of responders can generate data for surveillance. The variables collected include demographics (such as age, sex, and race/ethnicity), signs and symptoms, diagnostic codes, laboratory results, weather conditions, environmental sampling results, level of training, PPE used, and location, duration, and type of work. This information can be collected on paper forms, on handheld electronic devices (such as tablets), or via electronic system transfers of data (such as electronic medical records). Electronic devices and electronic systems can automatically download data into a database for processing. This capability provides the benefit of bypassing manual data entry, saving time, and reducing errors. The challenges to using electronic devices and systems can include their cost, technical complexity, and need for an adequate power supply to function.

These surveillance data are collected to assess the responder population at regular intervals (usually hours to days) and are analyzed for unusual or unexpected patterns or trends in response-related illnesses and injuries. The empirical data are used to make evidence-based decisions regarding responder occupational safety and health, to assess the effectiveness of interventions, and to inform postdeployment decision-making. This information can also be used to keep the responders, leadership, and public informed about how the response is affecting the safety and health of responders.

Even a small incident can necessitate the handling of tremendous amounts of PII for participating responders. At each step of data collection, analysis, interpretation, and storage, procedures should be in place to provide confidentiality and protect PII during the deployment phase of the response. A data security plan should define which response personnel have access to responders' PII and which personnel can enter PII into the responders' files (eg, a report of an injury incurred while working on the response, recommended follow-up care

Scenario: Identifying a trend in responder health using medical visit data

The ongoing systematic review of response first aid station records for predetermined symptoms of concern by the ERHMS Unit indicates an increase in station visits for headache and nausea but no fever or upper respiratory infection symptoms in a group of responders working in the same location operating forklifts to transfer supplies. Rapid follow-up by response medical staff reveals the responders have elevated carboxyhemoglobin levels and/or sudden resolution of symptoms upon leaving the enclosed work area as the first indication that carbon monoxide (CO) from vehicle exhaust is reaching dangerous levels at the worksite. The healthcare provider arranges for further medical evaluation and treatment of the responders, and the Safety Officer suspends activities in the area where the affected responders worked. After the suspension of activities, an assessment of CO levels and ventilation in that work area would be conducted to find the cause of elevated CO levels in the environment and steps would be taken to mitigate the issue. The Safety Officer could then provide refresher "on the spot" training to responders working in the affected area and similar locations on the risks of CO exposure when operating gasoline-powered equipment in enclosed areas without adequate ventilation.

Implementation of responder surveys

In 2016, during the Hurricane Matthew response, the Georgia Department of Public Health (GA DPH) used the ERHMS framework and a web-based survey tool to quickly develop a novel responder health monitoring system called Responder Safety, Tracking, and Resilience (R-STaR). This enabled daily health checks (ie, the collection of self-reported information regarding duties, exposures, illnesses, and injuries) on 128 deployed GA DPH responders. This activity allowed GA DPH to identify and follow up on seven reported illnesses or injuries. The use of R-STaR was so successful that GA DPH also used it during Hurricane Irma, where they identified 48 illnesses, injuries, or exposures among the 472 daily health checks received. GA DPH continues to build upon and use R-STaR during all three phases of responses. For more information on GA DPH's implementation of R-STaR, see Grippo et al. (2018).

for a specific injury, or a responder's need to be discharged from the response due to behavioral health concerns). Additionally, it should be decided what entities will be responsible for archiving responder data, how long the data will be retained, and who will be responsible for giving responders copies of their deployment personnel records. Responders should give these deployment records to their primary healthcare providers for inclusion in their medical records.

During the deployment phase, ongoing data collection and analysis, interpretation of results, and recommended actions based on these results should be communicated to more than just the Safety Officer and the Incident Commander. Newly identified health, exposure, or safety issues should be shared immediately with the responders themselves. The Public Information Officer, a communications specialist who develops outward-facing, audience-specific messaging for the response, should provide briefings at regular intervals to all appropriate stakeholders about any relevant updates on the response. It is vital that the Public Information Officer works in conjunction with the appropriate subject matter experts to ensure scientific accuracy while creating plain-language messages for the media, elected officials, and the public. Public Information Officers can also lend their technical expertise to create concise talking points for Incident Command leadership on the immediate concerns arising from the response.

Postdeployment

Postdeployment is the third phase of a response in the ERHMS framework. The postdeployment phase of the deployment lifecycle begins when responders are preparing to leave response or recovery operations (ie, demobilizing). They could be returning to their nonresponse duties with no plans to return to the response or with the intention to redeploy later. Preparation for postdeployment activities should begin immediately after the decision to deploy responders to an incident, because demobilization of responders will take place throughout the entire course of the response and recovery phases. Demobilization can happen sooner than expected because of an injury or other health concerns or at the planned completion of a responder's deployment. The postdeployment phase consists of the following three key activities: (1) responder out-processing, (2) determining the need for health tracking, and (3) after-action reporting (Table 45–2).

Responders should complete out-processing during demobilization, in addition to returning equipment and any other administrative requirements. Responder out-processing is an activity typically led by the Safety Officer within the ICS structure or their designated representative. The Safety Officer or designee gathers information on the self-reported physical and behavioral health and exposure experiences of the responder during deployment and the physical and behavioral health status of the responder at demobilization. During out-processing, long-term contact information, ideally accurate for one or more years, is obtained from the responder. This information can be used to contact responders in the future to gather from them or provide to them further information regarding their health and the incident to which they responded.

The best way to conduct out-processing for an individual responder is face to face and on-site at the time of their demobilization, because this is the ideal time to maximize participation, assess the responder's physical and behavioral state, and ensure the most accurate recall of events. Depending on the hazards present during the response, it might be necessary to have healthcare professionals conduct the medical and behavioral assessments at out-processing. If it is not possible to conduct on-site, in-person out-processing, alternatives include a survey on paper or via the web or phone preferably within 2 weeks after demobilization. The timing would depend on any known need for postdeployment health monitoring.

There are many benefits to conducting responder out-processing, and the greatest benefits are realized when the activity is completed as soon as possible during the demobilization process. If a responder is in urgent need of additional medical or behavioral evaluation, then the interviewer can make an immediate referral. Additionally, information gathered during out-processing about self-reported health status and exposures during deployment and current health status at demobilization can be crucial for identifying ongoing physical and behavioral health trends within the responder population. This information can be used to determine the need for changes to job tasks or PPE for responders coming into or still deployed to the incident and can be added to the data used to make health-tracking decisions. Eliciting responder feedback about response-related problems they encountered or issues that could be addressed will also assist in improving current or subsequent responses.

The out-processing interview is also a good time to share written materials containing postdeployment resources. The information could include behavioral self-care and reintegration techniques, available postdeployment support programs, workers' compensation claim filing processes for response-related health issues, the potential for ongoing contact with incident staff, possible opportunities to participate in research studies about responders, and how the responder

---

ERHMS implementation during the postdeployment phase

The Roseburg, Oregon, mass shooting incident at Umpqua Community College in 2015 occurred when a 26-year-old student entered his classroom and began shooting. Nine people were killed (eight students and one faculty member) and nine students were injured before the shooter engaged with police and then took his own life. Recognizing that this tragedy called for more behavioral health services for the community and responders than the small city of Roseburg could provide, the Oregon Health Authority (OHA) deployed additional behavioral health clinicians who were part of the State Emergency Registry of Volunteers in Oregon (SERV-OR) to provide surge support. The SERV-OR volunteer clinicians stood up and staffed the Umpqua Wellness Center, a free counseling center for community members and responders affected by the incident. The SERV-OR organization, managed by OHA, follows ERHMS framework principles and serves as an example of good pre- and postdeployment practices. Although organizations often have well-developed practices for predeployment, they might not have the same for postdeployment. After the Roseburg mass shooting incident, the SERV-OR organization excelled in the area of postdeployment practices. Shortly after deploying the SERV-OR volunteers, OHA staff began creating their demobilization plan. Upon demobilization, SERV-OR volunteers participated in an out-processing session that consisted of a facilitated group discussion and individual debriefs with a clinician to assess their behavioral health and determine any need for additional resources at their home base. As a result of gaps identified in the after-action report, OHA developed an improvement plan and continues to exercise that plan with its SERV-OR behavioral health team. For more information on SERV-OR's implementation of the ERHMS framework, see Saito (2018).

information collected during the response will be protected and stored once the incident response is completed. Providing a welcome-home letter to all responders who are demobilized is often an effective way to share that information. This letter may also include a short summary of the disaster (event description, duration, documented hazards, etc.), so healthcare providers can better understand the context of any documented exposures to potentially hazardous substances and biological testing responders may have had during their participation in the response. Figure 45–5 is a basic letter template that can be customized to address any situation or include additional information. In addition to sharing resources and a welcome-home letter, during demobilization is an opportune time for out-processing staff to provide the responder with his or her deployment personnel file and assure them that their information will be treated securely and confidentially, no matter the phase of deployment. The deployment personnel files should contain documentation and sampling results of exposures encountered during deployment as well as tailored recommendations for medical monitoring follow-up, if appropriate. It is also important to impress on responders how essential it is to participate in postdeployment surveillance or monitoring (if necessary) after they return home.

The need to monitor responders postdeployment will vary from no need to self-reported monitoring to monitoring by a healthcare or public health professional as part of a health-tracking program. The level of monitoring needed is based on the hazards present, a responder's documented or potential exposures during response, and the potential for adverse health effects associated with exposure hazards. If self-reported monitoring is required, then responders should

---

[Place of Deployment] Post-Deployment Health Information for Responders

Welcome back and thank you for a job well done during your deployment! Please read the following document to familiarize yourself with illnesses that may be more common in individuals that have been to/involved in [Place of Deployment]. Information in this material will help alert you to health concerns (injury, illness, and mental health) that may need further evaluation.

Things to tell your doctor:

- If you are experiencing symptoms such as [symptoms of deployment disease of concern – if applicable – example: fever, flu-like illness, chills, headache, joint/muscle aches]
- If you were injured or have wounds that are not healing well while in/involved in [Place of Deployment]
- If you feel depressed, confused, have trouble sleeping, or have a hard time adjusting back into your home environment
- If you were bitten or scratched by an animal while in [Place of Deployment]
- If you believe you were exposed to hazards such as dust, pathogens, or chemicals and continue to have persistent health problems

What to watch for in the next few weeks:

If you experience symptoms or conditions discussed in this document or have other concerning symptoms not listed, please see your doctor as soon as possible.

[List of the symptoms you would most likely see with the diseases of concern for the location or incident personnel were involved in]

EXAMPLE

increased stress, difficulty adjusting to routine, sleeplessness, persistent sadness, depression

Illnesses More Common in Individuals Who Have Been to/Involved in [Place of Deployment]

[List potential exposures, illnesses, injuries, or mental health issues common to the locale or incident (examples: TB, Japanese encephalitis, dust/asbestos, mental health…). Here go into more detail about causes, latency periods, symptoms.]

▲ **Figure 45–5.** Welcome-home letter template.

receive information during out-processing on how to self-monitor for behavioral or physical signs and symptoms and how to report them if they occur. If it is necessary to establish health tracking, then responders can be given information on how to enroll in a short- or long-term health-tracking program.

Determining the need for health tracking and how long the tracking should be conducted is one of the critical decisions made during the postdeployment phase. Tracking can last for varying amounts of time, weeks to years, depending on the exposures experienced by a responder. The information gathered as part of responder out-processing during the postdeployment phase is combined with information collected during the predeployment and deployment phases (eg, demographics, predeployment health status, hazards and exposures encountered during deployment) to determine the length of time responders should be tracked. Short-term health tracking is typically used to follow responders for the incubation period of infectious diseases, such as avian influenza or Ebola virus disease. Though it can also be used to monitor short-onset behavioral health issues, environmental exposures causing short-lived conditions, and progress of injuries or illnesses that are expected to quickly resolve. Long-term health tracking is used to follow long-term adverse health effects or identify the delayed onset of health effects that could develop because of a responder's deployment experience. Some examples of adverse health effects that are long-term and/or can have delayed or variable onset are allergies, asthma, silicosis, specific cancers, and posttraumatic stress disorder.

To determine the need for postdeployment responder health tracking, the exposure and health data from all responders are analyzed. Often medical professionals (such as occupational physicians) work with statisticians and epidemiologists to analyze and interpret the data to determine if any responders might benefit from short-term or long-term health tracking. If the data are insufficient for this purpose, a gap analysis can determine what additional information is needed, and then that data should be sought. With enough information, a conclusion will be reached that health tracking will benefit no responders, a subset of responders, or all responders. If health tracking is needed, the duration (short- or long-term) will also be determined using the parameters previously mentioned.

Long-term health tracking can involve one or more of the following types of programs: medical surveillance, medical monitoring, responder research, and periodic health surveys. When long-term tracking is determined to be necessary, sometimes a registry is created. In the context of the ERHMS framework, a registry is a database of the select group of responders determined to need long-term tracking. Ideally, the decision to create a registry is made shortly after an incident has occurred; however, more often, this determination is made late in the response or recovery periods of a disaster, after many responders have been deployed or have completed their deployment. For this reason, the on-site responder roster, work tasks, and

How one registry has benefited responders, survivors, and the research community

The World Trade Center (WTC) Health Registry, based in the New York City Department of Health and Mental Hygiene, tracks 71,431 enrolled responders and survivors of the terrorist attacks in the United States on September 11, 2001 (9/11). The Registry has been able to communicate a wealth of information to responders, survivors, researchers, policy makers, and the public. It shares research findings and information on resources, such as the WTC Health Program that provides medical monitoring and treatment, with enrollees and the public. These resources help those affected by 9/11 make informed decisions about their health. Information is disseminated via multiple channels, including a comprehensive website, annual reports, e-newsletters, social media, targeted mailings, press announcements, and stakeholder meetings.

Communications with enrollees are designed to keep them engaged with the Registry for the long term and to obtain enrollees' updated contact information. This in turn enhances enrollees' participation in follow-up health surveys and nested studies to track and understand long-term changes in physical and mental health, quality of life, and gaps in care. Through such studies, it has been proven that select respiratory diseases, mental health disorders, cancers, and other conditions are associated with exposure to the events of 9/11.

The Registry works with community, labor, and other stakeholders to keep them informed and to acquire input on various research studies and surveys. Registry researchers disseminate findings at scientific conferences and through peer-reviewed journals. For over 15 years, Registry findings have helped to inform health and compensation policy for survivors and responders affected by 9/11. Additionally, the Registry helps thousands of enrollees and their families by linking them to healthcare through the WTC Health Program. More information about this Registry can be found on the WTC Health Registry website.

location information from the deployment phase and the long-term contact information collected during postdeployment are useful resources for determining who should be included in a registry.

The information usually collected as part of a registry can be used to provide postdeployment information (and sometimes care) to responders and others. It also can be used to conduct research to learn more about the effects of occupational and environmental exposures and to determine disease characteristics and risk factors. Though registries are challenging and can require a considerable amount of resources, when successfully implemented they have provided a wealth of information to the responders and the scientific research community. The World Trade Center Health Registry is a well-known example; it was created to track the long-term health and gaps in care of recovery workers and responders to the terrorist attacks of September 11, 2001, as well as people who lived, worked, or went to school in lower Manhattan. Registries should be undertaken only if necessary, because they are resource intensive regarding personnel, administrative oversite, participant privacy and confidentially, funding, and data storage, security, and management.

For any type of long-term health tracking of responders, additional considerations are program type, purpose, management, desired overall outcomes, and long-term funding. Other factors important to the success of these long-term programs must also be established:

- Duration and scope of data collection
- Clear ownership of data
- Data use policies
- Database management processes
- Rules for participant privacy and confidentiality
- Data security protocols
- Member and stakeholder communications

Regardless of the duration of use, all information and data collected in the postdeployment period should be handled with the same level of security and confidentiality mentioned for the previous phases of predeployment and deployment, ensuring that the rules surrounding PII and confidentiality are adhered to closely. Further considerations are long-term database ownership, management, and storage of the data collected during postdeployment. Small, local-level responses sometimes involve few data, only one or two response organizations, and a clearly established, standard data disposition protocol. However, for larger responses involving multiple or more complex exposures, a large amount of data, and numerous organizations, data-sharing agreements ideally should be established in advance of potential incidents or shortly after an incident has begun.

After a response has concluded, it is important to conduct a review and create an after-action report (AAR). More information on AARs can be found in the U.S. Department of Homeland Security document entitled *Homeland Security Exercise and Evaluation Program (HSEEP)*. An AAR will document successes, challenges, gaps, and lessons learned and establish recommendations for improving processes for subsequent responses. The individual or group within the response that conducts ERHMS activities should complete an internal AAR to create a detailed assessment of ERHMS activities. More than one AAR may be necessary to capture all of the information to make impactful recommendations for future responses. Overarching details of how an organization responded to a disaster and how the ERHMS activities related to the overall response should be included in the larger, response-wide AAR. The successes, gaps, and lessons learned can then be used to adjust how ERHMS activities are operationalized moving forward.

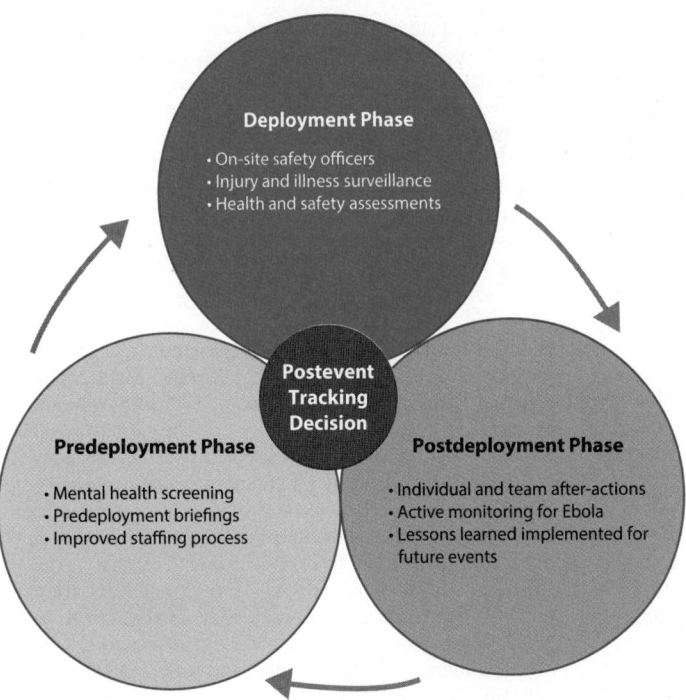

▲ **Figure 45–6.** ERHMS activities implemented during the Centers for Disease Control and Prevention response to the 2014 Ebola outbreak.*

*For more information on how CDC used ERHMS during this response, see Funk (2017).

Summary

Disasters vary in size and intensity, but response and recovery always involve a variety of workers to ensure success. These workers often operate in unstable environments with multiple OSH hazards. The ERHMS framework provides recommendations and tools that can help organizations ensure the safety and health of their responders when preparing for, responding to, and recovering from a disaster. The framework is scalable and flexible, so it can be implemented by both large and small organizations, and the activities listed in the framework are suggestions that organizations can adjust to fit their needs (Table 45–2). Figure 45–6 gives a brief description of the ERHMS activities that CDC conducted during all three phases of its response to the 2014 Ebola outbreak.

Disclaimers

The findings and conclusions in this chapter are those of the author(s) and do not necessarily represent the official position of the National Institute for Occupational Safety and Health, Centers for Disease Control and Prevention.

Mention of any company or product does not constitute endorsement by the National Institute for Occupational Safety and Health, Centers for Disease Control and Prevention.

In addition, citations to websites external to NIOSH do not constitute NIOSH endorsement of the sponsoring organizations or their programs or products. Furthermore, NIOSH is not responsible for the content of these websites. All web addresses referenced in this document were accessible as of the publication date.

REFERENCES

Centers for Disease Control and Prevention: Epi Info™. https://www.cdc.gov/epiinfo/index.html. 2018.

Centers for Disease Control and Prevention, National Institute for Occupational Safety and Health: Emergency Responder Health Monitoring and Surveillance (ERHMS). https://www.cdc.gov/niosh/erhms/default.html. 2018.

Federal Emergency Management Agency: National Incident Management System, 3rd ed. Funk R. In: J Horney, ed. *Applications: Emergency Responder Health Monitoring and Surveillance.* Salt Lake City, UT: Academic Press, 2018:121-128.

Gibbins J, West C, Dowell C, King B, Niemeier T: Health hazard evaluation of Deepwater Horizon response workers: NIOSH health hazard evaluation interim report #2. https://www.cdc.gov/niosh/hhe/pdfs/interim_report_2.pdf. 2010.

Grippo J, Edison L, Soetebier K, Drenzek C: Responder safety, tracking, and resilience—Georgia, 2016–2017. Online J Public Health Inform. 2018;10:e165. https://journals.uic.edu/ojs/index.php/ojphi/article/view/8958.

Jackson BA et al: Introduction, In: *Protecting Emergency Responders: Lessons Learned from Terrorist Attacks.* 3rd ed. Santa Monica, CA: Rand, 2002:1-4.

National Oceanic and Atmospheric Administration, National Centers for Environmental Information: U.S. Billion-Dollar Weather and Climate Disasters. https://www.ncdc.noaa.gov/billions/. 2019.

National Response Team: Emergency Responder Health Monitoring and Surveillance™ NRT Technical Assistance Document. https://www.nrt.org/sites/2/files/ERHMS_Final_060512.pdf. 2012.

Saito AM: Vignette from recent responses: Roseburg, Oregon mass shooting. In: J Horney J, ed. *Disaster Epidemiology: Methods and Applications.* Salt Lake City, UT: Academic Press, 2018:136-137.

ADDITIONAL RESOURCES

NIOSH Emergency Preparedness and Response Program Website at: https://www.cdc.gov/niosh/programs/epr/.

Online course FEMA IS-930: Emergency Responder Health monitoring and Surveillance (ERHMS) Training.

U.S. Department of Homeland Security's Homeland Security Exercise and Evaluation Program at https://www.fema.gov/emergency-managers/national-preparedness/exercises/hseep.

U.S. Federal Emergency Management Agency (FEMA) Training Website at: https://www.fema.gov/training-0.

World Health Organization Occupational safety and health in public health emergencies: A manual for protecting health workers and responders at https://www.who.int/occupational_health/Web_OSH_manual.pdf.

World Trade Center Health Registry website at: https://www1.nyc.gov/site/911health/about/wtc-health-registry.page.

■ SELF-ASSESSMENT QUESTIONS

Select the one correct answer for each question.

Question 1: Baseline and annual health screenings are
a. not interested in the responder's anticipated deployment activities or the deployment setting
b. primarily directed at requirements to wear masks and other protective equipment, a requirement of work in hazardous settings
c. generally more complete than predeployment screenings, which can be focused for a specific incident or concentrate on recent changes from a baseline or annual health screening
d. functions of the organization to which each responder belongs and his/her experience in work with government agencies

Question 2: Safety and health training

   a. need not include topics such as preparing for disasters

   b. does not depend on specific duties such as hazard communication

   c. should not be conducted online because documentation is required

   d. is the responsibility of the response organization

Question 3: The first step in the ERHMS deployment phase is

   a. to create an on-site responder roster to track the personnel who are deployed for the incident and to confirm that they were qualified to be dispatched

   b. the selection of responders to track the personnel who are deployed for the incident

   c. the development of a roster of participants based on expertise to complete various tasks

   d. issuing ID badges to clearly identify a responder's role on site

Principles of Environmental Health

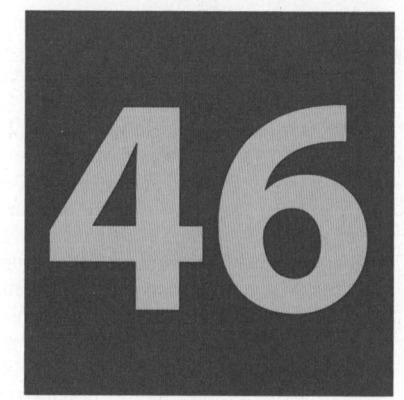

Gina M. Solomon, MD, MPH

Physicians are increasingly called upon to address questions related to environmental health. Pollution of air and water, contamination of food, releases from nearby activities such as industrial facilities or waste sites, and hazards in the home are all common causes for concern among patients, community members, the media, and public officials. All health care providers should understand how to approach clinical and public health problems in environmental health, as well as the similarities and differences between occupational health and environmental health.

Although environmental health issues are important worldwide, the severity and nature of the problem differs geographically. Many developed countries have taken significant steps to address pervasive problems such as air pollution and contamination of drinking water. These countries continue to face issues around the safety of chemicals in consumer products, legacy contamination from historic land uses, and emerging concerns about recently identified chemical hazards. Disasters, such as fires, floods, major wind events, and industrial upset conditions can bring environmental health issues to the forefront, even in developed countries.

Developing countries, in contrast, have faced enormous increases in pollution. The dramatic expansion in motor vehicles worldwide, the shift of industrial production to nations where environmental laws are less stringent and their enforcement is often nonexistent, and the practice of shipping hazardous waste to less-developed countries for recycling or storage, have all created massive and relatively new environmental problems around the globe. Mining and petroleum drilling operations have caused serious environmental contamination with heavy metals and hydrocarbons (HC), respectively. Indoor use of cookstoves is now recognized to be one of the most significant environmental health threats to women's and children's health globally. Overall, air pollution and contamination of the water and food supply are very serious concerns in the developing world. Global threats such as climate change, depletion of natural resources, loss of biodiversity, and the pervasive presence of persistent, bioaccumulative chemicals in the environment threaten health throughout the world.

Clinicians may encounter patients known to have been exposed to an environmental hazard, or who believe they may have sustained such an exposure. In some cases, an entire community may be affected by a natural or technologic disaster, or because of a discovery such as contaminants in the water supply or an apparent disease cluster. These situations require careful evaluation, including a thorough exposure history and quantification—where possible—of exposure levels. A basic understanding of major issues in environmental health can help to address individual patient and community issues, and can help identify public health threats if they exist.

AN APPROACH TO ENVIRONMENTAL HEALTH

Although workplace exposures to industrial chemicals are often far higher than environmental pollution levels, environmental exposures can be a significant concern. Lower-level exposures are an issue when the size of the exposed population is sufficient that even fairly rare or subtle health effects may have public health importance. For example, a chemical that confers a cancer risk, at environmental exposure levels, of one extra case per 100,000 people is of considerable importance when the base population exposed includes millions of people. Similarly, a 10 mcg/dL increase in blood lead is associated with a 2–3 point decrease in IQ of exposed children. A slight decrease in IQ may not seem significant on an individual basis, but across a population of children exposed to lead such a decrement shifts the entire distribution of child IQ scores downward, resulting in a substantial increase in the number of children falling into categories that require special education services.

Although environmental exposures are often lower than exposures in the workplace, there are many exceptions. For example, the populations most highly exposed to organic mercury compounds are heavy fish consumers, not industrial workers. Exposures to arsenic are frequently higher from naturally occurring arsenic contamination in drinking water worldwide than in workplace settings. Inhalation of radon gas is primarily a problem in the residential environment. In addition, the widespread popularity of chemical-intensive hobbies can lead to significant nonoccupational exposures. Art products, home-improvement products, automotive products, solders, dyes, adhesives, and solvents are often used in similar ways in workplace and home settings; in the home, people may be less likely to have adequate safety training, personal protective equipment, ventilation, and disposal practices, so exposures may be higher than in the workplace.

Many workers in chemically exposed industries are healthy adult males. In contrast, the general population includes pregnant women, young children, those with underlying disease or poor nutritional status, and the elderly. Each of these groups may face increased risk from environmental exposure. For example, toddlers engage in frequent hand-to-mouth activity, meaning that they consume more contaminants (such as lead, pesticides, polycyclic aromatic hydrocarbons [PAHs], or flame retardants) in house dust or soil. Fetuses and young children are more susceptible to long-term damage from neurotoxicants or endocrine disruptors because of the critical phases of brain and reproductive system development during gestation and infancy. The elderly, and those with underlying cardiovascular or respiratory disease, are more likely to suffer severe and sometimes fatal complications from exposure to air pollution.

Environmental exposures can therefore be important and can lead to disease for multiple reasons: They affect large numbers of people, the exposures are high to some subpopulations, and underlying vulnerabilities in the population increase susceptibility to health effects with lower-level exposures.

Data on Environmental Exposures and Hazards

Environmental health issues can be very difficult to assess. Exposures are often complex, cumulative, and difficult to quantify; diseases are often multifactorial with long latencies; important information is often patchy or absent. For example, due to Confidential Business Information (CBI) claims, it can be difficult or impossible to get full ingredients information for many consumer products. Current law in the United States does not mandate toxicity testing before chemicals are introduced into consumer products, so even if ingredients are known, little or no toxicity information may be available. Of the roughly 100,000 chemicals on the market today, of which about 3000 are produced and used in amounts over a million pounds per year, only a few hundred have been tested for toxicity using standard laboratory animal methods. Reporting of chemical releases to the environment from industry—in countries where reporting is mandated—includes several hundred toxic chemicals, and analytical chemistry testing of environmental media focuses on a similar subset of chemicals. The result is that many potentially hazardous chemicals have not undergone toxicity testing, and are not prioritized for emissions reporting or environmental monitoring, leading to insufficient information on the potential health risk from thousands of chemicals.

In addition to the above limitations, population-based studies in environmental health are difficult to perform. Retrospective studies almost universally suffer from very large exposure uncertainty, which tends to bias toward null results. Prospective studies are often prohibitively expensive because they require following a cohort of individuals for years or decades to assess health effects over time. Cross-sectional studies, which assess both exposure and health status at the same time, can be useful for generating hypotheses for future research, but are often subject to confounding by multiple variables and cannot demonstrate a temporal cause-effect relationship.

In recent years, the limitations of toxicity and exposure information, and the prohibitive expense of doing thorough testing on tens of thousands of chemicals, has led to an explosion of new scientific methods that focus on predicting the toxicity and exposure patterns of chemicals based on new types of data. For example, high-throughput cell-based assays can identify chemicals that have endocrine activity or exhibit cytotoxicity, mutagenicity, or other characteristics that may predict human toxicity. Chemical structure can be used to predict persistence, bioaccumulation potential, toxicity, and even chemical uses in commerce. The science of toxicogenomics allows tools that have been developed in medicine to be used to predict chemical toxicity. Nonmammalian models such as zebrafish embryos have been increasingly used as models of developmental toxicity and neurotoxicity, allowing rapid screening of thousands of chemicals in these organisms for complex endpoints. Clinicians who encounter new data streams, such as cell-based assays, informatics, or nonmammalian methods, may find them challenging to interpret. These types of data will become ever more common and will often be the only type of information available on chemicals. One advantage of the new methods is that they often screen a wide range of concentrations of chemicals, including levels that are relevant to environmental and occupational exposure. Many of these methods also use human cell cultures. For these reasons, some of the historical challenges with interpretation of high-dose rodent studies have been addressed with the emerging methods, only to be replaced with a new set of interpretation challenges.

The new science of toxicology focuses on the biological pathways that are perturbed by chemicals. This scientific effort has demonstrated that many of the same important biological pathways underlie multiple human diseases. For example, a chronic inflammatory state is associated with diseases ranging from asthma to diabetes, cardiovascular disease, cancer, and Alzheimer's dementia. The ultimate disease manifestation in an individual may depend on the timing, duration, and route of exposure, as well as multiple host and environmental factors. With this complexity in mind, it becomes possible to regard chemicals that activate important biological pathways at low concentrations as potentially hazardous, and develop guidance to minimize exposure based on this information.

THE MAGNITUDE OF ENVIRONMENTAL CONTAMINATION

Although about 90% of community drinking water systems meet health-based standards each year, nearly 21 million people in mostly rural parts of the United States are still served by one of the over 4000 drinking water systems that reported at least one violation of a health-based drinking water standard. About 10% of people in the United States obtain their water from private wells that are not regulated or tested for contamination. Air quality in the United States has significantly improved in recent years and air pollution emissions have dropped, but nearly 134 million people in 215 counties in the United States live in areas that exceed one or more of the primary air pollution standards.

In the United States in 2016 over 3.4 billion pounds of toxic chemicals were disposed of or released into the environment (ie, air, water, or land); releases to air have decreased over time, while disposal of waste on land has slightly increased. Over half the US population lives within 3 miles of one of the over 18,000 hazardous waste generators, storage, or clean-up sites that collectively occupy about 22 million acres of land. Nonwhite people are between 1.7 and 2.3 times more likely to live in a neighborhood with a hazardous waste facility compared with white residents of the United States. Significant racial and income disparities have also been reported for proximity to other environmental pollutants.

Globally, the situation is dire. According to the World Health Organization (WHO), air pollution from outdoor sources kills about 4.2 million people per year, with 91% of people on the planet breathing air that is unhealthy according to WHO guidelines. Indoor air pollution from use of solid fuels is estimated to cause over 3.8 million deaths annually. Ninety countries are facing water stress, with polluted or overdrawn water supplies. Globally, 663 million people lack clean water. In 2015, the WHO estimated that 2.4 billion people globally do not have access to sanitation facilities.

In 2018, the Lancet Commission reported that "Pollution is the largest environmental cause of disease and premature death in the world today." The Commission concluded that diseases caused by pollution cause an estimated 9 million premature deaths each year—16% of all deaths worldwide. The impacts of pollution are not homogenous, with some countries more severely affected. In the most polluted countries, pollution-related disease is responsible for more than a quarter of all deaths.

MAJOR ENVIRONMENTAL HEALTH ISSUES

Many significant environmental health issues are discussed elsewhere in this textbook. Preceding chapters on specific chemicals and diseases, surveillance, and biomonitoring contain issues relevant to environmental health, as do all the chapters that follow this chapter. Several issues of global importance cut across the various environmental health topics. Global energy use and transportation are major drivers of air pollution, resource depletion, global warming, and health. Global warming poses significant planet-wide human health challenges, including major disasters with severe and widespread health effects. Finally, principles of environmental justice and risk communication need to be considered in almost any context related to environmental health.

▶ Energy Use & Transportation

The world's environmental challenge is evident from the continued growth in energy demand, especially in Asian countries. Global oil consumption is increasing annually, reaching 99.3 million barrels per day in 2018. Coal consumption, on the other hand, has flattened in recent years, but it still accounts for 27% of global energy consumption. Coal is associated with the largest carbon emissions of any fossil fuel, as well as the largest emissions of air pollutants. Renewable forms of energy have been increasing dramatically in recent years. When hydropower is included, renewables accounted for nearly 25% of global electricity generation in 2017. Solar and wind power are growing particularly quickly and now account for one-third of the electrical power in Europe.

A 2015 working paper from the International Monetary Fund (IMF) estimated the global energy subsidies for fossil fuels—especially the damage air pollution imposes on human health. This study found that the "true cost" of fossil fuels is $5.3 trillion a year. The IMF projected that eliminating fossil fuel subsidies in 2015 could raise government revenue by $2.9 trillion (3.6% of global GDP), cut global carbon dioxide (CO_2) emissions by more than 20%, and cut premature air pollution deaths by more than half. After allowing for the higher energy costs faced by consumers, this action would raise global economic welfare by $1.8 trillion.

Transportation, which relies almost exclusively on oil, accounts for nearly 30% of US emissions of greenhouse gases. Vehicles are a major contributor to air pollution around the world, accounting for most of the carbon monoxide (CO), and a large share of the HC, nitrogen oxides (NOx), and particulate matter in major urban areas. Worldwide, there are over 1 billion cars on the roads; use of motor vehicles is increasing especially fast in industrializing countries, with resulting adverse effects on air quality and public safety.

▶ Climate Change

Certain gases effectively trap heat in the atmosphere and impair radiation of that heat into space. Although a certain amount of heat-trapping is essential to life on earth, the system has been in delicate balance for millennia, and the massive emissions of "greenhouse gases" released by human activities in the last century is disrupting that balance. Emissions of CO_2 have increased globally from about 2 billion tons in 1900 to 36 billion tons in 2015; as a result, the concentration of CO_2 in the atmosphere has increased from approximately 277 parts per million (ppm) at the beginning of the industrial era to 405 ppm in 2017, and the earth has already warmed by about 1°C. The top greenhouse gas emitters worldwide are China, the United States, the European Union (EU), India, the Russian Federation, Japan, and Canada. Together, these sources represent the vast majority of total global CO_2 emissions. The Intergovernmental Panel on Climate Change, a United Nations scientific group, issued a special report in 2018 warning that if the earth warms by a total of 1.5°C, climate-related widespread food shortages, wildfires, coastal flooding, and population displacement are projected by 2040 or sooner in many areas. The effects will be far more severe if warming exceeds that threshold.

Greenhouse gas emissions cause two main phenomena: overall temperature increases and greater variability in the weather due to the increased heat energy in the atmosphere, with resulting effects on other natural systems from phenomena such as drought and flooding.

Eighteen of the 19 warmest years on record have occurred since 2001. There is extensive research on the health effects of heat, extreme weather events, and infectious diseases; some studies have also looked at the effects of climate change on crop yields and resulting hunger and population displacement. Climate change is projected to result in significant sea level rise, and two-thirds of the world's largest cities are at risk because they are located in low-lying coastal areas.

Heat waves have significant effects on health, including substantial increases in mortality, hospitalizations, and emergency room visits during days of extreme heat. Areas that are normally cooler, where people and the built environment are less acclimatized, have larger increases in heat-related morbidity during extreme heat events.

Climate change and pollution are often caused by the same human activities, primarily extraction and combustion of petroleum. For this reason, health experts have called for global policy solutions that address these issues jointly, to protect human health from both the direct effects of pollution and the indirect effects that are related to a changing climate.

▶ Persistent, Bioaccumulative Toxicants

Numerous industrial chemicals and pesticides are a particular problem for human health and the environment due to their resistance to environmental degradation and propensity to bioaccumulate. Chemicals in this category are not only a hazard to workers and individuals who are directly exposed, but also to ecosystems and people far away from sites where these chemicals are used or emitted. Chemicals that fall in the category of persistent, bioaccumulative toxicants (PBTs) include some metals such as methyl mercury, cadmium, and lead; some halogenated organic chemicals such as PCBs, dioxins, and polybrominated diphenyl ethers (PBDEs); and organochlorine pesticides such as DDT. Other groups of chemicals such as perfluorinated chemicals (used as stain repellants, waterproofing agents, and in

Greenhouse Gases

- Carbon dioxide is produced through combustion of fossil fuels and biomass. It is removed from the atmosphere ("sequestered") when it is absorbed by plants, or into the ocean where it reacts to form carbonic acid, leading to acidification of the ocean and resulting threats to marine organisms. Although CO_2 is not the most potent greenhouse gas, it is the most important because it is emitted in the largest quantities and has a long half-life in the atmosphere.

- Methane has a global warming potential at least 28 times that of CO_2. Methane primarily comes from livestock, and from landfills, composting facilities, and sewage treatment plants. Emissions also come from natural gas drilling and pipeline transport. Methane is produced naturally from decaying vegetation in marshlands; melting of the arctic permafrost is expected to result in significant increases in methane production over the coming decades.

- Nitrous oxide has a global warming potential at least 265 times that of CO_2. It is emitted from fertilizer use and industrial activities, as well as during combustion of fossil fuels and solid waste.

- Hydrofluorocarbons, perfluorocarbons, and sulfur hexafluoride are synthetic, powerful greenhouse gases that are emitted from a variety of industrial processes. Fluorinated gases are sometimes used as substitutes for stratospheric ozone-depleting substances (eg, chlorofluorocarbons, hydrochlorofluorocarbons, and halons). These gases are typically emitted in small quantities, but because they are potent greenhouse gases, with global warming potential thousands of times that of CO_2, they are referred to as High Global Warming Potential gases ("High GWP gases").

- Although black carbon is not a gas, it is important because it directly absorbs sunlight and infrared radiation. It also deposits on and darkens snow and ice, increasing absorption of sunlight and accelerating snow melt. The major source of black carbon is diesel engines, but it also comes from wood smoke, power plants, and other industrial facilities.

grease-proof coatings), short-chain chlorinated paraffins (used as flame retardants, plasticizers, additives in metal working fluids, sealants, paints and coatings), and musk xylenes (used as fragrances) are also highly persistent in the environment.

Although some PBTs (such as most organohalogens) are lipophilic and tend to accumulate in fatty tissue of biota at increasing concentrations up the food chain, other PBTs (such as many metals) accumulate in muscle, bone, or other tissues. These chemicals can be transported globally in air, water, and biota, and have been detected at locations far from where they were manufactured or used. For example, many PBT chemicals are found at especially high concentrations in the arctic, and are major contaminants in marine mammals and polar bears. Inuit populations generally have among the highest exposures to these chemicals in the world, due to their dietary patterns, and adverse health effects in these populations have been associated with exposures to PCBs and other PBT chemicals in epidemiologic studies.

Dioxins, PCBs, and other lipophilic chemicals also concentrate in breast milk lipids, resulting in disproportionately large exposures among nursing infants compared to adults. The Institute of Medicine (IOM) reviewed dietary intakes of dioxins and related chemicals in the United States and concluded that although concentrations have been generally declining, the typical levels in women of reproductive age are still higher than advisable. Dioxins are potent endocrine disruptors and carcinogens, raising concerns about exposures during fetal development and infancy. The IOM panel recommended educational efforts directed toward young girls to encourage them to eat a diet low in animal fat as a way of reducing dioxin exposures. It is unclear that these recommendations have been followed. Dioxins are not produced intentionally, but are by-products of incineration, combustion, chlorine-based bleaching, and other industrial processes; some dioxins are also produced naturally in forest fires and volcanic eruptions.

Many PBT chemicals are on the list of substances subject to international reduction efforts under the Stockholm Convention on Persistent Organic Pollutants, effective in 2004. Although the United States has not ratified this treaty, it has been signed by 182 countries and has resulted in significant success in globally reducing or eliminating many persistent, bioaccumulative chemicals.

APPROACHING DIFFICULT ENVIRONMENTAL HEALTH PROBLEMS

▶ Environmental Justice

Low-income communities of color have become increasingly concerned about a disproportionate burden of environmental risk in their communities. Even a relatively small risk may be seen in the context of a history of racial and socioeconomic disparities in the distribution of environmental risks, and is perceived as adding to an already unacceptable background of health stressors. In the mid-1980s, a coalition between civil rights activists and environmentalists working for the rights of low-income communities of color to clean and healthy environments became known as the environmental justice movement.

A groundbreaking 1987 report by the United Church of Christ's Commission on Racial Justice found that three-fifths of African-Americans or Hispanics lived in communities with uncontrolled toxic waste sites, and that the most significant predictor for the location of hazardous waste facilities nationwide was the race of the local community. In the

intervening years, numerous studies have documented the presence of disproportionately large numbers of polluting industrial facilities, sewage treatment plants, busy roadways, and other undesirable land uses in low-income communities populated by racial or ethnic minorities. Such communities also frequently lack healthy food options, have greater numbers of fast food restaurants and liquor stores, few green spaces, degraded housing quality, and limited recreational opportunities. High levels of community violence and stress add further to the health risk profile in such neighborhoods.

Reviews of research in this area have shown that children of color suffer disproportionate burdens of disease with potential environmental aspects, ranging from lead poisoning to asthma and childhood cancer. In addition, African-American children are at greater risk of preterm birth or low birth weight. Although these health conditions may be caused or exacerbated by some environmental factors, the causes are multifactorial and cannot be attributed to any specific set of conditions.

The Presidential Executive Order on environmental justice, signed in 1994, mandates that every federal agency "make achieving environmental justice part of its mission." In an effort to help guide implementation of the Executive Order on environmental justice, the National Academy of Sciences (NAS) produced a report in 1999 offering guidance to government agencies, scientists, and the medical community. The NAS report identified a lack of knowledge among health care professionals, researchers, and communities about environmental hazards, and recommended "enhanced efforts in the training of health professionals and education of the public."

The NAS panel recommended that education and risk communication efforts be directed toward four main goals: (1) increasing individual and community awareness of environmental health issues and resources, (2) involving the community in the identification of problems related to environmental exposures, (3) soliciting community involvement in research approaches, (4) and improving links between community members, health care providers, and researchers.

Increasingly, the environmental justice perspective has come to illuminate important underlying themes in environmental health. In particular, the concept of cumulative health impacts from multiple chemical and nonchemical stressors has come to be recognized as critical for understanding health disparities both locally and globally. Intrinsic vulnerability and variability within the population due to genetics and other host factors is affected by multiple extrinsic occupational, environmental, nutritional, and other factors. Many of these intrinsic and extrinsic factors can be measured and even mapped, allowing patterns of population health disparities to be identified and potentially addressed.

▶ Risk Communication

Risk communication can be defined as the exchange of information about the nature, magnitude, significance, and control of a risk. Health care providers have emerged as one of the most trusted and credible sources of information about occupational and environmental health risks.

Understanding different perceptions of risk is important to help understand how to communicate about risk. If the person who is attempting to explain a risk does not realize that the audience or individual may perceive risks very differently, risk communication is less likely to be productive and effective. Failure to recognize these differences in perception and deal with them appropriately can cause risk communication to fail. Factors influencing risk perception include differences in the nature of the hazard itself, differences among individuals or groups in how they react to the hazard, and factors related to the social context in which the risk communication occurs.

In the patient care setting, environmental health concerns tend to focus on questions about individual risk. Because the science on environmental health does not pertain to individual risk but rather to population risk, the challenge to the health care professional is substantial. Even assuming that the health care provider is familiar with the scientific data relevant to the issue in question, there remains a challenge in translating a combination of complex and sometimes conflicting results from a variety of sources such as *in vitro* assays, laboratory animal studies, and limited human epidemiologic research to practical advice for a patient's individual situation. This problem is further complicated by difficulties in exposure assessment, the fact that individuals are exposed to mixtures and multiple health stressors, and differing effects of chemicals due to underlying vulnerabilities. The resulting conversation must therefore move away from a focus on trying to "answer the question" toward a more open discussion of scientific uncertainty, risk, and prevention.

Individuals may come to their health care provider after an adverse event (such as a miscarriage or cancer diagnosis), or they may have concerns about potential future harm. They may have had exposure to an occupational or environmental hazard, or there may be no obvious exposures. Patients who have already suffered from an adverse event may be focused on exploring causation. They may be trying to understand what happened, to assign blame, or to recover compensation for the event. Individuals who have suffered a known hazardous exposure, irrespective of dose or of whether an adverse event has occurred, may require counseling about their future risk and may have questions about biological monitoring for the chemical, and potential treatment or health screening options to reduce their risk.

Many patients believe that science "proves" or "disproves" links between potential environmental hazards and health effects. The many shades of uncertainty, data gaps, and data quality problems are not the issues most people have grappled with in their personal or professional lives. Yet communicating about risk requires the clinician to convey these uncertainties as a way of explaining why there are no clear answers to most questions.

Many scientific links between exposure and adverse effects are based on animal toxicology studies. People respond to rodent data based on their preconceptions about risk, with some people dismissing such results as irrelevant to humans, and others finding any positive results alarming, irrespective of data quality, consistency, and dose. The clinician can discuss the animal toxicology findings and offer interpretation appropriate to the situation, either to encourage precautionary action to reduce exposure, or to indicate the difficulty of establishing causation based on limited animal toxicology data.

Even when the hazard associated with an environmental agent is known, the dose a patient may have received is often unknown. Route of exposure, dose, and timing of exposure are important determinants of risk. Some people may be falsely reassured, for example, learning that an exposure was below the Occupational Safety and Health Administration Permissible Exposure Limit (PEL), even though these limits are generally outdated and are not designed to protect against all health effects in all populations. Other people may be extremely anxious about a single low-dose, short-term exposure and require extensive counseling and reassurance.

Even with well-understood toxicants such as lead and known blood lead levels, it remains difficult to communicate risk, since epidemiologic studies allow prediction of neurodevelopmental deficits on a population level, but are not predictive for an individual. For example, if a mother has a blood lead level of 10 mcg/dL, it is not possible to predict that her child will lose 3 IQ points and will be more hyperactive, inattentive, and prone to violent behavior, even though epidemiologic studies have shown these associations on a population level. Due to the multifactorial determinants of health, the child of such a mother could grow up to be a genius or could be profoundly developmentally delayed. Predicting or attributing risk on an individual basis must be done with great caution.

Some characteristics of a hazard serve to magnify apparent risk irrespective of the outcome of a risk assessment. Hazards that are seen as potentially catastrophic, although unlikely, are generally perceived as more serious than hazards that are more likely but would result in less serious or reversible outcomes. For example, the risk from a nuclear power plant is seen by most people as greater than the risk from coal power plants although the overall risk to health is much higher from coal plants. Similarly, the risk of a dreaded outcome (such as cancer, birth defects, or brain damage) is often seen as worse than the risk of a disease that is less universally dreaded (such as liver, lung, or kidney disease). Unfamiliar hazards are generally seen as riskier than familiar hazards, and manmade hazards may be perceived as riskier than those that occur naturally. For example, people are more likely to be concerned about radioactive waste than about naturally occurring radon, even though radon gas is among the top causes of lung cancer in the United States.

The population affected by the hazard is also important. For example, a hazard to children is often judged as worse than a similar hazard to adults. Finally, hazards that are involuntary are almost always judged more serious than hazards that are faced by choice. Thus, comparison of the risks associated with skiing or drinking alcohol with risks from a hazardous waste incinerator will not be seen as equivalent because the former are voluntary and under the control of the individual, whereas the latter is imposed from outside and not controlled by the individual.

Estimates of risk used for comparison and the order in which they are presented can affect how risks are perceived. Compression refers to the tendency to overestimate the frequency of risks that are rare and underestimate those that are frequent. Availability refers to the tendency to base the expected likelihood of an event on the ability to recall instances of a similar event. As a result, events that draw media attention tend to be perceived as more likely.

Different groups within the population often have different perceptions of risk. In particular, experts and scientists tend to view many risks as less significant than do nontechnically trained individuals. Among scientists and professionals, where one works is relevant to risk perception. For example, toxicologists who work for industry rate risks from chemicals significantly lower than toxicologists who work for universities. Men frequently rate risks lower than do women. This difference is not explained by differences in familiarity with scientific issues because the difference is present even between male and female toxicologists. Interestingly, the gender difference in risk rating is only seen in whites. Black men, black women, and white women all rate risks similarly, whereas white males tend to rate virtually all risks as less serious.

The social context of risk communication efforts is extremely important to perceptions of risk. If the individual or organization imposing the risk is trusted by the community (ie, a local company that has provided jobs in the community for many years and is well known to the community) the risk is often perceived as less than if the risk is imposed by an outsider. Similarly, the level of trust in government regulatory officials and in the risk communicator is important in the perception of risk. Risks seen as unfair are often seen as larger than risks seen as fairly distributed. For example, if an individual or community perceives significant benefits from submitting to a risk, that risk seems smaller than if the benefits will only accrue to a distant corporation. Human rights issues such as the right to personal integrity, to privacy, and to informed consent all play into risk perception.

▶ Disease Clusters

Sometimes a cluster of illnesses can signal a workplace or community hazard requiring attention. In the United States, physicians are legally required to report work-related illnesses or injuries, and some states have additional requirements. For example, the State of California requires that health care providers report all pesticide-related illnesses and that laboratories report blood lead levels to the state. Likewise, many industrialized countries require reporting of occupational illnesses and injury and some have occupational disease registries designed for capturing sentinel events. Cancer or birth defects surveillance programs can also sometimes be helpful in assessing disease patterns. There is no reporting or tracking system for potential environmental disease clusters, but these are often reported anecdotally to county or state health departments, or to the Centers for Disease Control and Prevention (CDC).

Due to a lack of resources for conducting investigations, epidemiologic limitations that make it difficult to investigate small communities or rare diseases, and a lack of tools for accurately measuring exposures retroactively, it has been difficult for state and federal agencies to shed light on the causes of most chronic disease and cancer clusters. Most cluster investigations that are done fail to provide clear answers for the community. Many disease clusters are likely to be due to chance; statistical probabilities show that events (such as rates of disease) vary around the mean, and some geographic areas will inevitably have rates that are significantly above the mean for some period of time due to chance alone. On the other hand, sometimes there will be reasons for unusually high rates of disease during a time period, or sometimes the rates are so high that chance is an unlikely explanation. It is often difficult to discern when a cluster represents a statistical fluke and when it represents a sentinel event that could provide an important clue to occupational or environmental factors and disease.

Many important chemical hazards were initially identified because of clusters of adverse events. For example, the pesticide dibromochloropropane (DBCP) was first identified as a potent testicular toxicant in 1977 when a group of workers at a chemical plant realized through word-of-mouth that they all had been unable to father children. Subsequent investigation revealed that most of the production workers had oligospermia or azoospermia, and that prior animal tests identifying this effect in rats had been disregarded. The teratogenic and neurotoxic effects of methyl mercury were first discovered in the 1950s when numerous severely developmentally disabled children were born in the fishing village of Minamata, Japan at the same time as cats in the town were exhibiting bizarre behavior, and some adults were experiencing neurologic symptoms. Initially an infectious disease was suspected, but the cause was ultimately discovered to be mercury discharged from a nearby chemical facility into Minamata Bay, methylated by bacteria in the sediment of the Bay, and concentrated in fish which was the dietary staple in that town. The reproductive toxicity of several glycol ethers was first identified due to reports of spontaneous abortions among women working in "clean rooms" at semiconductor manufacturing facilities. The link between n-methyl-2-pyrrolidone (NMP), a common solvent used in many consumer products, and stillbirth was first described in a case report.

Although it is often more difficult to identify carcinogens from disease cluster investigations due to the generally longer latency of cancer compared to reproductive effects, some carcinogens have famously been identified in this manner. For example, vinyl chloride was shown to cause cancer in humans because of a cluster of hepatic angiosarcoma in 1974 at a vinyl chloride production facility in Louisville, Kentucky. As with DBCP, there were previously published rodent toxicology studies demonstrating liver toxicity and liver tumors, but these were largely disregarded until the outbreak of liver cancers in workers was established and linked to vinyl chloride.

In more recent years, outbreak investigations have linked nylon flock exposure to interstitial lung disease, and diacetyl flavoring agent to bronchiolitis obliterans. A review of occupational disease clusters identified 87 reports that established new disease-agent connections from 1775 to 1990.

Some investigators, however, have pointed out that the limited number of workers at any given worksite, the latency period of many diseases, and the mobility of the workforce make it very difficult to identify sentinel outbreaks. For a disease to be noticed against the general background, it would generally need to be acute or rare, or the causative agent would need to be extremely potent. Chemicals or other substances that cause a subtle increase in a common disease would tend not to be identified through workplace clusters.

Clusters of environmental disease have historically been less likely to yield answers than in the occupational context. In community situations, exposure pathways are often more complex than in the workplace, exposures are generally lower, and it can be very difficult to do dose reconstruction in an investigation. One notable exception was the discovery in 1999 of a lung cancer and restrictive lung disease cluster associated with asbestos contamination at a vermiculite mining operation in Libby, Montana. This investigation uncovered the associated deaths of about 400 workers and community residents, prompted the first declaration of a public health emergency by the U.S. Environmental Protection Agency, and triggered a clean-up that has cost hundreds of millions of dollars.

Health care providers should remain alert to disease clusters, as they can sometimes be sentinel events. The decision to report a potential problem and to intervene may prevent many future adverse outcomes in the population. However, clinicians should also recognize that many clusters occur by chance alone, and even if there is an occupational or environmental cause, cluster investigations often end with no clear answers due to scientific limitations such as small sample size and difficulty categorizing exposure. As a community is engaged in working with researchers on a cluster investigation, these factors should be discussed early in the investigation and frequently during the course of the investigation, to prepare the community for the possibility of equivocal or negative results.

▶ Knowing the Community

Clinicians should learn about potential occupational and environmental hazards in the communities they serve so that they are better prepared to prevent and respond to potential issues that may arise. For example, clinicians who practice in agricultural communities should be aware of the crops grown in their area and the pesticides most commonly used on those crops, so they have the ability to recognize potential symptoms of overexposure to those pesticides. Familiarity with the major industries in a local catchment area can be helpful in appropriately diagnosing or treating both occupational and environmental exposures, including in emergency situations. Anticipatory guidance can also link to local issues. For example, clinicians who practice in areas where radon levels tend to be high should be aware of this public health threat and should advise patients to test for radon in their homes, thereby preventing many potential cases of lung cancer.

Water source is an important environmental health issue. In the United States, water utilities are required to distribute an annual report detailing the levels of regulated contaminants in the system. These reports are publicly available and health providers should check them for any contaminants that exceed the Maximum Contaminant Level Goal (MCLG), which is the health-based exposure limit and is generally lower than the enforceable legal limit.

It is also important to know what fraction of the community is supplied by private wells. If that fraction is significant, it will be important to identify whether there are any local or state agencies that offer free or subsidized testing of well water. Well water is not regulated by any government agency and it is difficult to know what contaminants it may contain. In many cases, individuals must pay for their own water to be tested by private labs; such testing should be done by labs that are state certified and it is reasonable to screen for total coliform, metals, and nitrates. Depending on local land uses, it may sometimes be advisable to also test for pesticides, chlorinated solvents, or other contaminants.

In some regions in the world, there is no universal standard for regulating drinking water contaminants or for reporting requirements. The WHO has recommended drinking water guidelines for use internationally.

Local industrial facilities may expose their workers to hazards and may also pollute the community. Routine emissions to air or water, storage and transport of hazardous materials, and accidental releases are all issues that can cause public health concerns. In the United States, facilities that emit any of over 650 federally listed toxic chemicals over certain quantity thresholds are required to report emissions; the approximately 20,000 sites around the country with significant releases are mapped and their emissions data are readily available online through the toxics release inventory (TRI). In the EU, the European Pollutant Release and Transfer Register (E-PRTR) reports emissions from industrial facilities into air and water, and maintains an online database. The EU report covers more than 90 pollutants and over 30,000 facilities.

Other air-quality issues relate to ambient pollutants that are not emitted from local industrial sources. For example, particulate matter, ozone, and other pollutants come from a variety of sources especially including motor vehicles. It is possible to sign up for alerts from the AirNow program in the United States or the European Air Quality Index, or to use any of a number of mobile apps for regular updates on local air quality. This information is very useful to clinicians, since many acute respiratory and cardiovascular health outcomes have been linked temporally to air quality.

Health care providers who are attuned to local environmental conditions are better positioned to identify patterns, anticipate potential issues, and respond quickly and appropriately when needed. Fortunately, there is extensive information available on the Internet to allow clinicians to gather significant information relatively quickly and easily.

REFERENCES

Dhesi S, Lynch Z: What next for environmental health? Perspect Public Health 2016;136(4):225-230 [PMID: 26438593].

Finn S, Herne M, Castille D: The value of traditional ecological knowledge for the environmental health sciences and biomedical research. Environ Health Perspect 2017;125(8):085006 [PMID: 28858824].

Iyer S, Pham N, Marty M, Sandy M, Solomon G, Zeise L. An Integrated Approach Using Publicly Available Resources for Identifying and Characterizing Chemicals of Potential Toxicity Concern: Proof-of-Concept With Chemicals That Affect Cancer Pathways. Toxicol Sci. 2019 May 1;169(1):14-24. PMID: 30649495.

Kabisch N, van den Bosch M, Lafortezza R: The health benefits of nature-based solutions to urbanization challenges for children and the elderly—a systematic review. Environ Res 2017 Nov;159:362-373 [PMID: 28843167].

Landrigan PJ et al: The Lancet Commission on pollution and health. Lancet 2018;391:462-512 [PMID: 29056410].

Landrigan P, Fuller R, Haines A, Watts N, McCarthy G: Pollution prevention and climate change mitigation: measuring the health benefits of comprehensive interventions. Lancet Planet Health 2018;2:e515 [PMID: 30526935].

Morello-Frosch R: Understanding the cumulative impacts of inequalities in environmental health: implications for policy. Health Aff (Millwood) 2011;30:879 [PMID: 21555471].

Solomon GM, Morello-Frosch R, Zeise L, Faust JB. Cumulative Environmental Impacts: Science and Policy to Protect Communities. Annu Rev Public Health. 2016;37:83-96. PMID: 26735429.

■ SELF-ASSESSMENT QUESTIONS

Select the one correct answer for each question.

Question 1: Oil
   a. accounts for less than half of global energy consumption
   b. consumption is exceeded by coal consumption
   c. creates the largest carbon emissions of any fossil fuel
   d. causes the largest emissions of air pollutants

Question 2: Transportation
   a. relies almost exclusively on oil
   b. accounts for nearly 50% of US energy demand
   c. produces 40% of US emissions of carbon dioxide
   d. by automobiles is on the decline

Question 3: Dioxins
   a. are suspected to be endocrine disruptors and carcinogens
   b. are produced intentionally
   c. are by-products of industrial processes
   d. are excluded from international reduction efforts

Question 4: Testicular dysgenesis syndrome
   a. is a result of disrupted pituitary development
   b. may include undescended testis but not hypospadias
   c. is an early form of testicular cancer
   d. has been associated with prenatal phthalate exposure

Question 5: A disease cluster was the very first indication of the link between
   a. DBCP and male infertility
   b. vinyl chloride and liver cancer
   c. diacetyl and bronchiolitis obliterans
   d. inorganic mercury and neurodevelopmental toxicity

Question 6: Risks are perceived as more serious if they
   a. are within individual control
   b. primarily affect otherwise healthy adults
   c. are imposed by a locally owned company
   d. are linked to a dreaded disease such as cancer

Question 7: Environmental justice is
   a. purely a social movement with no significant relevance to health care providers
   b. not based on any real data showing disproportionate environmental hazards in low-income and nonwhite communities
   c. not something US government agencies need to consider when they make decisions
   d. something the Institute of Medicine recommends for inclusion in education for all levels of health professionals

Question 8: Health care providers do not need to know
   a. whether the region may have elevated radon levels
   b. which homes have carbon monoxide detectors
   c. the source of local drinking water and contaminants that have been reported in the water
   d. major local industries and pesticide use patterns

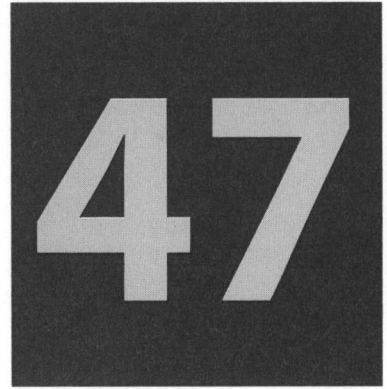

International Occupational & Environmental Health

Joseph LaDou, MS, MD

GLOBAL WORKING CONDITIONS

More than 1.4 billion people, most of them in developing countries, work in hazardous settings or occupations. Despite international efforts, the number of workers in vulnerable employment increases by around 11 million each year. Developing countries seldom have enforceable occupational and environmental regulations. Occupational health should have high priority on the international agenda, but occupational safety and health (OSH) regulations and laws cover only about 10% of workers in developing countries and do not include many major hazardous industries and occupations. Progress in bringing occupational health to the industrializing countries is painfully slow. In some of the poorest countries, there has been no progress at all.

The world's workforce sustains more than 370 million injuries every year, a figure that would be much higher if reliable reporting existed. Only 15% of workers worldwide have access to specialized occupational health services that provide for prevention of occupational risks, health surveillance, training in safe working methods, first aid, and consulting with employers on occupational health and safety. The global epidemic of occupational injury and disease is not new. It is inherent in the nature of industrial development that poorer countries adopt hazardous production. The resultant epidemic of injuries and illnesses is compounded by the rapid transfer of hazardous industries no longer compatible with developed country government regulation. While international standards appear to obligate employers to provide occupational health and safety procedures, and to pay for occupational injury and disease, inadequate prevention, detection, and compensation undermine these standards.

There are nearly 3 million workers known to die each year from occupational accidents and occupational diseases. More people die from traumatic work-related injuries in China than in any other country or region in the world. High workplace fatality figures are also seen in India and in sub-Saharan Africa. The vast majority of these deaths are avoidable and preventable. Occupational cancer is responsible for almost a third of all work-related deaths. Circulatory diseases are the second most common cause of death, accounting for almost a quarter of deaths. Acute traumatic injuries account for just under one-fifth of deaths attributable to work, followed by communicable diseases and respiratory diseases.

Occupational injuries and diseases have a profound effect on the health of the world's population. Occupational injuries and diseases play an even more important role in developing countries, where 70% of the working population of the world lives. Occupational injuries and diseases have a serious impact on the economy of all countries. Occupational injuries and diseases cause permanent disabilities and economic losses amounting to 4–6% of national incomes, costs to developing countries in excess of $10 trillion. These preventable injuries and diseases also have profound impacts on the work productivity, income, and social well-being of workers and their families. Often ignored is the reality that a single occupational injury or illness can tip an entire family into poverty.

Musculoskeletal disorders account for nearly half of the total cost. Other conditions that incur major costs include heart conditions, respiratory disease, central nervous system disorders, and mental disorders. Occupational illnesses attributed to hazardous exposures or workloads may be as numerous as occupational injuries.

SOCIAL PROTECTIONS

The labor force in developing countries totals around 1.8 billion, but it will rise to more than 3.1 billion in 2025—implying a need for 38–40 million new jobs every year. Adding to this burden, the technological revolution will automate more than one-third of jobs in developed countries over the next decade. Automation and advances in technology are not just affecting manufacturing workers in developed countries. They will have profound impact on developing countries as well. The UN forecasts that automation and machine learning innovations in the workplace will put 69% of India's existing jobs at risk, and 77% of China's jobs. Over 200 million workers worldwide are already unemployed.

In developing countries, nearly 780 million workers, about one in three, live in moderate to extreme poverty. These workers are less likely to have secure jobs with regular incomes and access to social protection. They are the world's workers most in need of a serious effort to assure worker protections and occupational health. Impoverished workers are in no position to make demands, and if they do make demands, they are not likely to be received. There is a virtual absence of organized labor around the world. This deficiency contributes to the overall problem of worker protections and occupational health. Unions provide a protective effect on workers' safety. Anti-union legislation increasingly advanced in populist governments has a deleterious effect on occupational health.

Developing countries are far behind industrialized countries in the development of workers' compensation programs. In many countries of Asia, Latin America, and Africa, only a small fraction of the workforce is covered by workers' compensation programs. In countries as large as Egypt, India, Pakistan, and Bangladesh, fewer than 10% of workers are covered by workers' compensation. In China, fewer than 15% of workers are covered, and in Venezuela and Colombia, fewer than 20%. In many developing countries, workers' compensation is little more than a paper program where the government works in concert with industry to minimize the provision and the costs of benefits.

GLOBALIZATION

Globalization, the fast-paced growth of trade and cross-border investment, is a selective phenomenon. Many countries benefit from globalization, and many do not. Indeed, the decline of some economies is linked to the advantages gained by others. In addition to inequities between countries, the benefits of trade are not fairly spread within countries. Globalization benefits countries that are competitive in the knowledge economy, which rewards skills and institutions that promote cutting-edge technological innovation, or the low-wage economy, which uses widely available technology to do routine tasks at the lowest possible cost.

Newly industrialized countries are eager for the financial benefits that foreign companies and foreign investors bring them. However, these benefits bring profound social and ecological problems. In the developed countries, industry provides jobs, pays taxes that support community services, and is subject to environmental and occupational health laws. As industrialized nations enact laws to limit the environmental hazards associated with many industrial operations, production costs rise and undermine competitive advantages. Thus, there is an incentive to avoid or subvert legislative controls.

Middle-income countries have not done nearly as well under globalized markets as either richer or poorer countries. These countries, notably countries in Latin America and Eastern and Central Europe, have been unable to compete in high-value-added markets dominated by wealthy economies because their workforces are not sufficiently skilled and their legal and banking systems are not adequately developed.

As a result, they have had little choice but to try to compete with China and other low-income economies in markets for standard products made with widely available and relatively old technologies. But because of their higher wages, the middle-income nations are not able to compete effectively.

▶ Multinational Corporations

The major multinational corporations account for one-third of all manufacturing exports, three-fourths of commodity trade, and four-fifths of the trade in technology and management services. Yet the human labor required for each unit of their output is diminished dramatically. During the last generation, the world's 500 largest multinational corporations grew sevenfold in sales. Yet the worldwide employment by these global firms remained virtually unchanged. Global foreign direct investment (FDI) is well in excess of $1 trillion per year. Developing and transition economies together attract more than half of global FDI flows.

All too many multinational corporations accept the reality of developing countries, including internal corruption, poor work practices, lack of regulation and enforcement of labor standards, and the local workers' inability to claim compensation for injuries and illnesses. Manufacturers may take advantage of the opportunity to move many of their hazardous operations to newly industrialized countries. They are welcomed because the creation of an infrastructure in many developing nations relies on industrial expansion by foreigners. When industry migrates to developing nations, companies not only take advantage of lower wages, but also benefit from the low tax rates in communities that are not spending much on such things as sewage systems, water treatment plants, schools, and public transportation. Developing countries may have a weak capacity to collect taxes, or to control tax avoidance. When companies establish plants in developing countries, their tax burden is a small fraction of what it would be in most developed countries.

Some migrating companies try to introduce their own corporate or home country's environmental and occupational health and safety standards in the host country. Unfortunately, less conscientious companies simply conform to the standards of the host country. Many companies often state that it is corporate policy not to have international "double standards" in health, safety, and environmental protection in their worldwide operations. In this age of multinational investment and global supply chains, corporate social responsibility for health and safety has to be looked at on a global scale. Workers in all countries are entitled to the basic benefits of federal labor and health and safety laws, including workers' compensation. At present, only a small minority of workers in Africa, Latin America, and Asia receive protection from social security programs.

There have been many efforts to influence the behavior of industry. The Organization for Economic Cooperation and Development (OECD) Guidelines for Multinational Enterprises, the UN Code of Conduct on Transnational Corporations, and the ILO (International Labor Organization)

Tripartite Declaration of Principles Concerning Multinational Enterprises and Social Policy (MNE Declaration) attempt to provide a framework of ethical behavior. The IOL MNE Declaration provides direct guidance to enterprises on social policy and inclusive, responsible, and sustainable workplace practices. It was adopted 40 years ago and amended several times, most recently in March 2017. Its principles are addressed to multinational and national enterprises, governments of home and host countries, and employers' and workers' organizations providing guidance in such areas as employment, training, conditions of work and life, industrial relations, and general policies.

The Coalition for Environmentally Responsible Economies (Ceres) advocates for ethical and environmentally sustainable business practices. Multinational corporations that sign on to the Ceres Principles agree to operate plants according to more strict home-based regulatory standards and thereby set the best example possible in the developing countries. When these corporations bring their home health and safety practices to the developing world, they are a force for improvement in working conditions in newly industrialized countries. They are also a force for raising the living standards and working conditions of women and child workers. Critics contend that these efforts are watered-down substitutes for a more aggressive regimen that would actually impose human rights obligations on corporations.

Influenced by public policy makers in the United States, such organizations as the World Bank, International Monetary Fund (IMF), and World Trade Organization have advocated policies that encourage reduction and privatization of health care and public health services previously provided in the public sector. Corporate strategies have culminated in a marked expansion of corporations' access to social security and related public sector funds for the support of privatized health services. The Global Agreement on Trade and Services (GATS) includes health services as a commodity subject to trade rules. International financial institutions and multinational corporations have influenced reforms that, while favorable to corporate interests, have worsened access to needed services and have strained the remaining public sector institutions.

SMALL & MEDIUM-SIZED ENTERPRISES

There are 19 million small- and medium-sized enterprises (SMEs) in the European Union (EU), operating in different sectors and employing nearly 75 million people. In the EU, SMEs account for 82% of all occupational injuries and 90% of fatal incidents.

The workforce of developing nations is accustomed to working in small industry settings. Small firms greatly predominate over large firms around the world, both in number and the share of the labor force they employ. Yet the problem is not a simple one. Between and within countries there may be large differences in SMEs. It is often asserted that attention to SMEs will solve problems of unemployment and underdevelopment in the poorer countries. The World Bank and

the IMF advise developing countries on how to support SME development in order to obtain donor aid. However, it is hard to find evidence to support what is essentially a dogma. In South Africa, the perceived need to facilitate SME growth threatens to roll back legislative gains made by the labor movement in the transition from apartheid. Some of these key gains are in employment and health and safety provisions.

Nonetheless, in every region studied, the smaller the industry, the higher the rate of workplace injury and disease. SMEs are characterized by unsafe buildings and other structures, old machinery, poor ventilation, noise, and with workers of limited education, skill, and training. Risk assessment capacity is not provided by government, with no clear emphasis of cleaner production methods and control of hazards at the source. Protective clothing, respirators, gloves, hearing protectors, and safety glasses are seldom available. The companies are often inaccessible to inspections by government health and safety enforcement agencies. In many instances, they operate as an "underground industry" of companies not even registered with the government for tax purposes.

Most SMEs in industrializing countries lack appropriate occupational health regulations and protective or control measures. It is the common world experience that small-scale enterprises do not provide basic occupational health services and other primary medical care. Moreover, many small factories are located in the middle of or near residential areas. Small-scale industrial hazards threaten the health of workers' families and the adjacent community.

INFORMAL SECTOR

In developing countries, the bulk of new employment is in the informal economy where workers become trapped in survival and subsistence activities. The informal sector is defined as all economic activities by workers and economic units that are—in law or in practice—not covered or insufficiently covered by formal arrangements, and are operating outside the formal reach of the law. The informal sector encompasses a large body of poor workers who are not recognized, recorded, protected, or regulated by the public authorities. The informal sector can no longer be considered a temporary or residual phenomenon. Ghana's employment is about 60% or more in the informal sector, making it a vital part of public policy. When Ghana introduced a National Health Insurance, its major concern was how to fund it with such a large pool of the workforce falling outside the tax net. The solution proposed was to fund it through a value-added tax (VAT). VAT can, however, be a very regressive tax, doubly unfair to the poor.

Much of the world's workforce is in the informal sector. The informal nonagricultural employment in Latin America is at about 60%. The informal sector is an integral part of the Mexican economy and includes unofficial self-employed workers whose activities range from hawking goods on the street to independent contracting and small family-run businesses. Approximately 18 million people and their families work in the informal sector in Mexico.

The Indian Ministry of Labor acknowledges that the informal sector comprises the bulk of the workforce. In India and Indonesia, the informal economy accounts for 90% of the women working outside agriculture, while in Benin, Chad, and Mali the proportion is 95%. In India, the informal economy generates about 60% of national income, 50% of gross national savings, and 40% of national exports.

MIGRANT WORKERS

The world's largest population migration is taking place at this time—one in seven of the world's people are on the move. A migrant worker is a person who either relocates within their home country or outside it to pursue work. Migrant workers do not usually intend to stay permanently in the country or region in which they work. Of the 1 billion migrants in the world today, 250 million are international migrants and 763 million are internal migrants. Moreover, 65 million of these people are forcibly displaced today, often by wars. In recent years, more than half of all refugees worldwide came from just three countries: the Syrian Arab Republic (3.9 million), Afghanistan (2.6 million), and Somalia (1.1 million).

According to Gallup, 700 million people—14% of the world's adults—would like to move permanently to another country. In sub-Saharan Africa the figure is 31%. High-income countries host more than two-thirds of all international migrants. Nearly two-thirds of all international migrants worldwide live in Europe or Asia. North America hosts the third largest number of international migrants, followed by Africa and Latin America. Only 30% of the world's migrants live in middle- or low-income countries. International migrants accounted for less than 2% of the population of Africa, Asia, and Latin America and the Caribbean. By contrast, in Europe, Northern America, and Oceania international migrants comprise at least 10% of the population.

Most of the world's migrants live in just 20 countries. The largest number resides in the United States: 47 million, equal to 19% of the world total. Germany and the Russian Federation host the second and third largest numbers of migrants worldwide, followed by Saudi Arabia, the United Kingdom, and the United Arab Emirates. Of the top 20 destinations of international migrants worldwide, 9 are in Asia, 7 in Europe, 2 in Northern America, and 1 each in Africa and Oceania. Women comprise slightly less than half of all international migrants. Most migrants worldwide are of working age. Of all international migrants, 72% are aged 20–64 years, compared to 58% of the total population. Thirteen percent of migrants worldwide were at least 65 years old.

There are many reasons why people migrate, such as globalization, conflict, poverty, climate change, urbanization, inequality, and to improve job prospects. Climate change-related hazards and disasters contribute to migration. Environmentally motivated migration and displacement may lead to the disruption of existing social ties, with potentially adverse consequences for migrant workers as

well as their family members who remain in places of origin. Syria accounts for the largest forcibly displaced population globally, with 12.6 million people, many of which are asylum seekers. Colombia, in 2017, had 7.9 million victims of conflict, the Democratic Republic of Congo 5.1 million, and Ukraine 2.0 million displaced citizens.

The wages that migrants earn abroad are far greater than what they would earn doing similar jobs in home countries. The World Bank reports that immigrants from the poorest countries, on average, experience a 15-fold increase in income, a doubling of school enrollment rates, and a 16-fold reduction in child mortality after moving to a developed country. Migrants from developing countries return an estimated $450 billion of their earnings to their home countries which provides a powerful incentive for many countries to encourage worker migration. In 2003, the United Nations adopted the International Convention on the Protection of the Rights of All Migrant Workers and Members of Their Families to guarantee equality of treatment and the same working conditions for migrants and nationals. Not one single migrant-receiving country in Western Europe or North America ratified the Convention.

Only 36 of the 187 ILO member states have ratified the five ILO Conventions related to international migrants and migration, and 14 member states have refused to ratify any of the five conventions.

Many nations have country-specific policies and regulations regarding the provision of health care services to regular and irregular immigrants. Enforcement is inconsistent at best and ignored in most countries. Access to public and private health care for migrant workers depends on national regulations, and the legal status of migrants in host countries. Access is also affected by poverty, stigma, discrimination, social exclusion, language and cultural differences, separation from family, and sociocultural norms. Efforts have been made to improve the rights for migrants in Europe with regard to health care, but seasonal migrant workers still remain largely outsiders where these measures are concerned.

Immigrant workers are a rapidly growing segment of the US workforce. Immigrant workers are over-represented in low-paying occupations. High-risk occupations in which a large proportion of immigrant workers are hired include agriculture, sweatshops, day laborers, and construction. In the United States, the number of on-the-job fatalities among Hispanic or Latino workers recently reached its highest level. Pesticide-related illness is an important cause of acute and chronic morbidity among migrant farm workers and their families.

The issues of a migrant workforce in some parts of the developing world take on even greater import. In Southern Africa, for example, migrant mining workers face the extraordinary multiplicative risks of silicosis, tuberculosis, and HIV diseases that are inextricably linked to workplace, housing, social, and economic factors. The migrant labor system drove the disastrous spread of HIV in the region. Migrant workers and asylum seekers are an expanding global population of growing social, demographic, and political importance.

The rise in migration for employment has had serious consequences for many Asian countries. Asian migrant workers tend to be young, male, married, and better educated than the average home population. Most of them come from rural areas and are predominantly employed in construction and labor. The most distinctive feature of these workers is their concentration in a few blue-collar occupations—carpenters, masons, electricians, plumbers, truck drivers, mechanics, and heavy equipment operators. These production and transport workers outnumber the professional and technical workers by anywhere from 3 to 1 in the Philippines to 17 to 1 in Pakistan and Sri Lanka.

Despite the efforts of governments to ensure that workers have satisfactory contracts on going abroad, many cases of "contract substitution" occur. An increasing number of women, especially Asian women, are migrating for overseas employment. These women are among the most vulnerable to exploitation and abuse, mainly because they are outside the legal protection of their home countries and because they work in jobs—as domestic servants, prostitutes, entertainers, contract manual laborers—that are not covered by labor legislation. Their situation is made worse by the fact that they are usually young and poor, living in fear of losing their jobs, do not speak the language of the host country, are unaware that their rights are being infringed, and normally do not know where to go for help. Many also end up in a situation of debt bondage, having borrowed money to pay for the costs of obtaining an overseas job. Upon return, former domestic workers often face social disapproval and marital problems.

CHILD LABOR

Children are the most easily exploited of all workers. Children account for 11% of the workforce in some countries in Asia, 17% in Africa, and 25% in Latin America. Worldwide, at least 250 million children, one in every six aged 5–17, are involved in child labor. Of these, some 180 million children are required to perform the worst forms of child labor, exposing them to work so hazardous that it endangers the child's physical, mental, or moral well-being. The ILO distinguishes child work from child labor, and proscribes the worst forms of child labor.

Most child labor occurs in developing countries, where poverty, traditions, and cultural differences thwart international efforts to stop it. Child labor in the agriculture sector accounts for 80% of child laborers in India and 70% of working children globally. A majority of child workers in India report physical and/or verbal abuse by their employers. Nearly a quarter of all Bangladeshi children are in the labor force even though the Bangladeshi laws prohibit child labor.

Poor or nonexistent enforcement of laws that attempt to prevent child labor creates conditions that allow children in some cases to be held in near slavery, often sexually and physically abused. Child labor is an economic and social reality in many developing countries. Children may provide 25% or more of a family's total income, and many traditional cultures include child labor as an integral part of the child's socialization and achievement of status in the local community. Governments may regard child labor as a key factor in keeping their economy competitive through the provision of cheap labor. Children who work full-time do not attend school and thereby lose any opportunity for an education.

In developing countries, the poorest and most vulnerable children are most often involved in work in order to earn money for survival. These children are also likely to already lack basic necessities of food and medical care, predisposing them to diarrhea, anemia, and dietary deficiencies. Children are more susceptible to the effects of toxic substances such as lead. Underlying health conditions add to the problem. Children are in occupations with exposures to hazards known to cause illness or injury in adults. Manual labor exposes children to injury, harmful fumes and dust, and poisoning from chemicals such as solvents, pesticides, metals, and caustic agents used on the job.

Over 1.5 billion people live in countries that are affected by conflict, violence, and fragility. Moreover, around 200 million people are affected by disasters every year; a third of them are children. Conflicts and disasters have a devastating impact on people's lives. They kill, maim, injure, force people to flee their homes, destroy livelihoods, push people into poverty and starvation, and trap people in situations where their basic human rights are violated. Children are often the first to suffer as schools are destroyed and basic services are disrupted. Many children are internally displaced or become refugees in other countries and are particularly vulnerable to trafficking and child labor.

Occupational illnesses and diseases are seldom if ever reported to governmental agencies when they occur in child workers. When occupational injuries are encountered, they are treated as accidental injuries since, officially, children are not workers. Children are exposed to physical and chemical hazards without proper training or personal protective equipment. Personal protective equipment is hardly ever designed with a child worker in mind, so even if properly used, it is likely to be ineffective. Moreover, relying on training to prevent injury or illness to child workers presupposes that children are able to translate training into safety practices. The more important health and safety deficiencies are poor or nonexistent safety standards and industrial hygiene, and inappropriate work practices.

In 1992, the ILO instituted the International Program for the Elimination of Child Labor (IPEC). IPEC seeks preventive approaches directed toward eliminating the underlying social and economic situations that produce child labor. It is now the ILO's largest technical cooperation program. Solutions that address the general problems of poverty, while developing alternative sources of education and employment, are most likely to be effective in reducing child labor in countries such as India. The cornerstone of the ILO program is to focus on eradicating the worst forms of child labor while recognizing that phasing out all forms of child labor may aggravate household poverty.

The ILO effort against child labor has had substantial legislative successes. The ILO Minimum Age Convention No. 138 sets the age below which children should not be in work at 15. Two years before they reach this minimum legal age, children can do "light work"—nonhazardous work for no more than 14 hours a week, work that does not interfere with schooling. The ILO Convention No. 138, Minimum Age for Employment, has been adopted in 170 member states. Children under the minimum working age who are engaged in more than light work are in child labor. Convention No. 182, Worst Forms of Child Labor, has received a record number of ratifications, adopted by 181 member states. Recent results show that child labor has declined worldwide since 2000. This may be an outcome of the enforcement of five key ILO conventions, but as well it may be the result of unreliable reporting. Inaccurate and fraudulent reporting plague ILO programs.

INTERNATIONAL AGENCIES

Most countries defer to the United Nations in the matter of responsibility for international occupational health. The UN's international agencies have had a very limited success in bringing occupational health to the industrializing countries. The lack of proper WHO and ILO funding severely impedes the development of international occupational health. There are 194 UN member states that support the activities of the WHO and the ILO. The WHO structure is designed to limit the power of any one member state to influence policy or direction. All member states contribute a proportion of the core WHO and ILO budget based on their wealth measured in GNP and population size. They have a duty to provide the support regardless of agency priorities or performance. However, member states do use rewards or punishments to influence the actions of WHO and ILO. The threat to quit UN membership is the option most feared by WHO and ILO. A less drastic method that member states use to influence the WHO and ILO is to propose changes to the budget.

The WHO and ILO receive additional funding from voluntary contributions from its member states, philanthropic foundations, corporations, NGOs, and private individuals. The importance of voluntary contributions to the operation of the WHO and ILO has increased dramatically over the past two decades. Voluntary contributions now comprise a large majority of the WHO overall budget. Most of these voluntary contributions are designated for specific purposes proposed by the donor. Unlike member assessments, these contributions require the WHO and ILO to work in the interests of a few states or organizations. Reliance on such nondemocratic funding leaves the WHO and ILO open to state-sponsored or corporate influence or outright control. The impact of the tobacco industry, asbestos, and other mining and manufacturing industries came to light after the donors had obtained the relief they sought. It is quite likely that the relatively little WHO and ILO funding and staffs in support of occupational and environmental health are the result of donor influence and control of governance.

▶ World Health Organization

The World Health Organization (WHO) is responsible for the technical aspects of occupational health and safety, the promotion of medical services and hygienic standards. The WHO addresses occupational health through a program in WHO headquarters, six WHO regional offices, and WHO country offices, with the support of a network of collaborating centers.

WHO is implementing a global strategy to:

- Provide evidence for policy, legislation, and support to decision makers, including work carried out to estimate the magnitude of the burden of occupational diseases and injuries
- Provide infrastructure support and development through capacity building, information dissemination, and networking
- Support the protection and promotion of workers' health

To encourage countries to support the protection and promotion of workers' health, particularly where occupational health services do not reach, WHO has recently introduced the healthy workplaces approach. Healthy workplaces not only reinforce occupational health and safety standards, but also provide physical, organizational (workload, management style, communication), and community environments that protect and promote health and safety of the workers.

The WHO Global Plan of Action on Workers' Health (GPA) has the following main objectives:

- Strengthen the governance and leadership function of national health systems to respond to the specific health needs of working populations.
- Establish basic levels of health protection at all workplaces to decrease inequalities in workers' health between and within countries, and strengthen the promotion of health at work. Ensure access of all workers to preventive health services and link occupational health to primary health care.
- Improve the knowledge base for action on protecting and promoting the health of workers and establish linkages between health and work.
- Stimulate incorporation of actions on workers' health into other policies, such as sustainable development, poverty reduction, trade liberalization, environmental protection, and employment.

Despite these efforts, there is a growing problem of credibility with the WHO, a problem exploited by the private sector to shift authority for key decision-making in occupational health and safety away from the WHO to other UN agencies and to the private sector itself.

The global asbestos cancer epidemic is an example of the failure by international organizations to protect the public health. The asbestos cancer epidemic may take as many as 10 million lives before asbestos is banned worldwide and exposures are brought to an end. The asbestos cancer epidemic would have been largely preventable if the WHO and the ILO had responded early and responsibly. The WHO was late in recognizing the epidemic and failed to act decisively after it was well underway.

▶ WHO Collaborating Centers

The WHO global policy on occupational health is primarily advanced by assisting, coordinating, and making use of the activities of existing institutions. The selection of WHO Collaborating Centers lacks academic and ethical rigor. Typical is the WHO Collaborating Centers' proposal for a WHO global strategy for "Occupational Health for All." In adopting the strategy, the centers recognized the urgent need to develop occupational health at a time when rapid changes in work are affecting both the health of workers and the health of the environment in all countries of the world. The overall accomplishments of the Centers are of marginal significance. The lack of impact of these global announcements and publications is never honestly presented.

The collaborating centers are asked to provide networks in developed and developing countries aimed at capacity building. The WHO unfortunately provides no funding for the work of the collaborating centers. Critics contend that very little can be achieved through the exhortations by volunteers to industry stakeholders to improve health and safety practices. The collaborating centers currently implement a large number of projects of dubious value. Many government and academic centers display the WHO collaborating center imprimatur for their own purposes, providing little or nothing to the agency endeavor.

▶ International Labor Organization

The International Labor Organization (ILO) is a tripartite organization of government, employer, and worker representatives that develops policy statements, conventions, recommendations, and guidelines. Representatives use a consensus process to develop policy. The adoption and supervision of international labor standards is the primary task of the ILO. The ILO adopts, at an annual International Labor Conference, two kinds of standards: conventions and recommendations. Only conventions can be ratified and thus become legally binding on member states. Recommendations are most frequently used to supplement conventions, either giving more detail on the contents of the standard or setting a higher standard than the convention.

The ILO is the logical starting point for constructing an international basis of OHS standards, starting with key standards and then including additional conventions, recommendations, and guidelines over time. A key aspect of the ILO Fundamental Principles and Rights at Work is that they are binding on all 187 member countries of the ILO, regardless of whether the country has specifically ratified all core conventions or not. The goal in establishing international OHS standards is that all countries will uphold the core conventions, combined with a progressive "upward harmonization" of standards over time, at a pace consistent with the socioeconomic standards of each country, and with financial and technical assistance from countries with more resources and experience.

The ILO conventions guide all countries in the promotion of workplace safety and in managing occupational health and safety programs. The ILO conventions and recommendations on occupational safety and health are international agreements that have legal force if they are ratified by the member country. More than half of the conventions adopted so far by the ILO have links to health and safety issues. Ratification by member countries is entirely voluntary. No sanctions are provided against member countries that do not ratify conventions, and there is usually no time limit set for ratification. Moreover, even if a country has ratified a convention, the ILO cannot enforce compliance. Nonetheless, once ratified, these conventions have relevance in member country legal systems.

These conventions should be key instruments of ILO policy. In reality, none of the ILO Occupational Safety and Health Conventions are included as part of the ILO's core labor standards. When the ILO adopted its declaration on fundamental principles and rights at work in 1998, eight conventions were rightly confirmed as core labor standards and became the subject of a major campaign. That prompted some of ILO's constituents, including the US government, to relegate other conventions to second-class status. Core (fundamental) conventions of the ILO cover only freedom of association, child labor, forced labor, and discrimination issues. In practice, it means that occupational safety and health is always given second or third priority when regular budget resources and issues such as international technical cooperation are discussed.

Economic development is a strong predictor of the ratification of ILO conventions. Ratification occurs much more frequently in more highly developed countries, presumably because these countries already have similar labor regulations. Among developing countries, it is the economic costs of ratification which most significantly affects the probability of ratification. Governments and trade unions in developed countries provide political support for ratification. In developing countries, this support is almost never achieved.

Convention No. 155 can be considered as the framework for occupational health and safety law at national and at company level. It contains fundamental principles on safety policies, work organization, and prevention of occupational injury and illness. The most important ILO Convention on Occupational Safety and Health has been ratified by only 66 of the 194 ILO member countries. Convention No. 187 (promotional framework for occupational safety and health) seeks to promote a preventive safety and health culture and a safe and healthy working environment. It requires ratifying States to develop, in consultation with representative organizations of employers and workers, a national policy and program on occupational safety and health. It has received only 43 ratifications.

Ratifications are made by a disappointingly small percentage of ILO member states. Conventions directed at managing occupational health and safety programs, such as Convention No. 161 (occupational health services), have only 33 ratifications, No. 167 (safety and health in construction) 31 ratifications, No. 170 (chemical safety) 21 ratifications, and No. 184 (safety and health in agriculture) a mere 16 ratifications.

▶ ILO safework

Safework, the ILO program on safety, health at work, and the environment, has been leading the ILO's efforts to promote occupational health, but in recent years has diminished greatly. Safework attempts to create worldwide awareness of the dimensions and consequences of work-related accidents and diseases; to place OSH on the international and national agendas; and to provide support to the national efforts for the improvement of national OSH systems and programs in line with relevant international labor standards.

Labor inspection departments in ministries of labor are seen in most countries as little more than a nuisance, commanding very little in the way of resources, powers, and respect. Labor inspection is increasingly troubled by obstacles placed by industry, a lack of facilities, and even harassment of inspectors. Recently, inspectors in Brazil and France were killed when carrying out their normal and fully justified duties. A labor inspector in Sao Paulo has been subjected to law suits by asbestos manufacturers and interruptions of her work by her own government because of her attempts to protect the health and safety of Brazilian workers.

The reliance on international agencies to promote health and safety in industrializing countries is not nearly adequate. Developing countries need more direct assistance to help them develop health and safety programs that welcome them into the family of countries that protect their workers. The international agencies have observed that most countries do not have concise legislation on occupational health, and provisions are often scattered in several separate laws and regulations. It is a significant lost opportunity that the developed countries and the international agencies do not fully provide this service.

▶ Consultation With Local Governments

The ILO's Tripartite Consultation (International Labor Standards) Convention (No. 144) requires governments to adopt procedures that ensure effective consultation with employers' and workers' representatives on measures entailed in ratified conventions.

The WHO and the ILO are required to provide direct consultation to developing countries when such countries request aid with their health and safety programs. In reality, the WHO and the ILO have limited budgets and staffs are unable to provide the required consultative services. Moreover, it is not clear that the WHO and the ILO could identify a model occupational health and safety program to recommend. Virtually all models of health and safety programs require trained and experienced personnel to institute them and to provide continuing leadership. The overwhelming

reality in the industrializing countries is that they lack trained personnel at every level.

The ILO Decent Work program has been a means of generating interest in and some action on worker protections in industrializing countries. The ILO is a major source of information for government, employers, and workers. The ILO Labor administration assists constituents in promoting Decent Work through the strengthening of labor administration machinery, including labor inspection. Yet employers and workers are also calling for better resources for Ministries of Labor and inspectorates to make Decent Work a reality.

The number of workplaces subject to inspection dwarfs the resources available to inspect them, leading to a situation in which workers are unprotected, violators operate with impunity, and unfair competition for compliant businesses pervades. ILO's strategic compliance model provides labor inspectorates with a methodology to achieve compliance outcomes in light of limited resources. Independent assessment of such programs will be needed to evaluate their full effectiveness.

▶ Basic Occupational Health Services

The Basic Occupational Health Services (BOHS) approach was advanced by WHO and ILO in 2005. The institution of a minimum occupational health system to meet the objectives of ILO Convention No. 161 (occupational health services) in developing countries is moving very slowly, if at all. No single system can be proposed that satisfies the particular preferences of various governments, industries, and institutions. Moreover, until a local government supports OHS and a legal system ensures regulation and enforcement of OHS laws, little progress can be made.

▶ Developed Country OSH Models

A convincing government OSH policy and close cooperation between social partners and the government are critical factors that guarantee sustainable OSH programs in a developing country over a long-term basis. There are a number of regional or national occupational health and safety programs that have served as models for the developing countries. None of these models has been entirely useful, given the complex problems posed by circumstances in developing countries and the great differences found in their levels of industrialization. No model of occupational health and safety transferred to a developing country will work properly if the local conditions are not taken into account.

The Scandinavian system of a powerful health and safety establishment sponsored by the government and welcomed by industry and labor has not provided a transferable model for industrializing countries. The Communist model of large, central Institutes of Occupational Health and Safety with regulations seldom enforced and heavy governmental controls imposed on the scientific agencies that regulate industry, although widely accepted by many developing countries, is of limited value to them.

The US and the UK models are often emulated, but with little direct consultative assistance. Malaysia provides an example of a successful OSH program development drawing on many sources. The EU criteria for diagnosis of occupational diseases have been employed as the basis for criteria documents and notification of occupational diseases, poisoning, and accidents. Being a former colony of Britain, most of the early legislation in Malaysia was based on that of the United Kingdom. However in the later years, legislation from other countries such as the United States and the United Kingdom has been used as a model. The American Conference of Governmental Industrial Hygienists (ACGIH) determines a protective standard, the threshold limit value (TLV). TLVs are not health-based standards, a deficiency shared by virtually all countries' protective standards. TLVs have largely been developed by industry experts and need more scrutiny than they have received. These standards have wide currency because there is little other guidance. The concept of safe is taken by the public and by workers to imply that government has all the appropriate information needed to conclude that harm will not occur as a result of chemical exposure. Protective standards seldom, if ever, are health based.

The EU provides grant support for economic transformation of Central and Eastern European countries, including occupational health and safety projects. The European Commission has expanded its development policy to include cooperation with African, Caribbean, and Pacific countries. The United States sponsors an international effort in occupational health through the Fogarty International Center and by other governmental agencies and academic institutions. These are primarily focused on research and capacity building, with limited policy reach. There are many other national and regional efforts, but in sum, they are far from adequate to meet the challenge.

Finland provides development collaboration in East African countries and in the Asian-Pacific region, and research and training opportunities in Finland's government and academic centers of occupational health. The Finnish Institute of Occupational Health (FIOH) works with the WHO and the ILO in producing the African and the Asian Newsletters on Occupational Health and Safety.

AGRICULTURE

Agriculture employs half the world's workforce. Agricultural workers account for a particularly high proportion of unprotected workers, especially in developing countries. Their work is generally heavy, their working hours can be very long, they are often exposed to difficult climatic conditions, and many are exposed to hazardous chemicals, especially pesticides. Workers and small farmers live where they work so workplace exposures all too easily migrate into the home. Living conditions are often extremely poor, and many have limited access to clean water, electricity, adequate shelter, and nutrition. Literacy is often low in agricultural workers causing an inability to read cautionary material.

These problems are compounded by poverty. Poverty is a multidimensional phenomenon, but agriculture plays a major role. More than 75% of the world's poor live in rural areas where the agricultural sector employs 40% of the workers and contributes to over 20% of their countries' gross domestic product (GDP). Moreover, agriculture has the greatest dominance of female employment in the poorest regions of the world. Therefore, a focus on this sector can also contribute to greater gender equality in the world of work.

In the recent past, researchers and policymakers largely neglected the agricultural sector, while favoring modernization through the development of the manufacturing and service sectors. Declining official investment in agricultural development provides evidence for this trend. This shift away from agriculture went hand in hand with a lower rate of poverty reduction. Poverty, whether relative or absolute, needs to be defined. Average GDP may improve but inequality may become worse. This has implications for what kind of agricultural development is needed.

▶ Pesticide Exposure

In the agricultural sector, the use of pesticides causes at least 7 million cases of acute and long-term nonfatal illness. Pesticides are essential to modern agriculture: more than 2 million tons of pesticides, derived from 900 active ingredients, are used annually worldwide. Pesticides are widely used both in developed and developing countries. They constitute a major risk to farm workers, and in some countries account for as much as 14% of all occupational injuries in the agricultural sector and 10% of all fatal injuries. Unintentional poisonings kill an estimated 355,000 people globally each year. Although developed countries have much more intensive use of pesticides than developing countries, the disease burden is disproportionately carried by developing countries.

Women and children are at considerable risk of pesticide poisoning in the household. Farm workers' contaminated clothes are washed by their wives or children, and are often mixed in with other laundry. Pesticides stored in the home create the risk of accidental poisoning, especially among children. Moreover, the use of pesticides for domestic vermin control leads to home poisoning. The sale of toxic pesticides typically occurs in the informal sector, resulting in many acute and chronic health consequences.

Monocrotophos was cited in the death of 23 school children in Patna, India in July 2013, when some of the pesticide was mixed into the school lunches. Monocrotophos is an organophosphate insecticide which works systemically and on contact. It is acutely toxic to birds and humans, and for that reason has been banned in the United States since 1988. The pesticide is still produced by at least 15 manufacturers. It is manufactured and exported by companies in India, China, Brazil, and Argentina.

In developing countries—where two-thirds of these deaths occur—such poisonings are associated strongly with excessive exposure to, and inappropriate use of, toxic pesticides. Virtually all deaths due to acute pesticide poisoning occur in developing countries.

Many developing country governments report fatalities from pesticides as suicides, thereby shifting responsibility for prevention to the individual, reducing corporate responsibility, and limiting policy options available for control. To be fair, it is often the employer who is responsible for this fiction, to avoid whatever feeble liability does exist in the country concerned. It is true that governments do not critically examine such reports. Whether this is the result of willful collaboration with industry or simply ineptitude or political bias is not clear.

Some widely used pesticides in developing countries are highly toxic. Many of these pesticides are banned or severely restricted in developed countries, yet still legally sold to farmers in developing countries. Pesticides are often applied in combinations or mixtures, a common practice in both developed and developing countries. Studies on pesticide poisoning in developing countries suggest that exposures to mixtures of pesticides are associated with higher rates of case fatality and morbidity. Farmers often mix different pesticides into one mixture for application. Because they do not understand the pesticides they were sold, nor the mechanisms by which the pesticides work, they end up mixing two agents with different trade names but identical active ingredient. This is neither efficient, nor safe, and it is a waste of money. But given the circumstances under which pesticides are sold, there is no stewardship or information to farmers to make rational decisions on whether to use chemicals for pest control, and, if so, what chemicals to use.

It is common for farmers in developing countries to apply hazardous pesticides while working barefoot. Their clothing is soaked with pesticides after spraying with a backpack tank, which further enhances absorption through the skin. Personal protective equipment is often neither available nor affordable in developing countries, nor is it practical to wear in tropical climates because of the heat, humidity, and potential to decrease farm workers' productivity. Washing facilities are rarely located close to agricultural fields. Dermal absorption continues until the farmer or farm worker can get home to wash. But farm workers spend long hours in agricultural fields and cannot take long breaks to go home. They eat, drink, and smoke with pesticide-soaked hands, ingesting pesticides orally as well as through dermal absorption.

International organizations provide the major sources of information, advice, and technical support on pesticide health and safety to developing countries. There is a lack of rigorous legislation and regulation to control pesticides. Moreover, there are too few training programs for personnel with the responsibility to inspect and monitor the use of pesticides. This is true at the ministry level, but only part of the problem. The farmers and farm workers have little information from any reliable source. What they do learn usually comes from peers in the form of pressure to maximize production, or private entrepreneurs whose business is to sell pesticides. Consequently, there is an incentive to provide only certain kinds of information, and to limit any health and safety information or advice on how to reduce pesticide usage.

There often is a mutually beneficial relationship established between the pesticide industry (not small salesmen or entrepreneurs running a village shop) and government beholden to these companies. Government in many developing countries allows industry a free hand to shape policy, information, and technical guidance for pesticides. For example, the South American government outsources training of new emergent farmers to the pesticide industry, a training program paid for with public funding.

CONSTRUCTION INDUSTRY

The construction industry accounts for at least 60,000 fatal workplace accidents each year worldwide. About 17% of all fatal workplace accidents occur in this sector. The construction industry accounts for around 10% of the world's economic activity and employs 180 million people.

The construction industry is one of the most hazardous occupations, and in some countries, the most hazardous. The construction industry accounts for around 7% of the world's employment but 30–40% of the world's fatal injuries. Falls from heights due to inadequate scaffolding and lack of basic protections, being buried in excavations, or being crushed by vehicles or building materials are the most common causes of fatal injuries.

Construction is a hazardous industry for almost all key risks—chemicals, dusts, manual handling, physical hazards, and psychosocial hazards. Construction industry exposures are routine and excessive. Moreover, poor access to care and benefits compounds the hazards. The vast majority of construction is taking place in developing countries, where health and safety laws are seldom if ever enforced. In most countries, construction is characterized by low status, low paid, short-term, unregistered, informal, and hazardous jobs in a highly fragmented industry. Many workers, in particular rural-urban migrants, are faced with exploitative employment practices, hardship, and hazards.

Worldwide, the cost of occupational injuries and illnesses across all sectors is estimated by the ILO at 4% of the GDP, making workplace prevention a development issue. Yet it is very common to find that even large construction projects have no safety policy or prevention program, no safety officer, no project-specific health and safety plan, no information or training on prevention, no collective measures to prevent accidents or illnesses, and not even the most basic personal protective equipment.

The employment relationship in construction is distinctive for the weak ties between contractors and trade workers and the limited supervision provided by the general contractor. These factors are exacerbated by social norms and power relationships characteristic of construction worksites, which create further difficulty in both studying and ameliorating construction site ergonomic risks. The absence of steady employment relationships in construction reinforces a climate in which workers are hesitant to complain about work conditions for fear that they will simply be replaced, and this same dynamic reinforces a culture in which it is assumed that working while injured is just part of the job.

Construction workers are potentially exposed to asbestos, wood dust, various oils, man-made mineral fibers, welding fumes, lead, organic solvents, silica, isocyanates, diesel exhaust, concrete dust, and asphalt vapors. Silicosis from exposure to cement and stone dust kills many thousands of workers. Respiratory diseases, skin problems, deafness, and chronic pain from heavy physical work, punishing workloads, and long hours are almost universal health complaints. The ILO estimates that 100,000 construction workers die annually from diseases caused by past exposure to asbestos. In some countries, deaths from asbestos-related diseases have now outstripped the number of deaths from occupational accidents.

Basic amenities, such as clean drinking water; latrines; facilities for washing, cooking, or eating; or first aid, are seldom provided on site. Proper accommodation is a basic problem and workers who migrate to the urban centers in search of day labor have no alternative but to live on or near the construction site. Malnutrition and diseases such as malaria, dengue, cholera, and tuberculosis are widespread among construction workers and their families. This vulnerability is most extreme when whole families migrate from rural areas in search of work.

THE COVID-19 PANDEMIC

The COVID-19 crisis began in early 2020, with a profound impact on occupational health throughout the world. The initial impact was in infections, work loss, and failure in most countries to properly address the public health needs of patient care, equipment, testing, and immunization. The pandemic later evolved into a prolonged economic crisis, with many job losses, and disruption of previously weak or deficient occupational health and safety programs. The impact on world economics affects the funding and enforcement of worker protection laws. The pandemic exposed inequalities and social fissures in societies that profoundly affect the most vulnerable and marginalized groups. Loss of employment means large income losses for workers, many of which become working poor, workers close to or below the poverty line. School closures and economic pressures caused by the pandemic increased child labor across the developing world. The limited reporting of international occupational health and safety has now decreased, and it will take many years before new assessments can be made. The international system of institutions has historically been inadequate to the tasks assigned to the United Nations to address global occupational health problems. The lack of resources for the WHO and the ILO to adequately respond to the COVID-19 pandemic further demonstrated this gap.

REFERENCES

ILO International Labor Standards on Occupational Safety and Health: http://www.ilo.org/global/standards/subjects-covered-by-international-labour-standards/occupational-safety-and-health/lang--en/index.htm.

ILO Labor Migration: http://www.ilo.org/global/topics/labour-migration/lang--en/index.htm.

ILO Occupational Safety and Health: http://www.ilo.org/safework/lang--en/index.htm.

ILO: Labor Administration and Labor Inspection, 2018. http://www.ilo.org/labadmin/lang--en/index.htm.

LaDou J. A World of False Promises: International Labour Organization, World Health Organization, and the Plea of Workers Under Neoliberalism. Int J Health Serv. 2020 Jul;50(3):314-323. PMID: 32276564.

LaDou J, London L, Watterson A: Occupational health: a world of false promises. Environ Health 2018;17(1):81 [PMID: 30463563].

NIOSH Global Outreach: http://www.cdc.gov/niosh/programs/global/.

WHO: e-GOHNET (Global Occupational Health Network) Newsletter: http://www.who.int/occupational_health/publications/newsletter/en/index.html.

WHO Workplace Health Promotion: http://www.who.int/occupational_health/topics/workplace/en/index1.html.

Workplace Safety and Health Institute. Global Estimates of Occupational Accidents and Work-related Illnesses, 2017. https://www.wsh-institute.sg.

World Health Organization. The 12th General Program of Work 2014–2019: Not merely the absence of disease © WHO 2014. http://apps.who.int/iris/bitstream/handle/10665/112792/GPW_2014-2019_eng.pdf?sequence=1.

■ SELF-ASSESSMENT QUESTIONS

Select the one correct answer for each question.

Question 1: Occupational health and safety laws in developing countries
  a. are highly developed and adequately funded
  b. apply to all workers
  c. cover only about 10% of the population
  d. ensure access to adequate occupational health services

Question 2: Global working conditions are
  a. largely the result of progressive practices of multinational corporations
  b. improving because of the controlled growth in the working population
  c. complicated by a small informal sector in developing countries
  d. affected by a large migrant workforce

Question 3: Child labor
  a. is controlled by international law
  b. is prevented by the International Labor Organization (ILO)
  c. is an economic and social reality in many developing countries
  d. is disappearing at a rapid rate

Question 4: Globalization benefits
   a. all countries equally
   b. China more than it does Pakistan
   c. countries that are competitive in the knowledge economy
   d. only corporate interests

Question 5: The World Health Organization (WHO)
   a. is solely responsible for occupational safety and health
   b. addresses occupational health through the promotion of medical services and hygienic standards
   c. has had no occupational health initiatives in recent years
   d. is not responsible for technical aspects of occupational health

Question 6: Occupational diseases
   a. have a profound effect on the health of the world's population.
   b. occur primarily in developed countries
   c. are diagnosed and compensated in all countries
   d. are diagnosed and compensated only in developed countries

Question 7: The ILO
   a. plays no role in promoting policies for occupational health and safety
   b. is under the WHO with respect to occupational health and safety
   c. is a tripartite organization of government, employer, and worker representatives
   d. conventions guide only a few occupational health and safety programs

Question 8: Global occupational injuries
   a. cause economic losses amounting to 4–6% of national incomes
   b. occur in about 1 in 20 workers each year

   c. seldom involve preventable fatalities
   d. occur most commonly in developed countries

Question 9: ILO conventions and recommendations
   a. are international agreements that have legal force if they are not ratified by the national parliament
   b. guide all countries in the promotion of workplace safety and in managing occupational health and safety programs
   c. leave occupational disease prevention to the WHO
   d. are approved by most member states

Question 10: Agriculture is
   a. the most prevalent type of employment in the world
   b. dominated by male employment in the poorest regions of the world
   c. no more dependent on a fair globalization than any other sector
   d. the development of the agricultural sector is not important to reducing poverty

Question 11: Global use of pesticides
   a. is hardly essential to modern agriculture
   b. affects only agricultural workers
   c. causes fatalities that are rare and largely accidental
   d. includes highly toxic pesticides banned in some countries

Question 12: Global construction industry
   a. is the fourth most hazardous industry
   b. accounts for about 30–40% of all fatal workplace accidents
   c. has only a minor problem with fatalities in the United States and Europe
   d. has overcome its problem with carcinogen exposures

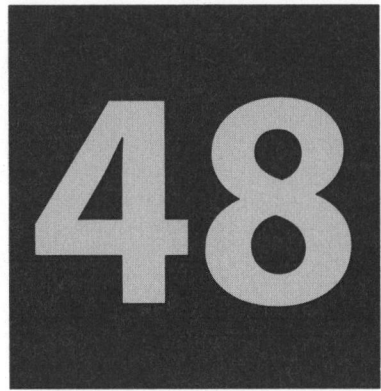

Pediatric Environmental Health

Stephanie M. Holm, MD, MPH

Mark D. Miller, MD, MPH

Vulnerability of Children to Environmental Hazards

Many of the physical differences in children compared to adults put them at increased risk from toxicants in their environments. Because children are growing, they have a higher metabolic rate relative to their size compared to adults. For this reason, children consume relatively more of all the things needed to sustain life and growth; they eat more food, drink more water, and breathe more air. Children thus get a higher exposure per kilogram of body weight to many pollutants. Moreover, children have a higher surface area to body mass ratio, so their potential for dermal absorption is also higher. Children are also at risk in utero. Toxicants which are either small molecules or fat-soluble cross the placenta easily, as do some metals. Children also have longer remaining life expectancy, meaning that exposures with long lead times before disease (such as many carcinogens) can be more problematic for children, who are more likely to live long enough to experience an adverse effect. Finally, crawling on the floor and children's short stature can increase their exposure to heavy airborne toxicants, such as mercury, which will be concentrated closer to the ground, in children's breathing zone. Metabolism of many pharmaceuticals and environmental contaminants differ by age. Cytochrome P450 (phase 1) and conjugating (phase 2) enzyme development during early life can result in slower detoxification and clearance of many chemicals in neonates and young children. For example, while conjugation by some UGT enzymes is mature by 2 months, for others adult activity is not reached until puberty. For some chemicals the metabolic pathways are age dependent; for example, acetaminophen is metabolized by sulfation rather than glucuronidation in the neonate.

Young children are in a period of rapid growth. In addition to implying a higher metabolic rate for their size, this means that they have many cells rapidly dividing, further increasing their susceptibility to environmental insults. As a result, though adults can generally be expected to have a predictable pattern of insults with exposure to toxicants, regardless of the timing of exposure, the same cannot be said for children. In children there are specific developmental windows of susceptibility. For example, it is well described that alcohol exposure in utero has differential effects based on the timing of that exposure. Lead exposure during childhood can result in long-term cognitive deficits at lower levels than in adults because the exposure affects children during a period of substantial learning. Adolescence represents another time period of rapid growth concentrated around the development of sexual organs. As in younger children, adolescents are uniquely susceptible to toxicants during this period of growth and differentiation.

Many childhood behaviors also contribute to an increased risk of environmental exposures. Young children go through an exploratory phase which involves mouthing behaviors, meaning that they may have significantly higher exposure via ingestion of toxicants that adults would not ingest. Similarly, by crawling (in young infants) or simply playing on the floor (older children) children have increased exposure to toxicants in dust, such as polybrominated diphenyl ethers (PBDEs). As the American Association of Poison Control Centers attests, children are also at risk for exposure to chemicals and pesticides because of their developmental inability to assess hazardous situations and chemicals. Finally, young children have a much more restricted diet than adults; for example, children eat many more apples and apple products putting them at increased risk of exposure to specific pesticides used on that crop.

The environmental exposures of the fetus and young child contribute not only to childhood illness and disability but also to disease in adulthood. For example, low birth weight has been associated with an increased risk of adult lipid profiles linked to cardiovascular disease and hypertension, impaired glucose regulation, and type 2 diabetes in later life. This "programming" in response to poor fetal nutrition illustrates that permanent changes in organ structure, metabolism, and function can result from early life exposure. Unique vulnerabilities may be found during development of the nervous, respiratory, and immune systems. Thus, the combination of physical factors that increase children's effective dose of exposure, behaviors that increase the risk of exposures, and windows of particular susceptibility during development, mean that children are a population particularly vulnerable to environmental health hazards.

Precautionary Principle

Designing public policy and laws to protect children is difficult, particularly due to often limited research as bioethics limits the types of exposure research that can be done with children. Consequently, if an environmental exposure has even the potential to cause harmful effects in children, it should be avoided or minimized, without delaying for further scientific inquiry. The precautionary principle provides justification for public policy actions in situations of scientific complexity, uncertainty and ignorance, where there may be a need to act in order to avoid, or reduce, potentially serious or irreversible threats to health or the environment, using an appropriate level of scientific evidence, and taking into account the likely pros and cons of action and inaction.

Pediatric Environmental Health History

The content of a pediatric environmental health history depends greatly on whether the history is being taken for screening purposes or in response to a direct and specific concern. A screening history should focus on the settings in which children spend time, with home and school usually taking up a large portion of that time. Specific guidance on questions to ask are in Table 48–1.

A helpful way to approach environmental exposures in children is to determine the routes of exposure: inhalation, ingestion, and dermal absorption, as all toxicants act through one or more of these routes. The clinician is tasked with elucidating the usual components of an HPI including details of where, when, and how the exposure occurred, as well as any estimate the parent has to the quantity of exposure. This should be explored in relation to the potential outcome in question; is there any literature supporting a potential link between this exposure and outcome, and does the time course of this child's exposure fit with what would be expected for causing disease. With the exception of acute poisonings, there are only a few environmental exposures for which laboratory measurement in the child is useful (eg, carbon monoxide or lead). Often, a potential exposure occurs over a long period of time, often long before the child is presenting for care, making it difficult to pinpoint the exact contribution of a specific exposure to a child's disease. Questions regarding testing options warrant consultation with a local pediatric environmental health specialist (such as at a Pediatric Environmental Health Specialty Unit), and in the setting of an acute exposure, the local poison control services. In the case of specific exposures at home or school, coordination with an industrial hygienist to assess the environment may be necessary.

Physicians are sometimes asked to interpret environmental laboratory tests from a laboratory that performs various assays without correlation with clinical findings. Interpretation of such tests should be approached with caution as test methods may not be validated and laboratories often set their own reference ranges. Hair testing in particular is not generally considered clinically reliable at this time and is used primarily in research settings.

Considerations by Age—Diet

Infants and children are at particularly high risk of toxicity from food or water contamination as they tend to have a much more restricted diet compared to adults.

The most extreme example of a restricted diet in childhood is in young infants (up to 4–6 months of life) who usually consume only 1–2 sources of nutrition: breastmilk and/or formula. Breastfeeding mothers should minimize their intake of fish that are high in mercury; safer fish choices include salmon, shrimp, tilapia, and cod. Most commonly formula is prepared by mixing a dried powder with water. The water used for formula preparation should be known to be safe either because the municipal water supply has been tested, or if the family uses well water, testing should be done for arsenic, nitrates, coliforms, and other local ground water contaminants. Families can minimize lead exposure, if lead pipes are definitively or possibly present, by running cold water for 1–2 minutes prior to preparing formula, which minimizes the use of water that has been sitting in the pipes leaching lead. Finally, as both breastmilk and formula can be given in bottles, polycarbonate bottles which can leech bisphenol A and other similar compounds should be avoided. Safer alternatives include colored or opaque plastics or tempered glass (which do not break as easily as regular glass).

Older infants and young children also often have restricted diets. For example, some toddlers may only consistently eat 1–2 fruits or vegetables, meaning that if these have high pesticide residues these children may be disproportionately exposed. For this reason, it is recommended that fruits and vegetables are washed and peeled, and when possible, purchased organic. Of particular concern, arsenic is high in multiple foods that have historically been popular with infants and young children, such as rice (and rice-based cereals) and apple products. Rice cereal was often used as a first food for infants, but given the arsenic concerns, it would be prudent for families to provide a variety of grains or select a different first food.

Surroundings—Home, Day Care, & School

Children have increased minute ventilation relative to their size compared to adults, with the highest relative minute ventilation occurring in the smallest children. Thus, infants and young children have proportionally higher exposures of airborne toxicants such as radon, second-hand tobacco smoke, particulate matter pollution, and aerosols from cleaning products.

Once children start crawling and walking, they are also at increased susceptibility for compounds occurring in

Table 48–1. Pediatric environmental health screening.

Area	Questions	Potential Exposures
Surroundings At home	What type of home does your child live or spend time in?	Indoor air pollutants, lead
	What are the age and condition of your home? Is there lead, mold, or asbestos?	Asbestos, indoor air pollutants, mold, lead (in household paint prior to 1978)
	Is there ongoing or planned renovation?	Asbestos, lead
	Do you have carbon monoxide detectors?	Carbon monoxide
	What type of heating/air system does your home have?	Indoor air pollutants
	Where and how do you use and store chemicals and pesticides?	Pesticides, cleaning products
	Do you use chemicals in the garden or spray the lawn with pesticides?	Pesticides
	Have you tested your home for radon?	Radon
	Do you think there is lead in your soil?	Lead
	Do you have a picnic table or playset made of treated wood?	Arsenic (in treated wood prior to 2004)
	How close is your home to major roadways?	Outdoor air pollutants
At school	Are there concerns about your child's school environment?	Indoor air pollutants, lead, asbestos, carbon monoxide, pesticides, radon, arsenic
In the community	Is there a source of pollution in your community?	Indoor air pollutants, outdoor air pollutants, hazardous waste
Tobacco Smoke Exposure	Do any of the adults who care for the child smoke? Do you or other caregivers allow smoking in the car?	Second-hand tobacco smoke exposure
Water Sources	Do you use tap water? Well water?	Lead, nitrates, arsenic, bacterial contamination
Exposures from Food	Does your family and your child eat fish? What kinds and how often? What kinds/how often does the child eat fruits and vegetables? How often does the child eat rice?	Mercury, PCBs, pesticides, arsenic
Sun and Other Exposure to Ultraviolet Radiation (UVB)	Is your child protected from excessive sun exposure? Do you visit tanning salons?	Ultraviolet radiation
Exposure Resulting from Household Members' Occupations and Hobbies	What jobs do household members hold, and are they exposed to any chemicals at work? What are the hobbies of household members?	Solvents, lead

Source: Adapted from American Academy of Pediatrics: *Pediatric Environmental Health*, 3rd ed. American Academy of Pediatrics, 2012:Table 5.2, pp. 42-43.

dust (lead, PBDEs). Ways to mitigate risk related to dust exposures include testing for/abating lead paint, and washing children's hands frequently and before eating. Household pest management strategies should use an integrated approach which minimizes the use of chemical pesticides and preferentially uses baits/traps/gels when needed rather than dusts or sprays.

Accidental ingestion of toxic compounds by young children is unfortunately a frequent occurrence. Families should keep as few chemicals in their homes as possible. Those present should be out of children's reach and in their original containers so that they can be easily identified in case of an ingestion.

Though young children do not have workplaces, many of them spend time outside the house. Environmental exposures in those locations, such as early childhood care settings, are important to consider. Early childhood education facilities may be sources of exposure from art and craft supplies (which should be low VOC whenever possible) as well as from disinfectants. Day care and early childcare facilities often have regulations requiring disinfection after particular activities (diaper changes, eating) making them one of the few places where disinfection is mandated with children present. Care providers should limit the use of sprays and use products without bleach or ammonia. Finally, older pressure-treating methods for wood often used compounds containing arsenic (such as CCA—chromated copper arsenate). Facilities with older wooden structures (prior to 2004 in the United States) such as play structures, picnic tables or decks, should not have children eat while in contact with these structures and should consider sealing or replacing the wood.

Teenagers who may be working can have workplace or hobby exposures similar to adults, with the added risk that they are often given less desirable, higher exposure tasks. For young children, any working individual in their household may bring home potentially toxic materials. All workers should be aware of what their workplace exposures are so that potential take-home exposures can be prevented. In many work settings, work clothes and shoes should be changed prior to coming home and laundered separately.

Exposures That Affect Children

▶ Endocrine Disrupting Chemicals

Prenatal and childhood exposures to endocrine disrupting chemicals are of greater concern than those in adults. The adult endocrine system is relatively resilient, with endogenous hormones generally at higher concentrations than the chemicals at issue, and feedback loops that regulate hormone levels. In early life, however, background levels of sex hormones are much lower and endogenous regulatory mechanisms are not fully developed. At the same time, hormonally sensitive organs, including the brain, are actively developing and therefore sensitive to permanent developmental damage from biological perturbations. As a result, fairly subtle endocrine fluctuations during fetal and child development may lead to permanent structural and functional deficits.

Endocrine disrupting chemicals alter the action of hormones in ways that may result in health effects. Some of the earliest examples of chemicals in this category were those that were found to activate the estrogen receptor in a manner that mimics estrogen itself, such as bisphenyl-A (BPA). BPA was ubiquitous in products using clear, hard plastics, many of which were used for food packaging. BPA interferes in hormone function, with a wide range of health effects including neurobehavioral deficits in children and obesity. In the United States, accumulating evidence of health effects from BPA led to changes in consumer preferences, creating a large market of "BPA-free" products. However, substitute chemicals (with similar chemical structures) may have similar estrogenic effects, and the safest option for families would be to avoid clear, hard plastics, particularly for products used by infants and young children (such as bottles, sippy cups).

Another category of endocrine disrupting chemicals is the phthalates. These are found in soft plastics and PVC products as well as many personal care products (such as shampoos, cosmetics, and lotions). Phthalates are also found in large quantity in food packaging as well as in processed foods, high-fat dairy and high-fat meat products. Phthalates are antiandrogenic and can impact androgen sensitive tissues, having lasting effects on testicular function and genital development. For example, phthalate exposure in-utero is associated with testicular dysgenesis syndrome and alterations in pubertal timing. Exposure to phthalates can be minimized by consuming low-fat dairy products, avoiding heating foods in soft plastics (to avoid leaching of phthalates), and minimizing the use of personal care products. There are many other known endocrine disrupting chemicals including pesticides, detergents, plasticizers, and combustion byproducts. Other well-established endocrine disruptors with widespread human exposures include alkylphenols, dioxins, polychlorinated biphenyls (PCBs), polybrominated diphenyl ethers (PBDEs), perchlorate, and triclosan. Several of these are known to effect thyroid hormone production or activity. Thyroid hormone is essential during many time windows for normal development.

▶ Heavy Metals

Lead

There is no safe level of lead in children. In the United States concentration of lead in blood at the 95th percentile in children aged 1 to 5 years declined from 29 mcg/dL in 1976–1980 to 2.8 mcg/dL in 2015–2016, a decrease of 90%. In response to decreasing childhood levels the Centers for Disease Control and Prevention (CDC) established a new "reference value" for blood lead levels (5 mcg/dL) in 2012, thereby lowering the level at which evaluation and intervention are recommended. Lead can affect children's brains and the developing nervous systems, causing reduced IQ, learning disabilities, attention problems, executive function disorders, and behavioral problems. Higher levels of exposure can also cause anemia and kidney problems, and as in adults, acute exposures can result in a variety of other effects. Lead readily crosses the placenta and has been detected in the fetal brain as early as the end of the first trimester and has been associated with neurobehavioral impacts in children.

Older houses may have been painted with lead-based paint, and lead-contaminated paint dust is the most common significant source of childhood lead exposure. Lead dust comes from deteriorating lead-based paint and lead-contaminated soil that is tracked into homes and schools, which can then be unintentionally ingested by children during normal hand-mouth behaviors. Less common sources of lead exposure include leaching from lead pipes, certain imported cosmetics, and ceramic ware; vinyl miniblinds made before 1997; certain candle wicks and crayons; soft vinyl lunch boxes; and some traditional/herbal remedies and foods. Occupations or hobbies like painting and refinishing, cleaning and shooting of firearms, battery production or recycling, stained glass making, and ceramics may result in take-home lead poisoning among children. As many as 2.5% of the elevated BLLs among US children younger than 6 years may be the result of take-home exposures.

Due to the potential for long-term developmental effects the CDC recommends that health departments develop a local strategy for lead screening based on the local housing risks, poverty rates, and knowledge of community elevated blood lead incidence. As a result, guidance varies from universal blood lead screening to determination of need by risk-assessment tools. US Federal policy states that all children enrolled in low-income insurance policies should have a blood lead test at age 1 and 2 and that children 36–72 months old have one if not previously tested. Children of all ages who are immigrants, refugees, or adoptees are at higher risk and should be screened at the earliest opportunity. The CDC and the American College of Obstetricians and Gynecologists recommend considering the possibility of lead exposure in pregnant and lactating women by evaluating risk factors as part of the initial examination. If any risk factors are identified blood lead testing is recommended. Key risk factors for lead exposure in pregnant and lactating women include emigration from areas with high ambient lead, working or living with worker in industry using lead, pica, use of alternative or complementary substances, herbs, or treatments, home renovation of older home without appropriate controls, use of imported lead glazed pottery, history of previous exposure or elevated blood lead, and high-risk hobbies such as stained glass or ceramic pottery. The *Guidelines for the identification and management of lead exposure in pregnant and lactating women,* published by the CDC, provides extensive guidance on screening and follow up of exposures resulting in blood lead greater than 5 mcg/dL. Though not concentrated, a fraction of blood lead enters breastmilk. Initiation of breastfeeding is recommended for maternal blood leads under 40 mcg/dL with continuation recommendations dependent on the infant's level.

Management of children with elevated blood lead levels is multifaceted including management of diet, environmental exposures, and referrals to community agencies and developmental specialists. Clinicians can be assisted by consultation with local public health programs and Pediatric Environmental Health Specialty Units. Chelation has not been demonstrated to provide improved outcomes for levels below 45 mcg/dL. For levels ≥ 45 mcg/dL, chelation should always be considered under management of a pediatrician/medical toxicologist experienced in treatment of lead poisoning. These clinicians can be identified through poison control centers, childhood lead poisoning programs at state health departments, or the Pediatric Environmental Health Specialty Units.

Fetal and child lead exposure, particularly in low- and middle-income countries, places a heavy cost on society. It has been estimated that as much as 12.4% of the global burden of intellectual disability can be attributed to lead. Mass poisonings from lead still occur with a recent example being in Nigeria in 2010. Over 400 children died of acute lead poisoning resulting from artisanal processing gold ore containing lead and thousands of others were left with disabilities. The common method included dust creating methods and

was conducted inside the family compounds. Public health interventions (including education and introduction of safer processing methods) resulted in dramatic decreases in exposure to children in the region. Exposures from a variety of activities including recycling of batteries, e-waste, continued use of lead containing paints, and industrial contamination continue to result in high exposures to children in many countries.

Exposures can be minimized by avoiding lead containing products where possible (some costume jewelry, some Ayurvedic medications, some imported foods and candies), running water from lead pipes for a few minutes before using, dusting frequently with a damp cloth to minimize lead dust, abatement of lead paints by a certified contractor, and finally by decreasing take-home exposures by having household members with lead exposures outside the home change clothing and shoes and do their laundry separately.

Mercury

Mercury exists in multiple forms: organic (ethyl and methyl mercuries), elemental mercury, and inorganic mercury salts. Ingestion of mercury-contaminated fish is the major source of human exposure to methylmercury. Elemental and inorganic mercury from industrial emissions are converted to methylmercury by bacteria, which then enters the food chain. Methylmercury is efficiently absorbed from the gastrointestinal tract and readily crosses both the placenta and blood-brain barrier.

High-level fetal exposures may cause psychomotor retardation, blindness, deafness, and seizures. In contrast, lower-level exposures, such as those that occur with typical maternal fish consumption, have been associated with language and memory deficits. Fish consumption should still be encouraged in children and pregnant women due to the healthy fats contained therein, but low-mercury options should be consumed (such as salmon, shrimp, tilapia, and cod).

In contrast, exposure to elemental mercury is mostly via mercury vapor, and inorganic mercury exposure can occur via imported products such as skin-lightening creams. These exposures result in very similar findings in children compared to adults but again with a predominance of neurologic findings. A pathognomonic finding of mercury exposure in children is acrodynia (peripheral neuropathy with a pink desquamating rash on the hands and feet, hypertension, and irritability), which occurs in a non–dose-dependent fashion.

Arsenic

Arsenic is a metalloid element that occurs naturally in the earth's crust. High concentrations are released into the environment by polluting industries. Worldwide, drinking water is the principal source of arsenic exposure, including some areas of the United States, but inhalation can be an important exposure route for people living near smelters. Inorganic arsenic is associated with several human cancers, including lung, bladder, and skin cancer. Perinatal exposures to arsenic in drinking water have been linked to increases in late fetal, neonatal, and postneonatal mortality, as well as to neurodevelopmental abnormalities, adult cancers, and bronchiectasis. The risks for lung and bladder cancer are 2–4 times greater for early life exposure than during later childhood or adulthood.

Inorganic arsenic is naturally concentrated in rice, particularly in the hull. Thus, brown rice has a higher content than white. Traditionally in the United States rice has been a common ingredient in infant diet during the transition to solid foods. Recent recommendations from the American Academy of Pediatrics include choosing first foods to vary the grains used to limit exposure. Young children should limit consumption of rice beverages and brown rice syrup which can be high in inorganic arsenic content.

▶ Flame Retardants (PBDEs)

PBDEs are a class of brominated hydrocarbon flame retardants that were phased out of commercial products in the United States in 2013. They were used in small appliances and foam products including furniture, baby and child products (strollers, car seats), and carpet underlay. However, even in areas where PBDEs have been phased out they are ubiquitous in the environment due to the prior widespread use and the persistence of these compounds both in the environment and in fatty tissues of humans and animals. The PBDE-laden foams break down into PBDE containing dust, which can both settle and become airborne and is the leading source of exposure. Because of young children's normative hand-to-mouth behaviors, they may have much higher exposures to such dust. Some dietary exposure also occurs because of the persistence of PBDEs in fatty tissues of meat and fish.

Children have higher serum levels of PBDEs than adults. Children show associations between prenatal or early life exposures and both attention and executive function deficits. Animal studies show associations between PBDEs and neurobehavioral, liver, and thyroid effects. Families should be encouraged to minimize fat consumption (by choosing lean meats and allowing fat to drain), replace older crumbling foam items, and avoid products treated with chemical flame retardants when purchasing new items. In addition, dusting with a damp cloth, wet mopping, and use of a HEPA vacuum air filters can decease dust levels.

Stress & Adverse Childhood Experiences

High levels of stress, such as during pregnancy, divorce, or death of a close family member, has been associated with altered/accentuated stress response, increases in inflammatory cytokines, and a more allergic prone Th1/Th2 balance in adult female offspring. The more adverse childhood experiences (ACEs) experienced during childhood, the higher the risk for lifelong negative impacts across a spectrum of health and behavioral outcomes including cancer, heart disease, diabetes, and respiratory diseases. Similarly, environmental chemicals (such as those found in air, water, and consumer products) can have a harmful influence on lifelong health. These impacts may be compounded by multiple exposures.

For example, children who experience both violence (at home or in their communities) and air pollution are at an increased risk for developing asthma, compared with children exposed to only one of these factors. Good nutrition, positive educational experiences, and high levels of social support may serve as mitigating factors.

Environmental Pollution

Pollution of the air, water, and soil is estimated to have resulted in 940,000 deaths in 2016 among children worldwide, with two-third occurring in children under the age of 5. The majority of pollution-related deaths in children occur in low- and middle-income countries, most due to respiratory and gastrointestinal diseases caused by polluted air and water. Pollution is also linked to low birth weight, asthma, cancer, and neurodevelopmental disorders in children.

REFERENCES

Agency for Toxic Substances and Disease Registry: Principles of Pediatric Environmental Health. What are Factors Affecting Children's Susceptibility to Exposures? https://www.atsdr.cdc.gov/csem/csem.asp?csem=27&po=6.

Bethell CD et al: Prioritizing possibilities for child and family health: an agenda to address adverse childhood experiences and foster the social and emotional roots of well-being in pediatrics. Acad Pediatr 2017;17(7S):S36-S50 [PMID: 28865659].

Caito S, Aschner M: Developmental neurotoxicity of lead. Adv Neurobiol 2017;18:3-12 [PMID: 28889260].

Centers for Disease Control and Prevention. Guidelines for the identification and management of lead exposure in pregnant and lactating women. Atlanta (GA): CDC; 2010. http://www.cdc.gov/nceh/lead/publications/leadandpregnancy2010.pdf.

Hauptman M, Bruccoleri R, Woolf AD: An update on childhood lead poisoning. Clin Pediatr Emerg Med 2017;18(3):181-192 [PMID: 29056870].

Korten I, Ramsey K, Latzin P: Air pollution during pregnancy and lung development in the child. Paediatr Respir Rev 2017;21:38-46 [PMID: 27665510].

Landrigan PJ et al: Pollution and children's health. Sci Total Environ 2019;650(Pt 2):2389-2394 [PMID: 30292994].

Lead screening during pregnancy and lactation. Committee Opinion No. 533. American College of Obstetricians and Gynecologists. Obstet Gynecol 2012;120:416-20 (https://www.acog.org/-/media/project/acog/acogorg/clinical/files/committee-opinion/articles/2012/08/lead-screening-during-pregnancy-and-lactation.pdf).

Miller MD, Marty MA, Landrigan PJ: Children's environmental health: beyond national boundaries. Pediatr Clin North Am 2016;63(1):149-165 [PMID: 26613694].

Pediatric Environmental Health Specialty Units. https://www.pehsu.net/. Washington, DC 2019.

Western States Pediatric Environmental Health: Pediatric Environmental Health Toolkit. https://peht.ucsf.edu/index.php San Francisco, CA 2016.

Pediatric Environmental Health Specialty Units, Pediatric Recommendations on Medical Management of Childhood Lead Exposure and Poisoning. https://www.pehsu.net/Lead_Resources.html.

■ SELF-ASSESMENT QUESTIONS

Select the one correct answer for each question.

Question 1: Endocrine disrupting chemicals
  a. alter the action of hormones in ways that may result in health effects
  b. stimulate estrogen production in children
  c. are harmless to children
  d. are seldom found in plastics

Question 2: Phthalates
  a. are the sole category of endocrine disrupting chemicals
  b. are found in soft plastics and PVC products
  c. are not found in processed foods
  d. are antiandrogenic and can impact androgen-sensitive tissues

Climate Change and Worker Health: Implications for Clinical Practice

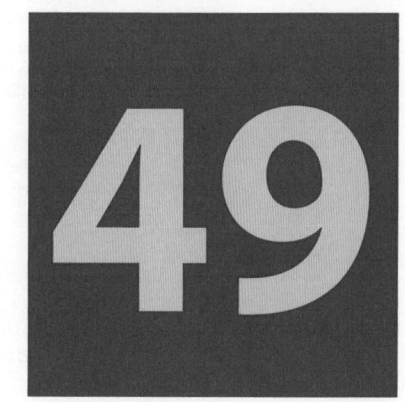

Cecilia J. Sorensen, MD

Margaret Cook-Shimanek, MD

Lee S. Newman, MD, MA

There is unambiguous scientific evidence that climate change is occurring and widespread scientific consensus that climate change is anthropogenic. In recent years, global climate change has resulted in increased frequency and intensity of adverse weather events including heat waves, droughts, wildfires, extreme weather events, and flooding. These events have affected all regions of the United States, resulting in economic costs in the billions of dollars and extensive health impacts that are projected to increase if environmental changes continue to occur with under-mitigated carbon release.

Climate change results from a process whereby increased production of carbon dioxide (CO_2), and other greenhouse gases (GHGs), leads to increased retention of heat energy in the planet's atmosphere and oceans. Trapped heat as well as increasing CO_2 result in a series of environmental changes including increased ambient temperatures, heavier and more variable precipitation, warmer oceans, increased frequency and intensity of extreme weather, melting of land-based snow and ice, ocean acidification, and a rise in sea level. These environmental changes drive exposure pathways (eg, extreme heat) (Table 49–1) that in turn have significant impacts on worker's physical, mental, and community health (Figure 49–1).

As of 2018, the average global temperature has risen approximately 2.7°F (1°C) above preindustrial levels. In October 2018, the Intergovernmental Panel on Climate Change (IPCC) released a *Special Report on Global Warming of 1.5°C,* that outlines the serious repercussions to human health and livelihoods should warming exceed 1.5°C. Currently, global commitments to curb carbon emissions put us on track for an alarming 3°C average rise in global temperatures by 2100. Representative Concentration Pathways (RCP) comprise a set of four GHG concentration trajectories used to model climate projections ranging from a best case to worst case scenario over the next century. Figure 49–2 demonstrates projected changes in average temperature and precipitation by the end of the century under lower (RCP 2.6) and higher (RCP 8.5) pathways of GHG emissions,

illustrating the difference between ambitious and effective interventions (left) versus weak (right) action, respectively.

Workers in a variety of geographic regions and occupations are especially susceptible to health hazards imposed by climate change. Fundamentally, climate change results in diseases of vulnerability (Figure 49–3). It affects human health by compounding existing medical conditions and health threats and by placing new stresses on housing, food, and water security, job security, and many determinants of stable livelihoods and safe workplaces. In this way, climate change acts as a threat multiplier, amplifying existing health and worker safety issues, and leading to new unanticipated hazards.

Worker populations are vulnerable to negative health impacts of climate change either due to the nature of their profession (eg, firefighters, emergency response workers) or due to preexisting underlying health conditions (eg, cardiovascular or respiratory disease). Workers are also at higher risk than the general population because they are disproportionately exposed to environmental conditions that the general public can elect to avoid, but that they must endure due to the nature of their work. Since the workforce is a potential sentinel population for climate-related health effects, occupational and environment (OEM) collaboration with public health infrastructure can be mutually beneficial. Surveillance systems, which are common in both OEM and public health, will allow for early detection and tracking of climate-related health events. Ideally, this will result in earlier preventive and mitigation efforts with positive impacts for both populations. Concerted development of early warning systems may help workers and the general population prepare for impending climate-related events or epidemics. OEM clinicians are at the forefront of emerging health issues pertaining to working populations and must be prepared to advise, recognize, respond to, and mitigate climate-related health risks in workers. They have a role to play in helping companies develop sustainability plans that help address these shifting environmental challenges.

Table 49–1. Impacts of climate change on worker health.

Exposure Pathway	Description	Health Effect	At-risk Occupational Groups
Extreme heat	Increasing frequency of extreme heat events and rising average seasonal temperatures	Heat illness, exacerbation of underlying cardiovascular, respiratory, renal, or psychiatric disease, increased risk of accidental and nonaccidental trauma, obstetric complications	Outdoor workers, agricultural workers, electricity and pipeline utility workers, factory workers, firefighters, manufacturing workers, military, migrant workers, athletes, workers with underlying cardiac, renal, or respiratory disease; older workers
Air pollution	Combustion of fossil fuels leads to fine particulate matter ($PM_{2.5}$) and ozone air pollution that is intensified by rising temperatures, resulting in poor air quality	Exacerbation of underlying respiratory disease (asthma, COPD, allergic disease), cardiovascular disease, premature mortality	Outdoor workers, agricultural workers, construction workers, delivery workers, workers with underlying respiratory and cardiac disease
Extreme weather events	Increasing frequency of weather-related disasters, including hurricanes, flooding and wildfires with resultant increased exposure to potentially traumatic events, forced migration and relocation secondary to disasters	Trauma, electrocutions, drownings, exposure to toxic chemicals, exposure to biologically contaminated waste, delays in treatment for chronic underlying medical conditions, mental health and trauma-related effects (eg, posttraumatic stress disorder, depression, anxiety, substance abuse)	First responders, medical workers, engineering/construction worker, those involved in recovery efforts, those with a history of depression, substance abuse or anxiety
Changes in vector, pathogen, and host characteristics	Changes in temperature, precipitation, and ecology are altering the geographic distribution of vector-borne diseases	Increased exposure to vector-borne diseases transmitted by mosquitos, ticks, fleas, and rodents	Sanitation workers, demolition workers, food/animal production workers, military/deployed populations, agricultural workers, landscapers, forestry workers, pregnant women, immunocompromised workers
Water quality impacts	Shifting rainfall patterns and increased rates of evaporation lead to heavy rainfall events in some places and drought in others, ultimately increasing the risk of waterborne disease	Increased exposure to waterborne pathogens and toxic fish/shellfish poisoning	Fishers, outdoor workers, sanitation workers, first responders, older workers, immunocompromised workers
Mental health	Increased exposure to potentially traumatic events, forced migration, and relocation secondary to disasters	Risk of posttraumatic stress disorders, depression, anxiety, substance abuse	First responders, displaced workers, workers involved in recovery efforts, those with a history of depression, substance abuse or anxiety

Increased Ambient Temperature and Heat-Related Illness in the Workplace

There is clear evidence that exposure to more frequent and intense heatwaves is increasing, with an estimated 125 million additional adults exposed to heatwaves between 2000 and 2016. In the year 2017 alone, the majority of Americans experienced temperatures that were well above average or the hottest ever recorded (Figure 49–4). Increased ambient temperature is associated with increased risk of mortality, particularly among vulnerable populations, due to heat illness and the effects of heat on underlying medical conditions. For example, heat is associated with an increased risk

of cardiovascular and cerebrovascular events, exacerbations of respiratory disease as well as cardiac dysrhythmias and acute renal failure. Additionally, increased ambient temperatures have been shown to increase the risk of injury, illness, and death for those working in hot environments.

Exposure to extreme heat is the leading cause of direct weather-related deaths in the United States, and is a major climate risk factor among workers who perform heavy labor in hot conditions. Each year, there are, on an average 30 reported heat stroke deaths among workers in the United States. Of these deaths, approximately 24% occur in workers employed in the agriculture, forestry, fishing, and hunting industries and 67% occur in workers employed in crop production or

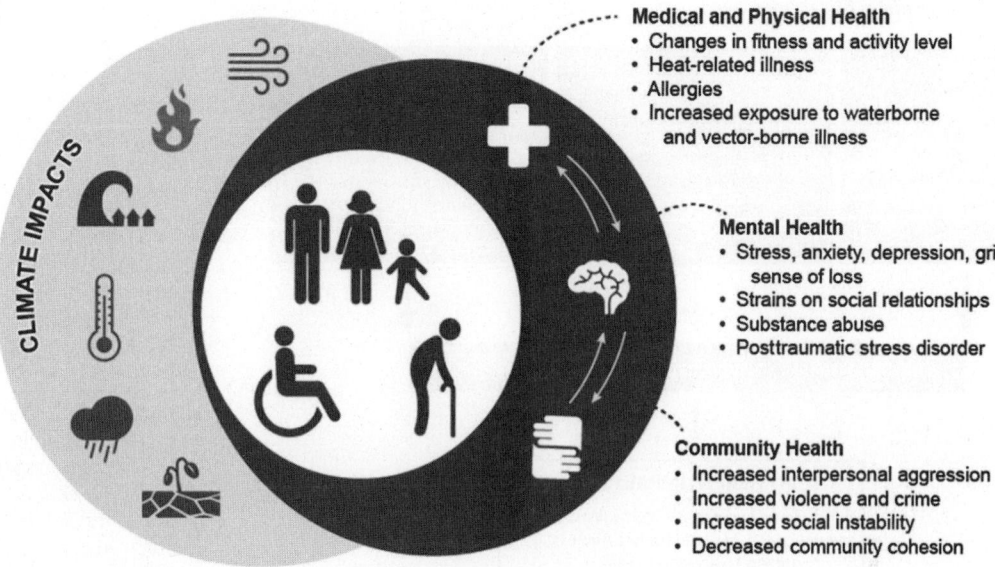

▲ **Figure 49–1.** Medical and physical health, mental health, and community consequences of climate change.

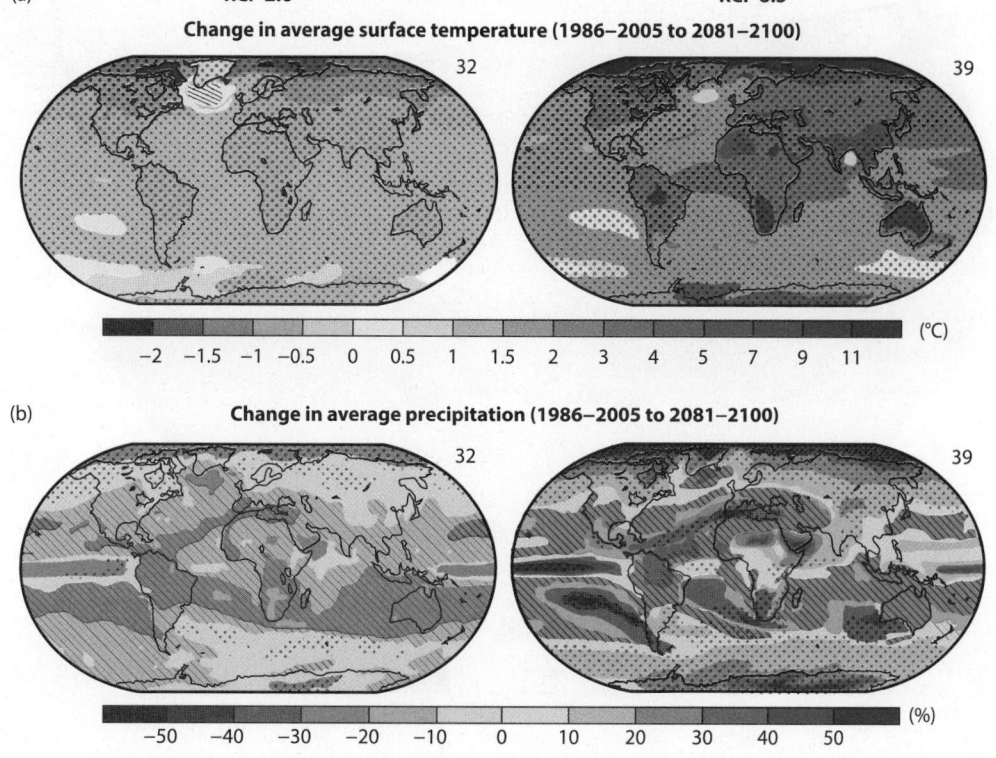

▲ **Figure 49–2.** Maps of projected changes in (a) average temperatures and (b) precipitation by the end of the century under two different scenarios of greenhouse gas emissions, assessed by the IPCC.

Determinants of Vulnerability

EXPOSURE	SENSITIVITY	ADAPTIVE CAPACITY
Exposure is contact between a person and one or more biological, psychosocial, chemical, or physical stressors, including stressors affected by climate change.	Sensitivity is the degree to which people or communities are affected, either adversely or beneficially, by climate variability or change.	Adaptive capacity is the ability of communities, institutions, or people to adjust to potential hazards, to take advantage of opportunities, or to respond to consequences.

VULNERABILITY of Human Health to Climate Change

HEALTH IMPACTS

Injury, acute and chronic illness (including mental health and stress-related illness), developmental issues, and death

▲ **Figure 49–3.** Determinants of vulnerability to health impacts associated with climate change. *(Source: United States Global Change Research Program, Climate Health Assessment, 2016.)*

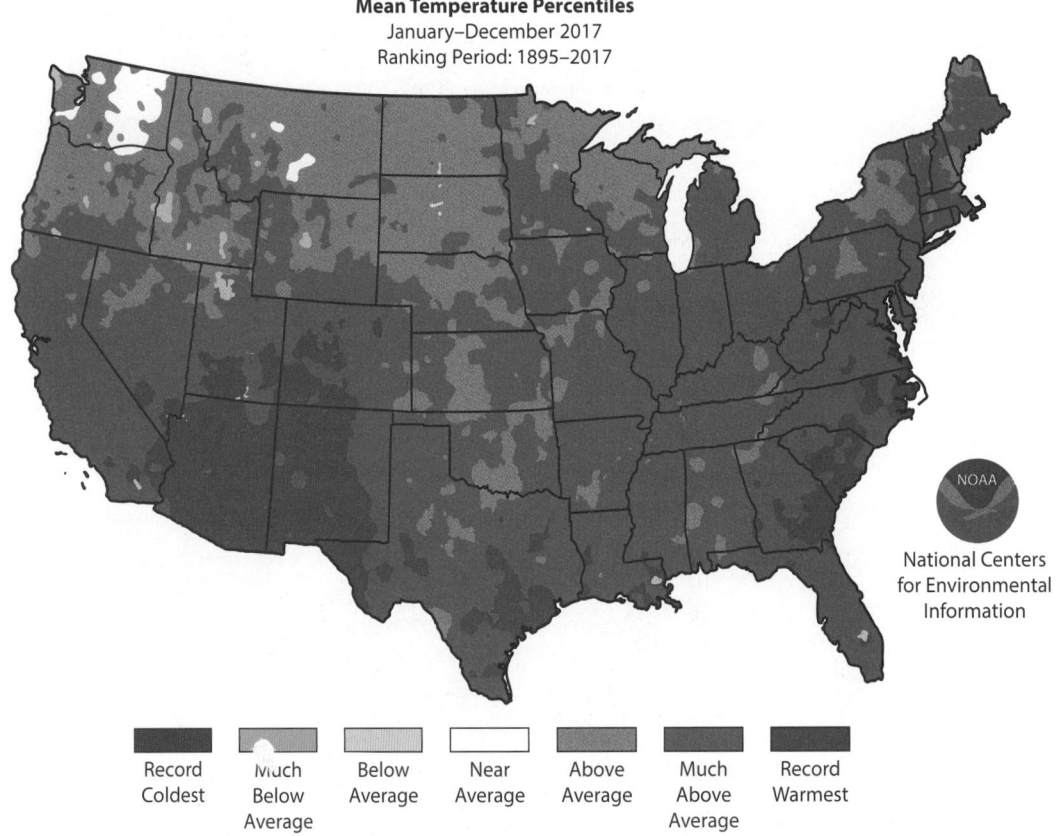

Mean Temperature Percentiles
January–December 2017
Ranking Period: 1895–2017

NOAA

National Centers for Environmental Information

Record Coldest | Much Below Average | Below Average | Near Average | Above Average | Much Above Average | Record Warmest

▲ **Figure 49–4.** Mean annual temperature percentiles as rankings compared to baseline data (1985–2017). *(Source: National Oceanic and Atmospheric Administration's National Centers for Environmental Information, 2018.)*

support activities for the agricultural sector. The Centers for Disease Control and Prevention report that crop workers die from heat stroke at a rate nearly 20 times greater than for all US civilian workers and that the majority of fatalities occur in adults aged 30–54 years, with a majority of victims being foreign-born workers.

However, these numbers are likely a gross underestimate of the true extent of heat-related illness (HRI). Comorbid diseases that are exacerbated by heat exposure are often erroneously reported as the primary diagnosis, thus concealing the role of heat as an inciting factor. Additionally, workers underreport heat effects for fear of losing their jobs, which is particularly true for undocumented workers. The Bureau of Labor Statistics relies on employer Occupational Safety and Health Administration (OSHA) Form 300 logs of injury when counting occupational injury and illness, but the Occupational Safety and Health Act of 1970 (OSHAct) does not apply to federal government agencies, self-employed persons, or household workers. Small farms with fewer than 11 workers are also exempted from this reporting requirement, potentially missing a substantial portion of HRI in agricultural workers. An absence of uniform diagnostic criteria for heat illness death resulting in misclassification and the fact that some workers with mild heat illness may not file claims also contribute to underreporting.

Many factors contribute to the risk of HRI in working populations including: direct exposure to heat (indoor and outdoor), extreme physical exertion, protective work clothing, job insecurity, and more (Figure 49–5). Workers have less control over their work environment and activities than nonoccupational groups, thereby affecting the normal behavioral response to the heat, which might include drinking water, resting or removing extra clothing or equipment.

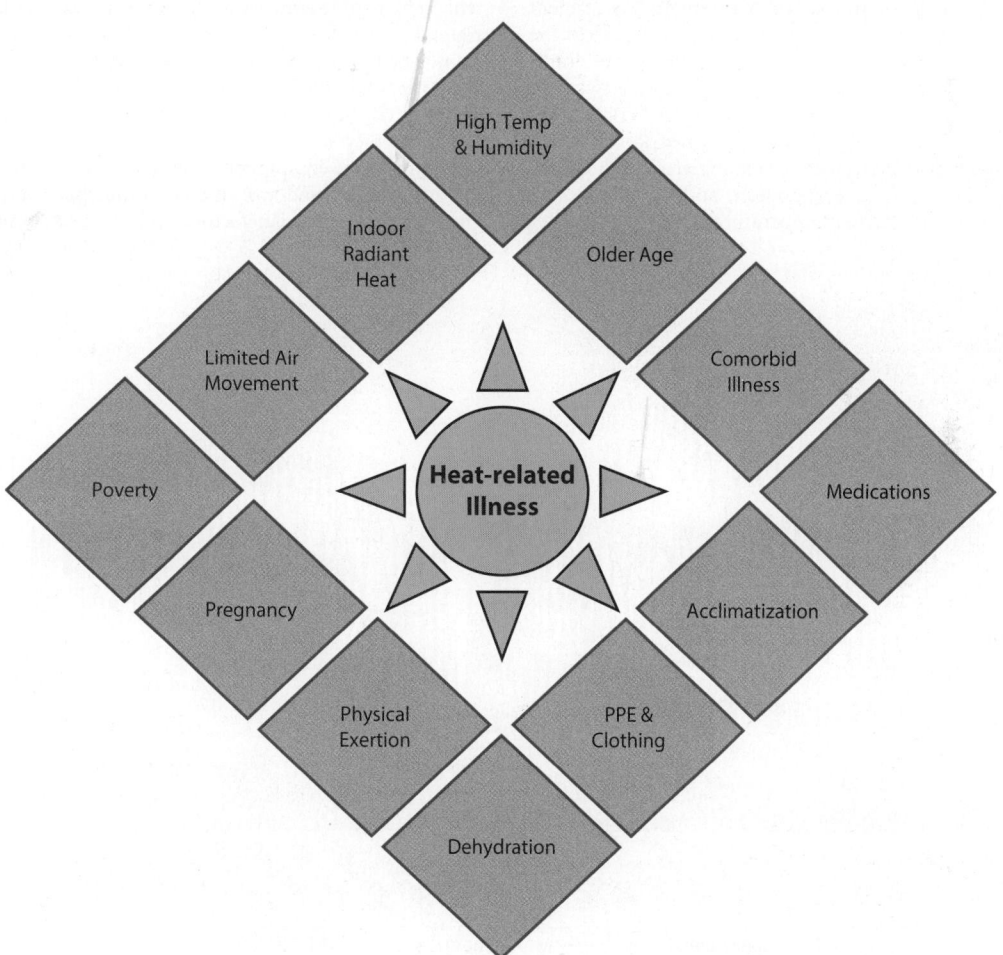

▲ **Figure 49–5.** Risk factors for heat-related illness. (*Modified from Occupational Safety and Health Administration technical manual on heat stress, 2018.*)

Physiologic Aspects of Body Temperature Regulation

The human body is designed to maintain a core temperature of 37°C. However, many basic metabolic reactions of the human body are exothermic in nature, meaning they create heat, which must be dissipated in order to maintain a safe core temperature. The basal metabolic rate of a 70 kg person amounts to approximately 100 kcal/h, which in absence of cooling mechanisms would lead to a 1.1°C hourly rise in core temperature. Furthermore, heat production can increase by 20-fold in the setting of strenuous physical activity. Therefore, physically active workers must dissipate large amounts of heat in order to keep their bodies in a safe state of thermal homeostasis.

Environmental heat can add to the total body heat burden as well as limit heat dissipation through radiation (heat transfer to surrounding environment), which is the primary form of heat regulation in cooler environments. As ambient temperatures rise, evaporation (conversion of liquid to the gaseous state) in the form of sweating, becomes the dominant form of heat dissipation. However, excessive sweating can result in dehydration, which in and of itself contributes to HRI. Lastly, heat can be lost through convection, in which heat transfers to air molecules circulating around the body. If cooling via radiation, evaporation, and convection are insufficient to keep the core temperature at 37°C, the worker needs to reduce metabolic heat generation (physical activity) in order to avoid heat illness. Therefore, there are limits to which workers can safely perform activities in heat that depend on local climatic factors as well as the occupational environment.

Vulnerable Worker Populations

Importantly, underlying individual biologic and behavioral factors as well as work-related factors put certain populations at higher risk (Figure 49–6). Biological factors include older age, lack of prior acclimatization, genetics, pregnancy status and medical comorbidities, including cardiovascular disease, kidney disease, diabetes, and more. Workers taking medications that interfere with salt and water balance and circulatory function are at even higher risk. These medications include but are not limited to: diuretics, anticholinergic agents, beta-blockers, as well as medications which interfere with centers of thermoregulation such as selective serotonin reuptake inhibitors (SSRIs) and anti-dopaminergic medications. The use of recreational drugs such as cocaine, ecstasy, and amphetamines can also interfere with heat regulation. Work-environment risk factors include direct exposure to high humidity and temperature, use of heavy clothing/personal protective equipment (PPE), work near indoor sources of radiant heat, and work in environments with poor air circulation. Other risk factors include citizenship status,

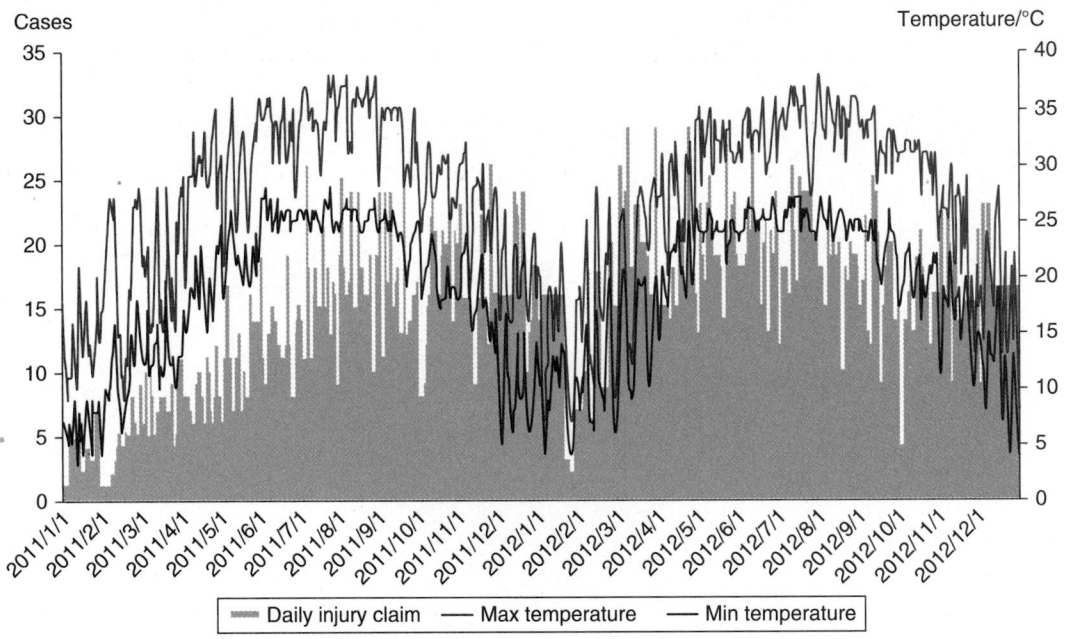

▲ **Figure 49–6.** The distribution of daily injury claims and daily maximum and minimum temperatures in Guangzhou, China between 2011 and 2012. The grey represents daily injury claims. *(From Sheng et al 2018.)*

socioeconomic background, hydration status, and degree of physical exertion.

For worker populations such as migrant workers and day laborers who may have inadequate housing or other social and economic constraints, the adverse health effects of exposure to heat-related hazards in the workplace could be exacerbated by exposure to similar environments in the home. Additionally, workers who perform heavy labor in outdoor and indoor hot environments and are paid a piece-rate, and those who have poor economic conditions with few or nonexistent bargaining possibilities, may also be particularly vulnerable to adverse effects. These workers may decline rest and water breaks if such breaks result in a negative effect on their earnings. Workers laboring in "unskilled" fields compared to the semi-skilled workforce have been found to suffer from higher rates of dehydration, potentially for the reasons mentioned earlier. Additionally, unacclimated new workers or workers with less employment tenure have been shown to suffer from higher rates of HRI. OEM providers must strategically prepare occupational heat plans, acknowledging and addressing these drivers, as they will likely impact adherence to and effectiveness of proposed engineering and work practice controls designed to minimize climate-related health effects.

Athletes are another population that is especially prone to heat illness. For example, the 2007 Chicago Marathon was cancelled mid-race after hundreds of heat-stricken runners required medical care. In 2016, 70% of the elite competitors in the US Olympic Team Trials Marathon in Los Angeles finished, in a race where peak temperature reached 25.6°C. In a recent study, authors predicted that secondary to climate change, by 2085, only 8 (1.5%) of 543 cities outside of western Europe will meet the low-risk category (< 10% probability of > 26°C wet bulb globe temperature [WBGT]) of summertime heat, bringing into question the future of outdoor athletic competitions, such as the summer Olympics.

▶ Clinical Aspects of Heat Illness

Workers performing physical activities in hot environments are at risk of developing a myriad of manifestations of heat illness that range from minor to life-threatening. Many workers spend their entire work shift in a variety of indoor and outdoor hot environments that may become hotter because of ambient rising temperatures, increases in extreme heat events, or shifting and expanding hot seasons. Thus, OEM providers should be prepared to recommend heat stress medical surveillance programs and to evaluate and treat HRIs. The occurrence of workplace HRI incidents, even when considered clinically minor, should prompt critical reevaluation of the current workplace heat controls and procedures in a deliberate effort to reduce the likelihood of future events.

A. Minor Heat Illness

1. Heat cramps—Heat cramps are intermittent and often severe skeletal muscle spasms that usually develop in the postexertion period in workers that are poorly acclimatized

and salt deficient from excessive sweating and subsequent replenishment with excessive hypotonic fluid such as water. Athletes, roofers, steel workers, coal miners, field workers, and boiler operators are the most frequently affected. Victims exhibit hyponatremia, hypochloremia, and painful peripheral muscle spasm, however rhabdomyolysis is uncommon. Symptoms are usually rapidly relieved by oral rehydration with electrolyte solution, however severe cases may require treatment with IV normal saline.

2. Heat edema—Heat edema is characterized by dependent swelling primarily in the feet and ankles in most commonly reported nonacclimatized individuals with no underlying cardiac, hepatic, or lymphatic disease. It is thought to result from increased cutaneous vasodilation coupled with orthostatic and hydrostatic pressure resulting in leakage of vascular fluid into the interstitium. Clinicians should be aware of heat edema in order to prevent unnecessary and costly work-ups for more serious medical causes of peripheral edema. Treatment is supportive, including rest, elevation of the affected limbs and support stockings. Symptoms usually resolve with acclimatization and diuretics are not indicated.

3. Prickly heat—Prickly heat is an inflammatory disorder of the epidermis that results from blockage of sweat glands followed by superimposed staphylococcal infection. The initial phase is associated with a severely pruritic superficial vesicular rash with a distribution confined to clothed areas. During the subsequent week, the obstructed ducts will rupture, producing deeper, dermal vesicles that can persist for weeks and become chronic. Treatment consists of application of antibacterial lotion during the acute phase (eg, chlorhexidine, erythromycin, salicylic acid) and avoidance of exacerbating factors including tight-fitted clothing and poorly ventilated/ hot environments.

4. Heat syncope—Syncope in the setting of heat exposure and exertion results from the body's competing needs to thermoregulate (shunt blood to cutaneous capillary beds), provide blood to metabolically active skeletal muscle, and maintain adequate blood pressure for an upright posture. Combined with volume depletion from sweating, a drop in cardiac output occurs, resulting in insufficient cerebral perfusion and loss of consciousness. Prodromal symptoms include tunnel vision, lightheadedness, diaphoresis, and bradycardia. Victims are most often normothermic or have a slightly elevated core temperature. Mental status usually quickly resolves with rest in the horizontal position and volume repletion. Clinically, heat syncope must be differentiated from general causes of syncope unrelated to heat and exercise including arrhythmias, cardiomyopathy, seizure, and more.

B. Major Heat Illness

1. Heat exhaustion—Under conditions of strenuous exercise and environmental heat exposure, intracellular and intravascular salt and water depletion can occur. Free water depletion results from inadequate rehydration in the setting of ongoing water losses. Those performing strenuous labor in hot environments may require over a liter of fluid per hour to replace sweat losses, and this is seldom logistically possible for workers. Salt depletion takes longer to develop and similarly results from excessive salt losses through sweating with inadequate electrolyte replacement. Clinically, this syndrome is characterized by hyponatremia or hypernatremia, volume depletion, and moderate core temperature elevation (usually below 40°C). Symptoms include fatigue, generalized weakness, vertigo, nausea, and headache. Treatment is aimed toward rest, cooling and fluid and electrolyte replacement, with attention to slow correction of sodium status.

Heat stroke—Heat stroke is a catastrophic, multisystem, life-threatening illness categorized by central nervous system (CNS) dysfunction, liver injury, renal injury and rhabdomyolysis, disruption of homeostatic thermoregulation, and elevation of body temperature above 40°C. Heat stroke is differentiated from heat exhaustion by a core temperature above 40°C in addition to CNS dysfunction. Permanent organ damage due to underlying cellular disruption is dependent on maximum core temperatures in addition to the duration of exposure and individual genetic factors and comorbidities. CNS dysfunction results from cerebral edema and accompanying pathologic changes in the cerebrum and cerebellum. In cases of exertional heat stroke, profound CNS dysfunction dominates the clinical picture and can manifest as delirium, coma, hallucinations, posturing, and more. Seizure occurs in a high proportion of patients. Patients often have hemodynamic instability due to profound volume loss, respiratory alkalosis due to hyperventilation, and coagulopathy (manifesting as petechia, purpura, hematuria, hematochezia, and hematemesis) due to protein dysfunction. Liver injury, pathologically classified as centrilobular necrosis and accompanying acute renal failure are very common.

Treatment is directed toward rapid cooling since death and disability are correlated with maximum temperature as well as duration of exposure to high core temperature. Removal from the hot environment occurs in the prehospital setting. In the emergency department, evaporative cooling is initiated with a combination of fans and atomized water. Cold intravenous fluids are given. Core temperature should be monitored to assess progress of resuscitation. Complications during resuscitation include seizures and encephalopathy with resulting need for airway control. Pulmonary edema can develop secondary to underlying multiorgan failure and excessive crystalloid administration. Arrhythmias are common as are electrolyte abnormalities and rhabdomyolysis, which should be treated with crystalloid and urinary alkalinization. Multisystem organ failure can be reversible yet survivors often manifest permanent personality changes, dementia, cerebellar deficits, and hemiplegia. Mortality rates range between 20% and 65%.

C. Other Heat-related Health Impacts

In addition to heat illness, heat exposure is associated with cardiovascular, respiratory, and renal complications that can result in significant morbidity and mortality. For example, heat exposure is associated with an increased risk of ischemic heart disease, cardiac dysrhythmias, and cerebrovascular disease. Mechanistically, heat activates inflammatory pathways, perturbs blood coagulability, and alters CNS regulation of the heart, which may contribute to the observed increased incidence. Respiratory distress, acute renal failure, and dehydration are also more common. Recent studies have shown that with only modest increases in seasonal temperature, the risk of emergency department presentations for the aforementioned conditions increase proportionally. Workers with preexisting cardiac, respiratory, and renal disease are at highest risk. Agricultural workers exposed to pesticides and other chemicals may experience increased dermal uptake in the setting of hyperthermic conditions accompanied by sweating and increased blood flow. Medical surveillance should identify those at greatest risk for work in hot environments due to comorbid medical conditions or concurrent environmental exposures and evaluate if working in such environments is medically appropriate or if accommodations are necessary.

▶ Heat Acclimatization

Adaption to labor conditions in hot environments results from both physiologic changes and behavioral modifications. Studies suggest that workers who are not physiologically well adjusted to a high ambient temperatures and higher exertion levels suffer a greater degree of HRIs and workplace injuries. For example, sudden and significant increases in daily maximum workplace temperatures (of 10°F or 5.5°C) were associated with approximately 42% of HRI claims in a study of workers in Washington state. Similarly, approximately 14% of HRI claims occur within the first week of a workers employment.

Acclimatization involves a series of physiologic changes and behavioral accommodations. Physiologic changes involve alterations in hormonal regulation, which ultimately increase the rate of sweating, as well as changes to the cardiovascular system which redirect blood flow to the periphery. These changes occur between 4 and 28 days of exposure to high ambient temperatures. However, acclimatization is not universal and is dependent on the individual. For example, in studies of South African mine workers, before acclimatization, 14% of new workers in the mines could cope with extreme heat conditions while carrying out heavy labor, and this increased to 29% after a systematic 2-week acclimatization process. Therefore, 71% of workers were still not able to cope with the heat conditions after physiologic acclimatization. OEM providers and safety professionals should be prepared to advise on and develop sample acclimatization plans.

When the limits of physiologic acclimatization have been reached, workers must rely on behavioral adaptations to avoid heat-related injury. This can be achieved via "self-pacing," taking more rest breaks, and avoiding work during hot hours of the day. These modifications may result in decreased short-term productivity goals, with potential balance by longer-term gains in sustained workforce health and productivity. The OEM provider or safety professional planning workplace heat policy should make every effort to design a sustainable plan that remains protective of health and minimizes disruption, thereby maximizing adherence and associated positive health outcomes.

Heat & Workplace Injuries

According to the International Labor Organization (ILO), approximately 317 million workplace accidents occur each year with accompanying economic costs estimated to equal 4–6% of the gross domestic product (GDP) for most countries. For many reasons, heat exposure is associated with an increased risk of workplace injuries. Heat exposure and early heat illness can manifest as CNS dysfunction that affects coordination, fine motor skills, and judgment and similarly result in fatigue and dizziness. Additionally, physical and behavioral factors such as slippery sweaty hands, foggy glasses, hot tools and working faster to avoid the heat may exacerbate injury risk. Commonly reported injuries under high heat conditions include slips, trips, falls, wounds, lacerations, and amputations. It is critical that the OEM provider understands the injury circumstances, documents and addresses a heat-related component, if present, and follows up with the employer to prevent additional events and recommend modifications to the workplace environment.

Several studies across a wide geographic range have found correlations between workplace heat exposure and injury. For example, in an analysis of work-related compensation claims between (2002–2012), one researcher found that the odds of injury increased by 1% for each 1°C increase in daily minimum temperature, and by 0.8% for each 1°C increase in daily maximum temperature. Both maximum and minimum temperatures have been significantly associated with work-related injuries and that a 1°C increase in maximum temperature was associated with a 1.4% (RR = 1.014, 95% CIs 1.012–1.017) increase in daily injury claims (Figure 49–6). The rate of injuries has been found to increase with rising temperatures until the threshold temperature of 37.7°C after which they drop off. This decline after a threshold temperature was attributed to workers halting work at such high temperatures. A recent systematic review with meta-analysis noted that individuals working in heat stress conditions were four times more likely to experience occupational heat strain during or at the end of a work shift compared to individuals working in thermoneutral conditions.

Studies have found that workers in occupations are at higher risk of heat-related work-place injury. These occupations include agricultural laborers, construction workers, laborers, manufacturing workers, intermediate production and transport workers, tradespersons, electricity, gas, and water workers. More than half of the planet's workforce works outdoors, primarily in construction and agriculture, which based on available data, is the most vulnerable outdoor worker population. Workers in the construction industry are one of the most affected by heat stress, second only to agricultural workers. Likewise, studies have shown

that construction workers in the United States are 13 times more likely to die from a HRI compared to workers in other industries, and within the industry, roofers and road construction workers face a particularly high risk of HRIs. In the United States, the construction industry accounted for 36.8% of the occupational heat-related mortality nationwide and the agricultural industry accounted for 21%. Risk factors include long working hours compounded by heavy workloads and vulnerabilities due to an immigrant worker status that limits access to healthcare resources. Additionally, those workers employed by smaller versus larger companies have been shown to be at higher risk, possibly due to less worker health oversight and/or absence of reporting requirements based on workforce size. OEM providers involved in surveillance and injury treatment have the opportunity for brief clinical preventive discussions regarding heat stress, with a focus on those at highest risk in agriculture and construction.

Workplace Injuries Among Indoor Workers

There has been significantly less attention paid to the effect of rising ambient temperatures on HRI and injuries among indoor workers. There is some evidence that outdoor temperatures can predict indoor heat exposures, making the threat of climate change also relevant to indoor working populations. The presence of local heat source (eg, laundry equipment, combustion engines, other machinery, etc.) can compound occupational heat stress and related adverse effects. Potentially due to lack of readily available public data or a lack of surveillance, there is currently significant bias in the literature, with most studies analyzing work-related injuries in high-income countries, and minimal evaluation of worker injuries in countries in which a large percentage of the workforce is employed in manufacturing and factory labor, such as in China and India. Among limited reports, a recent study in the Guangzhou province of China found that among all industrial sectors, the sector with the greatest increased risk of work-related injury in association with temperature was manufacturing. The authors suggest that outdoor heat may add to heat-generating industrial processes and be compounded by lack of effective cooling and ventilation systems in manufacturing facilities. They found that workers employed by small- and medium-sized companies were at higher risk. Similarly, a recent study of Chronic Kidney Disease of Unknown Origin (CKDu), a newly emerging, heat-related epidemic, found that factory workers involved in the sugarcane industry were at a higher risk of kidney disease than field workers.

More research and surveillance is needed to understand the risks to indoor workers, particularly in less-developed regions of the world, where enforcement of guidelines for workplace safety and building safety may be less consistent.

Heat & Worker Productivity

In recent years, climate change and resulting extreme temperatures have reduced global labor capacity and productivity as workers reach the physiologic limits of heat tolerance and adaptation. When exposed to high temperatures, workers may take more frequent breaks, reduce their workload or stop work entirely. Reductions in work capacity and productivity have significant implications for national economies, the health of economic sectors and household budgets. A recent systematic review with meta-analysis determined that 30% of individuals working in heat stress conditions demonstrated productivity losses, which increased by 2.6% for every degree increase beyond 24°C WBGT. In 2017 alone, it is estimated that 153 billion hours of labor were lost as a result of climate-driven increases in ambient temperature, an increase of 62 billion hours relative to the year 2000. Globally, 80% of the lost labor hours occurred in the agricultural sector in highly economically vulnerable geographic regions (southeast Asia, India, South America, and sub-Saharan Africa).

In the United States, increased heat exposure contributed to the loss of an estimated 1.1 billion labor hours in the United States between 2000 and 2017. These losses occurred in multiple sectors and geographic regions, including agriculture, tourism and fisheries; however industry was found to be the most highly impacted and rural communities were found to be most vulnerable.

Interestingly, while most studies on the subject have focused on modeling the impact on healthy workers, a study done in Guatemalan agricultural workers suggests that individuals who come to work with preexisting health conditions, such as kidney disease, are more severely affected by increasing temperatures, experiencing lower job performance (ie, tons of sugarcane cut per day) and greater job attrition. The combination of climate change and rising rates of workers who have chronic health conditions will result in potentially even more significant losses of labor capacity and productivity than suggested by existing models.

Without strict global GHG mitigation, extreme heat is projected to have a significant impact on future US labor hours, especially for outdoor industries. Under high emissions scenarios, almost 1.9 billion labor hours across the national workforce are projected to be lost annually by 2090 due to high ambient temperatures and resulting untenable working conditions. Such losses of labor would lead to an estimated total of over $160 billion in lost wages per year by 2090. In contrast, with strict mitigation efforts and a lower emission scenario, we would avoid the loss of more than 900 million labor hours and nearly $75 billion in wages in 2090 compared to a high emissions scenario. In communication with employers, the OEM provider should highlight the economic consequences of climate-related worker health and productivity effects and make employer-specific recommendations for prevention, adaptation, and mitigation efforts.

▶ Managing the Effects of Increased Ambient Temperatures on Workers

A. Federal Standards

Despite convincing evidence for negative health effects of increased workplace heat, there is no dedicated federal standard specifically addressing occupational heat exposure. The National Institutes for Occupational Safety and Health (NIOSH) develops recommendations for preventing disease and hazardous conditions in the workplace. These criteria documents are formal publications transmitted to the U.S. Department of Labor for use in promulgating legal standards. NIOSH has generated three criteria documents (1972, 1986, 2016) advising the OSHA to develop a heat standard, however no such standard has been created. In response to a 2011 petition for a heat standard, OSHA noted that the majority of workers with HRI experience mild and reversible effects and would not qualify as "compelling evidence of a serious health impairment involving incurable, permanent or fatal consequences," a requirement to statutorily support a permanent standard under Section 6(b) of the OSHAct. OSHA currently performs heat inspections and issues citations for heat stress violations under the OSHAct's General Duty Clause, Section 5(a)(1), which requires employers to provide a workplace free of recognized hazards likely to cause death or serious physical harm. Notably, between 2013 and 2017, the California state OSHA program performed 50 times more inspections resulting in one or more citations or violations for unsafe heat exposure practices as compared to OSHA nationwide. NIOSH estimates that two in 1000 workers are at risk of heat stress, suggesting that approximately 260,000 workers outside of California, Washington, and Minnesota, which have state-based heat standards, are at risk for HRI and death in the absence of a federal standard to protect them.

The NIOSH criteria address both environmental and metabolic sources of heat, mostly by means of work practice and engineering controls. Heat stress thresholds, which quantify risk in terms of Recommended Exposure Limit (REL) for acclimatized workers and Recommended Alert Limit (RAL) for unacclimatized workers, provide guidance for mandatory rest breaks, the use of personal protective equipment (eg, water-cooled garments, air-cooled garments, or cooling vests), and access to water and shade. Under the NIOSH model, employers are responsible for developing medical monitoring programs for workers exposed at or above the RAL/REL, developing a heat acclimatization plan, and monitoring for environmental heat exposure and employee workloads. NIOSH recommends posting language-appropriate high heat warnings and developing a heat alert program to improve worker knowledge and preparedness for anticipated high heat scenarios. Employers will use heat illness/fatality and workplace environmental/physiologic measurements to improve workplace safety. NIOSH also recommends independent whistleblower protection programs to report heat stress violations in an effort to curb one source of underreporting.

In 1976, the Mine Safety and Health Administration (MSHA) published *Heat Stress in Hot U.S. Mines and Criteria for Standards for Mining in Hot Environments* followed by a revised Safety Manual Number 6, *Heat Stress in Mining*, in 2001. The documents provide recommendations for acclimatization, a work/rest schedule, pacing tasks, timing of heavy task completion, personnel rotation, providing cooler rest areas and cool drinking water, and increasing dietary salt consumption for those not on salt-restricted diets. Recognition of the signs and symptoms of HRI, how to administer first aid, and how to reduce heat stress are also covered.

B. US State-based Standards

California, Washington, and Minnesota are the only three states with formal occupational heat standards. California adopted a heat stress standard (Title 8, Chapter 4 SS 3395, Heat Illness Prevention) in 2006, which applies to all outdoor places of employment. The regulation ensures provision of potable drinking water and access to shade, outlines high heat and emergency response procedures, acclimatization rationale, employee and supervisor training, and requires a Heat Illness Prevention Plan. Critique of the California standard includes the absence of a heat stress threshold which accounts for humidity and mandatory rest breaks. A 2019 draft standard *Heat Illness Prevention in Indoor Places of Employment* which will address heat in indoor workplaces is currently under review.

The Washington State Department of Labor and Industries enacted the Outdoor Heat Exposure Rule in 2008. This rule applies to those performing outdoor work from May 1 through September 30 if employees are exposed to temperatures $\geq 31.7°C$ (89°F); for those wearing double-layer woven clothes (eg, coveralls, jackets, and sweatshirts) in temperatures $\geq 25°C$ (77°F); or those wearing nonbreathing clothes (eg, vapor barrier clothing or PPE such as chemical resistant suits) in temperatures $\geq 11.1°C$ (52°F). The rule notes that the employer's written accident prevention program must include an outdoor heat exposure safety program, employers must provide training to workers and supervisors before beginning heat-intensive work and outlines criteria for provision of water and procedures when employees show signs or symptoms of HRI. The Minnesota OSHA heat stress standard applies to indoor workers only. The standard addresses hydration, acclimatization, heat stress monitoring, engineering controls to reduce exposure (eg, improved ventilation, installing local exhaust, proving heat shields, etc.), training for supervisors and employees on the hazards of heat stress, recognizing the signs and treatment of heat stress.

C. Other US Organizational Guidance

Other US organizations offer guidance regarding occupational heat exposure. In 2003, the U.S. Army and U.S. Air Force published *Heat Stress Control and Heat Casualty Management* which addresses the procedures for assessment, measurement, evaluation, and control of heat stress and the recognition, prevention, and treatment of HRI and injury. The document details heat stress and core temperatures, heat acclimatization, work-rest cycles, microclimate cooling methods, and fluid and electrolyte replacement. Due to an absence of recordkeeping requirements, it is unclear

how widely implemented this guideline is and to what extent it is enforced. In 1973, the U.S. Navy developed Physiological Heat Exposure Limit (PHEL) curves based on metabolic and environmental heat load and represent maximum allowable exposure limits. The Navy monitors WBGT rise, signified by colored flags flown at installations with all nonessential outdoor activity stopping at WBGT greater than 90°F. The U.S. Marine Corps has followed the Navy Guidelines since 2015. The American Conference of Governmental Industrial Hygienists (ACGIH) defines a heat stress threshold limit value (TLV) representing the heat stress conditions under which nearly all workers will avoid adverse health effects (ACGIH). The TLV goal is to maintain core body temperature within +1°C of normal (37°C) accounting for both environmental and metabolic sources of heat, with exceptions under certain circumstances.

D. International Guidelines

There are several international organizations that have developed and published standards, recommendations, and guidelines for limiting worker exposure to potentially harmful levels of occupational heat stress. The International Organization for Standardization (ISO) has members from 164 countries and develop standards by using a consensus-based approach, including several that address assessment of environmental and metabolic sources of heat and calculation of heat strain (eg, 7243, 7933, 8996, 9886, 9920). The Canadian Centre for Occupational Health and Safety outlines occupational exposure limits to protect industrial workers and provides thermal comfort limits for office workers. Some Canadian provinces have adopted heat stress standards as either rules or guidelines based on ACGIH TLVs. Canada's federal governments has established permissible temperature ranges for food service workers, workplace first aid rooms, and temperatures at which a heat barrier must be provided to protect the operator of motorized materials handling equipment. The Japan Society for Occupational Health sets heat and cold stress threshold limit values and the Ministry of Health, Labor and Welfare sets thermal standard for offices. The temperature exposure limits decline with increased workloads, which is similar to the NIOSH's recommended RELs for acclimatized workers.

E. Resources for OEM Providers

OEM providers have the opportunity to directly communicate the advantages of adopting heat policies and can use the NIOSH criteria in developing heat programs and procedures for employers. Mitigation and adaptive response to increasing ambient temperatures may prevent unnecessary workers' compensation expenses associated with heat illness and business expenses associated with decreased worker productivity. OEM providers are uniquely qualified to perform medical monitoring for workers exposed to heat, with attention to acclimatization, individual risk factors, and prior history of HRI.

Despite an absence of a specific heat standard, OSHA has incorporated the NIOSH criteria into the 2017 technical manual on heat stress and offers many valuable resources for safety and health professionals. In May of 2012, U.S. OSHA launched a nationwide education and outreach campaign *Water. Rest. Shade* to educate workers and employers about heat hazards and preventing HRIs. OSHA also adapted the State of California OSHA heat campaign materials for national purposes, with many materials targeting at-risk populations and those with limited English proficiency. OSHA partnered with the National Oceanic and Atmospheric Administration (NOAA) to incorporate worker safety precautions for distribution in weather service alerts for extreme heat. Safety and health professionals, supervisors, and workers have access to simple tools to evaluate heat index, including a smart phone application. The National Integrated Heat Health Information System (NIHHIS) is not specific to occupational populations, but provides a variety of resources to decision makers preparing for extreme heat event days and includes special sections on at-risk groups, including outdoor workers, athletes, and emergency responders. Heat Shield is a project that addresses the negative impacts of workplace heat stress on the health and productivity of the European Union workforce, providing adaptation strategies for manufacturing, construction, transportation, tourism, and agriculture. Taken together, there are a variety of resources available to OEM providers as they develop and optimize workplace heat illness prevention, surveillance, and mitigation strategies.

Air Quality & Cardiorespiratory Health

Poor air quality is intrinsically linked to climate change and has far reaching impacts on worker health. The combustion of fossil fuels directly increases ground level ozone (O_3) and fine particulate matter ($PM_{2.5}$), and increasing ambient temperatures accelerate the formation of O_3. There is robust evidence that climate change worsens ozone pollution through increased temperatures and drives $PM_{2.5}$ generation through increased frequency and intensity of wildfires, as well as from desertification and resulting dust generation. Climatologic and meteorologic factors, such as temperature, precipitation, cloud cover, and wind velocity can influence the concentrations of these pollutants in local ambient air and thus impact workplace exposure.

Particulate matter and ground-level ozone pose significant risks to human health. Mechanistically, inhaled particles can react with neural receptors resulting in alterations in normal functioning of the autonomic nervous system, can generate oxidative stress in alveolar-capillary cells resulting in local and systemic inflammation, and can cross the alveolar membrane resulting in endothelial injury within the cardiovascular system and prothrombic changes in blood proteins. Ultimately, these pathophysiologic changes can result in aggravation of normal respiratory and cardiovascular function and can lead to premature death and exacerbation of underlying cardiovascular and respiratory disease in vulnerable populations.

Outdoor workers in hot environments have increased respiratory rates and thus may be more affected by air pollution than other members of the general population. Additionally, while the general public can avoid poor air quality days by going inside, outdoor workers cannot take such health protective actions. Additionally, workers in many industries, such as agriculture, industry, transportation, wildland firefighting, mining, and manufacturing, have added exposures from inhalation of particulate matter from the nature of their work. Poor ambient air quality can worsen the negative health impacts. OEM providers educate and advise employers on the risk for cardiorespiratory issues in vulnerable workers and develop medical surveillance programs addressing the needs of those vulnerable to changes in air quality. The OEM provider must be prepared to identify, diagnose, and treat occupational or environmental disease that result from air pollution and manage associated work restrictions or accommodation.

Wildland firefighters and workers in forest management and land use sectors are a particularly vulnerable work group as they are subjected to frequent exposure to severely unhealthy air. Due to the nature of their shift work and residence in fire camp, they often sleep in similar air quality conditions as they work, eliminating appreciable periods of exposure relief. Currently, climate change is driving arid conditions in North America, which, in turn, is fueling more frequent and prolonged wildfire events. For example, the frequency and acreage burned by large wildfires in the western United States and Alaska has increased steadily since the 1980s and is projected to further increase over the course of the century under both low and high carbon emission scenarios. Each year, an average of 339,000 premature deaths worldwide are estimated to result from wildfire smoke, and emissions from wildfire smoke are projected to double by the end of the century in parts of the United States.

Evidence to date demonstrates that exposure to wildfire smoke has direct effects on human health, with consistent reports of negative respiratory health effects and increases in all-cause mortality. The literature contains mixed reports on the association between smoke exposure and cardiovascular disease and cerebrovascular disease, potentially due to the heterogeneity of the composition of wildfire smoke, the population exposed and/or the air quality variable investigated. There have been a relatively limited number of studies which directly assess the acute and long-term impacts of occupational exposure; however, several studies have demonstrated acute declines in lung function measured across the work shift. Wildland firefighters also work under extreme conditions with little rest for long periods of time that have gotten longer over the past two decades as the intensity and duration of wildfires has increased. Mental and physical fatigue places workers at risk of cognitive errors and slow reaction times which may predicate injuries. Wildland firefighters' exposures to air pollution continues to be an area of research and concern. Beyond fitness for duty determinations, wildland firefighter preemployment and surveillance examinations may also have value in tracking long-term occupational health effects and offer potential protective solutions for this exposed workforce. Knowledge of the unique environmental risks associated with wildland firefighting and how this might interact with underlying comorbidities is critical in making fitness for duty determinations, largely due to the lack of current exposure controls.

Climate-related Extreme Weather Events

Overall, the frequency of climate-related disasters, including hurricanes, droughts, heavy precipitation events and floods, has increased by 46% since 2000. These events present unique health hazards to workers, particularly emergency responders and those involved in rescue, medical relief, cleanup, and remediation. Between 1992 and 2006, a total of 307 workers died during response efforts to climate-related disasters. Wildfires, hurricanes, and floods accounted for the majority of these fatalities. The United States has experienced 241 weather and climate disasters since 1980 where overall damages and costs have reached or exceeded $1 billion. The United States in 2018, there were 14 weather and climate disaster events with losses exceeding $1 billion each and resulting in 247 deaths (Figure 49–7). Extreme weather events force workers to remain at the worksite for prolonged hours until replacements arrive,

triggering fatigue that increases the risk of accidents and death and mental health burdens.

Unique health risks exist for certain subgroups of workers. Workers who respond during and after hurricanes include search and rescue personnel, law enforcement, medical workers, chemical/hazardous waste cleaners, and utility and construction workers, among others. They are potentially exposed to contaminated flood waters, increased exposure to vector-borne diseases, electrical hazards, carbon monoxide exposure, and more. These exposures can result in acute medical emergencies, including drowning, electrocution, heat stress, carbon monoxide poisoning, injuries, infectious diseases, and in the long term, can contribute to significant respiratory disease. Additionally, the population level health impacts of extreme weather events leads to significant demands on local and regional health care system and often put health workers, including physicians, nurses, emergency medical responders, and support staff, under psychological pressure. Medical staff are expected to work longer shifts in difficult situations with limited resources. Staffing shortages and personal losses can compound these stressors.

The mental health impacts on workers responding to disasters are often underrecognized. Often, workers are exposed to highly traumatogenic experiences, including

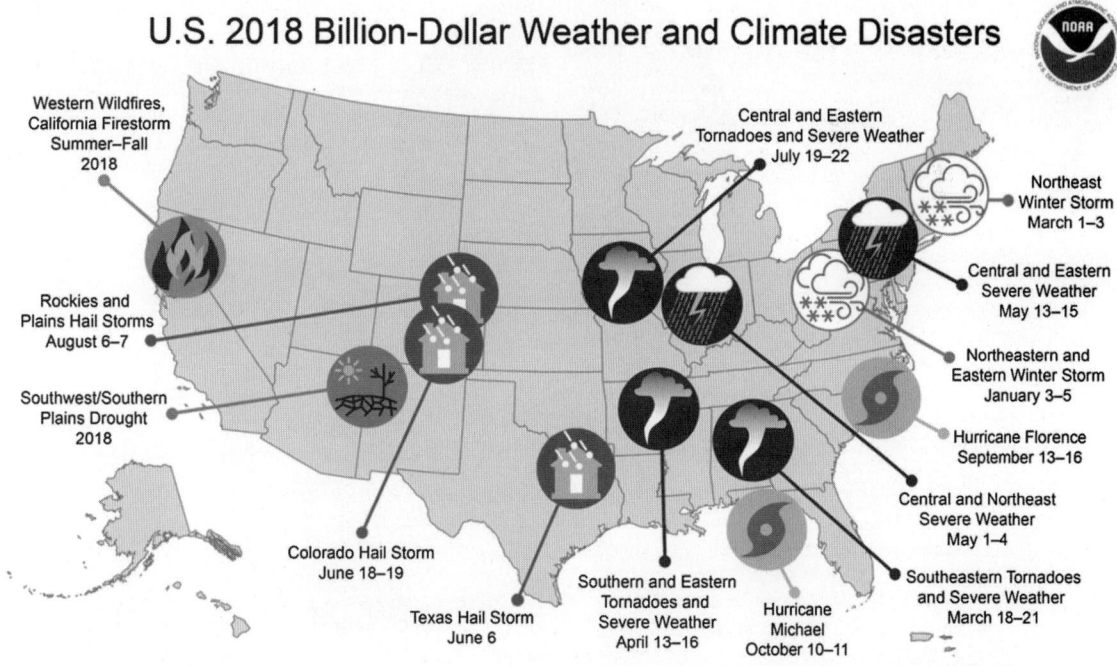

▲ **Figure 49–7.** 2018 Weather and climate disaster events with losses exceeding $1 billion each in the United States. *(Source: National Oceanic and Atmospheric Administration.)*

witnessing tragic loss of life and suffering of others. Furthermore, emergency workers face both personal and societal pressure to sacrifice their own personal well-being for the sake of the greater good, no matter the circumstances. These experiences place disaster responders at increased risk of depression, anxiety, and posttraumatic stress disorder, especially those with a prior history of underlying mental health disorders. Vulnerable worker populations include those with chronic health conditions, those of lower socioeconomic status with lower education, and those lacking social supports to manage a disaster's health impact.

Proper training for this workforce is essential and should include recognition of hazards, egress and evacuation, use of PPE, activation of emergency response system, incident command and skills specific to their response duties. Surveillance provides a means to track and address workforce health hazards associated with response efforts. The Emergency Response Health Monitoring and Surveillance (ERHMS) System represents a collaboration between NIOSH, federal agencies, state health departments, and unions with the express goal of monitoring emergency responder health and safety throughout the predeployment, deployment, and post-deployment phases of a response and is a valuable resource for OEM providers charged with monitoring this workforce.

Impacts of Environmental Change on Agricultural Communities

Agricultural communities are inherently dependent on a stable climate and stable soils in order to produce successful and dependable harvests. Rising temperatures, prolonged drought, heavy precipitation, flooding and resultant soil erosion, in addition to altered patterns of pests, directly threaten the livelihoods of over 2.6 million US workers in the agricultural sector and an additional 21 million workers whose livelihoods depend on agricultural-related sectors of the food supply chain. These impacts extend beyond national borders. Almost two billion of the world's farmers, as a result of endemic poverty, are vulnerable to impacts from climate change, mainly in Africa and Asia. Their subsistence living from agriculture is dependent on a specific range of temperature and rainfall and their capacity to adapt and protect themselves is limited. Additionally, because of increased growth, range, and duration of growth of pests and weeds, pesticide use is expected to increase, including use in areas where specific pesticides were not previously necessary, thus putting applicators and other workers at increased risk of exposure and potentially lead to increased risk of resistance.

Crop failure not only leads to economic poverty and malnutrition, but the experience translates to poor mental

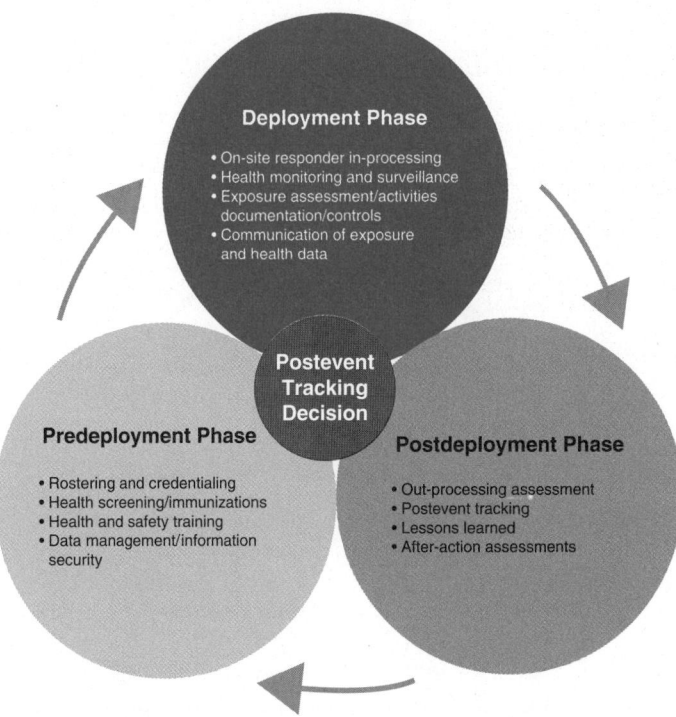

▲ **Figure 49–8.** Framework of the ERHMS program for emergency responder surveillance. *(Source: National Institute for Occupational Safety and Health, 2018 (111).)*

health. Unpredictability in resources due to circumstances completely out of a worker's control causes despair and ultimately may result in depression, anxiety, and substance abuse, which further impair a worker's ability to cope. Instances of suicide among farmers in relationship to drought, debt accumulation, and crop failure has become a growing concern over the past two decades and has been documented on almost every continent. It is estimated that climate change has contributed to over 60,000 farmer suicides between 1980 and 2013 in the subcontinent of India alone. More recently, the suicide rates among farmers has grown to 3000 per year (baseline 300/y) among farmers in Kenya in the setting of prolonged drought and soil contamination. OEM providers should be aware of an increased risk of climate-related mental health effects among agricultural workers and screen for these conditions, particularly in the setting of an unrelated occupational injury or illness that can potentially compound climate-related decreased productivity.

Vector-borne Disease & Worker Health

Microbial pathogens and their vectors are sensitive to climatic conditions, primarily through temperature extremes and precipitation patterns, which dictate their survival, geographic range, seasonality, and transmission rates. Recent evidence suggests that climate change may expose more people to endemic tick-borne and mosquito-borne illnesses, such as Lyme disease, West Nile virus, dengue virus, chikungunya, and others. Outdoor workers are primarily at risk, including those working in construction, landscaping, forestry, brush clearing, land surveying, farming, oil field and utility work, natural resources management, and more. The increased risk stems from increased contact with vectors, such as mosquitos, ticks, and fleas that transmit viruses, bacteria, and parasites. Furthermore, alterations in work patterns due to increased ambient temperatures, such as longer rest periods in the middle of the day and increased work when it is cooler at dawn and dusk, may coincide with the times when insect vectors are most active thus increase the likelihood of disease transmission.

Greater than 75% of reported vector-borne disease in the United States from 2004 to 2016 was tickborne disease, with a doubling of reported cases during the time period, in addition to an expanding geographic area at risk for Lyme disease. The number of US counties at high risk for Lyme disease has increased by more than 320% in northeastern states and more than 250% in northcentral states over the last 20 years (Figure 49–9). Outdoor workers have five-times the risk of contracting Lyme disease compared to indoor workers. The incidence of coccidioidomycosis also increased substantially in the past two decades. This climate-sensitive fungal disease, endemic in the Southwest United States, is associated with aridity and drought. Climate may be a contributing factor leading to the observed rise in cases. Outdoor workers in endemic regions are susceptible to breathing windborne dusts that contain these harmful organisms. Recent predictions are that the geographic range of *Aedes aegypti,* the mosquito which carries Zika virus, dengue virus, and chikungunya, will increase over the course of this century as a result of climate change, with some of the largest population increases in North America. Already, changes in this vector's distribution are apparent, however the impact on worker health is unknown. Vector-borne diseases can negatively impact worker health and are responsible for considerable losses in economic productivity every year, attributable to a less healthy and less physically capable workforce leading to increased work days lost to ill health. In the short term, infection leads to lost days of work, medical costs and additionally, physical weakness once the acute illness has passed. In the long term, repeated infections can result in job loss with resultant negative economic outcomes for workers and their families.

Of note, men and women have a different risk of acquiring VBD's because they hold different occupations and have different underlying biologic risks. For example, pregnant women are a notably vulnerable population. Physiologic

Reported Lyme Disease Cases in 1996 and 2014

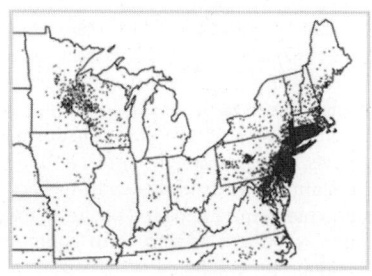
1996

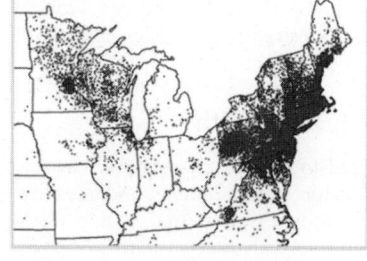
2014

▲ **Figure 49–9.** Reported Lyme disease cases in 1996 and 2014. *(Source: Environmental Protection Agency, climate change indicators, 2018.)*

changes during pregnancy, such as a higher respiratory rate and CO_2 production (a chemoattractant for mosquitos) coupled with increased peripheral blood flow and skin temperature together increase biting risk. Furthermore, hormonally induced changes in immunologic function may suppress host defenses resulting in higher intensity of viremia and parasitemia. These biologic factors coupled with workplace exposure place pregnant women and their children at high risk of obstetric complications. Zika virus is of particular concern for women who intend to become pregnant, pregnant women, and men who intend to have children in the near future, as men can also propagate Zika virus. The OEM provider should account for these vulnerable populations when designing prevention efforts.

Preventive interventions to curb vector-borne disease require coordination at the level of the employer and medical provider. This includes risk assessment methods adapted to address risks not typically included in occupational standards, such as exposure to ticks, poison ivy, mosquitoes, and waterborne diseases. There are simple environmental (eg, avoiding/clearing brushy work areas, insecticide application, removing standing water) and personal (eg, tick checks, long-sleeved clothing, tucking pant legs into boots, Permethrin-treated clothing) controls. Administrative controls, such as altering workday schedules to avoid vectors with strong temporal patterns; increasing the frequency and length of breaks; and developing methods to incentivize workers to use breaks can each reduce exposure. At times, the OEM provider will have to weigh competing climate-related risks (eg, heat versus vector exposure) to establish the safest administrative controls, depending on regional characteristics and balanced by other available prevention tools. OEM providers are uniquely qualified to perform research and educate employers about vector-borne disease risks unique to a particular job site, stay abreast of geographic distribution, and anticipate new pathogens that might occur in a particular region, which will become increasingly relevant in the clinical and travel medicine setting.

OEM and public health professions must be aware of and anticipate the additional risk of insecticide and drug resistance for vector-borne diseases and consider alternative approaches. Some feel that environmental and personal protective approaches are of limited practicality for outdoor workers. However, absent vaccination for certain vector-borne diseases, these measures remain the safest and most effective preventive methods.

Water Quality & Worker Health

Hydrologic factors related to climate change, such as the warming of the oceans and increased frequency and intensity of heavy downpours and droughts, alter marine and fresh water resources in a manner which affects the incidence of many disease-causing organisms. Climate-induced changes in water quality and availability as well as local temperature are closely linked to the spatial and temporal distribution of waterborne diseases. Cholera, shigella, salmonella, campylobacter, noroviruses, enteroviruses, rotaviruses, cryptosporidium, and giardia are all climate-sensitive and show variable abundance in relationship to temperature, rainfall, and distribution of host or reservoir species. For example, ocean warming and reduced salinity has resulted in a steady increase in the proportion of coastal habitats suitable for outbreaks of Vibrio infections, which result in an estimated 80,000 illness and 100 deaths in the United States each year. Similarly, campylobacter infections show seasonal differences in transmission rates with warmer winters correlated with increased transmission. A wide-range of workers are at risk of acquiring climate-sensitive waterborne infections as a result of their proximity to potentially contaminated water sources. These occupations include but are not limited to: fishers, outdoor workers, sanitation workers, first responders, natural resource managers, older workers, and immunocompromised workers.

Diarrheal disease is one of the primary clinical manifestations of waterborne disease and accounts for an estimated 1.4–1.9 million deaths worldwide on an annual basis and between 12 million and 19 million nonfatal illnesses annually in the United States alone. Diarrheal disease leads to insidious health impacts which erode the health of workers. For example, diarrheal disease can impair growth and cognitive development, cause malnutrition and anemia, and increase susceptibility to other infectious agents. Additionally, diarrheal disease may impair worker productivity and lead to illness which may necessitate the need for medical attention and ultimately result in lost work days and medical debt. Premature return to work may contribute to decreased productivity and disease spread. Furthermore, these negative impacts are incurred by the household regardless of which family member is sick, through the costs of health care and loss of income when caring for a sick child or relative. Older adults (primarily age 65 and older), pregnant women, and immunocompromised workers have higher risk of gastrointestinal illness and severe health outcomes.

Heavy downpours are already on the rise and increases in the frequency and intensity of extreme precipitation events are projected for all US regions (Figure 49–10). Analysis of long trends in heavy precipitation across the United States and Canada have demonstrated that in recent years, 68% of waterborne disease outbreaks in the United States were preceded by extreme precipitation events. Other studies have demonstrated the link between heavy precipitation events and hospital admissions for diarrheal illness. Mechanistically, heavy rainfall and flooding mobilizes pathogens from human and animal waste lying dormant in topsoil and transports these pathogens into surface waters which are later reclaimed for drinking water or become recreational waters downstream. Exposure occurs through ingestion, inhalation, or direct contact with contaminated water. Workers may preferentially come in contact with such contaminated waters as they perform municipal sanitation duties or use untreated surface water for agricultural irrigation. Emergency response workers are also at particularly high risk of infection due to close proximity to the source in the setting of

Projected Changes in Heavy Precipitation

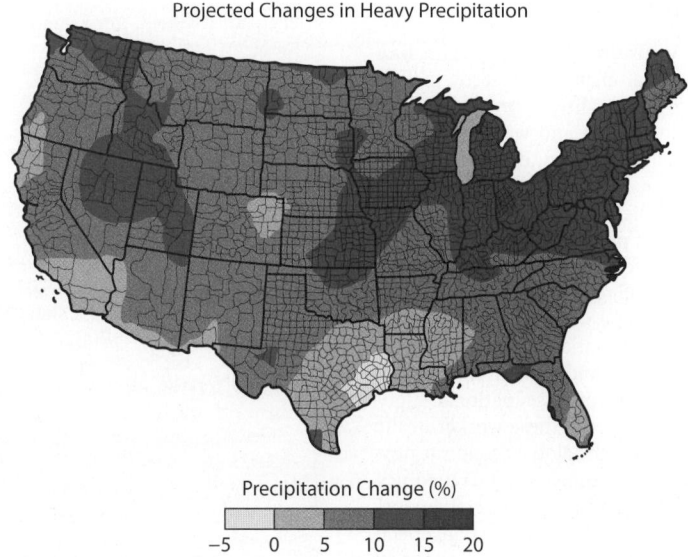

Precipitation Change (%)

−5   0   5   10   15   20

▲ **Figure 49–10.** Projected changes in heavy precipitation across the United States (2046–2065 compared to 1981–2085, multimodal average using RPC 8.5). *(Source: United States Global Change Research Program.)*

wading through stagnant flood waters during rescue efforts or repairing sanitation and water infrastructure.

Rising ocean temperatures, as well as extreme precipitation events and subsequent increases in runoff and nutrient loading in coastal waters, contribute to the growth of harmful cyanobacterial algae blooms. Workers laboring near coastal areas may become exposed to these aerosolized toxins which cause acute respiratory illness and eye irritation. Those with asthma or other underlying respiratory disease are at increased risk of negative health impacts. Harmful algae blooms may also lead to higher rates of ciguatera fish poisoning and paralytic shellfish poisoning, which may preferentially affect mariners. The projected 4.5–6.3°F increase in sea surface temperature in the Caribbean over the coming century is expected to increase the incidence of ciguatera fish poisoning by 200–400%. Additionally, projected increases in sea surface temperatures are expected to lengthen the seasonal window of growth and expand geographic range of *Vibrio* species in coastal waters. Vibrio infections result in eye, ear, and wound infections as well as diarrheal illness in those exposed. In the United States, reported rates of illness for all *Vibrio* infections have tripled since 1996, with *Vibrio alginolyticus* infections having increased by 40-fold.

Workers whose livelihoods depend upon oceanic fisheries are at a high risk of financial instability from changes in the distribution, timing, and productivity of harvests resulting from ocean warming, acidification, deoxygenation, and other aspects of climate change. The fishing sector alone contributes more than $200 billion in economic activity each year and supports 1.6 million US jobs. These workers are inherently at risk of cascading mental and physical health impacts.

Public Health & Policy for OEM Providers

OEM providers are, at times, in the unique position to advise employers on workforce health within the larger corporate context. This lends itself to consultation on more global company-driven strategies to address climate change and related effects. Implementing workplace sustainability measures results in increased efficiency for employers and also promotes the growing sustainable technologies workforce. Knowledgeable OEM providers will be aware of occupational hazards in "green" industries and those associated with mitigation strategies such as reforestation and carbon capture and sequestration, adding value during these transitions. Pursuing policy changes that positively impact both public health and worker health aligns available resources and skillsets of these disciplines, making substantive change more likely. The creation and enforcement of air pollution standards is an example of positive collaboration and addresses the "double burden" workers face with both community and workplace exposure to air pollution. Cooperation between public health and OEM will also bolster the ability to track and monitor climate-related health effects using surveillance systems. Sharing research across international borders will reduce duplicative data accumulation, focus research to issues most applicable regionally, and strengthen efforts to minimize occupational climate-related impacts.

Summary

Many workers are uniquely susceptible to the health hazards imposed by environmental changes. Hazards include increased heat, worsening air quality, extreme weather events, and exposure to vector-borne and water borne diseases. These hazards can result in injuries, death, lost labor, economic poverty, and poor mental health outcomes. Climate change is a threat multiplier, putting pressure on vulnerable worker populations and presenting a myriad of new challenges to OEM providers. Reducing and managing health risks over the coming decades will require modifying worker health systems to prepare for, cope with, and recover from the health consequences of climate variability and change.

Research is needed to better understand the climate change effects on workers and improve occupational safety, as well as to assess the consequences of these worker health impacts for business sustainability, the global economy, poverty, climate-related migration, and other societal outcomes. Areas of high priority include: identifying vulnerable work populations, identifying indicators of climate change effects on workers, identifying effective mitigation and exposure control interventions, and increasing worker health surveillance. With training in clinical and environmental health; hazard recognition, evaluation and control; public health and surveillance; disaster preparedness and emergency management; and toxicology, in addition to direct contact with the workforce and collaboration with employers, OEM providers are uniquely poised to become leaders in preventing, mitigating, and adapting to climate-related events.

REFERENCES

California Code of Regulations: Heat Illness Prevention, from California General Industry Safety Orders. https://www.dir.ca.gov/title8/3395.html 2018.

Centers for Disease Control and Prevention: The National Institutes for Occupational Safety and Health (NIOSH) Criteria for a Recommended Standard: Occupational Exposure to Heat and Hot Environments. See https://www.cdc.gov/niosh/docs/2016-106/.

Environmental Protection Agency: Climate Change Indicators in the United States: Heat-Related Deaths. www.epa.gov/climate-indicators 2016.

Flouris AD et al: Workers' health and productivity under occupational heat strain: A systematic review and meta-analysis. Lancet Planet Health 2018;2(12):e521-e531 [PMID: 30526938].

Johnson RJ, Wesseling C, Newman LS: Chronic kidney disease of unknown cause in agricultural communities. N Engl J Med 2019;380(19):1843-1852 [PMID: 31067373].

Levy BS, Patz JA: Climate change, human rights, and social justice. Ann Glob Health 2015;81(3):310-322 [PMID: 26615065].

Navarro KM et al: Wildland firefighter smoke exposure and risk of lung cancer and cardiovascular disease mortality. Environ Res 2019;173:462-468 [PMID: 30981117].

Perkison WB et al: Responsibilities of the occupational and environmental medicine provider in the treatment and prevention of climate change-related health problems. J Occup Environ Med 2018;60:e76-e81 [PMID: 29252921].

Reid CE et al: Critical review of health impacts of wildfire smoke exposure. Environ Health Perspect 2016;124:1334-1343 [PMID: 27082891].

Schulte PA, Chun H: Climate change and occupational safety and health: establishing a preliminary framework. J Occup Environ Hyg 2009;6(9):542-554 [PMID: 19551548].

Spector JT, Masuda YJ, Wolff NH, Calkins M, Seixas N: Heat exposure and occupational injuries: Review of the literature and implications. Curr Environ Health Rep 2019;6(4):286-296 [PMID: 31520291].

■ SELF-ASSESSMENT QUESTIONS

Select the one correct answer for each question.

Question 1: Exposure to extreme heat
- a. does not correlate with direct weather-related deaths
- b. is a major climate risk factor among workers who perform heavy labor in hot conditions
- c. is seldom a problem with crop workers
- d. can easily be prevented in the workplace

Question 2: Climate change and resulting extreme temperatures
- a. have little effect on work performance
- b. result in fewer work breaks and less work stoppage
- c. have reduced global labor capacity and productivity as workers reach the physiologic limits of heat tolerance and adaptation
- d. need not be considered at this stage of global warming

Air Pollution

John R. Balmes, MD
Stephanie M. Holm, MD, MPH

The dramatic air pollution episodes that occurred in the early part of the twentieth century in Belgium's Meuse Valley, Donora, Pennsylvania, and London, England, are not likely to occur in high-income countries today. These episodes were caused by the large-scale burning of coal in the presence of "ideal" meteorologic conditions—atmospheric inversion leading to a stagnant air mass. A clearly evident excess mortality was observed during and after these episodes. Current air quality standards in North America generally avoid the development of episodes of this magnitude today. Yet, in some Asian countries, where sulfur-containing fuels are burned without adequate air quality regulations, air pollution levels may be attained similar to those that occurred during the historic episodes listed above. Furthermore, catastrophic wildfires associated with climate change have begun to create pollution crises that could rival those historic events. In addition to air pollution crises, certain outdoor air pollutants, such as ozone and respirable particles, regularly reach levels that may cause chronic health effects. Thus, clinicians should be aware of factors contributing to high-level air pollution episodes around the globe, as well as the health effects that can be attributed to chronic, lower-level exposures.

REGULATION OF OUTDOOR AIR POLLUTANTS

The Clean Air Act (CAA) was passed by the U.S. Congress in 1970 and last amended in 1990. It is the principal US standard addressing outdoor air quality. It requires the U.S. Environmental Protection Agency (EPA) to list those pollutants for which there is sufficient scientific evidence documenting the risk to public health from unregulated exposure. To achieve this, the EPA periodically reviews a large body of scientific research dealing with the adverse health effects of the so-called criteria pollutants. These reviews do not involve a cost-benefit analysis. The subsequently produced integrated science assessment documents are used in the development of a National Ambient Air Quality Standard (NAAQS) for each of the criteria pollutants. Table 50–1 lists the six criteria air pollutants, their NAAQSs, and their principal adverse health effects.

The CAA mandates that the primary NAAQS be set to protect the health of all sensitive groups within the population. The EPA has identified children, people with a chronic respiratory disease such as asthma, and people with ischemic heart disease as constituting sensitive groups (ie, that demonstrate a response to a pollutant at a lower level or to a greater degree than the average response of the general population).

TYPES & SOURCES OF EXPOSURE

Outdoor air contains an array of naturally occurring pollutants, including soil, dust, pollens, and fungi. In addition, human activity generates complex mixtures of pollutants. Much of the regulatory effort and scientific research have concentrated on the individual components of these complex mixtures. This chapter discusses the criteria pollutants (see Table 50–1). It does not discuss highly toxic air pollutants, so-called air toxics, that are emitted from point sources and that are present in low concentrations in the environment.

The sources of outdoor air pollution usually are categorized as stationary or mobile. Stationary sources are primarily power or manufacturing plants and are responsible for most sulfur dioxide (SO_2) emissions, as well as considerable amounts of nitrogen oxides (NO_x) and particulate matter (PM). In the eastern United States and Canada, atmospheric acidity is caused largely by the oxidation of SO_2 to sulfuric acid (H_2SO_4) and other acid sulfate species; this problem has been ameliorated to a large extent as natural gas has been replacing coal for power generation. The combustion of fossil fuel is the most important cause of stationary-source emissions, although release of volatile organic compounds (VOCs) by various industrial facilities can contribute to the generation of ozone (O_3) in the atmosphere.

In contrast with the pollution from stationary sources that characterizes eastern North America, "smog" is derived primarily from automotive, or mobile-source, emissions. A large fraction of ambient O_3 is the product of complex photochemical reactions involving NO_x and VOCs emitted from automotive tailpipes. Nitric acid (HNO_3) is a more important

Table 50–1. Criteria air pollutants (U.S. National Ambient Air Quality Standards).

Air Pollutant	Standard	Principal Adverse Health Effect
Ozone	0.070 ppm as an 8-h average concentration	Increased respiratory symptoms Decreased lung function Airway inflammation Increased airway responsiveness to nonspecific stimuli
Nitrogen dioxide	0.053 ppm as an annual arithmetic mean concentration and 100 ppb as a 1-h average concentration	Increased respiratory symptoms and illnesses in children
Particulate matter (PM_{10})	150 mcg/m^3 as a 24-h average concentration	Increased respiratory symptoms Increased respiratory illnesses Increased respiratory morbidity in persons with asthma and COPD
($PM_{2.5}$)	12 mcg/m^3 as an annual arithmetic mean concentration and 35 mcg/m^3 as a 24-h average concentration	Increased cardiovascular morbidity in persons with ischemic heart disease Increased cardiopulmonary mortality in elderly persons Increased lung cancer incidence
Sulfur dioxide	0.5 ppm as a 3-h average concentration and 75 ppb as a 1-h average concentration	Increased respiratory symptoms Increased respiratory morbidity and mortality Decreased lung function in asthmatics
Lead	0.15 mcg/m^3 as a concentration quarterly average	Cognitive deficits in children
Carbon monoxide	9 ppm as an 8-h average concentration and 35 ppm as a 1-h average concentration	Increased adverse reproductive outcomes Decreased exercise capacity in healthy adults Shorter duration to onset and increased duration of angina in people with CAD

COPD, chronic obstructive pulmonary disease; PM_{10}, particulate matter less than 10 μm in diameter; $PM_{2.5}$, particulate matter less than 2.5 μm in diameter; ppb, parts per billion; ppm, parts per million.

contributor to atmospheric acidity than H_2SO_4 and is formed in the atmosphere from the reaction of NO_x with the hydroxyl radical (OH$^-$). Motor vehicle emissions are also responsible for much carbon monoxide (CO) and particulate pollution. A major success story in the control of the criteria pollutants involves the markedly decreased concentrations of lead in the ambient air of US cities achieved as a result of removal of tetraethyl lead from gasoline beginning in 1974.

PERSONAL EXPOSURE

Central stations monitor the ambient air for concentrations of the criteria pollutants. However, the regional average concentrations measured at such stations may not characterize personal exposures adequately. For example, local conditions will affect pollutant concentrations to the extent that areas downwind from major traffic congestion may have higher levels than those in the immediate vicinity of the congestion. Individuals who spend a lot of time outdoors, especially if they are increasing their effective dose by means of increased minute ventilation from exercise, may sustain relatively high exposures to pollutants such as O_3 and PM. There is a common misconception that indoor air is uniformly cleaner than outdoor air, but the concentration of NO_2, for example, may be higher in indoor air largely as a result of

natural gas–burning stoves. For all these reasons, total personal exposure should be considered; this is estimated by the summation of the products of the concentrations of the pollutant in various microenvironments with the duration spent in each.

▶ Principles of Inhalational Injury

For any one individual, the total potential dose of a pollutant can vary depending on the preceding factors. Furthermore, pollutants in inhaled air are either gases or aerosols—droplets of liquid or particles suspended in gas—and their site of deposition after inhalation is determined largely by their water solubility. Gases that are extremely water soluble, such as SO_2 and HNO_3 vapor, are deposited and removed primarily by the upper respiratory tract. Therefore, these water-soluble gases mainly induce toxic effects on the proximal airways and only damage the distal lung when inhaled in high concentrations. In contrast, gases that are of relatively low water solubility, such as NO_x and O_3, may injure the distal lung predominantly. The less soluble the gas, the greater is the potential for damage at the level of the terminal respiratory unit.

The deposition of aerosols is determined by a number of factors, including the size and chemical characteristics of the aerosol, the anatomy of the respiratory tract, and the breathing pattern of the exposed person. The size of the droplet or particle usually is the primary factor affecting deposition, although the chemical nature of the inhaled pollutant can be important, especially if it is a water-soluble acid aerosol that can be neutralized by oral ammonia, such as a H_2SO_4 mist.

The majority of inhaled particles with a mass median aerodynamic diameter (MMAD) of more than 10 μm are deposited in the nasopharynx and will not penetrate below the larynx. Particles in the range of 2.5–6 μm deposit primarily in the conducting airways below the larynx, and particles in the range of 0.5–2.5 μm deposit primarily in the distal airways and alveoli. Many particles with a MMAD of less than 0.5 μm do not deposit in the alveoli and actually are exhaled. Particles less than 0.1 μm are called *ultrafine*; these particles are of considerable interest because there is evidence that they are especially toxic, likely related to their increased surface area for a given mass and their potential ability to directly enter the bloodstream.

The site of particle deposition also is influenced by hygroscopic growth in the humidified environment of the airways, the shape and dimensions of the respiratory tree, the ventilatory pattern (respiratory rate and tidal volume), oral versus nasal breathing, and the amount and nature of respiratory tract secretions. Respiratory tract disease can affect particle deposition by altering airway dimension, airflow pattern, or respiratory secretions. Physiologic differences can also affect particle deposition; with periods of exercise in both children and adults, there are increases in oral breathing, bypassing the nasal scrubbing mechanism, and increases in minute ventilation, thereby increasing particle velocity and inertial impaction. Both these changes result in greater particle deposition in the lower airways.

Clearance of inhaled pollutants occurs by several mechanisms. In general, highly water-soluble particles and gases are absorbed through the epithelial layer into the bloodstream near where they have been deposited. The clearance of insoluble particles depends on where they impact. Those deposited in the anterior nasal cavity are expelled by sneezing or rhinorrhea, whereas the remainder of particles deposited in the nose are cleared posteriorly to the pharynx. Particles deposited in the trachea, bronchi, or bronchioles, where there are ciliated epithelium and a layer of mucus, are transported up the mucociliary escalator to be expelled by coughing or swallowing. Particles deposited distal to the terminal bronchioles are cleared by alveolar macrophages and/or dissolution. Alveolar macrophages will ingest particles and migrate to the mucociliary escalator or into lymphatics. A small fraction of particles deposited in the alveoli will migrate through the alveolar epithelial layer directly into the lymphatic circulation, and ultrafine particles may pass directly across the alveolar-capillary membrane.

SPECIFIC OUTDOOR AIR POLLUTANTS

In 2014–2016, approximately 40% of the US population lived in counties with measured air quality above the primary NAAQSs and/or in areas with exposures to heavy traffic.

Between 2015 and 2017, 6–8% of the urban population of the EU-29 were exposed to concentrations in excess of the EU limit value for fine particulate matter ($PM_{2.5}$), while 74–81% were exposed to concentrations above the World Health Organization (WHO) guideline value. For particulate matter (PM_{10}), the respective exposure estimates were 13–19% for the EU limit value and 42–52% for the WHO guideline value. For O_3, estimates were 12–29% for the EU target value and 95–98% for the WHO guideline value. For nitrogen dioxide (NO_2), estimates were 7–8% in both cases (EU limit value and WHO guideline value). Therefore, from a clinical and public health perspective, such exposures continue to be of relevance. The health effects of outdoor air pollutants are understood via interpretation of the combination of toxicologic studies (ie, animal studies, in vitro studies, and controlled human exposure studies) and epidemiologic studies (ie, ecologic, cross-sectional, and longitudinal designs). This section discusses each of the major air pollutants individually; however, it should be understood that exposures often occur to a mixture of pollutants, and separating out the individual contribution of each pollutant frequently is not possible.

▶ Ozone

O_3 is a colorless, pungent, relatively water-insoluble gas that occurs with other photochemical oxidants and fine particles to form "smog." Tropospheric O_3, or ground-level O_3, is an environmental air pollutant and is distinct from the stratospheric O_3 that occurs at altitudes of greater than 10 km (6.2 mi) above the earth's surface. O_3 is generated by a series of sunlight-driven reactions involving NO_x and VOCs from predominantly mobile (ie, motor vehicle) but sometimes stationary sources. The meteorologic conditions that tend to foster the generation of ozone typically are present from late spring to early fall. Peak concentrations of O_3 typically occur in midafternoon, after both the morning rush hour and several hours of bright sunlight. Indoor sources of O_3 include office equipment with electric motors or ultraviolet light, such as photocopy machines, and electrostatic devices, such as air purifiers and ion generators.

While O_3 has long been associated with southern California smog, many other areas of North America also experience high concentrations of this pollutant, especially Houston, Mexico City, and cities in the eastern United States and Canada during the summer months. In these areas, there are many days each year when the current NAAQS for O_3 is not attained.

Ozone is a potent oxidant and is capable of reacting with a variety of extracellular and intracellular molecules. When these molecules are unsaturated lipids, free radicals and toxic intermediate products are generated and can lead to cellular damage or cell death. Although direct cytotoxicity is clearly a necessary mechanism of O_3-induced tissue injury, secondary damage from the inflammatory response also may play a role.

Dosimetric studies indicate that much of the inhaled O_3 is deposited in the upper and proximal lower airways. However, because of its relative water insolubility, a considerable fraction does penetrate to the distal airways and alveoli, and the dose at the tissue level is highest at these sites. Increased inspiratory flow, such as with exercise, may overcome the upper airway "scrubbing mechanisms" and cause greater deposition of O_3 in the distal lung.

Most of the research on the health effects of O_3 has focused on short-term exposure. O_3 inhalation by healthy subjects causes mean decrements in forced expiratory volume in 1 second (FEV_1) and forced vital capacity (FVC) that correlate with concentration, exposure duration, and minute ventilation. These decrements in lung function are primarily a result of decreased inspiratory capacity rather than airways obstruction. The mechanism of the decreased inspiratory capacity appears to be neutrally mediated involuntary inhibition of inspiratory effort involving stimulation of C-fibers in the lungs. Somewhat surprisingly, older subjects and those who are cigarette smokers demonstrate lower O_3-induced decrements in pulmonary function than healthy subjects. In contrast, individuals who lack the antioxidant enzyme, glutathione S-transferase mu1 (GSTM1) appear to have increased sensitivity to the acute lung function effects of O_3. These acute decrements in lung function usually resolve within 24 hours.

Respiratory symptoms appear to be associated with these mean decrements in pulmonary function. There is a correlation between the decline in FEV_1 and the probability of developing lower respiratory tract symptoms (eg, substernal chest discomfort, cough, wheeze, and dyspnea). Another adverse effect of short-term exposure to O_3 is enhanced airway responsiveness to nonspecific stimuli such as methacholine and histamine. This effect may persist longer than the acute decrements in lung function and may occur in individuals who do not experience a decline in their FEV_1. Ozone levels have also been repeatedly associated with increases in healthcare utilization for respiratory illnesses.

Nasal inflammatory changes, type I alveolar and ciliated airway epithelial cell injury, infiltration of the airway mucosa by neutrophils, and increased bronchoalveolar lavage (BAL) fluid neutrophils and inflammatory mediators also have been observed after exposure. BAL evidence of inflammation has been demonstrated at effective doses allowable under the current NAAQS for O_3. Evidence of increased airway inflammation has been reported for GSTM1-null individuals.

Some other effects of short-term ozone exposures have also been described. There is a consistent relationship between increasing ozone levels and ischemic strokes. In the last two decades, several epidemiologic studies in both Europe and the United States that have linked ambient ozone with daily mortality have been reported. However, the mechanism underlying this association is unclear. Limited evidence from controlled human exposure studies suggests that exposure to O_3 can decrease heart rate variability and increase systemic oxidative stress and inflammation.

The effects of chronic O_3 exposure in humans have not been as well studied as acute effects from short-term exposures. However, work involving multiple large cohorts has suggested that the incidence of asthma in childhood is related to chronic ozone exposure, even at levels below the NAAQS. Finally, in a study of the American Cancer Society

cohort, chronic exposure to O_3 was reported to increase risk of death due to primarily respiratory disease. A massive cohort representative of the elderly population of the United States also found a 1% increase in mortality for every 10 ppb increase in chronic ozone exposure, even at levels well below the NAAQS.

Because of their tendency to experience bronchoconstriction on inhalation of noxious stimuli, persons with asthma usually are more sensitive to inhaled irritants. Although studies of asthmatic and atopic subjects have failed to show enhanced spirometric responses to short-term O_3 inhalation, there are indications that asthmatics may experience a greater inflammatory response to exposure. Furthermore, there are several epidemiologic studies that show that high ambient O_3 concentrations are associated with an increased rate of asthma attacks and increased hospital admissions/emergency department visits for respiratory disease, including asthma. In addition to the exacerbation of preexisting asthma, there is also evidence that playing outdoor sports in a high ambient O_3 environment can lead to the onset of asthma.

Ozone toxicity may be enhanced by co-exposure to other pollutants such as other oxidants, particulates, and atmospheric acidity commonly seen in urban smog. The mechanisms by which these cofactors may potentiate O_3 toxicity are poorly understood.

In summary, tens of millions of persons in the United States and globally are exposed to levels of O_3 above the current NAAQS. This exposure is capable of inducing both acute decrements in lung function and respiratory symptoms. Although these effects are transient, acute respiratory tract inflammation also can be induced by short-term exposure to ambient concentrations of O_3 with exercise. The long-term consequences of this type of acute inflammatory response are not well understood, but there is epidemiologic evidence consistent with airway remodeling. Because O_3 inhalation can induce both airway inflammation and enhanced airway responsiveness, it is reasonable to expect persons with asthma to have greater susceptibility to this pollutant. Evidence is accumulating that both short- and long-term exposures to ambient levels of O_3 are associated with increased risk of mortality. Ozone is rarely the sole pollutant of concern in urban smog, and it is likely that environmental cofactors enhance its toxicity.

▶ Nitrogen Dioxide

Most ambient nitrogen dioxide (NO_2) is generated by the burning of fossil-derived fuels, during which oxygen and nitrogen react to form nitrogen oxide (NO), which further reacts to form NO_2 and other NO_x. The principal source of NO_2 in outdoor air is motor vehicle emissions, but power plants and fossil fuel–burning industrial facilities also contribute. In most US urban areas, ambient levels of NO_2 vary with traffic intensity. Annual average concentrations range from 0.015 to 0.035 ppm, below the current annual NAAQS. A 1-hour NAAQS was promulgated in 2010 to protect people with asthma from experiencing acute exacerbations.

In contrast to other criteria pollutants, NO_2 is a common contaminant of indoor air, and indoor levels often exceed those found outdoors. Indoor sources of NO_2 include gas cooking stoves, gas furnaces, and kerosene space heaters. Because the majority of homes in the United States have gas cooking stoves and Americans spend a large proportion of time in their homes, the home environment is an important contributor to total NO_2 exposure. High concentrations may be generated in a kitchen with a gas stove in use, though the use of stove range hoods for ventilation can decrease exposure. Nitrous acid (HONO) and other NO_x are emitted by gas stoves, so health effects associated with the use of such appliances may not be a result of NO_2 alone.

Nitrogen dioxide, like O_3, is an oxidant, but it is less chemically reactant and therefore usually is considered less potent. Although both pollutants are relatively insoluble in water, the solubility of NO_2 is somewhat higher. When NO_2 is absorbed onto the moist surfaces of the respiratory tract, it can be hydrolyzed to evolve acidic species such as HONO and HNO_3. The potential for NO_2 to cause the local generation of hydrogen ions in the airways may be an important feature of its toxicity. Nitrogen dioxide and O_3 are frequent co-pollutants in southern California smog.

The results of controlled human exposure studies have demonstrated no significant decrements in pulmonary function in normal, healthy subjects after exposure to NO_2 at low concentrations. Controlled exposure studies of subjects with asthma, however, have demonstrated that NO_2 exposure can enhance airway responsiveness. Perhaps the most intriguing finding from controlled studies of asthmatic subjects is that of enhanced bronchoconstrictor responses to inhaled allergen following NO_2 exposure. There are also animal studies that support an adjuvant effect of NO_2 exposure on allergic airway responses.

The toxic effects of NO_2 exposure have been studied extensively. There are abundant animal toxicologic data and reports of accidental human exposure that indicate that short-term inhalation of high concentrations of NO_2 can produce terminal bronchiolar and diffuse alveolar injury; exposure of humans to very high concentrations (ie, > 150 ppm NO_2) typically results in death. However, in contrast to what is seen with O_3, short-term exposure to NO_2 at concentrations in the ambient range does not induce airways inflammation.

Chronic exposure of animals to high concentrations of NO_2 has been shown to cause structural damage to alveoli with airspace enlargement, which is somewhat analogous to human emphysema. The terminal lung unit is the site of greatest NO_2-induced injury. Animal infectivity studies after NO_2 exposure have shown that high concentrations may impair respiratory tract defenses against some bacteria and viruses. The mechanisms of NO_2-induced enhanced microbial infectivity are not clearly understood but likely are caused by alveolar macrophage dysfunction. While some epidemiologic studies have shown a positive association between indoor NO_2 and respiratory illness, others have failed to demonstrate this finding. A meta-analysis using 11 cross-sectional and prospective studies of residential NO_2 concentrations in children estimated a 20% increase in risk of respiratory illness per 15-ppb increments in long-term NO_2 exposure. A more recent study of indoor NO_2 levels and respiratory symptoms failed to show an association between these factors. The inconsistency of this association in epidemiologic studies may be partly a result of methodologic factors such as different statistical power, confounding, and misclassification.

Somewhat surprisingly, given its lower potency than ozone as an oxidant gas, ambient NO_2 was significantly associated with a slower rate of growth of lung function in a large longitudinal study of school children living in 12 communities in southern California. As described previously for ozone, several epidemiologic studies have shown associations between ambient NO_2 and hospital admissions and emergency department visits for asthma. An Institute of Medicine review has concluded that there is sufficient evidence of an association between brief high-level exposures to NO_2 and airway responsiveness in patients with asthma.

In summary, NO_2 is a pollutant that is a ubiquitous component of urban smog. It is generated by combustion of fossil-derived fuels from both mobile and stationary sources. Indoor exposures are also important because of the use of gas appliances. Inhaled NO_2 penetrates to the deep lung because of the relatively low water solubility of the gas. Perhaps the most important effect seen in controlled human exposure studies of NO_2 is enhanced bronchoconstriction to inhaled allergen in specifically sensitized asthmatic subjects. Chronic exposure of experimental animals to high concentrations of NO_2 has caused emphysema-like changes and decreased resistance to bacterial infection. The applicability of these findings to ambient exposure of humans is not straightforward. Multiple epidemiologic studies show associations between asthma exacerbations or reduced growth of lung function and ambient NO_2 levels. Some investigators currently feel that these associations reflect the adverse health effects of traffic-related pollution and that NO_2 is merely a good marker of such pollution.

▶ Sulfur Dioxide

Sulfur dioxide (SO_2) is generated whenever sulfur-containing fuels are burned and is a major air pollutant in many urban areas. The gas is emitted by coal- and oil-fired power plants and by industrial processes involving fossil fuel combustion. It leads to the secondary formation of acid aerosols. Because high-sulfur-content coal has remained a relatively cheap fuel in regions where it is mined, SO_2 emissions generally have been more of a problem in the eastern United States than in southern California, where smog is primarily a result of photochemical reactions involving motor vehicle emissions. Unfortunately, the building of tall smokestacks to reduce the local concentrations of SO_2 around midwestern and eastern US power plants led to the long-distance transport of sulfur oxide pollutants and their progeny, acid sulfates, to New England and Canada (so-called acid rain). Sulfur oxide emissions in the United States increased steadily during the twentieth century to a peak of 32 million tons in 1970. Fortunately, major progress has been made over the past several decades in reducing sulfur oxide emissions from US power plants due to both an EPA-sponsored sulfur oxides emissions trading program and the transition from coal to natural gas.

Exposure to high concentrations of SO_2 is highly localized to the vicinity (within 20 km [12.4 mi]) of major stationary sources. The initial clues that SO_2 might be an air pollutant capable of causing adverse respiratory effects came from the severe pollution episodes occurring earlier in this century. During these episodes, high ambient concentrations of SO_2, particles, and acid aerosols occurred and clearly were associated with increased mortality, primarily among persons with preexisting cardiopulmonary disease.

Sulfur dioxide is highly soluble in water and is absorbed mostly in the upper airways. Although the nose effectively removes much of the inhaled gas, significant amounts may penetrate to the large airways. Here, the irritant molecules may act directly on smooth muscle or via sensory afferent nerve fibers to cause reflex bronchoconstriction. At high concentrations, SO_2 can cause epithelial sloughing in the trachea and proximal airways, leading to a bronchitis-like pathology. Despite the irritant potential of SO_2, studies fail to demonstrate effects on respiratory mechanics (at levels up to 1.0 ppm) in healthy people. However, in asthmatics, low-level exposure causes bronchoconstriction. This acute bronchoconstriction is observed within minutes of exposure and resolves within 1 hour after exposure ceases. While the mechanism of SO_2-induced bronchoconstriction is not fully understood, a reflex mechanism involving vagal afferent and cholinergic efferent nerves is postulated.

▶ Particulate Matter

PM is a heterogenous group defined simply by size. Particles with an aerodynamic diameter of less than or equal to 10 μm (PM_{10}) are the focus of regulatory interest because particles of this diameter may penetrate into the respiratory tract. Particles between 10 and 2.5 μm in diameter ($PM_{10-2.5}$) or the coarse fraction of inhalable PM deposit in the airways of the lower respiratory tract; $PM_{2.5}$ or fine particles can be deposited in the gas-exchanging portions of the lung. Ultrafine particles (< 0.1 μm) are a component of $PM_{2.5}$. Particles of the coarse size range may be due to aerosolization of crustal materials that can include bioactive agents like pollens, endotoxin, and fungal spores as well as road dust that can contain toxic metals. Fine and ultrafine particles are usually from carbon-based fuel combustion.

During the 1952 severe air pollution episode in London, there were an estimated 4000 excess deaths attributed to emissions from coal-burning that contained large quantities of fine particles. More recently, multiple epidemiologic studies have demonstrated an association between lower levels of particulate pollution and increased daily mortality from cardiopulmonary disease. The consistent finding of this association in studies conducted at various times and in diverse geographic locations makes it likely that there is a true causal relationship between respirable PM and daily mortality. However, the biologic mechanism underlying this

association remains obscure, especially given the lack of toxicity of ambient levels of PM in animal studies.

Acute morbidity associated with lower-level particulate pollution has been examined using a variety of indicators, including measures of health care utilization by exposed populations, health status of exposed individuals, symptom questionnaires, and lung function tests. Exposure to PM has been associated with increased emergency room visits for respiratory illness, such as asthma and pneumonia; higher rates of hospital admissions for respiratory and cardiovascular illnesses; and increased daily mortality as a result of cardiovascular and respiratory diseases in elderly people.

Epidemiologic studies also show associations between exposure to particles and reports of respiratory symptoms severe enough to restrict activity. In smokers with Chronic obstructive pulmonary disease (COPD), declines in pulmonary function and daily emergency room visits for acute exacerbations have been positively associated with particulate air pollution. In children, studies have shown associations with particulate concentrations at levels commonly encountered today with respiratory illnesses, declines in pulmonary function, and aggravation of asthmatic attacks. In elderly people or patients with ischemic heart disease, decreased heart rate variability (a negative prognostic indicator), increased angina, and increased arrhythmias have been associated with ambient PM.

The chronic health effects of particulate air pollution are a more difficult endpoint to study. Despite this, a number of studies show an association between PM levels and the following: reports of chronic bronchitis, doctors' diagnoses of asthma, and in several prospective US studies, an increase in city-specific cardiopulmonary mortality rates. The same study of southern California school children that found an effect of NO_2 on growth of lung function also showed similar effects of PM and nitric acid vapor. A recent report of a prospective US study also showed an increased risk of lung cancer to be related to residence in metropolitan areas with higher particulate pollution. Newer associations between chronic exposures to PM and adverse health effects include increased risk for adverse birth outcomes such as low birth weight and preterm birth, metabolic disorders such as diabetes and obesity, decreased cognitive development of children, and increased risk of dementia in older adults.

The toxicity of inhaled particles is determined by the physical and chemical nature of the particles, the physics of their deposition and distribution in the respiratory tract, and the biologic effect(s) of exposure. Particle toxicity often is complicated by the presence of other air pollutants that may cause interactive effects. Particle size is thought to be a critical determinant of toxicity. After exposure of animals to ultrafine particles (those with a diameter of 0.2 μm or less), acute lung inflammation has been noted. In vitro studies of the cytotoxicity of particles collected from polluted urban air also have demonstrated that such particles can be highly toxic to alveolar macrophages. The relative toxicity of the particles studied depended on both the metal and the combustion-derived organic content of the particles.

A particular type of ambient particles, diesel exhaust particles (DEPs), has been the focus of considerable research attention. Several studies involving animal models of allergic airways disease document an adjuvant effect of DEPs on both inhaled antigen-induced airway hyperresponsiveness and airway inflammation. Nasal instillation of DEPs in humans with allergic rhinitis confirms enhancement of antigen-induced inflammation. Another controlled human exposure study also showed that a common genetic variation of an antioxidant enzyme (GSTM1) resulting in absence of the protein is a major determinant of this effect of DEPs. What is not clear about DEPs is the importance of exposure to ambient concentrations regarding allergies and asthma among the general population. In addition, there is considerable evidence that exposure to diesel exhaust can cause acute cardiovascular effects, such as myocardial ischemia and endothelial dysfunction.

In summary, ambient particles are a complex mixture of different sizes and chemical composition. Epidemiologic studies consistently have shown that they exert adverse health effects on both respiratory and cardiovascular morbidity and mortality. In vitro and in vivo studies have attempted to study the mechanism(s) of these effects, but their interpretation is complicated by the difficulty in separating out the individual contributions and the potential synergistic interactions of the components.

▶ Lead

Lead continues to be recognized as a significant toxicant and is known to have adverse health effects on humans of all ages. However, the phaseout of the additive tetraethyl lead from gasoline in the United States as a result of the CAA has been associated with declines in ambient lead concentrations and blood lead levels in the population. Thus, widespread airborne exposure to lead has ceased to be a major health problem in the United States. Airborne lead remains a serious problem in some developing countries.

▶ Carbon Monoxide

Carbon monoxide (CO) is a colorless, odorless, nonirritating gas that is generated by the incomplete combustion of carbon-containing fuels such as oils, gasoline, coal, and wood. Because of these described properties, exposure to CO may be insidious; in fact, exposure to high levels of CO is the leading cause of poisoning deaths in the United States. Ambient environmental air pollution levels are unlikely to cause acute toxicity and death, although low-dose exposure may be associated with adverse health effects. The most common source of exposure in nonsmoking individuals is from vehicle emissions. Engine exhaust may cause local accumulation of CO, especially during periods of heavy traffic. In transit exposure assessments, commuting individuals have been shown to be exposed to high levels. In fact, in one study of commuters, levels as high as 50 ppm with mean values of 10–12 ppm were recorded. Emissions from nonvehicular sources such as lawn mowers, chain saws, space heaters, and charcoal briquettes also contribute to ambient CO exposure.

The toxicity of CO lies in its ability to bind strongly to hemoglobin and interfere with the transport of oxygen from the alveoli to tissues. The degree of exposure to CO may be determined by measuring the blood carboxyhemoglobin level. Normal levels in nonsmokers range from 0.3% to 0.7%. The NAAQS is 9 ppm as an 8-hour average, not to be exceeded more than once a year.

Because CO has no direct effect on the lungs, its principal adverse health effects are through its ability to cause or exacerbate diseases associated with impaired oxygen delivery. Effects on fetal development, cardiovascular disease, chronic respiratory diseases, and nervous system disease have been described.

Animal studies show that low-level CO exposure during pregnancy may have developmental effects on the fetus. Low birth weight, fewer successful pregnancies, and increased fetal and neonatal mortality have been observed. A series of epidemiologic studies conducted in the Los Angeles area demonstrated associations between ambient CO concentrations and adverse birth outcomes (eg, low birth weight, preterm delivery, and cardiac malformations).

In healthy human subjects, controlled-exposure studies have shown that low-level CO exposure decreases exercise capacity. In individuals with ischemic heart disease, a shorter duration to onset and an increased duration of angina, as well as earlier ST-T changes (an objective measure of myocardial ischemia), have been observed with low-level CO exposure. Ambient levels of CO have not been shown consistently to cause ventricular arrhythmias. Several epidemiologic studies show an association between high ambient levels of CO and cardiorespiratory hospital admissions and cardiac deaths.

In summary, CO at ambient levels of exposure may exacerbate ischemic heart disease, increase cardiorespiratory morbidity and cardiac mortality, and lead to increased adverse reproductive outcomes.

INDOOR AIR POLLUTION

Forty percent of the world's population uses solid fuel for cooking and/or heating. This occurs predominantly in the rural areas of developing countries. The WHO has estimated 3.8 million deaths globally per year are attributable to indoor exposure to household air pollution from cooking or heating with solid fuels (wood, dung, crop residues, charcoal, coal) to household air pollution. This burden of disease places exposure to household air pollution as the leading environmental hazard for poor health on a global scale. Household air pollution also remains an important contributor to outdoor air pollution in many rapidly industrializing countries, such as India and China.

Because many families burn coal or biomass fuels in open stoves, which are highly inefficient, and inside homes with poor ventilation, women and young children are exposed to high levels of smoke on a daily basis. In these homes, 24-hour mean levels of fine PM ($PM_{2.5}$) have been reported to be 2–30 times higher than the NAAQS set by the U.S. EPA. The combustion of organically derived solid fuel is qualitatively similar to the burning of tobacco in terms of emissions of PM and gases, and the mechanisms by which solid fuel smoke causes adverse health effects in humans are likely similar. Acute lower respiratory infections in children, COPD and lung cancer in women, and cardiovascular disease among men and women have been associated with exposure to household air pollution.

Kerosene (similar to diesel fuel) is often used for lighting and sometimes cooking. Household exposure to kerosene has been associated with increased risk of pulmonary tuberculosis, but is increasingly a focus of studies on other outcomes.

REFERENCES

American Lung Association. State of the Air. http://www.stateoftheair.org.

Balmes JR. Household air pollution from domestic combustion of solid fuels and health. J Allergy Clin Immunol 2019;143(6):1979-1987 [PMID: 31176380].

Burnett R et al: Global estimates of mortality associated with long-term exposure to outdoor fine particulate matter. Proc Natl Acad Sci U S A. 2018;115:9592 [PMID: 30181279].

DeFlorio-Barker, Crooks J, Reyes J, Rappold AG: Cardiopulmonary effects of fine particulate matter exposure among older adults, during wildfire and non-wildfire periods, in the United States 2008-2010. Environ Health Perspect 2019;127:37006 [PMID: 30875246].

Rajagopalan S, Al-Kindi SG, Brook RD: Air pollution and cardiovascular disease: JACC State-of-the-Art Review. J Am Coll Cardiol 2018;72:2054 [PMID: 30336830].

Schraufnagel DE et al: Air pollution and noncommunicable diseases: A review by the Forum of International Respiratory Societies' Environmental Committee, Part 1: The damaging effects of air pollution. Chest 2019;155(2):409-416 [PMID: 30419235].

Schraufnagel DE et al: Air pollution and noncommunicable diseases: A review by the Forum of International Respiratory Societies' Environmental Committee, Part 2: Air pollution and organ systems. Chest 2019;155(2):417–426 [PMID: 30419237].

Turner MC et al: Long-term ozone exposure and mortality in a large prospective study. Am J Respir Crit Care Med 2016;193:1134 [PMID: 26680605].

U.S. EPA: National air quality standards. https://www3.epa.gov/airquality/.

■ SELF-ASSESSMENT QUESTIONS

Select the once correct answer for each question.

Question 1: The Clean Air Act (CAA)
a. is the principal international standard addressing outdoor air quality
b. requires all countries to list pollutants for which there is sufficient scientific evidence documenting the risk to public health from unregulated exposure
c. applies to countries with environmental protection agencies
d. is the principal federal standard addressing outdoor air quality in the United States

Question 2: The National Ambient Air Quality Standard (NAAQS) for a pollutant
a. is produced by the U.S. Environmental Protection Agency for all toxic pollutants
b. is set based on a cost-benefit analysis
c. limits protection to sensitive groups (ie, that demonstrate a response to a pollutant at a lower level or to a greater degree than the average response of the general population)
d. is set to protect the health of all sensitive groups within the population

Question 3: Stationary sources of air pollution
a. are primarily power or manufacturing plants
b. are responsible for a small portion of sulfur dioxide (SO_2) emissions
c. are responsible for trace quantities of nitrogen oxides (NO_x) and particulate matter
d. directly release ozone (O_3) into the atmosphere

Question 4: Ozone
a. is a colorless, pungent, relatively water-insoluble gas
b. reacts with other photochemical oxidants and fine particles to form "smog"
c. is found only in the stratosphere at altitudes greater than 10 km (6.2 mi) above the earth's surface
d. is released primarily by stationary sources

Question 5: Nitrogen dioxide
a. is a common contaminant of indoor air, and indoor levels often exceed those found outdoors
b. indoor sources may include electric stoves, furnaces, and space heaters
c. is an oxidant more potent than ozone
d. water solubility is somewhat lower than ozone

Question 6: Sulfur dioxide
a. is a major air pollutant in rural areas
b. is solely emitted by coal- and oil-fired power plants
c. leads to the secondary formation of acid aerosols
d. emissions from US power plants are steadily increasing

Question 7: Carbon monoxide
a. is a colorless, odorless, and irritating gas
b. has no direct effect on the lungs
c. causes or exacerbates diseases associated with hypertension
d. has no effect on fetal development

Water Pollution

Leslie Israel, DO, MPH

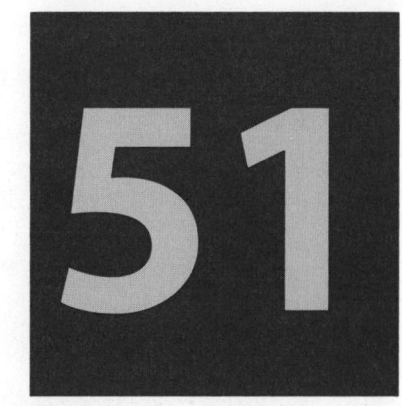

The availability of clean water is paramount to the sustainability of life and good health. Adequate supplies of water are essential for agriculture and societal development. Water availability is scarce, with less than 1% of global fresh water accessible while the global demand for water is increasing substantially. By 2050, feeding a planet of 9 billion people will require an estimated 50% increase in agricultural production and a 15% increase in water consumption.

The United Nations reports that billions drink polluted water that could be harmful to their health. Unsafe polluted water kills more people each year than war and all other forms of violence combined. Almost 80% of diseases in developing countries are associated with water, causing some three million early deaths. The World Health Organization (WHO) and many countries have established regulations and guidelines to protect water.

Factors impacting the global availability of water include climate change, and the contamination of water from biological agents, chemicals, and a wide range of substances that are detrimental to human, plant and/or animal life. These contaminants include fertilizers and pesticides from agricultural runoff; sewage, and food processing waste; plastic; chemical wastes from industrial discharges; chemical contamination from hazardous waste sites; and lead, mercury, and other heavy metals.

The earth's water is constantly in a cycle of evaporation and precipitation (Figure 51–1). Once deposited on the earth's surface, water may run off, be impounded, or percolate through various layers of soil, sand, and rock to become free-flowing water or confined water. Deep aquifers often are confined. Therefore, they do not participate in the evaporation and precipitation cycle unless the confining zone above them has been penetrated and fluids extracted. Evaporation from saline water sources, the oceans, and large salt marshes also contributes to the total airborne water vapor that eventually may precipitate to the earth's surface. The process of evaporation and precipitation has the potential to cleanse water of organic and inorganic contaminants, as does percolation of water through sand and soil and the action of soil microorganisms.

Climate change negatively impacts the water cycle by reducing the availability of drinking water. Precipitation in a warming world will not be uniform. In dry subtropical regions there is projected to be a reduction in mean precipitation crucially reducing renewable surface water and groundwater resources. While in mid-latitude land masses and wet tropical regions there is projected to be an increase in the intensity and frequency of precipitation. The interaction of increased temperature; increased sediment, nutrient and pollutant loadings from heavy rainfall; increased concentrations of pollutants during droughts; and disruption of treatment facilities during floods will significantly reduce drinking water quality and availability.

WATER USAGE

Water usage is based on geographic location, population density, and renewable water resources. Worldwide, agriculture accounts for 70% of all water consumption, compared to 20% for industry and 10% for domestic use. In industrialized nations, however, industries consume more than half of the water available for human use.

Since 1950, the U.S. Geological Survey (USGS) estimates total national water use every 5 years. Over the last 30 years, 90% of water is used by these three categories: thermoelectric power (225–350 million gallons/day), irrigation (approximately 200 million gallons/day), and public supply (approximately 75 million gallons/day). Withdrawals for thermoelectric power have been on a steady decline since 2005, which is attributed to plant closures, a shift from coal to natural gas as a fuel source, and new power plants using more water-efficient power generation and cooling-system technologies.

Public water systems provide drinking water to 90% of the US population. The remaining 10% obtain drinking water from private domestic wells. The distinction between

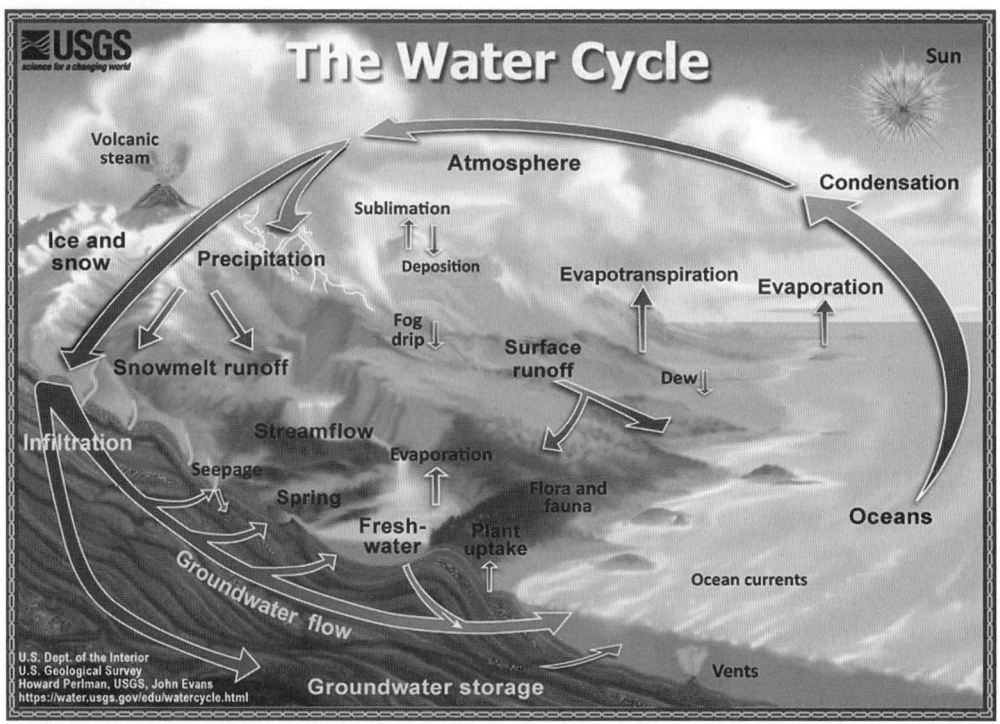

▲ **Figure 51–1.** The water cycle.

public water systems and private domestic wells has important implications in some countries like the United States since enforceable drinking water regulation typically only applies to public, not private, water supplies.

REGULATION OF WATER AND WASTEWATER

Water supply and quality significantly impact public health, which has contributed to the establishment of international, national, and state regulations and guidelines. WHO Guidelines for drinking water include recommendations for water system operations, management, surveillance, and treatment. They provide chemical fact sheets describing the occurrence, health effects of a large number of drinking water contaminants including microbial agents, organic and inorganic chemical, pesticides, and radionuclides. The WHO guidelines promote achievable regulations, applicable to low income, middle income, and industrialized countries. The United Nations General Assembly (2015) number six standalone goal was "Ensure the availability and sustainable management of water and sanitation for all." Several countries have established regulatory standards for maintaining the quality and safety of drinking water. Many of these are similar to or are based on recommended water quality guidelines developed by the WHO. The most recent edition (4th) of the WHO Guidelines for Drinking Water Quality is available at: https://www.who.int/water_sanitation_health/publications/

The WHO guidelines include valuable recommendations for water system operations, management, surveillance, and treatment, and provide chemical fact sheets describing the occurrence, health effects, along with values for a large number of drinking water contaminants including microbial agents, organic and inorganic chemicals, pesticides, and radionuclides. The WHO guidelines promote achievable practices and support the formulation of sound regulations, applicable to low-income, middle-income, and industrialized countries alike aiming to prevent health crises caused by the consumption of unsafe drinking water, against the backdrop of rapid urbanization, water scarcity, and climate change.

In the United States, regulatory standards for drinking water quality are guided primarily by the 1974 Safe Drinking Water Act (SDWA) authorized by the Environmental Protection Agency (EPA) to protect public health by regulating the nation's public drinking water supply. The SDWA differs from the 1972 Clean Water Act (CWA) in that the CWA is primarily aimed at limiting discharges of pollutants into surface water whereas the SDWA is focused specifically on the quality of water used for drinking. The SDWA was originally passed after widespread water quality problems and health risks from poor operating conditions and inadequate facilities and management of public drinking water supplies became apparent. The original 1974 law gave the U.S. Environmental Protection Agency (EPA) the authority to set minimum drinking water standards for contaminants in public water systems and require the owners or operators of these systems to comply with these standards. Major amendments to the SDWA included the 1986 amendments which required U.S. EPA to promulgate regulatory standards for additional contaminants beyond the 22 agents for which standards had previously been set, establish new regulations for disinfection and filtration of public water supplies, and ban the use of lead pipes and lead solder in new drinking water systems. The 1996 amendments established new standards requiring cost-benefit analyses when new regulatory standards are passed, new regulations regarding microbial contaminants and disinfection by-products, operator certification, funding for infrastructure or management

Table 51–1. Comparison of WHO drinking water guideline and EPA drinking water standard for selected substances.

Selected Substance	WHO (mg/L)	EPA (mg/L)
Arsenic	0.01	0.01
Benzene	0.01	0.005
Bisphenol A (BPA)	Not established	Not established
Cadmium	0.003	0.005
Chloramines	3.0	4.0
Chlorine	5.0	4.0
Chlorpyrifos	0.03	Not established
Chromium	0.05	0.1
Copper	2.0	1.3
Fluoride	1.5	4.0
Lead	0.01	0.015
Mercury (inorganic)	0.006	0.002
Methyl tert-butyl ether (MTBE)	Not established	Not established
Nitrate (measured as nitrate-nitrogen)	11.0	10.0
Nitrite (measured as nitrite-nitrogen)	0.9	1.0
Polynuclear Aromatic Hydrocarbons (PAH)	0.0007	0.0002
Polychlorinated biphenyls (PCBs)	Not established	0.0005
Perfluorooctanesulfonic acid (PFOS)	Not established	Not established
Toluene	0.7	1.0
Xylene	0.5	10.0

improvements, and requirements for Consumer Confidence Reports (CCRs). CCRs are prepared annually by the water suppliers and designed to inform consumers about the quality of the water they provide and the levels of various chemicals and other agents measured in the supplier's water.

The 1996 amendments to the SDWA also requires EPA to perform reviews every 6 years of existing National Primary Drinking Water Regulations (NPDWRs) and determine which, if any, are candidates for revision. The primary legal standards for contaminants in drinking water are referred to as the Maximum Contaminant Levels (MCLs). Through the SDWA, all public water systems in the United States need to follow the standards and regulations set by the EPA. The EPA has set MCLs and/or treatment technique requirements for over 90 different contaminants in public drinking water, including microorganisms, disinfectants, disinfections by-products, inorganic chemicals, organic chemicals, and radionuclides. In general, contaminants are selected to be considered for regulation based on their potential health risks and the extent to which they are found in public water supplies. States are allowed to establish their own drinking water standards, but they are required to be at least as strict as the national standards.

For noncarcinogens, the relevant data from this review are then used to identify a no observable adverse effect level (NOAEL), lowest observable adverse effect level (LOAEL), or a benchmark dose, and a maximum contaminant level goal (MCLG) is estimated after applying appropriate uncertainty factors (previously referred to as "safety factors") if needed. For carcinogens, there is no level that is entirely safe ("non-threshold"). That is, even at very low exposure levels of a carcinogen, there is always some associated risk, although that risk may be quite low at low exposures. For these agents, an acceptable risk level is established, commonly at one in one hundred thousand or one in one million excess risk of cancer, and dose-response data from the most relevant study or series of studies is used to estimate the concentration of the carcinogen that is likely to be associated with that acceptable risk. Overall, the goal of this process is to establish the enforceable MCL as close to the unenforceable MCLG as technically or feasibly possible, but for financial and technological reasons, the MCLs for many chemicals are above their respective MCLGs.

In recent years, dumping of agricultural and industrial chemicals has been reduced. In the future, new major US pollution problems may be prevented as a result of disposal practices by enforcement of the CWA. The right to discharge materials into the environment is granted under a permitting process that is administered by state, local, and federal authorities. The permits that are granted specify the quantities of pollutants that may be discharged, the conditions under which they may be discharged, and the time of discharge. They also establish the monitoring and other activities that must be carried out to ensure compliance with the permit. These National Pollutant Discharge Elimination System (NPDES) permits are designed to keep information flowing about environmental contamination. They help to ensure that a responsible standard is applied uniformly to all who discharge hazardous materials and who contaminate water resources, soil, or air.

WATER INTAKE AND RISK OF EXPOSURE TO CONTAMINANTS

Water intake in humans typically comes from one of three sources: drinking plain water (usually referred to as "direct" water consumption); consuming plain water that has been added to make other foods or beverages like tea, coffee, or soups (usually referred to as "indirect" water consumption); or water that is inherent in or produced in the metabolism of foods. The average acclimatized 70-kg (154.3-lb) human living in a temperate climate and at rest usually consumes about 1200 mL of plain water per day as either direct or indirect water, 500–1000 mL of water per day as water in food, and 300–400 mL of water per day is produced from oxidation of food. In a 70 kg adult, an intake of 1200 mL/d of direct and indirect water corresponds to a drinking water intake rate of about 17 mL/kg/d. To balance this intake, 800–1000 mL of water is insensibly lost in exhaled air, and approximately 200 mL is evaporated as sweat each day. A total of 100–200 mL of water is lost in the feces, and 1000–2000 mL of urine is produced per day. Thus, a balance at 2100–3400 mL of water intake and output is normal. However, heavy working conditions and hot humid climates may increase water loss from sweating and evaporation may increase intake by several liters per hour. In addition, pregnancy and lactation may increase water intake by 20–50%. The increased need for water intake in these women increases the exposure to higher doses of contaminants.

The amount of drinking water consumed by children is less than that in adults. For example, a child aged 0–12 months who is not breast-fed will typically consume less than 500 mL of direct and indirect water per day. However, drinking water *rates* (the amount of intake per body weight) in children are substantially higher than those in adults. For example, while an adult may have a drinking water rate of about 17 mL/kg/d, drinking water intake rates in young children are generally between 20 and 100 mL/kg/d depending on age (younger children have higher drinking water rates). The reasons for this are the increased physiologic requirements associated with the child's rapid growth and development. Therefore, children receive a higher dose of contaminants per kilogram of body weight than an adult, when drinking polluted water.

The developing fetus may be affected by toxic agents in the mother's drinking water. One of the roles of the human placenta is to protect the fetus from toxic insults occurring in the mother. However, many toxic chemicals in drinking water including arsenic, lead, and mercury have been shown to cross the human placenta, and these can potentially interfere with fetal development and health.

Exposure to water contaminants may also occur as a result of inhalation of water vapors, aerosols, and mists from showering, bathing, or other sources that use polluted water. In addition, small amounts of water on the skin may be absorbed. While these sources contribute relatively little to a person's total water intake, they may be an important route of exposure for some toxic chemicals.

WASTEWATER TREATMENT

The availability of safe and sufficient water supplies is inextricably linked to how wastewater is managed. Increased amounts of untreated sewage, combined with agricultural runoff and industrial discharge, have degraded water quality and contaminated water resources around the world. More than 80% of the world's wastewater flows back into the ecosystem without being adequately treated. According to the WHO, 1.8 billion people use a source of water contaminated with feces, putting them at risk of contracting cholera, dysentery, typhoid, and polio.

Monitoring of the results of urban water treatment is required under the SDWA in the United States and under various state and local regulations. In other countries, specific guidelines for monitoring treated water have been adopted. WHO recommends that public water supplies be sampled monthly. The number of recommended samples varies with the size of the water system.

Conventional wastewater treatment systems that employ sedimentation, activated sludge, biofiltration, aeration, and oxidation, combined with chemical disinfection, produce water with coliform counts that are very low. In the absence of a disinfection step, low coliform counts may not be achieved. Without slow-sand filtration of water and wastewater, protozoa, viruses, and other pathogens also may remain in the finished water. The use of slow-sand filtration should control the waterborne spread of the various hepatitis viruses, including hepatitis E, which is currently a major problem in many parts of the world.

The intensity of water treatment for a given supply and distribution area must depend on the nature and quality of the source. The degree of contamination will determine the required treatment. Multiple treatment barriers are recommended by the WHO for contaminated water sources to prevent the spread of pathogens.

The following description of a typical treatment process meets the multiple barrier requirements of WHO's Water Quality Guidelines which include:

- Impoundment and reservoir storage and if needed, predisinfection is applied during impoundment. Impoundment and storage in reservoirs may result in a 99% reduction in fecal indicator bacteria, *Salmonella*, and enteroviruses. During storage and impoundment, the microbiologic environment changes as a result of natural sedimentation, the lethal effect of ultraviolet light on the surface layers of the water, the deprivation of nutrients required by the organisms, and predation.

- Following impoundment and storage, coagulation, flocculation, and further sedimentation or flotation to remove solids are employed.

- Filtration and disinfection complete the cycle of typical urban water treatment. Aeration to improve the aesthetic quality of the final product also may be used.

In rural and remote areas, multiple barrier concepts also may be used. Typical protocols dictate impoundment and protection of the water, sedimentation and screening, gravel prefiltration and slow-sand filtration, and a final disinfection step.

A variety of smaller water filters are sold for home use and include carafe, faucet mounted, countertop, under sink, and whole house models. These use several different technologies to remove potentially toxic agents from water, and the effectiveness of each technology depends on the agents being targeted. Some technologies are more effective at removing some agents than others, and their effectiveness for any given agent can vary dramatically. As such, the most effective filter for any given household will largely depend on those agents of most concern to that specific household's water supply. Another crucial point is that many filters require routine maintenance, and lack of proper use and maintenance can dramatically impact filter effectiveness.

BIOCONTAMINATION OF WATER SUPPLIES

Biocontamination of water supplies used or intended for human drinking water represents the most immediate waterborne threat to human health. Nearly 80% of diseases in developing countries are associated with water, causing some 3 million early deaths. A growing understanding of the epidemiologic characteristics and patterns of disease associated with human pathogens distributed in drinking water has led to the development of infrastructure for potable and wastewater collection, storage, treatment, disinfection, and distribution in the urban areas of most developed countries. As the microbiologic integrity of the supply of potable water has improved, a significant reduction in human disease caused by waterborne pathogens has occurred. Nonetheless, potable water supply throughout the world is always at risk. Serious waterborne disease epidemics with recognized and new pathogens continue to occur in both developed and developing areas of the world.

Worldwide, explosive population growth, expanding poverty, urban migration, and increased international travel affect the risk of exposure to waterborne infectious disease. These diseases include waterborne cryptosporidial diarrheal disease and cholera, *Escherichia coli* 0157:H7 diarrheal disorders, *Mycobacterium avium* complex, *Legionella* species, *Helicobacter pylori*, and *Cyanobacteria* species. *Cyclospora* species, *Cryptosporidia*, and *Giardia* continue to be parasitic threats to potable water supplies. Coccidia and other protozoans are common food- and waterborne pathogens throughout the world. Toxoplasmosis has been identified as a result of waterborne *Toxoplasma gondii*. Hemorrhagic fevers, tuberculosis, and hantavirus infections may have waterborne sources. Municipal drinking water supplies can also be contaminated by viruses both from surface waters and from unidentified sources. These viruses include hepatitis A, enteroviruses, echoviruses, coxsackie viruses, Norwalk virus, rotavirus, caliciviruses, and adenoviruses.

The most common effect of waterborne biocontamination is acute diarrheal disease. This disease is characterized by loose or watery stools and is often accompanied by vomiting and fever. Many of these diarrheal episodes are the result of waterborne infection with bacteria, viruses, or parasites or the ingestion of their enterotoxins. Cholera, shigellosis, salmonellosis, coliforms, yersiniosis, giardiasis, campylobacteriosis, cryptosporidiosis, and viral gastroenteropathies produce diarrheal signs and symptoms. Careful evaluation of the patient and the water supply using newer laboratory tests permits the correct etiologic diagnosis of diarrhea in more than 70% of cases in developing countries. Unfortunately, the resources and equipment for such evaluations often are not available.

In less-developed countries, the proximity of human residence, agriculture, animal husbandry, and unprotected potable water sources typically are the cause of epidemic waterborne disease. Major climatologic changes, such as drought and flooding, also contribute to disruption of the normal supply of water in all countries. Abnormal events such as earthquakes, hurricanes, tornadoes, snowstorms, and similar phenomena cause disruption of normal potable water supplies and may result in epidemic disease in humans. In all such events, increased surveillance of water supplies and rapid response with appropriate public health measures are indicated. Such responses include "boil water" advisories, temporary shift of water supplies to uncontaminated resources, and microbiologic assessment of the supply for viral, bacteriologic, parasitologic, and helminthic contamination. In addition, facilities and supplies for the immediate assessment and treatment of victims of waterborne epidemics, which may include typhoid, cholera, hepatitis, and other diseases, should be prepared and put in place.

Effective methods of microbiologic and chemical treatment and surveillance of water supplies are in place in most public water supplies in developed countries. However, the water disinfection process is not without its risks. Although it is vital to the provision of pathogen-free potable water, water disinfection can produce by-products that may carry long-term risks of chronic illnesses. In less-developed and developing countries and in rural areas of developed countries where raw or untreated water from surface or groundwater sources is used as potable water, effective control of microbiologic water contamination is not always ensured. Despite the technological sophistication of civil engineering of water and wastewater supplies, outbreaks of waterborne disease occur frequently in both developed and developing countries. Epidemics of waterborne disease can be the result of technical flaws or unusual and unforeseen climatologic events that disrupt the normal potable water supplies. For example, in the Indian subcontinent, the substitution of tube-well technology for surface waters as the primary source of drinking water to reduce the risk of waterborne pathogen disease resulted in the use of large groundwater supplies with excessively high and toxic levels of naturally occurring arsenic.

In some areas, the use of wastewater containing human excreta as agricultural irrigation water greatly increases the risk of contamination of local drinking water supplies and the transmission of enteric and other diseases through the consumption of food crops contaminated with pathogens. The use of wastewater for irrigation purposes is recommended in certain areas of the world where water resources are very limited. Wastewater is applied to the fields, where natural biologic processes purify the water before it reached the rivers and reentered the potable water resources. As long as there is sufficient agricultural land in close proximity to large urban centers, this system is useful. However, as the proximity of agriculture and urban life diminishes, the usefulness of the sewage farming techniques also decreases.

CONTROL OF MICROBIOLOGIC WATER CONTAMINATION

Conventional management of potable water and wastewater supplies involves separation of the flow of the two fluid streams and protection of the potable water supply from contamination with the contents of the wastewater stream. Conventional wastewater treatment systems are developed to remove organic matter from wastewater on the basis of their biochemical oxygen demand (BOD) or chemical oxygen demand (COD). The BOD is a measure of the load placed on the oxygen resources of the receiving waters, usually as a result of microbiologic growth. Treatment efficiency is evaluated on the basis of BOD removal by the treatment facility. Unless otherwise stated, BOD signifies the biochemical oxygen demand for 5 days at 20°C (68°F).

The BOD is useful to determine the extent to which oxygen can be used by a supply of microbial life. The test is most important in the management of wastewater and in food manufacturing and drinking-water preparation facilities. High concentrations of dissolved oxygen predict that oxygen uptake by microorganisms is low and that the breakdown of nutrient resources in the water by microorganisms is also low. Low concentrations of dissolved oxygen signify high microorganism demands and imply contamination of the water.

COD is also employed in the assessment of water quality. This test determines the quantity of oxidizable material in the water. It varies with the composition of the water, temperature, concentration of the reagent, period of contact, and other factors. Generally speaking, the COD, BOD, and the total organic carbon (TOC), a quick method of estimating organic contamination of water, are correlated. Treatment facilities are also designed to remove total suspended solids (TSSs) to a level that is both microbiologically and aesthetically acceptable. Recently, tertiary treatments facilities have been designed that improve pathogen removal to produce finished water with very low pathogen counts.

CHEMICAL CONTAMINATION OF WATER SUPPLIES

Chemical contamination of water is a worldwide problem. Many water supplies contain toxic agents or toxic concentrations of agents that are otherwise benign at lower concentrations. Contaminants to drinking water resources include, but are not limited to agricultural chemicals, industrial chemicals, mining wastes, septic tank and landfill leakage, and direct sewage discharge to surface or groundwater. Contamination, whether from a small- or large-scale operation, has a far-reaching impact on drinking water.

In Henderson, Nevada, waste materials containing perchlorate released from a single chemical manufacturing plant made their way into nearby soil and eventually formed a plume of material that slowly spread from its original source to nearby water systems. This single source eventually resulted in 1000 lb of perchlorate per day entering Lake Mead and the Colorado River, which are major sources of drinking water for large parts of the southwest United States.

In 2014, Flint, Michigan's drinking water resource was switched from the Detroit Water to the Flint River to save costs. Shortly thereafter, residents reported that their tap water looked, smelled, and tasted foul. In 2015, a Virginia Tech study revealed elevated lead levels in drinking water, which was attributed to leaching from lead pipes. In September 2015, a pediatrician reported elevated blood-lead levels in children citywide, nearly doubled since 2014—and nearly tripled in certain neighborhoods, which was attributed to the lead contaminated drinking water. The switch from the Detroit water to the Flint River coincided with an outbreak of Legionnaires disease that killed 12 people and sickened at least 87 between June 2014 and October 2015. The switch in the drinking water resource also identified fecal coliform bacteria in the Flint drinking water. Unfortunately, the adding of more chlorine without addressing underlying issues created a new problem: elevated levels of total trihalomethanes (TTHM), cancer-causing chemicals that are by-products of the chlorination of water.

Smaller-scale backyard and garage contamination sources may be equally important. Although usually unrecognized and unreported, these releases will appear quite soon afterwards in the water supply of the local districts. Small-scale inputs of agricultural chemicals from domestic lawn and garden care with herbicides such as 2,4-dichlorophenoxyacetic acid (2,4-D) can pollute large quantities of drinking water. In the early 1970s, 2,4,5-trichlorophenoxyacetic acid (2,4,5-T), a phenoxy herbicide closely related to 2,4-D, which was a component of Agent Orange, the defoliant used in Vietnam by American military forces, was deregistered for domestic lawn care purposes because of its potential to contaminate water in or around homes with materials that were believed teratogenic or embryotoxic to humans. Halogenated solvents, paints and varnishes, carburetor cleaners, and gasoline may become troublesome if released to the groundwater or surface waters in quantities below those that are regulated and reportable. These chemicals can be a significant source of local and regional surface and groundwater pollution.

Extensive contamination of water resources with persistent organic chemicals is a worldwide problem. The North American Great Lakes and many local rivers and streams have been heavily polluted with polychlorinated compounds. These compounds include the polychlorinated and polybrominated biphenyls used extensively in twentieth century industrial processes. Huge expenditures to remove

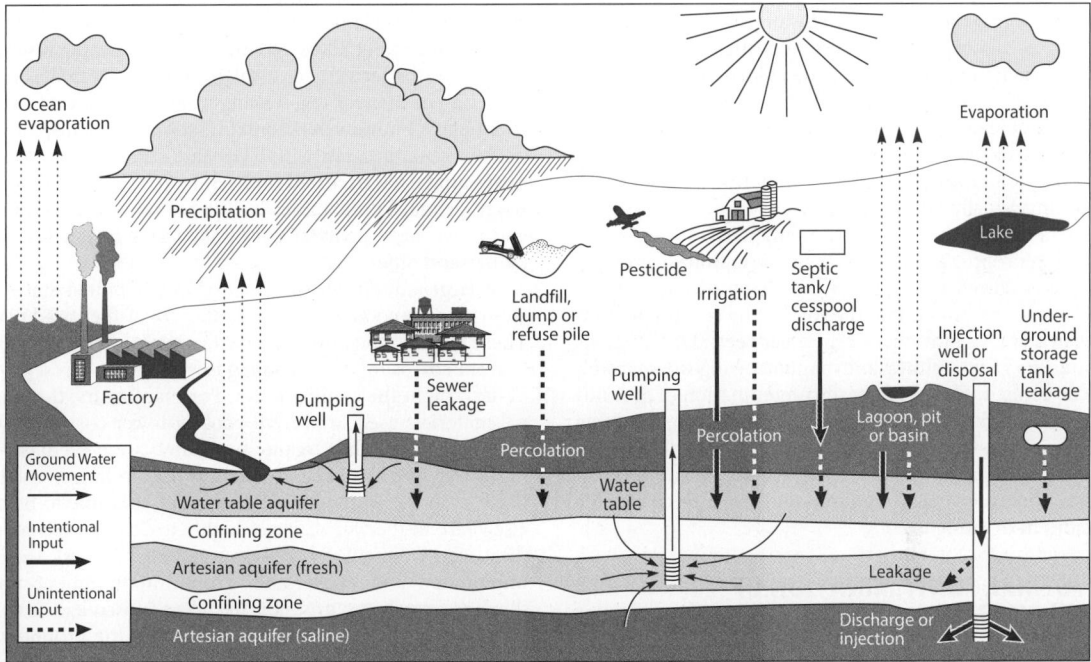

▲ **Figure 51–2.** How waste-disposal practices can contaminate the groundwater system.

and remediate these waters have been made, and more are underway. The ultimate removal of these materials from the environment will take many years. The problem is not confined to North America or Western Europe.

Airborne particulate matter, which is produced by the combustion of fossil fuels, may carry high loads of oxides of sulfur. These sulfur compounds are either adsorbed to the particulate's core or are dissolved in the aerosols that oxidative combustion produces. Acid particulates contribute an acid load to atmospheric water, which may become acid precipitation. Because these acidic materials are quite stable in water, they progressively acidify the surface and groundwater into which they are mixed. Smokes, aerosols, mists, and vapors all may contribute organic materials and inorganic substances of varying toxicologic significance to the air. In the vicinity of some coal-fired power plants and some other solid or beneficiated fuel-fired facilities, alkaline fly ash is deposited, which produces paradoxical alkalization of the soil and adjacent surface water and groundwater. Much of the particulate-bound load is partially water soluble. It will reprecipitate to the earth's surface as atmospheric conditions change and rain falls. Oxynitrogenated organics, partially soluble polynuclear organics, and metallo-organics may participate in the evaporation-precipitation cycle to contaminate surface and subsurface waters.

AGRICULTURE AND PESTICIDES IMPACT ON WATER SUPPLIES

Globally, agriculture accounts for 70% of all water consumption, compared to 20% for industry and 10% for domestic use. In industrialized nations, however, other uses such as cooling of thermoelectric power plants are larger consumers. Agriculture is the industry with the most direct access to surface and groundwater resources. The use of pesticides to control weeds, insects, and other pests has resulted in increased food production and reduced insect-borne disease, but because agriculture is universally chemically intensive and the chemicals generally are applied in solution, suspension, or as wettable concentrates and powders, agricultural chemicals can produce serious water pollution problems. In the past 50 years, the development of chemically intensive agriculture in every country has led to the contamination of water supplies with many evanescent and persistent chemicals.

Organic mercury contamination from seed-coating fungicides, paper-pulp fungicides, and cooling-tower biocides has been a major cause of water pollution in Japan, the Indian Ocean, and Scandinavia. Fungicides containing mercury are now banned in the United States and some other countries.

Perhaps of even greater significance currently is the widespread contamination of drinking and groundwater supplies of wells and rivers throughout Europe, Asia, and North America with herbicide chemicals. At least one pesticide is found in the majority of all groundwater sources, including one-third of all deep wells. Common pesticides detected in streams in agricultural areas include chlorpyrifos, azinphos methyl, atrazine, p,p′-DDE, and alachlor. In urban streams, common pesticides were simazine, prometon, metolachlor, diazinon, carbaryl, and fipronil.

Atrazine, a triazine herbicide used for weed control, appears in virtually every well in every area of the United States where it has been used. In many parts of the world, dibromochloropropane (DBCP) contamination of groundwater has occurred as a result of the direct injection of this carcinogenic compound into the soil for the control of nematodes in bananas, pineapples, and sugar beets. DBCP causes male sterility in agricultural and manufacturing workers who make or apply it. The widespread contamination of groundwater with this reproductive toxin has been reported in Costa Rica, Honduras, the Philippines, Ivory Coast, and California. In the home, point-of-use devices like charcoal and reverse-osmosis filters can also be used to remove or minimize some pesticides in drinking water.

INDUSTRIAL CONTAMINATION OF WATER SUPPLIES

Specific industries have been associated with local water contamination. For example, some mining operations have been associated with acid mine drainage. In addition, high concentrations of lead, zinc, nickel, vanadium, manganese, mercury, and iron have been demonstrated in surface and groundwater adjacent to and downstream from mines, mineral extraction facilities, or mine tailing piles. In the pulp and paper industry, discharge of 2,3,7,8-tetrachlorodibenzo-p-dioxin (2,3,7,8-TCDD) and its congeners from chlorine-based pulp bleaching plants has contaminated nearby streams and rivers in the United States. These highly persistent organics are transferred to silt, sediment, and biota. From the silt, toxics are transferred to fish in the stream ecosystem. These pollutants may then be concentrated many-fold within the fish before humans or animals consume the chemicals. When sportsmen or subsistence fishermen consume contaminated fish, they may further concentrate these toxins.

Leakage of gasoline products from underground storage facilities continuously inputs significant quantities of toxic and carcinogenic hydrocarbons such as benzene, toluene, xylene, and MTBE (methyl tert-butyl ether) into groundwater supplies that may be used for drinking. These volatile hydrocarbons are also released into the air of the homes of persons who live above contaminated ground-water plumes. Contaminant plumes could potentially be the cause of human illnesses such as immunologic impairment, neurologic and cognitive deficits, birth defects, and cancers characteristic of exposure to these substances at high levels.

High-technology industries such as semiconductor manufacturing plants use large quantities of halogenated organics such as trichloroethylene (TCE), trichloroethane, perchloroethylene, and carbon tetrachloride. Other chemicals used include complex organics and metals and metalloids such as arsenic, selenium, beryllium, cadmium, and lead. These materials may enter the wastewater discharge systems of the facilities or local groundwater supplies either by design or in error (eg, leaking from underground storage facilities). Groundwater contamination problems, in particular contamination with TCE and other volatile organic compounds, has occurred in the Silicon Valley of California. Based primarily on studies in highly exposed workers, several recent meta-analyses have linked TCE to cancers of the kidney and other organs.

A large amount of water is used in the United States and elsewhere for cooling coal- and other fossil-fuel-fired plants. These facilities treat this water with certain chemicals to help prevent corrosion of the cooling towers and to arrest growth of bacteria in the cooling water. For many years, the principal materials used to prevent cooling tower corrosion were Cr(VI) compounds. Organic mercurials were used as cooling-tower biocides. These materials are no longer used for these purposes in the United States but continue to be used elsewhere in the world. These highly toxic materials may be disposed of directly to the water systems. At best, they are impounded and evaporated. From impoundment ponds they may reach the groundwater after subsequent leaching caused by rain and runoff. In California, the groundwater supply of at least one community has been severely contaminated by the practice of disposing of cooling-tower wastes containing Cr(VI) from a natural gas compression plant into nearby unlined wastewater ponds.

Mercury is a naturally occurring element but industrial processes such as coal-fired power generation, waste incineration, and smelting can also release mercury into the air, and this mercury can eventually settle into lakes, rivers, and the ocean. Once in the water, bacteria in the sand or mud can convert it into methylmercury. Fish absorb this methylmercury when they eat smaller organisms. Because it is excreted only very slowly, methylmercury can build up over time, and bioaccumulate as larger and older fish eat smaller fish and other organisms. A consequence is that methylmercury levels are usually highest in those fish at the top of the food chain. Removal of mercury from contaminated waterways can take many years.

Methylmercury is toxic to the developing neurologic system and studies in heavy seafood-eating populations in the Seychelles Islands, the Faeroe Islands, and elsewhere have identified associations between mercury consumption in mothers and adverse cognitive development in the offspring including decreases in learning ability, language skills, attention, and memory. Based on these studies, many state and local agencies provide information about mercury levels in local fish and produce advisories regarding the maximum number of meals of fish that should be consumed per week, especially in pregnant women, and these local advisories can frequently be found online from the U.S. EPA or various state agencies.

Bisphenol A (BPA) is a man-made carbon-based synthetic compound used to make polycarbonate plastics used in food packaging and water bottles. In the United States, BPA is detected in the urine of 93% of all subjects tested. BPA has raised concerns because it appears to mimic the effects of estrogen. Some animal studies have identified links between BPA exposure and a variety of effects related to neural and behavior alterations, potentially precancerous lesions in the prostate and mammary glands, altered prostate gland and urinary tract development, and early onset of puberty in females. BPA continues to be used, but because of these concerns, some countries have banned the use of BPA for specific products such as baby formula bottles.

OTHER ENVIRONMENTAL AGENTS FOUND IN WATER SUPPLIES

Arsenic

The current regulatory standard for arsenic in water in many countries and the WHO recommendation is 10 mcg/L. Many countries do not follow or enforce this standard because of a lack of alternative water sources and the high cost of removing arsenic from water. Most ingested arsenic is excreted in the urine within 2 weeks of ingestion, and urinary concentrations of arsenic are the best metric for assessing exposure. Valid urine analysis should include inorganic arsenic and its major methylated metabolites, and exclude organic forms of arsenic which come predominantly from seafood and are mostly nontoxic. Most people receive some arsenic from foods such as rice, fruits, and vegetables, and urinary levels of inorganic arsenic and its metabolites in people without water contamination are usually less than 10 mcg/L. Treatment of arsenic exposure from water primarily involves removal from exposure. Chelation therapy has not been shown to reduce health outcomes in those with lower, more chronic and common drinking water exposures.

Chromium

Chromium (Cr) in the environment is present in several valence states but the ones considered the most biologically significant are Cr(III) and Cr(VI). Cr(III) is an essential nutrient found in dietary sources such as breads, cereals, and vegetables, while Cr(VI) is a carcinogen. Chromium can be released from industries that burn natural gas, oil, or coal or landfills and settle in soil and water supplies. Contamination of water by naturally occurring chromium leaching from topsoil and rocks can also occur. Most absorbed Cr(VI) is converted to Cr(III) and excreted in the urine within one day of ingestion. Chromium can be measured in the blood or urine but both represent only more recent exposure. Without obvious exposure sources, blood levels are generally less than 3.0 mcg/100 mL and urine levels are generally less than 10 mcg/L. For chronic low-dose exposures that typically occur with drinking water ingestion, no antidote is available and treatment primarily involves removal from exposure.

Nitrate & Nitrite

Nitrate and nitrite are nitrogen-oxygen chemical units whose chemical structures are NO_3^- and NO_2^-, respectively. Nitrate is formed naturally when nitrogen combines with oxygen or ozone. Nitrate is the more stable compound and is an important plant nutrient. In most people, food is the primary source of nitrate.

Nitrates in drinking water can result from either natural or manmade sources. Nitrogen from sources including fertilizer, animal and human waste, nitrogen oxides from utilities and automobiles, and some crops can be transformed to nitrate by various processes. The greatest industrial use of nitrates is as a fertilizer. Contamination of drinking water with nitrate can occur from runoff of agricultural fertilizer, leakage of wastes from septic tanks, improper sewage disposal, erosion of natural deposits, runoff from animal feedlots, industrial waste, food processing waste, or other routes. Private domestic groundwater wells, especially shallower ones, in rural agricultural areas seem to be especially vulnerable. In one European Union report, nitrate levels greater than the WHO recommended levels of 50 mg/L were reported in about 30% of all groundwater bodies for which measurements were available. In addition to being ingested in food and water, nitrate is also formed endogenously in the human body as part of normal metabolism.

Once ingested, nitrate is reduced to nitrite, which can bind to hemoglobin in red blood cells to form methemoglobin. Methemoglobin binds to oxygen more tightly than hemoglobin and is therefore less effective at releasing oxygen to tissues. In infants, elevated methemoglobin levels (usually exceeding 10%) can cause cyanosis and difficulty breathing, the so called "blue baby syndrome." Other symptoms can include tachypnea, vomiting, and diarrhea. Examination of the patient's blood reveals a chocolate brown color. Common risk factors for blue baby syndrome include age less than 3 months, a bottle-fed infant, glucose-6-phosphate dehydrogenase (G6PD) deficiency, gastrointestinal infections (which may increase conversion of nitrate to nitrite), private well use, and nitrate water levels greater than 50 mg/L.

Most regulatory standards for nitrate in drinking water are aimed at preventing blue baby syndrome, although increasing attention is being given to other possible adverse health effects, including cancer and thyroid deficiency. Nitrosating agents that arise from nitrite under acidic conditions, such as those found in the stomach, can react with secondary amines and amides and other nitrosatable compounds and form potentially carcinogenic N-nitroso compounds. The cancers most frequently studied include gastric, esophageal, brain, and urinary tract cancer, but to date, a clear causal association between nitrate in drinking water and cancer has not been established in humans.

About 60–70% of ingested nitrate is excreted in the urine within 24 hours and nitrate levels can be measured in either blood or urine. When evaluating nitrate levels in blood or urine it is important to consider that nitrate can come from multiple sources including food, water, and endogenous production. Treatment for blood baby syndrome due to nitrates can include methylene blue and supportive care. Methods of prevention include appropriate management of agricultural and farm animal practices to prevent runoff into nearby water supplies; careful placement, management, and maintenance of sewage facilities; and testing of groundwater supplies, especially in rural agricultural areas.

Perchlorate

The chemical structure of perchlorate is ClO_4^-. It has been used industrially as an oxidizer in solid rocket propellant, slurry explosives, road flares, and air bag inflation systems. Human environmental exposure can occur through food or water following industrial contamination from industries that use or manufacture perchlorate (eg, Colorado River water) or from perchlorate that is naturally occurring (eg, northern Chile). In two recent nationally representative surveys in the United States, detectable concentrations of perchlorate were reported in the urine of every person tested suggesting that essentially everyone has at least some exposure to perchlorate.

Concentrations of perchlorate in drinking water are typically orders of magnitude lower than those previously used to treat hyperthyroidism and decrease thyroid hormone production. However, several studies have reported links between perchlorate in drinking water and decreased thyroid hormone levels, especially in potentially susceptible groups such young children, those with low iodine intake. Urinary levels of perchlorate are the best metric for assessing recent exposure. In populations without an obvious exposure source, urinary perchlorate concentrations are usually 5–10 mcg/L.

Minerals in Drinking Water

Most drinking water contains mineral concentrations that are low enough that they do not adversely affect the health of most people and may actually provide some beneficial effect. For example, **calcium** and **magnesium** are important in bone health and other physiologic processes, **potassium** is important in regulating fluid balance and controlling the electrical activity of the heart and other muscles, **selenium** is important in general antioxidant function and in immune system health, and **sodium** is important for fluid balance. In some instances, minerals are intentionally added to water supplies in order to take advantage of their beneficial effects. Desalination of seawater is becoming an increasing source of drinking water in several areas lacking abundant freshwater supplies, such as very dry areas in Israel and northern Chile. This process can result in substantial demineralization of the water and a subsequent loss of any beneficial effects of the minerals normally present in other water sources. Mixing desalinated water with source water or the addition of minerals is sometimes done to achieve a balanced mineral content in desalinized water.

Fluoride often occurs naturally in drinking water sources and in some foods and beverages including those made with water from fluoridated municipalities. Elevated levels of fluoride are found in some teas, seafood, raisins, wine, grape juice, and other foods. Fluoride is also used in a number of dental products such as toothpaste and is frequently added to drinking water to help prevent dental caries. A number of studies have found neurologic effects in children possibly resulting from fluoride consumption. These studies may eventually lead to an end to the practice of fluoridating drinking water supplies. European countries do not add fluoride to drinking water and yet they have identical low rates of tooth caries to the United States.

Copper in drinking water can result from leaching from copper pipes. Copper is a required nutrient and deficiencies can lead to hematologic abnormalities (anemia, neutropenia, and leukopenia), osteoporosis, and myeloneuropathy. However, at higher exposures, copper in water has most commonly been linked with symptoms of gastrointestinal distress including nausea, vomiting, and abdominal pain, especially in young children.

Cadmium-induced nephropathies, and itai-itai ("ouch-ouch"), a cadmium-induced systemic disease, occurred in Japan as a result of the contamination of estuarine waters that provided most of the dietary fish to a large population. In Croatia, Serbia, and Bosnia, and some rural villages in Romania, Balkan endemic nephropathy is a chronic kidney disease associated with carcinomas of the upper urinary tract. In the past, it was thought to be the result of certain water contaminants. However, studies indicate that it is a chronic dietary poisoning by aristolochic acid, a chemical commonly found in Chinese herbal teas.

DISINFECTION BY-PRODUCTS

Gaseous or liquid forms of chlorine are commonly added to drinking water as a disinfection agent. In water, these agents react to form hypochlorous acid or hypobromous acid (in the presence of bromine) and these are very effective at killing harmful bacteria, protozoa, and viruses. The use of chlorine in this way has revolutionized water purification and reduced the incidence of waterborne infections and disease across the world, and chlorination and/or filtration of drinking water has been called one of the major public health achievements of the twentieth century. Other disinfection agents added to drinking water include chloramines, chlorine dioxide, and ozone. In the presence of organic material such as decaying plants or algae, a variety of potentially toxic agents can be formed when adding chlorine to water. The most common of these are trihalomethanes (THM) and haloacetic acids (HAAs), although many other compounds in smaller amounts can also be formed. Collectively these are known as disinfection by-products (DBPs) and hundreds of different ones may occur in chlorinated tap water, although most at very low levels. Common forms of HAAs in drinking water, and those five compounds regulated by the U.S. EPA, include monochloroacetic acid (MCA) ($CH_2ClCOOH$), dichloroacetic acid (DCA) ($CHCl_2COOH$), trichloroacetic acid (TCA) (CCl_3COOH), monobromoacetic acid (MBA) ($CH_2BrCOOH$), and dibromoacetic acid (DBA) ($CHBr_2COOH$). In the United States, an estimated 200 million or more people are served by water systems that apply a water disinfectant such as chlorine. In addition to ingestion, significant exposure to DBPs from water may also occur from showering or bathing as a result from inhalation or dermal absorption.

DBPs have been linked to a variety of health effects including anemia; liver, kidney, and central nervous system toxicity; reproductive and developmental effects; and cancer, although findings for some of these outcomes are not consistent across all studies and many may only be observable at exposure levels much higher than those commonly found in most drinking water sources. Based primarily on evidence from animal studies showing increases in kidney, liver, or other tumors, the International Agency for Research on Cancer has classified chloroform, bromodichloromethane, DBA, and DCA as possibly carcinogenic to humans (Group 2B). U.S. EPA does not regulate individual THMs or HAAs but rather regulates these agents as total THMs and total HAAs.

PHARMACEUTICALS FOUND IN WATER SUPPLIES

Another source of water pollution exists with pharmaceutical products for humans or animals, as well as their related metabolites. Human sources include intentional flushing of medications down the toilet, rinsing topically applied medications off in the tub or sink, or excretion of medications in urine or feces. Most wastewater treatment plants are not designed to remove these chemicals, and therefore they can pass through these treatment plants and eventually end up in downstream water sources. An example of this is Lindane. This is a topical treatment used to treat head lice and scabies and may cause skin irritation, dizziness, headaches, diarrhea, and other gastrointestinal symptoms at high exposures. Elevated levels of Lindane had been reported in the effluent of several large wastewater treatments plants in the Los Angeles area. Fortunately, these levels were shown to decline after state laws were passed banning the pharmaceutical use of this agent. Little is known about the health effects of long-term exposure to low concentrations of pharmaceuticals to humans or aquatic organisms. The precautionary principle—or possibly new scientific evidence—may give rise to more stringent demands on wastewater treatment in the future. A combination of biologic treatment with high sludge residence times and ozonation of the effluent seems to be the most promising technology to control pharmaceutical product contamination.

HEALTH EFFECTS FROM ENVIRONMENTAL CONTAMINANTS

EPA's Integrated Risk Information System (IRIS) is a human health assessment program that evaluates information on health effects that may result from exposure to environmental contaminants.

A summary of the EPA's NPDWRs for biological contaminants and their health effects is found in Table 51–2.

PLASTICS

Plastics in the aquatic environment are of increasing concern because of their persistence effect on the environment, wildlife, and human health. Plastic particles are generally the most abundant type of debris encountered in the marine environment, with estimates suggesting that 60–80% of marine debris is plastic. Although the media may focus on what is referred to as a "Pacific garbage patch," many other water bodies including lakes, coral reefs, rivers, estuaries, and beaches are polluted by plastics.

Since its inception in 2013, the EPA's Trash Free Waters (TFW) program has pursued a multipronged approach to reducing and preventing trash in US waters, including plastics. One may access the website link to their reports at: https://www.epa.gov/trash-free-waters/epa-reports

The EPA reports that approximately 90% of the plastics in the pelagic marine environment are microplastics (< 5 mm in diameter). Microplastics arise from the fragmentation of larger pieces as they weather from the effects of ultraviolet rays, and wind and wave action. Recent information on the use of tiny plastic abrasives (commonly called microbeads or nanobeads), especially in personal care products and home cleaning products, and synthetic fabrics shedding during laundering has shown the prevalence of micro- and nanoparticle size plastics as being pervasive in some water bodies. The plastics may not be removed as part of the wastewater treatment facility process and may pass through largely unchanged. Global trends suggest that accumulations are increasing in aquatic habitats, consistent with trends in plastic production.

RADIONUCLIDES

Radioactive mineral extraction used during cold war military activities and for the purposes of fueling nuclear power plants has led to surface and groundwater contamination with radionuclides. These radioactive materials include radium, uranium, and their decay products. In a number of areas, water has been significantly contaminated with tritium and alpha emitters as a result of these activities.

Erosion of natural deposits also leads to contamination of groundwater and drinking water sources. Drinking water contaminated by naturally radioactive derivatives of the uranium and thorium decay series accounts only for a very small portion of the total annual dose of radiation for most humans. In some situations, the risk of leukemia and other cancers may be elevated for those who live above or drink from groundwater sources that contain higher than normal radionuclide decay products including radon. Currently, the U.S. EPA current standards for drinking water are: Combined radium 226/228 of 5 pCi/L; a gross alpha standard for all alphas of 15 pCi/L (not including radon and uranium); a

Table 51–2. Biocontaminants summary.[a]

Contaminant	MCLG (mg/L)	MCL or TT[b](mg/L)	Potential Health Effects From Long-Term Exposure Above the MCL (Unless Specified as Short-term)	Sources of Contaminant in Drinking Water
Cryptosporidium	zero	TT[b]	Gastrointestinal illness (such as diarrhea, vomiting, and cramps)	Human and animal fecal waste
Giardia lamblia	zero	TT[b]	Gastrointestinal illness (such as diarrhea, vomiting, and cramps)	Human and animal fecal waste
Heterotrophic plate count (HPC)	n/a	TT[b]	HPC has no health effects; it is an analytic method used to measure the variety of bacteria that are common in water. The lower the concentration of bacteria in drinking water, the better maintained the water system is.	HPC measures a range of bacteria that are naturally present in the environment
Legionella	zero	TT[b]	Legionnaires Disease, a type of pneumonia	Found naturally in water; multiplies in heating systems
Total Coliforms (including fecal coliform and *E Coli*)	zero	5.0%	Not a health threat in itself; it is used to indicate whether other potentially harmful bacteria may be present[c]	Coliforms are naturally present in the environment; as well as feces; fecal coliforms and *E coli* only come from human and animal fecal waste[c]
Turbidity	n/a	TT[b]	Turbidity is a measure of the cloudiness of water. It is used to indicate water quality and filtration effectiveness (such as whether disease-causing organisms are present). Higher turbidity levels are often associated with higher levels of disease-causing microorganisms such as viruses, parasites, and some bacteria. These organisms can cause symptoms such as nausea, cramps, diarrhea, and associated headaches.	Soil runoff
Viruses (enteric)	zero	TT	Gastrointestinal illness (such as diarrhea, vomiting, and cramps)	Human and animal fecal waste

[a]From EPA National Primary Drinking Water Regulations (NPDWR).
[b]Treatment Technique (TT): A required process intended to reduce the level of a contaminant in drinking water.
[c]Fecal coliform and *E coli* are bacteria whose presence indicates that the water may be contaminated with human or animal wastes. Disease-causing microbes (pathogens) in these wastes can cause diarrhea, cramps, nausea, headaches, or other symptoms. These pathogens may pose a special health risk for infants, young children, and people with severely compromised immune systems.

combined standard of 4 mrem/year for beta emitters and the MCL for uranium is 30 mcg/L.

HYDRAULIC FRACTURING FOR OIL AND GAS

Large deposits of shale containing oil and natural gas are buried deep underground in several parts of the United States and in other countries. Historically, these deposits were difficult and very costly to access. However, around 2000, the combination of directional drilling technologies and hydraulic fracturing (or "fracking") expanded oil and gas production to oil- and gas-bearing rock (eg, shale, sandstone, carbonate, and coal) formations previously considered uneconomical. This use of "fracking" significantly increased US production of domestic oil 50% and domestic gas almost 70% in 2015.

Fracking activity may take place in the same watershed or different watersheds and close to or far from drinking water resources. Specific activities in the "Wastewater Disposal and Reuse" include (a) disposal of wastewater through underground injection, (b) wastewater treatment followed by reuse in other hydraulic fracturing operations or discharge to surface waters, and (c) disposal through evaporation or percolation pits.

This process has led to several environmental concerns, including the tremendously high water usage, the production of large amounts of wastewater containing a variety of potentially toxic materials, and the possible contamination of local groundwater used for drinking by the residents living near the wells. A large number of chemicals are added to fracking fluid in order to help initiate cracks in the rock, keep fractures open, prevent pipe corrosion, decrease pumping friction, and as gelling agents, bactericides, biocides, clay stabilizers, scale inhibitors, and surfactants. Chemicals found in fracking fluid or wastewater include hydrochloric acid, ethylene glycol, xylene, methanol, metals, as well as several known carcinogens like formaldehyde and benzene. Over 600 different chemicals have been identified as being used in fracking fluid. For the most part, however, the chemicals used in any particular well are considered by some companies to be proprietary information and are not disclosed. There have been concerns about contamination of the local groundwater from the salts, chemicals, and naturally occurring radioactive material present in flowback, which is usually temporarily pumped into wastewater ponds and then moved off-site, where it is reinjected back into the ground or transferred to wastewater treatment facilities for treatment and disposal. The majority of flowback that is not disposed of in injection wells is treated at centralized waste treatment (CWT) facilities that are designed to treat industrial wastewater, and which may then discharge into sewers or surface water bodies.

Currently there are no federal regulations requiring natural gas companies to disclose information about the chemicals used in hydraulic fracturing fluids. Hydraulic fracturing and reporting of the chemicals used in fracturing fluids exempt from the U.S. Emergency Planning and Community Right-to-Know Act (EPCRA). Section 313 of EPCRA created the Toxic Release Inventory (TRI), which requires companies that manufacture and/or use toxic chemicals to report information on chemicals, including identities and quantities that are stored, released, transferred, or "otherwise used." In 2005, Congress passed the Energy Policy Act exempting fracking from regulation under the 1974 SDWA. Some states are attempting to regulate the fracking industry but to date the effectiveness of these efforts are unclear.

REFERENCES

Benedict KM et al: Surveillance for Waterborne Disease Outbreaks Associated with Drinking Water—United States, 2013-2014. MMWR Morb Mortal Wkly Rep 2017;66(44):1216-1221 [PMID: 29121003].

Levallois P, Barn P, Valcke M, Gauvin D, Kosatsky T: Public health consequences of lead in drinking water. Curr Environ Health Rep 2018;5(2):255-262 [PMID: 29556976].

Microplastics Expert Workshop Report. Trash Free Waters Dialogue Meeting Convened June 28-29, 2017 EPA Office of Wetlands, Oceans and Watersheds. Primary Author: Margaret Murphy, AAAS S&TP Fellow Report Date: December 4, 2017. https://www.epa.gov/sites/production/files/2018-03/documents/microplastics_expert_workshop_report_final_12-4-17.pdf.

National Institute of Environmental Health Sciences Water Pollution, 2019. https://www.niehs.nih.gov.

National Toxicology Program. Fluoride: Potential Developmental Neurotoxicity, 2016. https://ntp.niehs.nih.gov/pubhealth/hat/selected/fluoride/neuro-index.html.

United States Environmental Protection Agency Hydraulic Fracturing for Oil and Gas: Impacts from the Hydraulic Fracturing Water Cycle on Drinking Water Resources in the United States EPA-600-R-16-236ES Dec2016 www.epa.gov/hfstudy.

United States Environmental Protection Agency Six-Year Review 3 – Health Effects Assessment for Existing Chemical and Radionuclide National Primary Drinking Water Regulations-Summary Report EPA-822-R-16-008, 2016. www.epa.gov/waterscience. www.epa.gov/sites/production/files/2016-12/documents/822416008.pdf.

United Nations World Water Development Report 2019: Leaving No One Behind. Paris, UNESCO. https://en.unesco.org/water-security/wwap/wwdr/2019#resources.

World Health Organization. Guidelines for Drinking-Water Quality. 4th ed. Water Sanitation Health, 2011. http://www.who.int/water_sanitation_health/publications/2011/dwq_guidelines/en/index.html.

■ SELF-ASSESSMENT QUESTIONS

Select the one correct answer for each question.

Question 1: Biochemical oxygen demand (BOD)
   a. is the measure of algal growth in water
   b. signifies the BOD for 5 days at 20°C (68°F)
   c. predicts the oxygen uptake by microorganisms
   d. implies irreversible contamination of the water

Question 2: Chemical oxygen demand (COD)
   a. is superior to BOD in the assessment of water quality
   b. determines the quantity of oxidizable material in the water

   c. varies with the composition of the water, not its temperature
   d. differs from the total organic carbon (TOC)

Question 3: Hydraulic fracturing (fracking) fluids
   a. amount to between 2 and 7 million gallons of water per well
   b. are mixed with sand but are isolated from chemicals
   c. are decreasing in quantity with improved regulations
   d. have no demonstrated environmental and health impacts

Question 4: The Safe Drinking Water Act
  a. is focused on limiting discharges of pollutants into surface water
  b. establishes regulations that apply to private domestic wells
  c. allows the U.S. EPA to establish regulations for chemicals in drinking water
  d. makes it optional for water companies to publish Consumer Confidence Reports

Question 5: Maximum contaminant level goal (MCLG)
  a. is set at a concentration that is expected to cause adverse health effects over a lifetime of consumption of water
  b. has a substantial safety margin
  c. is an enforceable standard
  d. has a financial penalty assessed for violation of the MCLG concentration

Question 6: Disinfection by-products include
  a. arsenic, fluoride, calcium, and magnesium
  b. trihalomethanes and haloacetic acids
  c. microorganisms such as bacteria, protozoa, and viruses
  d. only agents that clearly do not cause cancer

Industrial Emissions, Accidental Releases, & Hazardous Waste

Christina Armatas, MD, MPH

Over 150 million organic and inorganic chemicals are uniquely identified by the Chemical Abstracts Service. Although only a small fraction of these are active in commerce, newly developed chemicals are continuously entering the market. In the United States, just more than 40,000 chemicals are in commercial production and use, and the U.S. Environmental Protection Agency (EPA) has approximately 300 chemicals awaiting review for market release at any given time. The full lifecycle of chemicals from production to eventual disposal contains vulnerabilities for accidental releases that can cause significant human exposure and adverse acute and chronic health effects. Additionally, industrial processes release chemical byproducts of energy production and waste that have the potential to harm large populations around these sites over long periods of time.

No industrial disaster has matched the catastrophic release of methyl isocyanate in Bhopal, India in 1984 that killed an estimated 7000 people within days of the exposure and sickened hundreds of thousands more. Still, large scale chemical disasters continue to cause fatalities and lingering health effects. In 2019, a pesticide plant explosion in eastern China killed at least 78 people and injured hundreds. The disastrous health effects of this type of acute incident are dramatically visible. However, the health impacts of emissions with longer releases to the environment are difficult to quantify and may take years after discovery to understand, such as the long-term morbidity and mortality from the 2011 Fukushima Daiichi nuclear plant release following a tsunami in Japan.

▼ ROUTINE INDUSTRIAL EMISSIONS

Industrial facilities produce chemical goods and use chemicals as part of processes to make a vast array of end products. Chemical releases into the soil, indoor and outdoor air, and water can occur during many processes at a facility, including loading and unloading, manufacturing, storage, and transport preparation. Public health officials must understand the types and location of routine industrial emissions occurring in their jurisdictions. Characterizing routine emissions helps officials prepare for large quantity accidental releases and facilitates their understanding of the individual and community level factors that make certain residents particularly vulnerable to industrial pollution.

Industrial emissions include an array of chemicals, radionuclides, and biologicals. The chemicals released from industrial sources are numerous, and relatively few are well characterized toxicologically. The emitters of airborne chemicals are varied and range from large facilities, such as oil refineries, to small sources, such as gas stations, auto body shops, and dry-cleaning operations. Emissions are somewhat characteristic for specific industrial processes and source types. While epidemiologic studies have been useful for characterizing toxicity and the public health impacts of several air pollutants and a number of chemicals in the occupational setting, the most information on potential health effects of industrial chemicals comes from animal toxicology studies. Animal studies generally involve exposures of a genetically homogeneous population of rodents to one chemical at a time. Thus little direct knowledge exists about the interactions of chemicals or the consequences of exposure to many chemicals simultaneously in heterogeneous human populations.

AIR EMISSIONS & RELEASE SOURCES

The World Health Organization (WHO) has published air quality guidelines for release limits of particulates, ozone, nitrogen dioxide, and sulfur dioxide, which are four of the major air pollutants that impact human health. These contaminants contribute to cardiovascular and respiratory conditions, including ischemic heart disease, stroke, chronic obstructive pulmonary disease, respiratory infections, and lung cancer. Although it is not possible to differentiate the health impacts of traffic pollution from industrial pollution, the WHO estimates that combined outdoor air pollution accounted for 4.2 million premature deaths in 2016.

Table 52–1. World Health Organization 2005 guidelines for air quality.

Pollutant	Averaging Time	Guideline Value (mcg/m³)
PM$_{2.5}$	Annual mean	10
	24 h	25
PM$_{10}$	Annual mean	20
	24 h	50
Ozone	8 h	100
NO$_2$	Annual	40
	1 h	200
SO$_2$	24 h	20
	10 min	500

Source: WHO air quality guidelines for particulate matter, zone, nitrogen dioxide, and sulfur dioxide. Global update 2005.

Countries are not obligated to follow the WHO guidelines and may adopt individual standards. Table 52–1 summarizes the WHO guidelines for air pollutants.

In the United States, air pollutants are characterized for regulatory purposes into two basic categories: criteria air pollutants (CAPs) and hazardous air pollutants (HAPs). Both categories of emissions are toxic, and there may be other toxic chemicals emitted from industrial facilities that are not on the list of CAPs or HAPs.

Criteria Air Pollutants

CAPs are six typical components of smog that are regulated in the United States through the Clean Air Act of 1970, which charges the EPA to set limits for the emissions of these pollutants. The CAPs are ground-level ozone, carbon monoxide, sulfur dioxide, particulate matter (< 10 and 2.5 μm in diameter, or PM$_{10}$ and PM$_{2.5}$), lead, and nitrogen dioxide. These pollutants are the focus of regulations in both the United States and abroad due to their high prevalence and decades of research showing both acute and chronic adverse health outcomes, such as premature death and hospital visits for chronic disease exacerbation.

Hazardous Air Pollutants

Over time, Congress has amended the Clean Air Act to expand the reach of the EPA in emissions regulation. HAPs are 187 chemicals emitted into the air that are not CAPs and for which the EPA has regulatory authority. The included chemicals are hazardous pesticides, herbicides, radionuclides, and volatile organic compounds. Research studies attribute both cancer and other health effects to HAPs, including neurologic, reproductive, immune, and developmental harm. Humans may additionally be exposed to HAPs through ingestion of contaminated plants and animals.

Sources of Air Pollution

For regulatory purposes, the origins of airborne chemicals are divided into stationary and mobile sources. Stationary sources are fixed physical structures, and mobile sources are primarily cars, trucks, and buses.

A. Stationary Sources

Major stationary emissions sources include large industrial complexes, such as refineries, aerospace facilities, and chemical manufacturing plants. Onsite fuel combustion for energy requirements contributes to significant CAP emissions from major stationary emitters. Minor stationary sources have lower emission rates than major sources, yet their emissions can still be hazardous to health. For example, small dry-cleaning shops may emit tetrachloroethylene (perchloroethylene, PCE or PERC), a volatile organic compound (VOC) that is a probable human carcinogen. Incinerators, which can be found at both large and small facilities, emit an array of products of incomplete combustion ranging from carbon monoxide to complex chlorinated compounds such as 2,3,7,8-tetrachlorodibenzo-p-dioxin (TCDD, "dioxin"), which is associated with human sarcoma, lymphoma, stomach cancer, and a severe skin irritation called chloracne. Ground-level ozone formation is the result of industrially produced nitrogen oxides reacting with sunlight and hydrocarbons, whereas the other CAPs are released directly.

B. Mobile Sources

Engines in ships, trains, and trucks are major mobile emitters of the solid material in diesel exhaust known as diesel particulate matter (DPM). The tiny particles of DPM are considered a subset of PM$_{2.5}$, making DPM responsible for the same adverse health effects as other particulate matter, such as cardiopulmonary hospitalizations and premature deaths.

EMISSIONS TRACKING & TRENDS

Governments around the world use Pollutant Release and Transfer Registers (PRTRs) to collect data on emissions from fixed industrial sources. For countries with PRTR programs, facilities emitting chemicals report the location, type, and quantity of chemicals released. There is variability in the specifics of what triggers reporting by an emissions producer in each country. In the United States, the EPA collects this data in the Toxics Release Inventory (TRI) program. Both the Canadian and Mexican governments have established a PRTR, and all North American countries collaborate on reports of their combined release data through the Commission for Environmental Cooperation. The most recent European Union (EU) registry (E-PRTR) includes reporting from the EU member states, Lichtenstein, Iceland, Norway, Serbia, and Switzerland.

Trends

From 2007–2017, US air emissions decreased 57%, which is largely attributed to utility sources that have shifted away

Table 52–2. Top 5 TRI chemicals by volume of reported air emissions, 2017.

Chemical	Reported Total Air Emissions (million lb/y)
Ammonia	119
Methanol	100
Sulfuric acid	64
n-Hexane	36
Hydrochloric acid	34

from coal-fired power production. Many chemicals that top the list of highest volume releases in Table 52–2 have decreased the most since 2007, including hydrochloric acid, sulfuric acid, methanol, and ammonia. The Occupational Safety and Health Administration (OSHA) maintains a list of chemicals classified as carcinogens, which are reportable to the TRI program when present in air emissions. There was a 37% decrease in air releases of reportable carcinogens between 2007–2017, mostly due to the plastics and rubber industries reducing styrene release.

The TRI program created an online repository of pollution reduction practices implemented by facilities in various industries to replace, reduce, or eliminate pollutants. The success stories from this program are searchable online by its name *TRI P2 (pollution prevention) Spotlight Series.* Although chemical releases are declining, the United States remains the second-largest emitter of greenhouse gases after China. The key greenhouse gases are carbon dioxide, methane, nitrous oxide, and fluorinated gases, which are released from energy production and industrial processes.

EMERGENCY PREPAREDNESS

Facilities that manufacture, use, or store chemicals have an inherent risk for a chemical air release or spill that is beyond the routine emissions from day to day operations. In 1990, amendments to the Clean Air Act expanded regulations to prevent chemical accidents by requiring facilities to create and submit a risk management plan (RMP) to the EPA. The RMP is useful to local law enforcement, fire, emergency, and public health personnel, because it contains information on the hazards specific to the chemicals used at the facility, the processes in place by the facility to prevent an accident, and emergency plans in case of a chemical accident. Additionally, the OSHA has the Process Safety Management of Highly Hazardous Chemicals standard, which requires employers to conduct and train their employees on the dangers of operational processes involving chemicals and the administrative and engineering control mechanisms in place to mitigate the risk. This regulation enhances safety for the employees handling the chemicals and also contributes to prevention of chemical accidents that can have a broader public health impact.

Public health emergency preparedness for chemical accidents relies on understanding the facilities and industrial processes that are vulnerable to chemical releases, fires, or explosions from human error or secondary to natural disasters. Emergency preparedness practices for all hazards in a community can be applied to chemical incident preparedness. The Centers for Disease Control and Prevention (CDC) established a framework of 15 capabilities that form a national standard for public health emergency preparedness. The capabilities are organized into six domains, as seen in Table 52–3. This framework defines the necessary components for jurisdictional preparedness and response capacity to all hazards and requires collaboration across multiple disciplines and levels of government.

Public health officials must collect and analyze reports of the chemicals and quantity of emissions from industrial facilities to understand how continuous low-level releases may impact nearby populations, particularly those community members who are most at risk for an accidental large-scale release. As part of the *Community Preparedness* capability, public health emergency managers are charged with determining the risks and hazards within a jurisdiction, identifying populations with access and functional needs who may be disproportionately impacted by an incident, strengthening

Table 52–3. Public Health Emergency Preparedness and Response Capabilities, 2018. Centers for Disease Control and Prevention.

Domains	Capabilities
Community Resilience	Community preparedness Community recovery
Incident Management	Emergency operations coordination
Information Management	Emergency public information and warning Information sharing
Countermeasures and Mitigation	Medical countermeasure dispensing and administration Medical material management and distribution Nonpharmaceutical interventions Responder safety and health
Surge Management	Fatality management Mass care Medical surge Volunteer management
Biosurveillance	Public health laboratory testing Public health surveillance and epidemiologic investigation

Adapted from: Public Health Emergency Preparedness and Response Capabilities. National Standards for State, Local, Tribal, and Territorial Public Health. Centers for Disease Control and Prevention. October 2018, page 5.

stakeholder partnerships for preparedness, using nongovernmental community networks to improve resilience, and coordinating training and support for preparedness.

The first step in building community preparedness is the process of a jurisdictional risk assessment (JRA). A JRA informs local emergency managers of the historic and future risks to individuals within their jurisdiction, the effective use of limited resources during an emergency response, the vulnerabilities of populations within the community, and available partnerships in planning and response. All hazards must be considered for potential community impact. In the United States, the 1986 Emergency Planning and Community Right-to-Know Act (EPCRA), required facilities to report their use of chemicals and releases, which is helpful in emergency planning for industrial accidents.

A community's social vulnerability is a measure of the populations within a community that may be disproportionately impacted by an incident and require additional consideration for emergency preparedness. This includes individuals with access and functional needs, chronic health issues, mobility or transportation limitations, mental or behavioral health challenges, unique cultural and language barriers to communication, and baseline financial struggles. The CDC/Agency for Toxic Substances and Disease Registry (ATSDR) has developed a Social Vulnerability Index (SVI) to identify and rank all U.S. Census tracts on 15 social factors across four themes: socioeconomic status, household composition and disability, race/ethnicity and language barriers, and housing and transportation. The SVI can help emergency managers identify and map the communities that will most likely need support before, during, and after a hazardous event. During planning and preparation, emergency managers may use the SVI in conjunction with a mapping platform that identifies toxic release and hazardous waste sites. Both governmental agencies and private companies offer mapping products that visualize layers of information relevant to emergency planning within a jurisdiction. For example, the TOXMAP tool maps toxic releases and hazardous waste sites from three sources: emissions from stationary industrial and waste sites reported to the EPA's TRI database, hazardous waste sites on the EPA's Superfund National Priorities List (NPL), and facility emissions from Canada's National Pollutant Release Inventory. For community vulnerability planning around chemical releases, industrial facilities that are mapped near sites such as hospitals, elder care facilities, and schools may be locations of interest to invest additional planning resources. Emergency planning personnel in a community use all components of a JRA along with mapping tools, vulnerability information, and industry data to coordinate preparedness efforts with jurisdictional partners.

ACCIDENTAL RELEASES

The expertise of health care providers, first responders, and public health agencies is necessary for responding to any large-scale accidental chemical release. It is essential

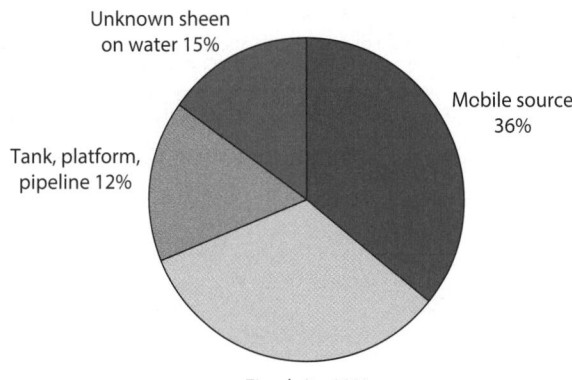

▲ **Figure 52–1.** Sources* of hazardous substance releases reported to the U.S. Coast Guard National Response Center. *Figure does not include nonrelease and continuous release reports.

for clinicians to be familiar with how to assess an exposed individual for health consequences, the steps involved in the public health assessment of chemical releases, and mechanisms to prevent injury in responders.

TRACKING & TRENDS

The storage and transportation patterns of hazardous chemicals contribute to the high potential for accidental releases. Annually, billions of pounds of hazardous chemicals are generated and stored at manufacturing plants and transported to offsite destinations for use. In 2018 alone, there were 23,516 release incidents recorded by the National Response Center, which is an emergency call line maintained by the U.S. Coast Guard for reporting pollution events. Figure 52–1 depicts the origin of these accidental releases, the largest proportion of which are from mobile sources during transport, such as rail, aircraft, and vessel. The manufacturing sector, which includes chemical and petrochemical production, accounts for the highest rates of releases from fixed sources in both US and European release reports.

When spills or releases occur, facilities are required to report to local, state, and federal authorities based on the type and quantity of the released substance, the presence of human health hazard, level of control over the release, clean-up implications, and potential for continued effects on the public and environment. For a snapshot of incidents in the United States, the National Toxic Substances Incidents Program (NTSIP) collected detailed incident data from several US states and produced a number of reports and publications. Tables 52–4, 52–5, and 52–6 display pertinent findings from the most recent NTSIP report on accidental release incidents from the participating states. As displayed in Table 52–4, the most frequent chemical releases from stationary sites differ from those released during transportation.

Table 52–4. Chemical releases.

Five Most Frequently Released Chemicals From Fixed Facility Incidents	Five Most Frequently Released Chemicals From Transportation Incidents
Natural gas	Alkaline hydroxide
Ammonia	Natural gas
Chemicals for methamphetamine production	Sulfuric acid
	Hydrogen peroxide
Carbon monoxide	Acetone
Mercury	

Based on incidents reported to the National Toxic Substances Incidents Program 2013-2014. https://www.atsdr.cdc.gov/ntsip.

Chemicals released less frequently or in smaller quantity can be more hazardous to human health than some larger releases due to their toxicologic profiles or the vulnerability of populations near the site of release. For example, air releases of hydrogen fluoride (hydrofluoric acid in its liquid form), most notably from oil refineries, can cause serious respiratory problems or death, depending on the level of exposure. In April 2018, an explosion and fire at a refinery in Texas resulted in a release of 974 lb of hydrogen fluoride. That same month and year another explosion and fire involving hydrogen fluoride occurred at a refinery in Wisconsin. Although hydrogen fluoride is not released in the highest quantities compared to other chemicals, the high health risk from hydrogen fluoride prompted dozens to seek medical attention, and a large portion of the surrounding community was evacuated.

Table 52–5 shows five of the chemicals that contribute to nearly half of injuries from releases. Carbon monoxide can be particularly toxic due to its lack of color and odor that make awareness of exposure nearly impossible to the victim. The additional chemicals on the list of most injurious are highly flammable, corrosive, or volatile, contributing to increased risk for injury on exposure.

Accidental chemical releases do not only occur as a result of the industrial lifecycle of product development and transportation. Improper storage and handling in homes and small business or malfunctioning equipment can lead to smaller releases that have real health impacts. In 2015, a chlorine gas

Table 52–5. Five substances responsible for the most injuries in release events.

Carbon monoxide
Chemicals for methamphetamine production
Sulfuric acid
Natural gas
Ammonia

Source: National Toxic Substance Incidents Program 2013–2014.

Table 52–6. Four most frequently reported health effects following accidental releases of hazardous substances.

Respiratory system
Burns
Dizziness or other central nervous system symptoms or signs
Trauma

Source: National Toxic Substances Incidents Program 2013-2014.

release at a recreational swimming pool in California led to 17 swimmers requiring emergency medical care after contact with the chlorine gas plume while in the pool. This release was due to mechanical malfunction in the pool chemical controller and human error in managing the malfunction. The incident prompted a public health investigation into similar incidents. Multiple additional reports of chlorine gas releases at swimming pools across the state had common root causes of inadequate or improper human response to malfunctions in pool mechanical equipment. Cumulatively, these incidents resulted in 121 swimmers exposed to chlorine gas who required medical evaluation in an emergency department over a 7-year period.

RESPONSE TO ACCIDENTAL RELEASES

Chemical emergency planning is most effective when industry, government, the medical community, local community organizations, and public interest groups have established working relationships and coordinate their efforts to mitigate the effects of an accident. Principles of decontamination, sheltering, and evacuation are relevant to both response professionals and members of the public who may participate in these harm mitigation strategies during an emergency.

▶ Incident Management

A standardized system called the National Response Framework (NRF) is the basis for coordination of stakeholder roles in the response effort, regardless of the size of the incident. The NRF relies on the concepts and terminology used in the National Incident Management System (NIMS), which outlines various incident operations systems and a standardized set of incident command roles. The Incident Command System (ICS) is run by an incident commander who coordinates the work of four subsections: operations, planning, logistics, and finance. The use of this structured approach to incident management has been adapted for use in a multitude of public health incidents globally by both governmental agencies and nongovernmental organizations.

▶ Sheltering-in-Place versus Evacuation

In general, a decision to institute protective actions immediately following a spill or air release is made by the emergency response incident commander, typically from a fire, hazmat, or a law-enforcement agency, in conjunction with local health personnel and elected officials. Few options are available for the protection of community residents after accidental releases. In the case of a release into water, residents may be cautioned to avoid contact with or consumption of the contaminated source. Following releases into air, the two alternatives for protective action are sheltering-in-place or evacuation. The decision to evacuate or shelter-in-place involves weighing many factors. Officials consider the characteristics of the chemical; the estimated concentration as a function of time; the source, size, and duration of the release; meteorologic conditions; and the tightness and infiltration rates of the structures used for protection. Finally, officials account for the proximity of institutions that might require special attention during both evacuation and sheltering-in-place, such as schools, hospitals, elder care facilities, and prisons.

Sheltering-in-place should be the initial response while any situation is being assessed. It is of greatest benefit when the chemical's peak concentration, rather than its cumulative dose, presents the greater toxicity. Buildings with ventilation systems turned off and with intact doors and windows closed may reduce exposure significantly to those taking shelter indoors. Evacuation may be the preferred choice when there is the threat of a release, though none has yet occurred, or when the release may create an explosion or fire hazard. Evacuation is usually a time-consuming and confusing process and is the safest alternative only when it can be completed prior to the time that a toxic cloud reaches a populated area in chemical incidents. Both in-place protection and evacuation are most effective in protecting individuals from toxic exposure when the local population has received prior education about the proper procedures to follow in the event of an accidental release and an alert system is in place to disseminate information quickly.

▶ Decontamination

To minimize contamination of response personnel and most efficiently treat exposed individuals, the incident commander at a hazardous materials incident typically establishes a command post and creates hazard zones (Figure 52-2). The hot zone, also known as the "exclusion zone," is closest to the spill, and only responders wearing personal protective equipment (PPE) should be allowed to enter. Entry and exit is controlled through one entry point and a separate point of exit. Only rudimentary first aid is provided in this area. The warm zone, or "decontamination area," provides a systematic way to lessen the exposure to the chemical hazard for those who have been in the hot zone and also serves to control the spread of contamination into the cold zone.

The cold zone is also termed the "support zone." This area is theoretically safe from the chemical hazard and is usually set up a considerable distance upwind of the spill. Command and control activities, first aid, and planning take place in the cold zone. Plume modeling may be used to map expected chemical concentrations to determine the distance each zone should be from the spill site.

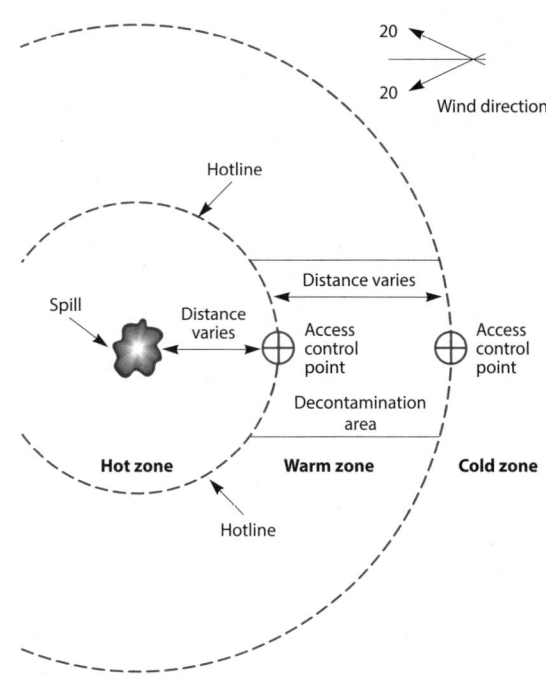

▲ **Figure 52–2.** Schematic of hot, warm, and cold zones at a hazardous spill site.

The highest level of PPE for entering a hot zone includes a positive-pressure supplied-air respirator or self-contained breath apparatus, full chemical protective suit, and chemical-resistant gloves and boots. Responders may adjust to less protective PPE, which may be more comfortable, if the identity and air concentration of the released substance are known and do not require the highest level of PPE to maintain safety. When exiting a hazard zone, emergency personnel must undergo decontamination to prevent spread of the chemical to others and to decrease their personal exposure time to the substance. Depending on the contaminant, cleaning may require the use of wet or dry methods. The exterior of chemical protective suits is typically decontaminated before removal by the responders.

Appropriate decontamination techniques are specific to an individual substance and may not be immediately intuitive to a contaminated person. Seeking toxicologic expertise or referring to the corresponding safety data sheets are the best ways to get accurate information on the correct method for cleaning. Decontamination with water may be harmful in some cases. For example, in the presence of water, metal phosphides such as aluminum, zinc, and magnesium phosphides hydrolyze to produce the toxic gas phosphine.

Health care facilities and workers can be at risk for secondary contamination from toxic materials on the skin or clothes of accident victims or from vomitus. Substances that are the highest risk for causing secondary contamination include those that are most toxic and easily transferred from clothing and skin. These may include potent pesticides, biological agents, radioactive materials, and strong acids or bases. Secondary contamination is of lower concern from gases and vapors, such as chlorine, which do not stay on the victim.

▶ Roles of Response Professionals

Emergency responders, health care providers, hospitals, and public health agencies are essential to chemical release response. Unique aspects of their roles will be covered in this section.

A. Emergency Responders

Emergency first responders are usually the first to arrive on the scene of a hazardous incident. The responders may include firefighters, emergency medical technicians, police officers, and local trained hazardous materials (HAZMAT) personnel. First responders will evaluate the situation, control the release, and depending on the nature and scale of the incident, will issue orders for shelter-in-place or evacuation of the surrounding community. They will also decontaminate the exposed individuals, provide necessary care in the field, and transport the injured victims to health care facilities. During a response, the safety of emergency personnel is of utmost importance to ensure the best management of the hazard scene.

Emergency responders are vulnerable when they do not immediately understand the cause of patient illness as related to a chemical or agent that carries the risk for secondary contamination. For example, in the United States, symptoms of opioid toxicity have been reported in first responders caring for victims of opioid overdose prior to and during transportation to an emergency department. The first responders were not adequately protected against the possibility of imperceptible secondary contamination by aerosolized opioids in the environment. Responders can be similarly susceptible to contaminants at hazardous spill sites that are not readily noticeable and identifiable. A comprehensive review of responder safety is found in the chapter *Responder Safety and Health*, which covers the necessary considerations for protecting responders pre-, during, and post-deployment in a disaster response.

B. Health care Providers

Exposure to accidental chemical releases may cause a variety of health effects. The information gathered from health care providers can help identify the released substance, if not immediately known, and provide symptoms to include in a case definition for patients who may subsequently present for care due to the same release. Prior to directly evaluating an exposed patient, health care personnel must consider and take precaution against secondary contamination if there is concern that a patient was not adequately decontaminated in the field. When a victim of a hazardous substance exposure is evaluated, the following information should be recorded in the medical record. Additional details may be relevant based on the specific exposure incident.

- Subjective complaints
- General medical history
- Smoking history
- Occupational history, including potential workplace exposures unrelated to the release that might contribute to health complaints
- Identity of the substance(s) released
- Location of the individual relative to the site of the release
- The estimated duration of time spent at any given location relative to the release
- Activities that may affect the exposure dose of chemical, such as strenuous exercise in the area of the chemical release or consumption of contaminated water or food
- Timing of symptom onset relative to the potential exposure
- Whether fires or explosions occurred as a result of the accident, which could indicate exposure to combustion or pyrolysis products
- Whether other persons appeared to be exposed at the same time
- Physical examination
- Results of laboratory tests, imaging, and spirometry as appropriate

Health care providers may play multiple roles following accidental releases of hazardous substances. In order to adequately assist the response effort, health care providers should:

- Rely on general principles of emergency management that can be applied to any natural or man-made incident.
- Be familiar with presentations of the chemical, biological, radiologic, nuclear, and explosive (CBRNE) agents that have greatest potential for harm.
- Report syndromes, illnesses, and exposures to public and environmental health agencies.

Online resources, safety data sheets, and regional poison control centers should be consulted for substance identification and medical treatment options. If these sources do not have appropriate toxicity information, it may be necessary to contact the manufacturer directly. Manufacturers are allowed to withhold trade secrets about hazardous chemicals from the public, but they are required to provide this information to physicians or nurses who need it for the purpose of treating victims of exposure. Specific proprietary information can be legally obtained in order to render appropriate medical care, but the person receiving this information must agree to maintain the information confidential.

C. Hospitals

Following major chemical incidents, local hospitals may be overwhelmed by the volume of patients seeking acute care. To optimize response to these emergencies, hospitals should plan for surge due to chemical hazards and establish policies and procedures specifying the scope and conduct of patient care to be provided at the facility. Planning may vary by the hospital due to the available capacity and capabilities. The goal of planning is to provide efficient and quality care for a potentially large number of victims while preventing injury to hospital staff and patients who were not initially exposed to the hazardous substance. Hospital officials can minimize the risk of secondary contamination of the medical facility, staff, and bystanders by ensuring that plans are in place for prehospital or prompt decontamination of victims on presentation. Examples of components in a hospital's preparedness plan include: the method and location of patient decontamination, if not done prior to transport to the hospital; protocols to triage patients into mild, moderate, and severe injury categories; establishing treatment guidelines; and coordinating with other area hospitals and local and state agencies. Current toxicologic reference materials, including online databases and telephone numbers of the regional poison control center should be readily available, some examples of which are included in Table 52–7. Information on referral and consultation services should be regularly updated.

Hospitals and health care systems in the United States participate in the Hospital Incident Command System (HICS) as a standardized method for incident management during large-scale emergencies. HICS follows the framework of the ICS, which is applicable to all public health emergencies (Table 52–8). The HICS system provides both preparedness information for a variety of potential incidents and protocols to follow during response operations. Hospitals, emergency responders, and public health stakeholders should coordinate drills and simulations to ensure optimal response during a large-scale emergency.

D. Public Health

Public health agencies work together with emergency responders and hospital systems to coordinate response to a chemical release. Some jurisdictions also have an environmental health department that takes on the majority of the responsibility alone or in conjunction with the public health department. Officials of these departments play a central role in collecting and disseminating information to response stakeholders, providing subject matter expertise, and participating in incident management during the response effort.

In the United States, communication of critical information in a public health response can be distributed rapidly through the Health Alert Network, a communication platform maintained by the CDC to disseminate information nationally to health officials at all levels of government, clinicians, and laboratories. Many states administer and maintain similar programs.

The Laboratory Response Network (LRN) is a critical partner to chemical incident preparedness and response. The LRN is a collaboration of laboratories with different specialties overseen by the CDC that have the capability to test specimens for the presence of substances of interest during public health

Table 52–7. Resources for hazardous material identification, response, and health effects.

Managing Hazardous Materials Incidents. Volumes I–III ATSDR *http://www.atsdr.cdc.gov/MHMI/index.asp*	Planning guides for emergency medical services, hospital emergency departments, and acute chemical exposure management guidelines for clinicians
Publication: *Primary Response Incident Scene Management (PRISM): Guidance for the operational response to chemical incidents* *https://www.medicalcountermeasures.gov/barda/cbrn/prism/*	A comprehensive strategic and tactile guide for mass casualty decontamination measures
New Jersey Hazardous Substance Fact Sheets *http://web.doh.state.nj.us/rtkhsfs/indexfs.aspx*	Summarized information on hazards, safe storage, control, first aid, and emergency procedures for common chemicals
Integrated Risk Information System (IRIS) *http://www.epa.gov/iris/*	Health risk assessment information on chemicals from the U.S. EPA
Poison control centers *(800) 222-1222* *http://www.poison.org*	Provides information on immediate health effects, need for decontamination, protective gear, and specific treatment
U.S. Department of Transportation placards	Warning placards for vehicles carrying hazardous materials
Chemical Hazard Response Information System (CHRIS)	Emergency response information from the U.S. Coast Guard for transportation accidents on water involving hazardous chemicals
National Fire Protection Agency labels	Labeling system for describing chemical hazards

Table 52–8. Guidance for emergency response and preparedness.

Response Plan	Description	Website
Hospital Incident Command System (HICS)	Crisis management plan for hospitals to coordinate their own response to emergencies or disasters	http://www.emsa.ca.gov/hics/
National Incident Management System (NIMS)	Federal system that establishes standard protocols and procedures for incident managers and responders to work together to prepare for and respond to all incidents, including natural disasters and acts of terrorism	http://www.fema.gov/national-incident-management-system
National Response Framework (NRF)	Establishes an all-hazards approach to manage domestic incidents; integrates best practices and procedures from disciplines, such as emergency medical services, law enforcement, first responders, public health, and worker health and safety into a unified structure	http://www.fema.gov
Health Alert Network (HAN)	Rapid communication system for the dissemination of vital public health information from the Centers for Disease Control and Prevention (CDC) to governmental jurisdictions, clinicians, and laboratory stakeholders	https://emergency.cdc.gov/han/
Technical Resources, Assistance Center, and Information Exchange (TRACIE)	An online resource gateway by the U.S. Department of Health and Human Services Assistant Secretary for Preparedness and Response. The platform contains technical resources and supports information sharing for health care and public health stakeholders and their partners in emergency preparedness	https://asprtracie.hhs.gov/

emergencies and investigations for both chemical and biological threats. Fifty-three laboratories make up the chemical testing sector, which is known as LRN-C. There are three levels of LRN-C laboratory designation that indicate the capacity and breadth of testing available, Level 1 being the most expansive. Level 1 laboratories have the capability to test human specimens for a multitude of agents, including those potentially used for chemical warfare and industrial chemicals.

▶ Risk Assessment

Following a major toxic release, public health officials assess the ongoing and future risk to public health through hazard identification, dose-response assessment, exposure assessment, and risk characterization. This four-step process is called health risk assessment and is described in detail in the chapter of the same name. In the case of an unplanned release, the steps may occur simultaneously by subject matter experts in order to guide the response and public messaging.

In the United States, the ATSDR offers the Assessment of Chemical Exposures (ACE) program to assist state and local public health officials in evaluating a chemical incident. The ACE personnel can provide technical assistance to local officials and connect stakeholder agencies for collaboration. The ACE program provides the structure for conducting interviews of first responders, hospital staff, and impacted members of the public; reviewing medical charts for relevant information; and conducting laboratory testing. The local health officials use this information to evaluate the response to the incident, understand the effects on the local population, and plan for further follow-up and future emergency preparedness.

▶ Incident Reporting

The accurate and timely reporting of accidental chemical releases is required by law in many countries to support chemical response and planning efforts. However, there are no global uniform reporting requirements nor a common database for incidents. The Comprehensive Environmental Response, Compensation, and Liability Act (CERCLA) requires that the U.S. EPA issues a reportable quantity (RQ) for extremely hazardous substances, which is a level that prompts the reporting of release events to both the National Response Center and authorities within the state. The EPA establishes the RQ based on the health risk from the substance's physical, chemical, and toxicologic properties. States may have more stringent reporting requirements than the federal RQs. In the EU, member States must report both chemical accidents and near misses to the Major Accident Hazards Bureau. The data collected facilitates communication between member States on the lessons learned from a chemical release to improve future planning and prevention efforts.

NUCLEAR & RADIOLOGICAL ACCIDENTS

There is overlap in the comprehensive emergency planning and response principles for chemical releases and radiological exposure accidents. Nuclear and radiological accidents may occur during the use, storage, or transport of radioactive materials at a wide variety of sites, including power plants, industrial sites, roadways, and research laboratories. As radioactive materials have a broad range of applications, preparedness for accidental exposure incidents is paramount to prevention and quick management of injuries.

Multiple scientific organizations and governmental agencies provide best practice guidance related to the use of radiological materials and emergency preparedness.

▶ Nuclear Response Organizations & Guidance

Nuclear regulation and cooperation occurs both at the level of individual countries and through collective global efforts. The International Atomic Energy Agency (IAEA) is a cooperative organization on the use of nuclear technology with 171 global member States. The IAEA provides expertise in multiple areas, including safety, nuclear applications, and sustainable development. The IAEA maintains reporting registries of incidents at nuclear power plants, research reactors, and fuel cycle facilities that impact human safety. The Emergency Response and Preparedness framework created by the IAEA outlines the organization's response during incidents and provides guidance on structuring emergency response capabilities in member States. The 33 member countries of the Organisation for Economic Cooperation and Development (OECD) have established the Nuclear Energy Agency, which has initiatives and work groups that focus on peaceful nuclear uses, sound nuclear policy, and sustainability.

In the United States, various federal agencies share responsibility for incidents involving radioactive materials under the Radiological Emergency Preparedness Program implemented by the Federal Emergency Management Agency (FEMA). This program covers planning and policies for commercial nuclear power plant incidents licensed by the U.S. Nuclear Regulatory Commission (U.S. NRC). Facility licensing and regulation is done at the national level. Some states have "agreement state" status with the U.S. NRC, allowing them to maintain a state-level radiation control program. The Department of Energy is responsible for emergencies and transportation accidents involving radiologic material in its custody. The EPA is the lead agency in emergencies involving radioactivity originating in a foreign country or in a domestic accident involving unregulated radioactive material. State and local governments are responsible for the health and welfare of the general public during an emergency.

The IAEA and OECD have collaborated on an internationally accepted tool to classify the health significance of releases, called the International Nuclear and Radiological Event Scale (INES), depicted in Figure 52–3. The scale is useful in communicating the safety concern of a particular event to the public. Seven levels make up the scale with increasing severity from bottom to top. The three bottom tiers of lower severity events are considered *incidents* and the four upper tiers of higher severity are called *accidents*. Classification of an event is based on the radiation doses to people and the environment near the release, the impact on radiologic barriers and controls within nuclear facilities, and failure of the safety measures intended for prevention. Every increase in one level on the scale indicates ten times greater severity of the event.

The EPA has developed a system of protective action guides (PAGs) to help officials make critical decisions that safeguard human health during and immediately after an accident with radioactive material based on the projected dose to be avoided. The PAGs identify three phases of an emergency: early, intermediate, and late. In the early phase, which usually lasts from several hours to several days, evacuation and sheltering are the principal actions to shield the public from exposure to radiation. Stable iodine can protect the thyroid against radioactive iodine if it is administered prior to exposure. The intermediate phase begins when the active release has been contained and can last from weeks to months. Actions in the intermediate phase include protective measures to avoid the ingestion of contaminated food and water and relocating people to minimize radiation exposure. In the late phase, which can last from months to years,

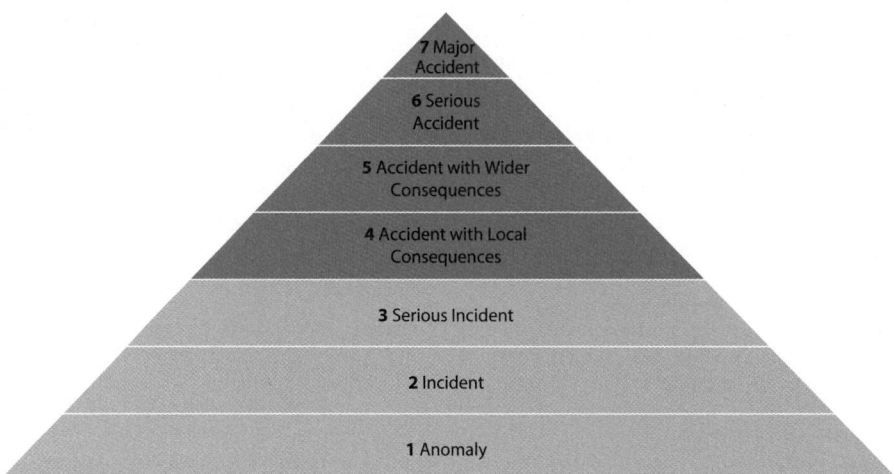

▲ **Figure 52–3.** Adaption of The International Nuclear and Radiological Event Scale from the International Atomic Energy Agency (IAEA).

the PAGs address the control of exposures and reoccupation of contaminated property. In an actual emergency, protective actions in addition to those addressed by the PAGs may be needed.

Clinicians responsible for the evaluation and treatment of victims exposed to radiation must be familiar with the clinical syndrome and management of these patients, which is discussed in earlier chapters. The Radiation Emergency Assistance Center/Training Site (REAC/TS) of the U.S. Department of Energy can provide subject matter expertise to global health and emergency professionals during a radiological event through telephone consultation and deployment.

▼ HAZARDOUS WASTE

The following material includes an overview of common hazardous wastes, the use of exposure assessment to study the health impact of hazardous waste, and a synopsis of waste management and regulation. The focus is on chemical waste; however, given their particular interest to the health care community, pharmaceutical, regulated medical waste (biohazardous), and radioactive waste are also briefly addressed.

DEFINITION OF HAZARDOUS WASTE

There are as many possible types of hazardous wastes as there are possible combinations of toxic substances. In the United States, the definition and regulation of hazardous waste is limited to solid waste, which can include physical solids, sludge, certain liquids, and containerized gases. Some substances are excluded from hazardous waste regulation even though they would appear to meet the criteria of solid waste (Table 52–9). Hazardous waste excludes chemicals discharged directly into the air or water, such as releases allowed by permits under other federal pollution-control statutes such as the Clean Air Act and the Clean Water Act.

Most household chemicals are also excluded from hazardous waste categorization, although there are many toxic chemicals in today's commercial products. Universal waste is a special category of hazardous waste found in some household and businesses waste that is not permitted to be discarded with municipal solid waste. Universal waste includes substances that can become toxic, corrosive, or flammable, such as batteries and mercury-containing equipment,

pesticides, and lamps. Some states have added items to the list of universal waste, such as aerosol cans, antifreeze, electronics, and pharmaceuticals. Universal waste must be collected separately, thus making it easier to send for recycling or proper disposal.

In the United States in 2017, a total of 25,548 hazardous waste generators produced 35 million tons of hazardous waste, which is about 1 ton per 9 people. Chemical and petroleum/coal producers were responsible for most of the hazardous waste generation with a combined total of nearly 26 million tons. The states generating the most hazardous waste were Texas and Louisiana, which accounted for 65% of the national total quantity generated.

The EPA maintains the NPL of sites contaminated with hazardous waste that are of highest priority for investigation and clean-up due to the presence of contaminants highly toxic to human health and the environment. The process for site clean-up of NPL listings is known as Superfund. This program includes site assessments, remedial feasibility and design studies, and site reviews post-cleanup. The EPA estimates that as many as 450,000 abandoned hazardous waste sites exist in the United States.

Given the magnitude of hazardous materials that are produced and discarded, a comprehensive list and review of each is not possible within this chapter. Table 52–10 lists commonly used online resources that contain information on the facilities that are required to report hazardous waste products that they release, known hazardous waste sites, and the chemical properties of substances released as waste from industrial processes.

STUDYING THE HEALTH IMPACTS OF HAZARDOUS WASTE

▶ Exposure Assessment

The U.S. EPA estimates that 53 million people, or 16% of the US population, live within three miles of an EPA NPL site that is targeted for hazardous waste cleanup, and 15 million of those residents live within just one mile of a site. However, residence near a hazardous waste site or a facility that handles hazardous waste does not necessarily translate to human harm if there is not a viable pathway for human exposure to the toxic substances. A complete exposure pathway between a released toxin and humans consists of the following five elements: a source of contamination, an environmental medium, a point of exposure, route(s) of exposure, and a receptor population. Exposure assessment is the process of identifying the population exposed to a hazardous agent and modeling the route and magnitude of exposure. This process allows for an understanding of the types of human health impacts that could result from a hazardous waste site. A detailed explanation of conducting an exposure assessment is available in the chapter *Health Risk Assessment*. The path between a hazardous waste release and human contact is a target for interventions to mitigate human exposure.

Table 52-9. A partial list of substances excluded from federal hazardous waste regulation in the United States.

• Domestic sewage	• Agricultural waste
• Radioactive waste	• Household waste
• In-situ mining waste	• Mining waste
• Pulping liquors from paper production	• Combustion of fossil fuel and
• Wood preservatives	oil, gas, and geothermal waste

Table 52–10. Hazardous waste databases.

Database Name/Location	Description of Database
Agency for Toxic Substances & Disease Registry (ATSDR) www.atsdr.cdc.gov	A database of reports known as Public Health Assessments, on the public health impact of environmental contaminants at sites on the U.S. EPA National Priority List for hazardous site clean-up. The ATSDR also provides toxicologic profiles of hazardous substances and surveillance of populations with certain known exposures.
Toxic Release Inventory (TRI) U.S. EPA www.epa.gov/trinationalanalysis	Self-reported information on chemical releases and handling by industrial facilities in the United States
Biennial Report Summary U.S. EPA	U.S. EPA's database of large-quantity generators and transporters of hazardous waste viewable by state and territory.
Superfund Enterprise Management System (SEMS) U.S. EPA	U.S. EPA's database of sites assessed for the NPL to undergo clean-up.
U.S. Nuclear Regulatory Commission	Database of nuclear reactors, radioactive waste, and emergency preparedness in the United States
European Chemicals Agency	Database culminating reports from companies that manufacture or import chemicals to the EU, which contain the chemical properties and human and environmental safety profile in accordance with the Registration, Evaluation, Authorisation, and Restriction of Chemicals (REACH) regulations
Hazardous Substances Data Bank (National Institutes of Health)	Database containing a breadth of information on hazardous chemicals, including chemical properties, health effects, and industrial hygiene considerations

The ATSDR publishes a biannual substance priority list (SPL) of the hazardous materials of greatest health threat from sites on the NPL awaiting cleanup. Table 52–11 lists the top 20 substances out of 275 on the SPL.

The prioritization of the substances on the SPL is based on three criteria: frequency of occurrence of a toxic substance at NPL sites, the substance's toxicity, and the potential for human exposure. Of note, many hazardous waste sites are contaminated with a mixture of chemicals rather than a single chemical, and very little toxicologic information is available on combined substances.

▶ Biological Monitoring

The standard method for identifying and quantifying chemical exposures in humans is through biological monitoring or biomonitoring, which is the measurement of chemicals in human body fluids and tissues. Biological monitoring measurements, or biomarkers, are indicators of contact with a toxic substance in body tissues, blood, urine, serum, or saliva. Biomarkers are used in two ways for studying health effects. Biomarkers *of exposure* are measured biochemical indicators, typically from the blood or urine, that provide evidence that contact with a chemical or other substance of interest has occurred. Biomarkers *of effect* are processes that can be measured through biochemical or radiographic testing that suggest physiologic changes occurring due to an exposure, which can be an early sign of clinically significant disease to come. These measurements are used in health risk assessment, which is a process usually undertaken by public health professionals or scientists to characterize the health risks of exposures to chemicals and other environmental contaminants. Biomarkers of exposure are increasingly used in studies of human contact with toxic substances and help avoid many of the exposure assumptions and animal-to-human extrapolations that are used in traditional exposure/risk assessment. However, depending on the pharmacokinetics of the chemical, biological monitoring might not provide the needed information about chronic exposure to chemicals from a hazardous waste site. For instance, volatile organic compounds and their metabolites can have short half-lives on the order of hours, limiting the utility of testing for exposure. The chapter *Biological Monitoring* provides more information on these types of measurements and includes a table of chemicals and their properties for which reliable data exist. Unlike public health standards for allowable concentrations of a chemical in drinking water or soil, there are no accepted guidelines for the interpretation of biological monitoring levels, and concerns about reproducibility may impact clinical utility in some cases.

Interpretation of biological monitoring samples for individuals or communities surrounding a hazardous waste sites is facilitated by the availability of large databases on the background levels of chemicals in the general population. The CDC publishes biomonitoring data as part of the National Health and Nutrition Examination Survey (NHANES), an ongoing survey of the general US population that randomly selects about 7000 people per year for participation. The blood and urine of participants are sampled and tested for

Table 52–11. Top 20 hazardous substances at CERCLA sites.

2017 Rank	Hazardous Substance
1	Arsenic
2	Lead
3	Mercury
4	Vinyl chloride
5	Polychlorinated biphenyls
6	Benzene
7	Cadmium
8	Benzo(*a*)pyrene
9	Polycyclic aromatic hydrocarbons
10	Benzo(*b*)fluoranthene
11	Chloroform
12	Aroclor 1260
13	*p,p′*-Dichlorodiphenyltrichloroethane (DDT)
14	Aroclor 1254
15	Dibenzo(*a,h*)anthracene
16	Trichloroethylene
17	Chromium, hexavalent
18	Dieldrin
19	Phosphorous, white
20	Hexachlorobutadiene

Source: ATSDR: http://www.atsdr.cdc.gov/spl.

over 350 chemicals and organic pollutants. This national reference information is useful in finding correlation patterns between chemical elevations in the biological samples and residence near hazardous sites or other health comorbidities. For example, a study using the NHANES data found a correlation in patients with elevated fasting glucose or diabetes and elevated urinary cadmium, which is a known environmental contaminant.

In general, little is known about long-term exposure to low levels of environmental contaminants. Useful data to study health outcomes may be drawn from morbidity and mortality databases, birth statistics, medical records, tumor and disease registries, and surveillance databases. Reviewing such information for the small population around one site could not discriminate the risk from an environmental

exposure unless the relative risk is high. However, reviewing available data sources over a larger area, called an *ecologic study*, has identified significant effects from hazardous waste sources, such as increased risk of low birth weight with maternal residency near a PCB-contaminated hazardous waste site and increased rates of hospitalization for coronary heart disease near sites contaminated with polychlorinated biphenyls (PCB), dioxins/furans, and pesticides.

There are limitations to biomarker-based approaches for health risk assessment of chemical pollutants, and most hazardous waste site studies are restricted by the small size of the exposed community. For the general population, the scientific explanation why or why not health studies are appropriate in certain situations is very difficult to understand. A helpful tool for communities is the website: http://communityhealthstudies.cdph.ca.gov, which is aimed at lay audiences and provides background information on epidemiologic principles that illustrates the challenges in designing such a study.

HEALTH IMPACTS OF HAZARDOUS WASTE

Despite the growing interest in biomarkers and the availability of data related to exposed populations, the challenges of studying hazardous waste impacts remain, making it difficult to use the results of past studies to predict the future health impacts of exposures. Limitations include study design, properties of the chemicals released, unknown exposure level, varying baseline characteristics and confounders in the population, varying latency periods for physiologic outcomes, reporting bias, and inconsistent exposure time to the populations at risk. Both studies with positive and negative findings of health effects from hazardous waste sites are reported in the literature. Health impacts based on specific substances released from waste sites may be postulated from their toxicologic profiles, the most common of which are covered in earlier chapters of this book.

Systematic reviews of the literature on health effects surrounding hazardous waste sites have been conducted by multiple research groups. The most recent systematic review concluded that the quality of evidence for chronic outcomes related to cancers and congenital abnormalities is limited and the data are inadequate for drawing conclusions on other health endpoints. A synopsis of the long-term health impacts described in published reviews is described below. Information specific to certain chemical or heavy metal exposures and organ systems is found in the preceding chapters.

A. Fetal Health and Children

In the late 1970s, the environmental disaster site known as Love Canal came to national attention following years of concerns by impacted residents in New York State. Love Canal was an abandoned canal used by a chemical company to dump hazardous waste materials. The chemicals found in environmental testing of the Love Canal site included chlorinated hydrocarbons and organic solvents. Studies on fetal development found lower birth weights of infants born to mothers living near the site. Additional studies from developed countries on pregnancies near hazardous waste sites have shown evidence for low birth weight and preterm birth. Despite a trend toward excess risk for congenital abnormalities, statistical significance was not reached in several studies observing this outcome. No compelling evidence for increased fetal or infant mortality risk has been found.

Further health consequences have been identified in pediatric populations. Love Canal studies found lower statures of children living near the site. Exposure to metals such as lead, arsenic, cadmium, and manganese has been documented near hazardous waste sites in both the developed and developing world, including communities with rudimentary electronic waste recycling practices. Heavy metal exposure in childhood is known to impact behavior and intellectual development. Other correlated effects include lower scores on intelligence quotient (IQ) testing, tests of verbal memory, and temperament assessment.

In Israel, children living near an industrial park and hazardous waste treatment site had increased rates of hospitalization for respiratory disease diagnoses than case-matched controls. Also, compromised pulmonary forced vital capacity has been found in children with elevated blood concentrations of heavy metals living near electronic waste recycling sites.

B. Cancer

The overall evidence for excess cancer risk from exposure to hazardous waste sites is inadequate, often due to incomplete exposure assessment and limitations with cancer surveillance data. Several solid organ and hematologic cancers have been studied for links with hazardous waste. Examples of single-site studies that have suggested associations with certain malignancies include: excess incidence of pancreatic and skin cancers in men living in homes built on an industrial dump site in Finland; excess mortality from laryngeal cancer near a hazardous waste incineration site in Italy; increased hospitalization rates for hematologic malignancies near benzene waste sites in New York; and increased bladder cancer mortality in men near an industrial chemical dump site in Pennsylvania.

C. Chronic Disease

Correlations but not a causal link have been identified between hazardous waste sites and noncancer chronic disease in adults. Studies of residents in areas containing or abutting hazardous waste sites with persistent organic pollutants found increased rates of metabolic syndrome and diabetes mellitus as a primary or secondary diagnosis during hospitalizations. The diagnosis of metabolic syndrome includes a grouping of metabolic conditions that include insulin resistance, abdominal obesity, dyslipidemia, and hypertension. The known persistent organic pollutants in the studied geographic area included dioxins, furans, PCB, and chlorinated pesticides. These findings warrant further investigation into the link between residential exposure to persistent organic pollutants and chronic health conditions.

D. Behavioral Health

Behavioral health effects can occur among people regularly exposed to hazardous waste. However, the intersection between physical symptoms, behavioral health effects, and anxiety over health concerns might complicate studies of specific exposures and outcomes. An example of a condition with both physical and behavioral symptoms is Multiple Chemical Sensitivity, which is covered in detail in the chapter of the same name. This syndrome encompasses both physical health effects and reported impacts on mood, which can be due to exposure to a vast number of potential toxins.

Psychological or behavioral health impacts may have a considerable effect on individuals living near hazardous waste sites. While there has been some effort to study the physical health effects from living near hazardous waste facilities, the psychological effects remain inadequately defined and quantified, possibly due to hurdles in understanding the behavioral health effects from chronic exposure to toxicants. Many chemicals have neurotoxic effects that may impair mood and memory, and it is difficult to differentiate symptoms due to the stressful living conditions near hazardous waste sites from the direct chemical impacts on the brain. Additionally, evidence exists that residents who express worry about a hazardous site or perceive toxic odors from the site are more likely to report the presence of symptoms compared to others with similar exposure. Although not exclusively from hazardous waste sources, ecological studies have found correlations between geographic areas with higher air lead levels or elevated aggregate blood lead levels and rates of violent and property crime.

While studies of the psychological effects in acute disaster exposures have found increased incidence of clinical behavioral health diagnoses, further research is necessary to understand the long-term impacts of chronic hazardous waste exposure.

HAZARDOUS WASTE REDUCTION

Hazardous waste management is necessary to minimize the environmental and health impact of the byproducts of an industrialized society. Management of hazardous waste involves recycling, treating the waste to reduce its volume or hazardous level, and disposal. While all these activities are regulated, accidents still happen leading to releases. Historically absent or lax regulations on hazardous waste also contribute to health impacts from ongoing exposure to these materials.

Two important pieces of legislation guide US hazardous materials regulation and hazardous waste site clean-up today: the Resource Conservation and Recovery Act of 1976 (RCRA) and the Comprehensive Environmental Response, Compensation, and Liability Act of 1980 (CERCLA or Superfund). The RCRA requires that hazardous waste be identified and tracked through its lifespan by the party that generates it (ie, "cradle-to-grave" hazardous waste management). There are relevant regulations that guide waste handling from generation to transport and, ultimately, its recycling, treatment, and disposal.

Following the discovery of the Love Canal dump site in the 1970s, the public became concerned about past mismanagement of hazardous waste. Health authorities and public health professionals were pressured to identify the actual and potential health problems associated with abandoned hazardous waste sites. CERCLA was created in 1980 to address clean-up of inactive or abandoned sites. This requires that the parties responsible for the site contamination be required to pay for or perform remediation. Most generators now endeavor to minimize waste, and many manufacturers even factor waste management into the life cycle of their products.

Material reduction, reuse, and recycling in industrial processes are means to reduce waste impact. One mechanism for applying these principles is through "green chemistry," which is the invention, design, and application of processes that minimize or eliminate hazardous substance generation in the lifecycle of chemical products. Many companies and academic institutions in a variety of industries have been acknowledged for their efforts to reduce hazardous waste production by the EPA.

TREATMENT & DISPOSAL OF HAZARDOUS WASTE

▶ Treatment

Treatment of hazardous waste that cannot be reused or recycled and remediation of contaminated hazardous waste sites involve a variety of methods. Physical, chemical, biological, and thermal treatment options exist for various types of waste. These methods are described in Table 52–12.

▶ Disposal

Disposal of hazardous waste refers to long-term storage in landfills, underground injection wells, or ocean dumping. Regulations require hazardous waste storage sites to have mechanisms that prevent leaching of chemicals into the environment. Waste must meet certain criteria related to its toxicity and reactivity before disposal in a landfill, meaning that the waste may need to be treated first, potentially though one of the methods described in Table 52–12.

Table 52-12. Methods of hazardous waste treatment.

Methods and Examples	Description
Physical Treatment	Does not reduce the toxicity of the waste but does transfer the waste into another medium or prevents the waste from migrating.
Air Stripping	Air stripping is one of the most common physical processes used for remediating groundwater contaminated with volatile organic compounds (VOCs). Air forced through contaminated water enhances evaporation of the compounds.
Soil Vapor Extraction	Contaminated soils may be cleaned using soil vapor extraction, which involves passing an air stream through soil to raise VOCs to the surface for treatment.
Chemical Treatment	Alters the chemical structure of the waste constituents, thereby reducing the material's toxicity.
Chemical Oxidation	Uses oxidants such as ozone, hydrogen peroxide, and chlorine to destroy a wide range of organic molecules by causing a breakdown reaction to less harmful components.
Biological Treatment (Bioremediation)	The degradation of organic waste by the action of microorganisms, such as bacteria and fungi, with the aim of changing the molecular structure to create less toxic metabolites or completely breaking down the molecule to harmless residuals.
In Situ	The soil or water is treated by applying microorganisms directly to the polluted site and enhancing contaminant degradation by application of additional components like air injection and hydrogen peroxide.
Ex Situ	The contaminated material is excavated from the site and treated in aboveground beds, enclosures, or tanks where microorganisms and materials that enhance degradation are added.
Thermal Treatment	Involves the use of heat to clean contaminated soil.
Incineration	Uses very high temperatures between 871°C and 1371°C (1600°F and 2500°F) to alter the molecular structure to ideally reduce the toxicity of soil contaminated with chemicals but does not work to treat metals. Because of the tight regulations on incineration air emissions and concern from communities, on-site incinerators rarely are chosen as a remedy at hazardous waste sites.
Thermal Desorption	Uses temperatures between 93.3°C and 537.8°C (200°F and 1000°F) to evaporate low-volatile compounds from contaminated soil. The compounds are then trapped, cooled, and recovered for proper disposal. Sometimes the gas vapors require further treatment or oxidation. Unlike incineration, the soil remains intact with thermal desorption.

The treatment method also may generate a byproduct that must be disposed of as hazardous waste, such as incineration dust. As a result, even though landfilling of hazardous waste is discouraged, there always will be the need for some hazardous waste landfills.

Waste injection into deep underground wells is also used for disposal of hazardous waste. Injection usually occurs below the deepest drinking-water aquifer, 1000–10,000 ft. (304.8–3048 m) down.

In the earlier part of the twentieth century, ocean dumping was a method of choice for disposing a variety of hazardous materials internationally, including dredge spoils, industrial waste, sludge from wastewater treatment plants, and radioactive waste. In the mid-twentieth century, concern rose on the health and ecologic impacts of this unregulated dumping. That led to the London Convention, or The Convention on the Prevention of Marine Pollution by Dumping of Wastes and Other Matter of 1972, to encourage dumping control. An update to this agreement called the London Protocol was made in 1996, and, to date, 87 countries have signed.

PHARMACEUTICAL WASTE

Pharmaceutical waste contains discarded prescription and nonprescription drugs from health care facilities and private homes. Hospitals and long-term care facilities waste an estimated 62,000 tons of pharmaceuticals per year. In private homes, pharmaceuticals that are not used are often flushed down the toilet or poured down the drain. Since water treatment plants are not designed to remove these substances, this type of improper disposal has led to detectable concentrations of pharmaceuticals in surface water in many countries. Other potential sources of groundwater and drinking water contamination with pharmaceuticals include livestock operations and manufacturing.

▶ Health Effects of Pharmaceutical Waste

Pharmaceuticals impact aquatic life in waterways by disruption of endocrine pathways, which can have implications for reproduction. The concentrations of pharmaceutical metabolites in water and fish is very low and no direct human health impacts have yet been reported from ingestion of contaminated water or seafood. However, the level of water contamination in some countries or regions may exceed the levels at which no adverse effect would be expected, called the predicted no-effect concentrations (PNEC). Further study is needed to characterize and quantify potential human health effects of pharmaceutical agents in drinking water.

▶ Disposal of Pharmaceutical Waste

In December 2018, the U.S. EPA enacted a new rule on management of pharmaceutical waste produced by the health care sector, which prohibits dumping pharmaceuticals into the sewer system. This is projected to decrease the amount of pharmaceuticals that end up in US waterways by about 2000 tons every year. The U.S. Food and Drug Administration recommends that some controlled substances with a high risk for adverse health effects if taken incorrectly can be flushed down the toilet in private homes when no longer needed. Many developed countries have programs for consumers to take-back unused pharmaceuticals to pharmacies or other collection sites to be destroyed. The website medsdisposal.eu allows residents of the European Union to see how their country recommends pharmaceutical waste disposal through an interactive map. For example, residents of Germany are instructed to dispose of pharmaceuticals with their household trash, as all waste there is incinerated or pretreated before being placed in a landfill. Additionally, the WHO provides guidance for disposing pharmaceutical waste that was collected during an emergency event and is unwanted, expired, or unused.

REGULATED MEDICAL WASTE

Regulated medical waste is often called "biohazardous," as it refers to waste that is potentially infectious or contaminated with blood, body fluid, or tissue. Regulated medical waste is generated or produced as a result of any of the following: diagnosis, treatment, or immunization of human beings or animals; research dealing with infectious agents; serums, vaccines, antigens, and antitoxins; waste that is biohazardous; or "sharps," which are devices having acute rigid corners, edges, or protuberances capable of cutting or piercing, including needles, blades, and broken glass. Regulated medical waste is generated by medical and dental clinics, hospitals, skilled nursing facilities, research facilities, research and clinical laboratories, illicit drug users, and patients with insulin-dependent diabetes mellitus or other health conditions that require injections. As dependence on disposable supplies increases in health care, there is an increase in the amount of regulated medical waste produced.

▶ Health Risks of Medical Waste

The primary health risks associated with infectious health care wastes are a result of occupational exposure for those who handle the waste, not for the general population. The biggest concern is for the transmission of infectious material through medical waste, especially the hepatitis B and C viruses and HIV. Sharp objects pose the greatest concern because of their ability to puncture the skin and provide a portal of entry for disease transmission. The risk for viral transmission after a needle stick containing blood from an infected patient is approximately 6–30% for hepatitis B, 1.8% for hepatitis C, and 0.3% for HIV. The general public is at greatest risk from cuts and infectious transmission through medical sharps due to improper disposal outside of a designated sharps bin at home or in the community.

▶ Disposal of Medical Waste

Historically, over 90% of medical waste in the United States was incinerated for disposal. Incineration is no longer a recommended nor permitted way to manage medical waste from health care facilities and laboratories due to the production of HAPs such as particulate matter, carbon monoxide, and heavy metals. Dioxin production is of particular health concern, which has prompted the promotion of alternative disposal methods. The prevalence of chlorine-containing polyvinyl chloride (PVC) plastic products in health care waste is largely responsible.

Not all countries have prioritized moving away from incineration of medical waste, which remains prevalent especially in health care systems in the developing world. Alternative strategies for medical waste treatment include steam sterilization or autoclaving, microwave heating, and chemical application. In 2014, the WHO published the updated manual *Safe management of wastes from health care facilities*, which describes multiple aspects of medical waste, including alternate treatment and disposal strategies.

RADIOACTIVE WASTE

Radioactive waste is classified by the type and amount of radioactivity it contains. High-level waste is the byproduct of nuclear reactors and fuel used in the production of nuclear power and weapons. Low-level radioactive waste is typically generated by routine radiological uses in hospitals, universities, biomedical research, pharmaceutical development, and other industrial sources. Civilian nuclear waste (eg, contaminated trash, sludge, resins from the reactor, and irradiated reactor parts) is generated by about 450 nuclear power plants in over 31 countries worldwide. Decommissioning civilian reactors and military bases results primarily in remnant low-level nuclear waste.

▶ Health Effects of Radioactive Waste

Leaking waste from storage facilities at production sites can contaminate the surrounding environment. Although clusters of pediatric leukemia near nuclear plants have been reported worldwide, larger studies have not found convincing evidence for causation with residential proximity to nuclear plants. More detailed information on radiation injuries and acute radiation syndrome are covered in the chapter *Injuries Caused by Physical Hazards*.

▶ Disposal of Radioactive Waste

Radioactive waste does not respond sufficiently to stabilization by chemical, physical, or biological processes. Only time can render radioactive waste inactive. At present, storage appears to be the only means for disposal. Spent fuel from nuclear reactors can be reprocessed, but this involves extracting the uranium and plutonium and results in concentrated fission products that also require disposal. The United States has discontinued reprocessing due to the concern that the extracted plutonium could be diverted for the production of nuclear weapons. However, reprocessing is done in other countries producing nuclear energy in Europe and Asia.

Low-level waste disposal typically occurs in near-surface disposal facilities that are topped with an impermeable cover to prevent emissions and keep rainwater from filtering through the waste. There are not yet any permanent storage facilities for high-level fuel storage facility worldwide. The quantities produced so far are being stored temporarily in cooling pools or dry casks near the generating facilities. In the United States, the development of a long-term storage facility at Yucca Mountain in Nevada has been studied and politically debated since 1987 with still no final resolution. Currently, the Waste Isolation Pilot Plant in New Mexico is the designated location for long-term disposal of low-level transuranic waste from the US nuclear defense program. The waste is stored deep in stable salt beds at the site.

INTERNATIONAL PERSPECTIVES

All countries face hazardous waste issues. The response to these concerns varies according to the social, political, and economic policies of the nation's government and acceptance of international agreements on hazardous waste. Spreading industrialization brings increased locations, quantities, and types of waste production.

▶ Developed Nations

Most industrialized nations have established a national regulatory program that is aimed at protecting human health and the environment from the mismanagement of hazardous waste. Countries may differ in the split of roles between the national government and regional municipalities and how hazardous waste is defined. It is difficult to compare quantities of industrial or hazardous waste in different countries because of varying definitions and surveillance mechanisms. The major elements in a national control system for hazardous waste management are:

- Developing an administrative definition for identifying and classifying hazardous waste to the particular level of detail necessary to support legal procedures
- Defining the responsibilities placed on the waste generator
- Registering or licensing those involved in collection, transport, intermediate storage, treatment, and disposal of hazardous wastes
- Controlling transport, including importing and exporting, using a cradle-to-grave theory
- Developing a national strategy or plan for establishing waste management facilities
- Addressing old or abandoned sites

▶ Developing Countries

Developing countries struggle with management of hazardous waste due to infrastructure hurdles and inadequately enforced laws on dumping. Waste management suffers from poorly regulated industrial production internally and is compounded by shipment of waste from other countries for final disposal in some parts of the world. The practice of moving hazardous waste across borders for disposal disproportionately impacts developing countries. Although global efforts have been made to curb this transboundary waste movement, not all countries have ratified or upheld the agreements. In the late 1980s, the Basel Convention was formed to protect underdeveloped countries from the unjust transmission of hazardous waste into their borders. The Convention now includes 187 parties globally. The initial Convention agreement allowed the movement of waste as long as the receiving countries provided informed consent prior to transfer. An early amendment to the Convention to ban all hazardous waste transfers has not yet been ratified by the number of parties formally required for entry into force.

Electronic waste (e-waste) management is a growing issue as demand and turnover of electronic devices increases. It is estimated that nearly 50 million tons of electronics are discarded annually worldwide. Although Asian countries contribute most to the gross production of e-waste by weight, the per capita generation is highest in Europe. E-waste is considered a hazardous waste, as the metals used to make these devices can have severe consequences on environmental and human health if leached into the environment or handled incorrectly by humans. Some countries have banned dumping of electronics in municipal waste landfills due to the potential for environmental contamination.

The e-waste recycling industry is based on repurposing the valuable metal components in the devices. Although safe methods for the collection and recycling of discarded electronics exist, less than half of the produced e-waste is managed responsibly. Reputable processing facilities conduct recycling of e-waste collected from retail drop-off sites and municipal or commercial pick-up programs in some countries. However, some e-waste collectors ship the devices to developing countries where they are often dismantled by hand using primitive tools, heating, and chemical application. The individuals doing the disassembly work are exposed to heavy metals and other contaminants like lead, cadmium, mercury, chromium, polycyclic aromatic hydrocarbons, PCB, and components of flame retardants. The regions of the world most impacted include communities in Southeast Asia, Africa, and Latin America. Studies of towns conducting significant amounts of e-waste dismantling have found negative health effects on children and fetal health, including preterm birth, impaired growth, decreased cognitive ability, and abnormal temperament.

An inventory of the hazardous waste sites in the developing world is needed to understand the health impacts of these areas. An international nonprofit organization called Pure Earth, formerly the Blacksmith Institute, has taken on the assessment of contaminated locations by training stakeholders in academia and public health to conduct hazardous waste site identification. So far, over 3100 hazardous locations in more than 50 countries have been identified as posing a public health risk. Further understanding of the scope of hazardous waste worldwide is an important step towards meaningful intervention.

REFERENCES

ATSDR. Agency for Toxic Substances and Disease Registry. Case Studies in Environmental Medicine. https://www.atsdr.cdc.gov/csem/csem.html.

CDC. Centers for Disease Control and Prevention. Public Health Emergency Preparedness and Response Capabilities: National Standards for State, Local, Tribal, and Territorial Public Health. October 2018, updated January 2019. https://www.cdc.gov/cpr/readiness/capabilities.htm.

Fazzo L et al: Hazardous waste and health impact: a systematic review of the scientific literature. Environ Health 2017;16(1):107 [PMID: 29020961].

FEMA. Federal Emergency Management Agency. National Incident Management System. https://www.fema.gov/national-incident-management-system.

Occupational Safety and Health Administration. United States Department of Labor. Decontamination. https://www.osha.gov/SLTC/hazardouswaste/training/decon.html.

US EPA. United States Environmental Protection Agency. Superfund: CERCLA overview. https://www.epa.gov/superfund/superfund-cercla-overview.

US EPA. United States Environmental Protection Agency. Toxics Release Inventory (TRI) National Analysis 2017. March 2019. https://www.epa.gov/trinationalanalysis.

Zimmerman JB, Anastas PT, Erythropel HC, Leitner W: Designing for a green chemistry future. Science 2020;367(6476):397-400 [PMID: 31974246].

■ SELF-ASSESSMENT QUESTIONS

Select the one correct answer for each question.

Question 1: Criteria air pollutants (CAPs)
- a. make up all the components of smog
- b. pose few public health risks
- c. include carbon monoxide (CO), sulfur oxides (SOx), and nitrogen oxides (NOx)
- d. are chemicals for which there are no regulatory standards

Question 2: Hazardous air pollutants (HAPs)
- a. are CAPs emitted into the air
- b. are chemicals for which there is no regulatory concern
- c. are formally identified by the EPA
- d. circumvent specific regulatory requirements

Question 3: Superfund Amendments and Reauthorization Act (SARA)
a. replaced the Emergency Planning and Community Right-to-Know Act (EPCRA)
b. gave states the authority above that of the EPA
c. authorizes citizens to block the use of toxic materials in their communities
d. mandates emergency planning for chemical accidents

Question 4: Health impacts of HAPs
a. cannot be inferred from occupational epidemiologic studies
b. cannot be inferred from toxicologic studies in experimental animals
c. do not involve respiratory irritants or systemic toxicants
d. include respiratory disease, systemic toxicity, and carcinogenicity

Question 5: The federal Clean Air Act of 1990
a. fails to reduce overall exposure to toxic air pollutants
b. ignores the stratospheric ozone layer
c. places a cap on the deposition of acidic constituents of air pollution
d. provides for use of market-based principles and other innovative approaches to reducing air pollution

Question 6: Hazardous materials (HAZMAT) teams
a. are licensed by OSHA
b. respond to hazardous materials incidents
c. prefer to perform decontamination in hospitals
d. first remove clothing and rinse the skin with water

Question 7: Emergency response action levels
a. are used to guide shelter-in-place or evacuation decisions
b. determine when it is safe for HAZMAT teams to enter the area

c. define the fatal doses to which individuals are exposed
d. offer absolute safety for officials in charge

Question 8: Protective action guides (PAGs)
a. help officials make critical decisions following a nuclear accident
b. designate the state and local officials who will take actions to safeguard human health during a nuclear accident
c. establish EPA authority in the event of nuclear accident
d. discourage protective actions other than those addressed by the PAGs

Question 9: Hazardous waste
a. is internationally defined to include solids, sludges, liquids, and containerized gases
b. includes domestic sewage, certain nuclear waste, and in situ mining waste
c. exclusions include agricultural wastes used as fertilizers
d. includes most household chemicals

Question 10: Agency for Toxic Substances Disease Registry (ATSDR)
a. was established to reimburse populations exposed to hazardous wastes for their associated health effects
b. has developed several specialized registries to study the long-term health effects of exposure to specific chemicals at hazardous waste sites
c. has selected four hazardous substances for the chemical-specific registries: trichloroethylene, dioxin, benzene, and PCBs
d. has established registries to monitor miners living in Montana and individuals most directly affected by the Love Canal chemical contamination

Building-Related Illness

Rajan Puri, MD, MPH

Richard Wittman, MD, MPH

Indoor air quality (IAQ) can cause or contribute to a variety of symptoms, or even illness, in building occupants, negatively impacting their health and productivity. Americans, on average, spend 90% of their time indoors, where air quality is dependent on local ventilation and conditions. Climate change, extremes of heat and cold, and changes in seasonal conditions impact IAQ, both directly due to changes in moisture and dust content in the air, as well as indirectly due to increased reliance on recycled/conditioned air. In such scenarios, concentrations of some endogenous pollutants inside buildings may exceed standards established for outdoor concentrations.

Building-related illness (BRI) encompasses health problems that develop in nonindustrial settings that are customarily considered nonhazardous, such as homes, schools, and offices. In such settings, indoor air contamination has been linked to a wide variety of building materials and consumer products. In contrast, *sick-building syndrome* (SBS) has been a popular misnomer in past decades, with the label "*sick-building*" previously defined as the occurrence, in more than 20% of the building occupants, of a variety of nonspecific symptoms with minimal or no objective findings that are not linked to a specific diagnosis. Current literature has seen the SBS term drop out of favor, and is considered more part of the nonspecific BRI type.

NATURE, SOURCES, & CONCENTRATIONS OF EXPOSURES

Potential indoor air contaminants can be classified as: (1) contaminants released from the building or its contents, including asbestos, formaldehyde, and radon; (2) contaminants generated by such diverse human activities as cooking, heating, cigarette smoking, and cleaning; and (3) infiltrated contaminants, or agents that enter the house or building along with the outside air, but in lower concentration (typically by 25–75%).

Contaminant concentration is influenced not only by the exposure source but also by the exchange rate between indoor and outdoor air. The introduction of outdoor air into a home or building occurs either by implemented ventilation or by infiltration. Infiltration occurs through cracks or other leaks in the structure or through open doors and windows. The amount of infiltration depends on the type of building, the amount of insulation, and other weather-proofing and climatic conditions. Implemented ventilation, for example, forced-air heating or air-conditioning systems, may provide substantial amounts of outdoor air but also may be designed to recirculate preconditioned air with minimal fresh-air intake.

The amount of air exchange often is expressed in air changes per hour (ACH). ACH may vary from 0.2 in tightly sealed homes to 0.7 in an average home to 60 or more in some industrial settings with implemented ventilation. Alternatively, with implemented ventilation, the amount of outdoor air supplied may be expressed in cubic feet per minute (cfm) per occupant or liters per second per occupant.

The concentration of contaminants at any location within a building will be influenced by the location of the source and the degree of air mixing. In the case of reactive or particulate contaminants, the concentration will be affected by the rate of chemical reaction or the rate of deposition, respectively.

TYPES OF BUILDING-RELATED ILLNESSES & HEALTH CONCERNS

The planning and construction process for buildings typically prioritizes economic, regulatory, and aesthetic drivers, with often limited consideration given to potential health consequences of new building materials and processes. Although demand is increasing for "green" or "organic" materials, most furniture and floor/wall coverings are typically selected without close review of local circulation patterns within a building and without knowledge of the individual health status of its occupants. As such, indoor air concerns are addressed after occupancy has already occurred, which may necessitate a retrofit for improvement.

BRIs are (1) specific, those linked to a known and/or codified exposure or illness; or (2) nonspecific, those for which

Table 53–1. Types of building-associated illness.

Short-latency illnesses
  Sick-building syndrome (SBS) or nonspecific building-related
    illness (nsBRI)
  Mass psychogenic illness
  Building-associated hypersensitivity pneumonitis
  Dampness-associated asthma exacerbations
  Building-associated infections
    Legionnaires disease
    Pontiac fever
    Q fever
  Illnesses associated with specific contaminants
    Formaldehyde
    Carbon monoxide
Possible long-latency illnesses
  Lung cancer
  Chronic nonmalignant respiratory disease

the exposure source and illness is unclear or unknown. Table 53–1 depicts a classification scheme for BRIs, with the principal focus on acute and short-latency illness.

The short-latency illnesses include specific medical conditions resulting from identifiable sources of noxious materials, including certain infectious diseases (such as Legionnaires), building-associated hypersensitivity pneumonitis, dampness-associated asthma exacerbations, and mass psychogenic illness. These conditions are characterized by relatively acute-onset symptoms, closely related in time to the individual's presence within the building, and often relieved or mitigated by their removal from further exposure.

In contrast, the long-latency illnesses include cancer and chronic pulmonary diseases, perhaps resulting from long-term low-level exposure to contaminants in indoor air. The relationship of these long-latency illnesses to indoor air pollution is typically predicated on the basis of mathematical extrapolations from high-dose industrial or animal experimental exposures to substances encountered in much lower doses in building environments. Because of the long induction-latency periods for these conditions and their multifactorial origin, it is much more difficult to establish a causal link to the building exposure.

Agents in indoor air that may be responsible for such illnesses include cigarette smoke, asbestos, radon gas, oxides of nitrogen, polycyclic aromatic hydrocarbons (PAHs), and chlorinated hydrocarbon insecticides. Exposure to tobacco smoke and to indoor asbestos typically occurs at very low levels unless the insulation materials are disturbed or improperly removed. Radon gas from building materials and soil underlying basements or foundations can result in low-level exposure to radioactive elements, increasing lung cancer risk. PAH are released into indoor air from wood-burning fireplaces and other sources and can have carcinogenic effects despite their low-level acute toxicity. Prolonged exposure to certain products of combustion, such as oxides of nitrogen from unvented gas appliances, may increase risk

of respiratory infections and symptomatic asthma as well as reduce performance on pulmonary function testing.

EVALUATION OF BUILDING-RELATED ILLNESS

A guideline prepared by National Institute for Occupational Safety and Health (NIOSH) and U.S. Environmental Protection Agency (EPA) presents approaches to prevention, investigation, and management of IAQ problems. The Indoor Air Quality Building Education and Assessment Model (I-BEAM) updates and expands EPA's Building Air Quality (BAQ) guidance, and is designed to be a comprehensive guidance for managing IAQ in commercial buildings.

Proper assessment of illnesses relating to IAQ involves both evaluation of the symptoms, usually by a physician, and assessment of the physical work environment, usually by an industrial hygienist. A symptom questionnaire may be helpful in establishing the nature, chronology, and frequency of complaints; the temporal relationship to an individual's presence in the building; the locations at which complaints arise; any incidents or activities that preceded the complaints; and the coexistence of any medical problems or risk factors that might account for some of the symptoms. Analysis of the symptom data, with grouping of symptoms into categories and a search for factors associated with symptom occurrence across the population, is essential.

Industrial hygiene evaluation usually begins with gathering of background information on the building, such as its age, type of construction, ventilation system design, and history of problems, renovations, and repairs. A walk-through survey will give a deeper understanding of the floor plan and the physical locations at which symptoms have occurred, as well as inspection of the ventilation system and any possible point sources of air contaminants. These sources may include 3D- printers, blueprint machines, cleaning supplies, areas of microbial growth, and cafeteria equipment and exhaust (including cooking odors). Water intrusion history, which could lead to mold growth, should always be included in the survey.

ENVIRONMENTAL MONITORING

Targeted environmental monitoring may be helpful in assessing the adequacy of ventilation, including the extent of fresh versus recirculated air, and temperature and humidity control. Minimal equipment is required for this monitoring— a room thermometer and relative humidity (RH) meter, smoke tubes to assess air movement, and direct-reading carbon dioxide colorimetric detector tubes. Because carbon dioxide is a product of respiratory metabolism, its accumulation in office buildings reflects a balance between generation by building occupants and removal through ventilation and introduction of fresh outdoor air. Measurement of CO_2 levels aids in evaluating whether sufficient quantities of fresh air are being introduced into the building.

The outdoor concentration of CO_2 varies typically from 250 to 500 parts per million (ppm), with increased levels in urban/industrial setting, reflective of contaminant sources and/or combustion. Both the American National Standards Institute (ANSI) and the American Society of Heating, Refrigerating, and Air Conditioning Engineers (ASHRAE) have issued consensus standards regarding the relationship between indoor and outdoor CO_2 levels, with 2016 guidance supporting that steady-state indoor CO_2 concentrations less than or equal to 700 ppm above outdoor air levels will dilute odors and other irritants to satisfy 80% of indoor visitors. This approximates a ventilation rate of 7.5 L/s/person (15 cfm/person), which generally will keep CO_2 levels below 1000 ppm.

In prior building investigations, levels above 1000 ppm often were associated with perceptions of poor air quality and complaints of headache and mucous membrane irritation. Although the CO_2 itself is not responsible for these symptoms, a high concentration suggests that other air contaminant levels are likely to be increased; in other words, the CO_2 level serves as a surrogate measure for the adequacy of fresh air ventilation and the presence of other as yet unidentified contaminants likely to be the cause of these symptoms.

IAQ complaints occur occasionally with concentrations of CO_2 as low as 700–800 ppm, which is not surprising as CO_2 levels are not impacted by volatile organic compound offgassing from furniture and other materials. Increasing the fresh-air ventilation rate to 25 cfm per person will reduce the CO_2 concentration below this level, often resulting in subsidence of symptoms. Table 53–2 lists some guidelines for factors having an impact on IAQ.

In 2017, ASHRAE issued its most recent guidelines for temperature and humidity control. These describe six conditions that impact thermal comfort for most indoor space occupants: (1) metabolic rate, (2) clothing insulation, (3) air temperature, (4) radiant temperature, (5) air speed, and (6) humidity. The first two conditions represent characteristics of the occupants and can be impacted by underlying medical conditions and choice of clothing, respectively. The latter four, which represent occupant environment characteristics of the local environment, are not independent conditions, as the acceptable temperature range varies with the RH.

ASHRAE also has issued guidelines for provision of adequate amounts of fresh outside air. In the current 2016 ventilation guideline, outside air should be provided in office areas at a rate of 17 cfm per occupant (remains slightly reduced from prior guidelines of 20 cfm per occupant), which amounts to about 8.5 L/s per occupant of outside air. Recent consensus recommendations recommend much higher fresh air intake in offices, up to 25 L/s.

In 2018, the project "Health-Based Ventilation Guidelines for Europe" proposed new ventilation guidelines that can be used as a foundation on which to improve exposure control and achieve IAQ goals by utilizing explicit health criteria. This new approach to the built environment advocates different strategies for controlling IAQ that examines not only the building but also its surroundings, whether rural or urban. This approach recognizes that the IAQ of a given indoor space is the result of interactions between the outdoor

Table 53–2. Relevant guidelines for indoor air quality.

Factor	Guideline/Study Finding	Comment
Temperature	See text 72°F	ASHRAE Standard 55, 2017 Reduced prevalence of sick-building syndrome symptoms
Relative humidity	30–60%	ASHRAE Standard 55, 2017
Fresh outside air (ventilation)	17 cfm per occupant or 8.5 L/s Up to 25 L/s	ASHRAE Standard 62.1, 2016 Sundell, 2011
Carbon dioxide	≥ 1000 ppm, or ≥ 700 ppm differential between indoors and outdoors ≤ 650 ppm	Perception of poor air quality and increased symptoms Improved occupant satisfaction
Carbon monoxide	9 ppm (8 h)	Outdoor air standard from NAAQS/EPA
Total volatile organic compounds (TVOCs)	No guideline	Indoor Air Quality Guidelines for selected Volatile Organic Compounds (VOCs) in the UK
Formaldehyde	0.1 ppm 0.05 ppm	Residential air quality guideline from Health Canada Residential level to avoid irritation in allergic and asthmatic individuals from California Air Resources Board
Particulates < 2.5 μm < 10 μm	65 mcg/m³ over 24 h 150 mcg/m³ over 24 h	Outdoor air standard from NAAQS/EPA

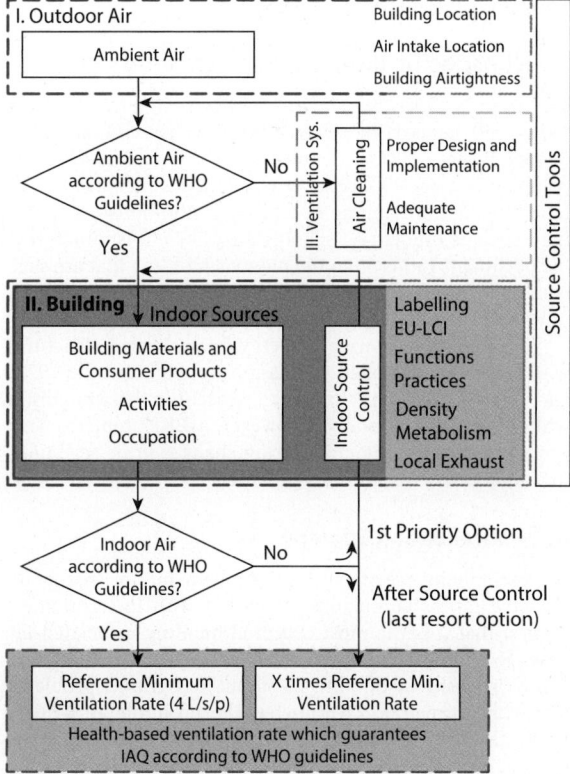

▲ Figure 53–1. Decision diagram for deriving the adequate health-based ventilation rate for a specific building.

air, the building itself, and the system that provides ventilation, Figure 53–1. Their approach references the WHO air quality guidelines, with a base ventilation rate of 4 L/s.

In many cases where environmental monitoring is considered, conducting these simple evaluations and measurements will be sufficient to assess likely sources of problems. Further and more specific air sampling should be performed if significant sources of air contaminants are identified or suspected. In the absence of such point sources, however, it may be unlikely that extensive untargeted industrial hygiene sampling will identify an unrecognized contaminant in concentrations sufficient to cause symptoms. Moreover, in part because of the very high sensitivity of available analytic methodology, sampling invariably detects some contaminants, often in the low-ppb range. These results may raise concerns in building occupants and may not explain symptoms or identify the cause of the building problem. A transparent and balanced risk-communication approach, with frequent updates to the concerned parties, reduces the anxiety and helplessness that building occupants might feel when concerned about a harmful exposure.

RESULTS OBTAINED FROM BUILDING INVESTIGATIONS

Analysis of accumulated experience from multiple IAQ investigations facilitates an understanding of the relative frequency of different causal factors, permitting prioritization of building investigation approaches. In a landmark compilation of building air quality investigations, the NIOSH reported the results of approximately 500 evaluations conducted during the 1980s of buildings with IAQ problems. Although they recognized that some of the problems may have had multiple causes, the NIOSH investigators classified the results by the primary identified cause, as follows:

- Inadequate ventilation: 52%
- Contamination from inside building: 16%
- Contamination from outside building: 10%
- Microbial contamination: 5%
- Contamination from building fabric: 4%
- Unknown sources: 13%

In 32% of the evaluations, building ventilation was found to be inadequate, as evidenced by inadequate fresh-air intake, poor air distribution and mixing, draftiness, poor temperature and humidity control, pressure differences between office spaces, or air filtration problems. Inside contamination from various types of wet copiers, improper pesticide application, improper use of cleaning agents such as rug shampoo, tobacco smoke, combustion gases (eg, from food preparation areas), and the like accounted for ~16% of the problems. Such contaminants were present at levels above the normal background but far below any permissible exposure limits. Building materials were the source of contaminants in 3% of the investigations, including such things as particle board, plywood, and some glues and adhesives.

Outside contamination sources were the primary factor in ~10% of the investigations, generally a result of entrainment of contaminated outside air as a result of improperly located exhaust and intake vents or contaminant generation near intake vents. A commonly identified source was the entrainment of vehicle exhaust fumes from parking garages into the air intake vent. Other contaminants included boiler gases, previously exhausted air, and asphalt from roofing operations.

Although they did not list it as a primary cause, the NIOSH investigators indicated that tobacco smoke may have been a major contributor to IAQ problems largely because it contains numerous odoriferous and irritant compounds. Because of nonsmoking policies implemented in many workplaces and other locations in recent years, environmental tobacco smoke is now a less frequent contributor to IAQ problems in nonresidential buildings.

Microbiological contamination accounted for 3% of the problems, resulting from standing water in ventilation system components or from water damage to carpets or other furnishings. A variety of disorders—including hypersensitivity pneumonitis, humidifier fever, allergic rhinitis, asthma, and allergic conjunctivitis—can arise from microbial contaminants.

MICROBIAL CONTAMINATION

As referenced earlier, certain infectious diseases that are noncommunicable may be transmitted in indoor air. Legionnaires disease—a multisystem disease dominated by pneumonia—is caused by the bacterial organism *Legionella pneumophila* and occasionally other *Legionella* species. Pontiac fever, also caused by *L pneumophila*, is an influenza-like illness characterized by fever, chills, headache, myalgias, and sometimes cough and sore throat. Most reported cases are sporadic, with only about 11% of cases associated with an outbreak of illness.

Most commonly, building-associated outbreaks result from contaminated aerosols, usually disseminated in the ventilation system from cooling towers, evaporative condensers, humidifiers, and air-conditioning systems. Other sources of aerosols include decorative fountains, whirlpool hot tubs, and produce misters in grocery stores. *Legionella* species can be cultured in up to 40% of cooling towers, although infections stemming from exposure to the aerosols are reported uncommonly. *Legionella* bacteria thrive in water systems maintained at warm temperatures between approximately 26.7°C (80°F) and 48.9°C (120°F). Proper cleaning and maintenance of these potential sources is critical in preventing outbreaks of Legionnaires disease.

The appropriate investigation and management of a building and its occupants, when one or more individuals are found to have *Legionella* infection, may find the source of exposure to be in the community outside the workplace. Nevertheless, it is appropriate to begin a building investigation and to inquire about compatible illnesses in other building occupants, referring those with symptoms for medical care. Investigation of the building involves identification of relevant elements in the water and ventilation systems, particularly those from which aerosolization could occur, and testing the water by culture for *Legionella*. Any likely source then should be cleaned properly and decontaminated with chlorine or other biocides. If such decontamination can occur promptly, the facility typically can remain open and operational while the investigation proceeds. Characterization of isolated organisms from water systems and from the case patient by species and serogroup may provide evidence for or against a link with the building.

Q fever, caused by the rickettsial organism *Coxiella burnetii*, has been responsible for several building-associated outbreaks. The animal reservoirs for this infection typically are sheep, goats, and cattle, and less commonly cats, dogs, and rabbits. Airborne transmission of organisms from animal excreta and products of parturition to humans has occurred via ventilation systems in animal-handling and medical research facilities.

SHORT-LATENCY ILLNESSES

▶ Nonspecific Building-Related Illness

The term *sick-building syndrome* was first termed in the 1970s and henceforth referred to as *nonspecific building-related illness (nsBRI)*, denotes a spectrum of nonspecific complaints, typically headache and mucous membrane irritation, recognized among occupants of nonindustrial buildings, such as offices and schools. In a likely misnomer, it is the occupants rather than the physical building that are sick, with symptoms often temporally related to the occupant's physical proximity to the implicated office space.

In an effort to conserve energy, many sealed structures with centrally controlled ventilation were built in the 1970s and 1980s. Initially, nsBRI tended to occur in these buildings without operable windows. However, nsBRI problems continue to occur despite engineering changes in newer buildings to improve outside air ventilation.

A. Occurrence and Etiology

The exact incidence of nsBRI is unknown, but the frequently reported illness complaints consistent with this condition suggest that it is the most common building-associated illness. Symptoms that occupants relate to a building are common, even in buildings without recognized problems and with normal IAQ parameters. For example, in a questionnaire study of four nonproblem state-owned buildings in Washington State, 55% of the 646 respondents reported recent upper respiratory symptoms temporally related to being at work, including dry eyes, nasal symptoms, and dry or sore throat. Forty-eight percent reported central nervous system symptoms, including commonly headache, unusual tiredness, tension, and mental fatigue. These symptoms were associated with such factors as perception of the air as too dry or too stagnant and the workspace as too noisy. Symptoms were not correlated with measured air contaminant levels.

There are a variety of known and suspected contributing factors to the development of nsBRI, including physical and chemical factors as well as biological and host considerations.

1. Physical factors

VENTILATION—It is commonly held that natural ventilation no longer provides optimal distribution of fresh air. Thus, building designers place great emphasis on adequate heating, ventilation, and air-conditioning (HVAC) and mechanical ventilation systems. However, it is this common feature present in most afflicted buildings that is of interest due to air recirculation possibly shifting pollutants. Historically, these buildings often had low outdoor air ventilation rates, below 20 cfm per occupant (or about 10 L/s per occupant). However, nsBRI does occur in buildings that meet current ventilation and temperature control standards. A widely held theory is that suboptimal ventilation, in some cases below ventilation standards, permits the accumulation of low levels of many contaminants—volatile organic compounds (both nonreactive, such as toluene, and reactive, such as formaldehyde, ozone, cigarette smoke, dust-including ultrafine particles, microbial contaminants, and the like) that together induce the symptoms. Contaminants with low odor threshold may particularly contribute to symptoms, even when air concentrations are well below irritation thresholds.

Increasing fresh-air ventilation rates reduces the frequency and intensity of nsBRI symptoms. Further, lower ventilation rates appear to be associated with airway inflammation, respiratory infections, asthma symptoms, and sick-leave absences. At low outdoor-air ventilation rates, increases in the outdoor-air ventilation rates will reduce levels of contaminants, symptoms, and potentially respiratory conditions. The presence of an air-conditioning system is often associated with increased reporting of nsBRI symptoms when compared with naturally or other mechanically ventilated buildings. A study by NIOSH of 80 buildings found an association between dirty HVAC systems and nsBRI symptoms. The NIOSH study also emphasized that improperly maintained ventilation systems increase the adverse health effects among the occupants, particularly amongst asthmatics, due to exposure of accumulated indoor pollutants and microbiological growth.

TEMPERATURE AND HUMIDITY—There is largely consistent evidence supporting an association of increased room temperature and nsBRI symptoms, including eye and mucous membrane dryness and irritation, with a strong relationship between temperature increases, even within the "comfort zone," and symptoms. One large study suggested that temperature elevations in winter may be particularly problematic. However, the authors also found that symptoms increased and thermal comfort decreased when buildings were over-cooled in summer. Thus, there is a need to consider the impact of temperature in all observational and experimental studies evaluating IAQ.

Dryness of the indoor air, both perceived dryness and actual dryness, may contribute to some of the symptoms of nsBRI. The sensation of dryness in many cases actually reflects the presence of higher air temperature and probably dust and air contaminants, with a lesser impact from lower RH. In some cases, increasing air humidity when the RH is low has reduced the sensation of dryness and symptoms related to dryness. Dryness of indoor air appears to interact with work activities, such as prolonged computer/monitor usage, to increase the frequency of eye complaints. Given that RH often falls in indoor environments during the heating season, low humidity may play a significant role in the induction of symptoms of nsBRI (particularly mucous membrane symptoms) in some situations. On the other hand, high RH may lead to the apparent adverse impacts noted in some studies due to increased fungal, other microbial, and dust-mite growth, which could contribute to nsBRI symptoms and other problems. Humidifiers provide a potential site for microbial growth. Thus moderate levels of RH, in the range of 35–45%, appear most desirable.

For office workers working at a RH of 30%, the acceptable temperature lies between 20.5°C and 25.5°C (69°F and 78°F) during the heating season and between 24.5°C and 28°C (76°F and 82°F) in the cooling season. In an office environment, the desired RH is between 30% and 60%. RH levels below 20% often result in drying of mucous membranes, with associated discomfort, whereas levels above 60% support mold growth. Depending on the ventilation system design, there may be localized areas within buildings that fall outside the comfortable range even though the rest of the building is controlled adequately.

The role of sunlight cannot be underscored. Sunlight is known to be bactericidal and mutagenic to a variety of potential airborne organisms including *staphylococci*, *streptococci*, and *Mycoplasma tuberculosis*. Sunlight from building windows contributing to solar radiation is usually lethal to potential sources of infection within a few hours. Thus, the addition of windows to existing and new buildings should be a welcome addition not only for cosmetic and psychological reasons, but also for documented infection prevention.

2. Chemical factors—It appears that low levels (below ACGIH- and NIOSH-recommended indices) of chemical contaminants present in indoor air do contribute, in some cases, to nsBRI. Despite extensive measurements for a wide variety of possible contaminants, however, few substances have been found to be consistently implicated in different nsBRI environments in concentrations judged sufficient to induce symptoms.

An exception to these findings may be the presence of formaldehyde (and potentially other biologically and chemically reactive contaminants). Formaldehyde is present in, and will evaporate from, resins in particle board and plywood (used in furniture and construction materials) and furnishings (including carpets and draperies), as well as from urea-formaldehyde foam insulation used previously to insulate homes. Indoor air concentrations as low as 50–100 ppb have been shown to cause mucous membrane irritation, including in epidemiologic studies in mobile homes and other structures.

Although the majority of indoor emissions generally come from interior surfaces such as ceilings, walls, and floors, there are a number of other potential sources for air contaminants in the office environment. Volatile organic compounds (VOCs) may evaporate from carpet glues and drying paints or from adhesives used on the contact surfaces of building products. Releases from photocopiers, including ozone, and other office equipment also may contribute to the symptoms. Chamber studies suggest that complex mixtures of VOCs at relatively low concentrations can lead to symptoms of mucous membrane irritation and perhaps other symptoms such as headaches. Some building studies have suggested a correlation between exposure to low-level VOC mixtures, particularly for those chemically and biologically reactive VOCs, and irritant symptoms. There is evidence that these reactive VOCs, including formaldehyde and terpenes (released from furniture and citrus and pine oils used in cleaning products), react chemically with ozone and oxides of nitrogen in indoor air to form more irritating oxidized chemicals.

Moreover, odors from chemicals, including VOCs, and from other sources, including mold or other microbial growth (including microbial VOCs), may contribute independently to nsBRI symptoms. Unpleasant odors are reported frequently by occupants of problem buildings. Odors are known to be capable of causing irritation, headaches, nausea, and other symptoms in the absence of toxicologically significant concentrations, with mechanisms that may include odor annoyance, anxiety about their source and potential associated hazards, and conditioned responses. Unlike the induction of irritation caused by indoor VOCs or other contaminants, for which there is a latency requiring prolonged exposure, odors may induce symptoms immediately on entering an environment.

The presence of increased dust in the indoor environment has been associated with increased reporting of nsBRI symptoms in some studies. There is some suggestion that symptoms may be associated with inadequate cleaning practices, as well as some evidence that thorough office cleaning may reduce nsBRI symptoms. However, some interventions to reduce dust, such as HEPA filtration of air, have not been shown to reduce symptoms.

Carbon monoxide in buildings may be the cause of mild symptoms, such as headache and nausea, or more severe, potentially life-threatening intoxication. Incomplete combustion in defective gas furnaces or unvented gas stoves and other appliances, typically in residences, may be the source of significant indoor emissions of carbon monoxide. In addition to the potential for acute intoxication, long-term low-level exposure can cause recurrent subacute symptoms, such as headaches. Attentiveness to these symptoms, when temporally related to presence in a building, may help to identify and eliminate previously unrecognized CO exposure sources. Less commonly, carbon monoxide may be entrained from the outside via air intakes in the vicinity of vehicle loading docks.

3. Biological factors—There is some evidence that exposure to damp buildings and to molds may be a contributor to symptoms of nsBRI. Some studies indicate an association between dampness and certain nonspecific symptoms, such as headache and fatigue. There has been some study of the potential role of exposure to mold and mold products—fungal glucans and microbial VOCs (responsible for some of the mold odor)—in the induction of nsBRI symptoms. These findings suggest a possible role for dampness and mold in the induction of symptoms, at least in buildings with moisture problems. However, the role of mold exposures, including the role of mycotoxins and microbial VOCs, remains unclear.

4. Host factors—Individuals with atopy appear to develop more mucosal irritation symptoms, an observation supported by chamber studies demonstrating reactions to lower concentrations of irritants than for non-atopics. Contact lens wearers tend to be more prone to eye irritation. With regard to gender, studies have reported that women have a higher prevalence of nonspecific BRI than men. This may be due to a variety of exposures in the office environment from different work tasks, or differences in personality traits. Interestingly, age has not been demonstrated to show a consistent association with nonspecific BRI.

Personal interviews and physical examinations of affected employees may be useful to elucidate other disease contributors to the ascribed symptoms, including autoimmune conditions, thyroid abnormalities, obstructive sleep apnea, work stress, general environmental allergy, and insomnia.

5. Work organization and psychosocial factors—A variety of work organization and psychosocial characteristics, including absence of varied work, dissatisfaction with the supervisor, little influence on the organization, high work speed, and reported general and work stress, are associated with the prevalence of symptoms, both mucosal irritation and general symptoms. Other factors that have been identified as affecting the perception of the indoor environment include noise, overcrowding, the degree of management response to IAQ complaints, and the sense of empowerment to be heard or effect change.

There is likely to be a complex interaction of these various factors in the induction of the symptoms of nsBRI, for example, the concurrent presence of low humidity levels, higher temperature, low levels of multiple air contaminants (for prolonged time periods), and odors, as well as work organization factors and psychological factors. Table 53–3 lists possible causative factors for the nsBRI.

B. Clinical Findings

Atopic subjects, with a history or findings consistent with allergic rhinitis or asthma, in general seem to be more prone to develop symptoms in association with indoor air-quality problems. The most common symptoms are those associated with mucous membrane irritation and headaches. Eye irritation, difficulty in wearing contact lenses, nasal and sinus irritation and congestion, throat irritation, chest tightness or burning, nausea, headache, dizziness, and fatigue are common complaints. As noted above, some symptoms may be psychophysiological in origin. Physical findings are minimal, consisting perhaps of mild injection of the oropharyngeal or conjunctival mucous membranes. Laboratory studies, including spirometry and chest radiographs, are typically normal.

Often symptoms occur shortly after entering the building and are relieved soon after leaving. It should be emphasized that while many of these symptoms are nonspecific with multiple potential causes (including host and nonbuilding factors), a temporal association of symptoms with presence in the work environment suggests that there are etiologic factors worthy of consideration.

C. Building Evaluation, Treatment, and Prevention

An understanding of potential contributing factors provides the rationale for a targeted multidisciplinary approach to

Table 53–3. Postulated causative or contributing factors to sick-building syndrome.

Category	Factor

Building factors	Contaminants
	   Volatile organic compounds
	   Formaldehyde
	   Odors
	   Dust
	   Microbial agents
	   Other contaminants
	Inadequate fresh air ventilation
	Central ventilation system with no operable windows
	Elevated or reduced relative humidity
	High temperature
	Carpeting
	Noise

Host factors	Atopy (hay fever/asthma) Contact lens use Female gender Psychological conditions
Work factors	Job stress Lack of control of work/environment Dissatisfaction with the supervisor Absence of varied work Job satisfaction diminished by quantity of work High work speed Little influence on the organization

building evaluation. The proper approach in an individual problem building involves an iterative approach. One should start with the simplest activities, such as interviews of affected employees and a building walk-through to assess ventilation and to look for potential sources of exposure, as discussed in the section on building evaluation.

For the individual patient, treatment consists of explanation of the possible sources and removal from the environment until the source of symptoms is determined. Follow-up with the employer to determine if the building materials may be a source of indoor contamination, with investigation of the heating and ventilation system is usually warranted. Fear about potential exposures and uncertainty about their health significance may cause anxiety that may amplify symptoms.

Building interventions, such as reduction in room temperature to the lower end of the comfort zone, should be considered. If the outdoor-air ventilation rate is low (below 10 L/s, or about 20 cfm per occupant), efforts to increase outdoor-air intake could be considered. Recommendations for the optimal outdoor-air ventilation rate vary. There is some support for conducting thorough cleaning of office areas, ideally during periods of low occupancy, and using cleaning materials with low volatility and odor. Especially with new or newly renovated buildings, there is some empirical support for "purging" the building, that is, maximizing ventilation with

the system set for maximum fresh-air intake and raising temperatures in the building, while the building is unoccupied. In addition to reducing the occurrence of symptoms, there is evidence that interventions to improve air quality have led to improvements in productivity. The occurrence of building-related symptoms tends to reduce subjective and objective measures of productivity and to increase absenteeism. This suggests that interventions to improve air quality may be justifiable not only to increase occupant comfort but also on cost-benefit grounds.

Depending on the nature of the problem identified, other changes may be necessary, such as relocation of air-intake vents or alteration in cleaning or pesticide application practices. Prevention would appear to require balancing energy-conservation concerns with the need to provide adequate fresh-air intake rates when designing ventilation systems. Open communications of findings and any remediation plans to the group and responsiveness to employee concerns should be considered important interventions for nsBRI. One should attempt to follow general recommendations for health risk communication in these situations.

BUILDING-ASSOCIATED HYPERSENSITIVITY PNEUMONITIS

Hypersensitivity pneumonitis (HP) is a form of interstitial lung disease characterized pathologically by lymphocytic and granulomatous infiltration of alveolar walls that results from inhalation of a variety of organic dusts. HP has been reported in a number of individuals in homes or offices where mold or bacteria had been allowed to grow on humidifiers or air conditioners. Attack rates in such outbreaks have varied from up to 70% of the exposed population.

A. Occurrence and Etiology

HP is an immunologic disorder triggered by repeated inhalation exposures to a foreign antigen that probably results from a combination of immunopathogenic mechanisms. In building-associated HP, a number of agents and antigens are implicated, including bacteria (thermophilic actinomycetes such as *Thermoactinomyces vulgaris* and *Micropolyspora faeni*), fungi (*Aspergillus, Penicillium, Alternaria,* and others), and amebas (*Naegleria* and *Acanthamoeba*). Pigeon antigen has also been reported to cause acute and chronic HP in homes and workplaces. The source of antigens usually is contaminated ventilation systems. Less commonly, persistently moist carpets, furnishings, and surfaces from water leaks in occupied areas are implicated.

B. Clinical Findings

The symptoms, signs, and laboratory and imaging findings in building-associated HP are not different than in other types of HP, other than the observation that symptoms and signs in acute HP are temporally related to presence in the affected building.

C. Diagnosis

The presence of serum-precipitating antibodies to suspected microbial antigens is of limited usefulness in that it documents intense and extensive exposure but does not indicate the presence of clinical pulmonary disease. Such antibodies may be seen in asymptomatic individuals, and some individuals with HP may have negative precipitin tests.

In a study of HP in office workers exposed to a contaminated air cooling system, shortness of breath and fever were present in all the affected individuals. If the onset of these two symptoms was in close temporal association with exposure to the workplace, this finding was even more suggestive of HP. Because dyspnea and fever are uncommon in nsBRI, the presence of these symptoms in one or more individuals in a building should trigger concern about possible HP. Similarly, abnormal findings on chest imaging procedures or pulmonary function tests (particularly reductions in the diffusing capacity for carbon monoxide) in individuals whose respiratory symptoms are temporally related to presence in a building should strongly suggest this diagnosis. Such findings would not be expected with most other types of building-associated illness, including nsBRI.

D. Treatment

Avoidance of further exposure by removal from the building environment usually results in resolution of symptoms and abnormalities, unless the disease has progressed to a chronic stage. In some outbreaks, extensive cleanup efforts, including removal of contaminated items and alteration of ventilation systems, have allowed the return of affected workers without recurrence of symptoms.

MOLD & DAMP INDOOR ENVIRONMENTS

Dampness in buildings results in conditions that favors the growth of dust mites and mold. Exposure to dust mite allergens, primarily in homes, is associated with the occurrence of inhalant allergies in susceptible individuals. Molds are ubiquitous in the outdoor and indoor environment, including in the air. There has been a considerable amount of interest in the possible health effects of building dampness and indoor mold in buildings. *Cladosporium, Penicillium, Aspergillus,* and *Alternaria* are the most common genera of mold identified indoors during building investigations, all of which arise from outdoor sources but which proliferate indoors on some surfaces in the presence of dampness or water damage.

Exposure to fungi in indoor environments can elicit IgE antibodies to certain molds, and an IgE-mediated hypersensitivity response may cause allergic symptoms, including upper airway irritation, eye irritation, rhinitis, sinusitis, and asthma. There is strong evidence that exposure to mold and damp indoor spaces cause and/or aggravate allergic disease in children, and probably in adults. Epidemiologic studies indicate significant associations between visible dampness or mold and upper respiratory symptoms, cough, wheeze, and asthma exacerbations. Under certain circumstances,

many molds produce mold toxins or mycotoxins, which sometimes may become airborne—this includes a number of common indoor fungi, including *Aspergillus, Cladosporium, Penicillium,* and *Stachybotrys* species. There has been considerable scientific inquiry and speculation, news media attention, and litigation regarding the relationship between exposure to mycotoxins in buildings and alleged illness. In particular, exposure to *Stachybotrys* species (black mold or "toxic" mold) has generated considerable interest, although it is identified in buildings and homes less commonly than the above mold species. If discovered to be notably present in an indoor setting, where it typically is found on drywall and fiberboard in the presence of moisture, *Stachybotrys* removal is generally recommended, if not in part due to multiple animal studies reporting its relationship to lung inflammation, allergic sensitization, and pulmonary cytotoxicity.

A. Building Evaluation for Mold Exposure

A high level of scrutiny is important when investigating dampness, water damage, and mold growth issues. The initial approach involves a thorough walk-through of the building, searching for sources of water intrusion and visible evidence of mold growth on surfaces, such as walls. Sampling of suspect contamination, for example, on wall surfaces, can confirm the presence and type of fungi present. Further investigation may not be necessary, especially if the factors leading to water intrusion can be corrected and mold growth can be readily identified and remediated.

While air sampling can be performed, it is not generally required. There are two primary methods of air sampling, nonviable and viable testing, results of which are expressed in spores and colony-forming units (CFUs) per cubic meter of air, respectively. Air sampling may be useful to confirm a source for documented hypersensitivity in an individual. In general, a health hazard is present if the indoor level of airborne mold species is greater than an outside control sample. Higher concentrations of fungi indoors compared with concurrent outdoor sampling suggests that there is a source of biomagnification/growth within the building that requires remediation.

B. Clinical Findings and Diagnosis

The clinical findings and diagnosis of allergic respiratory disease (and potentially de novo asthma) related to dampness and exposure to mites and mold are identical to those for other types of allergic disorders. In addition, some individuals may report symptoms of headache, fatigue, and cognitive impairment in association with mold exposure. Diagnosis may be aided by performance of skin prick tests to detect IgE specific to fungal allergens or serologic testing for IgE antibodies to fungal allergens, although such testing is limited by the availability of standardized fungal antigens, cross-reactivity among fungi, and the occurrence of false-positive and false-negative tests. These tests need to be interpreted carefully in conjunction with the history and physical findings. Inflammatory markers and other diagnostic studies of immunological of systemic disease have not been well correlated with mold exposure and should not be used for clinical decision-making.

C. Treatment and Building Remediation

Treatment for mold-related allergic disease is similar to that for other allergic conditions. When mold or damp conditions are demonstrated, removal from exposure is essential—either by environmental remediation or removing the individual from the environment. Given the evidence that mold and damp conditions may cause allergic disorders in children, removal from the source of exposure is especially important if children are present in the home. After remediation is performed, repeat assessment by an environmental specialist may be useful to determine if return to the environment can be advised. Generally, allergic disorders caused or aggravated by mold improve and/or resolve within several weeks after exposure ceases.

Mold prevention measures for new buildings should include (a) minimizing moisture accumulation in construction materials, (b) maintaining the integrity of building impermeable envelope, and (c) ensuring the effectiveness of the HVAC system to control thermal comfort and RH. For existing buildings, corrective measures could include (a) repair and maintenance of water leakage in ceilings, walls, and draining systems, (b) deep cleaning of building interiors and HVAC systems, (c) control of the reservoirs of visible mold in ceiling and carpets, and (d) periodic assessment of IAQ. In any highly suspicious case of mold intrusion, a plan should include (a) rectifying the underlying moisture problem, (b) mitigating contamination spread by cleaning ventilation pathways and enhancing ventilation to remove any indoor pollutants, and (c) removing visible moldy materials by excising large areas around the concerned site, for example, drywall, ceiling tile, ensuring a clean border.

MASS PSYCHOGENIC ILLNESS

Mass psychogenic (or sociogenic) illness is an illness of psychophysiologic origin occurring simultaneously in a group of individuals. Less-satisfactory terms include *mass hysteria* and *behavioral contagion*.

A. Occurrence and Etiology

Episodes felt to represent building-associated mass psychogenic illness have rarely occurred in office buildings, light industrial facilities, and electronics plants. The incidence of these illnesses is unknown. The precise cause, though unknown, would appear to involve the occurrence of an appropriate stimulus or trigger in a psychologically susceptible or anxious population. The trigger often is an unexplained odor. Concern that the odor represents a toxic gas or other threat may initiate psychophysiologic symptoms in some individuals. Individuals must perceive the threat to be credible in order to be affected. Because the trigger may be low levels of a respiratory irritant or an irritating odor,

symptoms of nonspecific BRI may occur concurrently. Thus, nonspecific BRI and mass psychogenic illness may occur simultaneously or sequentially in the same building incident. While nonspecific BRI symptoms tend to occur in individuals who appear to be most exposed to the suspected environmental causal factors, building-associated mass psychogenic illness is transmitted within specific social networks in the workplace.

Episodes of mass psychogenic illness have occurred in groups of workers in jobs they perceive as stressful, often with repetitive work and physical stress. Some evidence suggests that individuals who have lived and worked under high levels of stress and anxiety, often long prior to the illness outbreak, may be more prone to the development of mass psychogenic illness. These individuals attribute their symptoms of psychophysiologic origin to a possible toxic hazard from a problem building or a noxious odor.

B. Clinical Findings

Symptoms commonly reported in investigations of outbreaks felt to represent mass psychogenic illness include headaches, dizziness, light-headedness, drowsiness, and nausea; dry mouth and throat; eye, nose, and throat irritation and chest tightness; and weakness, numbness, and tingling. There are few or no physical or laboratory findings. Of note, the illness in the index case or cases may be a result of actual exposure to an unpleasant odor or noxious substance or to a nonoccupational cause, for example, a viral syndrome.

In contrast to nsBRI, symptoms often do not resolve promptly when the individual leaves the building. One should use caution in applying the label of mass psychogenic illness to an outbreak of building-related symptoms, given the similarity of symptoms to those of nsBRI and the frequent occurrence of psychophysiologic symptoms in nsBRI.

Certain features strongly suggest the diagnosis of mass psychogenic illness. The symptoms are difficult to explain on an organic basis and are not consistent with the toxicologic properties of any suspected contaminants. There is a high level of anxiety in the group. The attack rate generally is higher among women than among men. There is a visual or auditory chain of transmission. Despite apparent severity and sudden onset of illness, the illnesses are consistently benign and without sequelae.

C. Treatment

Investigation of the building is indicated to exclude the presence of significant contaminants, with the investigation scope dependent on the potential sources of exposure. Because it may take a few weeks to conduct an investigation and obtain results of air or ventilation system performance, it may be necessary to consider closure of the building or area. Removing employees from the area of concern also may reduce anxiety and transmission of symptoms to others. Early, open, and frequent communication with concerned individuals is important.

REFERENCES

Caillaud D, Leynaert B, Keirsbulck M, Nadif R, mould ANSES working group: Indoor mould exposure, asthma and rhinitis: findings from systematic reviews and recent longitudinal studies. Eur Respir Rev 2018;27(148):170137 [PMID: 29769295].

California Department of Public Health Indoor Air Quality Section. https://www.cdph.ca.gov/Programs/CCDPHP/DEODC/EHLB/IAQ/Pages/Mold-FAQs.aspx.

Cox-Ganser JM: Indoor dampness and mould health effects—ongoing questions on microbial exposures and allergic versus nonallergic mechanisms. Clin Exp Allergy 2015;45(10):1478-1482. [PMID: 26372722].

Lawrence Berkeley National Laboratory's Indoor Air Quality Scientific Findings Resource Bank. https://iaqscience.lbl.gov/.

Mendell MJ, Macher JM, Kumagai K: Measured moisture in buildings and adverse health effects: a review. Indoor Air. 2018;28(4):488-499 [PMID: 29683210].

Sauni R, Verbeek JH, Uitti J, Jauhiainen M, Kreiss K, Sigsgaard T: Remediating buildings damaged by dampness and mould for preventing or reducing respiratory tract symptoms, infections and asthma. Cochrane Database Syst Rev 2015;(2) [PMID: 25715323].

Shrubsole C, Dimitroulopoulou S, Foxall AK, Gadeberg B, Doutsi A: IAQ guidelines for selected volatile organic compounds (VOCs) in the UK. Building and Environment, 2019.

US Environmental Protection Agency—Indoor Air Quality. https://www.epa.gov/indoor-air-quality-iaq/indoor-air-quality-building-type.

WHO Guidelines for Indoor Air Quality—Selected Pollutants, 2010. See http://www.euro.who.int/__data/assets/pdf_file/0009/128169/e94535.pdf.

Wolkoff P: Indoor air humidity, air quality, and health—an overview. Int J Hyg Environ Health. 2018;221(3):376-390 [PMID: 29398406].

■ SELF-ASSESSMENT QUESTIONS

Select the one correct answer for each question.

Question 1: Short-latency illnesses
  a. include nonspecific building-related illness, mass psychogenic illness, but exclude specific illnesses resulting from identifiable sources of noxious materials
  b. include certain infectious diseases, building-associated hypersensitivity pneumonitis, but exclude dampness-associated asthma exacerbations
  c. are characterized by a relatively slow onset
  d. are closely related in time to the individual's presence within the building and often relieved by removal from further exposure

Question 2: Long-latency illnesses
  a. include cancer and chronic pulmonary diseases, perhaps resulting from long-term low-level exposure to contaminants in indoor air
  b. usually have exposure histories that clearly establish a causal link to the building exposure
  c. present little difficulty in establishing a causal link to the building exposure if industrial hygiene data are available
  d. may be caused by agents in indoor air such as cigarette smoke, asbestos, radon gas, and carbon dioxide

Question 3: Molds found in buildings
  a. are often easily identifiable upon inspection
  b. often lead to a variety of respiratory symptoms, auto-immune conditions, and sometimes death
  c. can lead to IgE-mediated hypersensitivity which may be detected by serum testing to specific fungal allergens
  d. are easily remediated after building inspection with little no long-term health consequence

Question 4: Mass psychogenic illness
  a. is not to be confused with sociogenic illness, mass hysteria, or behavioral contagion
  b. is an illness of psychophysiologic origin occurring simultaneously in a group of individuals
  c. has occurred in office buildings, but not in light industrial facilities and electronics plants
  d. is triggered solely in a psychologically susceptible or anxious population

Question 5: Carbon monoxide in buildings
  a. may be the cause of mild symptoms, such as headache and nausea, but is never life-threatening
  b. results solely from incomplete combustion in defective gas furnaces
  c. does not cause recurrent subacute symptoms
  d. may be entrained from the outside via air intakes in the vicinity of vehicle-loading docks

Multiple Chemical Sensitivity

Robert J. Harrison, MD, MPH

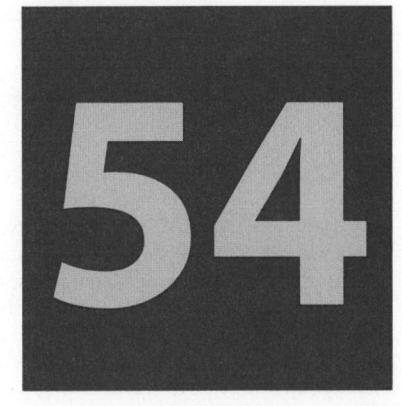

Clinicians have been challenged by the individual with multiple complaints relating to low-level occupational or environmental exposures. Patients report respiratory, central nervous system, musculoskeletal, gastrointestinal, and systemic symptoms after exposure to common environmental irritants such as perfumes, cigarette smoke, home or office furnishings, household cleaners, and a host of other petrochemical products. Upper respiratory (eg, nasal congestion, dryness, or burning), central nervous system (eg, concentration problems, memory difficulties, insomnia, drowsiness, irritability, and depression), and vegetative (eg, fatigue, headache, arthralgias, and myalgias) symptoms predominate. Symptoms occur with exposures well below thresholds permitted by federal or state regulatory agencies as causing acute adverse effects in humans, resulting in significant impairment, lost work time, complete job loss, or major alterations in social and family functions. Individuals may report symptom onset following acute or chronic low-level occupational or environmental exposures, with persistent symptoms that are triggered by subsequent environmental contaminants. Often patients seek help from multiple health care providers who suggest psychiatric etiologies or treatment, obtain toxicologic or immunologic test batteries, or initiate a variety of empirical treatments. Workers' compensation or disability claims often are disputed, and employers may have difficulty accepting or accommodating clinician or patient requests for alternative work environments. As a result, frustration, anger, hostility, and suspicion may confront the clinician when significant impairment continues despite lengthy and expensive consultations.

Some controversy continues to surround the etiology, case definition, diagnosis, and treatment of individuals with *multiple chemical sensitivity* (MCS). The specialty of clinical ecology that emerged in the 1960s adopted theories of causation that differ from those of traditional allergy, immunology, and toxicology, thereby laying the basis for medical and legal disputes regarding legitimate or acceptable forms of treatment, medical or workers' compensation insurance reimbursement, and disability benefits. As a result, some clinicians believe that etiologic theories, diagnosis, and the clinical management of MCS are inconsistent with sound medical science. In more recent years, however, important progress has been made in elucidating and defining the nature of this condition. The combined efforts of several disciplines, including toxicology, psychology, and physiology, have suggested a multifactorial explanatory model for this condition. To guide the clinical evaluation of individuals with this disorder or to respond to requests for epidemiologic investigation, the health care practitioner should be aware of current controversies, including knowledge gaps and the need for further research.

EPIDEMIOLOGY & CASE DEFINITIONS

The term *multiple-chemical sensitivity* was defined in 1987 as an acquired disorder characterized by recurrent symptoms, referable to multiple organ systems, occurring in response to demonstrable exposure to many chemically unrelated compounds at doses far below those established in the general population to cause harmful effects. These seven criteria should be met:

1. The disorder is acquired in relation to some documentable environmental exposure(s), insult(s), or illness(es).

2. Symptoms involve more than one organ system.

3. Symptoms recur and abate in response to predictable stimuli.

4. Symptoms are elicited by exposures to chemicals of diverse structural classes and toxicologic modes of action.

5. Symptoms are elicited by exposures that are demonstrable (albeit at low level).

6. Exposures that elicit symptoms must be very low, by which is meant standard deviations below "average" exposures known to cause adverse human responses.

7. No single, widely available test of organ function can explain the symptoms.

Previous terms for this disorder included *environmental hypersensitivity and environmental illness (EI)*. *Environmental hypersensitivity* was defined as a chronic (ie, continuing for more than 3 months) multisystem disorder usually involving symptoms of the central nervous system and at least one other system. Affected persons are frequently intolerant to some foods and react adversely to some chemicals and to environmental agents, singly or in combination, at levels generally tolerated by the majority. Affected persons have varying degrees of morbidity, from mild discomfort to total disability. On physical examination, the patient usually is free from any abnormal objective findings. Improvement is associated with avoidance of suspected agents, and symptoms recur with reexposure. The term EI has been described as an acquired disease characterized by a series of symptoms caused and/or exacerbated by exposure to environmental agents. Symptoms involve multiple organs in the neurologic, endocrine, genitourinary, and immunologic systems.

A panel of the World Health Organization (WHO) recommended that the terms MCS and EI be replaced by *idiopathic environmental intolerance* (IEI), arguing that use of the word sensitivity may be construed as connoting an allergic cause and that the link between symptoms and exposure is unproven. Other names for this disorder have been used in the published literature, including *chemical intolerance* and *toxicant-induced loss of tolerance*. However, none of these terms has been adopted universally.

Patients with MCS should be distinguished from those with acute occupational diseases such as acute solvent intoxication, occupational asthma, and allergic rhinitis/sinusitis. In these conditions, there usually are objective findings, and the relationship between the condition and exposure is more readily apparent. Several medical organizations, including the American Academy of Allergy and Immunology, the American College of Physicians, the American College of Occupational and Environmental Medicine, and the Council of Scientific Affairs of the American Medical Association, have issued position statements about the causal etiology of MCS. These organizations have not found evidence to link MCS with toxic chemical exposures and have suggested that MCS is primarily a psychological or behavioral disorder.

The epidemiologic and clinical case definitions for MCS have been refined by researchers over the past few years, and certain subsets of questions can provide high specificity for the diagnosis. In one study, combinations of four symptoms (having a stronger sense of smell than others, feeling dull/groggy, feeling "spacey," and having difficulty concentrating) successfully discriminated MCS patients from controls. In another study, self-reported reactions to copy machine emissions, marking pens, aftershave, window cleaner, nylon fabric, pine-scented products, and Rayon material were significant in a discriminant matched-pair analysis of MCS cases and controls. Other studies report overlap between these symptoms and those reported by patients with other conditions of unexplained etiology, such as chronic fatigue syndrome, fibromyalgia, irritable bowel syndrome, and temporomandibular disorder. The Quick Environmental

Exposure and Sensitivity Inventory (QEESI) can be used to assess chemical intolerance. In one study of a primary care population, one of five respondents met criteria for chemical intolerance using the QEESI. These individuals had significantly higher rates of comorbid allergies and possible major depressive, panic, generalized anxiety, alcohol abuse, and somatization disorders. The Idiopathic Environmental Intolerance Symptom Inventory (IEISI) has also been suggested as a reliable, valid, and fast tool for the study of specific symptom prevalence in IEI.

A population-based survey in California found that 6.3% reported physician-diagnosed "environmental illness" or "multiple chemical sensitivity," and 15.9% reported being "allergic or unusually sensitive to everyday chemicals." Hispanic ethnicity was associated with physician-diagnosed MCS, and female gender was associated with self-reported sensitivity. Significant functional impairment in terms of physical, occupational, and social functioning was reported among individuals with MCS. This prevalence is similar to that found in Australia. Another population-based survey in Georgia found that 12.6% reported increased sensitivity. Among these individuals reporting hypersensitivity to common chemical products, the most common triggers of symptoms were cleaning products, tobacco smoke, perfume, pesticides, and car exhaust. Lifestyle modifications were reported frequently, including change in household cleaning/personal hygiene products, home water- and/or air-filtration systems, and location of residence. Self-reported chemical sensitivity was found among 9% of respondents in a population-based survey in Germany. A nationally representative cross-sectional population-based sample of adult Americans found that 12.8% reported medically diagnosed MCS and 25.9% chemical sensitivity.

No single chemical exposure or workplace process is more prevalent in association with the onset of MCS. Records-based reports from an allergy practice, academic occupational medicine clinic, and environmental health center suggest that individuals with MCS are predominantly women (70–80%) in the 30- to 40-year-old age range, with a disproportionate number from service industries. MCS patients in these reports tend to be of higher socioeconomic status, more highly educated, and had a diversity of both occupational and environmental exposures. In a Canadian survey, symptoms such as difficulty concentrating, fatigue, forgetfulness, and irritability were reported at the start of illness. Symptoms related to respiratory irritation such as sneezing, itchy or burning eyes, and hoarseness or loss of voice were reported commonly after subsequent exposure to environmental irritants. Several populations have been identified that may develop symptoms of MCS, including industrial workers, occupants of "tight buildings" such as office workers and school children, residents of communities whose air or water is contaminated by chemicals, and individuals with unique, personal exposures to various chemicals in domestic indoor air, pesticides, drugs, or consumer products. Workplace exposures to poor indoor air quality, pesticide exposure, and remodeling have been associated with the onset of MCS. Other diagnostic subsets have been reported among individuals with solvent-associated psycho-organic syndrome, chemical headaches, and intolerance to solvents. One study has found an association between MCS and birth by caesarian section.

Symptoms of MCS also resemble those of sick-building syndrome, a constellation of excessive work-related symptoms related to an indoor office environment (eg, headache; eye, nose, and throat irritation; fatigue; and dizziness) without an identifiable etiology. MCS has been reported to follow pesticide exposure among employees in a casino and among several office workers following a large-scale outbreak of sick building syndrome. Several symptoms included in the Centers for Disease Control and Prevention (CDC) case definition of chronic fatigue syndrome (ie, fatigue, confusion, memory loss, sleep difficulties, myalgias, and headaches) also are common among individuals with MCS, and affected individuals may be concerned about occupational or environmental etiologies for chronic fatigue syndrome. Aside from symptom overlap, there is currently no evidence linking chronic fatigue syndrome to occupational or environmental chemical exposures.

A number of epidemiologic surveys have been performed among symptomatic veterans of the Gulf War and Cambodian peacekeeping operations. In most studies, veterans report poorer general health, more cognition difficulties, and a higher prevalence of chronic fatigue syndrome, posttraumatic stress disorder, irritable bowel syndrome, and MCS. One study reported a prevalence of symptoms consistent with MCS in 13.1% of Gulf War veterans. Another study of Gulf War veterans found a higher prevalence of MCS than among non–Gulf War military personnel (5.4% versus 2.6%), with greater sensitivity to organic chemicals, vehicle exhaust, cosmetics, and smog. The prevalence of MCS among British Gulf War veterans was significantly associated with exposure to pesticides. Among Cambodian peacekeeping operations veterans, significantly more MCS subjects reported having used insect repellants that contained N,N-diethyl-metatoluamide (DEET). However, the proportion of Cambodia peacekeeping veterans with symptoms of MCS was relatively low.

In a prospective panel survey of a Swedish population sample, elevated subjective health complaints, high stress in daily life, and a strained work situation increased the risk of developing annoyance to environmental factors. These results of this survey suggest that reduced subjective health, over the course of time, may be attributed to environmental factors. Several clinical surveys also demonstrate marked functional impairment in MCS patients, consistent with reported difficulties working and caring for their homes and families, and support the concept of comprehensive assessment, medical management, and social and financial support to avoid the deterioration of function associated with prolonged illness.

▼ ETIOLOGY

The major theories of pathogenesis of MCS can be divided into those that center on a physiologic or toxicologic mechanism and those that ascribe MCS to psychological or behavioral determinants.

▶ Toxicologic Mechanisms

Studies of symptoms in MCS patients are focused on responses below those seen with classic higher-dose exposures as workplace or environmental exposures in this population are considerably lower than those expected to cause end-organ toxicity based on known dose-response relationships. In some studies, no specific reactions to the type or level of chemical exposures have been found in controlled environments, suggesting that autonomic arousal mechanisms in response to odors may play an important role in mediating symptoms. In these studies, MCS subjects do not demonstrate lower olfactory threshold sensitivity or enhanced ability to identify odors accurately. This suggests that nonsensory factors (eg, attention, bias, and personality) can alter the self-reported impact of exposure to volatile chemicals. In a recent study of Gulf War veterans with chemical sensitivity compared with healthy veterans, MCS subjects exposed to low levels of chemicals (ie, diesel vapor with acetaldehyde) reported significantly increased symptoms such as disorientation, respiratory discomfort, and malaise.

To examine genetic and metabolic parameters in MCS, MCS patients and population controls were divided into four severity groups of chemical sensitivity. When genotyping was performed for variants in the genes encoding cytochrome P450 2D6, arylamine N-acetyltransferase 2, paraoxonase 1, methylene tetrahydrofolate reductase, and the cholecystokinin 2 receptor, no significant differences were consistently confirmed.

▶ Psychiatric Mechanisms

Several studies suggest that anxiety and depression are significant contributors to the physical and cognitive symptoms of MCS subjects. Data from some clinical and epidemiologic studies show an association between lifetime psychiatric disorder, particularly mood, anxiety, somatoform, and personality disorders. Many patients with MCS are reported to have psychiatric conditions (eg, psychoses, affective or anxiety disorders, or somatoform disorders—somatization, conversion, and hypochondriases) with symptoms well before their diagnosis of environmentally related illness. Some patients with persistent or recurrent medically unexplained symptoms may have an atypical posttraumatic stress disorder, where specific and recurrent somatic symptoms follow acute or chronic chemical exposures, with subsequent experience of symptoms repeatedly triggered by low-level environmental irritants.

Patients with MCS display high anxiety sensitivity and in response to laboratory carbon dioxide inhalation tend to experience heightened anxiety and panic attacks. Patients with self-identified chemical sensitivity exhibited a positive symptomatic response to sodium lactate compared with placebo infusion, suggesting that MCS may have a neurobiologic basis similar to that of panic disorder. MCS subjects in one study scored significantly higher than controls on standardized psychological questionnaires for agoraphobic conditions and agoraphobia. One study has shown a significantly higher prevalence of the panic disorder–associated CCK-B allele 7 in subjects with MCS. In a recent Danish study, there were positive and statistically significant associations between psychological distress and IEI, which remained statistically significant after adjusting for major life events and social support. Prolonged physical symptoms and sensitivity to common environmental irritants have been described as a behavioral conditioned response or an "odor-triggered panic attack." Several authors suggest that the development of MCS in some individuals may be a result of, at least in part, Pavlovian conditioning processes in which the expression of overt symptoms to certain substances reflects classically conditioned responses to previously neutral olfactory and contextual stimuli. Specific cognitive and behavioral interventions such as systematic desensitization, relaxation techniques, self-hypnosis, and biofeedback have been suggested as treatment strategies for these patients. Some MCS patients have been described as primarily ideational (obsessive-compulsive) or phobic in character, requiring a different psychotherapeutic approach focusing on the effect of physical symptoms on psychological function, stress associated with physical and interpersonal isolation, or the frustration of multiple physician consultations.

Neuropsychologic measures (eg, electroencephalography [EEG], scalp electromyography, and skin resistance) during relaxation in individuals who attribute medical and psychological symptoms to chemical exposures have been compared with subjects with primary psychological disorders and with a control group. MCS patients did not differ from psychological subjects, and both were significantly different from controls, suggesting that individuals with MCS may have primary emotional, anxiety, attentional, or personality disorders. The MCS group had a higher somatization score on a standard self-report symptom inventory, and a subset of these patients had a history of early childhood sexual abuse. Patients recruited from the practice of a community allergist with a reported diagnosis of chemical sensitivity were compared with control patients from a university-based occupational musculoskeletal and back-injury clinic. Patients with MCS reported a higher prevalence of current psychological distress (ie, depression, anxiety, and somatization) and somatization symptoms preceding the onset of sensitivity symptoms. Neuropsychologic performance did not differ when adjusted for the level of psychological distress.

In one case series of patients referred for outpatient evaluation for MCS, three-quarters met DSM-IV criteria for at least one psychiatric disorder, and over one-third had somatoform disorders. Subjects with a diagnosis of EI had a higher prevalence of affective disorders (particularly major depression), anxiety, and somatoform disorders compared with controls, and more EI subjects met lifetime criteria for a major mental disorder. Both asthmatics and MCS subjects performed significantly higher than controls on scales of chemical odor intolerance and anxiety sensitivity, and anxiety and depression were significant contributors to the physical and cognitive symptoms of MCS subjects. Individuals with EI filing workers' compensation claims had a greater prevalence of prior psychiatric morbidity (ie, anxiety, depression, and somatization trait) and higher self-reported measures of somatization and hypochondriasis.

Although many studies find that MCS is a psychological disorder with a belief system characterized by the toxic attribution of symptoms and disability, some studies suggest that psychiatric and psychological disorders may be a consequence, rather than a cause, of MCS. Among subjects referred to an occupational medicine clinic who met the case definition for MCS, psychiatric evaluation did not suggest any premorbid psychiatric diagnosis or a premorbid tendency toward somatization. Clinically significant psychiatric symptoms of depression and anxiety were present among most subjects, with a subset performing poorly on tests of verbal performance. Despite a preponderance of psychiatric symptoms among MCS patients, psychiatric diagnoses were uncommon, and most did not suffer from a diagnosable psychiatric disease. In a population-based survey of Georgia residents, among individuals reporting hypersensitivity to common chemicals, only 1.4% had a history of prior emotional problems, whereas 37.7% developed these problems after physical symptoms began. In a study designed to test the hypothesis that IEI symptoms result from learning via classical conditioning of odors to fear, the fear conditioning account of IEI was only partially satisfactory as an explanation of symptoms. In a Canadian community survey, individuals with MCS had significantly greater odds of major depressive disorder, generalized anxiety disorder, and severe distress.

▶ Immunologic Mechanisms

Environmental and occupational chemical exposures may affect the immune system, with a variety of cellular and cell-mediated immunologic effects established in both animals and humans. Xenobiotics may produce immunosuppression and alter host resistance in experimental animals following acute or subchronic exposure, and immunologic effects in humans have been reported in association with dusts (eg, silica and asbestos), polyhalogenated aromatic hydrocarbons (eg, dioxins, furans, and polychlorinated biphenyls), pesticides, metals (eg, lead, cadmium, arsenic, and methyl mercury), and solvents. However, neither experimental immune dysfunction nor epidemiologic evidence of altered immunity has been correlated with clinical disease.

MCS has been postulated to be an immunologic disorder, with generalized immune dysregulation as a result of free-radical generation and alkylation, structural alteration of antigens, or hapten/carrier reactions. Chemicals are hypothesized to alter immune responses, triggering lymphokines and leading to clinical symptoms of cell-mediated immune response. Chemically sensitive patients are reported to have altered T- and B-lymphocyte counts, abnormal helper-suppresser ratios, and antibodies to a variety of chemicals. Patients with building-related illness have been reported to have an abnormal antibody response and altered cellular immunity to formaldehyde, although these findings have not been confirmed using controls, and clinical correlation is absent. MCS also has been hypothesized to be the result of an interaction between the immune and nervous systems.

Studies of patients with MCS have found no consistent abnormalities in immunoglobulins, complement, lymphocytes, or B- or T-cell subsets. A study of patients with MCS found no evidence of increased autoantibodies, lymphocyte count, helper or suppresser cells, B or T cells, or TAI- or interleukin-2-positive cells compared with control subjects. Absence of objective evidence for immunologic abnormality distinguishes patients with MCS from those with other allergic disorders, autoimmune diseases, and congenital or acquired immunodeficiencies.

▶ Respiratory Mechanisms

Many individuals with MCS report a heightened sense of smell or develop symptoms at low levels of environmental irritant exposure. MCS has been hypothesized to represent an amplification of the nonspecific immune response to low-level irritants. Altered function of C-fibers, respiratory epithelium, or neuroepithelial interaction is postulated to result in increased symptom reporting correlated with physiologic abnormality. Neurogenic inflammation mediated by cell-surface enzymes could play a role in upper respiratory symptoms reported by MCS patients. Subjects with MCS were reported to have a significant decrease in flow values with anterior rhinomanometry, independent of substance or doses, compared with controls. Subjects with MCS showed greater respiratory symptom scores with controlled exposures to test irritants. Capsaicin inhalation provoked more respiratory symptoms in subjects with MCS than controls, suggesting that neurogenic factors may be of importance. Patients with MCS were found with rhinolaryngoscopy to have marked cobblestoning of the posterior pharynx, base of the tongue, or both. In a study of environmental chemosensory responsivity (CR) and the relationship to personality traits, affective states, and odor perception, CR and odor thresholds predicted perceptual ratings of odors and high CR was associated with nonchemosensory affective traits. To test the concept that MCS might be a function of symptom learning, experimental evidence on healthy volunteers suggested that conscious expectancy, which may be modulated by odor quality, determined whether learned symptoms develop in response to a specific odor or to the general context.

▶ Olfactory-Limbic Mechanisms

MCS has been postulated to be the result of environmental chemical exposure, with the triggering or perpetuation of affective and cognitive disorders as well as somatic dysfunction in vulnerable individuals via sensitization of the central nervous system. The neural sensitization model may incorporate both physical and psychological stressors that are elicited following chemical exposure. This theory proposes that MCS may result from neural sensitization, with excessive

or altered neurotransmitter activity and/or alterations of the blood-brain barrier. There are anatomic links between the olfactory nerve, limbic system, and hypothalamus that could explain how odor or irritation of the respiratory tract indirectly results in multiorgan symptoms. There is some evidence for altered neurologic processing of sensory information involving sensorial ascending pathways.

Animal models have been developed to study the effects of repeated formaldehyde exposure on the hypothalamus-pituitary-adrenal axis and behavioral sensitization. Interactions between environmental chemicals and the vomeronasal organ also have been postulated to play a role in altered chemosensory function.

Kindling is a type of time-dependent sensitization of olfactory-limbic neurons by drug or nondrug stimuli, with activation of neural structures such as the amygdala and hypothalamus. Limbic structures are among the most susceptible to kindling-induced seizures, and persistent cognitive and emotional sequelae have been associated with temporal lobe epilepsy in humans and kindling in animals. The vanilloid receptor also has been proposed a possible CNS target in MCS. In this model of MCS, sensitization to food or chemicals parallels the phenomenon of time-dependent sensitization from drugs or nondrug stressors, with heightened sensitivity to stimuli, gradual improvement following withdrawal, and reactivation of symptoms following reexposure. Time-dependent sensitization has been studied as a possible model for cacosmia (subjective sense of feeling ill from odors) among nonpatient populations, which may have relevance to similar symptoms reported by MCS patients. It also has been hypothesized that shy individuals may have hyperreactive limbic systems and may self-report greater symptoms of illness owing to chemical exposures. Laboratory studies have demonstrated sensitization in individuals with MCS for variables such as electroencephalographic activity and increased heart rate and blood pressure. In a small study, chemical exposure caused neurocognitive impairment, and Single-photon-emission computed tomography (SPECT) brain dysfunction particularly in odor-processing areas. In this model, low-level chemical exposure among susceptible individuals could result in affective spectrum disorders with various cognitive and somatic symptoms. This theory attempts to unify physiologic and psychological theories, suggesting that altered neurotransmitter activity may be the underlying mechanism for both affective and somatic symptoms seen among MCS patients.

CLINICAL MANAGEMENT

▶ History & Physical Examination

A careful, thoughtful, and compassionate exposure and psychosocial history is critical. Although the etiology of MCS is controversial, the patient may be suffering from disabling symptoms and frustrated by the lack of definitive answers from clinicians and sometimes is desperately seeking advice and counsel regarding treatment. Approaching the history with the suspicion that the patient with MCS is suffering from a psychiatric disorder, is malingering, or is seeking monetary benefits is not helpful in establishing a therapeutic relationship. Acknowledgment of symptoms and the establishment of a trusting relationship should not necessarily be avoided because the etiology is uncertain or patient motivation is suspect. Where the diagnosis is suspect or contested, an adversarial relationship sometimes may emerge in the provider-patient context that may erode trust, challenge the provider's capacity to treat the patient, and interfere with the therapeutic goals.

A history should be obtained of symptom onset in relationship to acute or chronic exposures. One standardized questionnaire called the Quick Environment Exposure Sensitivity Inventory (QEESI) has been developed that can assist clinicians in evaluating patients and populations for chemical sensitivity. Attention should be paid to respiratory, dermal, neurologic, and systemic symptoms. Most patients with MCS report general systemic symptoms such as difficulty concentrating, fatigue, lethargy, forgetfulness, and irritability. Myalgias, gastrointestinal complaints, headache, burning eyes, and hoarseness or loss of voice also are reported commonly. These various symptoms are provoked by exposure to low-level airborne contaminants such as perfumes, colognes, cleaning solutions, smoke, gasoline, exhaust fumes, and printing inks. Duration and severity of symptoms should be recorded, particularly in relationship to repeated exposures in the workplace or environment (eg, improvement away from work or on weekends/vacations with worsening symptoms at work). An occupational history should be obtained, including past employment and exposure to chemicals, dusts, or fumes. Recent and past chemical exposures should be identified by product names or material safety data sheets, and any environmental monitoring data should be reviewed if available.

Symptoms of headache, fatigue, lethargy, myalgias, and trouble concentrating may persist for hours to days or even weeks, with typical "reactions" reported after exposures to airborne chemicals. Often the individual with MCS will have already identified a variety of chemicals that result in symptoms and will have initiated an avoidance regimen. Varying degrees of restrictions in social and work activities may be reported, including problems driving an automobile, grocery shopping, wearing certain types of clothing, or staying away from office buildings or other workplaces.

The physical examination often is normal in patients with MCS, but particular attention should be paid to examination of the respiratory tract, skin, and nervous system.

▶ Diagnostic Tests

Although routine laboratory evaluations usually do not reveal any consistent diagnostic abnormalities, it is essential to rule out other nonoccupational diseases through a comprehensive history, review of previous records, and appropriate diagnostic studies. The presence of asthma and/or allergic disorders should be considered carefully and an appropriate workup undertaken. A few patients may have increased airway responsiveness and develop symptoms of chest tightness or shortness of breath on exposure to low-level environmental contaminants. Pulmonary function testing with nonspecific airway challenge testing may be indicated depending on history and symptoms. As suggested by the clinical history, confirmatory serologic and/or skin testing for common aeroallergens may be useful. If contact dermatitis is suspected, diagnostic level IV patch testing should be performed.

If a focal neurologic defect is suggested by history or physical examination, additional neurodiagnostic testing may be indicated. One patient with symptoms of altered odor sensitivity was found to have papilledema and a visual-field defect and was determined to have a treatable occipital lobe meningioma. SPECT or positron-emission tomographic studies of brain perfusion, computerized electroencephalographic analysis, or visual-evoked response and brain stem auditory-evoked response have not revealed consistent neurotoxic or neuroimmunologic brain changes in patients with MCS and should be used primarily to confirm clinical findings.

Additional psychological evaluation should be considered if the history suggests the presence of significant psychiatric disorder. Psychiatric consultation and/or treatment may be advised regardless of the etiology of MCS because many patients may have significant psychiatric morbidity with this disorder. Caution is advised in the interpretation of neuropsychologic test results because these techniques are very sensitive but not specific. Abnormal test results could be a result of a neurologic, medical, or neuropsychiatric disorder. Neuropsychologic studies have not shown significant differences between MCS patients and controls on tests of verbal learning, memory functioning, and psychomotor performance.

The capsaicin inhalation test has been used to assess sensory hyperreactivity in patients with MCS, but this test is not widely available for routine use, and its correlation with symptoms and response to treatment is not reliable for diagnosing MCS. The capsaicin concentration causing five coughs or more (C5) can be used to verify presence of lower airway symptoms related to odorous chemicals.

There is no convincing evidence that MCS is caused by a disturbance of heme synthesis, and tests for porphyrin metabolism in blood, urine, or stool specimens have not been correlated with clinical symptoms.

Several controversial techniques have been employed for the diagnosis of MCS, including provocation-neutralization testing, chemical and food challenges, inhalant challenges, serologic testing for Epstein-Barr virus antibodies and various autoantibodies, blood testing for organic hydrocarbon and pesticides, and hair testing for heavy metals. Many of these tests have no diagnostic utility. There is no evidence linking MCS to past infection with the Epstein-Barr virus. There is no association between MCS and levels of organic hydrocarbons or pesticides in blood or fatty tissue, and knowledge of minute residues of these chemicals may serve only to mislead and alarm the patient. Unless specific exposures are suspected, the use of biomarkers (eg, detailed profiles in serum of lipid-soluble toxins and their metabolites or heavy metals in the hair matrix) have little role in the diagnosis of patients with MCS. These tests have not been correlated with any pathologic consequences in MCS or control groups.

Blinded provocation testing has been employed in research studies but has not been evaluated rigorously as a useful diagnostic technique for individual patients. In a double-blind placebo-controlled trial, patients with MCS and controls underwent exposure sessions (solvent mixture and clean air in random order, double-blind) in a challenge chamber. There were no differences between the groups with regard to sensitivity, specificity, and accuracy were found. Cognitive performance was not influenced by solvent exposure, and did not differ between the groups. Likewise, immunologic testing has not been shown to be diagnostic for specific chemical exposure or associated illness.

In the absence of other concurrent medical conditions suggested by history, physical examination, or routine laboratory testing, the diagnosis of MCS relies on the patient's history of multiple symptoms triggered by low-level chemical exposures.

▶ Treatment

Patients with MCS should be advised that, as with a chronic illness, treatment is not directed at a "cure" but rather at accommodation. Care should emphasize relief of symptoms and a return to active work and home life. These treatment strategies entail a treatment alliance between patient and clinician without judgment regarding the etiology of MCS. Ethnographic studies have shown that many MCS patients manage their symptoms through a combination of prevention/avoidance, detoxification, and emotional self-care. In addition to symptoms and the ongoing difficulty in living with this condition, social relationships and daily life may be affected greatly. For some individuals, education regarding general principles of toxicology (eg, routes of exposure of toxic chemicals and routes of elimination) may be reassuring if they are concerned about long-term storage of chemicals in the body and the fear of ongoing damage. Elimination of exposures at home, workplace, or school through a variety of strategies (including room air filters) often is implemented by patients. In one case series of MCS patients from an occupational health practice, improvement in symptoms was associated with self-reported avoidance of specific substances or materials. Two of the three most highly rated treatments as reported by a large series of MCS patients were creating a chemical-free living space and chemical avoidance. While many patients report empirical improvement of symptoms, avoidance of low-level irritants has not been tested in controlled scientific studies. In some patients, avoidance may reinforce the notion of disability and lead to further isolation, powerlessness, and discouragement.

Although it is not clear whether psychological symptoms are the cause of MCS or simply accompany the diagnosis, specific cognitive and behavioral interventions may be most useful in the treatment of MCS. Evidence shows that MCS can significantly limit social and occupational functioning. A biopsychosocial model of illness conceptualizes a close correlation between physical and psychological diseases. MCS may be a heterogeneous disorder with more than one causal mechanism. Significant psychophysiologic symptoms may occur after exposure to low-level volatile compounds in persons with and without coexisting or preexisting psychiatric illness. Similar to techniques used in other functional syndromes, behavioral strategies such as response prevention, systemic desensitization, graduated exercise regimens, and progressive relaxation may help patients to regain normal activities, minimize role impairment, and curtail sick behaviors.

Improving the patient's understanding of the role of stress on illness and enhancing coping mechanisms for the impact on daily life may be helpful. Biofeedback-assisted relaxation training and cognitive restructuring have been reported with some success in MCS patients. Adults with MCS who completed an 8-week mindfulness-based cognitive therapy (MBCT) program generally reported benefiting in terms of improved coping strategies and sleep quality. Another study found that MBCT did not change overall illness status in individuals with MCS, but positively changed emotional and cognitive representations. Treatments with demonstrated efficacy in panic disorder also may be of benefit in MCS, and conversely, treatments that reinforce anticipatory anxiety and avoidance behavior may be detrimental.

Pharmacologic treatment for specific symptoms suggestive of depression or anxiety, in conjunction with other behavioral techniques, may offer some relief as part of an overall treatment program. In addition, antidepressants sometimes alleviate somatic symptoms (particularly pain and insomnia) and may improve the functional status of some MCS patients. One case report demonstrated dramatic improvement in a patient with MCS who received a selective serotonin reuptake inhibitor.

Patients in whom panic responses may be at least a contributing factor to symptoms might be responsive to intervention with psychotherapy to enable their desensitization or deconditioning of responses to odors or other triggers. These patients also may be helped by anxiolytic medications, relaxation training, and counseling for stress management.

A number of controversial methods have been used for the treatment of MCS, including elimination or rotary diversified diets, vitamins or nutritional supplements, oxygen, antifungal and antiviral agents, thyroid hormone supplement, supplemental estrogen or testosterone, transfer factor, chemical detoxification through exercise and sauna treatment, intravenous gamma-globulin, and intracutaneous or subcutaneous neutralization. A specially designed chemical-free environmental control unit has been used as a method to decrease blood pesticide levels and improve symptoms as well as intellectual and cognitive function. Controversial treatment methods offer hope of improvement to many individuals with MCS, and some patients do report symptom improvement over time. Many of these treatment methods are expensive and rarely are covered by health insurance. These treatment methods have not been validated through carefully designed controlled trials, may have unwanted side effects, and may serve to reinforce counterproductive behaviors. Patients should be advised that such treatments are controversial, have not been subject to controlled clinical trials, and are not recommended by most medical professional organizations.

Follow-up studies indicate that up to half of MCS patients may improve over a period of years, but the majority continue to remain symptomatic with a major impact on career, marriage or family and other common daily activities.

REFERENCES

Azuma K et al: Chemical intolerance: involvement of brain function and networks after exposure to extrinsic stimuli perceived as hazardous. Environ Health Prev Med 2019;24(1):61 [PMID: 31640568].

Driesen L, Patton R, John M: The impact of multiple chemical sensitivity on people's social and occupational functioning; a systematic review of qualitative research studies. J Psychosom Res 2020;132:109964 [PMID: 32114179].

Hauge CR et al: Mindfulness-based cognitive therapy (MBCT) for multiple chemical sensitivity (MCS): results from a randomized controlled trial with 1 year follow-up. J Psychosom Res 2015;79(6):628-634 [PMID: 26311155].

Johnson D, Colman I: The association between multiple chemical sensitivity and mental illness: evidence from a nationally representative sample of Canadians. J Psychosom Res 2017;99:40-44 [PMID: 28712429].

Karvala K, Sainio M, Palmquist E, Nyback MH, Nordin S: Prevalence of various environmental intolerances in a Swedish and Finnish general population. Environ Res 2018;161:220-228 [PMID: 29161654].

Pigatto PD, Guzzi G: Prevalence and risk factors for multiple chemical sensitivity in Australia. Prev Med Rep 2019;14:100856 [PMID: 29329146].

Steinemann A: National prevalence and effects of multiple chemical sensitivities. J Occup Environ Med 2018;60(3):e152-e156 [PMID: 29329146].

Viziano A, Micarelli A, Pasquantonio G, Della-Morte D, Alessandrini M: Perspectives on multisensory perception disruption in idiopathic environmental intolerance: a systematic review. Int Arch Occup Environ Health 2018;91(8):923-935 [PMID: 30088144].

■ SELF-ASSESSMENT QUESTIONS

Select the one correct answer for each question.

Question 1: Symptoms of multiple chemical sensitivity (MCS)
a. typically follow pesticide exposure
b. are helpful in the diagnosis of chronic fatigue syndrome
c. are invariably due to occupational or environmental chemical exposures
d. resemble those of sick-building syndrome

Question 2: Idiopathic environmental intolerance (IEI)
a. is a term favored over multiple chemical sensitivity by NIOSH
b. connotes an allergic cause
c. denotes that the link between symptoms and exposure is not caused by classic allergy
d. is a term that has been adopted universally

Question 3: The Quick Environmental Exposure and Sensitivity Inventory (QEESI)
a. can be used to assess chemical intolerance
b. finds that most respondents meet criteria for chemical intolerance
c. identifies individuals with low rates of comorbid allergies
d. misses somatization disorders

Health Risk Assessment

Jennifer B. Sass, PhD

Michael J. DiBartolomeis, PhD, DABT

INTRODUCTION

The community and workers are generally aware that voluntary or involuntary exposure to chemicals and other hazardous substances can cause harm to our health or to the health of our children and the unborn fetus. Industrial chemicals are made from the conversion of oil, natural gas, air, water, metals, and minerals into products that span almost all economic sectors including plastics, agrichemicals, medical products and pharmaceuticals, energy and transportation products, communication products, building materials, personal care products, and household goods.

Chemicals that are derived from methanol, ethylene, propylene, butadiene, benzene, toluene, and xylenes are based on carbon atoms, so they are called "organic" chemicals. Inorganic chemicals are not carbon based; they include metals like elemental lead and mercury, and minerals like silica and asbestos. Both inorganic and organic chemicals can be synthesized in a laboratory or extracted from the earth. But, in all cases they may be hazardous.

Taken at the minimum necessary dosages, however, some chemicals, such as medicines, are beneficial to human health. Manufacturing with chemicals has resulted in some new products and technologies that have, arguably, benefited society by creating new jobs, developing less costly and more durable consumer products and building materials, and improving communication and transportation. However, while the economic value of the chemical industry is readily measured, the true cost of the production, use, and disposal of these synthesized chemicals to the environment and human health is much more difficult to quantify. Furthermore, we know that workplace chemical exposures such as during product manufacturing are often much greater than the exposure to the finished consumer products or even environmental pollutants. On the other hand, workers are usually healthy adults, whereas consumer products may be in daycare facilities, nursing homes, hospitals, schools, and other places where exposures can impact vulnerable populations such as the very young and people with compromised health. Many other factors also play a role in risk considerations, including poverty and employment status which affect stress, nutrition and access to health care, residential proximity to polluting industrial facilities, co-exposures to multiple pollutants, violence, smoking, and drug use. Scientists and policymakers still do not know the exact degree to which human health problems can be attributed to environmental pollution, chemical exposures in consumer products, genetics, and lifestyle choices. However, we do know that the contribution from environmental exposures is significant because policies and practices to reduce harmful exposures can effectively reduce diseases and deaths.

In the early 1970s, the level of concern for the safety of the food supply, air, drinking water, and working environment intensified, and new laws were passed, and regulations promulgated to help control and restrict the level of pollutants released into the environment. Many of these regulations were based on observed or predicted human health effects of exposure to hazardous materials either in the environment, in the food or water supplies, or in the workplace. Despite these efforts, some contend that not enough is being done to clean up and maintain a healthy environment, whereas others believe that these concerns are exaggerated or unwarranted. In particular, the Toxic Substances Control Act (TSCA) of 1976 provides U.S. Environmental Protection Agency (EPA) with authority to regulate new chemicals before they are commercialized. In 2016 it was amended to require mandatory evaluation of existing chemicals, expanded authority to require premarket testing of new chemicals, and increased public access to chemical hazard information that EPA's regulatory decisions are based on. Notable exclusions from TSCA include chemicals used in food, drugs, cosmetics, and pesticides, all of which are addressed through other laws with varying strengths and weaknesses.

Given the scientific uncertainties involved in evaluating the impact of environmental stressors on human health, it is prudent public health practice to reduce or eliminate preventable exposures to hazardous substances when an activity raises the risk of harm to human health or the environment, even if cause-and-effect relationships have not been fully established. This is the guiding principle behind the precautionary approach to risk management, a familiar component of international and European environmental laws. Furthermore, environmental protection programs should affect empowerment within individuals and communities and raise the consciousness about their health, their environment, and multicultural issues. In the United States, these are particularly important given the rapidly changing demographic face of the nation, the ongoing problems associated with environmental pollution, and the increased production and use of chemicals.

RISK AS A DECISION-MAKING FACTOR

Environmental decision making is a multidimensional process. Policies and laws that are written to address concerns about environmental pollution, occupational hazards, and the protection of human health usually rely on information taken from a myriad of sources, some of which are process-based and others are value-based or based on a systematic analysis. Table 55–1 provides examples of some factors that might be considered in formulating a decision on an environmental problem.

Although it is only one tool that might be used in the overall decision-making process, government agencies often consider risk first when making decisions on mitigation, control, enforcement, or regulation of chemicals released

into the environment. By definition, *risk* is the probability or chance that a desired or unwanted action, circumstance, or event will result in loss or harm. It can apply to almost any activity or event, such as the likelihood for injury when playing a sport or driving a car, the chance for developing a disease from exposure to pathogens or chemicals, or the possibility for property damage from a natural catastrophe. This chapter focuses on human health risks and how to evaluate risk. Risk assessment methodology also has been developed and applied to evaluate the impact of pollution on the environment and ecosystems and, to a lesser degree, on quality-of-life issues. In the context of human health, risk is the probability that adverse health effects, ranging from death to subtle biochemical changes, may occur because of exposure to a hazardous substance. Risk also might be thought of as voluntary or involuntary. Smoking, for example, is both a voluntary and an involuntary risk. It is voluntary because the smoker might choose to begin smoking. It is involuntary because second-hand smoke can cause harm to nonsmokers and because nicotine is addictive, and it is difficult to stop smoking even if the user wants to.

Risk assessment is a means or methodology to quantify risk, but it is important to recognize that it is a process and not a science. The process of risk assessment uses scientific data, statistical and mathematical methodology, and expert judgment to characterize the probability for an adverse outcome. In its most basic form, risk assessment is the process

Table 55–1. Examples of decision-making factors that might be considered in formulating environmental policy.

Process	Value-Based	Analysis
Negotiation (consensus and compromise)	Popular opinion (eg, from media accounts and polls and surveys)	Availability of or lack of relevant scientific data
Voting (ie, number of votes, majority versus minority)	Cultural diversity (eg, traditions, religious beliefs)	Demographics of impacted area
Application of existing laws, statutory mandates or legal precedence	Ethical considerations (eg, who benefits and who is harmed?)	Geographic location of impacted area
Political pressure (eg, lobbying, campaign contributions)	Public perception	Quantified exposures (measurement of environmental levels, biomonitoring)
Precaution (take all necessary action to protect from known or potential harm)	Education (presentation of factual materials that raise the level of knowledge about a particular issue)	Risk (absolute, excess, or relative)
Sustainability (conserving resources for future generations)	Quality of life (eg, aesthetics, peace of mind, health status)	Economics (cost and benefit analysis)
Urgency (eg, response to an emergency)	Voluntary versus involuntary (in terms of use of exposure)	Technical feasibility (eg, laboratory capability, existence of efficient mitigation technology)
Unification (eg, labor and community activism)	Justice (application of laws and practices regardless of socioeconomic status, race, gender, etc.)	Prevention (eg, reduce or eliminate exposures)
History or convention (continue practices that have been used in the past)	Right to know (knowledge is powerful)	Development and use of alternative (safer) technologies

through which toxicology data collected from animal studies and human exposure studies are combined with information about the degree of exposure to predict the likelihood that an adverse response will occur in an individual or a population.

Historically, the results of risk assessments have been used to regulate chemical production, use, and release into the environment or food supply. For example, risk assessment methodologies have been used to set standards for pesticide residues in food, chemical contaminants in drinking water, indoor and ambient air standards, and exposure limits for contaminants found in consumer products and other media. However, risks might be assessed differently among agencies, and there are only a few "environmental agencies" that assess environmental or occupational health risks. These agencies attempt to make decisions based on data supported with scientific judgment. Some agencies also are mandated to consider future or multiple risks. Except for the application of pesticides in agriculture, risk assessment has not been used widely as a basis for setting workplace exposure standards.

GENERAL RISK ASSESSMENT PROCESS

▶ Elements of the Model

The risk-based model for environmental priority setting generally follows a two-tiered approach. The first tier is to evaluate the size and scope of the potentially hazardous situation and quantify the level of risk posed by the hazard (risk assessment). The National Research Council defines *risk assessment* as a four-step process developed to aid in the evaluation of the safety of synthetic chemical use or the exposure to humans from chemicals in the environment. The four steps of risk assessment are hazard identification, dose-response assessment, exposure assessment, risk characterization. In conducting health risk assessments, several representative questions about each environmental problem are asked (Table 55–2).

The results of a risk assessment then are used to help determine which risks need to be addressed or managed. This second tier is called *risk management*, and it uses a value-based approach to determine what level of risk to human health will be considered significant and to formulate options for identifying, selecting, and implementing actions to prevent, reduce, or maintain risks below that level. Risk management considers risk along with other technical (such as technical or methodological feasibility), economic, legal, and social factors.

A third tier of the risk assessment model, *risk communication*, was added later with the intent of linking risk assessors with the public by presenting information in the most effective way. In communicating risk to the public, some questions that might be asked include the following: Is the information clearly relevant to and understandable by the affected public? Does the information respond to the public's concerns? What are the limitations of the risk assessment? Despite the best efforts of the risk assessors to communicate the results of a risk assessment to the public, risk communication is unfortunately

Table 55–2. Standard steps to conducting a health risk assessment.

Risk Assessment Step	Examples of Questions Asked by the Risk Assessor
Hazard identification	What substances harm humans, and what kind of harm is it? Of all the substances involved in a problem area (eg, air pollution) which substances will we look at in this analysis?
Dose-response assessment	What could happen to humans if they are exposed to different levels of these compounds? What are the cancer-causing effects and non-cancer-causing effects?
Exposure assessment	What are the sources and duration of exposures to this substance? How many people are exposed to the hazardous substance? What range of doses do they receive?
Risk characterization	Given all we have learned so far, what are the human health impacts of current exposures? What is the risk to an individual? What is the risk to an entire population? Are any subpopulations more impacted than others? How confident are we in the overall analysis?

often an afterthought in the process. More recently, as the emphasis for addressing environmental pollution issues has been placed on the affected communities (ie, disproportionate risk and environmental justice), the importance of involving the public earlier in the process has been realized.

▶ Scope of Risk Assessment

Health risk assessments can be conducted for any hazard for which there is adequate hazard information (such as from animal toxicology studies, epidemiologic studies, or cellular studies) and either measured or estimated exposure information in an individual or population. The spectrum of health effects described in toxicologic and epidemiologic studies is quite broad and might include acute, subchronic, and/or chronic effects following exposure to a chemical or chemical mixture. Acute studies test exposures of hours to a few days, usually at high doses, and measure rapid onset effects like seizures and death. Subchronic studies test exposures of weeks to months in rodents or up to a year in humans, usually across a mid-range of doses. Chronic studies test repeated or continuous exposures over one or several years or longer and include chronic diseases or disabilities such as cancer. In addition to the dose, it is also important to consider the timing of an exposure during sensitive life-stages. For example, even low-dose and short duration exposures to lead or mercury during prenatal development can cause permanent neurologic deficits, whereas similar exposures to an adult may have no measurable effect on neurologic function.

Infants, children, and pregnant women are recognized as sensitive subpopulations to consider when conducting hazard evaluations and risk assessments.

Table 55–3 presents some typical toxicologic endpoints used for risk assessment. For some toxic effects, the length and level of exposure might not be limited to any one category, and in fact, there is some overlap. Generally, risk assessment does not exclude any toxicologic effect that is clearly caused by the chemical exposure. In cases when there is ambiguity in the data or the data are incomplete, it is generally a responsible approach to assume that the health effect is related to the chemical exposure until more data become available that clearly show an alternative cause of the adverse health effect.

This approach to toxicity testing is resource intensive, time consuming, and cannot effectively account for the toxicity of complex chemical mixtures. Furthermore, the results of whole animal toxicity testing provide little information on the variability in human susceptibility and the mechanism by which a chemical exerts its toxic effects. Because of these and other reasons, the demand for complete toxicity testing of tens of thousands of chemicals in commerce is not being met. Proposals to address the inadequacies of the current testing system include focusing on upstream biochemical events and cellular changes that might lead to the downstream observable effects in whole animal studies. Using predictive, high throughput *in vitro* assays, individual chemicals and chemical mixtures could be evaluated for relevant perturbations of key early biochemical and cellular changes that are thought to initiate "toxicity pathways" leading to gross pathological changes and disease. If this vision is implemented, current toxicity testing models would be phased out while new rapid, high-throughput methods are developed, hopefully resulting in the more efficient testing of all chemicals in a timely, cost-effective fashion, without sacrificing predictive accuracy.

RISK ASSESSMENT STEPS

▶ Hazard Identification

To begin a risk assessment, hazard identification is the step in which it is determined whether exposure to an agent could (at any dose) cause an increase in the incidence of adverse health effects (eg, cancer, birth defects, or neurotoxicity) in humans. Many factors are considered in this determination, and depending on the toxicologic endpoint of concern, there might be specific additional factors to consider. A compound's chemical and physical properties need to be known to be able to evaluate its fate in the environment and biological systems (eg, stability, half-life for elimination), the potential for bioaccumulation, possible routes of metabolism, and the likely toxicity of the compound. Also, factoring in the potential for human exposure and the likely routes of exposure is important to prioritize chemicals for hazard assessment.

If human exposures and toxicity are well documented, identification of a hazard is relatively easy; it can be more complicated when only experimental data in animals are available. In general, the criteria used in a risk assessment to identify a threat to human health from animal data include the number of animal species affected, the dose at which the animals are affected, the existence of a dose-response relationship, and the severity of the effect.

For individual chemicals and chemical mixtures, multiple health effects frequently are observed following dosing in animals or exposure to humans. For example, as required under the Federal Insecticide, Fungicide and Rodenticide Act (FIFRA), the U.S. EPA can require registrants to submit data from a standard battery of experimental toxicity tests that include acute, subchronic, and chronic studies for all pesticide active ingredients—although frequently there are data gaps, such as for chronic studies. Each pesticide usually exhibits some consistent toxicologic effects in different species that are related or unrelated to the pesticidal action of the chemical. In addition, there also might be either nonspecific toxicity or species-specific effects that occur at comparable doses or at higher or lower doses than the consistent toxicologic effects. The spectrum of toxicity exhibited by a chemical in a battery of tests can be considered a "hazard profile" that might or might not be consistent with other structurally related chemicals or chemicals that share common mechanisms of toxicity.

For some toxicologic endpoints, additional consideration needs to be given to fully characterize or profile the hazard. For carcinogens, it is also important to consider the number and types of tumors occurring in the animals, the target organs affected, the background incidence (usually regarded as historical controls), the time-to-tumor response, the formation of preneoplastic lesions, and the genotoxicity (including mutagenicity) of the chemical. For carcinogens, there might not be consistency among species for tumor type, and there might be positive data (showing effects) in one species and negative data (no observed effects) in another. Depending on the final use of a risk assessment, it is often prudent to accept the results from positive studies even if there are negative studies in order to take a precautionary approach to protect public health where governments and industries take protective action, human suffering may be avoided, and lives are saved.

A systematic review is a systematic and transparent method to evaluate the quality of data and to support evidence-based decision-making. A systematic review framework that comports with scientific best practices should be used to conduct chemical assessments based on an evaluation and integration of all the evidence. This can include whole animal studies, cellular and *in vitro* studies (test tube and petri dish studies), and wide-ranging human data. All these study types have strengths and limitations; a systematic way to collect all the relevant information, assess the quality and reliability of each study, and then integrate all the studies together will lead to the most accurate assessment. A systematic review framework would replace a weight of evidence (WOE) approach.

A meta-analysis may also be useful. This involves compiling data from comparable experiments (ie, similar experimental design, statistical power, reporting details, and overall quality) and evaluating the data set in a quantitative, statistical context. Epidemiologic data from several comparable

Table 55–3. Common toxicologic endpoints reported in animal and human exposure studies that are used for quantitative health risk assessment.

Toxicologic Endpoint	Exposure Duration		
	Acute	Subchronic	Chronic
Clinical signs and overall abnormal appearance of test animal (general malaise)	++	++	++
Clinical signs and symptoms (reported in human exposures)	++	++	+
Abnormal results of gross pathologic and histopathologic examinations	+	++	++
Neurologic effects: (a) Cholinergic signs, cholinesterase inhibition, tremor, incoordination (b) Delayed neuropathy[a] (c) Behavioral effects (eg, attention deficit, lethargy)	++	++	++
Changes in absolute body weight, or body weight gain	+	++	+
Respiratory airway dysfunction and/or irritation	++	±	±
Dermal or ocular abrasion or irritation	++	+	−
Sensitization (dermal or upper airway)	+	+	±
Change in absolute or relative organ weight	−	++	++
Developmental (eg, birth defect, frank toxicity, lower body weights, spontaneous abortion)	−[b]	++	±
Reproductive effects (eg, decreased fertility, testicular atrophy or degeneration)	−	++	++
Changes in normal physiology and function (eg, changes in hormone production, transient or irreversible effects on the immune system)	−	++	++
Altered clinical lab values: (a) Biochemical (eg, changes in hepatic enzyme levels) (b) Blood (eg, increased white blood cell count) (c) Urine (eg, proteinuria or hematuria)	−	++	++
Evidence for cellular degeneration, changes in cellular metabolic activity	−	+	++
Genotoxicity[c]	+	±	±
Increased incidence of tumors	−[d]	−[e]	++
Decreased survival: (a) Lethality studies (b) Increased morbidity, premature death (decreased survival)	++	+	+

Legend: + = Common part of examination and frequently observed result for this type of study; ++ = common part of examination and frequently observed result for this type of study and endpoint is often the most sensitive for risk assessment; ± = might be part of examination and result might be reported for this type of study but not frequently; − = not usually part of examination and not usually reported for this type of study.

[a]By definition, the effect is delayed but it is usually the result of an acute high-level exposure.

[b]Not usually reported/observed after an acute exposure, however, a single in utero exposure at a specific time during pregnancy can result in a birth defect.

[c]Genetic toxicity endpoints are often used in risk assessment as supplemental data but not as a quantitative end point. Nevertheless, there are numerous *in vitro* and *in vivo* assays to assess the genotoxic potential of a chemical that usually fall into three categories: (1) mutations in genes usually in mammalian cells, bacteria, fruit flies, or yeast; (2) chromosomal effects usually in mammalian cells; and (3) DNA damage (usually assayed by measuring rate of unscheduled DNA repair).

[d]Single-dose irradiation can be oncogenic (eg, leukemia in atom bomb victims in Hiroshima).

[e]Unusual occurrence, but might be early onset caused by, for example, in utero exposure to diethylstilbestrol (DES).

studies sometimes are examined using meta-analysis, as are data from multiple carcinogen bioassays in animals.

In the hazard identification phase of a health risk assessment, there is often a need to separate statistical significance from biologic significance. Statistical significance might exclude effects of biologic significance, and in the case where several studies demonstrate comparable biologic effects with varying statistical significance, the effect still might be considered for risk assessment. In the dose-response assessment step, other criteria would be applicable to help discern the mechanism of toxic action and the use of the data for quantitative purposes. Furthermore, there are toxicologic endpoints for which biologic relevance is not known or difficult to define (eg, increased or compromised immunologic activity that may not trigger obvious clinical signs of toxicity until the immune system is challenged). In another example, the measured toxicologic endpoint might be an upstream indicator or a precursor to significant adverse effects, such as a precancerous lesion. Therefore, the risk assessor might attempt to define the term *adverse effect* or at least segregate an effect that is clearly adverse from one for which the data are equivocal. The validity of this exercise is open to scientific debate, and there are many examples where the difference between adverse and nonadverse is not at all clear for a toxicity endpoint.

▶ Dose-Response Assessment

Dose-response evaluations define the relationship between the dose of an agent and the observance or expected occurrence of a specific toxicologic effect. A dose-response evaluation usually requires extrapolation from doses administered to experimental animals to the exposures expected from human contact with the agent in the environment or in the workplace. When evaluating toxicologic effects in animals, it is generally assumed that at a given dose the animal response to a chemical will be nearly identical to the human response. This approach is reasonably accurate for chemicals that exhibit a threshold dose-response curve, and which are eliminated from the body fairly rapidly (ie, short biologic half-life). If available, human exposure/dosing data from occupational or environmental exposures might be useful to better characterize the dose-response relationship of a chemical and its toxic effect. Data from human volunteer studies for exposure to hazardous substances are less desirable because of the generally poor study design, inherent bias of the subjects or the investigators, lower statistical power, and questionable ethical context.

Chemicals are thought to exhibit two types of dose-response relationships: those exhibiting a threshold for toxicity and those that do not. For chemicals that exhibit a threshold, the basic principle is that a specific dose level can be identified below which no toxic effect would be observed. The conventional approach to selecting dose levels for risk assessment of chemicals that exhibit a threshold for toxicity is to first identify the most sensitive endpoint from all studies and then to identify the highest no-observed-adverse-effect level (NOAEL) for that endpoint from the data collected

from comparable studies. If no NOAEL can be identified (ie, effects are observed at all doses tested), then the lowest observed adverse effect level (LOAEL) is substituted. In the case where a LOAEL and not a NOAEL is used for risk assessment, additional uncertainty is inherent in the calculation of risk that should be accounted for in the risk characterization step (see section "Risk Characterization").

Alternatively, a benchmark dose (BMD) methodology might be better suited with certain data sets in which a NOAEL cannot be clearly established. In this method, a toxicologic effect is first identified, such as a percentage of animals exhibiting a response or a percentage of decrease or increase in an enzymatic activity. Second, a benchmark response level is selected (eg, a response rate of 5% or 10%), and a mathematical model is applied to the data. The fitted curve then is used to designate the corresponding BMD. A lower limit on the BMD confidence level often is chosen as the NOAEL equivalent. This BMD confidence level then is used for risk assessment calculations by applying the appropriate safety/uncertainty factors.

The methods for dose-response extrapolation employed for carcinogens are different. It is presumed that for substances that cause cancer—including chemicals and radiation—no threshold for toxicity exists, that is, there is no "no risk" level. This is a particularly prudent presumption where vulnerable populations such as pregnant women and children may be exposed, or where populations are exposed to multiple chemical and nonchemical stressors. However, we do not fully understand the mechanism(s) of action for all chemical carcinogens. Chemical initiators and promoters have been identified in experimental studies, and for these, a postulated genotoxic mechanism of action appears to be reasonable. For other chemicals that induce tumorigenesis in laboratory animals, the evidence supporting a genotoxic mechanism of action is equivocal or negative, and other mechanisms, such as cytotoxicity or disruptions in physiologic processes that affect hormone levels or immunologic response, have been postulated. It is important to keep in mind that cancer may result from numerous mechanisms or adverse outcome pathways; for this reason, it may not be appropriate to downgrade or dismiss evidence of toxicity, exposure, or risk based on the absence of evidence of a particular mechanism or pathway being triggered.

To describe the dose-response curve for carcinogens at the low doses expected for human occupational or environmental exposures, it is often necessary to extrapolate from the relatively high doses used in cancer bioassays (typically in rodents).

Most low-dose extrapolation models are derived from assumptions of the statistical distribution of the data (eg, log-probit, Mantel-Bryan, logit, and Weibull), the postulated mechanism of carcinogenicity (eg, linear one-hit, gamma multihit, and Armitage-Doll multistage), or some other parameter (eg, time to tumor, pharmacokinetic, and biologically based). The carcinogenic process typically is described mathematically by a set of elementary biologic events, most often as part of a multistage process, and the effect of carcinogens on these processes is assumed to be the simplest possible (eg, described by a chemical reaction rate). Therefore, the dose-response relationship described by these mathematical models usually will be as arbitrary as the assumptions made for the biologic processes.

There are several mathematical models that usually will fit the animal cancer bioassay data. Because these models use different formulas and assumptions for predicting the chemical's carcinogenic potency, they might yield different results at the doses to which humans are exposed depending on the characteristics of the dose-response curve and the assumed mechanism of carcinogenicity (Figure 55–1). For most carcinogens, the one-hit and linearized multi-stage models are applied to the animal cancer bioassay data to estimate cancer potency in humans. These models were

developed based on our understanding that ionizing radiation and genotoxic chemicals exhibit a linear, or nearly linear, response in the low-dose region. When presenting the results of the dose-response assessment for carcinogens, the upper-bound risk from the cancer models are provided as well as the upper and lower bounds of the risk. The objective of the bounding techniques is to attempt to account for the statistical uncertainty in the results of the animal tests.

There are chemicals for which there are positive cancer bioassay data but negative or equivocal genotoxicity data. There is an ongoing debate in the scientific community as to the mechanism of tumorigenesis for these agents. For example, the chloro-*s*-triazine herbicides (eg, atrazine, simazine, and cyanazine) induce mammary tumorigenesis in rodent

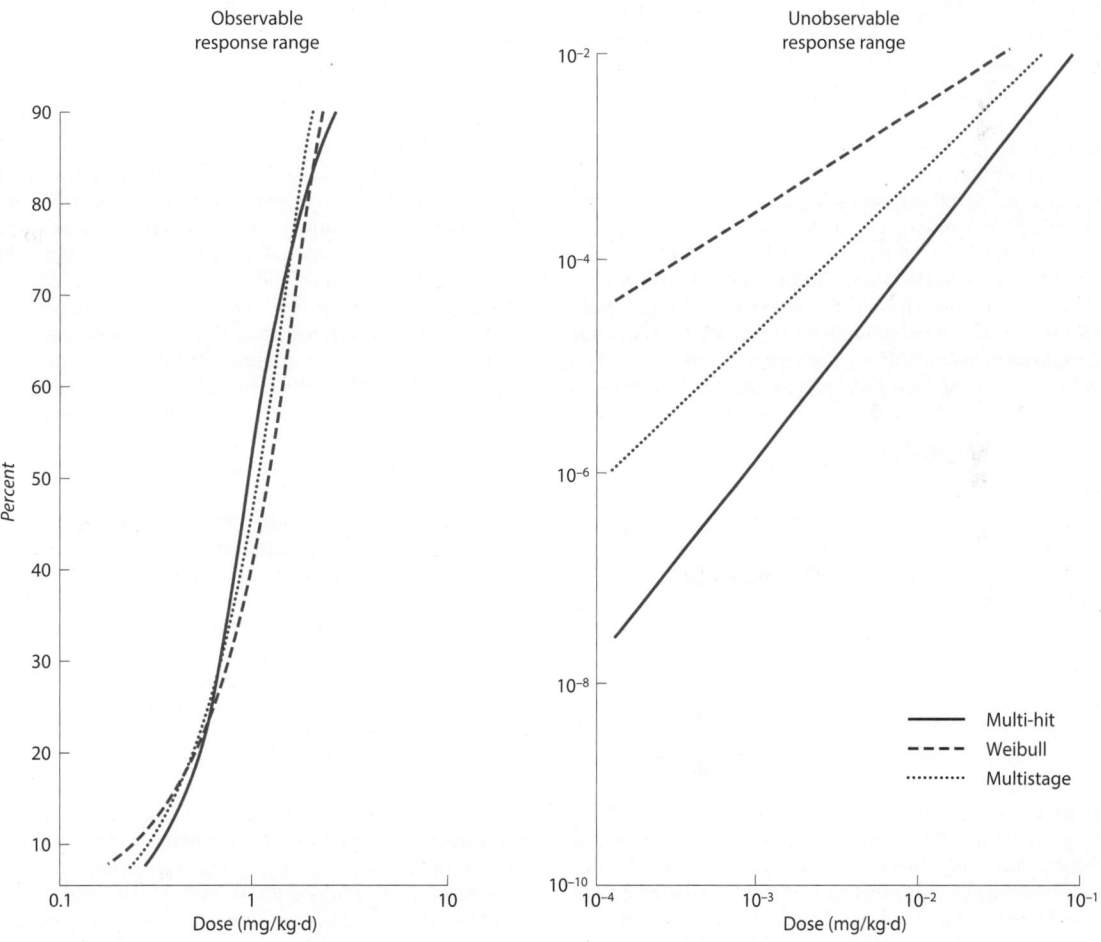

▲ **Figure 55–1.** The fit of most dose-response models to data in the observable range is generally similar (left plot). However, because of the differences in assumptions on which the equations are based, the risk estimates at low doses can vary dramatically between the different models (right plot).

studies, but the data for genetic toxicity are equivocal. There is some evidence that these chemicals disrupt endocrine systems, although they do not bind estrogen receptors. Therefore, a threshold dose-response for the triazine herbicides has been proposed, but no clear mechanism of action has been demonstrated. Other examples of chemical carcinogens for which there is ongoing debate as to the mechanism of action include chlorinated solvents such as chloroform and chlorinated polycyclic aromatic compounds such as 2,3,7,8-tetrachlorodibenzo-*p*-dioxin.

Physiologically based pharmacokinetic (PBPK) models are used by some risk assessors to predict the human response from rodent data. These models attempt to quantitatively account for differences between the test species and humans by considering body weight, metabolic capacity and products, respiration rate, blood flow, fat content, and other parameters (Figure 55–2). Confidence in the results of PBPK models often relies on some untestable assumptions, such as the delivered dose of an unstable metabolite to a target organ. While PBPK models have been developed for a variety of industrial chemicals (eg, chlorinated solvents) and pesticides (eg, malathion), application of the results of these analyses for risk assessment is still not clearly defined. Results from models are like a critical review of the overall scientific literature in that they incorporate the results of many studies to generate an overall summary of the data. As such, models can be highly subjective. The underlying assumptions that are used to build the model framework and define model parameters should be disclosed and carefully evaluated.

The results of human exposure (eg, epidemiology) studies also might provide useful data to supplement the animal cancer bioassay data or offer an independent assessment of the dose-response of a chemical and its effect in humans.

▶ Exposure Assessment

For there to be a health risk, there must be both inherent toxicity and exposure to a chemical. In other words, the prevention or elimination of the exposure to a toxic substance would result in zero risk. Because the total elimination of chemical exposure often is not feasible or practical, the exposure assessment step in a risk assessment is used to estimate the magnitude and probability of uptake from the environment by any combination of oral, inhalation, and dermal routes of exposure. The results of the exposure assessment are quantitative doses presented in the amount of the chemical per unit of body weight per unit of time (eg, mg/kg per day).

Early in the exposure assessment, the population at risk needs to be identified by determining who would be exposed to the chemicals of concern. The size of the exposed population depends on the proximity of the population to the source. For example, there is a high potential for exposing large numbers of people if the chemical is in drinking water or air. On the other hand, if the contamination is confined to an enclosed area (eg, indoor workplace), the population affected is likely to be smaller. In characterizing an exposed population, it is important to consider life stage and age, gender, health status, and race and cultural diversity within that population because individuals differ in sensitivity and susceptibility to a chemical hazard.

The primary routes of exposure to chemicals in the environment are inhalation of particulates, dusts, and vapors; dermal contact with contaminated surfaces (eg, soils or contaminated vegetation); use of consumer products (eg, paints and plastic containers); and ingestion of contaminated food, water, and contaminated surfaces (ie, hand-to-mouth transfer). Workplace exposures also result from inhaling, ingesting, and making contact not only with contaminated media but also with concentrated solutions or mixtures of industrial chemicals. Despite recent advances in protective clothing and gear, labeling instructions, and properly engineered ventilation systems, the potential for workplace exposures is still significantly higher than most environmental exposures.

Estimates of human exposure might be based on analytic measurements of samples taken from environmental or workplace monitoring, direct measurements of human exposure, or mathematical (predictive) models. Although direct measurements of human exposure are the most precise methods for detecting exposure in an individual or population, these methods are costly, require specialized instruments, and are time consuming. More frequently, exposure estimates are based on mathematical models. Numerous methodologies for estimating the human uptake of contaminants have been proposed and refined in recent years. Models have been developed and used to predict the movement of chemicals in the environment (eg, in air, groundwater, or surface water), transfer from contaminated surfaces (eg, carpet or clothing, hand-to-mouth), and deposition onto edible fruits and vegetables. PBPK models also are used to predict the rate of absorption, metabolism, and distribution of a chemical in the body.

In quantifying exposure doses, the number of exposed persons at each of the anticipated dose levels is described, as well as the upper and mean estimates of exposure. The best approach is to develop exposure scenarios that examine a range of potential or actual exposures for individuals, populations, and subpopulations. Depending on the use of the risk assessment, it might be adequate to estimate only doses from a single chemical exposure from a single source of the chemical. More often, multiple chemical exposures from multiple sources should be evaluated and aggregated, despite the relative complexity of doing this.

Formulas for estimating exposures from environmental and workplace chemicals can be applied to quantify dose levels for risk assessment. These formulas require entering values for physiologic and activity parameters such as breathing rate (resting and/or under exertion), daily water ingestion, food intake, body weight or size, and other factors that depend on the age, gender, physical well-being, and habits of the individual. Factors such as drug interactions, physical debilitation, stage in development (eg, fetus, perinatal, or infancy), and smoking status, for example, might increase susceptibility and sensitivity to a chemical exposure

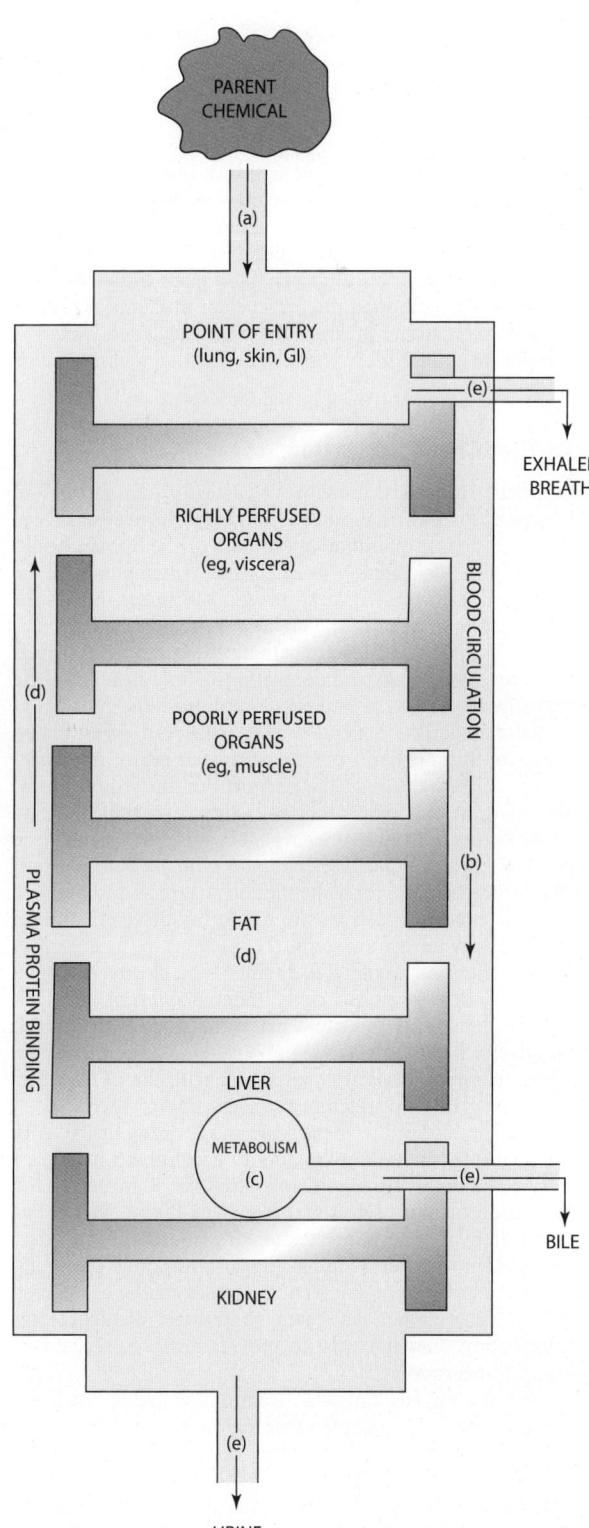

▲ **Figure 55–2.** Simplified diagram of a general compartmental physiologically based pharmacokinetic model. The (a) absorption, (b) distribution, (c) metabolism, (d) storage, and (e) elimination of an internalized xenobiotic are described by a series of mathematical interrelationships. Physiologically based pharmacokinetic models yield information such as the predicted change in the amount of a chemical in a given organ over time depending on the data input (eg, rate constants for transport, distribution, respiration, metabolism, and excretion, as well as the chemical and physical properties of the chemical). The compartments are intended to represent, as best as possible, actual anatomic structures, defined with respect to their volumes, blood flows (perfusion rate), chemical binding (partitioning) characteristics, and ability to metabolize and excrete the chemical of interest. For risk assessment purposes, these models are used primarily to predict and compare target tissue doses for different exposure situations in different animal species.

and should be documented and considered in the exposure assessment if possible. Values for body weight, breathing rate, and body size are obtained from tables that normalize the data and present mean and statistical bounds on the data. Often, values for parameters such as water ingestion and food intake are obtained from regional or even national surveys and therefore are not specific to a particular community, ethnicity, or lifestyle. For a more precise or defining exposure assessment for a specific population or individual, it is necessary to gather more specific data for entering the exposure formulas.

Application of statistical analyses to the exposure data set might be necessary to determine the distribution of data because environmental and occupational data might be lognormally distributed rather than conform to a Gaussian distribution.

Depending on the exposed population and the problem, exposure estimates might need to be made for different subpopulations (eg, children and infants, pregnant women, and the infirm) because these individuals are differentially susceptible, exhibit different activities patterns, or are particularly sensitive for a number of reasons. For a purely statistical description of a population, stochastic or "likelihood of risks" approaches were developed to characterize exposures using models that replicate randomness in exposure. The probabilistic techniques can characterize a range of potential exposures and their likelihood of occurrence.

Some chemicals persist for many years in the environment, whereas others degrade rapidly. The environmental fate of chemicals depends on several factors, for example, the chemical and physical properties of the substance, the potential for movement through various environmental media (eg, groundwater and porous soils) or storage (eg, binding of chemicals to sediments), the rate of degradation in the environment (eg, by sunlight, soil and water microbes, and evaporation), and the potential for bioaccumulation and biomagnification. Some chemicals such as chlorine and bromine-based chemicals can persist in the environment for 50 or more years (see for examples the Stockholm Convention list of Persistent Organic Pollutants), whereas other chemicals (eg, some organophosphorus pesticides) degrade within weeks or months, particularly when exposed to sunlight. Lipophilic chemicals (eg, methyl mercury) in the environment are stored in the tissues of animals, most notably fish and, through a process called *biomagnification,* increase (sometimes to concentrations hundreds of times greater than the original environmental levels) as the stored chemicals move up the food chain. Therefore, although direct human exposures to chemical contaminants might be reduced when chemicals are degraded rapidly, there is certainly significant exposure potential for even those chemicals that exist for only a few days in the environment (eg, to workers when manufacturing, formulating, or using chemicals) or that start out at low concentrations but bioaccumulate in the food chain (eg, contaminated fish).

New technologies and advances in analytic instrumentation and methodologies can detect very small quantities of exogenous (xenobiotic) chemicals in blood, urine, hair, feces, exhaled breath, and fat and other tissues (ie, biomonitoring). Measurement of chemical residues at parts per trillion (ppt) levels and even lower is now possible in biologic tissues (as well as in environmental media). For many chemicals, biomonitoring results represent a direct indicator of either acute or chronic exposure to a chemical. These direct measurements can offer a better alternative to assessing exposure than using mathematical models. Furthermore, environmental monitoring also has benefited from these advances in technology, although the presence of mixtures of chemicals and the matrices in which these chemicals reside tend to complicate and interfere with environmental measurements at low levels.

▶ Risk Characterization

In the risk characterization, the risk assessor summarizes and interprets the information collected from the previous three steps, presents a quantitative estimate of the human health risk(s), and identifies (and quantifies when possible) the uncertainties in these risk estimates. This process allows the risk assessor to identify the greatest individual and population health risks and promulgate health-based action levels to protect individuals and populations from further harmful exposure or to prevent immediate- or long-term injury.

Estimated risks depend on the measured or estimated exposure duration and can be calculated either retrospectively (ie, the release of the chemical or the exposure has already occurred) or prospectively (ie, to prevent a release or the exposure from happening). It is appropriate and often necessary in a risk characterization to estimate both noncancer and cancer risks for a chemical exposure and to evaluate multiple exposure scenarios to aid in the determination of the necessary mitigation steps.

For chemical toxicity endpoints that clearly exhibit a threshold dose-response curve, reference exposure levels (RELs), defined as threshold exposure levels below which no adverse health effects are anticipated, can be calculated. These reference levels are comparable with the EPA's reference doses (RfDs) or reference concentrations (RfCs).

RELs are derived by identifying and dividing the NOAEL (or BMD) by uncertainty factors to account for inadequacies in the database, incomplete scientific knowledge, and protection of more sensitive individuals (Table 55–4). The application of uncertainty factors offers a margin of safety to consider when developing mitigation options or regulatory standards. Some uncertainty factors can be considered default values when adequate physiologic or toxicologic information does not exist to provide a more precise estimate of uncertainty.

For carcinogens, unless a threshold for toxicity is clearly demonstrated, it is assumed that the dose-response is linear with no "no risk" level. For these chemical agents, a cancer potency is calculated, and the probability for excess individual cancer risk is estimated based on exposure estimates. The determination as to what is an "acceptable" (or *de minimis*)

Table 55–4. Uncertainty factors that may be applied in calculating risk-based exposure levels.

Data Gap or Methodologic Consideration	Uncertainty Factor (Range)
Data extrapolation from acute to chronic	100
Data extrapolation from subchronic to chronic	10
Human (intraspecies) variability	10
Animal to human (interspecies) variability	10
Increased sensitivity or susceptibility (eg, children)	(1–10)
Conversion of LOAEL to NOAEL	(3–10)
Evidence for genotoxicity (no cancer data)	(1–10)
Reported NOAEL may be a LOAEL	(1–10)
Extrapolation from subchronic to acute	1
Structure activity relationship	Varies with potency
Inadequate experimental design	(1–10)
Pharmacokinetic corrections	Varies with parameter measured or modeled

cancer risk is a value-based decision, and often a range of risk is presented for comparative purposes.

Documented differences in physiology and toxicology between species may be used to modify RELs and, to a lesser degree, cancer risk estimates to better reflect the human exposure and predicted response to the chemical. The concept of ensuring a margin of safety between exposure and toxicity still should apply, however, even when a more precise estimate of uncertainty can be made. Some subpopulations (eg, the developing fetus, infants, and children) may be more sensitive or differentially susceptible to a chemical exposure. It is difficult to predict with accuracy the effects of a chemical exposure to such an individual compared with the average, healthy adult in the population. Frequently, gender, race, other genetic traits, and social or economic stressors (such as access to medical care) also may affect an individual's sensitivity. The risk characterization step should account for differences in individuals and subpopulations and uncertainties in the data and methodology.

In general, a thorough characterization of risk also should discuss background concentrations of the chemical in the environment and in human tissue, pharmacokinetic differences between the animal test species and humans (the results of a PBPK or another biologically based model are useful here), the effect of selecting specific exposure parameters, the level of uncertainty in the methods (ie, calculations and statistical analyses), and other factors that can influence

the magnitude of the estimated risks. Furthermore, areas for which additional research is needed also should be identified (eg, data gaps).

EXAMPLE OF THE APPLICATION OF RISK ASSESSMENT METHODOLOGY

The general approach to calculating risk for noncancer and cancer endpoints is illustrated below for the pesticide and environmental contaminant dibromochloropropane (DBCP). California promulgates maximum contaminant levels (MCLs) for drinking water contaminants that are based in part on public health goals. In deriving an MCL, which is a regulatory standard, costs, benefits, and technical feasibility (eg, of detection or mitigation) must be considered. A public health goal is developed based on a risk calculation, consideration of the uncertainty in the methods and the data and accounting for the most sensitive or susceptible individuals (eg, infants and children). The public health goal is developed to protect public health, but it is not a regulatory standard like an MCL and therefore is not enforceable.

DBCP was used extensively as a soil fumigant and nematicide in the United States until 1977, when its registration as a pesticide was suspended. Although it is no longer manufactured commercially or used in this country, groundwater contamination still exists in the San Joaquin Valley and other agricultural regions in California. Exposure to DBCP occurs from the use of tap water as a source of drinking water, as well as in preparing foods and beverages. It is also used for bathing or showering and for washing, flushing toilets, and other household uses resulting in potential dermal and inhalation exposures.

▶ Noncancer Health Effects

DBCP induces testicular damage and infertility, as evidenced by numerous studies of occupational exposures, described as reduced (oligospermia) or no sperm counts (azoospermia), altered sperm motility, damage to the seminiferous tubules, and hormonal disruption. Testicular toxicity is reported most frequently and appears to occur at lower exposures than that of other noncancer endpoints (ie, it is the most sensitive noncancer toxicity endpoint). In experimental animal studies, the highest NOAEL of 0.025 mg/kg per day is identified for adverse testicular effects in the male rabbit. Using this information, the calculation of an REL (or public health goal), in this case defined as C mg/L for a noncarcinogenic effect of DBCP, follows the equation:

$$C = \frac{NOAEL \times BW \times RSC}{U \times W}$$

$$= \frac{0.025 \text{ mg/kg} \cdot d \times 70 \text{ kg} \times 0.8}{1000 \times 6 \text{ Leq}}$$

$$= 2.3 \times 10^{-4} \text{ mg/L} = 0.2 \text{ ppb (rounded)}$$

where NOAEL is no observed adverse effect level, BW is body weight (a default value of 70 kg [154.3 lb] for an adult male is used), RSC is relative source contribution (the sole anticipated source of exposure is groundwater, and therefore, 80% is used as input for DBCP), UF is the uncertainty factor (10 to account for interspecies extrapolation, 10 for use of subchronic NOAEL, and 10 for potentially sensitive human subpopulations), and W is daily water consumption rate (a daily water consumption rate of 6 liter equivalents [Leq] is used because direct ingestion accounts for approximately one-third of the total exposure from household use of DBCP contaminated water, and the remaining two-third is from dermal and inhalation exposure).

The risk of noncancer health effects from drinking DBCP-contaminated water can be determined by calculating the hazard index, which is the ratio of human exposure to the REL. If the hazard index is less than 1, an adequate margin of safety exists. If the hazard index is equal to or greater than 1, the estimated exposure is equal to or greater than the REL, and further examination of the public health implications is required. Applying this method for DBCP, a hazard index of greater than 1 would be achieved when drinking water levels exceed 0.2 ppb.

▶ Carcinogenic Effects

DBCP also causes cancer in experimental animals, and there is some evidence from human exposure studies—it is classified by the National Toxicology Program as "Reasonably Anticipated to be a human carcinogen" (NTP 2016), by EPA as a B2 carcinogen and by the World Health Organization as "probably" carcinogenic to humans (Group 2B, IARC 1999). For risk assessment purposes, the development of squamous cell carcinomas of the stomach in female mice is used to calculate a carcinogenic potency of 7 $(mg/kg \cdot d)^{-1}$. To calculate the cancer potency, the linear multistage model was fit to the animal carcinogenicity dose-response data, and the 95% upper confidence limit on the linear term ($q1^*$) was used. This estimate in animals is adjusted to a lifetime potency, assuming that potency tends to increase with the third power of the observation time in a bioassay. The estimate of lifetime animal carcinogenic potency is converted to an estimate of potency in humans by the factor (70 kg/animal body weight)$^{1/3}$. This conversion follows from the assumption that a dose rate calculated as daily intake of DBCP divided by (body weight)$^{2/3}$ has the same potency in rodents and humans. Using this cancer potency, the calculation of an REL (C) for DBCP in drinking water using the cancer endpoint follows the equation:

$$C = \frac{R \times BW}{CSF \times W}$$

$$= \frac{10^{-6} \times 70 \text{ kg}}{7 \text{ (mg/kg} \cdot \text{d)}^{-1} \times 6 \text{ Leq/d}}$$

$$= 1.7 \times 10^{-6} \text{ mg/L} = 1.7 \text{ ppt}$$

where BW is adult body weight (the default of 70 kg [154.3 lb] for an adult man), R is *de minimis* level for lifetime excess individual cancer risk (a default of 10^{-6}), CSF is cancer potency ($q1^*$) of 7 $(mg/kg \cdot d)^{-1}$ for the development of squamous cell carcinomas of the stomach in female mice, and W is daily volume of water consumed in liter equivalents (Leq) per day.

Therefore, for DBCP, an individual excess cancer risk of 1×10^{-6} (1 in 1 million) would be exceeded when drinking water levels are above 1.7 ppt. It is clear from the results of this risk assessment that the drinking water level considered more health protective is the one based on the cancer endpoint. The federal EPA identifies a health advisory for cancer risks at 0.003 mg/L DBCP in drinking water, which is associated with a 1 in 10,000 (10^{-4}) cancer risk (U.S. EPA 2018).

DISCUSSION

Quantitative risk assessment has been the foundation for environmental decision making in the United States for almost 40 years. If risk assessment and risk management are to remain the key factors in environmental decision making, "value" choices in the risk evaluation process should be made explicit, and policymakers must recognize the limitations of quantitative risk assessment. Furthermore, the design and results of the risk assessment must be described clearly in the context of the environmental problem. In other words, the context within which the "science" of risk assessment is performed should shape how scientific information is used and interpreted.

▶ Limitations of Using Risk Assessment for Environmental Decision Making

There is an ongoing debate concerning the limitations of using risk assessment results in environmental decision making. The primary complaints include the following:

1. Risk assessment is not solely "science based" but incorporates judgments and values that are limited by a high degree of uncertainty.

2. Conventional risk assessment methods do not account for the disproportionate risk burdens borne by certain communities, nor do they account for the impacts of cumulative and multiple exposures in toxic hot spots or to groups of people (eg, farm workers and their families).

3. Risk assessment as a two-tiered approach separates risk assessment from management as a means to insulate the "objectivity" of risk assessment from value-laden management decisions. This approach is criticized by scientists and philosophers of science for being unrealistic in that no practice of science is purely objective. Some social scientists argue that risk assessors cannot be completely immune to the political factors of the institutions within which they operate.

4. Risk assessment leads to regulatory delays; that is, "paralysis by analysis."

5. Focusing on the quantitative aspects of risk does not provide enough information on the qualitative aspects, such as anxiety about the future, involuntariness of exposure, and equity concerns.

6. Risk assessment is used primarily to justify certain amounts of pollution, whereas the goal should be pollution elimination, prevention, or environmental sustainability (eg, leaving sufficient resources and a clean environment for future generations).

7. The process is disempowering (undemocratic) and often neglects the public participation and social values needed to make good decisions about environmental priorities. Inclusion of "risk communication" in the latter stages of the risk assessment process not only is a poor use of an important information resource (eg, the affected community itself), but it also clouds the process, making it difficult to understand and reproduce.

8. Environmental decisions based on risk comparisons with regulatory benchmarks often are viewed with skepticism by those who are affected the most. This is particularly problematic when those who are at the greatest risk do not substantially benefit from the stressor.

▶ Does the Dose Really Make the Poison?

Students of toxicology will no doubt read somewhere in a textbook that "the dose makes the poison." While there are applications where this statement holds true, in general it oversimplifies what we know of the toxicity of chemicals in living organisms. This often leads to misunderstanding by laypersons or misuse by some in an attempt to downplay the impact of environmental pollutants and other chemicals on humans. Although the phrase "the dose makes the poison" has applicability for laboratory experiments where all variables are tightly controlled, there are some notable exceptions. The timing of exposure during pregnancy rather than the dose is more critical for chemicals that cause birth defects; therefore, it is the life stage of exposure that makes the poison for these chemicals. As noted previously, chemical carcinogens that cause genetic damage or mutations in DNA are thought to have no safe dose; therefore, any dose makes the poison for these chemicals. Other chemicals trigger receptors in cells at very low doses and can change the activities of the cell or the signals to other cells.

For humans, there are additional reasons why the statement "the dose makes the poison" does not adequately address the risk of health damage. For example, the statement does not account for the wide-ranging variations in the human population, including sensitive, susceptible, and vulnerable populations or individuals. For example, human defense and repair mechanisms will vary in individuals depending on factors such as age, physical state, gender, race and nutritional status. Therefore, the effective toxic dose will not only vary from person to person, it could also vary within an individual. Furthermore, no individual is exposed to a single chemical from a single source from a single route of exposure at the same dose over a lifetime. People are exposed to multiple chemicals in a limitless number of combinations and doses daily such that over a lifetime (starting at least at conception) it is likely the doses required for an individual chemical to exert toxicity will be highly variable.

Finally, carcinogens and some chemicals that cause noncancer health effects even at the lowest doses (eg, lead) do not exhibit thresholds for toxicity. For these chemicals, determining a level that "won't hurt anyone" requires a risk-based (probability-based) evaluation and by definition this is a subjective (not science-based) determination. It must account for the value system of the person being impacted. In other words, people will rightfully have different opinions regarding what level of risk is acceptable to them depending on their own values. Under these circumstances, the dose that "makes the poison" is subjective and dependent on an individual's own personal tolerance and acceptance levels.

▶ Individual Versus Population Risks

Some risk assessments or decisions based on risk assessments rely on measures of population risks; that is, measures of the additional incidence of some adverse impact in the affected population. In this situation, assessing and comparing risks for a potentially hazardous situation using population risks alone might not identify it as an environmental priority. For example, if arsenic were to leach from an abandoned toxic waste site into a nearby waterway, it could present alarmingly high individual risks. The total population risk associated with this situation, however, might be very small if only a small number of people depended on that water supply. A circular construct emerges: Waste sites and industrial facilities that often are located in poor communities and communities of color are not subject to stringent intervention or remedial action because the population risks (as opposed to individual risks of those exposed) are seen as minimal. By using population risk as the benchmark, policymakers might justify not taking action on the basis of the lesser benefits of mitigation to the overall population. Using average population risk for ranking without also looking at maximum individual risk is an economic or policy choice, not a "scientific" decision.

The use of aggregate statistics and population risk measures does not routinely account for "hot spots," that is, geographic areas where residents experience greater environmental risks or locations where multiple exposures to hazardous substances and associated risks occur over time. In addition, risk assessments do not routinely account for differences in individual susceptibilities to toxic substances and chemical-chemical interactions in mixtures. Some attempts have been made by the EPA to develop guidance to incorporate these and other considerations in the risk assessment process. Nevertheless, inclusion of these issues is not yet widely practiced.

▶ Public Involvement

Collaboration among the business community and industrial sector, impacted communities, workers and worker representatives, the general population, and government agencies is required for effective involvement of the public. Although public participation is now generally accepted in diverse policy fields, it is still not addressed adequately in science-based environmental decision making such as risk assessment and risk management.

Environmental agencies should develop and implement plans to involve the public in the decision-making process and recognize that public participation be a solution to some environmental problems in and of itself, but only when the public is involved as a full and equal partner, not as an adversary. This includes maximizing meaningful participation in the review of agencies' activities and progress in accomplishing the objectives of promoting long-term planning for sustaining a healthy environment and workplace. To accomplish this, public participation needs to be initiated early in the hazard evaluation process and incorporated into the decision-making process. Furthermore, education is a key component to effective public involvement, and therefore, technical information should be easily accessible to the public and translated, if necessary, into the residents' and workers' primary language(s).

▶ Research Needs

More research needs to be done to better understand the risks that environmental and workplace pollution poses, including the following:

1. Completing the toxicity database for many substances released in large quantities into the air, water, land, and workplace or as contaminants in food and other consumer products.

2. Making available data describing actual human exposures to most pollutants.

3. Developing risk assessment methods further. For example, methods to assess cumulative risk from multiple chemical exposures and the effects of chemicals on the endocrine, nervous, and immune systems are necessary to better understand the full spectrum of hazards posed by environmental pollutants and occupational hazards.

4. Considering subpopulations that bear disproportionate risks (ie, "hot spots"), which must be incorporated into any new and/or existing site-specific risk assessments.

5. Developing methods to assess the societal distribution of environmental and occupational health risks in the context of achieving environmental justice.

6. Devoting resources to measuring population exposures to toxicants, including from microenvironments, from accidental releases, and among highly exposed groups.

7. Increasing the capacity to identify and prevent future impacts on public health and the environment from emerging risks.

▶ Other Models for Environmental Decision Making

Applying scientific knowledge and judgment to address environmental issues requires universal strategies as well as some fundamental changes in the status quo of environmental decision making. In other words, more consideration should be given to alternative science or value-based processes proposed or used to address environmental and occupational hazards.

One alternative model used to support environmental decision making, predominantly in European countries, is the precautionary principle. This approach does not exclude making estimates of risk, but the burden of proof is levied on the polluter rather than the affected public. In fact, it has been argued that the precautionary principle should be viewed as a complement to science to be invoked when a lack of scientific evidence means that the outcomes are uncertain. In applying the precautionary principle, ethical and value-based aspects should be weighed equally with the science. The key element to the precautionary principle is that action should be taken in the face of uncertainty rather than delaying action until more "evidence" is generated.

Other options include technology-based approaches that require retooling or reformulating industrial processes to use fewer or lesser amounts of hazardous materials or by substituting them with safer alternatives. The EPA is already mandated to incorporate pollution prevention into its implementation plans under the TSCA and the Clean Air Act, whereas the reduction or elimination of hazardous pesticide use has lagged. These approaches apply the principles of hazard identification without necessarily relying on a risk-based assessment because the goal is to achieve elimination of hazardous materials and prevention of environmental and workplace exposures. In banning the chemicals DDT, polychlorinated biphenyl (PCB), and lead in gasoline, pollution prevention is achieved without allowing for some level of "negligible risk."

Public pressure, public right-to-know laws, and civil suits also have achieved a certain degree of success in influencing environmental decision making. For example, California's Proposition 65, approved by a wide margin in 1986 as an initiative to address growing concerns about exposures to toxic chemicals, is an example of a public right-to-know law that also empowers citizens to "blow the whistle" on polluters. Currently, there are approximately 900 chemicals listed as reproductive or developmental toxicants or carcinogens. California's Proposition 65 is an effective mechanism for reducing certain exposures that may not have been controlled adequately under existing federal or state laws. It also provides a market-based incentive for manufacturers to remove listed chemicals from their products. Furthermore, because of Proposition 65, information regarding the dangers of exposure to certain chemicals in more susceptible subpopulations is widely disseminated. The California Safe Cosmetics Act of 2005 is another right-to-know law, and the first in the country requiring manufacturers of cosmetic products to publicly disclose harmful ingredients used in their products. Almost 100 chemicals known or suspected to cause cancer, reproductive effects, and/or birth defects are used in cosmetic product formulations. Additionally, the California Safer Consumer Products regulations that took effect in 2013 aims to identify and reduce toxic chemicals in consumer products. Many other states have passed chemical-specific legislation to reduce harmful toxic chemicals including in consumer products and bans on certain pesticides. Where rules and regulations are failing to prevent harmful chemical exposures, many consumers are directly pressuring retailers and product manufacturers to fully disclose all ingredients, and provide products certified to be made without toxic ingredients.

REFERENCES

Krewski D et al: Toxicity testing in the 21st century: progress in the past decade and future perspectives [published online ahead of print, 2019 Dec 17]. Arch Toxicol 2019;10.1007/s00204-019-02613-4. doi:10.1007/s00204-019-02613-4.
See https://www.epa.gov/chemical-research/toxicology-testing-21st-century-tox21.

Krewski D et al: Toxicity testing in the 21st century: progress in the past decade and future perspectives. Arch Toxicol 2020;94(1): 1-58 [PMID: 31848664].
Madia F, Worth A, Whelan M, Corvi R: Carcinogenicity assessment: addressing the challenges of cancer and chemicals in the environment. Environ Int 2019;128:417-429 [PMID: 31078876].
State of California Office of Environmental Health Hazard Assessment. Public health goals for drinking water. https://oehha.ca.gov/water/public-health-goals-phgs.
State of California Office of Environmental Health Hazard Assessment, Proposition 65: https://oehha.ca.gov/proposition-65.
U.S. NTP (National Toxicology Program). Toxicology Testing in the 21st Century (Tox21).
U.S. NTP (National Toxicology Program). 2016. Report on Carcinogens, Fourteenth Edition; Research Triangle Park, NC: U.S. Department of Health and Human Services, Public Health Service. See https://ntp.niehs.nih.gov/whatwestudy/assessments/cancer/roc/index.html?utm_source=direct&utm_medium=prod&utm_campaign=ntpgolinks&utm_term=roc14.
U.S. Environmental Protection Agency, Cancer Risk Assessment Guidelines (2005): https://www.epa.gov/risk/guidelines-carcinogen-risk-assessment.
U.S. EPA Drinking Water Standards and Health Advisories Tables. (2018). See https://www.epa.gov/sites/production/files/2018-03/documents/dwtable2018.pdf.

■ SELF-ASSESSMENT QUESTIONS

Select the one correct answer for each question.

Question 1: Risk
a. is the anxiety that an event will result in loss or harm
b. may be thought of as voluntary but not involuntary
c. does not include the probability of adverse health effects
d. can apply to almost any activity or event

Question 2. Risk assessment
a. is solely "science based"
b. incorporates only values with a high degree of certainty
c. avoids regulatory delays
d. is a process and not a science

Question 3: Exposure assessment
a. is used to estimate the magnitude and probability of uptake from the environment by any combination of oral, inhalation, and dermal routes of exposure
b. presents results in qualitative, not quantitative, terms
c. identifies the population at risk by determining who has elevated blood levels of toxic chemicals
d. does not need to consider proximity of the population to the source

Question 4: A precautionary approach to decision making
a. avoids long delays in taking action when there is uncertainty in the existing data
b. supersedes risk assessment as a decision-making factor for federal regulators
c. requires government to prove harm before it acts
d. is supported by the chemical industry

Question 5: A risk management decision
a. involves evaluating the impact of risk assessment on medical research funding
b. is solely based on empirical data generated by impartial scientists and analysts
c. requires an impacted population or individual to assign an acceptable risk factor of their exposure
d. considers risk along with cost, technical feasibility, societal benefits, and political climate

Question 6: Reference exposure levels (RELs) are
a. defined as median exposure levels below which no adverse health effects are anticipated
b. derived by identifying and dividing the NOAEL (or BMD) by uncertainty factors
c. not modified by differences in physiology and toxicology between species
d. solely based on empirical data generated by impartial scientists and analysts

Appendix A: Biostatistics & Epidemiology

Stephanie M. Holm, MD, MPH

It is apparent to anyone who reads the medical literature today that some knowledge of biostatistics and epidemiology is a necessity. This is particularly true in occupational and environmental health in which many of the findings are based on epidemiologic studies of subjects exposed to low levels of an agent. Research has become more rigorous in the area of study design and analysis, and reports of clinical and epidemiologic research contain increasing amounts of statistical methodology. This Appendix provides a brief introduction to some of the basic principles of biostatistics and epidemiology.

▼ I. BIOSTATISTICS

DESCRIPTIVE STATISTICS

▶ Types of Data

Data collected in medical research can be divided into three types: nominal (categorical), ordinal, and continuous.

Nominal (categorical) data are those that can be divided into two or more unordered categories, such as gender, race, or religion. In occupational medicine, for example, many outcome measures, such as cancer rates, are considered separately for different gender and race categories.

Ordinal data are different from nominal data in that there is a predetermined order underlying the categories. Examples of ordinal data include clinical severity scores or socioeconomic status (SES).

Both nominal and ordinal data are examples of discrete data. They take on only integer values.

Continuous data are data measured on an arithmetic scale. Examples include height, weight, blood lead levels, or forced expiratory volume (FEV). The accuracy of the number recorded depends on the measuring instrument, and the variable can take on an infinite number of values within a defined range. For example, a person's height might be recorded as 72 in or 72.001 in or 72.00098 in depending on the accuracy of the measuring instrument.

▶ Summarizing Data

Once research data are collected, the first step is to summarize them. The two most common ways of summarizing data

are measures of location, or central tendency, and measures of spread, or variation.

A. Measures of Central Tendency

1. Mean—The mean ($\bar{x}$) is the average value of a set of data observations. It is computed using the following equation:

$$\bar{x} = \frac{\sum_{i=1}^{n} x_i}{n}$$

where n is sample size and x_i is a random variable, such as height, with $i = 1, \ldots, n$.

The mean can be strongly affected by extreme values in the data. If a variable has a fairly symmetric distribution, the mean is used as the appropriate measure of central tendency.

2. Median—The median is the "middle" observation, or 50th percentile; that is, half the observations lie above the median and half below it. When there is an odd number of observations, the median is merely the middle observation. For example, for the following series of observations of subjects' weights (in pounds): 124, 138, 139, 152, and 173, the median is 139. When there is an even number of observations, the median is the mean of the two middle numbers. Using a similar example of subject weights, for the following series of weights (in pounds): 124, 138, 139, 152, 173, and 179, the median is (139 + 152)/2 = 145.5. The median is not as susceptible as the mean to extreme values. If the variable being measured has a distribution that is asymmetric or skewed—that is, if there are a few extreme values at one end of the distribution—the median is a better descriptor than the mean of the "center" of the distribution.

3. Mode—The mode is the most frequently occurring observation. It is used rarely, except when there are a limited number of possible outcomes.

4. Frequency distribution—In discussing measures of location or spread, we often refer to the frequency distribution of the data. A frequency distribution consists of a series of predetermined intervals (along the horizontal axis) together with the number (or percentage) of observations whose values fall in that interval (along the vertical axis). An example of a frequency distribution is presented in Figure A–1.

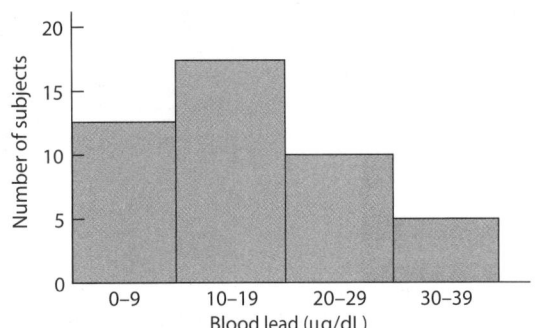

▲ Figure A–1. Frequency distribution of subjects by blood lead category.

B. Measures of Variation

1. Range—The range is the simplest measurement of variation and is defined as the difference between the highest and lowest values. Disadvantages of the range are that it is sensitive to a single extreme value, and it tends to increase in value as the number of observations increases. Furthermore, the range does not provide information about the distribution of values within the set of data. The interquartile range (25th–75th percentiles) is sometimes used because it is less influenced by extreme values.

2. Variance—The sample variance (s^2) is a measure of the dispersion about the mean arrived at by calculating the sum of the squared deviations from the mean and dividing by the sample size minus 1. The equation for deriving sample variance is as follows:

$$s^2 = \frac{\sum_{i=1}^{n}(x_i - \bar{x})^2}{n-1}$$

Variance can be thought of as the average of squared deviations from the mean, or more simply, variance tells you how spread out the distribution of the observations is.

3. Standard deviation—The sample standard deviation (s) is equal to the square root of the sample variance. Basically, it tells you how tightly clustered all the observations are around the mean of a set of data.

$$s = \sqrt{\frac{\sum_{i=1}^{n}(x_i - \bar{x})^2}{n-1}}$$

See Table A–1 for examples of the calculation of mean, median, mode, variance, and standard deviation.

Variability in data may be a result of the natural distribution of values or of random factors produced by errors in measurement. Neither the variance n or standard deviation distinguish between different sources of variability.

Table A–1. Calculation of mean, median, mode, variance, and standard deviation (n = 10 workers).

Worker	x_i = Number of Years of Exposure to Asbestos.		
	X_i	$(X_i - X)$	$(X_i - X)^2$
1.	$X_1 = 4.0$	−2.2	4.84
2.	$X_2 = 4.5$	−1.7	2.89
3.	$X_3 = 5.0$	−1.2	1.44
4.	$X_4 = 5.0$	−1.2	1.44
5.	$X_5 = 6.0$	−0.2	0.04
6.	$X_6 = 6.5$	+0.3	0.09
7.	$X_7 = 7.0$	+0.8	0.64
8.	$X_8 = 7.5$	+1.3	1.69
9.	$X_9 = 8.0$	+1.8	3.24
10.	$X_{10} = 8.5$	+2.3	5.29
Total:	$\Sigma X_i = 62.0$		$\Sigma(X_i - X)^2 = 21.6$

Mean: $\bar{x} = \dfrac{62.0}{10} = 6.2$

Variance $= \Sigma(x_i - x)^2/(n-1) = 21.6/9 = 2.4$

Standard deviation $= \sqrt{2.4} = 1.55$

Median:
1. Order the observation from lowest to highest.

2. Median $= \frac{1}{2}\left(\left[\dfrac{n}{2}\right]\text{observation} + \left(\left[\dfrac{n}{2}\right] + 1\right)\text{observation}\right) = 1/2$

(5th observation + 6th observation)

3. Therefore, median $= \frac{1}{2}(6.0 + 6.5) = 6.25$

Mode:
Most commonly occurring observation is 5, because it occurs twice and all other observations occur once.

▶ Sample Versus Population Descriptive Statistics

The descriptive statistics discussed thus far are sample estimates of true population values or parameters. Because we usually do not have the resources to measure the variable(s) of interest on entire populations, we instead select a sample from the population of interest and then estimate both the population mean and variance from the sample mean and variance. The population mean usually is represented by the Greek letter μ and the population variance by the Greek letter σ^2. One almost never knows the true population values

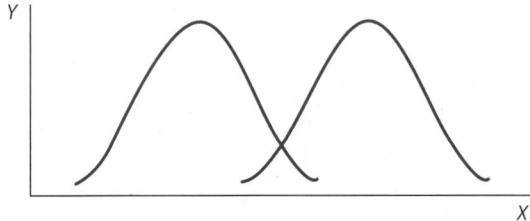

▲ **Figure A–2.** Two normal distributions with different means but identical standard deviations.

for these parameters and thus needs to take a sample of the population to estimate them.

▶ The Normal Distribution

The most important continuous probability distribution is the normal, or Gaussian distribution, also known as the *bell-shaped curve.* Many quantitative variables follow a normal distribution, and it plays a central role in statistical tests of hypotheses.

A particular normal distribution is defined by its mean and variance (or standard deviation). Two normal distributions with different means but the same variance will differ in location but not in shape (Figure A–2). Two normal distributions with the same mean but different variances will have the same location but different shapes or "spreads" about the mean value (Figure A–3). Note that the normal distribution is unimodal (has one value occurring most frequently), bell-shaped, and symmetric about the mean.

The population encompassed by one standard deviation (σ) on either side of the mean in a normally distributed population will include approximately 67% of the observations in that population (Figure A–4); the population between 2σ on either side of the mean will include approximately 95% of the observations; and that between 3σ on either side of the mean encompasses more than 99% of the observations in the population (see Figure A–4). This property of the normal distribution is particularly useful when a researcher or clinician is trying to identify patients with high or low values in

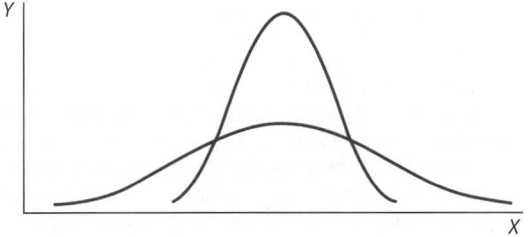

▲ **Figure A–3.** Two normal distributions with identical means but different standard deviations.

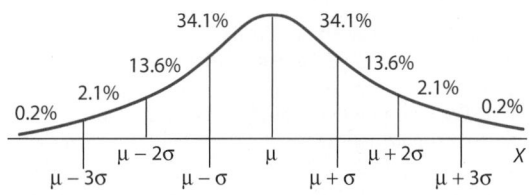

▲ **Figure A–4.** Standard normal distribution.

response to a certain test. If one knows the mean for that particular test and has a good estimate of what the standard deviation is, the range within which one would expect (let us say) 95% of patients to fall can be determined, and a patient with values outside this range might need to be examined further.

To use this property of the normal distribution, the sample should be large enough to provide reasonably certain estimates of the mean and standard deviation.

Example I: *If the mean hematocrit value in a clinical population is 42% with a standard deviation of 3%—and assuming hematocrit values follow a normal distribution—one would expect 95% of the clinic population to have hematocrit values between 42% ± (2 × 3%) or (36, 48)%. A patient falling outside this range could be identified for further testing.*

The normal distribution has several nice properties that make it amenable to statistical analysis, and because of this many common statistical tests (eg, *t*-tests, linear regression) make an assumption of a normal distribution. Such tests are often referred to as parametric tests. When the sample mean ($\overline{x}$) follows a normal distribution, parametric tests can be utilized.

There are two ways in which the sample mean can follow a normal distribution. When the underlying variable, *x*, has a distribution that follows a normal curve, the sample mean ($\overline{x}$) will also follow a normal distribution. We often transform data to make them more normal in distribution, so that the corresponding ($\overline{x}$) values will also have a normal distribution. For example, in occupational exposure studies, the log dose often is used rather than the actual dose because the log dose more closely approximates a normal distribution. Another principle relevant to the normal distribution is the central limit theorem, which holds that no matter what the underlying distribution of *x*, the particular variable of interest, the sample mean ($\overline{x}$) will have a normal distribution if the sample size (*n*) is large enough. Therefore, parametric tests are also appropriate for large sample sizes.

Because one is usually concerned with estimating the true population mean μ from the sample mean $\overline{x}$, it is important to know how good an estimate the sample mean is of the true mean. Every time a sample of size *n* is selected from the population and $\overline{x}$ is calculated, a different value for $\overline{x}$ will be obtained and thus a different estimate of μ. If this were done over and over again and many $\overline{x}$ values were generated, the $\bar{x}$ values themselves would have a normal distribution centered on μ with standard deviation equal to σ/√n. The standard deviation of $\bar{x}$ is called the *standard error of the mean* (SEM). In practice, one does not calculate several $\bar{x}$ values to estimate μ; only one is calculated. The SEM quantifies the certainty with which this one sample mean estimates the population mean. The certainty with which one estimates the population mean increases with sample size, and it can be seen that the standard error decreases as *n* increases. It also can be seen that the standard error increases as σ increases. This means that the more variability in the underlying population, the more variable will be the estimate of μ. The "true" SEM is σ/√n, and the sample estimate of the standard error of the mean is s/√n, where *s* is the sample standard deviation. An investigator wanting a more precise estimate of the mean (smaller SEM) could either increase the sample size *n* or try to decrease σ.

Many investigators incorrectly summarize the variability in their data with the standard error because it is smaller in value than the standard deviation. However, the standard error does not quantify variability in the population; it quantifies the uncertainty in the estimate of $\bar{x}$ the population mean. An investigator describing the population sampled should use the standard deviation to describe that population. The SEM is used in testing hypotheses about the population mean.

Example II: Suppose that blood lead is measured in 20 patients. Assume that the sample mean ($\bar{x}$) equals 20 μg/dL and that the sample standard deviation (s) equals 5 μg/dL with a sample size (n) of 20. If blood lead has a normal distribution in this sample, one would expect 95% of the population to lie within 2s of the mean. Thus, if the investigator's sample was a representative one, 95% of the population will have blood leads between 20 ± (2 × 5) (ie, between 10 and 30 μg/dL). These numbers quickly summarize the distribution and give the reader a range against which to compare the reader's own patients. However, investigators often summarize their data with the mean and the standard error of the mean and report, "Blood lead in this sample population was 20 ± [2 × (5/√ 20)]." This would lead a reader to believe that 95% of blood lead values are expected to fall between 17.8 and 22.2 μg/dL if one did not know the difference between the standard deviation and the standard error of the mean. The reader of the report usually wishes to compare a patient's blood lead with an expected range of values for blood lead, that is, the mean ±2s.

INFERENTIAL STATISTICS

In general, there are two steps to be followed in data analysis. The first is to describe the data by using descriptive statistics such as the mean, median, variance, and standard deviation. The second step is to test specific hypotheses that were formulated before conducting the research project. This is done by formulating a null hypothesis and an alternative hypothesis. An example of a null hypothesis might be, "There is no difference in pulmonary function between groups of underground miners and surface miners." The alternative hypothesis could be, "there is a difference between the two groups." Once the hypotheses are formulated, the appropriate statistical test can be performed. Basics of making inferences from statistical tests are explored and subsequently some of the most commonly used methods are discussed.

▶ Confidence Intervals, *P*-values & Statistical Significance

When sample means and variability are used to estimate the mean and variability of an underlying population distribution, statistical methods can be used to create a confidence interval (CI). The idea behind a CI is that if you choose a confidence level (such as 95% or 99%), you can calculate an interval that will contain the true mean 95% (or 99%) of the time. Many statisticians consider CIs to be the best tool for making inferences from statistical studies as they represent the estimate of the underlying data and are more intuitive for non-statisticians to understand.

However, CIs are often *incorrectly* interpreted. A common misconception is that a single 95% CI has a 95% chance of containing the true population mean, μ. This is not the case; the percentage refers to the behavior of this method over multiple repeated trials. If you took an infinite number of simple random samples from a distribution, and calculated a 95% CI for each sample, 95% of these intervals would contain μ, the true population mean.

The classic method for calculating CIs relies on assuming an underlying distribution for the population (such as the normal distribution, or the t-distribution), and multiplying the z-score obtained from that distribution by the standard error estimated from the sample (recall from earlier that this is s/√n). For example, using a normal distribution, z-scores of ±1.96 will contain 0.95 of all possible values. A 95% CI using the normal distribution would therefore be the sample mean ($\bar{x}$) plus or minus 1.96 × (s/√n). Modern computational power allows for researchers to utilize techniques that do not rely on an assumption of an underlying distribution. The most common of these is called "bootstrapping." In bootstrapping methods, the sample is repeatedly subdivided into subsamples and these subsamples are used to generate a CI. Similar to calculating a CI to estimate the mean of a single population, CIs are often calculated to estimate the mean difference between two populations.

It should be noted that the width of any CI will decrease as the sample size increases; that is, we are more confident of knowing the true population mean when it is estimated from a larger sample. The degree of certainty is also inversely related to the width of the CI. For example, we can be more precise (narrower CI) in estimating the 95% CI than the 99% CI for the same sample size.

Many studies in the scientific literature report *p*-values. The *p*-value is the probability of observing a study result as extreme as the one observed (eg, *t*-statistic calculated from study data) by chance alone when the null hypothesis is really true. For example, if you were studying the difference in blood lead levels among two different groups of workers, and in your sample, group A had blood lead levels 10 μg/dL higher than group B, the *p*-value gives the probability of finding a difference of 10 or more , when the true difference is zero. When the *p*-value is less than 5% ($p < 0.05$), the result is commonly referred to as being *statistically significant*. However, statistical significance may not be the same as clinical or public health significance because the former is affected by the size of the study population and may reflect differences that have no biological importance. Furthermore, simulations have demonstrated that the *p*-value can be quite variable, even when sampling from the same underlying distribution. Thus, though the medical field once relied nearly exclusively on *p*-values less than 0.05 to understand the importance of a statistical result, the savvy reader is encouraged to use CIs for statistical inference in their place.

A common mistake in statistical inference is known as the *multiple-comparison problem*. The problem arises when an investigator has several groups to compare and proceeds to compare them in groups of two, looking for a *p*-value of 0.05 each time. In other words, group 1 is compared against group 2, then group 2 against group 3, then group 1 against group 3, and so on. The problem with proceeding in this fashion is that overall there is *more* than a 5% chance of erroneously rejecting the null hypothesis even though there is only a 5% chance of making this mistake with each individual comparison. This increased probability of making a mistake occurs because multiple tests increase the likelihood that an error will occur. Thus, the chance of erroneously rejecting a null hypothesis is greater than the 5% risk of mistakenly rejecting each comparison taken by itself, even if all the hypotheses are true. There are many ways of adjusting for this situation, known as *multiple-comparison procedures*. What is important to remember is that if one does enough of such two-group comparisons, the probability of rejecting the null hypothesis incorrectly at least once increases with the number of such comparisons made and can be quite a bit greater than 5% unless the investigator uses an appropriate adjustment for multiple comparisons. Non-hypothesis testing methods of reporting uncertainty around estimates (such as confidence intervals) are best practice, but as hypothesis testing methods using p-values are still commonly used, the basics of these methods are presented here for your understanding.

▶ Type I Error

A type I error occurs if one decides to reject the null hypothesis and declare the two groups different when in fact they really are from the same underlying population. Type I error is equal to the significance level α, and the significance level must be established before the study is conducted. Thus, α equals the probability that one will reject the null hypothesis when the null hypothesis is true; that is, when the investigator decides what chance of making this kind of mistake is acceptable and sets the α level accordingly. For example, an investigator may decide that it is extremely important not to declare that a disease (eg, cancer) is associated with an exposure unless there is overwhelming evidence of an association from the study.

In this case, the α level might be set at 1% instead of 5%; however, in most studies the value used for α is 5%.

▶ Type II Error

A type II error occurs if a researcher decides not to reject the null hypothesis when, in fact, there is a difference between the two groups; that is, a true difference between the two groups has been missed. Type II error is usually designated by β.

▶ The Power of a Study

One of the most important quantities calculated for a research study is the power of a particular study. The power is the probability that one will correctly reject the null hypothesis when the null hypothesis is truly false. In other words, the power is the probability of correctly recognizing a true difference between the two groups. The power of a study is actually the complement of the type II error β, that is, power = $1 - β$. Thus, the power of a study is different for every different value of β that occurs. To calculate the power, one must specify a particular alternative. Power is particularly important when one is evaluating a negative study—a study that finds no difference between the groups.

Suppose that the power of a specific study is 40%. This means that the researcher has only a 40% chance of discerning that a true difference exists between the exposure groups. Therefore, if no difference between exposure groups is found and the power of the study is reported as 40%, a reader might wonder whether that particular study may have missed a difference between exposures even if the exposures were truly associated with the different outcomes. In practice, it is common to use 80% or 90% for the power of a study so that you have a reasonably good probability of detecting a difference between exposures if one truly exists.

The power of a statistical test is determined or affected by three quantities: (1) the magnitude of the type I error, α; (2) the size of the exposure effect, δ, the researcher is interested in detecting; and (3) the sample size of the study, *n*. Quantities (1) and (2) can be used to estimate the sample size needed in a study for a specified study power.

As the size of the type I error becomes smaller, the power of the study likewise becomes smaller. Remember, the type I error is the probability of incorrectly declaring a difference when none actually exists. As it becomes less likely to make this mistake (ie, α is smaller), it becomes less likely the null hypothesis will be rejected in general, and power involves correctly rejecting the null hypothesis.

When a study is set up to look for a very large exposure effect, δ, it is relatively easy to detect this large effect, and the chances are great that the null hypothesis will be correctly rejected. The opposite occurs when one is looking for a very small δ. Thus, power increases as δ increases.

As sample size increases, the variability of the measure of exposure effect decreases. Consequently, the test statistic increases in value, making it easier to exceed the cutoff point for rejecting the null hypothesis. This increases the chances of correctly rejecting the null hypothesis, and so power increases as sample size increases.

A handy table for remembering the quantities discussed in this section is shown below:

	H_0 true (no difference)	H_0 true (difference exists)
H_0 study (declare no difference)	Correct decision	Type II error β
H_0 reject (declare a difference)	Type I error α	Power 1–β

▶ The Case of Two Groups: The *t*-Test

In many instances, an investigator is interested in comparing two groups to determine whether they differ on average for some continuous variable. For example, an investigator might be interested in determining whether exposure to organic solvents has an effect on psychomotor performance such as reaction time. To do this, one would select a sample of a group of industrial painters who are exposed to such solvents and compare their test performances with those of a (otherwise similar) group of workers not exposed to such solvents. Obviously, even if there are truly no differences between two employee groups in how they perform on such a test, the sample mean test scores probably will be unequal simply because of random fluctuation.

The main question is, "Are the differences larger than one would expect by chance if there truly is no difference in the reaction times?"—that is, do the samples come from one underlying population, not two? The null hypothesis in this situation is that the true mean reaction time in the painter group equals the true mean reaction time in the non-painter group.

The alternative hypothesis is that the underlying true means are unequal. This is usually called a *two-sided* alternative hypothesis because we are not specifying the direction of the inequality. In the example, average reaction time in the painter group might be faster or slower than average reaction time in the non-painter group. Differences in either direction are examined by testing the null hypothesis.

The appropriate statistical test in this situation is the two-sample *t*-test. Two independent samples have been drawn; that is, the individuals in one sample are independent of the individuals in the other. The *t*-test has the following form:

$$t = \frac{\bar{x}_1 - \bar{x}_2}{SE(\bar{x}_1 - \bar{x}_2)}$$

where $\bar{x}_1$ is the sample mean in group 1 and $\bar{x}_2$ is the sample mean in group 2.

Note that the numerator is the difference of sample means, and the denominator is the standard error of this quantity. Dividing by the standard error standardizes the difference in sample means by the variability present in the data. If the difference in the means was very large but the data from which it was calculated were highly variable, the *t*-statistic would reflect this and would be adjusted accordingly.

Use of the *t*-statistic assumes that the two samples have the same underlying population variance s_p^2. Thus, a pooled estimate of the variance is calculated and substituted into the *t*-statistic. This pooled estimate s_p^2 has the following form:

$$s_p^2 = \frac{(n_1 - 1)s_1^2 + (n_2 - 1)s_2^2}{(n_1 + n_2 - 2)}$$

Therefore, the two-sample *t*-statistic is as follows:

$$t = \frac{\bar{x}_1 - \bar{x}_2}{\sqrt{\left(\frac{s_p^2}{n_1}\right) + \left(\frac{s_p^2}{n_2}\right)}}$$

Note that the pooled estimate of the variance is simply a weighted average of the variances from samples 1 and 2. Thus, for example, if sample 2 is much larger than sample 1, more weight would be given to s_2^2 (the sample 2 estimate of σ^2) because it is assumed to be more reliable given that it is based on a larger sample size. Note further that if the two samples are of equal size, the pooled variance is simply the sum of the two sample variances divided by 2. From the format of the *t*-test, one can see that if the two sample means are similar in value, the numerator of *t* will be close to zero—and consequently, the value of *t* would be small—leading to the conclusion that the null hypothesis is true and that there is probably only one underlying distribution from which the two samples come. If one obtains a large value for the *t*-statistic, it is likely that the two samples come from two different underlying distributions, and one therefore would want to reject the null hypothesis.

How large does *t* have to be to reject the null hypothesis? Tables of the *t*-statistic indicate what value of *t* would cause the null hypothesis to be rejected. Even when the null hypothesis is true and there really is no difference between the groups being compared, there is the possibility that a large value of *t* might occur owing to random chance alone. One would like the probability of this occurrence to be small, that is, less than 5%.

To find the proper cutoff value of *t* (to reject the null hypothesis) for a particular study, it is necessary to know the number of degrees of freedom. The degrees of freedom are equal to ($n_1 + n_2 - 2$). This may be thought of as the number of observations that are free to vary once the mean is known. Once the degrees of freedom are known, the value of *t* may be obtained from the *t*-table and compared with the *t*-statistic calculated in the study. If the study *t*-statistic is larger than the tabled cutoff value, one can conclude that this is unlikely to have happened under the null hypothesis, which is therefore rejected.

Bear in mind that the alternative hypothesis was the two-sided alternative, meaning that the means of the two groups were simply different but the direction of the difference was not specified. Consequently, in the *t*-table, two cutoff points actually are obtained because both very large negative and very large positive values of *t* are of interest. The *t*-distribution is symmetric, so the two cutoff points are simply ±t. If the study t-value is larger than +t or smaller than −t, the null hypothesis is rejected. (For a one-sided alternative hypothesis, a direction would be specified; the alternate hypothesis could be that one group would have a *larger* mean than the other, rather than simply different.)

Example III gives the flavor of the t-test and how it is used.

Example III: *Two-sample t-tests. The following tabulation presents the mean change in plasma cholinesterase concentration from baseline levels for 15 pesticide applicators and 14 unexposed controls.*

	N	Mean Decline (%)	Standard Deviation
Applicators	15	25	11
Controls	14	10	8

Do the data present sufficient evidence from which to conclude that the mean decline in cholinesterase is different for the two groups?

The null hypothesis is that there is no difference in cholinesterase change between the two groups. The alternative hypothesis is that there is a difference in cholinesterase change between the two groups.

First, calculate s_p^2:

$$s_p^2 = \frac{(n_1-1)s_1^2 + (n_2-1)s_2^2}{(n_1+n_2-2)}$$

$$= \frac{(15-1)11^2 + (14-1)8^2}{(15+14-2)}$$

$$= 93.56$$

Substitute into the formula for t:

$$t = \frac{\bar{x}_1 - \bar{x}_2}{\sqrt{\left(\frac{s_p^2}{n_1}\right) + \left(\frac{s_p^2}{n_2}\right)}}$$

$$= \frac{25-10}{\sqrt{\left(\frac{93.56}{15}\right) + \left(\frac{93.56}{14}\right)}}$$

$$= \frac{15}{\sqrt{6.24+6.68}}$$

$$= \frac{15}{3.59}$$

$$= 4.18$$

Therefore, t = 4.18 and df = $n_1 + n_2 - 2 = 27$.

The study t-value of 4.18 with 27 degrees of freedom is compared with the tabled t value of ±2.05, which has a 5% chance of occurring when the null hypothesis is true. Because +4.18 is larger than +2.05, the null hypothesis is rejected; that

is, there is a statistically significant difference in the mean change in plasma cholinesterase from baseline between the two study groups. In other words, this difference is unlikely to have occurred by chance.

This result also can be expressed as the CI of the difference in the means. As calculated above, the standard error of the difference in the means is 3.59. Using the t distribution with 27 degrees of freedom, the t score that corresponds to 0.95 is +/−2.05. Thus, the 95% confidence interval is 15 +/−2.05 × 3.59 or the 95% confidence interval for the difference in means between the two groups is 7.6–22.4. Stated another way, using these techniques to generate confidence intervals, the interval will contain the true mean difference in plasma cholinesterase concentration between the two groups 95% of the time. The range 7.6–22.4 is one such interval.

▶ Paired t-Test

The preceding discussion concerns the two-sample t-test and is appropriate for the situation in which two independent groups are being compared. Another common situation occurs when there are paired samples; that is, the two observations are not independent of one another.

For example, suppose that a researcher is measuring change in pulmonary function (eg, forced expiratory volume in 1 second [FEV_1]) over a work shift and there are 20 subjects in the study (see the example below). The researcher would measure FEV_1 among the subjects before and after the work shift. Clearly, the before and after measurements are not independent, and one would like to take advantage of the fact that all individual (nonexposure) characteristics have been controlled. To do this, the difference in FEV_1 (before–after) is calculated for each subject. Because the difference is the only observation made per subject, the data set now has gone from 40 observations (2 per subject) to 20 observations (1 per subject). If there is no effect of work shift on FEV_1, one would expect the difference in FEV_1 for each subject to be small in value or close to zero. If the null hypothesis is not true and work shift exposure does change FEV_1, the differences will not be close to zero. The t-statistic calculated in this situation is known as the *paired* t-statistic and has the following form:

$$t = \frac{\bar{D}}{(s_D/\sqrt{n})}$$

where $\bar{D} = \dfrac{\Sigma D_i}{n}$ = average difference and

s_D = standard deviation of differences

$$= \sqrt{\frac{\sum_{i=1}^{n}(D_i - \bar{D})^2}{n-1}}$$

The appropriate null hypothesis is that the true mean of the differences is zero, and the appropriate alternative hypothesis is that the true mean of the differences is not zero.

EXAMPLE: Paired t-test

A study of painters involved measuring pulmonary function (FEV, L) at the beginning (A) and end (B) of a work shift. The results were as follows:

Case #	A_1	B_1	$D_1 = (A_1 - B_1)$	$(D_1 - \bar{D})$	$(D_1 - \bar{D})^2$
1	3.14	3.01	0.13	0.10	0.010
2	2.85	2.80	0.05	0.02	0.000
3	2.50	2.30	0.20	0.17	0.029
4	3.01	3.15	−0.14	−0.17	0.029
5	1.55	1.55	0.00	−0.03	0.001
6	2.21	2.15	0.06	0.03	0.001
7	2.81	2.68	0.13	0.10	0.010
8	3.25	3.34	−0.09	−0.12	0.014
9	2.66	2.56	0.10	−0.07	0.029
10	1.95	1.90	0.05	−0.02	0.000
11	3.50	3.46	0.04	0.01	0.000
12	3.95	4.06	−0.11	−0.14	0.020
13	4.10	3.90	0.20	0.17	0.029
14	3.60	3.56	0.04	0.01	0.000
15	2.80	2.90	−0.10	−0.13	0.017
16	2.50	2.50	0.00	−0.03	0.001
17	2.10	2.16	−0.06	−0.09	0.008
18	3.70	3.61	0.09	0.06	0.004
19	2.92	2.86	0.06	0.03	0.001
20	3.31	3.42	−0.11	−0.14	0.020
			0.54		0.198

$$\bar{D} = \frac{\Sigma D_i}{n} = \frac{0.54}{20} = 0.027$$

$$s_D = \sqrt{\frac{\sum_{i=1}^{n}(D_i - \bar{D})^2}{n-1}}$$

$$= \sqrt{\frac{0.198}{19}} = 0.102$$

$$t = \frac{\bar{D}}{(s_D / \sqrt{n})} = \frac{0.027}{0.102 / \sqrt{20}} = 1.18$$

Compare the calculated t of 1.18 to the tabled t of 2.093. Since the calculated t is less than the t in the table, the null hypothesis (of no change in function over work shift) is not rejected.

Again, it is a two-sided alternative, and one is looking for large positive or large negative differences. Small absolute values of the t-statistic would indicate that the null hypothesis is probably true, and large absolute values of t would lead to rejection of the null hypothesis. One goes to the t-table or computer program to determine how large a value of t is needed to reject the null hypothesis. To obtain the correct value, one needs to know the appropriate degrees of freedom. In the paired t situation, there are $n - 1$ degrees of freedom, or the number of pairs minus one.

▶ Analysis of Variance

When the variables under study are continuous in nature and there are more than two groups being studied, the investigator usually is concerned with whether the means in the groups are different from one another. An appropriate statistical method to answer this question is to use *analysis of variance* (ANOVA).

Suppose that one were studying three groups of workers occupationally exposed to three different gases. One might want to test whether the particular gases affect mean FEV_1 levels differently in the three groups. In this example, individual FEV_1 values would be adjusted for nonexposure determinants (ie, age, gender, height, or race). The null hypothesis is that the group means for FEV_1 are equal, that is, a particular exposure has no effect on FEV_1 values. Obviously, there will be differences between the sample means in each group owing to random fluctuations in FEV_1 among individuals.

Are the differences observed in the sample means merely a result of random fluctuations, or are they a consequence of true differences in FEV_1 caused by the gas exposures? To answer this question, one examines whether the data are consistent with the assumption that the gas exposure has no effect and that the three groups are really random samples from the same underlying population. The null hypothesis assumes that any observed differences in the sample means and standard deviations are due simply to random sampling. ANOVA tests this null hypothesis by estimating the true population variance in two different ways and comparing these two estimates of the variance. If the three samples do indeed come from the same underlying population, these two estimates of the variance will be very close in value. If the three samples do not all come from the same underlying population, these two estimates will be further apart in value, and this variation is what one hopes to detect.

Certain statistical assumptions are made when an ANOVA test is performed on a set of data: (1) It is assumed that groups have been randomly assigned to receive the treatment or exposure and that the groups are independent; (2) the underlying variance (σ^2) in each group is assumed to be identical (even though the true group means may be different and the sample variances may differ slightly); and (3) the random variable under study—for example, FEV_1—has a normal distribution.

Conceptually, the method of ANOVA proceeds as follows: Once the null hypothesis is formulated, the sample variance (s^2) is computed within each exposure group, and each of these s^2 estimates is unaffected by differences among the group means. These s^2 estimates are averaged to obtain one "within group" variance estimate. The values of the individual exposure group means then are used to arrive at a second "between group" variance estimate of σ^2. In this "between group" estimate of σ^2, differences (or variability) among the group means will affect the overall estimate of σ^2. For example, if a particular gas exposure has no effect on FEV_1, both estimates of σ^2 should be similar. To test the null hypothesis, a statistic known as the F statistic is calculated. The value of F is simply the ratio of the "between group" variance estimate to the "within group" variance estimate. Because both numbers estimate the same parameter (σ^2), if the null hypothesis is true, the value of F should be close to 1. If F is significantly larger than 1, you should reject the null hypothesis and conclude that the exposure groups are different with regard to FEV_1.

How does one determine how large F must be in order to reject the null hypothesis? Because of random fluctuations in the data, it is possible that a large F statistic might result even when the null hypothesis is true. However, one would like the chance of this happening to be very small. Tables of the F statistic are available to assist the investigator in selecting a value of F against which the F statistic calculated from the data can be compared. The tabled value of F is one that would occur less than approximately 5% of the time if the null hypothesis were true. If the F statistic calculated from the researcher's data is larger than the one found in the table, the results are less than 5% likely to have occurred by random chance, even if the null hypothesis (no difference in sample groups) is true. Because the observed results therefore are very unlikely to have happened by chance under the null hypothesis, the researcher is justified in rejecting the null hypothesis and saying that there is a difference among the groups. The 5% cutoff point is an arbitrary one, and depending on the individual situation, one could set the cutoff at one or 10%; however, the conventional cutoff point is 5%.

When one is studying more than two groups and the data involved are continuous (eg, FEV_1 or blood lead concentration) and the question of interest is whether the groups all come from the same underlying population—that is, have the same mean for the variable of interest—ANOVA is the most appropriate method to use for initial testing of the null hypothesis. If one fails to reject the null hypothesis with the F statistic, no further tests of the null hypothesis are necessary. There are no differences among groups. On the other hand, if one performs ANOVA on the data and rejects the null hypothesis, then differences in the outcome (eg, FEV_1) among the study groups associated with the particular exposure may exist. One then can use multiple-comparison tests to identify exactly which group or groups are significantly different.

This is a simplified discussion of ANOVA meant only to introduce the concept of this important statistical method. We have not provided enough details for the reader to be able to perform this test accurately. The purpose is to identify

situations in which ANOVA is appropriate as an initial analytic procedure (see References).

▶ Analyzing Rates & Proportions: The Chi-Square Test

In preceding sections, we described methods of analysis for continuous types of data. This section begins a discussion of the analysis of categorical data. The following table of cigarette smoking history and lung cancer cases and controls (persons without cancer) presents an example of categorical data.

	Lung Cancer	**Controls**
Cigarette smokers	450	225
Nonsmokers	20	225
Total	470	450

It is immediately apparent, without doing any statistical tests, that there is an association of cigarette smoking and lung cancer. The row variable, cigarette smoking, is associated with the column variable, lung cancer. A simple calculation of the proportions of lung cancer cases and control cases who smoked confirms this association. Of the lung cancer cases, 450/470 = 95.7% smoked cigarettes, whereas 225/450 = 50% of the controls smoked cigarettes.

However, suppose that the table was of mesothelioma (a very rare type of lung cancer) and cigarette smoking, the following results were obtained:

	Mesothelioma	**Controls**
Cigarette smokers	80	200
Nonsmokers	40	104
Total	120	304

In this example, the ratios of cigarette smokers to nonsmokers among the mesothelioma cases (80/120 = 66.6%) and the controls (200/304 = 65.8%) are nearly the same, with approximately twice as many smokers as nonsmokers for both the case and control groups. In this case, one would say that there is no association between the column variable (mesothelioma) and the row variable (cigarette smoking). The null hypothesis in this example would be that there is no association between mesothelioma and cigarette smoking, and one could not reject the null hypothesis owing to the similarity of the proportions of smokers in the mesothelioma and the control groups.

Most situations with categorical data are not as clear-cut as these two examples. In most cases, one cannot simply eyeball the data to determine whether the two variables are independent or not. The statistical test one uses to determine whether or not there is an association in such data is known as the *chi-square test*. Example IV is a situation in which the chi-square test is applied.

Example IV: *Three groups of farm workers are studied for the occurrence of new skin rashes during the growing season. The three groups are involved in growing and harvesting (1) grapes, (2) citrus crops, and (3) tomatoes. The workers are followed for the growing season, and the occurrence of new rashes in the three groups is compared to determine if there is an association between exposure (crop) and outcome (rash).*

Crop 1, N = 100
Crop 2, N = 200
Crop 3, N = 200

Response	Exposure (Crop)			Total
	1	2	3	
Rash	30	40	32	102
No rash	70	160	168	398
Total	100	200	200	500

The null hypothesis in this situation is again the hypothesis of "no difference"; only it is phrased as no association between the row variable (rash) and the column variable (crop).

One can quickly compute from the table that the percentage working on crop 1 with a rash is 30/100 = 30%; on crop 2, it is 40/200 = 20%; and on crop 3, it is 32/200 = 16%. By just quickly observing the data, one might think that crop 1 is different from crops 2 and 3. However, the null hypothesis is that there is no association between crop worked and rash development. Thus, the question is whether the observed differences in response are simply a result of random variation in the data or are larger than one would expect by chance alone if the null hypothesis were true. To test this, a chi-square statistic is calculated. As with the *t*-test and *F*-test, one determines whether this chi-square value is unlikely to have occurred by chance alone under the null hypothesis. The calculation of the chi-square involves first determining an "expected" value for each cell in the table. The expected value is the value one would "expect" to see in the cell if there were no association between row (rash) and column (crop exposure) variables, that is, that value one would "expect" to see if the null hypothesis were true. The expected value is obtained as follows.

According to the null hypothesis, we would expect the same proportion to develop a rash in each group. If this is true, the best estimate of the expected proportion with rashes in each exposure group comes from the overall information given by the total number of workers with rashes divided by the total number of workers in the study; that would be 102/500 = 0.204. Then, for crop 1, one expects that 0.204 of the 100 people in crop exposure group 1 will develop rashes, that is, 20.4 people; for crop 2, one expects that 0.204 of the

200 people working with crop 2 will develop rashes, that is, 40.8 people; and for crop 3, one expects that 0.204 of the 200 people will develop rashes, that is, 40.8 people. In other words, because under the null hypothesis there is no association between exposure and percentage developing a rash, one expects the same percentage to respond favorably (or unfavorably) in each group. The expected proportion of workers not developing rashes is obtained in the same manner. The best estimate of the proportion not developing a rash in each group is the total number not developing a rash divided by the total number of workers, which equals 398/500 = 0.796. This gives an expected frequency of 100 × 0.796 = 79.6 working with crop 1 not developing rashes, 159.2 working with crop 2 not developing rashes, and 159.2 working with crop 3 not developing rashes. Putting the expected values in parentheses alongside the observed values, the table now looks like this:

Response	Exposure (Crop)			Total
	1	2	3	
Rash	30 (20.4)	40 (40.8)	32 (40.8)	102
No rash	70 (79.6)	160 (159.2)	168 (159.2)	398
Total	100	200	200	500

To test the null hypothesis, one looks at the observed and expected numbers in each cell to see how close together the two values are. If the values are close together, one may decide that the null hypothesis is true. If they are very different, one may decide that the null hypothesis is not true. To decide whether the observed and expected values are close together, the chi-square statistic is calculated. It has the following form:

$$\chi^2 = \sum_{i=1}^{n}\left[\frac{(O_i - E_i)^2}{E_i}\right]$$

where E_i is the expected value in cell i, O_i is the observed value in cell i, $i = 1, ..., n$, and n is the number of cells in the table.

Large chi-square values indicate a lack of agreement between observed and expected values; small chi-square values indicate close agreement.

How does one determine what constitutes a large chi-square value? As in the preceding discussions about *t*- and *F*-tests for continuous data, one consults a table of chi-square values. The table identifies the chi-square value that would occur less than 5% of the time if the null hypothesis (no association) were true, and this is compared with the study chi-square value. If the study-chi square is larger than the table cutoff value, the null hypothesis is rejected because this is known to occur less than 5% of the time when the null hypothesis is true. If the study chi-square value is smaller than the table cutoff value, the null hypothesis is not rejected. Alternatively, one could calculate the exact probability, or *P* value, of the study chi-square statistic. To use the chi-square tables, the degrees of freedom are needed to select the proper value from the table. The degrees of freedom in the chi-square situation are equal to (number of rows − 1) × (number of columns − 1). When there are two rows and three columns in a table, the degree of freedom is (2 − 1) × (3 − 1), which equals 2 degrees of freedom. One thing to remember is that the chi-square statistic works only when the sample is sufficiently large. A rule of thumb is that the chi-square test yields good results when the expected values in each cell are greater than or equal to 5.

Calculating the chi-square statistic for the preceding example, the following results are obtained:

$$x^2 = \frac{(70-79.6)^2}{79.6} + \frac{(160-159.2)^2}{159.2}$$
$$+ \frac{(168-159.2)^2}{159.2} + \frac{(30-20.4)^2}{20.4}$$
$$+ \frac{(40-40.8)^2}{40.8} + \frac{(32-40.8)^2}{40.8}$$
$$= 8.08$$

The tabled value of chi-square to which the calculated value is compared is 5.99. Because 8.08 is larger than 5.99, the null hypothesis is rejected.

Calculating the chi-square statistic is only one method for analyzing categorical data. It is, however, one of the most common statistical tests found in the medical literature.

▶ Other Statistical Tests

This section has touched on some of the simplest tests, including the chi-square for categorical data and a few parametric tests (*t*-tests and ANOVA). These are parametric meaning they rely on an assumption that the distribution of the sample means is normal. As described earlier, this assumption allows for calculation of statistics for many types of samples, including those with a normal distribution and those of large size.

Excluded from this chapter are two other kinds of tests: those involving multiple variables and tests for distributions which do not meet the assumption of normality. Multiple variable techniques, such as linear and logistic regression form the basis of many scientific studies and the reader is referred to an introductory statistics textbook for further exploration of these methods. Similarly, nonparametric methods (such as the Shapiro-Wilks test or permutation tests) are outside the scope of this chapter.

REFERENCES

Baldi B, Moore DS: *The Practice of Statistics in the Life Sciences.* 4th ed. New York, WH Freeman, 2018.
Cumming G: Dance of the p-values. https://www.youtube.com/watch?v=5OL1RqHrZQ8.

The R Project for Statistical Computing, R 3.5.2, www.r-project.org/ (R is a free software environment for statistical computing and graphics. It compiles and runs on a wide variety of UNIX platforms, Windows, and Mac OS).
Surfstat, https://onlinestatbook.com/2/calculators/normal_dist.html (Surfstat is an online tool for calculating probabilities from different distributions including the normal, t, chi-square and binomial distributions).

▼ II. EPIDEMIOLOGY

Epidemiology is the study of the distribution and determinants of health- and disease-related conditions in populations. It is concerned with both epidemic (excess of normal expectancy) and endemic (always present) conditions.

The basic premise of epidemiology is that disease is not randomly distributed across populations. Not only is it important to know what sort of disease a particular person has, but it is also necessary to know what sort of person has a particular disease. While the practice of much of occupational medicine is concerned with the pathogenesis (development) of disease and the treatment of individuals with diseases, the focus of occupational epidemiology is on groups of individuals—with or without diseases—in an attempt to infer the causes that precede specific disease conditions and to determine what occupational or other lifestyle factors can be manipulated to eliminate specific diseases or reduce the prevalence of the disease.

There are three major types of epidemiologic studies: descriptive, analytic, and experimental.

Descriptive epidemiologic studies characterize person, place, and time: (1) Person: What are the characteristics of people who get a particular disease (eg, age, race, gender, occupation, SES, immune status)? (2) Place: Where do they live, work, or travel (eg, international, national, and local comparisons; urban versus rural populations; climate; altitude)? (3) Time: When does the illness occur (eg, temporal variation, seasonal fluctuations)? Descriptive studies are not used to test hypotheses but nevertheless are powerful tools for characterizing disease distributions and associations.

Analytic studies attempt to determine the etiologic factors associated with a disease by calculating estimates of risk: (1) What exposures do people with the disease have in common (eg, smoking, exogenous hormone use, diet, exposure to radiation or asbestos)? (2) How much is disease risk increased by such exposures? (3) How many cases could be avoided if the exposures were eliminated? Analytic studies involve testing specific hypotheses.

Experimental studies involve a search for strategies for altering the natural history of disease. Examples of experimental studies are intervention trials to reduce risk factors, screening studies aimed at identifying the early stages of disease, and clinical trials of different treatment modalities to improve prognosis.

Table A–2. Measures of mortality.

$$\text{Crude death rate} = \frac{\text{Number of deaths in year (all causes)}}{\text{Total population}} \times 1000$$

eg, US 1977 = 8.8 ÷ 1000 population or 878.1 ÷ 100,000 population

$$\text{Cause – specific death rate} = \frac{\text{Number of deaths from specific cause in year}}{\text{Total population}} \times 100,000$$

eg, cancer in US 1977 = 178.7 ÷ 100,000 population

$$\text{Age – specific death rate} = \frac{\text{Number of deaths among persons of specified age group in year}}{\text{Population in specified age group}} \times 100,000$$

eg, cancer in age group 1–14 years = 4.9 ÷ 100,000

$$\text{Infant mortality rate} = \frac{\text{Number of deaths among children younger than 1 year age in year}}{\text{Number of birds in year}} \times 1000$$

eg, US 1977 = 14.1 ÷ 100,000 live births (12.3 for whites; 21.7 for blacks and others)

MORTALITY & MORBIDITY

The two basic measures of disease in a population are mortality (death) rates and morbidity (disease) rates. Table A–2 provides examples of different types of mortality rates and how each is calculated. Morbidity is measured by calculating either prevalence or incidence. *Prevalence* is the number of existing cases of a disease at a given time divided by the population at risk for that disease at that time. This result is commonly multiplied by 100,000 to derive the prevalence rate per 100,000 population.

For purposes of etiology, the *incidence* is a more important measure of morbidity and is equal to the number of new cases of a disease occurring over a defined interval divided by the population at risk for that disease (multiplied by 100,000). The population at risk over an interval can be calculated in multiple different ways, one of the simplest is to use the mid-interval population at risk.

While worldwide mortality data are available—at various degrees of precision depending on the quality of death registration systems—incidence can be calculated only for those diseases for which there are population-based registries or for which special studies have been conducted. The National Cancer Institute has a program of cancer registries around the United States that provides information on cancer incidence covering approximately 10% of the US population. Accurate enumeration of the population at risk—available from Census data—is vital for deriving valid estimates of both mortality and morbidity rates. Rates can be specific to any subgroup of interest, defined by age, gender, race, or other characteristics. For example, the age-adjusted incidence for cervical cancer among white women in the United

States was 8.7 per 100,000, compared with 11.1 per 100,000 among black women and 15.8 per 100,000 among Hispanic women. One must remember that in calculating a rate, the events in the numerator must be drawn from the population specified in the denominator; that is, those in the denominator must be at risk for the disease. Thus, for cervical cancer, men would not be included in the denominator.

Some problems to keep in mind about current disease data sources include the following:

1. The only complete cause-specific disease registry is for deaths, and the cause-of-death assignment on the death certificate is often inaccurate. In addition, for a disease whose case-fatality ratio is low (ie, a disease unlikely to result in death when it occurs), the death rate is a gross underestimate of the incidence of the condition in the community. An example of this is nonmelanoma skin cancer, which has a high incidence but low mortality rate.

2. Morbidity reports, even when legally mandated, as is the case for certain infectious diseases (eg, tuberculosis and sexually transmitted diseases), often are incomplete because of severe underreporting.

3. Complete and accurate population-based morbidity registries are limited in geographic coverage.

ADJUSTMENT OF RATES

In attempting to compare disease rates across population groups or assessing changes in rates over time, the effect of differential distributions of confounding factors in two populations whose rates are being compared should be taken into account. For example, disease risk is often a function of age; differences in crude rates (ie, rates not adjusted for age) across populations may reflect age differences rather than differences in occupational or environmental factors of interest.

Standardization of the observed rates provides a summary measure of disease risk for an entire population that is not influenced by variations in the distribution of a factor, such as age. There are two methods for adjustment: a direct method, which applies the observed factor-specific rates of death or disease to a standard population, and an indirect method, which applies factor-specific rates of death or disease from a standard population to the age distribution of the observed population. In discussing the methods for adjusting rates, cancer will be used as the disease of interest, and age will be the factor of interest.

The direct method of age adjustment is appropriate when each of the populations being compared is large enough to yield stable age-specific rates. For example, the direct method is used for comparison of cancer rates over time in the United States. Crude mortality rates showing a dramatic increase in cancer over the past few decades would seem to provide strong evidence of a cancer epidemic. It needs to be ascertained, however, to what extent the aging of the country's population has contributed to the apparent epidemic or to what extent other factors, such as an increase in cancer-causing agents in the environment, might be responsible.

The first three columns of Table A–3 show the actual age distributions of the US population in 1940 and 1970, the percentage of the population in each group in the two periods, the corresponding number of actual cancer deaths, and the age-specific death rates. Crude death rates per 100,000 population were 120.2 for 1940 and 163.2 for 1970, an increase of more than 30%. Comparison of the age-specific rates, however, shows only minor increases between the two time periods. It should be noted that the percentage of the population in all age groups over 40 was higher in 1970 than in 1940.

To remove the variable effect of age using the direct method of adjustment, a "standard" population is chosen. The number of people in each age group of the standard population then is multiplied by the appropriate age-specific rate in each of the study populations. This generates the number of deaths or cases of disease one would expect in each age group if the populations had similar age distributions. The expected number of deaths or disease cases then is summed over all age groups, the sum is divided by the total standard population, and the result is multiplied by 100,000. The choice of a standard population is arbitrary; it might be the combined population of the two groups whose rates are being compared, only one of those populations, or any other population.

In our example, the standard was the combined population of the United States in 1940 and 1970, shown in column 5 of Table A–3. The age-specific death rates for each period (column 4) were applied for each age group to the standard population, yielding the expected number of deaths shown in column 6. Age-adjusted rates then are calculated by dividing the sum of expected deaths for each period by the total standard population. The resulting adjusted rates are 139.8 per 100,000 for 1940 and 149.9 per 100,000 for 1970. Thus, the magnitude of the increase in the crude rates has been reduced from about 30% to 7%. It can be concluded that age is an important factor in the increased cancer rates in the United States, although age alone does not entirely explain changes over time.

When the group of interest is relatively small and thus likely to have unstable age-specific rates, it is more appropriate to use the indirect than the direct method of age adjustment. This is commonly the situation with investigation of cause-specific mortality in an occupational cohort. The indirect method is employed frequently to compare the cancer incidence or follow-up experience of a study group with that expected based on the experience of a larger population or patient series. With the indirect method, the standardized mortality ratio (SMR) is calculated. In calculating an SMR, the age-specific rates from a standard population (eg, county, state, or country) are multiplied by the person-years at risk in the study population (eg, industry employees) to give the expected number of deaths in that study population. The observed number of deaths divided by the expected number (times 100) is the SMR (see the example in Table A–4). The SMR gives information about how the individual population compares to what would be expected within that population *only*. Two SMRs from different populations cannot be compared.

Thus, the equation for an SMR is as follows:

$$SMR = \left[\frac{\Sigma\, a_i}{\Sigma\, E(a_i)} \right] \times 100$$

$$= \left[\frac{\text{Observed}}{\text{Expected}} \right] \times 100$$

where a_i is the number of people with a specific cause of death in the ith stratum of the factor being standardized, and $E(a_i)$ is the expected number of deaths based on the factor-specific rates in the reference population.

The result is multiplied by 100, so when observed deaths equal expected deaths, the SMR is 100, and the differences from 100 represent the percentage difference in mortality in the study population compared with that of the reference population.

Indirect standardization also may be used to adjust incidence rates (rather than mortality rates) for age or other factors. Thus, incident cases of a disease within a workplace could be expressed as the standardized incidence ratio (SIR), as follows:

$$SIR = \left[\frac{\text{Observed number of new cases}}{\text{Expected number of new cases}} \right] \times 100$$

Although it is most common to adjust rates for age and time, the direct and indirect methods of adjustment can be

Table A–3. Age adjustment by direct method, using cancer mortality data for the United States, 1940 and 1970.

Age Group	Actual Population (1)	(2)	Number of Cancer Deaths (3)	Age-specific Death Rates Per 100,000 (4)	Standard Population (5)	Expected Number of Cancer Deaths (6)
1940						
< 40	87,737,829	66.7	10,283	11.72	217,093,330	25,443
40–49	17,053,068	13.0	18,071	105.97	41,149,961	43,607
50–59	13,100,511	10.0	33,279	254.03	34,177,557	86,821
60–69	8,534,997	6.5	43,686	511.85	24,143,606	123,579
70–79	4,073,514	3.1	38,160	936.78	13,352,179	125,080
80+	1,139,143	0.9	14,721	1,292.29	4,934,355	63,766
Totals	131,639,062	100.0	158,200[b]		334,850,988	468,296[b]
1970						
< 40	129,355,501	63.7	16,096	12.44	217,093,330	27,006
40–49	24,096,893	11.9	26,075	108.21	41,149,961	44,528
50–59	21,077,046	10.4	61,143	290.09	34,177,557	99,146
60–69	15,608,609	7.7	90,099	577.24	24,143,606	139,367
70–79	9,278,665	4.6	88,826	957.31	13,352,179	127,821
80+	3,795,212	1.9	49,333	1,299.87	4,934,355	64,140
Totals	203,211,926	100.0	331,572[a]		334,850,988	502,008[a]

[a]Crude death rate = [sum of column 3/sum of column 1] × 10^5 = 163.2 per 100,000 population. Age-adjusted death rate = [sum of column 6/sum of column 5] × 10^5 = 149.9 per 100,000 population.
[b]Crude death rate = [sum of column 3/sum of column 1] × 10^5 = 120.2 per 100,000 population. Age-adjusted death rate = [sum of column 6/sum of column 5] × 10^5 = 139.9 per 100,000 population.

Table A–4. Age adjustment by indirect method in computation of standardized mortality ratio (SMR).

Age (Years)	Observed Deaths (1)	Person Years (2)	US Population Rates (per 10⁵) (3)	Expected Deaths = (2) × (3)
20–29	1	500	20.6	0.1
30–39	0	1500	22.7	0.3
40–49	4	6000	45.3	2.7
50–59	2	4000	94.3	3.8
60–69	12	7000	224.4	15.7
Σ Obs = 19				Σ Exp = 22.6

SMR = [Σ Obs/Σ Exp] × 100 = [19/22.6]100 = 84.

used to adjust for population differences in other factors as well, such as gender, race, SES, and stage of disease.

▶ **Design Strategies for Analytic & Experimental Studies**

Descriptive epidemiology provides disease rates for different groups. It identifies segments of the population—by age, gender, occupation, marital status, geographic area of residence, or other parameters—whose unique experience suggests etiologic hypotheses worthy of pursuit through rigorous analytic studies. Descriptive epidemiology tells who gets the disease where and when and is the basis of analytic epidemiology, which, in turn, focuses on specific questions, such as the following:

- What exposure do people with the disease have in common as compared with people without the disease?
- Why does exposure induce or promote disease?

- How much is disease risk increased by such exposure?
- How many cases might be avoided were the exposure eliminated?

The last question addresses the ultimate objective of epidemiologic research: to identify risk factors so that intervention might either prevent the occurrence of the disease (primary prevention) or lead to early detection (secondary prevention).

The three basic strategies for analytic epidemiology are (1) the cohort study, (2) the case-control study, and (3) the experimental study (including clinical trials). Cohort and case-control studies are observational: The investigator does not control exposure or modify behavior of the study subjects. In the experimental study, the investigator intervenes by introducing treatment or other exposures to study their impact on the disease experience. However, in order to make inferences from any study, the researcher needs to be aware of possible sources of bias.

SOURCES OF BIAS

Bias must be acknowledged as a potential issue for nearly every type of epidemiologic study design. It is defined as a systematic error in the design, execution, or analysis of a study that results in an erroneous estimate of the effect of an exposure of interest to the risk of an outcome or disease.

Historically many clinicians have been more concerned with bias in case-control studies, yet it may occur in any kind of study. For example, in a cohort study information about outcome measures may be obtained differently in exposed and unexposed subjects. However, the underlying principle is the same: Any difference in the way information is obtained from the study groups, or in the way those groups are recruited and enrolled, may bias the results of the study.

There are three main categories of bias to be aware of: selection bias, information bias (or measurement error), and confounding.

A. Selection Bias

Selection bias occurs when the probability of being included in a study is related to either the probability of having the exposure or disease of interest. In a case-control study, subjects are intentionally chosen based on disease status, but if inclusion in the study sample is related to exposure, selection bias has been induced. Conversely for cohort studies, subjects are enrolled based on exposure status, but if inclusion (or retention) in the study sample is related to exposure, selection bias has been induced. In either case, the distributions of exposure and outcome in the study sample will not be reflective of that in underlying population.

An example of selection bias could occur when doing a case-control study looking at the association between lung cancer and smoking. Case patients with lung cancer may have been recruited while in the hospital. However, if control patients are also recruited from hospitalized inpatients, those

controls would be more likely to be smokers than the general population (since smoking is a well-known risk factor for many diseases). The high rate of smoking in the control group could then cause you to *underestimate* the association between smoking and lung cancer. This is an example of the exposure (smoking) being related to the probability of control enrollment in a case-control study.

There is a well-known example of selection bias in cohort studies that is particular to occupational medicine; *the healthy worker effect.* People who are able to actively maintain employment tend to be healthier than the general population, as those who are ill are unable to continue working. Thus, a cohort study which compares a group of exposed workers to the general population, has inadvertently selected exposed persons who are more likely to be healthy, that is less likely to have disease. This could then *underestimate* the deleterious effects of an occupational exposure. This is therefore an example of selection into a cohort study being related to disease status.

B. Information Bias

Information bias is bias that is related to flawed definition of, or flawed measurement of study variables. For example, in interviewing study subjects about past exposures or events, the interviewer who knows the disease status of the individual (case or control) may pose questions unconsciously or probe for answers in a different manner (a specific information bias commonly referred to as *interviewer bias*.)

Another source of information bias can occur when a study subject is asked to recall past exposures or events because recall might depend on the person's current disease status. For example, a person with lymphoma is more likely to recall remote exposure to pesticides than a control subject without cancer. To minimize recall bias in this instance, one might try to obtain independent verification of previous exposure. It is also advantageous to use information recorded before the time of diagnosis wherever possible.

Misclassification of study subjects also can bias study results owing to inaccuracies in the methods by which data are gathered from study subjects or methods by which information is abstracted from various sources. Misclassification bias comes in two forms—differential and nondifferential. Differential misclassification that is related to disease or exposure status can lead to the appearance of a relationship between exposure and disease where one does not truly exist, or perhaps more unsettling, it can mask a true association. Nondifferential misclassification is not related to exposure or disease status and tends to attenuate any association between exposure and disease.

C. Confounding

The phenomenon of *confounding* is another explanation for an altered association between an exposure and a disease. As with other types of bias, confounding may occur in any type of analytic epidemiologic study. By definition, a confounder is a factor that is associated with the exposure of interest, is an independent cause of the disease being studied, but is not on the causal pathway for the exposure. (For a factor to be on the causal pathway between an exposure and an outcome, some or all of the effect of the exposure on the outcome would have to occur through that factor.) When confounding occurs, an observed association between an exposure and a disease is in fact due wholly or in part to the association of the exposure with the confounding factor.

An example of a confounding factor is cigarette smoking in a study of an occupational exposure and lung cancer. Cigarette smoking is a known cause of lung cancer. If the cigarette smoking prevalence were greater (or less) in the population exposed to the occupational exposure agent, then it would also be associated with the exposure. However, cigarette smoking is not on the causal pathway—the occupational exposure does not cause lung cancer by causing people to smoke. Thus, failure to control for smoking in the study design or analysis would lead to an apparently greater (or lesser) association between the occupational exposure and lung cancer.

TYPES OF EPIDEMIOLOGIC STUDIES

1. The Cohort Study

In the design of a cohort study, a disease-free group of individuals (a cohort) characterized by a common experience or exposure of interest is identified and followed over time to determine whether disease occurs at a rate different from that in a cohort without the exposure. The relative risk (RR) of disease associated with the exposure then can be calculated:

$$RR = \frac{\text{Incidence rate in the exposed group}}{\text{Incidence rate in the nonexposed group}}$$

A frequently cited example of the prospective cohort design is the follow-up study of British physicians whose smoking habits were ascertained by means of a mailed questionnaire. The doctors were grouped according to smoking habits, and their deaths were subsequently monitored. Lung cancer rates for those exposed to various levels of smoking were compared with the rates for nonsmokers by means of the RR. Other examples of cohort studies include investigations of long-term cancer incidence among atomic bomb survivors exposed to varying degrees of radiation, deaths among British coal miners and monitoring for disease among firefighters exposed to the 9/11 site.

Theoretically, the prospective cohort study is ideal because the hypothesized cause or exposure precedes the effect or disease. It is also valuable because disease rates and RRs can be calculated directly, provided that a suitable comparison group is built into the study or is otherwise available for calculation of rates in the nonexposed population. In addition, when cohorts are followed prospectively the exposure of interest can be recorded accurately at the time of exposure; it is not based on recall of past events. This approach has been popular in occupational studies in which the disease experience of workers exposed to putatively hazardous substances has been compared with that of other workers without the exposure or compared with that of the general population.

In practice, however, because of the expense, the time involved, and the number of subjects required, the model prospective cohort study is relatively rare. To avoid some of these constraints, a historical cohort study might be done, whereby a group of persons who in the past experienced an exposure of interest is identified, and their disease record up to the present is investigated. An example is the follow-up of mortality among insulation workers exposed to asbestos. The population of union insulation workers in the 1940s was identified, and their cause-specific mortality rates through the 1970s were determined. Mortality rates for lung cancer and other causes in this population were tabulated and compared with those expected on the basis of mortality rates for all US men. Because the historical cohort study is a retrospective approach, the terms *cohort study* and *prospective study* should not be used synonymously.

▶ Measures of Association in a Cohort Study

Measures of association illustrate the statistical relationship between two or more variables, and three important measures of association will be discussed using the symbols and numbers provided in Tables A–5 and A–6. Let us assume that one is doing a study of smokers and nonsmokers and following them to see who develops lung cancer over a defined period of time.

A. Relative Risk

Relative risk (RR) is the risk of disease among people exposed to a factor relative to the risk among people not exposed and is a measure of the strength of association between an exposure and a disease.

$$RR = \frac{\text{Disease rate in the exposed population}}{\text{Disease rate in the nonexposed population}}$$

$$= \frac{\dfrac{a}{a+b}}{\dfrac{c}{c+d}} = \frac{\dfrac{63}{10^5}}{\dfrac{7}{10^5}} = 9$$

An RR greater than 1 implies a positive association of the disease with the exposure of interest; an RR less than 1

Table A–5. Presentation of data from a cohort study.

		Disease		
		Present	Absent	
Exposure	Yes	a	b	$a+b$
	No	c	d	$c+d$

Table A–6. Example of data collected in a cohort study of lung cancer and smoking.

	Develop Lung Cancer	Do Not Develop Lung Cancer	
Smokers	63	99,937	100,000
Nonsmokers	7	99,993	100,000

implies a negative association (or protective effect) between the disease and the exposure.

The results in the preceding example suggest that the risk of lung cancer among smokers is nine times greater than the risk for nonsmokers. RR is important for testing etiologic hypotheses.

B. Attributable Risk

Attributable risk (AR) is the rate in the exposed population minus the rate in the nonexposed population.

$$AR = \frac{a}{a+b} - \frac{c}{c+d}$$

$$= \frac{63}{10^5} - \frac{7}{10^5} = \frac{56}{10^5}$$

It indicates the rate of occurrence of death or disease that is caused by a specific exposure factor.

Of the 63 lung cancer deaths that occur annually among 100,000 smokers, 56 (89%) are attributable to smoking. Because a disease may have multiple risk factors that interact with each other, the sum of ARs may be greater than 100%.

AR can be an important tool for counseling individuals with specific risk factors because it helps give an idea about the amount of disease that could be avoided by reducing risk factors in individuals.

C. Population Attributable Risk Percentage

Population attributable risk (PAR) *percentage* is the proportion of a disease in a population related to (or "attributable to") a given exposure.

$$PAR = \frac{P_e(RR-1)}{P_e(RR-1)+1}$$

where P_e is the proportion of the population exposed to the risk factor, and RR is relative risk.

Assuming that 40% of the population smokes (P_e) and that the RR of lung cancer associated with smoking is 9, then

$$= \frac{0.4(9-1)}{0.4(9-1)+1} = \frac{3.2}{4.2} = 76.2\%$$

That is to say, 76% of cases of lung cancer in the general population are attributable to smoking. PAR is important

for public health policy and planning, that is, in estimating what percent of cases in a population could be eliminated by removing an exposure.

2. Case-Control Study

The case-control study is a frequently used design in analytic epidemiology. It determines the risk factors associated with a particular disease by comparing a group of subjects who have the disease (cases) with one or more groups composed of subjects who do not have the disease (controls). Risk factors studied may be permanent, such as gender or race; they may be current, such as present drug use; or they may be historical, such as previous employment. The difference in the frequency distribution of the risk factors between the case and control groups is examined, and the magnitude of the association of these factors with the disease under study is estimated.

Case-control studies are a commonly used design in occupational epidemiology to evaluate either rare diseases or multiple exposures associated with a single outcome. For example, an investigator may be interested in the many occupational and nonoccupational causes of lung cancer. Conversely, a study of a common health outcome, or many health outcomes associated with a single exposure or workplace would best be investigated using a cohort design.

The case-control study is always retrospective. The investigator starts by identifying diseased and non-diseased individuals (ie, the effect) and looks backward for the presence or absence of exposures (ie, the causes) in these individuals.

For example, to study the relationship between asbestos exposure and mesothelioma, a case-control study would compare the history of asbestos exposure in a group of mesothelioma patients with the history of asbestos exposure in a group of subjects who do not have mesothelioma. A cohort study of the relationship between asbestos exposure and mesothelioma first would classify a group of non-diseased persons according to their asbestos exposure and follow them to determine whether the asbestos-exposed subjects had a higher incidence of mesothelioma over time than the nonexposed subjects.

Case-control studies generally can be done more rapidly and less expensively than cohort studies. The time required to complete the study is the time needed to assemble the necessary data; the investigator does not need to wait for cases of the disease to appear. This usually results in lower costs because fewer study personnel and subjects are necessary to test a hypothesis.

For example, suppose that half the general population is exposed to a risk factor (eg, cigarette smoking) and half is not. If a disease (eg, lung cancer) has an annual incidence rate of 100 per 100,000 in the exposed population and 10 per 100,000 in the nonexposed population, a study of 100 cases and 100 controls probably would reveal the increased risk of disease associated with exposure to the factor. Uncovering 100 cases of disease in a cohort study would mean following 10,000 exposed people for 10 years. The rarer the disease, the greater the relative advantage of the case-control study.

Source & Selection of Cases

In defining a case, the diagnostic criteria should be clear and permit selection of a homogeneous group of cases. For example, in cancer studies, microscopic confirmation of the presence of disease and clearly defined criteria for classification by a pathologist of the type of cancer greatly enhance the validity and generalizability of the study findings. The case group usually is composed of (1) all persons with the disease seen at a particular medical facility or group of facilities in a specified period or (2) all persons with the disease found in a community or in the general population in a specified period. Whatever the source of the cases, they should be newly diagnosed (or incident) cases of the disease. Inclusion of prevalent (diagnosed in the past) cases will increase the sample size but can complicate analysis and interpretation of results. Prevalent cases are "survivors" and therefore may not be representative of all people who develop a given disease. Inclusion of prevalent cases inadvertently may identify factors that result from the disease rather than factors that are causally related to its development.

Source & Selection of Controls

The most important principle when selecting controls for a case-control study is that the controls should be from the same study base that produced the cases. An intuitive way to think about this is to consider for the group of controls whether they would have been detected as cases had they developed disease. A population of controls which is systematically different than the cases is a common source of bias in case-control studies and can undermine the findings of the study as differences between the groups may be the result of factors other than the exposure being studied. Four common sources of the control group are (1) the general population, (2) hospital patients, (3) relatives of cases, and (4) associates or friends of cases, but again the most important thing to consider is whether these controls are from the same study base as the cases.

The general population control group may be appropriate if all or most cases occur in a specific geographic area—for example, a county—because in this situation the controls represent the same target population as the cases. Using general population controls, however, presents certain problems: potentially lower response rates than from other types of control groups and from the case group, differing quality of information if the interview setting differs for the cases and the controls, and higher costs for obtaining information.

The hospital patient control group is selected from patients at the same hospital or clinic that the cases attended. This control group may share the selective factors that influenced the cases to come to a particular hospital or clinic, such as residence, ethnicity, or income. These patients (the controls) are readily available, often have the time to accommodate study interviewers, and can be more cooperative. The disadvantage of the hospital control group is that it is composed of people with an illness who may differ from the general population with regard to factors often associated with disease, such as smoking habits and/or drug use.

In addition, the factors that cause patients to attend a particular hospital may not be the same for all diseases. For example, a hospital with a national reputation for treating Hodgkin disease may have patients with this disease from all over the country, whereas its population of coronary disease patients may come only from the region surrounding the hospital; thus, the two patient groups may differ greatly. Similarly, healthy people attending a hospital screening clinic may differ markedly in ethnic, socioeconomic, or other factors from the inpatient population of that hospital.

Spouses and siblings are the relatives used most commonly as controls because of similarity in ethnicity and environment with the case group. Moreover, sibling controls genetically are similar to the cases. Spousal controls are appropriate if there is an approximately equal number of male and female cases, and the age range of cases is such that a high proportion of spouses are likely to be alive. When siblings are the controls, one sibling should be selected per case; using all available siblings would result in the control group having many characteristics related to family size, which may confound any observed associations between the exposure factor and the disease. In contrast, cases with no siblings would have to be excluded from the study (for lack of an equivalent control), which may result in biased study results.

A control group of associates of cases such as neighbors, coworkers, friends, or schoolmates has the advantage of being composed of generally healthy individuals who are similar to the case group with regard to lifestyle characteristics; for example, neighborhood controls are usually of the same SES as the cases. However, such associates might be more similar to cases than members of the general population with respect to risk factors under investigation, thus impairing the ability of the study to detect true differences in exposure between people with and without disease. Other disadvantages of associates as controls are the effort necessary to identify them, a response rate different from that of cases, and probable variations in the quality of information obtained from cases and controls.

Analysis of Case-Control Studies

Data from the case-control study are conventionally arrayed so that cases and controls can be compared on exposure to a hypothesized etiologic factor:

			Disease Status	
			Cases	Controls
Exposure	Yes		a	b
	No		c	d
			$a + c$	$b + d$

The incidence of disease among the exposed and nonexposed cannot be calculated by using case-control data because the cases and controls in the study rarely reflect the true proportions of diseased and nondiseased persons in the population. (The investigator often selects roughly equal numbers of cases [a + c] and controls [b + d] in the study, whereas there are likely to be many more non-diseased than diseased people in the general population.) Therefore, the RR of disease associated with exposure cannot be calculated directly in a case-control study, as it was for the cohort study. However, the *odds ratio* (OR) can be calculated, and the OR approximates the RR under certain circumstances. One of the most common situations in which the OR can approximate the RR is if the proportion of diseased people in the general population is small compared with the proportion of non-diseased. Recall that the true RR using data from a cohort or incidence study is as follows:

$$RR = \frac{\frac{a}{a+b}}{\frac{c}{c+d}}$$

where *a* is the number of cases among the exposed group in a cohort study, *b* is the number of noncases among the exposed group, *c* is the number of cases among the nonexposed group, and *d* is the number of noncases among the nonexposed group.

In a cohort study, as in the general population, *a* is very small relative to *b*. Similarly, *c* is very small relative to *d*. Thus, in the general population (and the usual cohort study), $a/(a + b) \approx a/b$ and $c/(c + d) \approx c/d$. Consequently, in a situation with a rare disease the formula for RR reduces to

$$\frac{\frac{a}{b}}{\frac{c}{d}} = \frac{ad}{bc} = \text{odds ratio (estimated relative risk)}$$

Example: One hundred men with lung cancer and 100 controls are interviewed regarding smoking history:

	Cases	Controls
Smokers	80	30
Nonsmokers	20	70
	100	100

$$\text{Odds ratio} = \frac{ad}{bc} = \frac{80 \times 70}{30 \times 20} = \frac{5600}{600} = 9.3$$

Because lung cancer is rare, the OR is an estimate of RR, and one can conclude that these data show a nine-fold increased risk of lung cancer in smokers compared to nonsmokers.

▶ Matched Case-Control Studies

Controls frequently are selected in a case-control study so as to be individually matched to the cases as to characteristics

such as age, gender, race, or SES that are known to be related to the disease. Matching helps to make the two groups similar with respect to factors other than the exposure of interest in the study and thus serves to reduce the likelihood of spurious associations. The investigator must be careful not to overmatch, that is, to match cases and controls on factors related to the exposure of interest. Overmatching can artificially reduce—and may even eliminate—true exposure differences between diseased and nondiseased individuals in the study. It should be obvious that cases and controls cannot be compared in the analysis with respect to any characteristics on which they have been matched.

The data in a matched-pairs analysis are organized as shown below:

		Controls	
		Exposed	Nonexposed
Cases	**Exposed**	*r*	*s*
	Nonexposed	*t*	*u*

where *r* is the number of pairs in which both case and control are exposed to the factor (concordant), *s* is the number of pairs in which the case but not the control is exposed to the factor (discordant), *t* is the number of pairs in which the control but not the case is exposed to the factor (discordant), and *u* is the number of pairs in which both case and control are not exposed to the factor (concordant). The total number of subjects, *n*, would thus equal 2 times the sum of *r*, *s*, *t*, and *u*.

To compute the OR for a matched-pairs study, only the discordant pairs enter into the calculation:

$$\text{Odds ratio} = \frac{s}{t}$$

$$\text{where } t \neq 0$$

Example: One hundred seventy-five children aged 5–15 years admitted to hospital in 1968 with acute asthma were matched on age, gender, race, and date of admission to 175 controls. All children in the study or their parents were interviewed regarding personal habits and home characteristics during the month preceding the admission. The results regarding second-hand tobacco smoke (SHS) exposure were as follows:

		Controls		
		Yes SHS	No SHS	Totals
Cases	**Yes SHS**	10	57	67
	No SHS	25	95	108
		35	152	187

$$\text{Odds ratio} = \frac{s}{t} = \frac{57}{25} = 2.3$$

These data show that children who had asthma had a 2.3 times greater odds of second-hand tobacco smoke exposure than did children without an acute asthma admission.

3. The Experimental Study

The experimental study is the type of design most familiar to clinical investigators, but it is rarely encountered in occupational epidemiology. Unlike the cohort and case-control studies, which are observational in nature—that is, the investigator observes exposed individuals for the development of disease or diseased individuals for past exposures—in an experimental study, the investigator manipulates exposures and studies the impact on disease. The intervention can occur at different points in the natural course of the disease. Subjects are normally randomly assigned to the different interventions in an experimental study. Ideally, study outcomes also should be determined by individuals blind to the exposure status of the subjects.

Experimental clinical trials often are undertaken among individuals with the same disease who are assigned to different treatment groups. An example is the Carotene and Retinol Efficacy Trial (CARET) study, in which men with asbestos exposure, who are at increased risk of lung cancer, were randomly assigned to receive beta-carotene or a placebo. The study was undertaken to determine whether beta-carotene decreases the risk of developing lung cancer.

Alternatively, intervention might occur in the form of a screening program offered to one group of people at risk of disease and not to another similar group. An example of this type of intervention study is the National Cancer Institute's Cooperative Screening for Early Lung Cancer Program. Men aged 45 years and older with a history of heavy cigarette smoking were assigned to a dual-screened group receiving chest radiographs and sputum cytologic testing or to a group receiving only chest radiographs. The objective was to determine whether the addition of sputum cytologic testing to regular chest radiography resulted in earlier detection and improved lung cancer survival.

CAUSAL ASSOCIATION

An epidemiologic study may demonstrate an association that is not valid because of chance, bias, or confounding, as discussed previously. If the association is believed to be valid—that is, the disease occurrence is in fact not equal among the exposed and unexposed subjects—and the observed association cannot be explained by chance, bias, or confounding, the investigator must consider whether the data support a cause-and-effect association.

This process involves consideration of the study itself and all existing data on the subject. Factors that should be considered in evaluating whether an association is causal include (1) the strength of the association, (2) whether dose-response relationships are present, (3) consonance with existing knowledge (ie, other studies demonstrating the same finding), (4) biologic plausibility (ie, whether there is a proposed biologic mechanism), and (5) the temporal sequence of events (ie, cause precedes effect).

While uncertainties always will exist following an epidemiologic study, action on the findings of a study will depend in part on how strongly the data support a causal association and on the need for action versus the consequences of obtaining more data.

REFERENCES

Lash TJ, VanderWeele TJ, Haneuse S and Rothman K: Modern Epidemiology, 4th ed. Philadelphia, Wolters Kluwer, 2021.
The R Project for Statistical Computing, R 3.5.2, www.r-project.org/ (R is a free software environment for statistical computing and graphics. It compiles and runs on a wide variety of UNIX platforms, Windows, and Mac OS).

Appendix B: Answers to Self-Assessment Questions
(The one correct answer for each question)

Chapter 1

1. c. Occupational injuries and illnesses are among the five leading causes of morbidity and mortality in the United States and in most other countries.

2. b. Occupational physicians play an important role in prevention, recognition, and treatment of injuries and illnesses.

3. c. Independent medical examiners often provide the highest level of evaluation the worker will encounter.

4. a. Board-certified physicians generally have more diverse practice activities and skills, with greater involvement in management, public health-oriented activities, and toxicology.

Chapter 2

1. a. Occupational/environmental history should include information about current and previous jobs in a systematic manner.

2. b. Safety data sheets provide information on the properties of hazardous chemicals and how they affect health and safety in the workplace.

3. d. SHE(O) may trigger regulatory or public health investigations that can lead to prompt control of new hazards.

Chapter 3

1. d. The employer is responsible for providing medical treatment and compensation benefits to the injured employee.

2. c. A work injury that activates or aggravates a preexisting condition is compensable. Recurrence of an earlier compensable injury is also compensable.

3. a. The vast majority of occupational injuries are minor in nature. Well over 90% of occupational injuries are temporary disability cases.

4. c. There is a waiting period for this type of compensation, but it is paid retroactively if the worker cannot work for a certain number of days or if hospitalization is necessary.

5. b. Permanent total disability covers workers who are so disabled that they will not be able to work again in an open labor market.

6. b. Insurers in many states ask the physician to determine the degree of "impairment" (measured by anatomic or functional loss), which the insurers will give to disability raters, workers' compensation judges, commissioners, or hearing officers.

7. c. Occupational disease claims for workers' compensation benefits are increasingly common.

8. c. Apportionment applies only to permanent disability.

9. b. Compromise and release settlements allow the payment of benefits in a lump sum, rather than a series of payments over longer periods of eligibility.

Chapter 4

1. b. The main and legal authority for employee protections are OSHA-issued health standards addressing toxic materials or harmful physical agents.

2. a. Protection of the health of employees might be either *generic* for a workplace or *specific* to particular individuals found to be at risk.

Chapter 5

1. d. A small but important group develop long-term work disability. Although these persons are just a few percent of all workers with health-related work limitations, they account for the majority of total days lost from work due to health conditions.

2. c. The two most widely used methods of determining functional capacity are performance-based tests, often using specific equipment and physical measurement instruments or job simulation, and self-assessments using questionnaires.

3. d. Vocational rehabilitation can address work instability and incongruity, where there may be a mismatch between the skill of the individual and the duties required by the job description.

4. d. A comparative outcome study that examined a work-focused CBT intervention and a regular CBT intervention among employees on sick leave due to common mental disorders (including depression and anxiety) concludes that employees who received work-focused CBT resumed work earlier than those who received regular CBT.

5. c. Two methods to identify blue and black flags in the context of low back pain include: (1) using the clinical interview scenario or (2) using questionnaires, such as the Orebro Musculoskeletal Pain Questionnaire (OMPQ).

Chapter 6

1. c. The head follows the visual target. Therefore, location of the visual target determines head rotation and flexion.

2. c. The risk-assessment tools like ACHIG TLV for HAL or the strain index estimate the risk for musculoskeletal disorders of the hand, wrist, forearm, and elbow.

3. d. The most important physical design rule for a sedentary job at a desk or workbench is that the operator be able to reach all frequently used items (eg, parts, supplies, keyboards, tools, and controls) without leaning, bending, or twisting at the waist.

4. b. To avoid contact stress in the hands, tool handles should be designed so that the force-bearing area is as large as practicable and there are no sharp corners or edges.

5. a. Bifocal wearers will look at the screen through just the bottom of their glasses. Therefore, in order to prevent head extension, the screen should be lower than is usually recommended.

6. c. The NIOSH lifting equation aims to provide recommended weight limits (RWLs) that are protective of at least 75% of working women and 99% of working men.

7. a. The ACGIH TLV for lifting recommends upper limits for repetitive lifting, with the goal of allowing the majority of workers to perform the task without developing back and shoulder disorders.

8. a. HAVS involves damage to the small blood vessels and nerves of the fingers.

9. c. The maximum lift allowable by the NIOSH lifting equation is 51 lb.

10. a. Primary visual targets (screens and hard copy) should be located in front of the operator, between 0 and 30 degrees below eye level, and approximately 48–72 cm (20–30 in) away.

11. c. Repeated grip forces of greater than 10 N (1 kg) are associated with a greater risk of carpal tunnel syndrome.

12. d. Women of average dimensions (50th percentile) can reach horizontally only about 74 cm (29 in), and short women (5th percentile) can reach horizontally only about 68 cm (27 in), as measured from the backrest of the chair when they are seated in an upright position.

Chapter 7

1. a. Functional testing, including simple tasks performed during activities of daily living, is useful to assess injury severity.

2. a. CT scans are the most effective method for visualizing any bony pathology, including morphology of fractures.

3. b. Arthrocentesis must be performed promptly to rule out an infection when acute knee pain with effusion and inflammation are present and the patient is unable to actively flex the joint.

4. d. Cumulative trauma may involve the extremity (commonly the hand, wrist, elbow, or shoulder) or the trunk (low-back strain).

Chapter 8

1. a. The glenohumeral joint is surrounded by a fibrocartilagenous rim that helps to deepen and stabilize the joint. Tears that occur over the superior part of the labrum are known as "SLAP" lesions, or superior labral anterior to posterior lesions, and are often seen in throwing athletes such as pitchers.

2. a. Excessive force applied in any direction may cause a shoulder dislocation.

3. a. Acromioclavicular joint injuries may result from falls or from direct trauma to the arm or shoulder.

4. b. Thoracic outlet syndrome is a set of symptoms and signs caused by compression of the neurovascular structures passing out of the chest and neck and beneath the clavicle to the axilla.

5. c. Lateral humeral epicondylitis can occur among workers who perform repeated forceful pinching or power grasps.

6. d. Radial nerve entrapment at the elbow also called radial tunnel syndrome can be considered in cases of resistant lateral epicondylitis.

7. c. Compression of the nerve in the canal may be related to old elbow injuries with enlarging osteophytes, cubitus valgus, or subluxation of the nerve out of the groove.

8. d. De Quervain tenosynovitis involves the first dorsal compartment of the wrist. The onset is usually associated with overuse of the thumb and wrist particularly with radial deviation, as in repetitive hammering, lifting, or pipetting.

9. d. Stenosing tenosynovitis of the flexor tendon to a finger or of the flexor pollicis longus to the thumb may produce pain when the digit or thumb is forcibly flexed or extended.

10. d. Repeated or sustained forceful gripping or repetitive wrist and finger movements involved in work have been associated with carpal tunnel syndrome.

11. d. The diagnosis of carpal tunnel syndrome is confirmed by median nerve electrodiagnostic studies (nerve conduction studies and EMG).

12. c. Ulnar neuropathy at the wrist can be caused by a space-occupying lesion in the area of Guyon canal.

13. a. Hand arm vibration syndrome (HAVS) involves both neurologic and vascular signs and symptoms associated with the use of electric and pneumatic vibrating hand tools.

Chapter 9

1. b. Approximately 80% of episodes of low back pain resolve within 2 weeks and 90% resolve within 6 weeks.
2. d. Spinal stenosis may present with neurogenic claudication symptoms with walking.
3. d. The L5–S1 disk is affected in 90% of cases of lumbar disk herniation.
4. a. Hip fractures should be surgically repaired as soon as possible (within 24 hours).
5. c. Osteoarthritis involves a degeneration of the joint cartilage.
6. d. Anterior cruciate ligament injury leads to acute swelling immediately (or within 4 hours).
7. a. Collateral ligament injury is caused by a valgus or varus blow or stress to the knee.
8. a. Inversion ankle sprains may result in chronic instability.

Chapter 10

1. c. Pain has a felt, sensory quality and an affective aspect, demands our mind's attention, and includes a strong behavioral drive toward homeostasis.
2. d. As pain persists, pain circuits develop a hypersensitive state, with pain itself being a pain predictive conditioning cue.
3. b. Opioid pain medications, in addition to their pain relief, particularly effective for acute pain, are both rewarding and behaviorally reinforcing.
4. a. Depression is more common in chronic pain patients than in healthy controls, and pain is more common in depressed patients than in nondepressed individuals.
5. c. Pharmacologic treatments for chronic pain are usually most effective when combined with other treatment strategies.
6. c. The goal of CBT is to help patients identify destructive thought patterns and learn to generate more constructive thought patterns.
7. a. Pacing techniques prevent these periods of over- or underactivity by teaching patients to measure out task in advance and plan the amount of time they intend to spend on an activity.

Chapter 11

1. a. Open-angle glaucoma accounts for most cases of glaucomatous visual loss (90%).
2. c. Visual fields should be tested, especially in patients with suspected head injury or a significant decrease in visual acuity.
3. b. Strong alkalis and acids can cause the most severe and damaging chemical injuries to the eye and eyelids.
4. a. Iridoplegia is caused by damage to the pupillary sphincter.

5. b. Secondary hemorrhage frequently continues until the anterior chamber is completely filled with blood, during which time the intraocular pressure may rise to 50–60 mm Hg (normal 12–20 mm Hg).
6. c. This radiation is generated by the welder's arc and damages the exposed corneal and conjunctival epithelium.
7. d. Sympathetic ophthalmia can cause complete loss of vision in both eyes if unrecognized and untreated early in its course.

Chapter 12

1. d. In a clinical audiogram, conductive losses are indicated by an "air-bone gap," in which the air-conduction threshold exceeds the bone-conduction threshold.
2. c. The speech reception threshold (SRT) is the intensity (in decibels) at which the listener is able to repeat 50% of balanced two-syllable words known as *spondee words*. The normal range for young adults is between 0 and 20 dB.
3. b. Tests like this are attractive because they use more realistic speech than conventional speech tests (sentences rather than isolated words) and incorporate background noise, which is important in some jobs.
4. d. ARHL has a large genetic component; heritability is close to 50%.
5. a. ISSHL is differentiated by its sudden onset, usually developing within 24 hours, in the absence of precipitating factors.
6. a. NIHL results mechanically from trauma to the sensory epithelium of the cochlea and metabolically from the generation of reactive oxygen species.
7. d. Because the acoustic reflex is neurally mediated, it is delayed in onset for a period ranging from 25 to 150 ms, depending on the intensity of the sound.
8. a. OSHA regulates exposure to noise at or above an 8-hour time-weighted average (TWA) of 85 dBA, the approximate biologic threshold above which permanent shifts in hearing are possible.
9. a. When 8-hour TWA noise levels are equal to or greater than 85 dBA (a 50% noise dose) but below 90 dBA (a 100% noise dose), HPDs *must* be made available to the exposed workers.
10. a. Ototoxic hearing loss is the result of exposure to chemical substances that injure the cochlea.

Chapter 13

1. a. Systemic hypothermia is reduction of the body's core temperature below 35°C (95°F).
2. d. Heat stroke morbidity or mortality can result from cerebral, cardiovascular, hepatic, or renal damage.

3. c. A sudden exposure to intense electrical energy can cause not only tissue destruction and necrosis from heat and burning but also depolarization of electrically sensitive tissues such as nerve and heart.

4. d. Some patients with acute radiation syndrome pass through four phases: prodrome, latent phase, illness, and recovery.

5. d. Most cases of decompression sickness have occurred after rapid ascension from sea depths in excess of 9 m (29.5 ft) or after sudden cabin pressure loss at altitudes in excess of 7000 m (22,966 ft).

6. d. Class 3b and stronger lasers present two forms of risk: the power level can damage the eye before a blink reflex offers any protection, and even the diffuse reflection of an errant beam can cause eye damage.

7. c. High-pressure injection injuries often require extensive debridement with delayed closure.

Chapter 14

1. a. Nanoparticles are engineered structures that are less than 100 nm in size.

2. d. Toxicity is affected by atmospheric pressure, temperature, and humidity.

3. b. G6PD deficiency is an X-linked recessive disorder.

4. a. Biotransformation occurs in the liver by hydrolysis, oxidation, reduction, and conjugation.

5. d. Clearance is a measure not of how many milligrams of toxin is being removed but rather of the volume of fluid that is freed of the toxic agent per unit of time.

6. d. The results of hair analysis are difficult to interpret as hair samples are subject to external contamination.

7. a. Management of acute toxicity consists of removal from exposure, symptomatic treatment, and supportive care.

Chapter 15

1. c. Lymphocytes are responsible for the initial specific recognition of antigen.

2. b. Cytotoxic or "killer" T cells are responsible for defense against intracellular pathogens (eg, viruses), tumor immunity, and organ graft rejection.

3. c. Macrophages are involved in the ingestion, processing, and presentation of antigens for interaction with lymphocytes.

4. a. Eosinophils play both a proactive and a modulating role in inflammation.

5. a. Type I anaphylactic or immediate hypersensitivity reactions are initiated by the interaction of antigen with specific IgE antibodies bound to mast cells and basophils with the subsequent release of inflammatory mediators.

6. b. Reactive airways dysfunction syndrome (RADS) is a syndrome characterized by the acute emergence of bronchial hyperreactivity and symptoms of asthma, after an acute exposure to high levels of respiratory irritants, usually toxic chemicals, smoke, or particulates.

7. d. Allergic contact dermatitis (ACD) is a type IV delayed hypersensitivity disorder, caused by a variety of agents in the occupational setting including latex, nickel, formaldehyde, potassium dichromate, thiurams, epoxy resins, mercaptos, parabens, quaternium-15, ethylenediamine, and cobalt.

8. a. The late-reacting systemic syndrome ("TMA flu") is characterized by cough, occasional wheezing, dyspnea, and systemic symptoms of malaise, chills, myalgia, and arthralgia.

9. b. Patch tests are useful in evaluating skin contact sensitivity (type IV delayed hypersensitivity).

10. a. Inhalation challenge tests are conducted by exposing the worker to the suspected antigen.

Chapter 16

1. a. Hepatitis A is a viral hepatitis transmitted through the fecal-oral route.

2. a. Hepatitis B core antibodies indicate past or present HBV infections.

3. d. Hepatitis C is transmitted rarely following mucous membrane exposure, with no apparent transfer following exposures to intact skin.

4. d. Tuberculin skin test is considered positive in high-risk occupational groups with a reaction of 10 mm or more.

Chapter 17

1. a. Irritant contact dermatitis is a common form of occupational skin disease and, in the United States, accounts for nearly 80% of all occupational dermatitis.

2. d. ICD is a nonimmunogenic skin reaction to toxic substances either in low or high concentrations.

3. b. Numerous systemic drugs can cause phototoxic reactions.

4. c. The initial site of leukoderma is usually the hands and forearms.

5. d. ACD is an immunologic reaction classified as a delayed type IV or cell-mediated hypersensitivity. This distinguishes it from type I reactions, which are immediate and antibody mediated.

6. c. ACD results in considerable variation in the intensity of reaction depending on the body area affected.

7. a. ACD sensitization requires at least 4 days to develop.

8. a. The key to diagnosis of allergic contact dermatitis is diagnostic patch testing.

9. b. Photoallergic reactions are immunologically based.

10. b. With sufficient provocation, nearly all exposed individuals will develop nonallergic contact urticaria. Previous sensitization is not necessary.

11. c. Allergic contact urticaria reactions are immunoglobulin E (IgE)–mediated type I immediate hypersensitivity reactions and appear to be more common in atopics.

12. d. Peripheral neuritis and hepatotoxicity may occur with chloracne, suggesting systemic toxicity.

13. d. Employment of persons with active atopic dermatitis in food service industries and hospital patient care may need to be restricted.

14. c. Treatment of atypical mycobacterial infections with rifampicin or ethambutol is usually effective.

15. a. Avoidance, substitution with less-allergenic chemicals, modification of work activities, and protective measures are the best approach to management.

16. c. Prevention of occupational skin disorders requires close cooperation between the employee, employers, company physicians, dermatologists, and other relevant stakeholders such as workers unions.

Chapter 18

1. b. A growing body of evidence links the development of rhinitis with that of asthma, making the prevention (and early recognition) of upper airway inflammation a priority.

2. d. Workplace allergens producing allergic rhinitis may be either commonly encountered allergens, exposure to which may be incidental to the work environment (eg, grass pollen exposure in a landscaping gardener), or unusual agents encountered only in industrial environments (eg, trimellitic anhydride exposure in a plastics worker).

3. c. High-grade nasal obstruction (a reflex response to irritants and allergens) predisposes to oral breathing, bypassing the filtration and air-conditioning functions of the upper airway. This may be one of the mechanisms whereby rhinitis and asthma severity are linked.

4. d. Nasal hyperreactivity is a defining characteristic of vasomotor rhinitis, but can also be found in a subset (~40%) of allergic rhinitis.

5. a. Sinusitis has been linked to asthma incidence and severity.

Chapter 19

1. b. The diffusing capacity of the lung for carbon monoxide (DLCO) is closely correlated with the capacity of the lungs to absorb oxygen.

2. a. Bronchoprovocation tests are useful in the diagnosis of occupational asthma.

3. b. The site of deposition of an inhaled gas is determined primarily by water solubility.

4. a. Occupational asthma caused by such diverse agents as diisocyanates, snow crab, and western red cedar show persistence of symptoms and the presence of nonspecific airway hyperresponsiveness for periods up to 6 years after removal from the offending agent.

5. c. Hypersensitivity pneumonitis, also known as extrinsic allergic alveolitis, refers to an immunologically mediated inflammatory disease of the lung parenchyma that is induced by inhalation of organic dusts that contain a variety of etiologic agents (eg, bacteria, fungi, amoebae, animal proteins, and several low-molecular-weight chemicals).

6. b. Silicosis is a parenchymal lung disease that results from the inhalation of silicon dioxide, or silica, in crystalline form.

7. c. Coal workers' pneumoconiosis may lead to progressive massive fibrosis, identical to that of silicosis.

8. a. In reflex bronchoconstriction, neuroreceptors in the airway are stimulated by agents such as cold air, dusts, mists, vapors, and fumes.

Chapter 20

1. a. Chronic exposure to carbon disulfide appears to accelerate atherosclerosis and/or precipitate acute coronary ischemic events.

2. d. Carbon monoxide exposure may aggravate or induce cardiac arrhythmias.

3. d. Case-control studies suggest a 2.5- to 4-fold increase in the risk of cardiovascular death in workers handling explosives.

4. a. Intoxication with organophosphate and carbamate insecticides can produce diverse cardiovascular disturbances, including tachycardia and hypertension, bradycardia and hypotension, heart block, and ventricular tachycardia.

5. a. Arsine gas causes red blood cell hemolysis.

Chapter 21

1. a. Direct hepatotoxins or their metabolic products injure the hepatocyte and its organelles by a direct physicochemical effect, such as peroxidation of membrane lipids, denaturation of proteins, or other chemical changes that lead to destruction or distortion of cell membranes.

2. a. Indirect hepatotoxins are antimetabolites and related compounds that produce hepatic injury by interference with metabolic pathways.

3. b. The strategic role of the liver as the primary defense against xenobiotics depends largely on cellular enzyme systems (mixed-function oxidases [MFOs]).

4. d. Renal failure may ensue a few days after the carbon tetrachloride hepatic damage becomes manifest and in fact has been the cause of death in most fatal cases.

5. b. TASH has recently been used to describe hepatic steatosis, inflammation, and fibrosis among vinyl chloride production workers.

6. a. While contaminated food and water are common epidemic sources, hepatitis A is transmitted primarily by person-to-person contact, generally through fecal contamination.

7. b. Transmission occurs via percutaneous or permucosal routes when exposure to blood or potentially infectious body fluids occurs; HBV is not transmitted via the fecal-oral route or by contamination of food or water.

8. c. HCV is spread primarily through parenteral exposures from blood transfusions or intravenous drug abuse.

9. c. In the occupational setting, measures of hepatic functional capacity have been used epidemiologically to demonstrate liver dysfunction in the absence of clinical or serologic abnormalities.

10. a. The use of Cytokeratin 18 (CK18) has recently been explored as a tool to assess occupational liver disease.

Chapter 22

1. a. The kidney is especially vulnerable to occupational and environmental exposures.

2. d. In acute kidney injury, patients may require dialysis until the renal function recovers.

3. d. Most chronic kidney diseases associated with exposure to agents such as lead or cadmium present with chronic interstitial nephritis characterized by tubular proteinuria (usually < 2 g/24 h) and a urine sediment usually lacking any cellular elements.

4. a. Balkan-endemic nephropathy (BEN) is now considered a form of aristolochic acid nephropathy.

5. c. Lead nephropathy renal ultrasonography typically shows small, contracted kidneys.

6. a. Overt lead nephropathy is one of the few preventable renal diseases.

7. b. Once a critical concentration of 200 mcg/g of renal cortex is achieved, the renal effects of cadmium, such as Fanconi syndrome, become evident.

8. a. Heavy exposure to silica can result in a generalized systemic disease resembling collagen-vascular disease, such as systemic lupus erythematosus.

9. c. The cause of the epidemic of chronic kidney disease in Central America is unknown. It disproportionately affects agricultural workers at lower, warm weather altitudes.

10. c. Toluene inhalation (glue sniffing) is a classic cause of distal renal tubular acidosis.

Chapter 23

1. c. Encephalopathy is a general term that denotes a diffuse dysfunction of the central nervous system. The clinical manifestations may be diverse. Depressed level of consciousness is common, as are cognitive and psychiatric symptoms. Other manifestations depend on the selectivity of the injury. For instance, some toxins may cause more selective injury to the vestibular system or cerebellum resulting in dysequilibrium, vertigo, and gait or limb ataxia. Others may affect the basal ganglia causing an extrapyramidal syndrome of bradykinesia, tremors, and rigidity.

2. a. Evaluation of cognitive complaints should include at least a mini–mental state examination.

3. b. Peripheral nervous system disorders lead to sensory disturbances and weakness, often accompanied by impairment of the deep tendon reflexes on physical examination.

4. c. The hallmark of most polyneuropathies is the distal distribution of the clinical symptoms and signs.

5. c. Peripheral neuropathy may result from a wide range of systemic conditions. Despite continuing advances, the causes of many neuropathies remain elusive despite testing.

6. a. Focal neuropathy is a condition in which a single nerve is affected. Symptoms arise from the motor and sensory fibers in the affected nerve, typically resulting in weakness and sensory loss in a restricted anatomic distribution.

7. c. A neuropathy may develop as a delayed manifestation a few weeks after acute acrylamide exposure or insidiously after chronic exposure.

8. d. Chronic exposure leads to a more insidious sensorimotor polyneuropathy, although there is no agreement for a threshold limit.

9. a. Like many other toxins, mercury poisoning causes a diffuse encephalopathy.

10. b. Severe organophosphate intoxication may cause convulsions, coma, muscle paralysis, and respiratory arrest occur with severe intoxication.

Chapter 24

1. d. Methemoglobin is dangerous because of its inability to bind oxygen and because it increases the oxygen affinity of the remaining heme groups in hemoglobin tetramer, thereby decreasing oxygen delivery to the tissues.

2. d. Clinically, symptomatic porphyria can occur either as a result of inadequate enzymatic function along any step in heme biosynthesis or as a result of inappropriate overstimulation of δ-aminolevulinic acid synthetase, usually in the setting of decreased heme concentration.

3. c. The major differences between the two diseases are (1) an increase in neuropsychiatric signs in acute intermittent porphyria compared with lead intoxication and (2) anemia, which is present in lead intoxication but virtually absent in porphyria.

4. c. Aplastic anemia, or medullary aplasia, is an acquired abnormality of the pluripotent hematopoietic stem cells resulting in pancytopenia (anemia, neutropenia, and thrombocytopenia).

5. b. The myelodysplastic syndromes are a group of acquired genetic disorders of the blood-forming cells similar to cancer and characterized by ineffective hematopoiesis, clinically resulting in anemia, neutropenia, thrombocytopenia, or a combination of cytopenias.

6. c. Multiple myeloma is characterized by anemia, painful lytic and osteopenic bone disease, monoclonal immunoglobulin production (in serum or urine or both), hypogammaglobulinemia, and short survival.

Chapter 25

1. c. In both experimental animal models of cancer and human cancers with known causes, a significant interval of time is required from first exposure to the responsible agent to the development of malignancy. This interval is referred to as the induction-latency (or sometimes just latency) or incubation period.

2. a. Epidemiologic studies provide the strongest evidence for human carcinogenicity.

3. d. One of the best-studied and most commonly performed short-term tests is the Ames test, which uses a mutant strain of *Salmonella typhimurium* that is deficient in the enzymes required to synthesize histidine and which will not grow unless histidine is added to the growth medium.

4. a. Tests for DNA repair can demonstrate that DNA damage has occurred following exposure to a chemical.

5. a. DNA or protein adducts are a potentially valuable tool in the measurement of levels of specific carcinogens covalently bound to DNA or proteins.

6. c. Lung cancer is a major asbestos-related disease, accounting for 20% of all deaths in asbestos-exposed cohorts.

7. d. Diesel-engine exhaust contains a number of nitroarenes, which are nitro-substituted derivatives of polycyclic aromatic hydrocarbons (arenes).

8. d. Many different occupational exposures are linked to cancer of the nasal cavity and paranasal sinuses.

9. d. NIOSH has concluded that all benzidine-derived dyes should be considered to be potential human carcinogens.

10. d. Skin cancers from arsenic exposure tend to be multiple and occur in younger patients than those attributable to UV light.

11. b. The two major forms of leukemia that have been linked to occupation are acute nonlymphocytic leukemia (ANLL)—including myelodysplasia and preleukemia—and chronic myelogenous leukemia (CML).

Chapter 26

1. c. Mutagenicity refers to induction of alterations in the DNA sequence that can be transmitted to daughter cells during cell division.

2. a. DNA can be modified by reactive chemicals, including metabolically activated xenobiotics, as well as by reactive oxygen and nitrogen species (ROS and RNS) generated as byproducts of oxidative phosphorylation and other cellular processes or during xenobiotic metabolism.

3. b. A proto-oncogene is a normal cellular gene that will not transform cells without an alteration, such as a mutation, that activates it to an oncogene.

Chapter 27

1. a. Chemical exposures during weeks 1 and 2 after conception may cause early pregnancy loss if they interfere with tubal transport, implantation, or endocrine control or if they are cytotoxic to the fetus itself.

2. c. Chemical exposures after the first trimester may induce minor morphologic abnormalities or growth deficits.

3. b. Endocrine-disrupting chemicals are hormonally active agents.

4. c. Solvents such as perchloroethylene, methylene chloride, toluene, xylene, and glycol ethers have been associated with concurrent elevation in SAB risk.

5. d. Tobacco smoking is associated with infertility, menstrual disorders, and menopause at earlier age.

Chapter 28

1. d. Semen abnormalities can include azoospermia (complete absence of sperm), oligospermia (decreased sperm count), teratospermia (abnormally shaped sperm), and asthenospermia (sperm showing decreased motility).

2. d. Most occupational events involving high-level exposures and documented adverse reproductive effects have occurred in male workers with exposure to DBCP and exogenous estrogens.

3. d. Decreased fertility was experienced among workers with testicular changes, and the most extreme FSH elevations were found in workers who did not recover after a period of no exposure.

4. c. Inorganic lead presents in some males as endocrine changes (decreased testosterone and increased LH levels).

5. d. Phthalates may cause human male reproductive damage at levels found in the general population.

Chapter 29

1. d. Chronic arsenic inhalation may cause lung cancer, and chronic arsenic ingestion may cause cancer of the skin, lung, and bladder.

2. b. Chronic berylliosis may develop after months or years of exposure or following a single acute exposure.

3. a. The beryllium lymphocyte proliferation test (BeLPT) confirms sensitization.

4. c. Renal tubular dysfunction resulting from chronic exposure to cadmium can result in nephrolithiasis and osteomalacia.

5. c. Cough, chest pain, and dyspnea may indicate exposure to irritant levels of soluble chromium compounds or the development of chromium-induced asthma.

6. a. Acute high-dose lead exposure may induce a hemolytic anemia (or anemia with basophilic stippling if exposure has been subacute).

7. c. Approximately 95% of all elevated blood lead levels among adults in the United States are work related.

8. d. In 2010, the CDC issued guidelines recommending medical removal from workplace exposure of any woman with a prenatal blood lead level of equal to or greater than 10 mcg/dL.

9. c. Exposure to manganese may lead to a clinical syndrome that is similar to idiopathic parkinsonism, with slow speech, masked facies, bradykinesia, gait dysfunction, and micrographia.

10. d. The release of mercury into the atmosphere from both natural sources, such as volcanoes, and industrial emissions has led to global distribution of this element.

11. b. Nickel is a common cause of allergic contact dermatitis.

Chapter 30

1. a. Hydrofluoric acid (hydrogen fluoride) occupational exposure can occur both by direct skin contact and by inhalation of fumes.

2. d. Formaldehyde is a by-product of the incomplete combustion of hydrocarbons and is found in small mounts in automobile exhaust and cigarette smoke.

3. a. Symptoms of acute nitroglycerine illness include loss of consciousness, severe headache, difficulty breathing, weak pulse, and pallor.

4. a. PCP is used as a wood preservative, herbicide, defoliant, and fungicide.

5. c. PCBs have an efficient transplacental transfer, and adverse reproductive effects of PCBs have been reported in many animal species.

6. b. Styrene chronic exposure may cause weakness, headache, fatigue, poor memory, and dizziness.

7. a. Vinyl chloride disease is a syndrome consisting of Raynaud phenomenon, acro-osteolysis, joint and muscle pain, enhanced collagen deposition, stiffness of the hands, and scleroderma-like skin changes.

Chapter 31

1. c. Solvents may be classified as aqueous (water-based) or organic (hydrocarbon-based).

2. b. Skin absorption rates vary widely among individuals by at least a factor of 4.

3. a. One isomer of hexane, n-hexane, causes peripheral neuropathy.

4. d. Aromatic hydrocarbons cause acute anesthetic effects, respiratory tract irritation, and dermatitis and are associated with neurobehavioral dysfunction.

5. c. Respiratory tract and eye irritation usually occurs at lower concentrations than central nervous system depression and thus serves as a useful warning property.

6. c. Methylene chloride is unique in that it is metabolized to carbon monoxide, with formation of carboxyhemoglobin.

Chapter 32

1. a. High-intensity exposure to toxic gases and other airborne toxicants may result in clinical findings that develop abruptly or in a delayed manner.

2. d. Simple asphyxiants include methane gas, argon, carbon dioxide, and nitrogen.

3. c. Methane is also released in coal and other fossil fuel extraction settings and in the presence of organic material breakdown (including landfills).

4. d. Although carbon dioxide is considered a simple asphyxiant, at high concentrations it also acts as a potent central nervous system depressant.

5. a. Carbon monoxide competes with oxygen for binding sites on hemoglobin, thereby reducing the oxygen-carrying capacity of the blood.

6. a. Major current industrial use of cyanide is in metal plating operations and in the extraction of silver and gold salts from ores.

7. a. Like cyanide, hydrogen sulfide exerts its toxicity by blocking oxygen utilization through the cytochrome oxidase pathway.

8. d. Clinical findings in smoke inhalation injury can include features of both asphyxiant and irritant injury.

9. a. Arsine gas has been used as a dopant in the microelectronics industry.

10. d. With lower-level exposure of phosphine gas, pulmonary toxicity may be the primary manifestation, marked by dyspnea, cough, chest pain, and delayed-onset pulmonary edema in the hours following the exposure.

Chapter 33

1. a. In the United States, the Environmental Protection Agency (EPA) regulates the registration, sale, and conditions of use of all pesticides.
2. b. Organophosphates potency depends on their ability to bind with the cholinesterase molecule.
3. c. Carbamates differ from organophosphates in causing reversible rather than irreversible cholinesterase inhibition and typically have a short clinical course.
4. d. The initial diagnosis can be made on clinical grounds alone, samples sent to the laboratory, and a test dose of atropine delivered. A dose of atropine sulfate produces signs of mild atropinization in a normal adult; it has no effect in an individual with organophosphate poisoning.
5. a. The fumigants have in common innately high vapor pressures or by-products with high vapor pressure.

Chapter 34

1. b. A crucial aspect of diversity management involves avoidance of stereotyping based on age, gender, sexual orientation, and racial or ethnic status.
2. d. A significant benefit to remote workers is that their choice of employers is greatly expanded.

Chapter 35

1. a. Total Worker Health (TWH) seeks to identify and control exposures to hazards that impact worker safety.
2. d. The first step in implementing a TWH approach is the elimination of workplace conditions that cause or contribute to worker illness and injury.

Chapter 36

1. d. The hallmark of major depression is a severely depressed mood lasting at least 2 weeks.
2. a. Bipolar disorder is a cyclical mood disorder involving at least one episode of abnormally elevated energy level and mood which usually alternate with one or more episodes of depression.

Chapter 37

1. c. The majority of individuals subject to shiftwork or jet travel–related time shifts in their sleep-wake schedules commonly report some degree of depressive symptoms.
2. b. Extensive disruption in circadian function is known to occur among patients with bipolar disorder.

Chapter 38

1. c. OSHA provides the principles of a comprehensive occupational health and safety injury prevention program.
2. a. Type I violence is prevalent among late night retail workers and taxi drivers, who are at risk of injury from violence committed during an attempted robbery.

3. a. Determining whether or not an employee may become violent has less to do with a static profile of that person than a series of dynamic variables (behaviors).

Chapter 39

1. c. Certified Safety Professional (CSP) is the highest professional designation recognized by the BCSP.
2. b. The safety and health management system guides the organization to (1) prevent work-related injuries and illnesses, (2) comply with applicable health and safety regulations, and (3) minimize injury/illness, regulatory, and related compliance costs and violations.
3. a. Injury and Illness Prevention (IIP) programs are universal interventions that can substantially reduce the number and severity of workplace injuries and alleviate the associated financial burdens on workplaces.
4. c. Hazard assessment procedures should be part of an effective IIP program.
5. a. OSHA and often other regulatory agencies require employers in nearly all cases to prepare and implement an EAP for emergency situations.
6. b. All employers with hazardous chemicals in their workplaces must have labels and safety data sheets for their exposed workers, and train them to handle the chemicals safely and appropriately.
7. d. Exposure records consist of safety and/or industrial hygiene air and exposure monitoring data, and biological monitoring data.
8. b. Hazard prevention and control ensures that hazard correction procedures are in place.
9. b. Job safety analysis (JSA) uncovers the inherent hazards in the work environment, a task or activity, and recommends control strategies.

Chapter 40

1. a. The walk-through survey is the first and most important technique used to recognize occupational health hazards.
2. d. The current OSHA Workers' Right-to-Know regulation makes explicit (and subject to governmental investigation) the commonsense duty of the employer to inform workers of the nature and hazards of materials to which they may be exposed.
3. b. Sampling and analysis of airborne contaminants is a definitive function of the industrial hygienist.
4. d. Phase-contrast microscopy gives an imperfect index of exposure to all asbestos fibers.
5. c. Wipe sampling may be a useful adjunct to programs used to evaluate the effectiveness of housekeeping measures, particularly in manufacturing facilities where separation of manufacturing areas from cafeterias, offices, or dressing rooms is important.

6. b. Sound-level meters typically contain filtering circuits that permit evaluation of exposures to components of the noise spectrum weighted in accordance with their effects on hearing.

7. a. TLVs—or the OSHA PELs and the NIOSH RELs—represent *maximum allowable* time-weighted exposure levels.

Chapter 41

1. a. Public health surveillance systems seek to assess the burden and distribution of occupational diseases in the population.

2. d. To address the lack of uniformity in coding, a large collaborative initiative established a number of programs aimed at the standardization and routine recording of industry and occupation on death certificates.

3. b. The National Health and Nutrition Examination Survey (NHANES) is a program of studies of children and adults whose primary purpose is to assess the health and nutrition status of US residents.

4. d. The CDC administers the National Program of Cancer Registries (NPCR), which supports central cancer registries in 45 states representing 96% of the US population.

5. d. Even for injuries, there is concern that the SOII substantially undercounts work-related events.

6. c. Occupational disease surveillance utilizes hazardous material registries.

Chapter 42

1. c. Medical surveillance entails compiling and analyzing the health data from workers over a period of time.

2. d. Medical surveillance is the process of identifying, quantifying, and removing causative factors that increase the risk of occupational diseases or injuries.

3. a. Primary prevention methods are intended to minimize employee exposure to hazards and risk of injury or occupational disease.

4. d. Health-based regulations apply to hazardous substances such as lead, asbestos, and benzene.

5. c. The compliance plan must be reviewed and reevaluated at regular intervals at least annually.

6. b. Action level (AL) initiates medical surveillance.

7. d. OSHA health standards are codified as regulations such that employers may assume that all doctors are trained and knowledgeable for any problem or service that they or their facility offers.

8. d. The physician has a duty to protect confidential information learned about the company and its processes and methods. Usually, this information is protected in a contractual agreement between the employer and the physician or medical practice.

9. d. OSHA health standards only require that physicians evaluate health effects and risks of employees on an individual basis, not as a group.

10. c. Temporary removal of an employee from an exposure can be based upon the physician's assessment of the employee's medical condition which places the employee at increased risk of adverse health effects resulting from exposure.

Chapter 43

1. b. Biological markers are measurement of a chemical, its metabolite, or a biochemical effect in a biological specimen.

2. d. Measurements of chemicals in whole blood can be a valuable matrix for measuring adducts of hemoglobin, albumin, or DNA.

3. c. Biomonitoring of chemicals in exhaled air may be used to assess airway inflammation.

4. c. Health-based values for interpreting biomonitoring results may incorporate safety factors.

5. b. BEIs are based on studies that address minimal or no adverse health effect levels in exposed workers and animals.

6. a. Biologic monitoring in the occupational setting may be a voluntary or required component of routine medical surveillance.

Chapter 44

1. b. Nerve agent ocular effects include miosis, lacrimation, conjunctival injection, pain, and blurred or dim vision.

2. b. Mustard is a highly reactive molecule and acts as an alkylating agent to cause cellular tissue damage.

3. a. Anthrax is an infectious disease that affects animals and humans.

4. a. Inhalational anthrax begins with nonspecific symptoms of malaise, fatigue, myalgia, and fever.

5. a. Cutaneous anthrax first appears as a small papule that progresses to a vesicle containing serosanguinous fluid.

6. b. Gastrointestinal anthrax presents with nonspecific symptoms of nausea, vomiting, and fever.

7. d. Botulinum toxin attacks the presynaptic terminal of the peripheral nerves blocking the release of acetylcholine and inhibiting muscle contraction.

8. c. Ricin is a cellular toxin that inhibits protein synthesis by binding to and catalytically modifying ribosomes.

9. d. After inhalation of ricin, hemoptysis and pulmonary edema may develop over the next 18–6 hours leading to respiratory failure and death.

Chapter 45

1. c. Baseline and annual health screenings are generally more complete than pre-deployment screenings, which can be focused for a specific incident or concentrate on recent changes from a baseline or annual health screening.

2. d. Safety and health training is the responsibility of the response organization.

3. a. The first step in the ERHMS deployment phase is to create an on-site responder roster to track the personnel who are deployed for the incident and to confirm that they were qualified to be dispatched.

Chapter 46

1. a. Global oil consumption reached 88 million barrels per day in 2011, which accounts for 33.1% of global energy consumption.

2. a. Transportation, which relies almost exclusively on oil, accounts for nearly 30% of US energy demand and 20% of US emissions of carbon dioxide.

3. c. Dioxins are not produced intentionally, but are byproducts of incineration, combustion, chlorine-based bleaching, and other industrial processes. Dioxins are known human carcinogens and are well-established endocrine disruptors.

4. d. Prenatal phthalate exposure has been associated with testicular dysgenesis syndrome, an entity first described in 2001 is a result of disrupted gonadal development during fetal life, resulting in poor semen quality and higher rates of undescended testis, hypospadias, and testicular cancer.

5. c. Although the DBCP and vinyl chloride cancer clusters in workers were the first evidence in humans, both of these clusters were preceded (in some cases over a decade earlier) by significant evidence from animal toxicology tests of male infertility and liver cancer, respectively. The link between diacetyl (artificial butter flavoring) and bronchiolitis obliterans was first identified in the workplace. The disaster in Minamata, Japan involved methyl (organic) mercury poisoning.

6. d. Risks tend to be perceived as more serious if they are outside individual control, less familiar, and linked to a dreaded disease and affect children. If the benefit is seen as going to a distant corporation rather than a local and familiar company, the risks also tend to be seen as more serious.

7. d. The Institute of Medicine's consensus report, "Toward Environmental Justice: Research, Education, and Health Policy Needs," recommended environmental education relevant to environmental justice for all health professionals. Environmental justice is a social movement that is based on empirical evidence and that is very relevant to health providers because it relates to health disparities and to risk communication.

8. b. Although clinicians should recommend that patients have carbon monoxide detectors in their homes, they do not need to keep track of which homes have them.

Chapter 47

1. c. Occupational health should have high priority on the international agenda, but occupational health and safety laws cover only about 10% of the population in developing countries.

2. d. The rise in migration for employment has had serious consequences for many countries. The world's largest population migration is taking place at this time—one in seven of the world's people are on the move.

3. c. Child labor is an economic and social reality in many developing countries. Children may provide 25% or more of a family's total income, and many traditional cultures include child labor as an integral part of the child's socialization and achievement of status in the local community. Governments may regard child labor as a key factor in keeping their economy competitive through the provision of cheap labor.

4. c. Globalization benefits countries that are competitive in the knowledge economy, which rewards skills and institutions that promote cutting-edge technological innovation, or the low-wage economy, which uses widely available technology to do routine tasks at the lowest possible cost. Middle-income countries have not done nearly as well under globalized markets as either richer or poorer countries.

5. b. The World Health Organization (WHO) is responsible for the technical aspects of occupational safety and health and the promotion of medical services and hygienic standards.

6. a. Occupational injuries and diseases have a profound effect on the health of the world's population. Occupational injuries and diseases play an even more important role in developing countries where 70% of the working population of the world lives.

7. c. The ILO is a tripartite organization of government, employer, and worker representatives that develops policy statements, conventions, recommendations, and guidelines through a consensus process that all agree are the "minimum standard" for occupational health and safety.

8. a. Occupational incidents cause permanent disabilities and economic losses amounting to 4–6% of national incomes, costs to developing countries in excess of $10 trillion.

9. b. ILO conventions guide all countries in the promotion of workplace safety and in managing occupational health and safety programs. The ILO conventions and recommendations on occupational safety and health are

international agreements that have legal force if they are ratified by the national parliament.

10. a. Agricultural work is the most prevalent type of employment in the world. In developing countries especially, the performance of the agricultural sector often depends on conditions outside policymakers' reach.

11. d. Pesticides are essential to modern agriculture—more than 2 million tons of widely used pesticides in developing countries are highly toxic. Many of these pesticides are banned or severely restricted in developed countries, yet still legally sold to farmers in developing countries.

12. b. The construction industry accounts for around 7% of the world's employment, but 30–40% of the world's fatal injuries. Falls from heights due to inadequate scaffolding and lack of basic protections, being buried in excavations, or being crushed by vehicles or building materials are the most common causes of fatal injuries.

Chapter 48

1. a. Endocrine disrupting chemicals alter the action of hormones in ways that may result in health effects.

2. d. Phthalates are antiandrogenic and can impact androgen sensitive tissues, having lasting effects on testicular function and genital development.

Chapter 49

1. b. Exposure to extreme heat is a major climate risk factor among workers who perform heavy labor in hot conditions.

2. c. Climate change and resulting extreme temperatures have reduced global labor capacity and productivity as workers reach the physiologic limits of heat tolerance and adaptation.

Chapter 50

1. d. The Clean Air Act (CAA) is the principal federal standard addressing outdoor air quality in the United States.

2. d. The CAA mandates that the primary NAAQS be set to protect the health of all sensitive groups within the population.

3. a. Stationary sources of air pollution are primarily power or manufacturing plants and are responsible for most sulfur dioxide (SO_2) emissions, as well as considerable amounts of nitrogen oxides (NOx) and particulate matter.

4. a. Ozone is a colorless, pungent, relatively water-insoluble gas.

5. a. In contrast to other criteria pollutants, NO_2 is a common contaminant of indoor air, and indoor levels often exceed those found outdoors.

6. c. Sulfur dioxide leads to the secondary formation of acid aerosols.

7. b. Because CO has no direct effect on the lungs, its principal adverse health effects are through its ability to cause or exacerbate diseases associated with impaired oxygen delivery.

Chapter 51

1. b. Unless otherwise stated, BOD signifies the biochemical oxygen demand for 5 days at 20°C (68°F).

2. b. COD determines the quantity of oxidizable material in the water.

3. a. During hydraulic fracturing (fracking), a fluid mixture is pumped deep underground where it fractures the rock to liberate trapped natural gas. Fracking fluids amount to between 2 and 7 million gallons of water per well.

4. c. The Safe Drinking Water Act authorizes the U.S. EPA to establish and enforce regulations for chemicals and other toxic agents in drinking water.

5. b. The U.S. EPA sets two standards for each regulated pollutant. The first standard, called a maximum contaminant level goal (MCLG), is set at a concentration that is not expected to cause adverse health effects over a lifetime of consumption of water at that concentration. A substantial safety margin for this MCLG is included in each unenforceable standard.

6. b. The most common disinfection by-products are trihalomethanes and haloacetic acids and some studies have linked these to cancer.

Chapter 52

1. c. CAPs include chemicals emitted in large quantities and from many sources such as carbon monoxide (CO), sulfur oxides (SOx), nitrogen oxides (NOx), and particulate matter (< 10 and 2.5 μm in diameter, or PM 10 and PM 2.5).

2. c. The United States maintains a list of chemicals that have been formally identified as HAPs.

3. d. Superfund Amendments and Reauthorization Act (SARA) mandates emergency planning for chemical accidents.

4. d. Exposure to HAPs may contribute to respiratory disease, systemic toxicity, and carcinogenicity.

5. d. The Clean Air Act provides for use of market-based principles and other innovative approaches to reduce air pollution.

6. b. Many local jurisdictions have developed hazardous materials (HAZMAT) teams, trained to identify and respond to hazardous materials incidents.

7. a. Emergency response action levels are used to guide shelter-in-place or evacuation decisions; if evacuation has

occurred, these levels may be used to determine when it is safe for community members to reenter the area.

8. a. The EPA has developed a system of protective action guides (PAGs) to help officials make critical decisions following a nuclear accident.

9. c. Hazardous waste exclusions include agricultural wastes used as fertilizers.

10. b. ATSDR has developed several specialized registries to study the long-term health effects of exposure to specific chemicals at hazardous waste sites, with the intention of combining data from several sites where similar exposures have occurred to achieve populations large enough that the associated health effects can be detected.

Chapter 53

1. d. Short-latency illnesses are characterized by a relatively acute onset, closely related in time to the individual's presence within the building and often relieved by removal from further exposure.

2. a. Long-latency illnesses include cancer and chronic pulmonary diseases, perhaps resulting from long-term low-level exposure to contaminants in indoor air.

3. b. The term sick-building syndrome (SBS; previously referred to as closed-building syndrome or tight-building syndrome and sometimes referred to as nonspecific building-associated illness) denotes a characteristic set of symptoms, typically headache and mucous membrane irritation, recognized among occupants of nonindustrial buildings such as offices and schools.

4. b. Mass psychogenic (or sociogenic) illness is an illness of psychophysiologic origin occurring simultaneously in a group of individuals.

5. d. Carbon monoxide in buildings may be entrained from the outside via air intakes in the vicinity of vehicle loading docks.

Chapter 54

1. d. Symptoms of MCS resemble those of sick-building syndrome, a constellation of excessive work-related symptoms related to an indoor office environment (eg, headache; eye, nose, and throat irritation; fatigue; and dizziness) sometimes without an identifiable etiology.

2. c. A panel of the World Health Organization (WHO) recommended that the terms MCS and EI be replaced by idiopathic environmental intolerance (IEI), arguing that use of the word sensitivity may be construed as connoting an allergic cause and that the link between symptoms and exposure is unproven.

3. a. The Quick Environmental Exposure and Sensitivity Inventory (QEESI) can be used to assess chemical intolerance.

Chapter 55

1. d. Risk can apply to almost any activity or event, such as the likelihood for injury when playing a sport or driving a car, the chance for developing a disease from exposure to pathogens or chemicals, or the possibility for property damage from a natural catastrophe.

2. d. Risk assessment is a means or methodology to quantify risk, but it is important to recognize that it is a process and not a science.

3. a. The exposure assessment step in a risk assessment is used to estimate the magnitude and probability of uptake from the environment by any combination of oral, inhalation, and dermal routes of exposure.

4. a. The key element to the precautionary principle is that action should be taken in the face of uncertainty rather than delaying action until more "evidence" is generated.

5. d. Risk managers use a value-laden approach to consider risk, along with other factors, in determining what level of risk is acceptable and in developing measures that would prevent, reduce, or maintain risk at those levels.

6. b. RELs are derived by identifying and dividing the NOAEL (or BMD) by uncertainty factors to account for inadequacies in the database, incomplete scientific knowledge, and protection of more sensitive individuals.

Index

Note: Page numbers followed by *f* and *t* indicate figures and tables, respectively.